Clinical Pharmacology & Therapeutics

VOLUME 38, JULY-DECEMBER 1985
THE C. V. MOSBY COMPANY, ST. LOUIS

Volume 38

Printed in the United States of America

JULY 1985

CLINICAL PHARMACOLOGY & THERAPEUTICS

VOLUME 38 NUMBER 1

MOSBY

TABLE OF CONTENTS

1 **A note from the Co-Editor**

COMMENTARY

2 **The discipline of clinical pharmacology**
Marcus M. Reidenberg, M.D., New York, N. Y., Cornell University Medical College

ORIGINAL ARTICLES

6 **Salicylate kinetics in old age**
Patrick Netter, M.D., Gilbert Faure, M.D., Marie Christine Regent, M.D., Josephine A. Procknal, B.A., and Gerhard Levy, Pharm.D., Nancy, France, and Amherst, N. Y., Laboratoire de Pharmacologie, Clinique Rhumatologique, Clinique Medicale B, CHU de Nancy-Brabois, Nancy, and Department of Pharmaceutics, School of Pharmacy, State University of New York at Buffalo, Amherst

12 **Atropine serum concentrations after multiple inhaled doses of atropine sulfate**
Wayne A. Kradjan, Pharm.D., Robert C. Smallridge, M.D., Robin Davis, Pharm.D., and Pritam Verma, Ph.D., Seattle, Wash., Washington, D. C., and Aurora, Colo., Department of Pharmacy Practice, University of Washington School of Pharmacy, Seattle; Department of Clinical Physiology, Walter Reed Army Institute of Research, Walter Reed Army Medical Center, Washington; and Department of Biochemistry, Clinical Investigation Branch, Fitzsimmons Army Medical Center, Aurora

16 **Reassessment of verbal and visual analog ratings in analgesic studies**
Gary S. Littman, Ph.D., Barry R. Walker, M.D., and Bruce E. Schneider, Ph.D., Philadelphia, Pa., Wyeth Laboratories

24 **Labetalol and hydrochlorothiazide in hypertension**
Labetalol/Hydrochlorothiazide Multicenter Study Group

Continued on page 2A

28 **Endoscopic evaluation of slow-release potassium chloride preparations**
Colin Kendall, M.D., Kenneth D. Krantz, M.D., Ph.D., Arthur Berger, B.S., and Tessa Sharp, M.S., Princeton, N. J., and Kansas City, Mo., Ellis Pharmaceutical Consulting, Inc., Princeton, and Quincy Research Center, Kansas City

31 **Cefotaxime and desacetyl cefotaxime kinetics in renal impairment**
Gary R. Matzke, Pharm.D., Paul A. Abraham, M.D., Charles E. Halstenson, Pharm.D., and William F. Keane, M.D., Minneapolis, Minn., Drug Evaluation Unit, Hennepin County Medical Center and College of Pharmacy and School of Medicine, University of Minnesota

37 **Kinetics and dynamics of disopyramide and its dealkylated metabolite in healthy subjects**
Wen-Teh Chiang, M.D., Christer von Bahr, M.D., Berit Calissendorff, M.D., Rune Dahlqvist, M.D., Hakan Emilsson, Pharm.D., Anita Magnusson, B.S., and Karin Schenck-Gustafsson, M.D., Huddinge, Sweden, Departments of Clinical Pharmacology, Internal Medicine, Ophthalmology, and Pharmacy, Huddinge University Hospital

45 **Clinical pharmacology of 5-iodo-2′-deoxyuridine and 5-iodouracil and endogenous pyrimidine modulation**
Raymond W. Klecker, Jr., B.S., Jean F. Jenkins, M.S.N., Timothy J. Kinsella, M.D., Robert L. Fine, M.D., John M. Strong, Ph.D., and Jerry M. Collins, Ph.D., Bethesda, Md., Clinical Pharmacology and Radiation Oncology Branches, Clinical Oncology Program, Division of Cancer Treatment, National Cancer Institute

Volume 38, Number 1, July 1985. CLINICAL PHARMACOLOGY AND THERAPEUTICS. Published monthly by The C. V. Mosby Company, 11830 Westline Industrial Drive, St. Louis, MO 63146. POSTMASTER: Send address changes to The C. V. Mosby Company, 11830 Westline Industrial Drive, St. Louis, MO 63146.

1985 Annual subscription rates	*U.S.A.*	*International (surface mail)* *All regions*	*International (airmail)** *Region 1*	*Region 2*	*Region 3*
Institutional†	$93.00	$109.00	$127.10	$145.60	$164.05
Individual‡	$58.00	$ 74.00	$ 92.10	$110.60	$129.05
Student, resident‡	$46.40	$ 62.40	$ 80.50	$ 99.00	$117.45

Single copies are $6.50. Remittances should be made by check, draft, post office or express money order, in U.S. funds drawn through a U.S. bank, payable to this JOURNAL.

**Airmail breakdown—Domestic:* First-class and Priority rates for the U.S. and possessions are available upon request. *Region 1:* Central America, islands, and mainland colonies of European countries in The Americas. *Region 2:* South America, Europe, Egypt, Africa (bordering the Mediterranean). *Region 3:* Asia, Australasia, Africa (other than Mediterranean), Middle East, Far East, The Pacific, U.S.S.R. (and constituent Republics).

†Institutional (multiple-reader) subscriptions are available to public and private libraries, schools, hospitals, and clinics; city, county, state, provincial, and national government bureaus and departments; and all commercial and private institutions and organizations.

‡Individual subscriptions and all student-rate subscriptions must be in the names of, billed to, and paid by individuals. All student-rate requests must indicate training status and name of institution.

Subscriptions may begin at any time.

Second class postage paid at St. Louis, MO, and at additional mailing offices. Printed in the U. S. A.

52 Effect of acute alcohol consumption on lithium kinetics
Raymond F. Anton, M.D., Joseph A. Paladino, Pharm.D., Alex Morton, Pharm.D., and Russel W. Thomas, Pharm.D., Charleston, S. C., and Rochester and Buffalo, N. Y., Veterans Administration Medical Center and Medical University of South Carolina, Charleston; Rochester General Hospital, Rochester; and Millard Fillmore Hospital, Buffalo

56 Treatment of recurrent herpes simplex labialis with topical butylated hydroxytoluene
Donna J. Freeman, M.D., Gay Wenerstron, R.N., and Spotswood L. Spruance, M.D., Salt Lake City, Utah, Center for Infectious Diseases, Diagnostic Microbiology and Immunology and the Division of Infectious Diseases, Department of Medicine, University of Utah School of Medicine

60 Effects of chronic nitrendipine on casual (office) and 24-hour ambulatory blood pressure
William B. White, M.D., Vivienne-E. Smith, M.D., Ellen J. McCabe, R.N., and Moideen K. Meeran, M.D., Farmington, Conn., Divisions of General Internal Medicine (Hypertension Clinic) and Cardiology, Department of Medicine, University of Connecticut School of Medicine

65 Nonsteroidal anti-inflammatory effect of sulindac sulfoxide and sulfide on gastric mucosa
David Y. Graham, M.D., J. Lacey Smith, M.D., Geoffrey I. Holmes, B.A., and Richard O. Davies, M.D., Ph.D., Houston, Tex., and West Point, Pa., Digestive Disease Section, Veterans Administration Medical Center, Baylor College of Medicine, Houston, and Merck Sharp & Dohme Research Laboratories, West Point

71 Effects of d,1-verapamil on atrioventricular conduction in relation to its stereoselective first-pass metabolism
Hirotoshi Echizen, M.D., Barbara Vogelgesang, M.PSc., and Michael Eichelbaum, M.D., Bonn, West Germany, Department of Medicine, University of Bonn

77 Food-induced changes in theophylline absorption from controlled-release formulations. Part I. Substantial increased and decreased absorption with Uniphyl tablets and Theo-Dur Sprinkle
Aziz Karim, Ph.D., Thomas Burns, M.S., Lorraine Wearley, B.S., Janice Streicher, B.S., and Michael Palmer, M.S., Skokie, Ill., Searle Research & Development, a Division of G. D. Searle & Co.

84 Hemodynamic and respiratory effects of dezocine, ciramadol, and morphine
Robert L. Rothbard, M.D., Bernard F. Schreiner, M.D., and Paul N. Yu, M.D., Rochester, N. Y., Cardiology Unit, Department of Medicine, University of Rochester School of Medicine and Dentistry and Strong Memorial Hospital

Continued on page 4A

89 **Temporal variation in the disposition of theophylline and its metabolites**
Marie V. St-Pierre, M.Sc.Phm., Michael Spino, Pharm.D., Alan F. Isles, M.D., M.Sc., A. Tesoro, and Stuart M. McLeod, M.D., Ph.D., Toronto, Ontario, Canada, Faculties of Pharmacy and Medicine, Departments of Pediatrics and Pharmacology, University of Toronto and Division of Clinical Pharmacology, Research Institute, The Hospital for Sick Children

96 **Effects of the calcium antagonist tiapamil on pulmonary gas exchange in patients with chronic obstructive pulmonary disease who receive salbutamol**
Matthias Gugger, M.D., A. Marco Crivelli, M.D., Renato L. Galeazzi, M.D., and Hans Bachofen, M.D., Berne, Switzerland, Department of Medicine, University of Berne

101 **Myocardial ischemia induced by prostacyclin and iloprost**
Raffaele Bugiardini, M.D., Marcello Galvani, M.D., Donatella Ferrini, M.D., Claudio Gridelli, M.D., Daniela Tollemeto, M.D., Lucio Mari, M.D., Paolo Puddu, M.D., and Sergio Lenzi, M.D., Bologna, Italy, Clinical Medica II, Università di Bologna

109 **Effects of smoke deprivation interval on puff topography**
James P. Zacny, Ph.D., and Maxine L. Stitzer, Ph.D., Baltimore, Md., Department of Psychiatry, Francis Scott Key Medical Center and The Johns Hopkins University School of Medicine

ASCPT 116 **Notes of the American Society for Clinical Pharmacology and Therapeutics**

15 **Future meeting dates and sites of the ASCPT**

119 **ASCPT abstract form**

USAN COUNCIL 117 **USAN List No. 262**

Information to authors on pages 8A and 9A

AUGUST 1985

CLINICAL PHARMACOLOGY & THERAPEUTICS

VOLUME 38 NUMBER 2

MOSBY

TABLE OF CONTENTS

ORIGINAL ARTICLES

121 **Effect of probenecid on the formation and elimination of acyl glucuronides: Studies with zomepirac**
Philip C. Smith, Ph.D., Pim N. J. Langendijk, M.S., John A. Bosso, Pharm.D., and Leslie Z. Benet, Ph.D., San Francisco, Calif., Department of Pharmacy, University of California, San Francisco

128 **Metabolism of methoxyphenamine in extensive and poor metabolizers of debrisoquin**
Samir D. Roy, B.Pharm., Edward M. Hawes, Ph.D., Gordon McKay, Ph.D., Elarien D. Korchinski, M.D., and Kamal K. Midha, Ph.D., Saskatoon, Saskatchewan, Canada, Colleges of Pharmacy and Medicine, University of Saskatchewan

134 **Clinical pharmacology of timentin (ticarcillin and clavulanic acid)**
Gerald P. Bodey, M.D., Edna Yeo, M.D., Dah Hsi Ho, Ph.D., Kenneth Rolston, M.D., and Barbara LeBlanc, B.S., Houston, Tex., Division of Medicine, The University of Texas M. D. Anderson Hospital

140 **Isosorbide dinitrate bioavailability, kinetics, and metabolism**
Peter Straehl, Pharm.D., and Renato L. Galeazzi, M.D., Berne, Switzerland, Department of Medicine, University of Berne

150 **Moxalactam epimer disposition in patients undergoing continuous ambulatory peritoneal dialysis**
Gene Morse, Pharm.D., David Janicke, Pharm.D., Robert Cafarell, Pharm.D., Katherine Piontek, B.S., Michael Apicella, M.D., William J. Jusko, Ph.D., and John Walshe, M.D., Buffalo, N. Y., Departments of Pharmacy and Medicine, State University of New York at Buffalo, Erie County Medical Center

Continued on page 2A

157 **The effects of several weeks of ethanol consumption on ethanol kinetics in normal men and women**
Jordan L. Holtzman, M.D., Ph.D., Roger L. Gebhard, M.D., John H. Eckfeldt, M.D., Ph.D., Linda R. Mottonen, B.S., Denise K. Finley, R.N., and Fred N. Eshelman, Pharm.D., Minneapolis, Minn., and Research Triangle Park, N. C., Veterans Administration Medical Center and the Departments of Medicine, Pharmacology, and Laboratory Medicine and Pathology, University of Minnesota, Minneapolis, and Glaxo Inc., Research Triangle Park

164 **Cigarette smoking as a risk for cardiovascular disease. Part VI. Compensation with nicotine availability as a single variable**
N. J. Haley, Ph.D., D. W. Sepkovic, Ph.D., D. Hoffman, Ph.D., and E. L. Wynder, M.D., Valhalla, N. Y., American Health Foundation, Naylor Dana Institute, Division of Nutrition and Endocrinology

171 **Pentosane polysulfate: The effect on hemostasis of a continuous 3-day infusion**
Dominique de Prost, M.D., Ph.D., Claude Guérot, M.D., and Florence Karsenty, M.D., Paris, France, Laboratoire d'Immunologie et d'Hématologie and Service de Cardiologie, Centre Hospitalo-Universitaire Xavier Bichat, Université de Paris

176 **Oral ciramadol in the treatment of postoperative pain**
Louis Lasagna, M.D., and Jose F. Calimlim, M.D., Boston, Mass., and Rochester, N. Y., Tufts University Medical School, Boston, and University of Rochester School of Medicine and Dentistry, Rochester

Volume 38, Number 2, August 1985. CLINICAL PHARMACOLOGY AND THERAPEUTICS. Published monthly by The C. V. Mosby Company, 11830 Westline Industrial Drive, St. Louis, MO 63146. POSTMASTER: Send address changes to The C. V. Mosby Company, 11830 Westline Industrial Drive, St. Louis, MO 63146.

1985 Annual subscription rates	*U.S.A.*	*International (surface mail)* All regions	*International (airmail)** Region 1	Region 2	Region 3
Institutional†	$93.00	$109.00	$127.10	$145.60	$164.05
Individual‡	$58.00	$ 74.00	$ 92.10	$110.60	$129.05
Student, resident‡	$46.40	$ 62.40	$ 80.50	$ 99.00	$117.45

Single copies are $6.50. Remittances should be made by check, draft, post office or express money order, in U.S. funds drawn through a U.S. bank, payable to this JOURNAL.

**Airmail breakdown—Domestic:* First-class and Priority rates for the U.S. and possessions are available upon request. *Region 1:* Central America, islands, and mainland colonies of European countries in The Americas. *Region 2:* South America, Europe, Egypt, Africa (bordering the Mediterranean). *Region 3:* Asia, Australasia, Africa (other than Mediterranean), Middle East, Far East, The Pacific, U.S.S.R. (and constituent Republics).

†Institutional (multiple-reader) subscriptions are available to public and private libraries, schools, hospitals, and clinics; city, county, state, provincial, and national government bureaus and departments; and all commercial and private institutions and organizations.

‡Individual subscriptions and all student-rate subscriptions must be in the names of, billed to, and paid by individuals. All student-rate requests must indicate training status and name of institution.

Subscriptions may begin at any time.

Second class postage paid at St. Louis, MO, and at additional mailing offices. Printed in the U. S. A.

183 **A study of adverse reaction algorithms in a drug surveillance program**
Carol Louik, Sc.D., Peter G. Lacouture, M.S., Allen A. Mitchell, M.D., Ralph Kauffman, M.D., Frederick H. Lovejoy, Jr., M.D., Sumner J. Yaffe, M.D., and Samuel Shapiro, M.B., Boston, Mass., Detroit, Mich., and Bethesda, Md., Division of Clinical Pharmacology and Toxicology, Children's Hospital, Harvard Medical School and the Drug Epidemiology Unit, School of Public Health, Boston University School of Medicine, Boston; Children's Hospital of Michigan, Wayne State University, Detroit; and National Institute of Child Health and Human Development, Bethesda

188 **Treatment of arterial hypertension with ketanserin in mono- and combination therapy**
Anders Pettersson, M.D., Bengt Persson, M.D., Göran Berglund, M.D., and Thomas Hedner, M.D., Göteborg, Sweden, Hypertension Unit, Department of Medicine I and Department of Clinical Pharmacology, Sahlgren's Hospital

195 **Losulazine, a new antihypertensive**
Randall Gore, M.D., David Musselman, M.D., Edwin Micalizzi, B.A., and Michaline Slomka, M.A., Portland, Ore., and Kalamazoo, Mich., Heart Research Department, Providence Medical Center, Portland, and The Upjohn Company, Kalamazoo

199 **Enalaprilat, an intravenous angiotensin-converting enzyme inhibitor, in hypertensive crises**
Donald J. DiPette, M.D., James C. Ferraro, D.O., Robert R. Evans, Pharm.D., and Marcus Martin, M.D., Pittsburgh, Pa., Department of Medicine, Allegheny-Singer Research Institute and Departments of Medicine, Pharmacy, and Surgery, Allegheny General Hospital

205 **Felodipine kinetics in healthy men**
Boo Edgar, B.Sc., C. G. Regårdh, Ph.D., G. Johnsson, M.D., Ph.D., L. Johansson, B.Sc., P. Lundborg, M.D., Ph.D., I. Löfberg, M.Sc., and O. Rönn, Ph.D., Mölndal and Göteborg, Sweden, Research Laboratories, AB Hässle, Mölndal, and Department of Medicine, University of Göteborg, Östra Hospital, Göteborg

212 **Nitrendipine kinetics in normal and impaired renal function**
George R. Aronoff, M.D., and Rebecca S. Sloan, R.N., Indianapolis, Ind., Nephrology Section, Department of Medicine, Indiana University Medical Center

219 **Self-administration of clonidine, oxazepam, and hydromorphone by patients undergoing methadone detoxification**
Kenzie L. Preston, Ph.D., George E. Bigelow, Ph.D., and Ira A. Liebson, M.D., Baltimore, Md., The Johns Hopkins University School of Medicine and Francis Scott Key Medical Center

Continued on page 4A

228 **Effects of age and disease on the pharmacokinetics and pharmacodynamics of sulindac**
D. S. Sitar, Ph.D., J. A. Owen, Ph.D., B. MacDougall, M.D., T. Hunter, M.D., and P. A. Mitenko, M.D., Winnipeg, Manitoba, Canada, Geriatric Clinical Pharmacology and Rheumatic Disease Units, Departments of Medicine and Pharmacology and Therapeutics, University of Manitoba

ASCPT 235 **Notes of the American Society for Clinical Pharmacology and Therapeutics**

127 **Future meeting dates and sites of the ASCPT**

239 **ASCPT abstract form**

USAN COUNCIL 237 **USAN List No. 263**

Information to authors on pages 8A and 9A

SEPTEMBER 1985

CLINICAL PHARMACOLOGY & THERAPEUTICS

VOLUME 38 NUMBER 3

TABLE OF CONTENTS

ORIGINAL ARTICLES

241 **Dose-dependent absorption of amoxycillin and bacampicillin**
Jan Sjövall, Ph.D., Gunnar Alván, M.D., and Douglas Westerlund, Pharm.D., Södertälje and Huddinge, Sweden, Clinical Pharmacology and The Research and Development Laboratory, Astra Läkemedel, Södertälje, and the Department of Clinical Pharmacology, Huddinge Hospital, Huddinge

251 **The pharmacokinetics of baclofen derived from intestinal infusion**
Gregory M. Kochak, Ph.D., Ashok Rakhit, Ph.D., William E. Wagner, M.D., Frank Honc, M.S., Lorraine Waldes, B.S., and Richard A. Kershaw, Ph.D., Ardsley, N. Y., and Columbus, Ohio, Pharmaceuticals Division, CIBA-GEIGY Corporation, Ardsley, and Department of Pharmacology, College of Medicine, The Ohio State University, Columbus

258 **Sulindac is not renal sparing in man**
Douglas G. Roberts, M.D., John G. Gerber, M.D., John S. Barnes, B.S., Gary O. Zerbe, Ph.D., and Alan S. Nies, M.D., Denver, Colo., Division of Clinical Pharmacology, Departments of Medicine and Pharmacology, and Department of Preventive Medicine and Biometrics, University of Colorado School of Medicine

266 **Circulatory effects of intravenous and oral acebutolol in acute myocardial infarction**
Bernard Silke, M.D., Gregory Nelson, M.B., Satya Prakash Verma, M.D., Janet Clarke, M.B., Ganesh Baliga, M.B., and Stanley H. Taylor, M.D., Leeds, United Kingdom, University Departments of Cardiovascular Studies and Medical Cardiology, The General Infirmary

273 **Prostaglandins and nicotinate-provoked increase in cutaneous blood flow**
Jonathan K. Wilkin, M.D., Glenn Fortner, B.S., Linda A. Reinhardt, M.D., Otero Vogt Flowers, M.D., S. James Kilpatrick, Ph.D., and W. Carson Streeter, Richmond, Va., Dermatology Section, McGuire Veterans Administration Medical Center and Departments of Pharmacology, Dermatology, and Biostatistics, Medical College of Virginia

Continued on page 2A

278 **Pharmacokinetics of transdermally delivered clonidine**
Thomas R. MacGregor, M.Sc., Kandace M. Matzek, M.Sc., James J. Keirns, Ph.D., Rudolf G. A. van Wayjen, M.D., Abraham van den Ende, Ph.D., and Rudolf G. L. van Tol, Ph.D., Ridgefield, Conn., and Amsterdam and Alkmaar, The Netherlands, Boehringer Ingelheim Pharmaceuticals, Inc., Ridgefield; Vereeniging voor Ziekenverpleging and Slotervaart Hospital, Amsterdam; and Boehringer Ingleheim b.v., Alkmaar

285 **Pharmacokinetics of intravenous and intraperitoneal cefotaxime in chronic ambulatory peritoneal dialysis**
H. C. Albin, M.D., F. M. Demotes-Mainard, Ph.D., J. L. Bouchet, M.D., G. A. Vincon, Ph.D., and C. Martin-Dupont, M.D., Bordeaux, France, Departments of Clinical Pharmacology and Nephrology, Hôpital Pellegrin

290 **A new dosing regimen in renal insufficiency: Application to cephalexin**
Ryohei Hori, Ph.D., Katsuhiko Okumura, Ph.D., Hiromi Nihira, M.D., Hiroshi Nakano, M.D., Kazuyoshi Akagi, M.S., and Akira Kamiya, Ph.D., Kyoto and Hiroshima, Japan, Department of Pharmacy, Kyoto University Hospital and Faculty of Medicine, Kyoto University, Kyoto, and Department of Urology, Hiroshima University School of Medicine, Hiroshima

296 **Cyclosporine kinetics in renal transplantation**
Richard J. Ptachcinski, Pharm.D., Raman Venkataramanan, Ph.D., J. Thomas Rosenthal, M.D., Gilbert J. Burckart, Pharm.D., Rodney J. Taylor, M.D., and Thomas R. Hakala, M.D., Pittsburgh, Pa., Departments of Pharmacy Practice, Pharmaceutics, and Surgery, University of Pittsburgh School of Pharmacy and Medicine

Volume 38, Number 3, September 1985. CLINICAL PHARMACOLOGY AND THERAPEUTICS. Published monthly by The C. V. Mosby Company, 11830 Westline Industrial Drive, St. Louis, MO 63146. POSTMASTER: Send address changes to The C. V. Mosby Company, 11830 Westline Industrial Drive, St. Louis, MO 63146.

1985 Annual subscription rates	*U.S.A.*	*International (surface mail)* *All regions*	*International (airmail)** *Region 1*	*Region 2*	*Region 3*
Institutional†	$93.00	$109.00	$127.10	$145.60	$164.05
Individual‡	$58.00	$ 74.00	$ 92.10	$110.60	$129.05
Student, resident‡	$46.40	$ 62.40	$ 80.50	$ 99.00	$117.45

Single copies are $6.50. Remittances should be made by check, draft, post office or express money order, in U.S. funds drawn through a U.S. bank, payable to this JOURNAL.

**Airmail breakdown—Domestic:* First-class and Priority rates for the U.S. and possessions are available upon request. *Region 1:* Central America, islands, and mainland colonies of European countries in The Americas. *Region 2:* South America, Europe, Egypt, Africa (bordering the Mediterranean). *Region 3:* Asia, Australasia, Africa (other than Mediterranean), Middle East, Far East, The Pacific, U.S.S.R. (and constituent Republics).

†Institutional (multiple-reader) subscriptions are available to public and private libraries, schools, hospitals, and clinics; city, county, state, provincial, and national government bureaus and departments; and all commercial and private institutions and organizations.

‡Individual subscriptions and all student-rate subscriptions must be in the names of, billed to, and paid by individuals. All student-rate requests must indicate training status and name of institution.

Subscriptions may begin at any time.

Second class postage paid at St. Louis, MO, and at additional mailing offices. Printed in the U. S. A.

301 **Influence of transdermal scopolamine on motion sickness during 7 days' exposure to heavy seas**
W. F. van Marion, M.D., M. C. M. Bongaerts, M.D., J. C. Christiaanse, M.D., H. G. Hofkamp, M.D., and W. van Ouwerkerk, M.D., Overveen, The Netherlands, Department of Internal Medicine, Marine Hospital

306 **Oral triamterene disposition**
Fritz Sörgel, Ph.D., Jiro Hasegawa, Ph.D., Emil T. Lin, Ph.D., and Roger L. Williams, M.D., San Francisco, Calif., Department of Pharmacy, School of Pharmacy, University of California

313 **Controlled trial of acifran in type II hyperlipoproteinemia**
Donald B. Hunninghake, M.D., K. David G. Edwards, M.D., Ph.D., George S. Sopko, M.D., and Robert L. Tosiello, M.S., Minneapolis, Minn., and New York, N. Y., Lipid Research Clinic, University of Minnesota, Minneapolis, and Ayerst Laboratories, New York

318 **Kinetics of cocaine distribution, elimination, and chronotropic effects**
May J. Chow, M.D., John J. Ambre, M.D., Ph.D., Tsuen Ih Ruo, Ph.D., Arthur J. Atkinson, Jr., M.D., Dennis J. Bowsher, M.D., and Marian W. Fischman, Ph.D., Chicago, Ill., Clinical Pharmacology Center and Departments of Medicine and Pharmacology, Northwestern University Medical School, and the Department of Psychiatry, Pritzker Medical School, The University of Chicago

325 **Lack of pharmacokinetic interaction between cimetidine and pirenzepine**
F. Jamali, Ph.D., V. Mahachai, M.D., Paul A. Reilly, Ph.D., and A. B. R. Thomson, M.D., Edmonton, Alberta, Canada, Boehringer Ingelheim (Canada) Ltd. and Faculty of Pharmacy and Division of Gastroenterology, Department of Medicine, University of Alberta and University of Alberta Hospital

331 **Gastrointestinal absorption as a function of age: Xylose absorption in healthy adults**
Stephen L. Johnson, Ph.D., Michael Mayersohn, Ph.D., and Kenneth A. Conrad, M.D., Tucson, Ariz., Colleges of Pharmacy and Medicine, The University of Arizona

336 **Efficacy of clonidine and of methadone in the rapid detoxification of patients dependent on heroin**
Jordi Camí, M.D., Santiago de Torres, M.D., Lluís San, M.D., Àngels Solé, D.Psychol., Diana Guerra, D.Psychol., and Balbina Ugena, R.N., Barcelona, Spain, Division of Clinical Pharmacology, Hospital Nuestra Señora del Mar, Autonomous Univesity of Barcelona

Continued on page 4A

342 **Lack of interaction between verapamil and cimetidine**
Darrell R. Abernethy, M.D., Ph.D., Janice B. Schwartz, M.D., and Elizabeth L. Todd, Ph.D., Houston, Tex., Section on Hypertension-Clinical Pharmacology, Department of Medicine, Baylor College of Medicine

350 **Lack of effect of oral activated charcoal on imipramine clearance**
Mark J. Goldberg, M.D., Glen D. Park, Pharm.D., Reynold Spector, M.D., Lawrence J. Fischer, Ph.D., and Ross D. Feldman, M.D., Iowa City, Iowa, Departments of Internal Medicine and Pharmacology, College of Medicine and the Division of Clinical/Hospital Pharmacy, College of Pharmacy, The University of Iowa and the Veterans Administration Medical Center

ASCPT **354** **Notes of the American Society for Clinical Pharmacology and Therapeutics**

USAN COUNCIL **356** **USAN List No. 264**

BOOKS RECEIVED **358** **Books received**

ERRATA **317** **Errata to Hicks et al., "Tolrestat Kinetics," and to White et al., "Alpha-Methyldopa Disposition in Mothers with Hypertension and in Their Breast-Fed Infants"**

Information to authors on pages 10A and 11A

OCTOBER 1985

CLINICAL PHARMACOLOGY & THERAPEUTICS

VOLUME 38 NUMBER 4

TABLE OF CONTENTS

COMMENTARY

359 **The computerized on-line Medicaid pharmaceutical analysis and surveillance system: A new resource for postmarketing drug surveillance**
Brian L. Strom, M.D., M.P.H., Jeffrey L. Carson, M.D., M. Lee Morse, Pharm.B., and Aida A. LeRoy, Pharm.D., Philadelphia, Pa., Camden, N. J., and Arlington, Va., The Clinical Epidemiology Unit, Section of General Medicine, Departments of Medicine and Pharmacology, University of Pennsylvania School of Medicine, Philadelphia; Department of Medicine, University of Medicine and Dentistry of New Jersey/Rutgers Medical School, Camden; and Health Information Designs, Inc., Arlington

ORIGINAL ARTICLES

365 **Morphine-induced skin wheals: A possible model for the study of histamine release**
Roberto Saucedo, M.D., and Sergio Erill, M.D., Granada, Spain, Department of Pharmacology, University of Granada Medical School

371 **Interactions between ethanol and oral contraceptive steroids**
Joy Hobbes, M.Sc., John Boutagy, Ph.D., and Gillian M. Shenfield, D.M., St. Leonards, Australia, Department of Clinical Pharmacology, The Royal North Shore Hospital

381 **The acute effects of acrivastine (BW825C), a new antihistamine, compared with triprolidine on measures of central nervous system performance and subjective effects**
A. F. Cohen, M.D., M. Hamilton, Ph.D., R. Philipson, and A. W. Peck, Ph.D., Kent, United Kingdom, The Wellcome Research Laboratories

387 **Sulindac metabolism: The importance of an intact colon**
H. A. Strong, B.Sc., N. J. Warner, A. G. Renwick, Ph.D., and C. F. George, M.D., Southampton, United Kingdom, Clinical Pharmacology Group, Faculty of Medicine, University of Southampton

Continued on page 4A

394 **A family study of genetic and environmental factors determining polymorphic hydroxylation of debrisoquin**
E. Steiner, M.D., L. Iselius, M.D., G. Alván, M.D., J. Lindsten, M.D., and F. Sjöqvist, M.D., Stockholm, Sweden, Department of Clinical Pharmacology, Huddinge University Hospital and the Department of Clinical Genetics, Karolinska Hospital, Karolinska Institute

402 **Interethnic differences in genetic polymorphism of debrisoquin and mephenytoin hydroxylation between Japanese and Caucasian populations**
K. Nakamura, M.D., F. Goto, M.D., W. A. Ray, Ph.D., C. B. McAllister, M.S., E. Jacqz, M.D., G. R. Wilkinson, Ph.D., and R. A. Branch, M.D., Nashville, Tenn., and Tsukuba, Japan, Departments of Pharmacology and Preventive Medicine, Vanderbilt University, Nashville, and Department of Anesthesiology, University of Tsukuba, Tsukuba

409 **Pharmacokinetics and beta-blocking effects of timolol in poor and extensive metabolizers of debrisoquin**
John C. McGourty, M.B., Joseph H. Silas, M.D., Jude J. Fleming, Ph.D., Alan McBurney, M.Phil., and John W. Ward, M.B., Merseyside and Leicester, United Kingdom, Hypertension Unit, Clatterbridge Hospital, Merseyside, and Department of Clinical Pharmacology, Glenfield General Hospital, Leicester

414 **Stereoselective mephobarbital hydroxylation cosegregates with mephenytoin hydroxylation**
A. Küpfer, Ph.D., and R. A. Branch, M.D., Nashville, Tenn., and Bern, Switzerland, Division of Clinical Pharmacology, Vanderbilt University, Nashville, and Department of Clinical Pharmacology, University of Bern, Bern

Volume 38, Number 4, October 1985. CLINICAL PHARMACOLOGY AND THERAPEUTICS. Published monthly by The C. V. Mosby Company, 11830 Westline Industrial Drive, St. Louis, MO 63146. POSTMASTER: Send address changes to The C. V. Mosby Company, 11830 Westline Industrial Drive, St. Louis, MO 63146.

1986 Annual subscription rates	*U.S.A.*	*International (surface mail)* All regions	*International (airmail)** Canada & Mexico	Region 1	Region 2	Region 3
Institutional†	$103.00	$119.00	$137.10	$139.75	$158.95	$178.15
Individual‡	$ 62.00	$ 78.00	$ 96.10	$ 98.75	$117.95	$137.15
Student, resident‡	$ 45.00	$ 61.00	$ 79.10	$ 81.75	$100.95	$120.15

Single copies are $6.50. Remittances should be made by check, draft, post office or express money order, in U.S. funds drawn through a U.S. bank, payable to this JOURNAL.

**Airmail breakdown—Domestic:* First-class and Priority rates for the U.S. and possessions are available upon request. *Region 1:* Central America, islands, and mainland colonies of European countries in The Americas. *Region 2:* South America, Europe, Egypt, Africa (bordering the Mediterranean). *Region 3:* Asia, Australasia, Africa (other than Mediterranean), Middle East, Far East, The Pacific, U.S.S.R. (and constituent Republics).

†Institutional (multiple-reader) subscriptions are available to public and private libraries, schools, hospitals, and clinics; city, county, state, provincial, and national government bureaus and departments; and all commercial and private institutions and organizations.

‡Individual subscriptions and all student-rate subscriptions must be in the names of, billed to, and paid by individuals. All student-rate requests must indicate training status and name of institution.

Subscriptions may begin at any time.

Second class postage paid at St. Louis, MO, and at additional mailing offices. Printed in the U. S. A.

419 **Effects of long-term therapy with naltrexone on body weight in obesity**
Richard L. Atkinson, M.D., Lisa K. Berke, M.S.N., F.N.P., Charles R. Drake, M.D., Mary Lynn Bibbs, M.S.N., F.N.P., Frederick L. Williams, M.D., and Donald L. Kaiser, Ph.D., Charlottesville, Va., Department of Internal Medicine, University of Virginia Medical Center

423 **Terazosin kinetics after oral and intravenous doses**
Sean E. Patterson, Ph.D., Abbott Park, Ill., Department of Drug Metabolism, Abbott Laboratories

428 **Ventilatory effects of atenolol and bevantolol in asthma**
Jan-Willem J. Lammers, M.D., Hans T. M. Folgering, M.D., and Cees L. A. van Herwaarden, M.D., H. Landstichting, The Netherlands, Department of Pulmonary Diseases and Pulmonary Function Laboratory, University of Nymegen, Medical Centre Dekkerswald

434 **Antihypertensive and cardiovascular effects of nitrendipine: A controlled study vs. placebo**
Liberato Aldo Ferrara, M.D., Maria Luisa Fasano, M.D., Giovanni de Simone, M.D., Stefano Soro, M.D., and Renato Gagliardi, B.Sc., Naples, Italy, Institute of Internal Medicine and Metabolic Disease, Clinica Medica, Second Medical School, University of Naples, and Medical Department, Bayer Italia S.p.A.

439 **Pefloxacin kinetics in cirrhosis**
Gaby Danan, M.D., Guy Montay, Rober Cunci, M.D., and Serge Erlinger, M.D., Clichy and Alfortville, France, Service d'Hépatologie and Unité de Recherches de Physiopathologie Hépatique (INSERM U-24), Hopital Beaujon, Clichy, and Centre de Recherches du Laboratoire Roger Bellon, Alfortville

443 **Inhibition of prostaglandin synthesis by indomethacin interacts with the antihypertensive effect of atenolol**
Pauli Ylitalo, M.D., Timo Pitkäjärvi, M.D., Maija-Liisa Pyykönen, M.D., Anna-Kaisa Nurmi, M.Sc., Erkki Seppälä, M.D., M.Sc., and Heikki Vapaatalo, M.D., Tampere, Finland, Department of Biomedical Sciences, University of Tampere and the Community Health Centre

450 **Transdermal nicotine reduces cigarette craving and nicotine preference**
Jed E. Rose, Ph.D., Joseph E. Herskovic, Ph.D., Yvonne Trilling, and Murray E. Jarvik, M.D., Ph.D., Los Angeles, Calif., Psychopharmacology Unit, Veterans Administration Medical Center and Department of Psychiatry and Biobehavioral Sciences, The Neuropsychiatric Institute, University of California School of Medicine

Continued on page 6A

457 **Pharmacokinetics of high-dose pentobarbital in severe head trauma**
Charles D. Bayliff, Pharm.D., Michael L. Schwartz, M.D., and Brian G. Hardy, Pharm.D., Toronto, Ontario, Canada, Departments of Pharmacy and Surgery, Division of Neurosurgery, Sunnybrook Medical Centre, University of Toronto

462 **Pharmacokinetics of a new angiotensin I converting enzyme inhibitor (alacepril) after oral dosing in fasting or fed states**
Kaoru Onoyama, M.D., Hideki Hirakata, M.D., Hiroshi Tsuruda, M.D., Nobuaki Ohchi, M.D., Suguru Tomooka, M.D., Kenichi Motomura, M.D., Teruo Omae, M.D., Kouji Hayashi, Ph.D., and Masatoshi Fujishima, M.D., Fukuoka, Japan, Second Department of Internal Medicine, Faculty of Medicine, Kyushu University, National Cardiovascular Center, and Research Laboratories, Dainippon Pharmaceutical Co., Ltd.

469 **New insights into the pharmacokinetics of spironolactone**
Hans W. P. M. Overdiek, Pharm.D., Walter A. J. J. Hermens, B.S., and Frans W. H. M. Merkus, Ph.D., Sittard and Amsterdam, The Netherlands, Clinical Pharmacokinetics and Toxicology Laboratory, Hospital of Sittard, Sittard, and Department of Biopharmaceutics, University of Amsterdam, Amsterdam

LETTER TO THE EDITOR

475 **Concomittant food intake does enhance the bioavailability and effect of hydralazine**
A. Melander, M.D., H. Liedholm, M.D., and A. McLean, M.D., Dalby, Sweden, and Melbourne, Australia, Lund University Health Sciences Center, Dalby, and Monash University Department of Medicine, Melbourne

475 **Reply**
Alexander M. M. Shepherd, M.D., Ph.D., and Thomas M. Ludden, Ph.D., San Antonio, Tex., Divisions of Clinical Pharmacology and Pharmacy, Departments of Pharmacology, University of Texas Health Sciences Center

LIST OF REVIEWERS

477 **List of reviewers to volume 37**

ASCPT

478 **Notes of the American Society for Clinical Pharmacology and Therapeutics**

USAN COUNCIL

479 **USAN List No. 265**

Information to authors on pages 10A and 11A

NOVEMBER 1985

CLINICAL PHARMACOLOGY & THERAPEUTICS

VOLUME 38 NUMBER 5

MOSBY

TABLE OF CONTENTS

COMMENTARY

481 **Premarketing observational studies of population pharmacokinetics of new drugs**
Lewis B. Sheiner, M.D., and Leslie Z. Benet, Ph.D., San Francisco, Calif., Departments of Laboratory Medicine and Medicine, School of Medicine; Division of Clinical Pharmacology, Schools of Medicine and Pharmacy; and Department of Pharmacy, School of Pharmacy, University of California, San Francisco

ORIGINAL ARTICLES

488 **Mephenytoin hydroxylation polymorphism: Characterization of the enzymatic deficiency in liver microsomes of poor metabolizers phenotyped in vivo**
U. Thomas Meier, M.Sc., Pierre Dayer, M.D., Pierre-Jean Malè, M.D., Thomas Kronbach, Ph.D., and Urs A. Meyer, M.D., Basel, Switzerland, Department of Pharmacology, Biocenter of the University

495 **Evaluation and application of the linear variable differential transformer technique for the assessment of human dorsal hand vein alpha-receptor activity**
Assem O. Alradi, M.B., M.Sc., and S. George Carruthers, M.D., London, Ontario, Canada, Divisions of Clinical Pharmacology and Cardiology, Departments of Medicine and Pharmacology and Toxicology, University Hospital and the University of Western Ontario

503 **Pharmacodynamics of intravenous labetalol and follow-up therapy with oral labetalol**
Nicholas D. Vlachakis, M.D., Robert F. Maronde, M.D., James W. Maloy, Pharm.D., Milenko Medakovic, M.D., and Nadim Kassem, M.D., Los Angeles, Calif., Clinical Pharmacology Section, Department of Medicine, University of Southern California Medical Center

Continued on page 2A

509 **Biologic determinants of propranolol disposition: Results from 1308 patients in the Beta-blocker Heart Attack Trial**
Thomas Walle, Ph.D., Robert P. Byington, Ph.D., Curt D. Furberg, M.D., Kevin M. McIntyre, M.D., and Pantel S. Vokonas, M.D., Charleston, S. C., Houston, Tex., Bethesda, Md., and West Roxbury and Boston, Mass., Department of Pharmacology, Medical University of South Carolina, Charleston; BHAT Coordinating Center, University of Texas Health Science Center, School of Public Health, Houston; Clinical Application and Prevention Program, National Heart, Lung and Blood Institute, Bethesda; Veterans Administration Hospital, West Roxbury; and Boston University School of Medicine, Boston

519 **Pharmacologic reduction of sympathetic drive increases platelet alpha-2–receptor number**
Brent Egan, M.D., Richard Neubig, M.D., Ph.D., and Stevo Julius, M.D., Sc.D., Ann Arbor, Mich., Division of Hypertension, Department of Internal Medicine, University of Michigan Medical Center

525 **Pharmacodynamic evaluation of the benzodiazepine–oral contraceptive interaction**
Patricia D. Kroboth, Ph.D., Randall B. Smith, Ph.D., Gary P. Stoehr, Pharm.D., and Randy P. Juhl, Ph.D., Pittsburgh, Pa., and Kalamazoo, Mich., Departments of Pharmacy Practice and Medicine, University of Pittsburgh, Pittsburgh, and The Upjohn Company, Kalamazoo

533 **Fecal blood loss during isoxicam and piroxicam administration for 28 days**
John W. Hooper, Ph.D., June A. Anslow, B.Sc., William S. Martin, M.D., Pedro Araujo, B.Sc., and Andrew Darke, Ph.D., Montreal, Quebec, and Toronto, Ontario, Canada, Bio-Research Laboratories, Montreal, and Warner Lambert, Toronto

Volume 38, Number 5, November 1985. CLINICAL PHARMACOLOGY AND THERAPEUTICS. Published monthly by The C. V. Mosby Company, 11830 Westline Industrial Drive, St. Louis, MO 63146. POSTMASTER: Send address changes to The C. V. Mosby Company, 11830 Westline Industrial Drive, St. Louis, MO 63146.

1986 Annual subscription rates	*U.S.A.*	*International (surface mail)* All regions	*International (airmail)** Canada & Mexico	Region 1	Region 2	Region 3
Institutional†	$103.00	$119.00	$137.10	$139.75	$158.95	$178.15
Individual‡	$ 62.00	$ 78.00	$ 96.10	$ 98.75	$117.95	$137.15
Student, resident‡	$ 45.00	$ 61.00	$ 79.10	$ 81.75	$100.95	$120.15

Single copies are $6.50. Remittances should be made by check, draft, post office or express money order, in U.S. funds drawn through a U.S. bank, payable to this JOURNAL.

**Airmail breakdown—Domestic:* First-class and Priority rates for the U.S. and possessions are available upon request. *Region 1:* Central America, islands, and mainland colonies of European countries in The Americas. *Region 2:* South America, Europe, Egypt, Africa (bordering the Mediterranean). *Region 3:* Asia, Australasia, Africa (other than Mediterranean), Middle East, Far East, The Pacific, U.S.S.R. (and constituent Republics).

†Institutional (multiple-reader) subscriptions are available to public and private libraries, schools, hospitals, and clinics; city, county, state, provincial, and national government bureaus and departments; and all commercial and private institutions and organizations.

‡Individual subscriptions and all student-rate subscriptions must be in the names of, billed to, and paid by individuals. All student-rate requests must indicate training status and name of institution.

Subscriptions may begin at any time.

Second class postage paid at St. Louis, MO, and at additional mailing offices. Printed in the U. S. A.

538 Determinants of systemic availability of oral hydralazine in heart failure
Michael H. Crawford, M.D., Thomas M. Ludden, Ph.D., and Gemma T. Kennedy, M.S.N., San Antonio and Austin, Tex., Departments of Medicine and Pharmacology, University of Texas Health Science Center and Veterans Administration Hospital, San Antonio, and College of Pharmacy, University of Texas, Austin

544 Assessment of dezocine for morphine-like subjective effects and miosis
Donald R. Jasinski, M.D., and Kenzie L. Preston, Ph.D., Baltimore, Md., Department of Health and Human Services, Public Health Service, Alcohol, Drug Abuse and Mental Health Administration, and National Institute on Drug Abuse Addiction Research Center

549 Prilocaine in arthroscopy: Clinical pharmacokinetics and rational use
Danièle Debruyne, D.Chem., Maurice Moulin, M.D., Claude Thomassin, M.D., Bruno Locker, M.D., Jack Tartiere, M.D., Marie-Claire Bigot, B.S., Michel Besnard, M.D., Catherine Berthelin, M.D., and Jacques Beguin, M.D., Caen, France, Laboratory of Pharmacology, Department of Anesthesia, and Units of Orthopaedia B and Rhumatology, University Hospital Center of Caen

554 Effects of betaxolol, propranolol, and atenolol on isoproterenol-induced beta-adrenoceptor responses
James G. Riddell, M.D., and Robin G. Shanks, D.Sc., M.D., Belfast, Northern Ireland, Department of Therapeutics and Pharmacology, The Queen's University of Belfast

560 Effect of naloxone on the actions of captopril
Adesuyi A. Ajayi, B.Sc., M.B.Ch.B., Brian C. Campbell, M.D., Peter C. Rubin, D.M., and John L. Reid, D.M., Glasgow, United Kingdom, University Department of Materia Medica, Stobhill General Hospital

566 Oxidation of hydrazine metabolites formed from isoniazid
Bernard H. Lauterburg, M.D., Charles V. Smith, Ph.D., Elizabeth L. Todd, Ph.D., and Jerry R. Mitchell, M.D., Ph.D., Houston, Tex., Department of Internal Medicine and Institute for Lipid Research, Baylor College of Medicine

572 Excretion patterns of cannabinoid metabolites after last use in a group of chronic users
George M. Ellis, Jr., B.A., Marian A. Mann, B.A., Barbara A. Judson, M.S., N. Ted Schramm, M.A., and Agop Tashchian, CPT MC, USNR, San Diego, Calif., Treatment Department, Naval Drug Rehabilitation Center

Continued on page 4A

579 **Ultra-short-acting beta-blockade: A comparison with conventional beta-blockade**
Charles S. Reilly, M.D., Margaret Wood, M.D., Richard P. Koshakji, Ph.D., and Alastair J. J. Wood, M.D., Nashville, Tenn., Departments of Pharmacology, Medicine, and Anesthesiology, Vanderbilt University School of Medicine

586 **Pharmacokinetics of bupropion and its major basic metabolites in normal subjects after a single dose**
S. Casey Laizure, Pharm.D., C. Lindsay DeVane, Pharm.D., Jonathan T. Stewart, M.D., Cynthia S. Dommisse, Pharm.D., and Allen A. Lai, Ph.D., Gainesville, Fla., and Research Triangle Park, N. C., Colleges of Pharmacy and Medicine, University of Florida, Gainesville, and Wellcome Research Laboratories, Research Triangle Park

590 **The pharmacokinetics and bactericidal characteristics of oral cefixime**
David C. Brittain, Brian E. Scully, Toshiharu Hirose, and Harold C. Neu, New York, N. Y., Division of Infectious Diseases, Departments of Medicine and Pharmacology, College of Physicians and Surgeons, Columbia University

595 **Effect of alprazolam on digoxin kinetics and creatinine clearance**
Hermann R. Ochs, M.D., David J. Greenblatt, M.D., and Birgitt Verburg-Ochs, M.D., Bonn, Federal Republic of Germany, and Boston, Mass., Medizinische Universitätsklinik, University of Bonn, Bonn, and Tufts-New England Medical Center, Boston

ASCPT 599 **Notes of the American Society for Clinical Pharmacology and Therapeutics**

USAN COUNCIL 601 **USAN List No. 266**

Information to authors on pages 8A and 9A

DECEMBER 1985

CLINICAL PHARMACOLOGY & THERAPEUTICS

VOLUME 38 NUMBER 6

MOSBY

TABLE OF CONTENTS

COMMENTARY

603 **Clinical pharmacology: A personal perspective**
Elliot S. Vesell, M.D., Hershey, Pa., Department of Pharmacology, The Pennsylvania State University College of Medicine

ORIGINAL ARTICLES

613 **Inadequate aldosterone response to hyperkalemia during angiotensin converting enzyme inhibition in chronic renal failure**
M. Teresa Zanella, M.D., Edilio Mattei, Jr., M.D., Sérgio A. Draibe, M.D., Claudio E. Kater, M.D., and Horácio Ajzen, M.D., São Paulo, Brazil, Divisions of Nephrology and Endocrinology, Escola Paulista de Medicina

618 **Polymorphic dextromethorphan metabolism: Co-segregation of oxidative O-demethylation with debrisoquin hydroxylation**
B. Schmid, Ph.D., J. Bircher, M.D., R. Preisig, M.D., and A. Küpfer, Ph.D., Berne, Switzerland, Department of Clinical Pharmacology, University of Berne

625 **Effect of tolrestat on red blood cell sorbitol levels in patients with diabetes**
Philip Raskin, M.D., Julio Rosenstock, M.D., Patricia Challis, R.N., Steven Ryder, M.D., John F. Mullane, M.D., Ramona Gonzalez, Ph.D., David Hicks, Ph.D., Theodore Smith, Ph.D., and Dushan Dvornik, D.Sc., Dallas, Tex., Princeton, N. J., and New York, N. Y., Department of Internal Medicine, The University of Texas Health Science Center at Dallas, Dallas, and Departments of Biochemistry and Clinical Research, Ayerst Laboratories, Princeton and New York

631 **Epidural and intrathecal opiates: Cerebrospinal fluid and plasma profiles in patients with chronic cancer pain**
Mitchell B. Max, M.D., Charles E. Inturrisi, Ph.D., Robert F. Kaiko, Ph.D., Patricia Y. Grabinski, Ph.D., Choh Hao Li, Ph.D., and Kathleen M. Foley, M.D., New York, N. Y., and San Francisco, Calif., Department of Neurology and Analgesic Study Section, Memorial Sloan-Kettering Cancer Center and Departments of Neurology and Pharmacology, Cornell University Medical College, New York, and Hormone Research Laboratory, University of California Medical Center, San Francisco

DECEMBER 1985
INDEX ISSUE

Pharmacy

CLINICAL PHARMACOLOGY & THERAPEUTICS

VOLUME 38 NUMBER 6

OFFICIAL PUBLICATION OF THE
American Society for Clinical Pharmacology and Therapeutics
American Society for Pharmacology and Experimental Therapeutics

APPEARING IN THIS ISSUE

Clinical pharmacology: A personal perspective
Aldosterone response to hyperkalemia
Polymorphic dextromethorphan metabolism
Tolrestat and RBC sorbitol
Epidural and intrathecal opiates
Food-induced changes in theophylline absorption
Ibuprofen and H_2-blockers
Cimetidine, ranitidine, and midazolam
Computerized assessment of human neurotoxicity
Renal function and enalapril
Calcium blockers and digitoxin excretion
Etodolac and renal function
Estimation of GFR with gentamicin
Aminoglycosides and the thyroid
Sulbactam in breast milk
Nitrazepam disposition
ASCPT preregistration forms on pp 723-724

PUBLISHED AT ST. LOUIS, MISSOURI 63146 BY THE C.V. MOSBY COMPANY
ISSN 0009-9236

642 **Food-induced changes in theophylline absorption from controlled-release formulations. Part II. Importance of meal composition and dosing time relative to meal intake in assessing changes in absorption**
Aziz Karim, Ph.D., Thomas Burns, M.S., Denis Janky, M.S., and Aryeh Hurwitz, M.D., Skokie, Ill., and Kansas City, Kan., Searle Research & Development, Division of G. D. Searle & Co., Skokie, and Division of Clinical Pharmacology, University of Kansas Medical Center, Kansas City

648 **Interaction of ibuprofen with the H-2 receptor antagonists ranitidine and cimetidine**
Hermann R. Ochs, M.D., David J. Greenblatt, M.D., Rita Matlis, B.S., and Jutta Weinbrenner, M.D., Bonn, Federal Republic of Germany, and Boston, Mass., Medizinische Universitätsklinik, University of Bonn, Bonn, and the Division of Clinical Pharmacology, Tufts-New England Medical Center, Boston

652 **Effect of single doses of cimetidine and ranitidine on the steady-state plasma levels of midazolam**
Ulrich Klotz, Ph.D., Pentti Arvela, Ph.D., and Bernd Rosenkranz, M.D., Stuttgart, Federal Republic of Germany, Dr. Margarete Fischer-Bosch-Institut für Klinische Pharmakologie

656 **Computerized assessment of human neurotoxicity: Sensitivity to nitrous oxide exposure**
Benjamin D. Greenberg, Ph.D., Paul A. Moore, D.M.D., Ph.D., Richard Letz, Ph.D., and Edward L. Baker, M.D., M.P.H., Boston, Mass., Interdisciplinary Programs in Health and the Occupational Health Program, Harvard School of Public Health and Forsyth Dental Center

Continued on page 2A

Volume 38, Number 6, December 1985. CLINICAL PHARMACOLOGY AND THERAPEUTICS. Published monthly by The C. V. Mosby Company, 11830 Westline Industrial Drive, St. Louis, MO 63146. POSTMASTER: Send address changes to The C. V. Mosby Company, 11830 Westline Industrial Drive, St. Louis, MO 63146.

1986 Annual subscription rates	*U.S.A.*	*International (surface mail)* All regions	*International (airmail)** Canada & Mexico	Region 1	Region 2	Region 3
Institutional†	$103.00	$119.00	$137.10	$139.75	$158.95	$178.15
Individual‡	$ 62.00	$ 78.00	$ 96.10	$ 98.75	$117.95	$137.15
Student, resident‡	$ 45.00	$ 61.00	$ 79.10	$ 81.75	$100.95	$120.15

Single copies are $6.50. Remittances should be made by check, draft, post office or express money order, in U.S. funds drawn through a U.S. bank, payable to this JOURNAL.

**Airmail breakdown—Domestic:* First-class and Priority rates for the U.S. and possessions are available upon request. *Region 1:* Central America, islands, and mainland colonies of European countries in The Americas. *Region 2:* South America, Europe, Egypt, Africa (bordering the Mediterranean). *Region 3:* Asia, Australasia, Africa (other than Mediterranean), Middle East, Far East, The Pacific, U.S.S.R. (and constituent Republics).

†Institutional (multiple-reader) subscriptions are available to public and private libraries, schools, hospitals, and clinics; city, county, state, provincial, and national government bureaus and departments; and all commercial and private institutions and organizations.

‡Individual subscriptions and all student-rate subscriptions must be in the names of, billed to, and paid by individuals. All student-rate requests must indicate training status and name of institution.

Subscriptions may begin at any time.

Second class postage paid at St. Louis, MO, and at additional mailing offices. Printed in the U. S. A.

661 **The effect of renal function on enalapril kinetics**
D. T. Lowenthal, M.D., J. D. Irvin, M.D., Ph.D., D. Merrill, B.A., S. Saris, M.D., E. Ulm, Ph.D., S. Goldstein, M.D., M. Hichens, Ph.D., L. Klein, D.O., A. Till, Ph.D., and K. Harris, M.S., Philadelphia and West Point, Pa., Hahnemann University, Philadelphia, and Merck Sharp & Dohme Research Laboratories, West Point

667 **Effects of verapamil, diltiazem, and nifedipine on plasma levels and renal excretion of digitoxin**
J. Kuhlmann, M.D., Ph.D., Würzburg, Federal Republic of Germany, Department of Internal Medicine, Medical Clinic of the University of Würzburg

674 **Effect of etodolac in patients with moderate renal impairment compared with normal subjects**
D. Craig Brater, M.D., Shirley A. Anderson, R.N., Debbie Brown-Cartwright, P.A., Robert D. Toto, M.D., Andrew Chen, M.S., and Ginette B. Jacob, M.D., Dallas, Tex., Department of Internal Medicine and Pharmacology, The University of Texas Health Science Center at Dallas, and Ayerst Laboratories

680 **A simple method for the estimation of glomerular filtration rate by gentamicin pharmacokinetics during routine drug monitoring in the newborn**
Gideon Koren, M.D., Andrew James, M.D., and Max Perlman, M.D., Toronto, Ontario, Canada, Divisions of Clinical Pharmacology and Neonatal Intensive Care Unit, The Research Institute, The Hospital for Sick Children and Departments of Pediatrics and Pharmacology, University of Toronto

686 **Effect of aminoglycosides on the disposition of thyroid hormones and thyroglobulin**
Patrick du Souich, M.D., Ph.D., Cesar Pison, M.D., Louise Pedneault, M.D., Pierre Larochelle, M.D., Ph.D., Richard Morisset, M.D., Carlos Vega, M.D., Denis Phaneuf, M.D., and Michel Poisson, M.D., Montreal, Quebec, Canada, Division of Clinical Pharmacology, Service of Nuclear Medicine and Service of Infectious Diseases, Departments of Medicine, Radiology, and Pharmacology, Hôpital Hôtel-Dieu de Montréal and University of Montreal

692 **Sulbactam kinetics and excretion into breast milk in postpartum women**
George Foulds, Ph.D., R. David Miller, M.D., Anthony K. Knirsch, M.D., and Lauri D. Thrupp, M.D., Groton, Conn., and Orange, Calif., Central Research Division, Pfizer, Inc., Groton, and University of California Irvine Medical Center, Orange

697 **Age, sex, and nitrazepam kinetics: Relation to antipyrine disposition**
David J. Greenblatt, M.D., Darrell R. Abernethy, M.D., Ph.D., Ann Locniskar, B.S., Hermann R. Ochs, M.D., Jerold S. Harmatz, B.A., and Richard I. Shader, M.D., Boston, Mass., Houston, Tex., and Bonn, Federal Republic of Germany, Division of Clinical Pharmacology, Tufts-New England Medical Center, Boston; the Section on Hypertension/Clinical Pharmacology, Baylor College of Medicine, Houston; and the Medizinische Universitätsklinik, University of Bonn, Bonn

ASCPT 704 **Notes of the American Society for Clinical Pharmacology and Therapeutics**

723 **Preregistration forms**

USAN COUNCIL 705 **USAN List No. 267**

INDEX 707 **Index to Volume 38**

Information to authors on pages 6A and 7A

CLINICAL PHARMACOLOGY & THERAPEUTICS

CLINICAL PHARMACOLOGY & THERAPEUTICS
VOLUME 38 NUMBER 1 JULY 1985

A NOTE FROM THE CO-EDITOR

As the editorial transition from Dr. Modell's 25 years of leadership of CLINICAL PHARMACOLOGY AND THERAPEUTICS proceeds, I would like to bring some new policies and practices to the attention of our readers.

First, readers of our Information to Authors page may have already noticed that manuscripts should now conform to the "Vancouver" style. This is a uniform style for manuscripts that has already been adopted by many biomedical journals. We hope that by adopting this uniform style for manuscripts, we will make the mechanical part of manuscript preparation easier for our contributors.

Second, we have adopted a priority ranking system for manuscripts to aid in the editorial decision-making process. Valid, acceptable manuscripts, of which we receive more than we can publish, are ranked on the basis of novelty and importance as judged by the reviewers and editors. The degree of importance relates to the kinds of questions asked and the information and results obtained by the investigation. This aspect of our evaluation will consider whether the research has broad significance or has implications that are very narrow and relevant only to the specific phenomenon observed.

Third, we wish to reemphasize the broad scope of the JOURNAL. It is devoted to publishing "articles of high quality dealing with effects of drugs in man." To help assure competence in evaluating articles covering this broad field, the three Associate Editors were selected to span the range of areas in clinical pharmacology, including drug disposition and pharmacokinetics, drug epidemiology and clinical trials, and pharmacodynamic studies in man. The Editorial Board has members expert in many different fields and subspecialties to aid in manuscript evaluation and selection. Readers are invited to submit manuscripts describing research results dealing with any aspect of effects of drugs in man that they think present new and important findings. In addition, nominations of people to serve as outside reviewers are welcome. It is from the outside reviewers that new members of the Editorial Board will be appointed.

Fourth, we plan to start a small Letters to the Editor section for brief comments on papers published in the JOURNAL. Letters should be submitted in the same form as original articles, including copyright permission, and be limited to a maximum of 400 words including references. In addition, we would like to receive papers for the Commentary section. These should be brief, thoughtful essays on topics relevant to clinical pharmacology. Acceptance for publication will be at the discretion of the Editor.

For symposia to be published, three criteria must be met: (1) The subject of the symposium must be relevant to clinical pharmacology and therapeutics, (2) the symposium cannot be commercially oriented, and (3) each paper to be published must pass an independent peer review.

With these small changes, we hope to continue to keep CLINICAL PHARMACOLOGY AND THERAPEUTICS in the forefront of our discipline.

Marcus M. Reidenberg, M.D.
Co-Editor

COMMENTARY

The discipline of clinical pharmacology

Marcus M. Reidenberg, M.D. *New York, N. Y.*

In the last few years, it seems to have been fashionable for some people to take a rather pessimistic public stand about the future of clinical pharmacology. The late Prof. Franz Gross presented an "Editors' Headache"[10] that was rebutted by Sjoqvist[25] but restated by Gross.[11] We have been told clinical pharmacology has lost its way[1]; we have even been told no one needs clinical pharmacology.[16] Clearly there is a need for analysis of this issue.

Our predecessor, the American Therapeutic Society, was founded in 1900; thus our Society is 85 years old as of this annual meeting. If we look at the state of therapeutics when our Society was founded at the beginning of this century, and then consider some key factors in its progress since then, I think it will be clear that the discipline of clinical pharmacology is both vigorous and headed in the right direction.

Many of the early presidents of the American Therapeutic Society were surgeons who wrote papers about advancing therapeutics through new surgical techniques. Perhaps this was the principal way to improve therapeutics at that time. In the *Journal of the American Medical Association* in 1900, there is an article presenting the rational treatment of delirium tremens. The recommended management includes tincture of capsici in hot milk every 3 to 4 hours for nourishment, the sedating effects of a mixture of chloral hydrate, potassium bromide, and tincture of hyoscyamine if the patient is still awake, physical restraint, strichnine sulfate every 2 to 4 hours if there are signs of impending exhaustion of the heart, tincture of digitalis if the heart is weak and the patient sweating, and injection of aromatic spirits of ammonia or camphorated oil in the event of sudden collapse.

In 1908, 8 years after the founding of our Society, the American Society for Pharmacology and Experimental Therapeutics was formed. The first issue of its journal, the *Journal of Pharmacology and Experimental Therapeutics,* appeared in June 1909. The opening announcement of this new journal stated:

> Without rigidly defining the scope of the new journal, it may be stated that its pages will be open not only to pharmacologists and workers in experimental therapeutics, but also to the representatives of any of the biological or medical sciences who may wish to offer papers that have a close relationship to pharmacological or therapeutical questions.

It was clear even then that students of any of the biologic or medical sciences might be doing research in experimental therapeutics worthy of publication in this journal devoted to the discipline of pharmacology.

Another formal step on the path toward rational therapeutics was taken in 1937, when Dr. Harry Gold, the father of modern clinical pharmacology, began the Cornell Conferences on Therapy. He began publishing these conferences in book form in 1946; the following is from the preface of the first volume:

> It is the rare medical curriculum in which pharmacology and therapeutics are so arranged as to weave their teachings into a single and permanent design. The courses of pharmacology are isolated in a term or two in advance of the bulk of therapeutics and, to a considerable extent, clinicians continue to build the structure of therapeutic teaching with indifferent regard for the base already set for its support.
>
> . . . It is also clear that there is urgent need for a forum where pharmacologists and clinicians may come together and talk these things over. That, in essence, is the purpose of the Conferences on Therapy.

From the Cornell University Medical College.

Presented at the Annual Meeting of the American Society for Clinical Pharmacology and Therapeutics, March 28-30, 1985. (Presidential Address.)

Received for publication April 1, 1985; accepted April 7, 1985.

Reprint requests to: Dr. Marcus M. Reidenberg, Department of Pharmacology, Cornell University Medical College, 1300 Yale Ave., New York, NY 10021.

Thus in 1937 Dr. Gold described the need for the interface between pharmacology and clinical medicine that we now call clinical pharmacology.

In 1941, Drs. Louis S. Goodman and Alfred Gilman published the first edition of their now famous textbook of pharmacology titled *The Pharmacologic Basis of Therapeutics*. The title articulated the theme of the interface developing between medical science and medical practice.

In 1957, Dr. Walter Modell, who had perceived the need for a journal in the discipline of clinical pharmacology, began discussions that led to the founding of CLINICAL PHARMACOLOGY AND THERAPEUTICS in 1960. In his opening editorial Dr. Modell wrote:

> Because of the tremendous number of new drugs now being regularly introduced into medicine, problems of their pharmacologic and therapeutic evaluation have now become matters of great practical importance. As a result, clinical pharmacology, which has been some fifteen years in maturing, is now being recognized as a proper discipline in medical science . . . . much is still published about drugs and therapeutics in outstanding journals which is neither good nor acceptable. This is largely because most medical journals have no editorial standards for investigations of drug actions in man and their editorial boards are not properly geared to screen or edit publications resulting from them. By virtue of the specialized knowledge of its editorial board, a journal specializing in problems of drug evaluation in man would exclude poor papers. While this editorial screening by specialists in therapeutics as well as clinical pharmacology would, by itself, insure high standards of publication, the focalization of papers in the field would tend to elevate the standards of the field in general. It would tend to improve methods of investigation, to add insights into the subject, and to lead to more incisive analysis of the data. It would not only make the comparison of one paper with another easier, it would make it unavoidable, and would thereby encourage the critical examination of methods of investigation or analysis of results.

It was evident to Dr. Modell what the discipline of clinical pharmacology was and what purpose it served: It was to deal with the problems and the process of the evaluation of drugs in man.

Now let us look at how far our discipline has come and how slowly it has travelled until recently.

The idea of the comparative trial was described in the Bible. In First Kings, 21-24:

> And Elijah came near unto all the people and said: How long halt ye between two opinions? If the Lord be God, follow Him; but if Baal, follow him. And the people answered him not a word. Then said Elijah unto the people: I, even I only am left a prophet of the Lord; but Baal's prophets are four hundred and fifty men. Let them, therefore, give us two bullocks; and let them choose one bullock for themselves, and cut it in pieces, and lay it on the wood, and put no fire under; and I will dress the other bullock, and lay it on the wood, and put no fire under. And call ye on the name of your god, and I will call on the name of the Lord, and the God that answereth by fire, let him be God.

The Bible goes on to describe the failure of Baal to start a fire under his bullock. When Elijah called upon the Lord, a fire promptly started, consuming the offering and proving to the assembled people which was the true God.

The idea of a comparative trial was thus described in the time of Elijah in the ninth century B.C. Twenty-five hundred years later, in 1747, James Lind carried out his famous comparative therapeutic trial of scurvy, showing that oranges were effective treatment while a host of other standard remedies of the day were not.[28] This comparative clinical trial was published 6 years later, but Lind's discovery was not implemented until 1804, a drug lag of 57 years.

Evans and Hoyle introduced the placebo-controlled trial in 1933,[6] and Harry Gold was the first to emphasize placebo-controlled studies to differentiate the placebo effect from the pharmacologic effect of a dose of medicine. One of his early papers on this subject was published in 1937,[7] and he introduced the concept of and term "double blind" in 1950.[9]

In 1962, with the passage of the Kefauver-Harris amendment to the U.S. food and drug law, properly controlled clinical trials became the law of our land and a uniform requirement for new drugs, not merely an idealistic goal of a small fraternity of scientists. The discipline of clinical pharmacology, as defined and practiced by Lind, Gold, and Modell, had become the universal standard and was now part of the mainstream of American medical science.

But during this time the discipline of clinical pharmacology was expanding to other areas of drug effects in man, in addition to the area of the scientific evaluation of drug efficacy.

In 1951, two American hematologists, Wintrobe and Sturgeon, each noted a small number of patients with aplastic anemia who had taken chloramphenicol. They checked with their colleagues and learned of a few more cases. This led to the establishment of the Committee on Blood Dyscrasias of the American Medical Association in 1955, the formation of the Association's blood dyscrasia registry, and the start of systematic concern about adverse drug reactions.

The thalidomide tragedy of 1960 and 1961 focused the attention of the world on the subject of adverse drug reactions. The discipline of epidemiology, so successfully applied to uncover the cause of phocomelia in Germany in 1961,[27] was applied to the more general problem of adverse drug reactions. An observation in such studies was that two clinical factors appeared to predispose to adverse drug reactions. These were the absolute number of different drugs the patient was taking and the presence of preexisting impaired renal function. The first led to the burgeoning interest in drug interactions, a subject that had its earlier scientific basis in studies of factors that modified drug metabolism.[4,5] In the early 1970s, handbook collections of information about drug interactions were published,[2,12,15,26] and by the mid 1970s major international symposia were being held and published on the subject.[3,8,17]

The second factor, preexisting renal failure, also got further attention. Originally, antibiotic doses in renal disease were the focus of attention.[14] Attention later widened to the broad area of drug action in patients with poor renal function.[20,22,23]

At the same time as the blood dyscrasia program was developing, it was noted that two unrelated rare adverse drug reactions, prolonged apnea after succinycholine and hemolytic anemia after primaquine therapy, were due to specific enzymatic defects that were genetically determined. This started the line of study that inheritance might account for some of the individual differences in drug response[18] that Vogel subsequently named pharmacogenetics[19] and Werner Kalow established with his book.[13]

Thus we see that, starting in the 1950s, systematic attention to drug responses in specific individuals became a new theme of clinical pharmacology. This was anticipated by the work of Shannon, Brodie, and coworkers in the antimalarial program at Goldwater Memorial Hospital in the 1940s.[24] Clinical pharmacology had now begun to address how and why individuals differ in their response to drugs, in addition to how groups of similar patients treated with different regimens such as active drug and placebo, compare with each other. Developments in analytic chemistry permitted the measurement of a large number of drugs and metabolites in biologic fluids and enabled development of the fields of drug metabolism and pharmacokinetics. The concentrations of drugs associated with therapeutic efficacy and with toxicity were described. A new theme of clinical pharmacology emerged: the individualization of drug therapy.[21]

The discipline of clinical pharmacology concerns the scientific evaluation of drugs and their rational use in man. Its first theme has focused on the drugs: What do they do? Are they effective? What are their toxicities? The second theme has focused on the people: In what ways do they differ from each other? What are the causes of these differences? How can allowance for these differences be made in therapeutics? This theme, like the earlier one, has already been incorporated into the mainstream of medicine. Drug level monitoring has become commonplace, and individualization of drug dosage is now the rule rather than the exception.

Thus we see over the lifetime of our Society the development of the discipline of clinical pharmacology. It has identified, articulated, and moved two broad themes into the mainstream of medicine. These are the use of scientific method to study the effects of drugs in people and the individualization of drug therapy. The first focuses on learning about the drug; the second focuses on learning about the individual person. The first is essential for rational treatment of diseases; the second, for rational therapy of patients.

So much for the past. Where is our discipline now? I have reviewed most of the issues from October through December 1984 of the *Annals of Internal Medicine, New England Journal of Medicine, Lancet,* and *Journal of the American Medical Association.* With a definition of clinical pharmacology articles as those describing the effects of drugs in man, 26% to 31% of the original articles in these four journals were clinical pharmacology articles. Clearly our discipline is part of the mainstream of medicine, and the two themes of our discipline—the scientific study of drug effects in man and the individualization of drug therapy—have made possible the miraculous therapeutic progress of modern times.

Why, then, are people troubled about the future of clinical pharmacology? In my view, it is because they are confused. They are confused not about the discipline of clinical pharmacology, but about its practice.

We must all recognize that the concepts and techniques of clinical pharmacology are so basic, so fundamental, so important to all areas of medicine that they rapidly become incorporated into the mainstream of medicine and lose their identities with our separate discipline of clinical pharmacology. We have no fiber optic clinical pharmacologoscope that we can restrict to use by bona fide clinical pharmacologists. Yet even without a procedure requiring our personal services, we are doing reasonably well.

Our Society has 1,705 active members who are proud to be identified with our discipline. Our annual meeting attendance is excellent and the science presented is good and gets stronger each year. Clinical pharmacologists must be doing something right! What we are doing, what we are each concerned about, what we profess as a profession, is the scientific study of drugs in man and the individualization of drug therapy for the sick.

From this analysis, from tracing the roots of our discipline from biblical times to the present, it is evident that despite vigorous objections and obstacles, our discipline has permeated all of medicine and all of medical thought and is part of the mainstream of medicine. Furthermore, it is my belief that this is where the discipline of clinical pharmacology belongs, right in the mainstream of all of medicine.

And about the clinical pharmacologists, what is their specific role? It is to advance, to teach, and to practice our discipline. It is to be innovative and lead the mainstream of medicine in the scientific study of drugs in man and in the individualization of drug therapy for the sick. It is to teach about the importance and practice of the scientific evaluation of therapeutic regimens, and about individualizing drug therapy. It is to evaluate scientifically drugs in man and to individualize therapy for the sick. As clinical pharmacologists carry out these traditional functions of research, teaching, and practice in our discipline, it should be obvious that the pessimism of the present is unwarranted and that the future looks very bright indeed.

References

1. Bonati M, Tognoni G: Has clinical pharmacology lost its way? Lancet **1:**556-558, 1984.
2. Cadwallader DE: Biopharmaceutics and drug interactions. Nutley, NJ, 1971, Roche Laboratories.
3. Cluff LE, Petrie JC, editors: Clinical effects of interaction between drugs. Amsterdam, 1975, Excerpta Medica.
4. Conney AH, Burns JJ: Factors influencing drug metabolism. Adv Pharmacol **1:**31-58, 1962.
5. Cucinell SA, Conney AH, Sansur M, Burns JJ: Drug interactions in man. I. Lowering effect of phenobarbital on plasma levels of bishydroxycoumarin (Dicumarol) and diphenylhydantoin (Dilantin). CLIN PHARMACOL THER **6:**420-429, 1965.
6. Evans W, Hoyle C: The comparative value of drugs used in the continuous treatment of angina pectoris. Quart J Med **26**(vol 2 of new series):311-338, 1933.
7. Gold H, Kwit NT, Otto H: The xanthines (theobromine and aminophylline) in the treatment of cardiac pain. JAMA **108:**2173-2179, 1937.
8. Grahame-Smith DG, editor: Drug interactions. Baltimore, 1977, University Park Press.
9. Greiner T, Gold H, Cattell M, et al: A method for the evaluation of the effects of drugs on cardiac pain in patients with angina of effort. Am J Med **9:**143-155, 1950.
10. Gross F: Editors' headache. Eur J Clin Pharmacol **21:**443-444, 1982.
11. Gross F: Editor's reply. Eur J Clin Pharmacol **23:**473, 1982.
12. Hartshorn EA: Handbook of drug interactions. Cincinnati, 1970, Donald E. Francke.
13. Kalow W: Pharmacogenetics. Philadelphia, 1962, WB Saunders Co.
14. Kunin CM: A guide to the use of antibiotics in patients with renal disease. Ann Intern Med **67:**151-158, 1967.
15. Martin EW: Hazards of medication. Philadelphia, 1977, JB Lippincott.
16. Mitchell JRA: Who needs clinical pharmacology? Br Med J **289:**1119-1120, 1984.
17. Morselli PL, Garattini S, Cohen SN, editors: Drug interactions. New York, 1974, Raven Press.
18. Motulsky AG: Drug reactions, enzymes, and biochemical genetics. JAMA **165:**835-837, 1957.
19. Motulsky AG, Vogel F, Buselmaier W, et al, editors: Human genetic variation in response to medical and environmental agents: Pharmacogenetics and ecogenetics. Hum Genet (suppl 1):1-192, 1978.
20. Reidenberg MM: Renal function and drug action. Philadelphia, 1971, WB Saunders Co.
21. Reidenberg MM, editor: Individualization of drug therapy. Medical Clinics of North America. Philadelphia, 1971, WB Saunders Co.
22. Richet G, Fabre J, de Freudenreich J, Podevin R: La tolerance medicamenteuse des uremiques. Nouv Presse Med **74:**2339-2340, 1966.
23. Schreiner GE, Maher JF: Drugs and the kidney. Ann NY Acad Sci **123:**326-332, 1965.
24. Shannon JA: The study of antimalarials and antimalarial activity in the human malarias. Harvey Lectures **41:**43-89, 1946.
25. Sjoqvist F: The future of clinical pharmacology—Rebuttal of an editor's headache. Eur J Clin Pharmacol **23:**471-473, 1982.
26. Swidler G: Handbook of drug interactions. New York, 1971, Wiley-Interscience.
27. Taussig HB: A study of the German outbreak of phocomelia. The thalidomide syndrome. JAMA **180:**1106-1114, 1962.
28. Thomas DP: Experiment versus authority. James Lind and Benjamin Rush. N Engl J Med **281:**932-933, 1969.

ORIGINAL ARTICLES

Salicylate kinetics in old age

Salicylate kinetics were determined in 28 subjects 25 to 92 years old who received single, oral doses of sodium salicylate (1 gm/1.73 m²). The serum AUC_∞ of total salicylate did not correlate with age. There was a weak positive correlation between the AUC_∞ of free (unbound) drug and age, but there was no apparent difference between the AUC_∞ values of the 15 women and 13 men. Seven of the 16 subjects >70 years of age cleared salicylate at about the same rate as the younger subjects. A comparison of these seven subjects with the nine >70 years old who were slow eliminators of salicylate revealed that the latter group consisted of more bedridden patients and that these patients had somewhat lower serum albumin concentrations, but they did not differ from the more rapid eliminators with respect to serum creatinine or urea nitrogen levels, SGOT, average age, female/male ratio, and average body weight. The serum protein binding of salicylate decreased with increasing age, apparently due mainly to decreasing serum albumin concentrations. (CLIN PHARMACOL THER 38:6-11, 1985.)

Patrick Netter, M.D., Gilbert Faure, M.D., Marie Christine Regent, M.D., Josephine A. Procknal, B.A.,† and Gerhard Levy, Pharm.D.
Nancy, France, and Amherst, N. Y.

The proportion of the elderly in the population is increasing. About one of every three elderly people has arthritis or rheumatism[11] and is therefore a candidate for chronic salicylate therapy. Because the therapeutic salicylate plasma or serum concentration range in the treatment of inflammatory diseases is relatively narrow,[7,8] salicylate dosage regimens must be carefully adjusted on the basis of kinetic characteristics of the individual patient. Advanced age is associated with various physiologic changes that can alter the absorption, distribution, metabolism, and excretion of drugs. These changes include decreases in renal function, cardiac output, lean body mass, total body water, serum albumin concentration, and drug metabolizing enzyme activity.[3,6,13] It is desirable, therefore, to assess the effect of age on salicylate kinetics.

Salicylic acid is eliminated from the body by biotransformation to salicyluric acid, salicyl acyl and phenolic glucuronides, and gentisic acid and by renal excretion of unmetabolized drug. Two of these parallel pathways (the formation of salicyluric acid and salicyl phenolic glucuronide) are of limited capacity in man and exhibit Michaelis-Menten kinetics.[10] The serum protein binding of salicylic acid is concentration dependent in the usual therapeutic concentration range, which introduces an additional type of nonlinearity into the kinetics of salicylic acid. To facilitate interpretation of data in our comparative study, the test dose of salicylate was normalized on the basis of estimated body surface area and the effect of age was assessed on the basis of the concentration-time profile of free (unbound) drug.

METHODS

Our subjects were 15 women and 13 men ranging in age from 25 to 92 years. Most were hospitalized for various reasons but had no gastrointestinal, hepatic, renal, or inflammatory disease. None had received sa-

From the Laboratoire de Pharmacologie, Clinique Rhumatologique, Clinique Médicale B, CHU de Nancy-Brabois, Nancy, and Department of Pharmaceutics, School of Pharmacy, State University of New York at Buffalo, Amherst.

Supported in part by Grant No. GM 19568 from the National Institute of General Medical Sciences of the National Institutes of Health and by grants from Conseil Scientifique Université Nancy I and INSERM ATP 69.78.101.

Received for publication Nov. 5, 1984; accepted Jan. 14, 1985.

Reprint requests to: Dr. Gerhard Levy, Department of Pharmaceutics, School of Pharmacy, State University of New York at Buffalo, Amherst, NY 14260.

†Deceased.

licylates for at least 1 week before the study. Four were smokers and six drank alcohol regularly. Their serum creatinine concentrations were ≤1.5 mg/dl, the serum urea nitrogen level was <27 mg/dl, and the serum albumin concentration ranged from 2.50 to 4.57 gm/dl.

A single oral dose of sodium salicylate (1 gm/1.73 m^2; body surface area determined by nomogram[4]) was taken as an aqueous solution (100 ml and a rinse) in the morning on an empty stomach. Food was permitted after 1 hour. Blood samples were collected in glass syringes before dosing and about 0.5, 1, 2, 4, 6, 8, 10, and 12 hours thereafter. Serum was separated and stored in a freezer or in dry ice. Salicylic and salicyluric acid concentrations in serum were determined by HPLC after extraction. A mixture of 0.5 ml serum and 0.5 ml 6N hydrochloric acid was extracted with 6 ml ethyl ether. Four milliliters of the ether phase was then extracted with 0.5 ml 0.13 mol/L phosphate buffer at pH 7.4 containing *o*-methoxybenzoic acid as internal standard. The concentration of the internal standard was between 0.02% and 0.05%, depending on the anticipated concentration of salicylate. An aliquot (20 to 30 μl) of the buffer phase was injected onto a C-18 μ-Bondapak column (Waters Associates). The mobile phase consisted of methanol and 1.6% acetic acid (22/78, v/v). Flow rate was 2.5 ml/min and the effluent was monitored spectrophotometrically at 254 nm.

Salicylate serum protein binding was determined by equilibrium dialysis. Serum from blood drawn before dosing was dialyzed at 37° C for 4 hours against an equal volume of 0.13 mol/L isotonic phosphate buffer at pH 7.4 that contained 5 or 30 mg salicylic acid per deciliter. A part of the serum phase was then deproteinized by adding three parts absolute alcohol containing *o*-methoxybenzoic acid, mixing on a vortex, and centrifuging. The salicylic acid concentration in the supernatant was determined by HPLC. The buffer phase was assayed in a like manner, but the internal standard was dissolved in water rather than ethanol and the centrifugation step was omitted. A serum sample drawn after dosing containing about 5 mg/dl salicylic acid, constituted by combining in appropriate proportion serum containing salicylic acid in concentrations above and below 5 mg/dl, was also subjected to equilibrium dialysis. Results are reported as percent free fraction values (i.e., 100 × drug concentration in buffer phase divided by drug concentration in serum phase). Total protein concentrations in serum were determined by the method of Gornall et al.[5] with crystalline human albumin as the standard. The albumin fraction was quan-

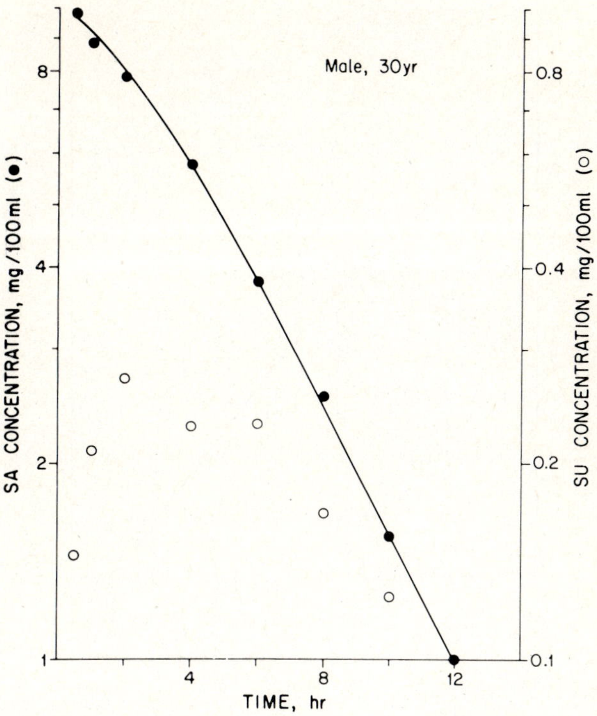

Fig. 1. Serum concentrations of salicylic acid *(SA)* and salicyluric acid *(SU)* in a 30-year-old man after a single, oral dose of sodium salicylate, 1 gm/1.73 m^2 body surface area.

titated by electrophoresis. Determinations were made from the zero-time and 12-hour serum samples and results were averaged. The same pairs of serum samples were assayed for urea nitrogen with a commercial kit.

The total serum salicylate and free serum salicylate AUCs from zero to 12 hours were determined by the trapezoidal method; the AUC from zero to infinity was estimated by adding to the AUC_{0-12} value the remaining area, calculated by dividing the salicylate concentration at 12 hours by the apparent terminal elimination rate constant. The concentrations of free (unbound) salicylate (C_f) used for the area calculations were the product of total concentration (C_t) and free fraction. Free fraction values at different salicylate concentrations were calculated by use of individual estimates of the constants a and b of the empiric equation of Behm and Wagner,[1] who found a linear relationship of the type $(C_f/C_t) = a + bC_t$ for salicylate protein binding determined by equilibrium dialysis. We confirmed this linearity over a salicylate concentration range of at least 5 to 30 mg/dl. Values of a and b for individual subjects were calculated from C_f/C_t ratios and C_t obtained by equilibrium dialysis of zero-time serum samples against

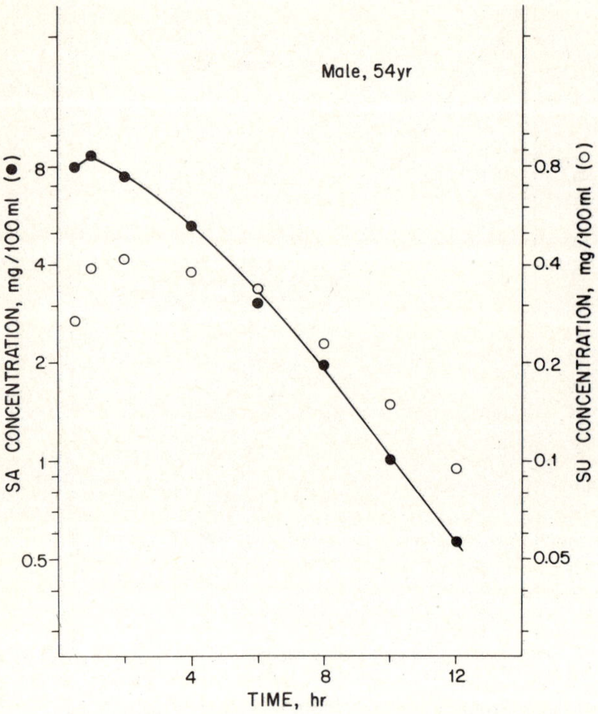

Fig. 2. Serum concentrations of salicylic acid *(SA)* and salicyluric acid *(SU)* in a 54-year-old man after a single, oral dose of sodium salicylate, 1 gm/1.73 m² body surface area.

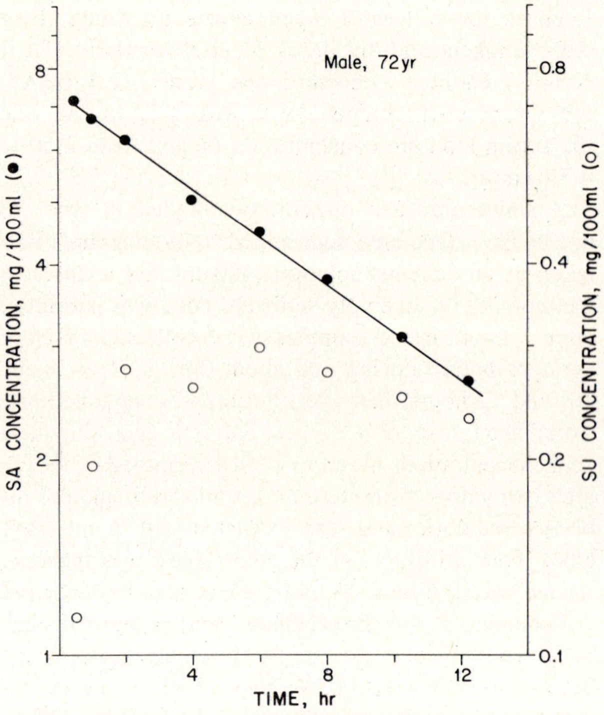

Fig. 3. Serum concentrations of salicylic acid *(SA)* and salicyluric acid *(SU)* in a 72-year-old man after a single, oral dose of sodium salicylate, 1 gm/1.73 m² body surface area.

buffer solutions containing 5 and 30 mg/dl salicylic acid, respectively.

RESULTS

Typical serum salicylic acid and salicyluric acid concentration-time curves over the age range of our subjects are shown in Figs. 1 to 4. Because the drug was taken in solution on an empty stomach, absorption was rapid, such that the first (30-minute) serum sample usually had the highest salicylic acid concentration. The salicylate concentration profile of the younger subjects exhibited the typical downward curve characteristic of Michaelis-Menten kinetics (Figs. 1 and 2), while most of the elderly subjects showed exponentially declining concentrations (Figs. 3 and 4), sometimes with an initial distribution phase (Fig. 4). Salicyluric acid concentrations were very low and tended to be higher in older subjects.

The relationship between the serum AUC_∞ for total (free plus protein bound) salicylic acid and age is shown in Fig. 5. There was no discernible difference between women and men and no apparent correlation between AUC_∞ and age, but AUC_∞ values for subjects >70 years of age varied more than those of the younger subjects. The mean (±SD) estimated AUC values from 12 hours (the time of the last blood sample) to infinity were 22% ± 12% (n = 28) of AUC_∞.

The relationship between the AUC_∞ for free (unbound) salicylate and age is shown in Fig. 6. There is a weak but significant ($r = 0.36$; $P < 0.03$) positive correlation between these AUC_∞ values and age. Seven of the 16 subjects >70 years of age had AUC_∞ values in the same range as those of the younger subjects, whereas nine of the subjects >70 years of age had significantly higher AUC_∞ values indicative of slower salicylic acid clearance. Characteristics of these two groups are compared in Table I. There were no significant differences between the groups with respect to serum creatinine and urea nitrogen levels, SGOT, female/male ratio, age, and body weight, but the relatively slow eliminators of salicylic acid had somewhat lower serum albumin concentrations and a larger proportion of these subjects were bedridden.

Salicylate serum protein binding was variable and concentration dependent, with no significant difference in the free fraction at comparable concentrations of total salicylate between serum samples drawn after dosing and the zero-time serum samples with salicylate added

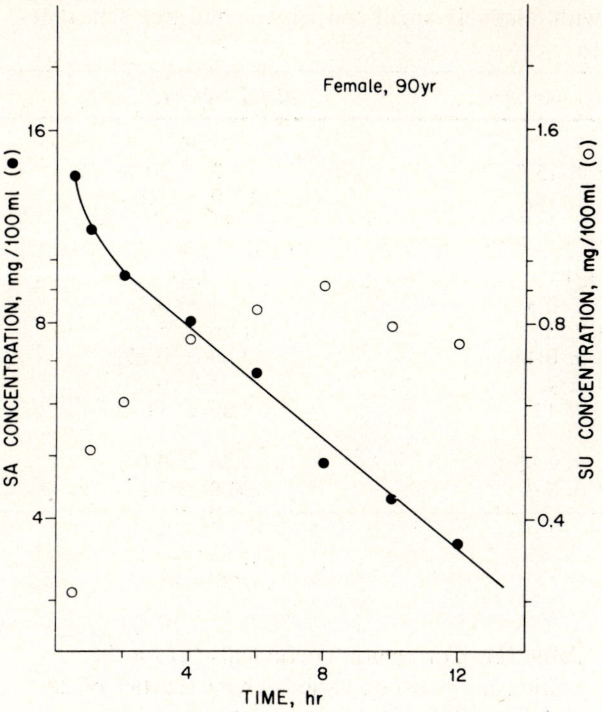

Fig. 4. Serum concentrations of salicylic acid *(SA)* and salicyluric acid *(SU)* in a 90-year-old woman after a single, oral dose of sodium salicylate, 1 gm/1.73 m^2 body surface area.

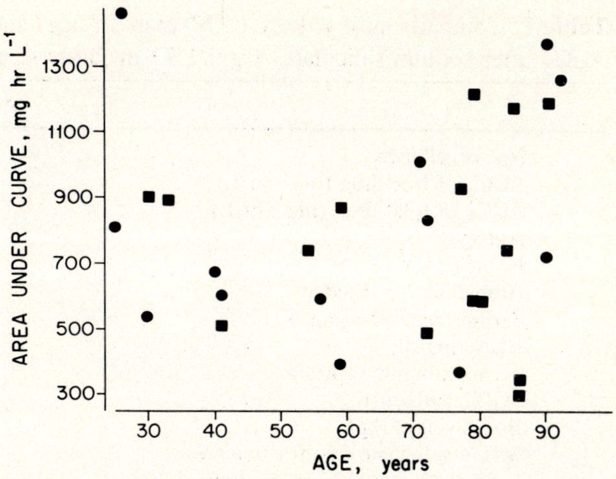

Fig. 5. Relationship between total salicylic acid serum AUC_∞ and age in subjects receiving a single, oral dose of sodium salicylate, 1 gm/1.73 m^2 body surface area. ■ = Women; ● = men.

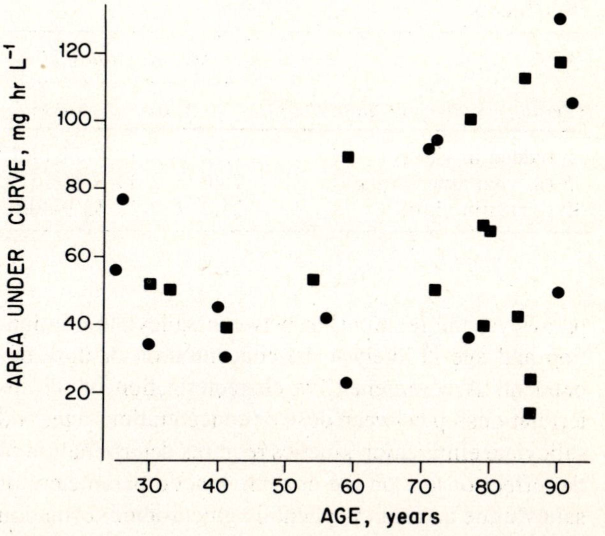

Fig. 6. Relationship between free (not protein bound) salicylic acid serum AUC_∞ and age in subjects receiving a single, oral dose of sodium salicylate, 1 gm/1.73 m^2 body surface area. ■ = Women; ● = men.

in vitro (Table II). The free fraction at an initial serum salicylate concentration of 5 mg/dl rose with increasing age ($r = 0.533$; $P < 0.005$) and the serum albumin concentration decreased with increasing age ($r = -0.528$; $P < 0.005$). In the elderly (>70 years of age), the slow eliminators of salicylate tended to have higher serum free fractions of the drug than did the more rapid eliminators, but the differences were not significant (Table I). The constants a and b of the equation relating the free fraction to total salicylate concentration in serum (see Methods) negatively correlated with serum albumin concentration and age and were independent of serum levels of creatinine and urea nitrogen (Table III).

DISCUSSION

Because of the capacity-limited kinetics of salicylate, its body clearance decreases with increasing concentration or dose.[9,10] To permit direct comparison of salicylate serum concentration–time profiles, we used doses normalized on the basis of estimated body surface area. The relative contributions of the five important pathways of salicylate elimination (see Introduction) to its body clearance change with dose or concentration. Relatively small single doses, including the dose we used, are eliminated mainly by conjugation of salicylic acid with glycine to yield salicyluric acid.[14] Renal excretion of salicylate and formation of salicylic acid glucuronides become relatively more important elimination pathways for large single doses and for multiple doses that produce high plasma salicylate concentrations. Because age may have different effects on each of these

Table I. Comparison of elderly (>70 years of age) subjects with relatively small and large serum free salicylate AUC_∞ after sodium salicylate, 1 gm/1.73 m² body surface area

	AUC_∞ <60 mg · hr/L	*AUC_∞ >60 mg · hr/L*
No. of subjects	7	9
AUC_∞ of free drug (mg · hr/L)	37.0 ± 13.5	99.3 ± 20.9
AUC_∞ of total drug (mg · hr/L)	505 ± 181	1070 ± 246
Age (yr)	82 ± 6	82 ± 8
Female/male	5/2	5/4
Ambulatory/bedridden	6/1	3/6*
Serum creatinine (mg/dl)	1.1 ± 0.3	1.3 ± 0.2
BUN (mg/dl)	18.9 ± 3.8	17.6 ± 5.6
Serum albumin (gm/dl)	3.43 ± 0.44	3.00 ± 0.35†
SGOT (mU/ml)	19 ± 4	21 ± 6
Body weight (kg)	51 ± 13	50 ± 11
Serum salicylate free fraction (%)		
50 mg/L initial concentration	8.22 ± 1.95	9.59 ± 3.00
300 mg/L initial concentration	27.3 ± 5.3	30.9 ± 7.5

Data are $\overline{X}$ ± SD.
*$P < 0.05$ by a test comparing two success probabilities.
†$P = 0.05$ (two-tailed t test).

Table II. Serum free fraction of salicylate in 28 subjects

	Free fraction (%)	
Predialysis concentration (mg/dl)	*$\overline{X}$ ± SD*	*Range*
5 (added in vitro)	7.76 ± 2.55	4.34-14.1
5 (in vivo after dosing)	7.46 ± 2.80	3.77-15.5
30 (added in vitro)	25.2 ± 7.2	13.9-40.6

Table III. Correlation coefficients (n) for the relationship between various characteristics of 28 subjects and the constants a and b for serum protein binding of salicylate*

Correlate	*a*	*b*
Serum albumin concentration	−0.651†	−0.861†
Serum creatinine concentration	0.094	0.133
Serum urea nitrogen concentration	0.094	0.003
Age	0.420‡	0.637†

*$C_f/C_t = a + bC_t$ (see Methods).[1]
†$P < 0.002$, ‡$P < 0.02$.

pathways, the relationship between salicylate elimination and age is likely to be concentration or dose dependent. A comprehensive characterization of the interrelationship between dose or concentration, age, and salicylate elimination kinetics requires determination of the effect of age on the enzyme kinetic parameters of salicylurate and salicyl phenolic glucuronide formation processes and on the kinetic constants of the other, apparently linear parallel elimination processes. Such studies necessitate intensive blood and urine sampling, which is very difficult in elderly subjects. Our investigation was designed to assess the need for such comprehensive studies by determining the magnitude of the effect of age on the elimination of a single salicylate dose. The size of the dose was such that most of it (about 90%) would be expected to be metabolized rather than excreted unchanged.[14]

As expected, the older subjects in our study had lower serum albumin concentrations, which probably accounted in large part for the decreased serum protein binding of salicylate with increasing age. Because the pharmacologic activity of salicylate appears to be a function of free drug concentration,[12] the effect of age on salicylate kinetics will be discussed relative to the free salicylate concentration data summarized in Fig. 6. It is evident that there is no strong distinct relationship between AUC_∞ (an index that is inversely proportional to body clearance) and age, nor is there any apparent sex difference. However, salicylate kinetics were more variable in the elderly. About half of the 16 subjects >70 years of age had AUC_∞ values of the same order as those of the 25- to 70-year-old subjects. The other half had much higher AUC_∞ values, reflecting a lower time-averaged body clearance of salicylate.

The two groups of subjects >70 years of age showed no evidence of differences in biochemical indices of renal and liver functions, but on the average the slow eliminators of salicylate had lower serum albumin concentrations, and relatively more of these subjects were bedridden. Bedridden subjects included those with cancer, tuberculosis, and hypertension, but the study group was too small to assess the effects of specific diseases and concurrent drug therapy.

Our results suggest that a substantial percentage of individuals >70 years of age may be relatively slow eliminators of salicylate. This conclusion is limited by the relatively small number of subjects and by the possibility that they may not be representative of the general elderly population. It appears, however, that advanced age per se does not have a pronounced effect on salicylate kinetics. It is more likely that certain pathophysiologic perturbations that affect salicylate kinetics are more frequent or become more severe in old age. These considerations indicate a special need for clinical and kinetic monitoring of salicylate therapy in the elderly.

References

1. Behm HL, Wagner JG: Parabolic equation relating free and total drug concentrations in cases of nonlinear plasma protein binding. J Pharm Sci **70:**802-804, 1981.
2. Brown BW, Hollander M: Statistics—A biomedical introduction. New York, 1977, John Wiley & Sons Inc., chap 8.
3. Crooks J, O'Malley K, Stevenson IH: Pharmacokinetics in the elderly. Clin Pharmacokinet **1:**280-296, 1976.
4. Diem K, Lentner C: Documenta Geigy Scientific Tables, ed 7. Basel, Switzerland, 1970, J.R. Geigy S.A., p 537.
5. Gornall AG, Bardawill CJ, David MM: Determination of serum proteins by means of the biuret reaction. J Biol Chem **177:**751-766, 1949.
6. Gorrod JW: Absorption, metabolism and excretion of drugs in geriatric subjects. Gerontol Clin **16:**30-42, 1974.
7. Levy G: Clinical pharmacokinetics of aspirin. Pediatrics **62:**867-872, 1978.
8. Levy G: Clinical pharmacokinetics of salicylates: A reassessment. Br J Clin Pharmacol **10:**285S-290S, 1980.
9. Levy G, Tsuchiya T: Salicylate accumulation kinetics in man. N Engl J Med **287:**430-432, 1972.
10. Levy G, Tsuchiya T, Amsel LP: Limited capacity for salicyl phenolic glucuronide formation and its effect on the kinetics of salicylate elimination in man. CLIN PHARMACOL THER **13:**258-268, 1972.
11. Moore SR: Prescription drug information for the elderly. Pharmacy Int **2:**283-289, 1981.
12. Reynolds RC, Cluff LE: Interaction of serum and sodium salicylate: Changes during acute infection and its influence on pharmacological activity. Bull Johns Hopkins Hosp **107:**278-290, 1960.
13. Triggs EJ, Nation RL: Pharmacokinetics in the aged: A review. J Pharmacokinet Biopharm **3:**387-418, 1975.
14. Tsuchiya T, Levy G: Biotransformation of salicylic acid to its acyl and phenolic glucuronides in man. J Pharm Sci **61:**800-801, 1972.

Atropine serum concentrations after multiple inhaled doses of atropine sulfate

Atropine may be given by inhalation for bronchodilation. Intravenous atropine at doses of 0.32 to 1 mg yields serum levels of 2 to 6 ng/ml, with an elimination $t_{1/2}$ of about 4 hours. Efficient inhalation of large single doses leads to similar concentrations in some individuals, but under clinical conditions drug delivery may be less efficient. Of concern is accumulation of the drug in the body with multiple-dose therapy. We measured serum levels of atropine after single inhaled doses and again after 48 to 72 hours of inhalation every 4 to 6 hours in 11 subjects. The drug was administered by therapists at doses and techniques commonly used in the clinical setting. Serum concentrations of atropine were negligible after the first dose in all subjects but were detectable in six of nine subjects who received the drug for more than 48 hours. Three of the subjects had levels >2 ng/ml. (CLIN PHARMACOL THER 38:12-15, 1985.)

Wayne A. Kradjan, Pharm.D., Robert C. Smallridge, M.D., Robin Davis, Pharm.D., and Pritam Verma, Ph.D. *Seattle, Wash., Washington, D. C., and Aurora, Colo.*

When given by nebulization, atropine and other anticholinergic drugs are effective bronchodilators.[2] Inhalation of a large single dose of atropine sulfate from a controlled delivery device (dosimeter) can result in serum atropine concentrations that can induce systemic side effects.[5] An important unanswered question is whether inhalation of more conventional doses under typical clinical conditions will also lead to significant systemic absorption, especially after several days of therapy. The purpose of our study was to measure serum atropine levels after single and multiple doses of inhaled atropine sulfate in hospitalized patients receiving the drug for acute respiratory distress.

METHODS

Patients were admitted to the study if they were inpatients in either the medical or intensive care units at our hospital and if their physician ordered inhaled atropine sulfate as part of their therapy. All subjects had severe bronchospasm secondary to acute exacerbation of asthma or chronic obstructive pulmonary disease. Most were also taking oral or parenteral theophylline derivatives and some form of inhaled sympathomimetic bronchodilator. The only subjects receiving enzyme-inhibiting or -inducing compounds were subjects 2 and 6, both of whom were receiving parenteral cimetidine. No attempt was made to alter the prescribed dose or dosing interval of atropine as long as it was appropriate for the subject's age and weight.[6] Exclusion criteria included the use of inhaled or parenteral atropine or other anticholinergic drugs within the last 7 days or a history of abnormal liver function test results, glaucoma, dysrhythmias, prostatic hypertrophy, or other known causes of urinary retention.

All doses of atropine (as atropine sulfate) were diluted to a total volume of 2.5 ml and administered by nebulization over a period of 10 to 15 minutes. For subjects in the intensive care unit the drug was always administered by a respiratory therapist, while administration to subjects in the medical wards was either by a therapist or (in two cases) by self administration. No attempt was made to modify the therapist's usual techniques. Subjects who administered the drug themselves had been instructed in proper inhalation techniques and had experience with home nebulizer equipment. In subjects who had a tracheostomy tube in place, the drug was either nebulized directly into the trachea or through the respirator. Details on the method of drug administration for each subject are listed in Table I.

Immediately before the first dose of atropine and 60 minutes after the end of nebulization, 5 ml blood was drawn into a heparinized tube either by direct venipuncture or through an indwelling venous access line

From the Department of Pharmacy Practice, University of Washington School of Pharmacy, Seattle; Department of Clinical Physiology, Walter Reed Army Institute of Research, Walter Reed Army Medical Center, Washington; and Department of Biochemistry, Clinical Investigation Branch, Fitzsimmons Army Medical Center, Aurora.

The opinions or assertions contained herein are the private views of the authors and are not to be construed as official or reflecting the views of the Department of the Army or the Department of the Defense.

Received for publication Jan. 8, 1985; accepted Jan. 15, 1985.

Reprint requests to: Wayne A. Kradjan, Pharm.D., Associate Professor, Pharmacy Practice, School of Pharmacy SC-69, University of Washington, Seattle, WA 98195.

Table I. Subject data and serum atropine levels

Subject No.	Age (yr)/ sex	Dose: mg	Dose: mg/kg	Dosing interval	Administration method	Serum atropine concentration (ng/ml): First dose: Pre	First dose: Post	Steady state: Pre	Steady state: Post
1	58/M	1	0.012	q. 4 hr	Trach	<0.50	<0.50	1.76	2.03
2	75/M	0.5	0.013	q. 4 hr	Therapist	<0.50	<0.50	NA	NA
3	58/M	1	0.015	q. 4 hr	Trach	<0,50	<0.50	NA	NA
4	77/F	1	0.016	q. 6 hr	Therapist	<0.50	<0.50	0.96	1.61
5	72/M	1	0.016	q. 4 hr	Self	NA	NA	0.69	1.13
6	70/M	1	0.018	q. 6 hr	Trach	<0.50	0.65	<0.50	<0.50
7	72/M	1	0.019	q. 4 hr	Therapist	NA	NA	4.30	5.23
8	61/M	1	0.020	q. 4 hr	Self	<0.50	<0.50	1.44	2.36
9	59/M	1	0.021	q. 4 hr	Trach	<0.50	<0.50	<0.50	<0.50
10	45/M	1.5	0.021	q. 6 hr	Therapist	<0.50	<0.50	<0.50	<0.50
11	73/F	1	0.025	q. 4 hr	Therapist	<0.50	<0.50	<0.50	0.63

M = Male; Trach = administered directly into tracheostomy tube of ventilated subject; NA = not applicable; F = female.

(heparin lock). The first 3 ml of samples drawn through the heparin lock was discarded to avoid contamination by saline solution or heparin. After a minimum of 48 hours of therapy (with dosing every 4 to 6 hours), a second set of blood samples were drawn. Samples were centrifuged at 2,000 rpm within 1 hour after collection and serum was stored at −20° C until assayed. Blood pressure and pulse were measured at each blood sampling, at which time the subject was questioned and the chart reviewed about possible side effects (confusion, agitation, urinary retention, or blurred vision).

The plasma atropine concentration was measured by radioimmunoassay. The antibody was raised in rabbits according to the method of Wurzburger et al.[7] and was used at a final dilution of 1:10,000. This antibody does not cross-react with tropine or D,L-tropic acid. The intra-assay and interassay coefficients of variation are 9.0% and 12.8%, respectively. Sensitivity of the method is 1 ng/ml when run with a sample volume of 50 μl. Many of the samples were also run with a sample volume of 100 μl, which increased the assay sensitivity to 0.5 ng/ml.

RESULTS

A total of 11 subjects (nine men and two women) were enrolled in the study. Their age ranged from 45 to 77 years and they weighed from 39.4 to 85.9 kg. The dose of atropine sulfate was 0.5 to 1.5 mg (0.012 to 0.025 mg/kg) given every 4 to 6 hours. Two of the subjects (nos. 2 and 3) failed to complete the study; one died shortly after the study began as a result of complications after suicidal carbon monoxide inhalation, and the other failed to respond to the drug. In both of these subjects the serum atropine concentration after the first dose was undetectable and neither had any pulse or blood pressure changes attributable to the drug. For technical reasons, two of the subjects (nos. 5 and 7) were not entered into the study until after they had received their first dose. For these subjects, only the concentrations after 48 hours are reported.

As seen in Table I, none of the subjects had any measurable atropine in their serum before or after the first dose. In contrast, samples drawn at later times contained highly variable amounts of atropine, ranging from essentially no drug up to levels as high as 5.23 ng/ml. Six of the nine subjects who had blood samples drawn after multiple doses had detectable serum concentrations. In four of these subjects the levels were high both before and after the inhaled dose.

Other than complaints of dry mouth from most of the subjects, there were no subjective side effects. Blood pressures and pulse rates varied considerably from day to day in several of the subjects, but no consistent pattern of change could be detected. In some subjects blood pressure or pulse increased after receiving atropine, while in others these values decreased. None of the changes were considered clinically significant. Subject 7, who had the highest serum atropine concentration, also showed the largest single rise in pulse rate (14 bpm). However, he consistently had high pulse rates even when not receiving atropine inhalation.

DISCUSSION

After an initial rapid distribution phase, a 0.32 mg iv dose of atropine yields a serum concentration of approximately 2 ng/ml, with an elimination $t_{1/2}$ of 2.5 to 3 hours.[3] A 1 mg iv dose in normal subjects gives proportionally higher plasma concentrations of 4 to 6 ng/

ml, with a $t_{1/2}$ of about 4 hours.[1] Because common therapeutic doses of parenteral atropine range from 0.4 to 1 mg, one would expect pharmacologic effects if plasma or serum levels of atropine exceed 2 to 3 ng/ml.

In previous investigations of inhaled atropine at a dose of 0.05 mg/kg (3.2 to 4.9 mg) administered by a dosimeter,[5] peak plasma levels >2 ng/ml were observed within 30 to 90 minutes in three of six subjects. More importantly, two of those subjects had measurable serum levels of the drug for up to 6 hours, possibly as result of slow, continuous absorption from the airway or gastrointestinal tract. While these previous findings are of concern, it is difficult to extrapolate them to clinical use, because the doses used clinically are generally smaller and the techniques of administration are often less efficient.[2,4,6]

Our results confirm that single-dose therapy poses little potential for significant drug absorption in the clinical setting, but that continued administration of the drug at 4- or 6-hour intervals can result in drug accumulation. This accumulation is a function of the rate of clearance of the drug from the body as well as possible prolonged absorption from the respiratory tree or the gastrointestinal tract.[5] If one assumes an atropine elimination $t_{1/2}$ of 2 to 4 hours,[1,3] steady-state plasma levels should be reached within 24 hours. We chose to wait at least 48 hours before drawing the second set of blood samples, to assure that steady state had been reached. None of the subjects had any detectable drug in their serum after the first dose, but six of nine subjects who had steady-state levels sampled had measurable amounts of the drug in the serum. These levels were highest 60 minutes after the dose, which corresponds to the time to peak plasma levels after single inhaled doses.[5] In two of these subjects the serum concentrations approximated those after a 0.32 mg parenteral dose of atropine, and in one subject the levels (4.3 to 5.2 ng/ml) were similar to those after a 1 mg iv dose. The levels in this one subject are high enough to possibly cause cardiovascular or central nervous system side effects. The only side effect noted in this subject was a heart rate that rose from 98 bpm before dosing to 112 bpm after dosing. It is not certain that this rapid heart rate was drug induced, because he had an underlying history of paroxysmal atrial tachycardia and atrial flutter that led to heart rates ranging from 85 to 105 bpm before atropine dosing. None of the subjects showed signs of blurred vision, urinary retention, or mental changes while participating in the study. Dry mouth was a frequent complaint, but this is more likely due to local effects of the drug on salivary secretion rather than to a systemic effect. Two of the subjects could not be fully evaluated because they were intubated and catheterized throughout the study.

No single factor can be identified to help predict which patients will have high atropine serum levels. As seen in Table I, arrangement of the dose administered (as milligrams atropine per kilogram body weight) in ascending order shows no correlation between dose and observed serum concentrations. The subject with the smallest dose had one of the highest serum levels, while the subject with the highest dose had one of the lowest serum concentrations. Comparison of 4-hour vs. 6-hour dosing shows a trend for those subjects receiving the drug every 4 hours to have higher serum concentrations. While this relationship is expected based on kinetic principles, the data are limited by the small number of subjects (three) who were dosed every 6 hours. Cimetidine, a well-described enzyme inhibitor, could possibly prolong atropine clearance and cause drug accumulation in serum, but neither of the two subjects who were receiving cimetidine showed measurable atropine levels in their serum at any time. Likewise, none of the subjects had laboratory or clinical signs of liver dysfunction or congestive heart failure to explain impaired drug clearance. The method of administration also has no clear relationship to the amount of drug absorbed. It would seem reasonable to predict that direct nebulization into the trachea would be the most efficient method of drug delivery, allowing more drug to enter the body and subsequently be absorbed. However, two of three subjects who were given the drug through this route had no drug detectable in their serum at any time during the study. Conversely, the two subjects who self administered the drug had measurable amounts of drug in their serum. Observation of these subjects showed that they inhaled the drug properly but that considerable loss of the dose occurred because the nebulizer continued to run even when they were not actively inspiring the drug.

In conclusion, atropine is absorbed into systemic circulation after multiple-dose inhalation therapy with common clinical administration techniques. The extent of absorption is highly variable and unpredictable. While it was not possible in our sample population to identify specific side effects attributable to atropine, the serum levels achieved in some of the subjects were high enough to lead to systemic anticholinergic effects.

We thank Carolyn Umstott for technical assistance.

References

1. Adams R, Verma P, Jackson A, Miller R: Plasma pharmacokinetics of intravenously administered atropine in

normal human subjects. J Clin Pharmacol **22:**477-481, 1982.
2. Gross N, Skorodin M: State of the art. Anticholinergic, antimuscarinic bronchodilators. Am Rev Respir Dis **129:** 856-870, 1984.
3. Hayden P, Larson S, Lakshminarayan S: Atropine clearance from human plasma. J Nucl Med **20:**336-337, 1979.
4. Kradjan W, Lakshminarayan S: Efficiency of air driven compressor nebulizers. Chest. (In press.)
5. Kradjan W, Lakshminarayan S, Hayden P, Larson S, Marini J: Serum atropine concentrations after inhalation of atropine sulfate. Am Rev Respir Dis **123:**471-472, 1981.
6. Pak C, Kradjan W, Lakshminarayan S, Marini J: Inhaled atropine sulfate: Dose response characteristics in adult patients with chronic airway obstruction. Am Rev Respir Dis **125:**331-334, 1982.
7. Wurzburger R, Miller R, Boxenbaum H, Spector S: Radioimmunoassay of atropine in plasma. J Pharmacol Exp Ther **203:**435-441, 1977.

Future meeting dates and sites of the ASCPT

March 20-22, 1986	Sheraton Washington Hotel, Washington, D.C.
March 25-28, 1987	Marriott Orlando World Center, Walt Disney World, Fla.
March 9-11, 1988	Town and Country Hotel, San Diego, Calif.

Call for scientific program abstracts forms for 1986 meeting in Washington, D.C., March 20-22, are included in this issue of the JOURNAL and will also appear in the June and August issues. Additional forms are available on request to Elaine Galasso, 1718 Gallagher Rd., Norristown, PA 19401; (215) 825-3838.

Reassessment of verbal and visual analog ratings in analgesic studies

The relative performance of three analgesic rating scales—visual pain analog, verbal pain intensity, and verbal pain relief—was assessed in clinical trials with 1,497 patients and a variety of pain models. The scales correlated strongly with one another, with inconsistent and generally minimal differences in sensitivity. Overall, the verbal relief scale tended to be slightly more sensitive than the pain analog rating, which in turn showed a small advantage over the verbal pain intensity assessment. When the scores derived from the categorized ratings 1 hour after drug dosing (generally the time of peak effect) were analyzed, there was little difference whether a parametric or nonparametric approach was taken. When the cumulative measures of overall effect over 6 hours were considered, however, the nonparametric approach was decidedly more powerful. There was a similar pattern when the analog scores were analyzed. This unanticipated finding appears to be due to the cumulative measures (from all three scales) being more skewed toward the lower end of their respective ranges than are the 1-hour scores. A composite efficacy variable was defined, incorporating data from the three primary scales; this measure was found to be generally comparable in sensitivity to the individual scales and may be useful as a global summary of response. While our investigation provides evidence that any of the ratings considered will accurately reflect analgesic response, the verbal relief scale was the most sensitive and might be the best choice if a single measure is desired. (CLIN PHARMACOL THER 38:16-23, 1985.)

Gary S. Littman, Ph.D., Barry R. Walker, M.D., and Bruce E. Schneider, Ph.D.
Philadelphia, Pa.

Visual analog scales have been proposed as alternatives to categorized pain intensity and pain relief ratings in the assessment of analgesic efficacy. In use in psychometric research since the early part of the century, analog scales were introduced into the evaluation of analgesia early in the 1960s[6,7]; since then, they have been compared with the verbal assessments used since the late 1940s.[2] It has been hypothesized, and in some situations demonstrated,[6,7,14,16,19] that the measurement continuum of an analog scale allows for greater sensitivity than the several descriptive terms available with a verbal scale. In clinical trials involving 1,497 patients, we assessed the efficacy of an analgesic through an analog pain intensity scale and the classic pain intensity and pain relief ratings, thus providing a large data base from which the relative performance of the three scales could be investigated.

These data were from the phase III clinical investigation of dezocine, a parenteral mixed agonist-antagonist analgesic. Patients with postoperative pain, chronic cancer pain, acute orthopedic trauma, and renal or ureteral colic were studied; morphine, butorphanol, and meperidine, as well as placebo, were used as control drugs. In planning these studies, which were conducted betwen 1980 and 1983, we decided to incorporate a pain analog scale because of its established reliability[7,13] and potential advantages over the verbal ratings. However, because of a lack of first-hand experience with the scale, along with regulatory guidelines that did not place analog scales at the same level of unquestioned acceptability as the verbal scales,[18] the classic pain intensity and pain relief ratings were also used.

The investigation of relative performance will first examine the degree to which the scales correlate with one another. Next, we will determine if any of the scales seem more sensitive than the others. In the traditional sense, the sensitivity of a rating system pertains to its ability to detect change in an underlying stimulus (e.g., pain). In comparisons of analgesic rating scales, sensitivity has often been portrayed in the literature as the ability to detect statistically significant differences between groups or as a narrow confidence interval for a relative potency estimate.[7,12,19] Although this distinction is important, the latter property—which might more technically be described as power, or the ability to dis-

From Wyeth Laboratories.
Received for publication Oct. 18, 1984; accepted Feb. 1, 1985.
Reprint requests to: Dr. Gary S. Littman, Wyeth Laboratories, P.O. Box 8299, Philadelphia, PA 19101.

Table I. Correlations among the cumulative 6-hour SPID, SPAID, and TOTPAR scores

Patient group	*No. of patients*	*Correlation coefficients (r)*		
		SPID vs. SPAID	*SPID vs. TOTPAR*	*SPAID vs. TOTPAR*
All patients	1330	0.933	0.909	0.896
Study drug				
Dezocine	696	0.927	0.894	0.882
Morphine	196	0.891	0.889	0.860
Butorphanol	133	0.977	0.926	0.903
Placebo	296	0.970	0.941	0.934
Study type				
Postoperative intramuscular	634	0.958	0.929	0.894
Postoperative intravenous	460	0.937	0.910	0.898
Renal colic	138	0.876	0.869	0.819
Orthopedic trauma	48	0.897	0.913	0.875
Chronic cancer	50	0.982	0.937	0.933

criminate between treatments—would appear to be most relevant, and our investigation will examine sensitivity in this context. In conjunction with this question, the issue of parametric vs. nonparametric analysis of the ratings will be addressed. Finally, the use of a composite efficacy variable, incorporating data from all the scales, will be discussed.

METHODS

Data were collected from 23 studies conducted under 14 protocols; all studies were double blind and of parallel design, and protocols differed with respect to pain model, control drugs, and the dose levels of dezocine. In 10 of the studies, patients were given a single dose and observed for 6 hours (at 15 and 30 minutes, 1 hour, and hourly thereafter). In the other studies, doses were given for up to 7 days; in all cases, the most detailed observations and analyses pertained to the 6-hour period after the initial dose, and we restricted our investigation to data from this 6-hour period.

Pain intensity was rated at baseline as none (0), mild (1), moderate (2), or severe (3); in the renal or ureteral colic studies, very severe (4) was added as a fifth category. Patients had at least moderate pain on entry. Randomization of patients to treatments was blocked on initial pain severity. Pain intensity was also assessed by means of an analog scale. The scale was linear, 100 mm long, and horizontally positioned; the extremes were "no pain" and the "worst pain I've ever felt," with no intermediate divisions or descriptive terms. A score from 0 to 100 was determined by measuring the distance from the left end, which represented no pain. At each scheduled observation time after drug dosing, pain intensity was rated on both the verbal and analog scales; in addition, the degree of relief (relative to pain at the start of the study) was assessed as complete (4), a lot (3), moderate (2), a little (1), none (0), or worse (−1).

For purposes of description and derivation of additional assessment parameters, the ordinal scores indicated above were assigned to the verbal pain intensity and pain relief categories. Pain intensity difference (PID) and pain analog intensity difference (PAID) scores were calculated by subtracting the score after dosing from that at baseline. Sum of the pain intensity difference (SPID), sum of the pain analog intensity difference (SPAID), and total pain relief (TOTPAR) scores were determined as cumulative measures of overall effect by taking weighted sums of the respective PID, PAID, and pain relief scores (the weights equaled the proportions of an hour since the preceding observation). In the determination of efficacy scores, patients who required additional analgesic medication were considered treatment failures and assigned scores corresponding to the baseline pain intensity (both scales) and to no relief for the observation points beyond the time of remedication, in line with standard conventions for handling such cases.[5,10] To assess the consistency of the measurements from the three scales, Pearson product-moment correlation coefficients were determined, with primary attention given to the cumulative SPID, SPAID, and TOTPAR scores. Consideration was also given to the scores at 1 hour; this was chosen as a time of generally maximal response, before remedication (and the assignment of scores) became too frequent.

The PID, PAID, and pain relief ratings, as well as the derived SPID, SPAID, and TOTPAR scores, were compared among the therapy groups in each study in two ways to assess the impact of the parametric vs. nonparametric choice. The parametric analysis of co-

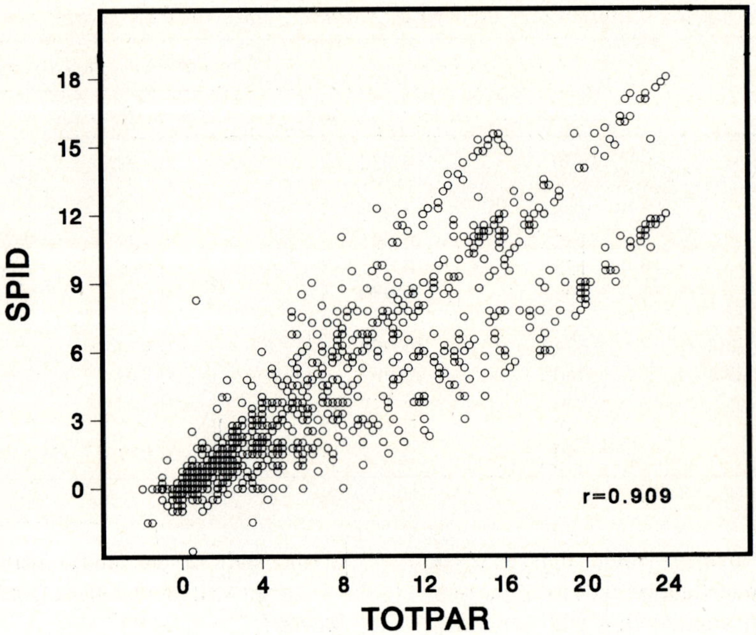

Fig. 1. Individual display of SPID vs. TOTPAR scores for all patients in all studies.

variance, with the inital pain score as the covariate, was contrasted with the nonparametric Cochran-Mantel-Haenszel (CMH) procedure.[8,9] In the latter, the analysis was based on a ranking of the response categories. Among groups, comparisons of the average ranks were first done within the initial pain categories (equivalent to the Kruskal-Wallis test); the overall test statistic was then determined through weighting the within-pain-level results (thus providing a direct generalization of the Kruskal-Wallis test).

To investigate a summary measure of response that might prove more sensitive than individual ratings, a composite efficacy parameter was determined as a weighted sum of the scores from the primary scales, with the weights chosen so that the three scales would contribute equally. Because the relief scores can range to 4, whereas the PID scores can range only to the score assigned to the inital pain severity, the PID scores were adjusted by dividing them by the initial severity score and then multiplying by 4. Similarly, the PAID scores were adjusted by dividing them by the baseline analog score and then multiplying by 4. Composite scores were analyzed by the methods outlined above.

RESULTS

Of the 1,497 patients evaluated, 1,330 had a complete set of observations on all scales; this group was the focus of our investigation. Of interest is the fact that 93 (56%) of the 167 patients excluded because of missing data were missing an observation on all scales, but most of the rest (63, or 38%) were missing only analog scale data. This relative difficulty in collecting analog scale data in certain situations (e.g., very near the time of surgery) has been reported by others.[16] Correlations among the cumulative SPID, SPAID, and TOTPAR scores for all 1,330 patients and also by study drug and by pain model are shown in Table I. There were consistently high correlation coefficients between each pair of scales and across therapy groups and pain models. When correlations among the 1-hour PID, PAID, and pain relief scores were considered, correlation coefficients remained high, although not quite as high as those for the cumulative measures (among all 1,330 patients: r = 0.881 between PID and PAID, r = 0.861 between PID and relief, and r = 0.842 between PAID and relief).

The relationships among the cumulative efficacy measures are shown in three scatter diagrams of individual responses. Fig. 1 shows the SPID vs. TOTPAR scores for all 1,330 patients (r = 0.909). There is generally a good correlation throughout the entire range of responses, with few outliers; it is apparent, however, that there is a particular cluster around 0 on both scales and a slight divergence from the linear relationship as the scores increase.

Fig. 2 shows the individual responses associated with the smallest correlation coefficient included in Table I (r = 0.819), that for the SPAID vs. TOTPAR com-

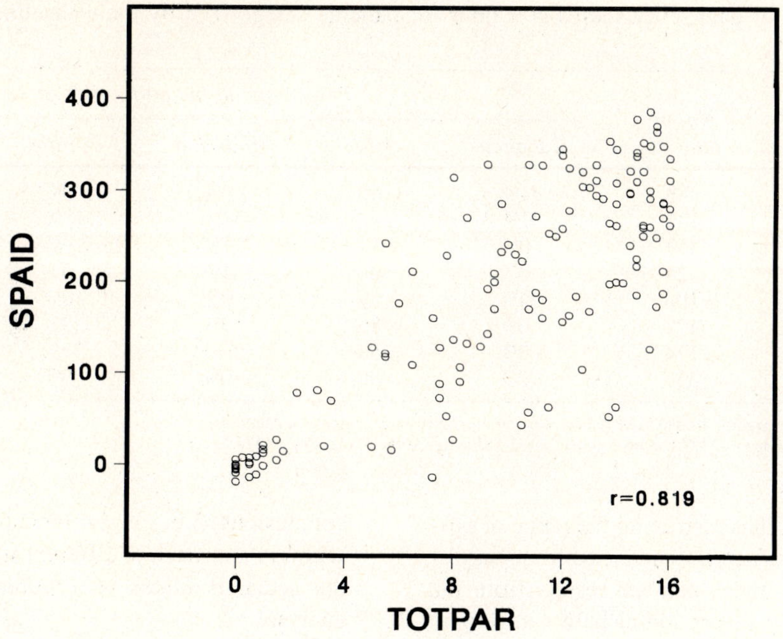

Fig. 2. Individual display of SPAID vs. TOTPAR scores in patients with renal colic.

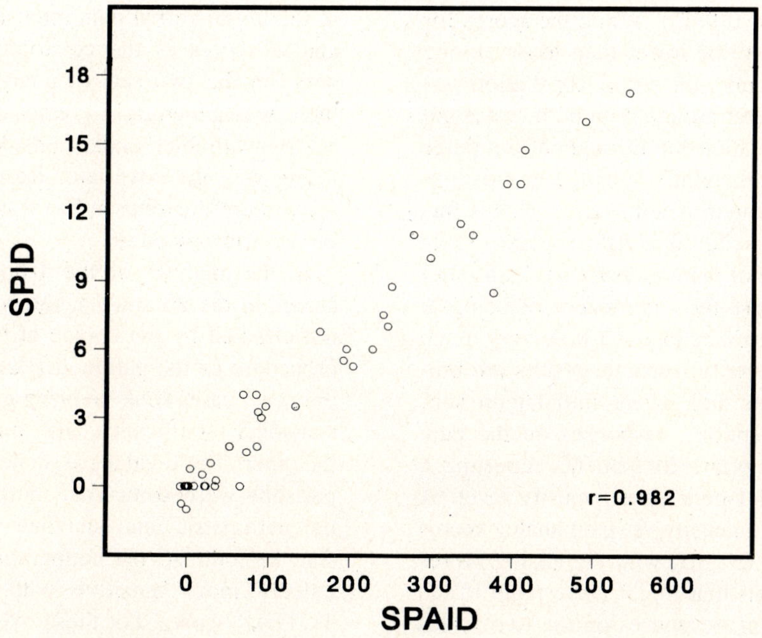

Fig. 3. Individual display of SPID vs. SPAID scores in patients with chronic cancer pain.

parison among the 138 patients with renal colic. Two factors appear to contribute to the relatively low degree of correlation. First, the efficacy scores in these studies (which did not involve a placebo) tended to be higher than those in the other pain models: thus there are few points near the cluster at 0 on both scales (where the correlation, to some extent, is forced by the assignment of scores after a short period of little or no response) and most responses are in the region where some divergence from a linear relationship was also seen in Fig. 1. The second factor is that there are several outliers, with low SPAID scores relative to their TOTPAR scores. These were found to be associated with unusually low baseline analog scores relative to their cate-

Table II. Distribution of pain relief scores at 1 hour for patients categorized by their baseline and 1-hour pain intensity scores

Pain intensity at		*No. of*	*Percentage in the pain relief category*					
Baseline	*1 hr*	*patients*	*Complete*	*A lot*	*Moderate*	*A little*	*None*	*Worse*
Moderate	→ none	83	94%	6%	0%	0%	0%	0%
Moderate	→ mild	182	1%	54%	32%	13%	0%	0%
Moderate	→ moderate	157	0%	1%	11%	19%	65%*	3%
Moderate	→ severe	24	0%	0%	4%	0%	38%	58%
Severe	→ none	105	94%	5%	0%	0%	1%	0%
Severe	→ mild	177	0%	78%	19%	3%	0%	0%
Severe	→ moderate	174	0%	5%	56%	37%	2%	0%
Severe	→ severe	357	0%	0%	0%	8%	66%†	25%

*Of the 102 patients in this category, 70 had been remedicated and assigned their scores (see Methods).
†Of the 236 patients in this category, 177 had been remedicated and assigned their scores (see Methods).

gorized pain intensity, thus restricting the range of possible SPAID scores; perhaps the increased frequency of such instances among these patients results from the availability of the very severe initial pain category in this pain model. At the other extreme, Fig. 3 displays the SPID vs. SPAID scores among the 50 patients with chronic cancer pain (associated with the highest correlation coefficient [r = 0.982]). While the scores for this pain model tended to be lower than those among the patients with renal colic, the strong correlation was not due merely to a cluster around 0 on both scales but to a consistent linear relationship throughout the range of scores reported for this relatively small group.

The consistency of response across the scales is further demonstrated in two additional data displays. Table II gives the distribution of pain intensity vs. pain relief scores at 1 hour. Because the significance of being in a particular pain intensity category at 1 hour very much depends on baseline severity, separate results are presented for the moderate and severe initial pain subgroups. With few exceptions, responses on the pain relief scale were appropriate for patients reporting a particular baseline and 1-hour pain intensity level. A comparison of the pain intensity vs. pain analog scores at 1 hour is given in Table III, with the analog scores aggregated into intervals that might correspond to the verbal categories. Again, responses on the two scales were generally consistent, although it was noted that a substantial proportion of patients (24%) with no pain on the verbal scale reported an analog score slightly above 0 (but no greater than 5).

The question of the relative sensitivity of the three scales was examined in 20 studies with sample sizes ranging from 15 to 152 patients. To compare sensitivity between rating scales or methods of analysis, consideration was first given to differences in the statistical conclusions (i.e., a significant difference found only with one approach or different significance levels); then, the actual P values were compared between the two analyses.

For the 20 separate studies, analysis of covariance was applied to the 1-hour PID and pain relief scores and the 6-hour SPID and TOTPAR scores, with each of the initial verbal pain intensity and the baseline pain analog scores as the covariate. Although differences between the two sets of analyses were not dramatic, there was generally a greater degree of sensitivity for all four variables under consideration when the verbal rating was the covariate. Results from this approach were therefore chosen for comparison with the nonparametric procedure.

In the analysis of the 1-hour PID and pain relief scores in the 20 studies, the conclusion was generally not affected by the choice of the nonparametric CMH procedure or the parametric analysis of covariance. In only two cases (one favoring each approach) was there statistical significance with one method but not with the other. The P values associated with the 1-hour comparisons were somewhat more frequently lower with the parametric analysis than with the nonparametric test. In contrast, the nonparametric procedure was decidedly more sensitive with the 6-hour SPID and TOTPAR scores. For these overall scores, the P values were generally lower with the nonparametric procedure, and in 30% of the cases the conclusion of the statistical comparison differed in favor of the CMH procedure (usually, there was significance with both tests but the difference was in significance level).

Preliminary investigation seems to indicate that the difference between the 1-hour scores and the cumulative measures is because the overall scores are skewed to a greater degree toward the lower end of the respective

Table III. Distribution of pain analog scores at 1 hour for patients categorized by their baseline and 1-hour pain intensity scores

Pain intensity at		*No. of*	*Percentage with pain analog score of*			
Baseline	*1 hr*	*patients*	*0-5*	*6-45*	*46-75*	*76-100*
Moderate →	none	83	89%	11%	0%	0%
Moderate →	mild	182	10%	80%	10%	0%
Moderate →	moderate	157	0%	11%	77%	12%
Moderate →	severe	24	0%	0%	29%	71%
Severe →	none	105	91%	9%	0%	0%
Severe →	mild	177	6%	84%	11%	0%
Severe →	moderate	174	1%	21%	70%	9%
Severe →	severe	357	<1%	1%	10%	89%

ranges than are the 1-hour assessments. Perhaps this is because there is another group between patients with no response at all and others with a good response for several hours that have some response for a short period. This middle group could be clearly separated from the group with no response when scores near the time of peak effect were considered, but would have scores that appear relatively close to 0 when the cumulative measures with a wider potential range were examined. The skewed nature of the scores derived from the categoric scales has been reported by others[1] and addressed in their analysis by application of a ridit transformation. The approach of applying the CMH procedure, with scoring based on ranks determined within the initial pain categories, thus seems an appropriate choice as the primary method of analyzing these data.

Examination of the 1-hour PAID scores and, particularly, the 6-hour SPAID scores showed that they, too, tended to be skewed toward the lower end of their scales. The pattern of differences between the parametric and nonparametric methods of analysis was similar to that with the categoric ratings. There was no distinction in sensitivity of one approach over the other with the 1-hour data. The 6-hour SPAID scores showed greater sensitivity with the nonparametric approach; in five cases, the statistical conclusion differed in favor of the nonparametric procedure (with no differences in the other direction) and the P values tended to be generally lower.

In accordance with the above results, the P values associated with nonparametric comparisons among groups of the SPID, SPAID, and TOTPAR scores in the 20 separate studies were examined along with corresponding values from an analysis of a composite efficacy score. Consideration of the composite score (determined as a weighted average of the scores from the three individual scales, as described in Methods) was motivated primarily by the potential advantage of having such an overall summary of response. Such a measure could allow a more parsimonious presentation of the data and might also prove more sensitive than the individual scales.

In 17 of the 20 studies, the conclusion of the statistical comparison was the same for all four variables. In one case, statistical significance was detected with all variables except the SPAID; in two other cases, all four variables showed statistical significance but the significance levels differed. Regardless of the level of significance (ranking the four variables within each study and then looking at the average rank for each variable across the 20 studies), the TOTPAR variable was the most sensitive (i.e., had the lowest P values), followed by the composite score, the SPAID, and then the SPID. Differences among the variables were neither large nor consistent in direction. For the 1-hour scores, the relative positions of the PID, PAID, and pain relief variables were the same as the SPID, SPAID, and TOTPAR scores, although the differences were slightly larger.

The issue of sensitivity was also explored from another direction. For most patients, an overall evaluation of treatment (as poor, fair, good, or excellent) was available; the cumulative efficacy parameters were examined within the four overall evaluation categories. Judged by the mean scores and the tightness of the confidence intervals around them, the clearest separation between categories was provided by the TOTPAR and composite scores, followed by the SPAID and then the SPID scores.

DISCUSSION

Comparisons of verbal pain intensity and pain relief assessments with visual analog ratings led to a consensus that such measurements generally correlate well with one another.[3,11,14] This observation of consistency among scales has been extended to include other assessments, such as curvilinear analog[17] and 11-point numeric[3] ratings. Our results confirm and help to quantify this impression in a large group of patients studied at a number of different sites who have pain of various causes. Whether analog scales provide increased sensitivity is more controversial. Whereas a number of investigators have described studies demonstrating the greater sensitivity of an analog scale,[6,7,14,16,19] others have either not found a difference[17] or favored a verbal scale.[11] Downie et al.[3] found an advantage for an 11-point numeric scale over either a visual analog or a 4-point categoric scale. Even the correspondence of "lower P values" with "greater sensitivity" is controversial; Ohnhaus and Alder[12] found lower P values with a verbal than with an analog scale, but they described this not as greater sensitivity for the verbal scale but rather as an artificial augmentation of drug effects due to the discrete measuring system.

Analysis of our 20 studies supports the position that there is no consistent difference in sensitivity between the verbal and analog scales. Overall, the verbal pain relief scale seemed slightly more sensitive than the pain analog scale (i.e., the former tended to be associated with lower P values), which in turn was slightly more sensitive than the verbal pain intensity scale. This relationship among the scales was somewhat more apparent when the scores at 1 hour rather than the 6-hour cumulative measures were considered. It is not surprising that analyses based on the verbal pain severity categorization seemed the least powerful; only four categories are available with this scale, and for patients starting with moderate pain there is only one step available between the baseline pain category and no pain. Supplemental analyses restricted to patients with moderate initial pain did, in fact, magnify the relative lack of sensitivity of this assessment scale.

Whereas a parametric approach to analyzing data derived from categorized analgesic efficacy scales has often been taken, several nonparametric alternatives have also been used.[4] Problems with a parametric analysis (without any transformation of the data) might arise as a result of the noncontinuous nature of the variables under consideration, the questionable validity of the scores traditionally assigned to the categories (as differences between successive steps have been assumed to be equal), and the tendency for the scores to be skewed toward the lower end of the scale. Analyses of the 1-hour PID and pain relief scores through the nonparametric CMH procedure and the parametric analysis of covariance (with the baseline level as the covariate in both cases) showed no consistent advantage in power for any one approach. However, for the cumulative 6-hour SPID and TOTPAR scores, the nonparametric approach was decidedly more powerful. Examination of the respective distributions has revealed that the cumulative measures are skewed toward the lower end of the scale to a greater degree than are the 1-hour scores. Thus it appears that it is primarily the skewness (rather than the lack of continuity, which would have more of an effect on the 1-hour scores) that is associated with the loss of power for the parametric procedure.

Sriwatanakul et al.[15] have suggested an alternative method for measuring pain, in which each patient associates several verbal categories with positions on an analog scale and scores corresponding to each category would be assigned on an individual basis. Although this method addresses the continuity and scoring problems and thus to a degree validates a parametric approach, it is not clear a priori whether the critical factor of skewness will be diminished to a sufficient degree to allow a parametric analysis to equal the nonparametric approach in power. Consideration of the more continuous 1-hour PAID and 6-hour SPAID variables in our studies did reveal skewness toward the lower end of the scales, particularly for the cumulative measure. Moreover, an increase in power (relative to the parametric approach) was again seen with the CMH analysis of the cumulative scores. Thus this nonparametric procedure, which has particular intuitive appeal for analyzing the verbal ratings, seems at least as powerful as the parametric alternative for both the categorized assessments and the scores derived from the analog scale. Thus, along with its relaxed distributional assumptions, it may be a reasonable approach to analyzing all the analgesic efficacy variables under consideration.

Whether to use a composite efficacy measure incorporating data from the three scales seems to be a matter of individual preference. Had inconsistencies appeared among the primary scales (as a hypothetic example, if morphine tended to have more favorable responses on the verbal scales than on the analog scale, while dezocine showed its best response on the analog scale), then the composite efficacy measure might be considered a useful supplement that provides a fair overall summary. Also, had the composite measure proved to have better discriminatory ability than the individual scales, it would have a clear advantage. Since neither of these arguments can be made, one must subjectively decide whether presentation (or even emphasis) of these global summary scores is warranted, since they lack the familiarity and general acceptance of the standard scales.

Furthermore, the choice of what scale(s) should be used may not be particularly critical. Our analysis showed three scales to correlate strongly with one another, with differences in sensitivity that were rarely large. Whereas some investigators and patients may be most comfortable with the simplicity of a verbal categorization, others may prefer the freedom of choice provided by an analog rating. The traditional verbal pain intensity scale did appear to be somewhat less sensitive than the others, sometimes markedly so, and thus may be a poor choice as the sole efficacy measure. Analog scale data have proved to be relatively difficult to obtain in certain situations; thus unless there is sufficient prior experience to eliminate concern about this potential problem, it might be prudent to avoid the use of this assessment without other complementary measures. Overall, the verbal pain relief scale seemed to be the most sensitive measure and, as a general recommendation, might be the best choice if a single measure is desired.

References

1. Beaver WJ, Wallenstein MS, Houde RW, Rogers A: A comparison of the analgesic effects of pentazocine and morphine in patients with cancer. CLIN PHARMACOL THER **7**:740-751, 1966.
2. Beecher HK: Measurement of subjective responses. New York, 1959, Oxford University Press.
3. Downie WW, Leatham PA, Rhind VM, Wright V, Branco JA, Anderson JA: Studies with pain rating scales. Ann Rheum Dis **37**:378-381, 1978.
4. Green JW: Design and analysis of clinical trials of analgesic drugs. *In* Buncher CR, Tsay JY, editors: Statistics in the pharmaceutical industry. New York, 1981, Marcel Dekker, Inc pp 189-204.
5. Houde RW, Wallenstein SL, Beaver WT: Evaluation of analgesics in patients with cancer pain. *In* Lasagna L, editor: Clinical pharmacology. Section 6 of the International Encyclopedia of Pharmacology and Therapeutics. New York, 1966, Pergamon Press, Inc., pp 59-97.
6. Huskisson EC: Measurement of pain. Lancet **2**:1127-1131, 1974.
7. Joyce CRB, Zutshi DW, Hrubes V, Mason RM: Comparison of fixed interval and visual analogue scales for rating chronic pain. Eur J Clin Pharmacol **8**:415-420, 1975.
8. Landis JR, Cooper MM, Kennedy T, Koch GG: A computer program for testing average partial association in three-way contingency tables (PARCAT). Proc Stat Comput Sec Am Stat Assoc 1977, pp 157-162.
9. Landis JR, Heyman ER, Koch GG: Average partial association in three-way contingency tables: A review and discussion of alternate tests. Int Stat Rev **46**:237-254, 1978.
10. Lasagna L: The evaluation of analgesic compounds in patients suffering from postoperative pain. *In* Lasagna L, editor: Clinical pharmacology. Section 6 of the International Encyclopedia of Pharmacology and Therapeutics. New York, 1966, Pergamon Press, Inc., pp 51-58.
11. Linton SJ, Gotestam KG: A clinical comparison of two pain scales: Correlation, remembering chronic pain, and a measure of compliance. Pain **17**:57-65, 1983.
12. Ohnhaus EE, Alder R: Methodological problems in the measurement of pain: A comparison between the verbal rating scale and the visual analogue scale. Pain **1**:379-384, 1975.
13. Revill SI, Robinson JO, Rosen M, Hogg MIJ: The reliability of a linear analogue for evaluating pain. Anaesthesia **31**:1191-1198, 1976.
14. Scott J, Huskisson EC: Graphic representation of pain. Pain **2**:175-184, 1976.
15. Sriwatanakul K, Kelvie W, Lasagna L: The quantification of pain: An analysis of words used to describe pain and analgesia in clinical trials. CLIN PHARMACOL THER **32**:143-148, 1982.
16. Sriwatanakul K, Kelvie W, Lasagna L, Calimlim JF, Weis OF, Mehta G: Studies with different types of visual analog scales for measurement of pain. CLIN PHARMACOL THER **34**:234-239, 1983.
17. Stambaugh JE, Sarajian C: Analgesic efficacy of zomepirac sodium in patients with pain due to cancer. J Clin Pharmacol **21**:501-507, 1981.
18. U.S. Food and Drug Administration: Guidelines for the clinical evaluation of analgesic drugs. Washington, D.C., 1979, U.S. Government Printing Office.
19. Wallenstein SL, Heidrich G, Kaiko R, Houde RW: Clinical evaluation of mild analgesics: The measurement of clinical pain. Br J Clin Pharmacol **10**:319S-327S, 1980.

Labetalol and hydrochlorothiazide in hypertension

This study was a multicenter, randomized, double-blind, parallel comparison of labetalol vs. placebo added to hydrochlorothiazide (HCTZ) for the treatment of essential hypertension. The study consisted of 2 to 4 weeks of placebo and 3 to 7 weeks of HCTZ, 25 mg twice a day. Both of these first two phases were single blind. Subjects whose standing diastolic blood pressure remained >95 mm Hg while taking HCTZ were randomized to receive either labetalol or matching placebo in addition to the HCTZ. Labetalol was started at 100 mg twice a day; the dose was increased every 2 weeks to a maximum of 400 mg twice a day. Subjects continued taking their maximum tolerated labetalol dose for another 4 weeks during the final phase of the study. Blood pressure fell 10/9 mm Hg supine and 17/13 mm Hg standing after the addition of labetalol (n = 83) and 3/4 and 5/5 mm Hg, respectively, after placebo (n = 91). Labetalol was equally effective in blacks and whites. There was suggestive evidence that women responded better to the combined therapy than did men, and that people >55 years old responded better than those <55 years old. Five subjects receiving labetalol and one receiving placebo were dropped from the study because of side effects. Rhinitis was the only adverse effect reported significantly more often with labetalol than with placebo. We conclude that labetalol is a safe and effective step II antihypertensive for patients with moderate to moderately severe hypertension that does not respond adequately to HCTZ alone. (CLIN PHARMACOL THER 38:24-27, 1985).

Labetalol/Hydrochlorothiazide Multicenter Study Group*

Labetalol is a nonselective β-adrenergic blocker, an α_1-adrenergic blocker,[2,11] and it may also exert some intrinsic β_2-agonist activity.[3] Clinical trials have shown it to be at least as effective as conventional β-blockers in lowering blood pressure, and in some cases to be effective even when other drugs, including β-blockers, have failed.[4,10] Labetalol's α-blocking property also decreases afterload, better preserving cardiac output and possibly visceral and renal blood flow.[6] We evaluated the efficacy of oral labetalol in patients with essential hypertension not controlled by hydrochlorothiazide (HCTZ) alone.

METHODS

Our subjects, who were 19 to 70 years old, were recruited from the outpatient hypertension and medical clinics at the institutions participating in this study group. All subjects had asymptomatic essential hypertension and none had a previous stroke, myocardial infarction within the past 6 months, congestive heart failure uncontrolled by digitalis alone, serum creatinine levels >2.5 mg/dl, clinically significant liver or hematologic disorders, ethanol addiction, or contraindications to diuretic or β-blocker therapy.

The study was of a multicenter, randomized, double-blind, parallel design divided into four phases. The placebo and the HCTZ phases (phases 1 and 2) were single blind. Phase 1 lasted 2 to 4 weeks and was intended to minimize the effects of any prior medications and to establish baseline blood pressure levels. During phase 1, subjects were seen weekly for at least three visits to measure blood pressure and other vital signs and to record concurrent illnesses and adverse effects. Subjects were qualified for entry into phase 2 if their mean standing diastolic blood pressure was 105 to 119 mm Hg on two consecutive visits and if the two readings did not differ by more than −5 or +10 mm Hg. Phase 2 lasted 3 to 7 weeks and established the antihypertensive effect of HCTZ alone. During this phase, subjects received HCTZ, 25 mg twice a day. They were seen weekly for measurement of vital signs and questioning as in phase 1. After 3 weeks in phase 2, if their standing diastolic blood pressure was >115 mm Hg or did not decrease by more than 5 mm Hg from the final value in phase 1, the subject advanced to phase 3. Subjects also entered phase 3 if their stand-

Supported in part by a grant from the Schering-Plough Corp.
Received for publication Oct. 31, 1984; accepted Feb. 2, 1985.
Reprint requests to: J. T. Wright, Jr., M.D., Ph.D., Departments of Pharmacology and Medicine, Medical College of Virginia, MCV Box 613, Richmond, VA 23298.
*A list of participants may be found at the end of this article.

ing diastolic blood pressure was >95 mm Hg during any of the subsequent four visits.

Subjects qualifying for entry into phase 3 were randomized to receive either labetalol or placebo in a double-blind fashion added to the HCTZ regimen. The labetalol dose was started at 100 mg twice a day and, unless side effects or symptomatic hypotension were noted, the dose was progressively increased by 100 mg twice a day at 2-week intervals to a maximum dose of 400 mg twice a day. During phase 4, subjects continued their maximum tolerated dose established during phase 3 for another 4 weeks.

Subjects had a complete history and physical examination taken at the start of the study. On entry into phases 2, 3, and 4, physical examinations, ECGs, automated blood chemistry tests, urinalyses, and complete blood cell and differential counts were repeated. If indicated, a chest x-ray film was taken before entry into phase 2. Vital signs including supine and standing blood pressures and pulse rates, body temperature, and weight were recorded weekly in the first three phases and every 2 weeks in phase 4. Supine (after 5 minutes of quiet rest) and standing (2 minutes) blood pressures were measured with a standard mercury sphygmomanometer and an appropriate sized cuff. The Korotkoff phase 5 sound was used as the diastolic reading. Pulse rates (supine and standing) were recorded immediately after the blood pressure measurements. The time of day of the clinic visits was relatively constant for each subject. Subjects were questioned about adverse drug reactions at each visit. Compliance was verified by pill counts. Throughout the study, the subjects were instructed to take two capsules and one tablet twice a day. Tablets contained either placebo or HCTZ, 25 mg. The labetalol dose was adjusted by varying the strength of the capsules, which were identical in appearance.

The two treatment groups were compared by chi-square analysis, and ANOVA was used to analyze the efficacy data. Fisher's exact test was used to analyze the safety data.

RESULTS

A total of 316 subjects were enrolled in the study; 123 were dropped during phases 1 or 2 before randomization because they (1) failed to meet criteria for advancement to the next phase, (2) were lost to follow-up, or (3) failed to meet entry or exclusion criteria. Thus 193 subjects were randomized to enter phase 3. Of these, 174 were evaluable for efficacy (18 were invalidated because of protocol violations and the 19th had no follow-up blood pressure readings). Characteristics of the evaluable randomized subjects are listed in Table I. Success of the randomization is demonstrated by the blood pressures during phases 1 and 2 (Fig. 1).

Table I. Subject characteristics

	Labetalol	*Placebo*
Sex (M/F)	39/44	39/52
Race (W/B/O)	42/36/5	45/43/3
Age (yr) ($\bar{X} \pm$ SD)	50 ± 10	52.2 ± 11
Weight (kg) ($\bar{X} \pm$ SD)	183 ± 38	186 ± 46
Demographic values, B vs. W		
Age (yr)	52.4/47.5*	53.3/50.6
Weight (kg)	180.5/182.6	185.7/182.8

M = Male; F = female; W = white; B = black; O = other.
*$P < 0.05$.

When compared with the addition of placebo, the addition of labetalol to HCTZ induced a small but significant decrease in blood pressure (Fig. 1). This fall in blood pressure was dose related up to 300 mg twice a day, but the 400 mg twice a day dose induced no further significant effects. The hypotensive effect of labetalol was demonstrated not only by the absolute decrease in blood pressure, but also by the number of subjects who reached the blood pressure goal, defined as a diastolic blood pressure <90 mm Hg or a ≥10 mm Hg fall from phase 2 diastolic blood pressure. Sixty-one percent of the subjects taking labetalol and 30% of those taking placebo reached the goal. The maximum effect of a given dose of labetalol was evident after 1 week of dosing. For subjects maintained on a particular dose, there was no further decrease during the 2-week measurement or during the phase 4 follow-up visits. Furthermore, no loss of effect was evident during the 1-month follow-up while taking the maximally tolerated dose.

When added to HCTZ, labetalol decreased blood pressure 10/9 mm Hg (systolic/diastolic) supine and 17/13 mm Hg standing; addition of placebo to HCTZ induced a 3/4 mm Hg decrease in the supine and a 5/5 mm Hg decrease in the standing blood pressures. The effect of labetalol and HCTZ was significantly greater than that of placebo and HCTZ on supine and standing systolic and diastolic blood pressures. To determine if certain demographic subgroups responded uniformly to treatment, further analyses were made from the standing diastolic blood pressure data. For every subgroup, the response to HCTZ with labetalol was greater than that to HCTZ with placebo. There were no differences in antihypertensive responses in blacks and whites. There was a suggestion that women responded more than men (by 4.0 mm Hg) and that subjects >55 years old responded more than those <55 years old (by 4.9 mm

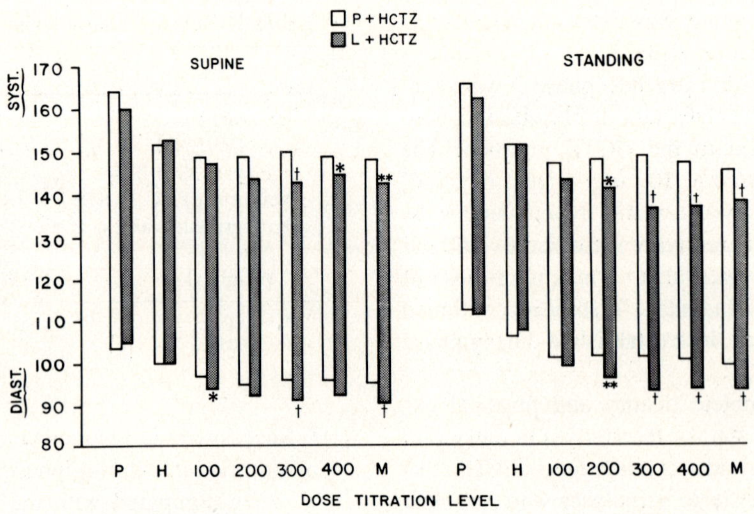

Fig. 1. Supine and standing diastolic *(diast)* and systolic *(syst)* blood pressures after 2 weeks at each dose level (100 to 400 mg twice a day) of labetalol. *P* = Placebo; *L* = labetalol; *HCTZ* = hydrochlorothiazide; *M* = maintenance dose of labetalol continued into phase 4. *P < 0.05, **P < 0.01, †P < 0.001.

Hg). At the end of phase 3, labetalol induced a net 8/5 mm Hg decrease in supine and 18/12 mm Hg decrease in standing blood pressures in blacks, whereas the corresponding decreases in whites were 13/10 and 15/13 mm Hg. The supine diastolic blood pressure response to labetalol was less in blacks during phase 3, but this difference was not evident by the end of phase 4. Supine heart rate decreased 8.1 bpm and standing heart rate decreased 7.9 bpm more after labetalol than after placebo. Almost all of the reduction in heart rate occurred by the end of the first week of the 200 mg twice a day dose titration.

Six subjects were dropped during phases 3 and 4 because of adverse reactions (five after labetalol and one after placebo). The five subjects who had been taking labetalol were dropped because of scalp paresthesias, bronchospasm, urinary retention, impotence, and elevated creatine kinase levels with chest pain. In this latter subject, no creatine kinase levels before labetalol dosing were measured and subsequent evaluation results including electromyography were normal. This subject's creatine kinase level remains 20% to 50% above the upper range of normal for women 1 year after labetalol discontinuation, and she has refused rechallenge with the drug. One subject taking placebo was dropped because of a transient ischemic attack. Also, two subjects taking labetalol and 11 taking placebo were dropped because of unacceptably high blood pressures. Adverse drug reactions not requiring discontinuance but reported more frequently after labetalol than after placebo included asthenia, dizziness, fatigue, headache, rhinitis, and gastritis. Only the incidence of rhinitis was significantly greater after labetalol.

DISCUSSION

Our data confirm the antihypertensive efficacy of labetalol as step II therapy in patients with essential hypertension not controlled by HCTZ alone. Labetalol was more effective than placebo in lowering systolic and diastolic blood pressures. The proportion of subjects not achieving control and the number of subjects dropped because of poor blood pressure response were significantly less for labetalol. For any given dose, maximal efficacy was evident within 1 week of dosing. This differs from convential β-blockers that may require several weeks before their maximal effect develops.[14] While the net fall in blood pressure after labetalol was in the range of 5 to 12 mm Hg, 11 subjects receiving placebo and only two subjects receiving labetalol were dropped as treatment failures. Thus our results may underestimate the actual effectiveness of the drug.

Our study confirms the efficacy of labetalol in blacks and fails to support the lack of efficacy of conventional β-blockers and labetalol that has been reported.[7,9,13,15,18] Our study, however, evaluated labetalol after subjects had been receiving chronic diuretic therapy; other studies evaluated their efficacy while dosed alone. This combined therapy may decrease the effect of differences in plasma volume and renin usually reported when comparing black and white patients with hypertension.[12] Both may affect the antihypertensive efficacy of β-blockers.[17,19] Furthermore, our study design preselected HCTZ responders, which would minimize differences between placebo and labetalol. These results will have to be confirmed in other studies.

Labetalol was well tolerated without significant adverse effects. Rhinitis was the only side effect reported significantly more often after labetalol than after placebo, but the incidence of other side effects may have been masked by the small sample size. Although five subjects taking labetalol were dropped because of suspected drug-related reactions, two deserve comment. While recently reported to be less likely after labetalol than after other β-blockers,[1,5,8] bronchospasm is an acknowledged risk of all β-blockers. Although elevations in creatinine kinase levels and myositis have been reported with labetalol,[16] there was insufficient evidence to incriminate the drug in our subjects.

In conclusion, labetalol is safe and effective as step II therapy for patients whose hypertension is not controlled by a diuretic alone. It has pharmacologic properties that may offer advantages over current therapy.

Study group participants

Jackson T. Wright, Jr., M.D., Ph.D., and Robert P. Goodman, M.D., Medical College of Virginia, Richmond, Va.; Jeffrey Gorwit, M.D., Escondido Cardiology Associates, Escondido, Calif.; Walter Flamenbaum, M.D., Beth Israel Medical Center, New York, N. Y.; William Mroczek, M.D., Hypertension Hemodynamics Research Lab, Alexandria, Va.; Robert L. Reeves, M.D., Puget Sound Medical Associates, Olympia, Wash.; Albert A. Carr, M.D., and L. Michael Prisant, M.D., Medical College of Georgia, Augusta, Ga.; Alastair J. J. Wood, M.B.Ch.B., and John Nadeau, M.D., Vanderbilt University, Nashville, Tenn.; and Philip Calderone, M.D., Shrish Jogklekar, M.D., and Renato Lenzi, M.D., Jewish Hospital and Medical Center of Brooklyn, Brooklyn, N. Y.

References

1. Adam WR, Meagher EJ, Barter CE: Labetalol, beta blockers, and acute deterioration of chronic airway obstruction. Clin Exp Hyperten **A4:**1419-1428, 1982.
2. Britain RT, Levy GP: A review of the animal pharmacology of labetalol, a combined α and β adrenoceptor blocking drug. Br J Clin Pharmacol **3**(suppl 3):681-694, 1976.
3. Carey B, Whalley ET: α-Adrenergic agonist activity of labetalol on isolated rat uteri. Br J Pharmacol **67:**13-15, 1979.
4. Dargie HJ, Dollery CT, Daniel J: Labetalol in resistant hypertension. Br J Clin Pharmacol **3**(suppl 3):751-755, 1976.
5. George RB, Manochak K, Burford JG, et al: Effects of labetalol in hypertensive patients with chronic obstructive pulmonary disease. Chest **83:**457-460, 1983.
6. Gross F: The place of α-adrenoceptor and β-adrenoceptor blockade in the treatment of hypertension. Br J Clin Pharmacol **3**(suppl 3):5S-11S, 1980.
7. Humphreys GS, Delvin DG: Ineffectiveness of propranolol in hypertensive Jamaicans. Br Med J **2:**601-603, 1968.
8. Jackson SHD, Beaver DG: Comparison of the effects of single doses of albuterol and labetalol on airway obstruction in patients with hypertension and asthma. Br J Clin Pharmacol **15:**553-556, 1983.
9. Jennings K, Parson V: A study of labetalol in patients of European, West Indian, and West African origin. Br J Clin Pharmacol **3**(suppl 3):773-775, 1976.
10. Kristensen BO, Petersen ELC: Effects of long-term high dose labetalol on blood pressure in patients with severe hypertension resistant to previous therapy. Postgrad Med J **56**(suppl 2):57-59, 1980.
11. MacCarthy PG, Bloomfield MB: Labetalol: A review of its pharmacology, pharmacokinetics, clinical uses, and adverse effects. Pharmacotherapy **3:**193-219, 1983.
12. Mitas JA, Holle R, Levy SB, Stone RA: Racial analysis of the volume-renin relationship in human hypertension. Arch Intern Med **139:**157-160, 1979.
13. Olivier LR, Retief JH, Buchel EH, et al: Evaluation of labetalol hydrochloride (Trandate) in hospital outpatients. Clin Trials J **17:**75-80, 1980.
14. Prichard BNC, Gillam PMS: Treatment of hypertension with propranolol. Br Med J **1:**7-16, 1969.
15. Seedat YK: Labetalol hydrochloride in the treatment of Black and Indian hypertensive patients. Med Proc **25:**53-57, 1979.
16. Teicher A, Rosenthal T, Kissen E, et al: Labetalol-induced toxic myopathy. Br Med J **282:**1824-1825, 1981.
17. Vaughan ED Jr, Laragh JH, Gavras I, Buhler FR, Gavras H, Brunner HR, Baer L: Volume factor in low and normal renin essential hypertension: Treatment with either spironolactone or chlorthalidone. Am J Cardiol **32:**523-532, 1973.
18. Veterans Administration Cooperative Study Group on Antihypertensive Agents: Comparison of propranolol and hydrochlorothiazide for the initial treatment of hypertension. JAMA **248:**1996-2011, 1982.
19. Woods JW, Pittman AW, Pulliam CC, Werk EE Jr, Waider W, Allen CA: Renin profiling in hypertension and its use in treatment with propranolol and chlorthalidone. N Engl J Med **294:**1137-1142, 1976.

Endoscopic evaluation of slow-release potassium chloride preparations

In a double-blind, randomized, placebo-controlled clinical trial, 30 healthy subjects took one of two potassium chloride preparations or placebo three times a day for 1 week with concomitant oral glycopyrrolate dosing. The upper digestive tract was endoscopically examined immediately before and after the treatment period. One subject in both of the KCl treatment groups and six subjects in the placebo group developed submucosal lesions. All lesions were minor and of limited clinical significance. There may be reason to believe that glycopyrrolate plays a role in the production of such lesions. If so, the concomitant use of glycopyrrolate in clinical trials of KCl preparations may cloud the results of such studies. (Clin Pharmacol Ther 38:28-30, 1985.)

Colin Kendall, M.D., Kenneth D. Krantz, M.D., Ph.D., Arthur Berger, B.S., and Tessa Sharp, M.S. *Princeton, N. J., and Kansas City, Mo.*

In 1982 McMahon et al.[7] described a new clinical pharmacologic model of repeated endoscopic examination of healthy subjects to monitor changes in the mucosa of the upper gastrointestinal tract. Comparing the effects of two potassium preparations (a wax matrix slow-release tablet and a microencapsulated formulation), they found the wax matrix tablets to be associated with a higher incidence of mucosal lesions. Barkin et al.[3] reported similar results with the same protocol in a smaller study. McMahon et al.[8] repeated their study in more subjects and confirmed their original findings. In those studies, most subjects were given unusually high doses of potassium chloride (96 mEq/day) as well as glycopyrrolate (6 mg/day) to delay gastric emptying. Nevertheless, given manufacturers' claims that the frequency of small bowel lesions among patients receiving their wax matrix tablets was approximately one per 100,000 patient years,* these results were quite unexpected. Moreover, data from the Boston Collaborative Drug Surveillance Program argue strongly against a positive association between wax matrix KCl use and upper gastrointestinal bleeding over a short period.[2]

In an attempt to reproduce the results of McMahon et al.,[7,8] Patterson et al.[9] conducted two endoscopically monitored studies and reported that all types of solid potassium preparations could induce erosive gastrointestinal mucosal lesions when given in high doses with glycopyrrolate; thus their data failed to support the contention that subjects receiving the microencapsulated product were not subject to erosive or ulcerative lesions. In a similar study in slightly older subjects, Ernest et al.[4] reported no differences between the effects of wax matrix and microencapsulated KCl. Most recently, Alsop et al.[1] compared the effects of five different preparations of KCl on the upper gastrointestinal tract in 90 healthy subjects treated concomitantly with glycopyrrolate and found endoscopic evidence of mucosal damage in all subjects, including those who had received placebo. Except for one ulcer after microencapsulated KCl, all lesions were superficial.

We report an endoscopically monitored study to compare the effects on the gastric mucosa of two slow-release potassium chloride tablets (Klor-Con [Upsher-Smith Laboratories] and Slow-K [Ciba Pharmaceutical Co.]) and a placebo tablet during concomitant glycopyrrolate dosing.

METHODS

Ours was a double-blind, randomized, multiple-dose, parallel group study over 7 days with three treatment groups of 10 subjects each. Medical history, physical examinations, laboratory screening tests, and ECGs were made within 10 days of starting the medications and were repeated (with the exception of medical history) at the end of the study. Stool guaiac tests were done daily to monitor gross gastrointestinal safety. Endoscopic examinations were performed on study days −1 and 7. Subjects were sedated with intravenous di-

From Ellis Pharmaceutical Consulting, Inc., Princeton, and Quincy Research Center, Kansas City.

Received for publication Dec. 14, 1984; accepted Feb. 9, 1985.

Reprint requests to: Colin Kendall, M.D., Ellis Pharmaceutical Consulting, Inc., 913 State Rd., Princeton, NJ 08540-1484.

*Ciba Pharmaceutical Company: Data on file.

azepam and meperidine before introduction of the instrument. The endoscopist examined and photographed the mucosa at 10 sites: mid and lower esophagus, cardia, greater and lesser gastric curvatures, greater and lesser pyloric antrum curvatures, pylorus, and bulbar and postbulbar duodenum. To avoid the possibility of mistaking instrument-induced artifacts for treatment-induced lesions, the examiner made his observations in a strictly descending order from midesophagus to postbulbar duodenum. After endoscopy, subjects received intravenous naloxone to awaken them. Identical scoring methods (0 = no lesion, 1 = 1 submucosal hemorrhage, 2 = >1 submucosal hemorrhage) for mucosal lesions were used for all endoscopies before and after treatment by the same endoscopist who did not know what treatment subjects had received. Each subject's highest scores in three areas (esophagus, stomach, and duodenum) were the basis for intersubject comparisons of the endoscopic findings.

Thirty normal subjects participated in the study. No significant differences between the three treatment groups were found at baseline, but mean (±SD) ages of the groups differed as follows: Klor-Con group, 28.1 ± 8.94 years; Slow-K group, 26.4 ± 8.83 years; and placebo group, 31.9 ± 6.90 years. One subject (103) was 4 kg over the weight limit but was nonetheless accepted for enrollment.

In accordance with inclusion criteria (except for one subject whose baseline serum γ-glutamyl transpeptidase value was outside the normal range), baseline laboratory screening test results for all subjects were within normal limits or so slightly out of range as to be of no clinical significance. The following three code-labeled test drugs were dispensed according to a randomization schedule: Klor-Con tablets: 7 × 10 mEq tablets a day = 70 mEq KCl; Slow-K tablets: 9 × 8 mEq tablets a day = 72 mEq KCl; and placebo tablets: 9 tablets a day. Because of their respective dosage forms, it was not feasible to dispense exactly equal daily doses of the KCl tablets. All subjects also received three 2 mg glycopyrrolate tablets each day to delay gastric emptying. Tablets were taken three times a day, after meals with a drink of water, for 7 days (study days 1 through 7).

RESULTS

Table I (lesion score) summarizes the findings for each treatment group during the endoscopic examination on days −1 and 7. One subject in each of the KCl groups developed one submucosal gastric hemorrhage, whereas four subjects in the placebo group developed one submucosal hemorrhage and two others each developed two submucosal hemorrhages. The endoscopist's report stated that all the lesions were minor and of limited clinical significance, and that such lesions could occur in normal untreated subjects. Stool sample test results were negative for heme for all subjects throughout the study.

Table I. Endoscopic findings

	No. of subjects with lesions	*Site*	*Description**
Klor-Con			
Day −1	0/10	—	—
Day 7	1/10	Stomach	1
Slow K			
Day −1	0/10	—	—
Day 7	1/10	Stomach	1
Placebo			
Day −1	0/10	—	—
Day 7	6/10	Stomach	2
		Stomach	1
		Stomach	1
		Duodenum	1
		Duodenum	2
		Duodenum	1

*1 = One submucosal hemorrhage; 2 = more than one submucosal hemorrhage.

Mean serum potassium levels rose during the study in the Klor-Con (4.25 to 4.58 mEq/L) and in the Slow-K (4.18 to 4.45 mEq/L) groups but fell in the placebo group (4.32 to 4.24 mEq/L). The few out-of-range results in the daily observations of vital signs and blood pressure were transitory and were seen in all treatment groups. The investigator concluded that none of these changes was drug related or represented any risk to the subject. Twelve-lead ECGs were recorded before and after the study. All results were either normal or showed normal variant characteristics. There were no drug related-changes between baseline and final ECGs.

Six complaints of gastrointestinal symptoms among five subjects in the Klor-Con group, six complaints among three subjects in the Slow-K group, and seven complaints among three subjects in the placebo group were blindly assessed as possibly or remotely treatment related. Treatment-related symptoms all referred to the gastrointestinal tract (loss of appetite, stomach cramps, nausea, and vomiting). All symptoms were mild or moderate, did not indicate a risk to the subjects' safety, and resolved without medical intervention. Ten complaints (three with Klor-Con, five with Slow-K, and two with placebo), including nausea, sore throat, and sore arms, were not drug related but were attributed to the pre-endoscopy intravenous anxiolytic/anesthetic infusion and to the passage of the instrument.

Several outlying clinical laboratory findings were noted at the final examination. No finding indicated a risk to subject safety. Findings were considered possibly drug related in only two subjects (no. 119 in the Klor-Con group and no. 129 in the Slow-K group) who had minimally elevated serum potassium levels. Three laboratory urinalysis findings after treatment were considered significant but not drug related. Apart from the serum potassium levels, laboratory findings outside the reference range that were not significant were thought to have occurred randomly, representing normal variation and quite unrelated to study drug.

DISCUSSION

The earliest studies cited[3,7] included no placebo groups. A later study[8] did include one group that received placebo and glycopyrrolate. Of this group, three of 15 subjects developed lesions, one of which was an ulcer. The only other placebo group reported[8] received no glycopyrrolate; two of 11 subjects developed erosions. The incidence of lesions found at screening is not stated for either study. In the study of Patterson et al.,[9] 15 of 127 (12%) subjects were rejected at screening because of gastric lesions or abnormal liver function test results. The number of subjects in each category was not reported, but it is clear that <12% of the volunteers had gastric lesions. In the placebo-glycopyrrolate group, five of 15 (33%) subjects developed lesions after 1 week of treatment.

In our subjects, nine of 39 (23%) were rejected at endoscopic screening because of unsuspected lesions. After treatment, only one of 10 subjects (10%) in each of the KCl groups had lesions, while six of 10 (60%) subjects in the placebo group had lesions. Alsop et al.[1] reported comparable results. Whereas they screened out nine of 101 (9%) subjects at baseline, the incidence of mucosal lesions (erosions or ulcers) after treatment in their placebo group was four of 15 (27%), a higher incidence than in any of their five KCl treatment groups. In all these studies, the placebo treatment was associated with an incidence of mucosal lesions in the upper gut approximately threefold that of the population from which subjects were recruited. In other pharmacologic studies (of anti-inflammatory drugs), lesions of the gastric mucosa have developed in the placebo group, but their incidence has been lower than that in the groups receiving active drugs.[5,6]

In our study, results with the novel clinical pharmacologic model introduced by McMahon et al.[7] are unusual in that the subjects in the placebo group received an active drug, glycopyrrolate. To our knowledge there have been no clinical reports describing endoscopic findings after glycopyrrolate dosing alone. Thus it is not known whether glycopyrrolate tablets per se have a local harmful effect on the gastric mucosa. Nevertheless, it is apparent from the several studies of McMahon et al.[8] and Alsop et al.[1] that, whether because of local irritation or because of delayed gastric emptying, the incidence of mucosal lesions in both placebo groups and in KCl groups is increased when glycopyrrolate is also taken.

We thank J. A. Woltjen, M.D., for scoring of the mucosal lesions.

References

1. Alsop WR, Moore JG, Rollins DE, Tolman KG: The effects of five potassium chloride preparations on the upper gastrointestinal mucosa in healthy subjects receiving glycopyrrolate. J Clin Pharmacol **24:**235-239, 1984.
2. Aselton PJ, Jick H: Short-term follow-up study of wax matrix potassium chloride in relation to gastrointestinal bleeding. Lancet **1:**184, 1983.
3. Barkin JS, Harary AM, Shamblen CE, Lasseter KC: Potassium chloride and gastrointestinal injury. Ann Intern Med **98:**261-262, 1983.
4. Ernest D: Report to the Cardiovascular and Renal Drugs and Gastrointestinal Drugs Advisory Committees of the Food and Drug Administration. Bethesda, March 2, 1983.
5. Lanza F, Royer G, Nelson R: An endoscopic evaluation of the effects of non-steroidal anti-inflammatory drugs on the gastric mucosa. Gastrointest Endosc **21:**103-105, 1975.
6. Lanza F, Nelson RS, Rack MF: A controlled endoscopic study comparing the toxic effects of sulindac, naproxen, aspirin, and placebo on the gastric mucosa of healthy volunteers. J Clin Pharmacol **24:**89-95, 1984.
7. McMahon FG, Ryan JR, Akdamar K, Ertan A: Upper gastrointestinal lesions after potassium chloride supplements: A controlled clinical trial. Lancet **1:**1059-1060, 1982.
8. McMahon FG, Ryan JR, Akdamar K, Ertan A: Effect of potassium chloride supplements on upper gastrointestinal mucosa. CLIN PHARMACOL THER **35:**852-855, 1984.
9. Patterson DJ, Weinstein GS, Jeffries GH: Endoscopic comparison of solid and liquid potassium chloride supplements. Lancet **2:**1077-1078, 1983.

Cefotaxime and desacetyl cefotaxime kinetics in renal impairment

Cefotaxime and desacetyl cefotaxime kinetics after a single, 1 gm intravenous dose were evaluated in five groups of subjects: group I, normal creatinine clearance (CL_{CR} >90 ml/min); group II, mild renal insufficiency (CL_{CR} 30 to 89 ml/min); group III, moderate renal insufficiency (CL_{CR} 16 to 29 ml/min); group IV, severe renal insufficiency (CL_{CR} 4 to 15 ml/min); and group V, end-stage renal disease requiring maintenance hemodialysis (CL_{CR} <6 ml/min). The steady-state volume of distribution (V_{ss}) ranged from 10% to 55% of body weight but was not related to CL_{CR}. The terminal $t_{1/2}$ values of cefotaxime and desacetyl cefotaxime were 0.79 and 0.70, 1.09 and 3.95, 1.55 and 5.65, 2.54 and 14.23, and 1.63 and 23.15 hours in groups I to V, respectively. There were no significant changes in V_{ss} or $t_{1/2}$ after multiple dosing, but there were significant correlations between CL_{CR} and cefotaxime total body clearance, cefotaxime and desacetyl cefotaxime renal clearance, and cefotaxime nonrenal clearance. Dosage regimens for the use of cefotaxime in patients with renal impairment are proposed. (Clin Pharmacol Ther 38:31-36, 1985.)

Gary R. Matzke, Pharm.D., Paul A. Abraham, M.D., Charles E. Halstenson, Pharm.D., and William F. Keane, M.D. *Minneapolis, Minn.*

Cefotaxime is a semisynthetic cephalosporin with a broad range of activity, including effectiveness against most clinically relevant gram-positive and gram-negative bacteria.[3,12,14] Kinetic studies of cefotaxime in normal subjects indicate that 40% to 60% of a single intravenous dose is excreted unchanged in the urine.[5,11] The kinetics of the active metabolite, desacetyl cefotaxime, after a single intravenous dose of the parent have also been assessed.[1,10,18] Multiple-dose studies indicate that there is no cumulation of cefotaxime in healthy subjects,[5] but kinetic data for cefotaxime and the desacetyl metabolite during multiple dosing of cefotaxime in patients with renal impairment are few.[11,21] Our study was designed to characterize the disposition of cefotaxime and its desacetyl metabolite after single and multiple intravenous doses in subjects with varying degrees of renal function, to compare the kinetics in subjects with normal and impaired renal function, and to propose dosing guidelines for cefotaxime in patients with varying states of renal function.

From the Drug Evaluation Unit, Hennepin County Medical Center and College of Pharmacy and School of Medicine, University of Minnesota.

Supported in part by a grant from Hoechst-Roussel Pharmaceuticals, Inc., Somerville, N. J.

Received for publication Nov. 6, 1984; accepted Feb. 14, 1985.

Reprint requests to: Gary R. Matzke, Pharm.D., Drug Evaluation Unit, Division of Nephrology, Department of Medicine, Hennepin County Medical Center, 701 Park Ave., Minneapolis, MN 55415.

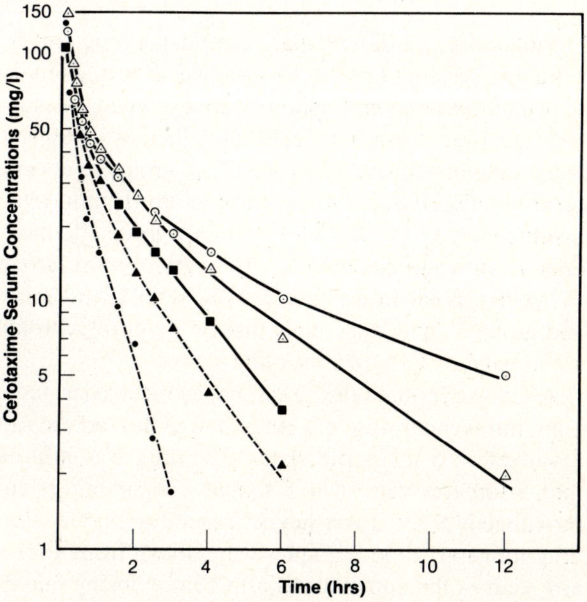

Fig. 1. Mean serum concentration–time profile of cefotaxime in groups I (●), II (▲), III (■), IV (○), and V (△). All subjects received cefotaxime, 1 gm iv over 5 minutes.

METHODS

Forty-two subjects underwent a medical history, physical examination, chest radiograph, and ECG, hematologic and biochemical tests, and two 24-hour creatinine clearance (CL_{CR}) determinations before participating in the study. Patients with major disorders of the

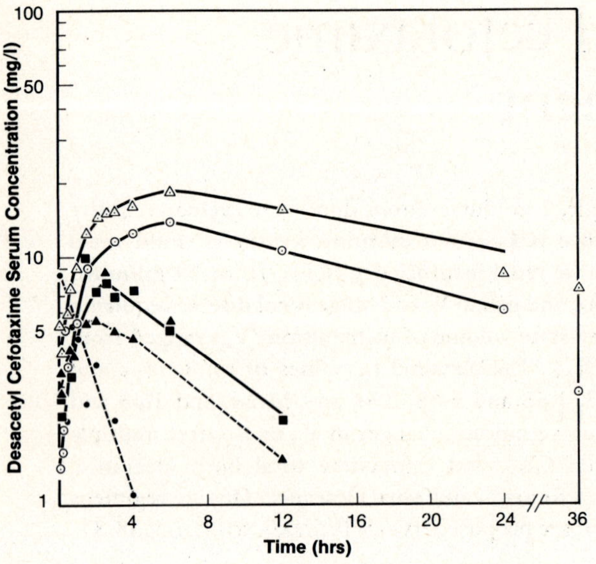

Fig. 2. Mean serum concentration–time profile of desacetyl cefotaxime in groups I (●), II (▲), III (■), IV (⊙), and V (△). All subjects received cefotaxime, 1 gm iv as a 5-minute infusion.

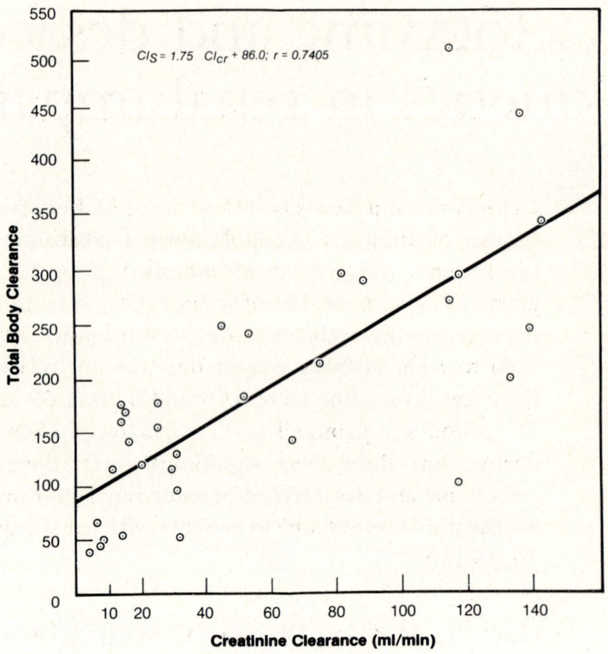

Fig. 3. Relationship between cefotaxime CL and CL_{CR}.

hepatobiliary, cardiovascular, central nervous, or respiratory systems or who had known hypersensitivity to penicillins or cephalosporins were excluded. No subject received concurrent antibiotic therapy. Subjects were categorized according to CL_{CR}: group I, normal renal function (CL_{CR} >90 ml/min); group II, mild renal insufficiency (CL_{CR} 30 to 89 ml/min); group III, moderate renal insufficiency (CL_{CR} 16 to 29 ml/min); group IV, severe renal insufficiency (CL_{CR} 4 to 15 ml/min); and group V, end-stage renal disease requiring chronic hemodialysis (CL_{CR} <6 ml/min).

After an overnight fast, each subject received a single 1 gm intravenous dose of cefotaxime as the sodium salt dissolved in 5 ml sterile water. The drug was infused into a forearm vein over 5 minutes beginning at approximately 8 AM. Each subject fasted for 2 hours after drug infusion. Blood samples were drawn from a forearm vein in the contralateral arm before dosing and 5, 10, 15, 30, and 45 minutes and 1, 1.5, 2, 2.5, 3, 4, 6, 12, 24, and 36 hours after the start of the infusion. Urine samples were collected before drug dosing and for the intervals 0 to 2, 2 to 4, 4 to 6, 6 to 12, 12 to 24, and 24 to 48 hours after the start of the infusion.

Subjects in groups I to IV received 1 gm cefotaxime sodium intravenously at 6-hour intervals for 5 days and a final dose on the morning of day 6. Multiple blood samples were drawn for 6 and 36 hours after starting the first and last infusion at the times indicated. On days 2 to 5, blood samples were drawn immediately before and after a 5-minute intravenous infusion at 8 AM. On day 1, urine samples were collected before drug dosing and for the intervals 0 to 2, 2 to 4, 4 to 6, 6 to 12, and 12 to 24 hours after the start of the infusion. On days 2 to 5, the total 24-hour urine output was collected. After the last dose, urine samples were collected according to the single-dose schedule. Serum and urine samples were stored at −70° C until assayed.

The concentrations of cefotaxime and desacetyl cefotaxime in serum and urine were determined by a modification of the HPLC technique of Chamberlain et al.[2] Between-day precision of the method ranged from 11.8% to 13.4% over the concentration range of 5 to 100 μg/ml, while the within-day precision ranged from 0.2% to 5.4% over the same concentration range for cefotaxime and desacetyl cefotaxime. Cefotaxime serum concentration–time data were analyzed based on minimization of the residual sum of squares: $C = Ae^{-\alpha t} + Be^{-\beta t}$, where C is the serum concentration at time t, A and B are the intercepts, and α and β are the disposition rates obtained from the first and second phases, respectively, of the plot of log serum cefotaxime concentration–time. Final estimates of the parameters were obtained by a standard curve stripping and nonlinear regression analysis program (AUTOAN/

Table I. Subject characteristics

Group	*n*	*Sex (M/F)*	*Age (yr)*	*Height (cm)*	*Weight (kg)*	*Serum creatinine (mg/dl)*	*CL_{CR} (ml/min)*
I	8	8/0	27.0 ± 3.3	180.5 ± 7.1	77.3 ± 7.6	1.0 ± 0.1	127.4 ± 12.2
II	8	7/1	39.6 ± 14.9	172.8 ± 13.6	68.4 ± 10.4	1.5 ± 0.5	61.8 ± 19.4
III	8	7/1	45.6 ± 15.4	178.7 ± 7.2	82.5 ± 13.8	4.1 ± 1.8	23.8 ± 6.4
IV	8	6/2	50.0 ± 15.2	177.4 ± 3.6	66.3 ± 9.3	8.1 ± 3.5	9.8 ± 4.0
V	8	5/3	49.5 ± 16.0	178.9 ± 6.9	72.0 ± 21.7	9.7 ± 2.6	3.4 ± 2.7

Data are $\overline{X}$ ± SD.
M = Male; F = female.

NONLIN).[20] The coefficients of the biexponential equation were corrected to values reflecting a single intravenous bolus dose by the equations of Gibaldi and Perrier.[6] The model-dependent kinetic parameters (central compartment volume of distribution [V_c], steady-state volume of distribution [V_{ss}], and the $t_{1/2}$ of the α and β phases) were calculated from the coefficients and exponents of the fitted curve.[6] The serum AUC was calculated by the linear trapezoidal method. The AUC beyond the last measured data point was estimated by dividing the value for the last data point by the terminal elimination rate constant β. A model-independent approach was used to calculate Vd_{ss}, mean residence time (MRT), and total body clearance (CL).[15]

The peak serum concentration (C_{max}) and time to peak serum concentration (t_{max}) for desacetyl cefotaxime were determined by visual inspection of the serum concentration–time profile. For those subjects demonstrating formation rate–limited elimination of desacetyl cefotaxime, the $t_{1/2}$ was determined by the methods of Huston.[9] The $t_{1/2}$ of desacetyl cefotaxime for those subjects with elimination rate–limited elimination was determined by nonlinear regression analysis. The desacetyl cefotaxime serum AUC and MRT were also determined.[6,15] The renal clearance (CL_R) of cefotaxime and desacetyl cefotaxime was calculated by standard techniques.[6] Nonrenal clearance (CL_{NR}) of cefotaxime was calculated as the difference between CL and CL_R. The cumulation ratio of cefotaxime and desacetyl cefotaxime during multiple dosing of cefotaxime was estimated from the ratio of trough serum concentrations, i.e., immediately before the last multiple dose and 6 hours after the single dose.

Between-group differences in kinetics were evaluated by ANOVA and the two-tailed unpaired Student's t test. Statistically significant differences in cefotaxime and desacetyl cefotaxime kinetics after a single dose and last multiple dosing were evaluated by paired Student's t test. The relationships between kinetics and renal function were assessed by linear regression analysis.

RESULTS

Clinical characteristics of the 40 subjects who completed the protocol are listed in Table I. Two subjects did not complete the protocol because of intercurrent illness. The mean serum cefotaxime concentrations after the first dose are shown in Fig. 1. The cefotaxime $t_{1/2\beta}$ increased as renal function declined. The 48-hour cumulative urinary excretion of cefotaxime was 43.6% ± 5.6% ($\overline{X}$ ± SD) and 3.1% ± 1.9% of the dose in groups I and V, respectively. Desacetyl cefotaxime was detectable in 33 of the 40 subjects. The desacetyl cefotaxime C_{max}, t_{max}, and $t_{1/2}$ increased as renal function declined (Fig. 2). A smaller fraction of desacetyl cefotaxime than of cefotaxime was recovered in the urine of group I (15.7% ± 4.4%) but not of group V (4.9% ± 5.5%).

Between-group differences in the single-dose cefotaxime kinetics ($t_{1/2\beta}$, AUC, MRT, CL, and CL_R) were noted (Table II). The $t_{1/2\beta}$ in group V was shorter than that in group IV (nonhemodialysis). Although there was no significant difference in the V_c among the five groups, the Vd_{ss} in group IV was greater than that in group I. CL and CL_R were lower in the subjects with moderate and severe renal insufficiency (groups III and IV) than in the subjects in group I. The CL in group V was markedly higher than that in group IV, despite the fact that CL_R was significantly lower. Desacetyl cefotaxime kinetics after the first cefotaxime dose ($t_{1/2\beta}$, MRT, and AUC) increased as renal function declined (Table III). There was also a fall in CL_R. Three of the eight subjects in group I had formation rate–limited elimination of desacetyl cefotaxime, a pattern not observed in any of the subjects in groups II to V. The values for β and CL for cefotaxime and the CL_R for cefotaxime and desacetyl cefotaxime correlated well

Table II. Cefotaxime kinetics after first dose

Group	C_{max} (mg/L)	$t_{1/2\alpha}$ (hr)	$t_{1/2\beta}$* (hr)	k_{10}* (hr^{-1})	k_{12} (hr^{-1})	k_{21} (hr^{-1})
I	125.3 ± 32.6	0.089 ± 0.046	0.79 ± 0.66	2.69 ± 0.97	4.46 ± 2.50	2.98 ± 1.10
II	122.6 ± 40.7	0.236 ± 0.230	1.09 ± 0.89	1.99 ± 1.32	2.21 ± 2.12	2.41 ± 1.34
III	119.7 ± 23.2	0.111 ± 0.061	1.55 ± 0.27	1.24 ± 0.35	4.08 ± 2.28	2.75 ± 0.85
IV	109.3 ± 21.8	0.120 ± 0.056	2.54 ± 1.30	0.84 ± 0.5	3.45 ± 2.20	3.04 ± 1.00
V	139.5 ± 71.2	0.111 ± 0.055	1.63 ± 0.45	1.05 ± 0.61	4.03 ± 2.70	3.70 ± 0.80

Data are $\overline{X}$ ± SD.
k_{10}, k_{12}, k_{21} = Intercompartmental transfer rate constants.
*Significant difference ($P < 0.05$; ANOVA) between groups.

Table III. Desacetyl cefotaxime kinetics after first dose

Group	C_{max} (mg/L)	t_{max} (hr)	$t_{1/2}$* (hr)	k* (hr^{-1})	MRT* (hr)	Total AUC* (mg/hr/L)	CL_R* (ml/min)
I	7.9 ± 6.0	0.43 ± 0.41	0.70 ± 0.63	3.25 ± 3.96	1.75 ± 0.60	12.49 ± 10.21	234.6 ± 122.7
II	9.4 ± 6.1	1.36 ± 0.83	3.95 ± 0.77	0.181 ± 0.035	8.44 ± 5.11	87.26 ± 87.43	78.6 ± 87.1
II	8.8 ± 2.5	2.46 ± 1.68	5.65 ± 3.11	0.200 ± 0.179	10.00 ± 4.99	89.59 ± 47.56	23.2 ± 15.6
IV	14.7 ± 5.5	5.96 ± 3.58	14.23 ± 5.41	0.056 ± 0.025	23.00 ± 9.69	358.74 ± 80.77	7.6 ± 4.6
V	21.0 ± 4.1	5.89 ± 3.22	23.15 ± 15.96	0.046 ± 0.031	34.85 ± 22.78	729.24 ± 487.30	2.5 ± 0.6

Data are $\overline{X}$ ± SD.
k = Elimination rate constant.
*Significant difference ($P < 0.05$; ANOVA) between groups.

with CL_{CR} (Fig. 3). There was no significant relationship between C_{max} or V_{ss} and CL_{CR}.

After the last multiple dose, there were no significant differences in any of the cefotaxime kinetics, and only the AUC of desacetyl cefotaxime was higher in group III than after single dosing. There was, however, significant cumulation of cefotaxime and desacetyl cefotaxime in group IV and groups III and IV, respectively. The observed cumulation ratio of cefotaxime of 1.74 in group IV was greater than the predicted value of 1.13. The observed cumulation ratios of desacetyl cefotaxime in groups III and IV of 2.5 and 4.1 were also greater than the predicted ratios of 1.4 and 3.5, respectively.

Cefotaxime was well tolerated after single doses, but during the maintenance dose period and in the 72 hours after the last maintenance dose there were several adverse effects. These included mild to moderate gastrointestinal complaints (diarrhea, nausea, and constipation) from nine subjects, dysuria in two, and maculopapular rashes in five. Four of the five subjects who developed maculopapular rashes had a CL_{CR} value of approximately 30 ml/min or less. The rashes were generally distributed over the total body surface and were accompanied by pruritus. They were first observed in four of the five subjects during the 72 hours after the last maintenance dose. All subjects responded to antihistamines and the rashes resolved in 2 to 10 days.

DISCUSSION

Cefotaxime kinetics in our subjects with normal renal function are similar to those reported by Ings et al.,[11] Luthy et al.,[13] and Wise et al.[21] Although the serum concentrations of desacetyl cefotaxime were lower than the simultaneous cefotaxime concentrations, they declined at an apparent rate similar to that of cefotaxime. This apparent elimination rate of desacetyl cefotaxime, however, was an underestimate in three of the eight subjects who had formation rate–limited elimination of desacetyl cefotaxime.[9] This observation corroborates the report of Ings et al.[10] The mean desacetyl cefotaxime $t_{1/2}$ in these subjects was thus shorter than that of cefotaxime.

The $t_{1/2\beta}$, CL, CL_R, and CL_{NR} of cefotaxime, as well as the $t_{1/2}$ and CL_R of desacetyl cefotaxime, were altered in impaired renal function. The increase in $t_{1/2\beta}$ and decrease in clearance correlated with CL_{CR}. Although the degree of decrease in CL was of the order of that reported by Ings et al.[11] in subjects with mild and moderate renal impairment, the decline was much greater in our subjects with severely impaired renal function (group IV). The CL of cefotaxime in the subjects with

MRT (hr)*	*Total AUC* (mg/hr/L)*	V_c *(L/kg)*	V_{ss} *(L/kg)*	*CL* (ml/min)*	CL_R* *(ml/min)*	CL_{NR} *(ml/min)*
1.01 ± 0.80	67.7 ± 36.9	0.080 ± 0.022	0.174 ± 0.063	300.5 ± 129.0	138.4 ± 59.9	162.1 ± 74.0
1.28 ± 0.88	107.1 ± 87.9	0.115 ± 0.060	0.185 ± 0.068	207.9 ± 81.7	84.2 ± 46.9	123.7 ± 53.3
2.13 ± 0.49	125.8 ± 26.7	0.088 ± 0.031	0.209 ± 0.055	137.7 ± 28.3	20.5 ± 11.9	117.2 ± 35.5
5.51 ± 3.94	256.5 ± 127.4	0.122 ± 0.027	0.306 ± 0.123	88.0 ± 55.4	7.18 ± 3.15	80.8 ± 53.3
2.64 ± 1.15	193.4 ± 93.8	0.138 ± 0.061	0.205 ± 0.060	111.5 ± 69.6	2.47 ± 2.28	109.0 ± 70.9

renal impairment studied by Ings et al.[11] approximates the clearance in our subjects in group V who had been undergoing chronic dialysis. The reason for a difference in patients with severely impaired renal function who have not undergone dialysis is not known, but recent studies with bis(2-ethylhexyl)phthalate, a component of dialyzer tubing, indicate stimulation of hepatic microsomal enzyme activity.[16] The potential for this phthalate plasticizer to alter hepatic drug metabolism (i.e., increase CL_{NR}) in patients undergoing hemodialysis may need to be considered in future kinetic characterizations.

There were no significant differences in any of the kinetic parameters of cefotaxime, and only the total AUC of desacetyl cefotaxime in group III was significantly different after multiple doses. Trough desacetyl cefotaxime serum concentrations were significantly elevated after multiple doses in group III (8.8 and 22.3 mg/L) and group IV (14.7 and 66.0 mg/L). Although there was no cumulation of desacetyl cefotaxime in group II, the correlations between CL_{CR} and both CL_R and CL suggest that cumulation is a continuous phenomenon and may thereby be apparent in some patients with "mild" renal impairment.

Detectable serum concentrations of cefotaxime were maintained in subjects with normal renal function for only 3 to 4 hours after multiple doses of 1 gm every 6 hours. Because of the inherent activity of desacetyl cefotaxime and synergy with cefotaxime,[3,17] treatment of highly susceptible organisms (minimum inhibitory concentration <1 μg/ml) in these subjects may be possible with an intravenous 1 gm dose every 8 to 12 hours. The use of cefotaxime to treat moderately susceptible organisms—organisms for which desacetyl cefotaxime has minimal inherent activity and for which synergy has not been demonstrated—may require more frequent and larger doses to attain clinical success.

Although the impact of declining renal function on the elimination of cefotaxime is not as great as has been reported with some of the cephalosporins, dosage adjustment is indicated. High blood concentrations of cephalosporins have been associated with neurotoxicity and the development of a direct positive Coombs reaction that may lead to significant hemolysis.[4,8] Furthermore, the attainment of high concentrations of the microbiologically active desacetyl metabolite in patients with renal insufficiency may contribute to the ability of cefotaxime to inhibit and kill organisms beyond the period predicted from the cefotaxime serum concentration–time profile.[17]

There are several approaches to modify drug dosage in patients with impaired renal function.[7,19] Prolongation of the maintenance dosing interval (τ) may be preferred because of its simplicity and the combined benefits of less frequent dosing and the assurance of attaining a high C_{max}. Regardless of which method is used, because the V_c and V_{ss} of cefotaxime do not vary with renal function, the loading dose in patients with severe renal impairment will be of the order of that in subjects with normal renal function. The degree of change in the dosing interval may then be calculated by use of the relationship between CL and CL_{CR} (Fig. 3). From this relationship, a CL of 296 ml/min can be calculated for a normal CL_{CR} of 120 ml/min. Through use of the standard dose, the new dosing interval ($\tau_{failure}$) can then be estimated from the following equation: $\tau_{failure} = \tau_{normal}$ (296 ml/min ÷ 1.75 × CL_{CR} + 86 ml/min). This yields a $\tau_{failure}$ of approximately 1.5, 2.0, and 3.0 times the normal values (every 4 to 8 hours) for patients with a CL_{CR} of 60, 30, and 10 ml/min, respectively.

We acknowledge the analytic expertise of Ken Miller, Ph.D., Ron Sawchuk, Ph.D., and David Haughey, Pharm.D., the technical assistance of Barb Fischley, the statistical assistance of Irwin Ho, M.S., and the continuing support of Surendra Puri, Ph.D., and Ron Sabo.

References

1. Bergan T, Larsen EW, Brodwall EK: Pharmacokinetics of a new cephalosporin, cefotaxime (HR 756) in patients with different renal functions. Chemotherapy **28:**85-104, 1982.

2. Chamberlain J, Coombes JD, Dell D, Fromson JM, Ings RL, McDonald CM, McEwen J: Metabolism of cefotaxime in animals and man. J Antimicrob Chemother **6**(suppl A):69, 1980.
3. Chin N, Neu HC: Cefotaxime and desacetyl cefotaxime: An example of advantageous antimicrobial metabolism. Diagn Microbiol Infect Dis **2**(suppl):21-31, 1984.
4. Endreny RG, Chazan JA, King BP, Zipin SB: Cephalosporin induced neurotoxicity (NT) in patients with renal failure. Am Soc Nephrol 72A, 1983.
5. Esmiu F, Guibert J, Rosenkilde HC, Ho I, Le GO: Pharmacokinetics of cefotaxime in normal human volunteers. J Antimicrob Chemother **6**(suppl A)83-92, 1980.
6. Gibaldi M, Perrier D: Pharmacokinetics. New York, 1982, Marcel Dekker, Inc.
7. Gibson TP: Influence of renal disease on pharmacokinetics. *In* Evans WE, Schentag JJ, Jusko WJ, editors: Applied pharmacokinetics, principles of therapeutic drug monitoring. San Francisco, 1980, Applied Therapeutics Inc., pp 32-56.
8. Goodman LS, Gilman A: The pharmacological basis of therapeutics, ed 6. New York, 1980, McMillan Publishing Company.
9. Huston JB: Drug metabolite kinetics. Pharmacol Ther **15**:521-552, 1982.
10. Ings RMJ, Bax RP, Reeves DS, White LO, Bywater MJ, Holt HA: The influence of renal tubular secretion upon the pharmacokinetics of cefotaxime and its metabolites. Presented at the Thirteenth International Congress on Chemotherapy, Florence, Italy, July 1981.
11. Ings RMJ, Fillastre JP, Godin M, Leroy A, Humbert G: The pharmacokinetics of cefotaxime and its metabolites in subjects with normal and impaired renal function. Rev Infect Dis **4**(suppl):379-391, 1982.
12. Jones RN, Thornsberry C: Cefotaxime: A review of *in vitro* antimicrobial properties and spectrum of activity. Rev Infect Dis **4**(suppl):300, 1982.
13. Luthy R, Blaser J, Bonetti A, Simmen H, Wise R, Siegenthaler W: Comparative multiple dose pharmacokinetics of cefotaxime, moxalactam and ceftazidime. Antimicrob Agents Chemother **20**:567-575, 1981.
14. Neu HC: Antibacterial activity of desacetyl cefotaxime alone and in combination with cefotaxime. Rev Infect Dis **4**(suppl):374, 1982.
15. Perrier D, Mayersohn M: Noncompartmental determination of the steady state volume of distribution for any mode of administration. J Pharm Sci **71**:372-373, 1982.
16. Pollack GM, Shen D: Effect of renal failure and bis(2-ethylhexyl)phthalate pretreatment on the disposition and metabolism of antipyrine in the rat. J Pharm Sci **73**:29-33, 1984.
17. Quintiliani R, Nightingale CH, Tilton R: Comparative pharmacokinetics of cefotaxime and ceftizoxime and the role of desacetyl cefotaxime in the antibacterial activity of cefotaxime. Diagn Microbiol Infect Dis **2**:635-705, 1984.
18. Reeves DS, White LO, Holt HA, Bahari D, Bywater MJ, Bax RP: Human metabolism of cefotaxime. J Antimicrob Chemother **6**(suppl A):93-101, 1980.
19. Tozer TN: Nomogram for modification of dosage regimens in patients with chronic renal function impairment. J Pharmacokinet Biopharm **2**:13-28, 1974.
20. Wagner JG: Fundamentals of pharmacokinetics. Hamilton, Ill., 1975, Drug Intelligence Publications.
21. Wise R, Wright N, Wills PJ: Pharmacology of cefotaxime and its desacetyl metabolite in renal and hepatic disease. Antimicrob Agents Chemother **4**:526-531, 1981.

Kinetics and dynamics of disopyramide and its dealkylated metabolite in healthy subjects

The kinetics and dynamics of total and free (unbound) disopyramide (D) after dosing with D, 1.5 and 2 mg/kg iv, were compared with those of the dealkylated metabolite (MND) after dosing with MND, 0.5 and 1.5 mg/kg iv, in six healthy subjects. Dynamic parameters included ECG with measurement of the QT interval corrected for heart rate (QT_c), systolic time intervals, vitamin C–stimulated saliva secretion, pupil size, and maximum accommodation capacity. Mean values of total clearance, apparent volume of distribution, and elimination $t_{1/2}$ of MND were 5.9, 2.3, and 0.4 times those of total D, respectively. D significantly prolonged the QT_c and systolic time intervals and induced transient inhibition of stimulated saliva secretion. In contrast, MND induced no substantial change in either the QT_c or systolic time intervals, but did induce more persistent inhibition of salivary secretion. If anticholinergic potency is determined as the degree of inhibition of stimulated saliva flow per plasma concentration unit, MND was three times as potent as its parent when measured at maximum inhibition. There were no consistent drug effects on the ocular parameters. The effect of D on QT_c correlated with both total and free plasma concentrations. Furthermore, its transient salivary inhibitory effect paralleled its initial rapid decline in plasma concentration. There was no relationship between the MND plasma concentration and its salivary inhibitory effect. We conclude that disopyramide significantly affected the QT_c and systolic time intervals in healthy subjects, while MND in a similar dose had no such effects. MND more strongly inhibited stimulated saliva flow, indicating a more potent anticholinergic effect than D. (CLIN PHARMACOL THER 38:37-44, 1985.)

Wen-Teh Chiang, M.D.,* Christer von Bahr, M.D., Berit Calissendorff, M.D., Rune Dahlqvist, M.D., Håkan Emilsson, Pharm.D., Anita Magnusson, B.S., and Karin Schenck-Gustafsson, M.D. *Huddinge, Sweden*

Disopyramide (D) is an antiarrhythmic with electrophysiologic properties resembling those of quinidine and procainamide.[6,14,20,23,24,30,32,33] Its kinetics and dynamics in man are complex. About 45% of D is metabolized, and a major metabolite is mono-*N*-dealkylated disopyramide (MND).[18,24] In clinical practice, MND plasma concentrations are usually 10% to 20% those of disopyramide, but the ratio of MND to D may vary more than twentyfold between individuals during chronic dosing.[25] This ratio can be particularly high in patients with renal disease and in those receiving drugs that induce drug oxidation.[1] MND has been shown in guinea pigs to have 20 times the anticholinergic potency of D (ileum model)[3] and to be one-fourth as active as D in prolonging the atrial effective refractory period.[13] The metabolite is ineffective against ouabain-induced ventricular arrhythmias in dogs,[3] but the kinetics and dynamics of MND have not been investigated in man. The clinical role of this active metabolite thus remains unclear.

We investigated the kinetics of MND and compared its cardiac and anticholinergic effects with those of D in healthy subjects. Because the plasma protein binding of D can be affected by MND[17] and varies with the total concentration of D,[27] the relationships between total as well as free (unbound) concentrations of D and its effects were also studied.

From the Departments of Clinical Pharmacology, Internal Medicine, Ophthalmology, and Pharmacy, Huddinge University Hospital.

Supported by grants from the Swedish Medical Research Council (Nos. 04X-03902 and 14X-05677) and the Swedish National Association against Heart and Chest Diseases.

Received for publication June 23, 1984; accepted Feb. 20, 1985.

Reprint requests to: Dr. Rune Dahlqvist, Department of Clinical Pharmacology, Huddinge University Hospital, S-141 86 Huddinge, Sweden.

*Visiting professor from Shanghai First Medical College, People's Republic of China, and supported by World Health Organization Scholarship No. CHN PTR 80-002.

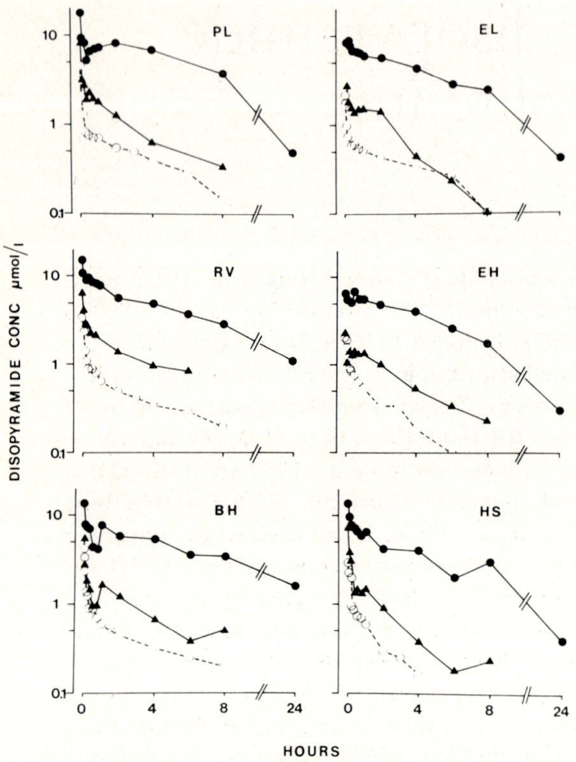

Fig. 1. Plasma concentration–time curves of total and unbound D and MND in six healthy subjects. D was injected (2 mg/kg iv) over 15 minutes; in a separate experiment, MND was injected (0.5 mg/kg iv) in the same subjects. Hour zero denotes the end of the infusion. ● = Total D; ▲ = unbound D; ○ = total MND.

METHODS

Our subjects were three healthy men and four healthy women. One woman was dropped from the study because of abdominal pain and nausea after the first dose of D (2 mg/kg iv). This coincided with her estimated ovulation time. The other six subjects completed the experiments. Age ranged from 22 to 30 years ($\overline{X}$ = 24.5 years) and body weight ranged from 55 to 82 kg ($\overline{X}$ = 69 kg). Neither drugs nor alcohol were allowed for 1 week before the study. None of the women were using oral contraceptives. Subjects did not eat breakfast on the morning of the studies and usually remained supine for the first 2 hours after drug dosing. Subjects were advised against participating in strenuous activities during the next 24 hours.

Our study consisted of two sets of experiments. The first was of an open design and was designed to follow the basic kinetics and dynamics of single intravenous doses of D and MND. Six subjects received D, 2 mg/kg iv, injected over 15 minutes. Four to seven days later, subjects received MND, which was prepared under sterile conditions. Because ours was the first dosing of MND in man, we determined the dose by a dose-increasing search starting from 0.2 mg/kg (i.e., one-tenth the dose of D). Because we found no obvious effects in two subjects, the dose was increased to 0.5 mg/kg iv, injected with the same volume and speed as D. The ECG was continuously monitored. Recordings of dynamic parameters were made simultaneous with blood samplings for drug analysis. Venous blood samples (10 ml into Venoject [Terumo Medical Corp.] glass tubes with heparin) were drawn before dosing, at the end of the injection, and then 5, 10, 20, 30, and 45 minutes and 1, 2, 4, 6, 8, and 24 hours thereafter. For MND, additional blood samples were drawn 2.5 and 15 minutes after dosing.

After the first experiment, five of the subjects participated in a double-blind study. Coded solutions of placebo (isotonic saline solution), D, and MND were made with an identical appearance and injection volume for each experiment, i.e., an intravenous dose of 0.15 ml/kg body weight. Treatment order followed a randomized block design. Blood was sampled for drug analysis and dynamic parameters were recorded before dosing, immediately after the injection, and then 20 minutes and 1, 2, and 4 hours thereafter. The intravenous doses of D and MND were the same (1.5 mg/kg body weight).

Plasma was frozen at −20° C until analyzed (within 1 week). Plasma D and MND concentrations were measured by an HPLC method slightly modified from Lagerström and Persson.[26] Unbound concentrations of D in plasma were determined by enzyme immunoassay after equilibrium dialysis for 6 hours. Dialysis was performed against phosphate-buffered saline solution at pH 7.4 in specially constructed chambers in which the volume of the plasma chamber was three times that of the buffer compartment, to minimize the effect on binding of decreased total plasma D concentrations. Free D was quantified to 0.1 μmol/L. At this concentration, the analytic error (within-assay coefficient of variation) was 9.8%. For the double-blind experiment the analysis was performed with the samples coded by an investigator not participating in the assay or data analysis.

A Siemens-Elema polychannel Mingograph was used to record simultaneously the ECG and systolic time intervals. The same experienced investigator measured all tracings from both the open and blind experiments without knowledge of the subject's name and the drug used. No significant differences in measurements were noted by an independent (also blinded) investigator. QT interval values corrected for heart rate (QT_c) were es-

Table I. Kinetics of MND and total and unbound D after a single intravenous dose (MND, 0.5 mg/kg; D, 2.0 mg/kg)

	Subjects							
	P. L.	*E. L.*	*R. V.*	*E. H.*	*B. H.*	*H. S.*	$\overline{X}$	*SD*
MND								
CL (L/kg · hr)	0.30	0.51	0.34	0.64	0.34	0.71	0.47	0.16
V_z (L/kg)	2.02	2.26	1.85	1.96	2.09	1.69	1.98	0.18
V_c (L/kg)	0.34	0.78	0.44	0.74	0.40	0.44	0.52	0.17
$t_{1/2}$ (hr)	4.4	3.2	3.7	2.1	5.2	1.6	3.4	1.4
Total D								
CL (L/kg · hr)	0.059	0.090	0.059	0.120	0.059	0.094	0.080	0.025
V_z (L/kg)	0.47	0.83	0.91	0.94	0.94	0.88	0.83	0.18
$t_{1/2}$ (hr)	5.3	5.9	10.2	5.5	12.2	6.5	7.6	2.9
Unbound D								
CL (L/kg · hr)	0.60	0.94	0.41	0.88	0.59	1.0	0.74	0.24
V_z (L/kg)	2.42	2.74	2.33	4.42	3.83	1.53	2.88	1.06
$t_{1/2}$ (hr)	*	2.0	*	3.4	*	*		

CL = Clearance; V_c = volume of the central compartment.
*In a few cases, the configuration of the terminal phase of the disposition curve did not permit accurate estimate of the $t_{1/2}$.

timated according to Bazett.[4] The systolic time intervals of QS_2, left ventricular ejection time (LVET), and pre-ejection period (PEP) were calculated from simultaneous recordings of the ECG, phonocardiogram, and carotid arterial pulse tracing during 10 consecutive beats according to the Weissler technique[9,34-36] and corrected for heart rate according to Wanderman et al.[34] Values after correction were abbreviated as QS_2-I, LVET-I, and PEP-I.

The examination of anticholinergic effects included inhibition of stimulated salivary secretion, pupil size, and maximum accommodation capacity. Salivary secretion was measured with slight modifications of a vitamin C stimulation test.[16] The subject swallowed his or her saliva and let a 500 mg vitamin C tablet dissolve in the mouth. After 30 and 60 seconds the subject spat into a cup. The total weight of the cup with the saliva was then measured and the net amount of salivary secretion was calculated. In the double-blind experiment, we compared the salivary inhibition induced by MND and D. The peak effect by MND and D occurred in 20 minutes after dosing, at which time a ratio between the drug effect and the plasma concentration was constructed and used as an index of potency.

Pupil size was measured (in millimeters) in a perimeter with standardized light. Accommodation was tested two ways: by the accommodation range and by near-point vision. The range of accommodation was determined by refraction and near-point vision was defined as the minimal reading distance (in centimeters) of a text with standard letters 0.35 mm wide. To avoid the interindividual error of measurers, these two optical parameters were measured by the same experienced ECG, and blood pressure were monitored continuously during drug dosing.

To identify symptoms in the open experiment, the subject's subjective feelings were recorded, whereas visual analog scales denoting change in general well being, dryness of mouth, and blurred vision were scored by the subjects themselves in the blind experiment. Changes in these symptoms were quantitated in terms of change (in millimeters) on the scale.

In the open experiment, all values after dosing were compared with control values. In the blind experiment, the values obtained during D and MND dosing were first compared with those during the placebo period and were then compared to each other. Paired t tests were used to test the statistical significance of differences between treatments and periods, and linear regression analysis was used to test relationships between concentration and effect. The plasma concentration–time data were fit to a polyexponential equation by weighted least-squares nonlinear regression with the computer program IGPHARM.[12] Data were weighted by the reciprocal of the square of the plasma level. Each solution was challenged with different initial parameter estimates to minimize the risk of obtaining a solution corresponding to a local minimum.

RESULTS

Individual plasma concentration–time curves of total D, unbound D, and MND in six healthy subjects are shown in Fig. 1. The plasma concentration of D declined continuously in three subjects, whereas in the other three (P.L., E.H., B.H.) there was an initial rapid decline during 20 to 30 minutes followed by a second

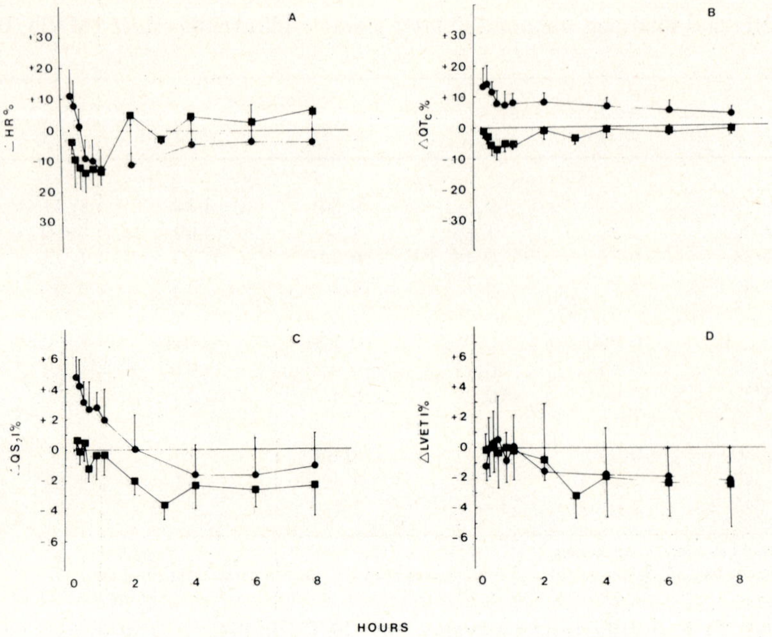

Fig. 2. Mean percent change in **(A)** heart rate, **(B)** QT_c, **(C)** QS_2-I, and **(D)** LVET-I after intravenous D (2 mg/kg) or MND (0.5 mg/kg) on separate occasions in six healthy subjects. Measurements before dosing serve as references. ● = D; ■ = MND.

peak occurring 30 minutes to 2 hours after dosing (Fig. 1). For unbound D, the terminal slope deviated from log linearity in four of the six subjects and thus $t_{1/2}$ values could not be calculated for them. After D, very low concentrations of MND (<0.3 μmol/L) were detected in the plasma (the disposition curves for MND in Fig. 1 are from the experiment in which MND, 0.5 mg/kg iv, was given separately).

Individual and mean kinetic parameters are listed in Table I. Total plasma clearance of MND was on the average almost six times that of D (0.47 and 0.080 L/kg · hr) and the volume of distribution (V_z) for MND was approximately twice that of D (1.98 and 0.83 L/kg; Table I). On the average, clearance of unbound D was almost 10 times that of total D and V_z for unbound D was 3.5 times that for total D (Table I). The unbound fraction of D in plasma was higher immediately after the end of dosing (34.6% to 52.3% [$\bar{X}$ = 42.9%]) than 8 hours after dosing (4.2% to 14.9% [$\bar{X}$ = 9.8%]).

There was a significant 11% increase in heart rate only 5 minutes after dosing with D, 2 mg/kg (Fig. 2, *A*). Between 30 and 60 minutes after injection, both D (2 mg/kg) and MND (0.5 mg/kg) decreased heart rate (Fig. 2, *A*), but a similar effect was also apparent after placebo (Fig. 3, *A*). In the open experiment, an intravenous bolus dose of D (2 mg/kg) prolonged the QT_c at all times measured after dosing, with a peak at 10 to 20 minutes (Fig. 2, *B*). MND (0.5 mg/kg) shortened the QT_c at 10 and 60 minutes and 3 and 6 hours, with peak shortening at 30 minutes. Results from the double-blind experiment were much the same (Fig. 3, *B*). Compared with the placebo effects, the smaller dose of D (1.5 mg/kg iv) still prolonged the QT_c. This lengthening was statistically significant 20 minutes ($P < 0.01$) and 2 hours ($P < 0.05$) after dosing, whereas the shortenings of QT_c by the same dose of MND were not significant at any recording time.

In the open experiment, D (2 mg/kg) prolonged both QS_2-I (Fig. 2, *C*) and PEP-I from 5 to 45 minutes after dosing, but there was no substantial effect on LVET-I (Fig. 2, *D*). In contrast, MND (0.5 mg/kg) induced no substantial effects on QS_2-I, LVET-I (Fig. 2, *C* and *D*), or PEP-I during the same early periods. During later recording periods, however, MND shortened QS_2-I at 30 minutes and from 2 to 6 hours, PEP-I at 2 hours, and LVET-I at 3 hours. In the double-blind experiment, compared with control values, the small increase in QS_2-I by a smaller dose of D (1.5 mg/kg iv) was significant 20 minutes after dosing (Fig. 3, *C*), and the increase in PEP-I was significant at 20 minutes to 2 hours. No significant effects on LVET-I were observed

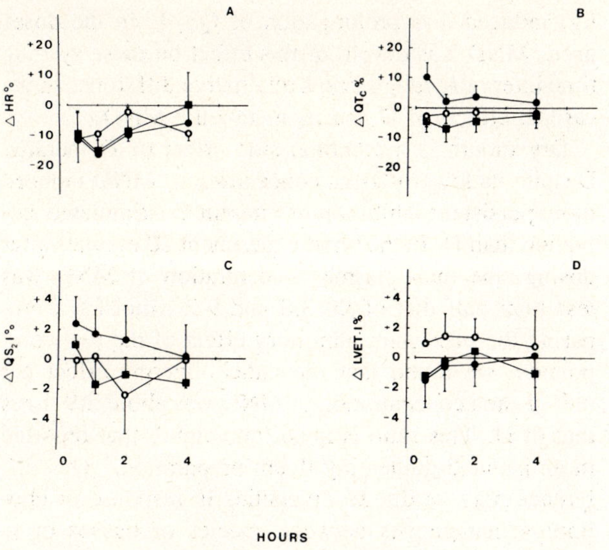

Fig. 3. Mean percent change in **(A)** heart rate, **(B)** QT_c, **(C)** QS_2-I, and **(D)** LVET-I after intravenous D (1.5 mg/kg), MND (1.5 mg/kg), or placebo in five healthy subjects. Measurements before dosing serve as references. ● = D; ■ = MND; ○ = placebo.

(Fig. 3, *D*). MND (1.5 mg/kg iv) did not induce effects on QS_2-I, LVET-I (Fig. 3, *C* and *D*), or PEP-I. The difference between the effects of D and MND on PEP-I was significant at 1 hour.

D induced transient inhibition of vitamin C–stimulated salivary secretion (Fig. 4). After D (2 mg/kg) in the open experiment, the decrease in stimulated saliva secretion was significant at 5 and 10 minutes, and in the double-blind experiment (Fig. 4) this effect was significant at 20 minutes. MND induced more persistent salivary inhibition (Fig. 4). There was significant inhibition from 5 to 30 minutes after MND, 0.5 mg/kg, and for 1 hour after MND, 1.5 mg/kg. The calculated index (see Methods) of maximal effect (in relation to drug concentration) of D was 2.9 ± 2.0 ($\overline{X}$ ± SD) and for MND it was 8.4 ± 5.0. The ratio between the inhibitory effects of MND and D was 2.9 at this point.

There was no significant change in the group mean values of pupil size after D or MND in either the open or the blind experiment. In the open experiment, after D all six subjects had improvement of the accommodation range that appeared consistent from 30 minutes after dosing and onwards. This effect was also occasionally seen after MND or placebo treatment and was probably at least partly due to an effect of training.

No significant treatment effect emerged from statistical analysis of the data from the visual analog scales for general well being, dryness of mouth, and blurred vision. Three subjects had slight paresthesias of the lips or the tip of the tongue during and a few minutes after D injection. Two subjects experienced transient dryness of the mouth and the eyes with both D and MND. One woman (not the excluded subject) also experienced slight abdominal pain suggestive of ovulation.

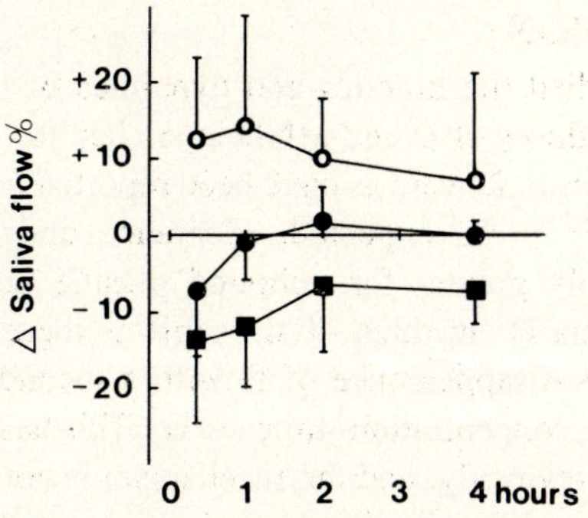

Fig. 4. Mean percent change in vitamin C–induced salivary secretion after intravenous D (1.5 mg/kg), MND (1.5 mg/kg), or placebo in five healthy subjects. Measurements before dosing serve as references. ● = D; ■ = MND; ○ = placebo.

The plasma concentration values of D were plotted against QT_c. In the subjects whose D plasma concentrations declined continuously, there were reasonably linear correlations between these two parameters during the 8 hours after dosing. For example, the correlation coefficients for total plasma concentration of D vs. QT_c were r = 0.87 for subject E.L. and r = 0.82 for subject R.V.; respective values for unbound concentration were r = 0.85 (E.L.) and r = 0.79 (R.V.). Those subjects whose plasma concentration–time curves had double peaks had poorer linear correlations between plasma D levels and QT_c. The group mean values of plasma D concentration and QT_c at each time point after dosing correlated with correlation coefficients for total and unbound concentrations (r = 0.86 and r = 0.91, respectively).

The inhibition of vitamin C–stimulated salivary secretion by D was transient. There was good correlation (r = 0.99) between the group mean D concentration and the decrease in stimulated saliva flow during the first 60 minutes after dosing. There was no such correlation after MND, 0.5 mg/kg, and neither was there any correlation between plasma MND concentrations after the higher dose (1.5 mg/kg), although its salivary inhibitory effect was more persistent.

DISCUSSION

We studied the kinetics and dynamics of single intravenous doses of D and MND in six healthy subjects. The kinetics of D were as have been reported for healthy subjects.[2,5,7,22] As expected, clearance and V_z were considerably greater for unbound plasma D than for total plasma D. In three of six subjects there was discontinuous disappearance of D with a second peak on the plasma concentration–time curve. This has not been reported previously, and the mechanism is not clear but may involve redistribution from tissues or gastroenteric and/or bilioenteric recirculation.

The main D metabolite, MND, was injected into man for the first time, which enabled characterization of its kinetics. MND had 400% higher total clearance, double the apparent V_z, and consequently a shorter $t_{1/2}$ than the parent drug. These differences are partly explained by the lesser degree of plasma binding of the metabolite.[1] Aitio et al.[2] estimated the MND elimination $t_{1/2}$ to be 13 hours after a single oral dose of D, in marked discrepancy with the average value of 3.4 hours after an intravenous dose of MND itself we report. The difference in estimated $t_{1/2}$ values can be explained by the continuous formation of MND from the parent drug in their experiment[2] and emphasizes that, in general, the plasma kinetics of metabolites are best resolved by administration of the metabolite itself. Thus after a single intravenous dose to healthy subjects, MND is more rapidly eliminated from the body than is D.

As has already been reported, D caused a slight, early, and transient acceleration of heart rate in the open experiment.[19,21] This change may be due to a vagolytic effect on the heart. No such effect was observed with MND, 0.5 mg/kg. With the higher dose of MND (1.5 mg/kg; Fig. 3, *A*), the earliest recording was after 20 minutes and there was no increase in heart rate for either MND or for D (1.5 mg/kg) at that time. It is possible because of an absence of early effect recordings that this design eliminated the possibility of determining a vagolytic effect of MND measured as increased heart rate. The QT_c lengthening induced by D in both sets of experiments agrees with the results of others.[5,20,]

Particularly after rapid intravenous injection, D has been reported to induce a negative inotropic effect demonstrated by an increase in PEP and the ratio PEP/LVET in patients with heart disease[21] and in healthy subjects[8] (although in one study rapid [1 minute] intravenous injection of the same dose did not depress myocardial function in healthy subjects[19]). Our results confirm a negative inotropic effect, as QS_2-I and PEP-I were prolonged by intravenous D. The smaller dose (0.5 mg/kg) induced less prolongation of QS_2-I. In the doses used, MND was devoid of this effect on these systolic time intervals, suggesting a qualitative difference in the cardiac effects of D and its metabolite MND.

Dry mouth is a common side effect of D therapy. Despite its lower plasma concentration, MND induced more persistent inhibition of vitamin C–stimulated salivation than D. In the blind experiment 20 minutes after dosing, the total plasma concentration of MND was less than half that of D (3.8 and 9.2 μmol/L). Comparing the maximum inhibitory effect of the two compounds, we found that the anticholinergic effect per unit plasma concentration of MND was about 2.9 times that of D. This ratio is about one-eighth that reported in an isolated guinea pig ileum preparation.[3] This difference may be due to diversities in response of cholinergic antagonists between species or tissues or to methods of recording. It is important to note that measurement of salivary inhibition at other times during the disappearance curve could well produce another potency ratio. However, the concentrations of D and MND were of the order of those that occur clinically during oral dosing with D, and the comparison should thus have some relevance. Because the characteristics of the concentration/effect curves for the two compounds at steady state are not known, the argument of a clinically important difference in anticholinergic potency should still be considered with caution. Moreover, it should be stressed that the above comparison of potency was based on total rather than free plasma concentrations, because free MND plasma concentrations were not determined. In view of the lesser average binding of MND,[1] a potency estimate based on unbound compounds would diminish the difference between D and MND. It should also be pointed out that inhibition of vitamin C–stimulated salivation is not with certainty synonymous with the sensation of dry mouth during D therapy.

Pupil size, accommodation range, and the visual analog scales did not reveal any consistent effects of either D or MND. Whether the absence of measurable effects was due to imperceptible drug effects or to insensitivity of the measurements remains to be established. In the open experiment, D and sometimes MND improved the accommodation range. This might be influenced by training, but such a "paradoxic" stimulating effect has sometimes been reported for anticholinergic drugs.[15] The inclusion of a placebo comparison was essential to control for period effects in dynamic variables during the experiment.

Our data complement those of Hinderling and Garret,[19] in that the effect of D on QT_c correlates with both the total and the unbound plasma concentrations of the drug. Better linear correlations were found in subjects with continuously declining plasma concentration–time curves than in those with discontinuous curves. This might be related to delay of this effect in relation to the plasma concentration, as has been reported after intravenous but not oral D.[19,37]

The assessment of concentration-effect relationships assumes that the compound assayed is identical to or bears a constant relationship to the pharmacologically active moiety. Thus one potentially perturbing factor is the presence of stereoisomers with differing dynamics and kinetics. Commercially available D as well as the MND we used exist as racemic mixtures of the *R*(−) and *S*(+) forms, and the biochemical analysis used measures the sum of these isomers. It has been shown that the *S*(+) isomer of D is a much more potent anticholinergic than the *R*(−) isomer.[10,28] Also, the *S*(+) isomer prolongs the duration of the action potential in Purkinje cells[29] and prolongs QT_c duration, whereas both isomers induced a negative inotropic effect.[31] In dogs, the plasma clearance of the *S*(+) isomer of D was about 50% greater than that of the *R*(−) isomer, whereas the apparent volumes of distribution did not differ.[11] The kinetic differences between the isomers have not been completely investigated in man.[31] It would be desirable in future investigations to account for the contribution of each of the stereoisomers of D and MND to pharmacologic effects.

In summary, MND at plasma concentrations comparable with those occurring during clinical therapy with D induce a pharmacodynamic pattern different from that of the parent drug. The metabolite elicits no substantial cardiac effects but could contribute to anticholinergic side effects. The conclusions drawn from this single-dose study in healthy subjects should not be extrapolated indiscriminately to the long-term therapy of cardiac patients.

We thank Professor Folke Sjöqvist for his valuable suggestions and Dr. Anders Grahnén for executing the IGPHARM procedure. The assistance of Diana Vuorisalo, nurse at the coronary care unit, is also gratefully acknowledged. D and MND were kindly supplied as base by L. Roussel Laboratories Ltd., England.

References

1. Aitio M-L: Plasma concentrations and protein binding of disopyramide and mono-*n*-dealkyldisopyramide during chronic oral disopyramide therapy. Br J Clin Pharmacol **11**:369-376, 1981.
2. Aitio H-L, Allonen H, Kanto J, Mäntylä R: The pharmacokinetics of disopyramide and mono-*n*-dealkyl-disopyramide in humans. Int J Clin Pharmacol Ther Toxicol **20**:219-226, 1982.
3. Baines MW, Davies JE, Kellett DN, Munt PL: Some pharmacological effects of disopyramide and a metabolite. J Int Med Res **4**(suppl):5-7, 1976.
4. Bazett H-C: An analysis of the time relations of electrocardiograms. Heart **7**:353-370, 1920.
5. Bryson SM, Whiting B, Lawrence JR: Disopyramide serum and pharmacologic effect kinetics applied to the assessment of bioavailability. Br J Clin Pharmacol **6**:409-419, 1978.
6. Dreifus LS, Morganroth J: Antiarrhythmic agents and their use in therapy. Pharmacol Ther **9**:75-106, 1980.
7. Dubetz DK, Brown NN, Hooper WD, Eadie MJ, Tyrer JH: Disopyramide pharmacokinetics and bioavailability. Br J Clin Pharmacol **6**:279-281, 1978.
8. Eliot HL, Sumner DJ, Bryson SM, Kelman AW, Campbell BC, Hillis WS, Whiting B: Evaluation of the cardiac effects following acute and steady state disopyramide. Br J Clin Pharmacol **14**:588P, 1982.
9. Garrard CL Jr, Weissler AM, Dodge HT: The relationship of alterations in systolic time intervals to ejection fraction in patients with heart disease. Circulation **42**:455-462, 1970.
10. Giacomini KM, Cox BM, Blaschke TF: Comparative anticholinergic potencies of *R*- and *S*-disopyramide in longitudinal muscle strips from guinea pig ileum. Life Sci **27**:1191-1197, 1980.
11. Giacomini KM, Giacomini JC, Swezey SE, Harrison DC, Nelson WL, Burke TR Jr, Blaschke TF: The stereoselective disposition of disopyramide in the dog. J Cardiovasc Pharmacol **2**:825-832, 1980.
12. Gomeni C, Gomeni R: IGPHARM: Interactive graphic package for pharmacokinetic analysis. Comput Biomed Res **11**:345-361, 1978.
13. Grant AM, Marshall RJ, Ankier SI: Some effects of disopyramide and its *N*-dealkylated metabolite on isolated nerve and cardiac muscle. Eur J Pharmacol **49**:389-394, 1978.
14. Heel RC, Brogden RN, Speight TM, Avery GS: Disopyramide: A review of its pharmacological properties and therapeutic use in treating cardiac arrhythmias. Drugs **15**:331-368, 1978.
15. Herxheimer A: A comparison of some atropine-like drugs in man, with particular reference to their end-organ specificity. Br J Pharmacol **13**:184-192, 1958.
16. Herxheimer A, Hefeli L: Human pharmacology of hyoscine butylbromide. Lancet **2**:418-421, 1966.
17. Hinderling PH, Bres J, Garrett ER: Protein binding and erythrocyte partitioning of disopyramide and its monodealkylated metabolite. J Pharm Sci **63**:1684-1690, 1974.
18. Hinderling PN, Garret ER: Pharmacokinetics of the antiarrhythmic disopyramide in healthy humans. J Pharmacokinet Biopharm **4**:199-230, 1976.

19. Hinderling PH, Garret ER: Pharmacodynamics of the antiarrhythmic disopyramide in healthy humans: Correlation of the kinetics of the drug and its effects. J Pharmacokinet Biopharm **4**:231-242, 1976.
20. Hulting J, Jansson B: Antiarrhythmic and electrocardiographic effects of single oral doses of disopyramide. Eur J Clin Pharmacol **11**:91-99, 1977.
21. Jensen G, Sigurd B, Uhrenholt A: Haemodynamic effects of intravenous disopyramide in heart failure. Eur J Clin Pharmacol **8**:167-173, 1975.
22. Karim A: The pharmacokinetics of Norpace. Angiology **26**(suppl 1):85-94, 1975.
23. Katz MJ, Meyer CE, El-Etr A, Slodki SJ: Clinical evaluation of a new antiarrhythmic agent, SC-7031. Curr Ther Res **5**:343-350, 1963.
24. Koch-Weser J: Disopyramide. N Engl J Med **300**:957-961, 1979.
25. Kumana CR: The therapeutic drug monitoring—Antidysrhythmic drugs. *In* Richens A, Marsk V, editors: Therapeutic drug monitoring. New York, 1981, Churchill Livingstone, p 370.
26. Lagerström P-O, Persson B-A: Liquid chromatography in the monitoring of plasma levels of antiarrhythmic drugs. J Chromatogr **149**:331-340, 1978.
27. Meffin PJ, Robert EW, Winkle RA, Harapat S, Peters FA, Harrison DC: Role of concentration-dependent plasma protein binding in disopyramide disposition. J Pharmacokinet Biopharm **7**:29-46, 1979.
28. Mirro MJ, Manalan AS, Bailey JC, Watanabe AM: Anticholinergic effects of disopyramide and quinidine on guinea pig myocardium. Circ Res **47**:855-865, 1980.
29. Mirro MJ, Watanabe AM, Bailey JC: Electrophysiological effects of the optical isomers of disopyramide and quinidine in the dog. Circ Res **48**:867-874, 1981.
30. Perrin A, Loire R, Rondelet J: Action de la disopyramide dans le traîtment des troubles du rythme cardiaque. Cah Med Lyonnais **44**:1487-1495, 1968.
31. Pollick C, Giacomini KM, Blaschke TF, Nelson WL, Turner-Tamiyasu K, Briskin V, Popp RL: The cardiac effects of D- and L-disopyramide in normal subjects: A noninvasive study. Circulation **66**:447-453, 1982.
32. Ross D, Vohra J, Sloman JG: Disopyramide in myocardial infarction. Lancet **1**:330, 1978.
33. Vismara LA, Mason DT, Amsterdam EA: Disopyramide phosphate: Clinical efficacy of a new oral antiarrhythmic drug. CLIN PHARMACOL THER **16**:330-335, 1974.
34. Wanderman KL, Hayek Z, Ovyshcher I, Loutaty G, Cantor A, Gussarsky Y, Gueron M: Systolic time intervals in adolescents. Normal standards for clinical use and comparison with children and adults. Circulation **63**:204-209, 1981.
35. Weissler AM, Harris WS, Schoenfeld CD: Systolic time intervals in heart failure in man. Circulation **37**:149-159, 1968.
36. Weissler AM, Schoenfeld CD: Effect of digitalis on systolic time intervals in heart failure. Am J Med Sci **259**:4-20, 1970.
37. Whiting B, Holford NHG, Sheiner LB: Quantitative analysis of the disopyramide concentration-effect relationship. Br J Clin Pharmacol **9**:67-75, 1980.

Clinical pharmacology of 5-iodo-2′-deoxyuridine and 5-iodouracil and endogenous pyrimidine modulation

We describe the clinical pharmacology and metabolism of 5-iodo-2′-deoxyuridine (IdUrd) during and after a 12-hour infusion. The kinetics of IdUrd were linear between 250 and 1200 mg/m^2. The plasma IdUrd concentration reached steady state in <1 hour. Total body clearance of IdUrd was 750 ml/min/m^2 and the disappearance $t_{1/2}$ at the end of the infusion was <5 minutes. The primary metabolite, 5-iodouracil (IUra), did not reach steady state during the infusion. At the end of the 1200 mg/m^2 infusion, the maximum plasma IUra concentration was 100 μmol/L, or about 10 times the simultaneous IdUrd plasma concentration. During the infusion there was at least a fifty- to 100-fold increase in uracil and thymine plasma concentrations. After the infusion, IUra disappearance from plasma was nonlinear, with an apparent Michaelis constant of 30 μmol/L. Plasma uracil and thymine levels slowly decreased after the IdUrd infusion until IUra fell to <30 μmol/L. There was subsequently a parallel and more rapid decrease in the plasma concentrations of uracil and thymine. Uridine, 2′-deoxyuridine, and thymidine plasma levels did not change significantly as a result of IdUrd therapy. These changes in endogenous pyrimidine pools are consistent with competitive inhibition of dihydrouracil dehydrogenase by IUra. An in vitro human bone marrow assay was used to determine the relative toxicity of IdUrd and IUra. Although exposure to IUra was tenfold higher than that to IdUrd, IdUrd was at least 100 times more cytotoxic to marrow cells. (Clin Pharmacol Ther 38:45-51, 1985.)

Raymond W. Klecker, Jr., B.S., Jean F. Jenkins, M.S.N., Timothy J. Kinsella, M.D., Robert L. Fine, M.D., John M. Strong, Ph.D., and Jerry M. Collins, Ph.D.
Bethesda, Md.

5-Iodo-2′-deoxyuridine (IdUrd; NSC 39661) was first synthesized in the late 1950s[18] and was used as an antitumor agent and a radiosensitizer in the early 1960s.[5,6] In the initial clinical trial,[6] IdUrd was infused intravenously at doses of 100 to 120 mg/kg over 2 to 3 hours for 5 to 6 days. Specific tumor-bearing areas were irradiated before and immediately after IdUrd treatment. The trial resulted in modest tumor inhibition in six of 16 patients. In four of the six patients the tumor inhibition was attributed to synergism of IdUrd and irradiation. IdUrd has also been successfully used as an antiviral drug.[20]

The van der Waals radius of the iodine moiety of IdUrd is similar to that of the methyl group of thymidine; thus IdUrd follows the same metabolic pathways as thymidine.[18,19] In vitro studies show fortyfold greater deoxyribonucleic acid (DNA) incorporation of thymidine than of IdUrd at equimolar concentrations.[19] In fact, an earlier clinical study used thymidine for regional protection from IdUrd-radiation therapy.[5] The uptake of the primary catabolite, 5-iodouracil (IUra), is much slower than that of IdUrd in mammalian DNA.[8] Prusoff and Goz[21] have extensively reviewed the biochemistry of halogenated pyrimidine deoxyribonucleosides.

Through urinalysis, Calabresi et al.[6] studied the pharmacology of IdUrd and found that IdUrd was rapidly catabolized to iodouracil and further dehalogenated to free iodide. Metabolism studies suggest that dehalogenation of IdUrd may occur before or after the hydrolysis of 5-iodo-5,6-dihydrouracil.[12,22] Other studies with rat and pig liver homogenates have shown that IUra as well as other halogenated uracil analogs inhibit the degradation of uracil and thymine[1,3,24] via dihy-

From the Clinical Pharmacology and Radiation Oncology Branches, Clinical Oncology Program, Division of Cancer Treatment, National Cancer Institute.

Received for publication Nov. 29, 1984; accepted March 1, 1985.

Reprint requests to: Raymond W. Klecker, Jr., National Institutes of Health, Bldg. 10, Rm. 6N119, Bethesda, MD 20205.

drouracil dehydrogenase (dihydrouracil, NADP oxidoreductase; EC 1.3.1.2). Earlier studies did not define the effect of IUra on endogenous pyrimidine pools.

Previous studies of the pharmacology of IdUrd did not include blood or plasma measurements. Our purpose was to investigate the pharmacology of IdUrd and IUra in plasma during a 12-hour infusion. The effects of IdUrd and IUra on the plasma concentrations of uracil, thymine, uridine, 2′-deoxyuridine, and thymidine were also studied. The radiosensitization properties, toxicity, and clinical results have been reported elsewhere.[13]

METHODS

IdUrd infusion. Each treatment cycle consisted of 14 days of chemotherapy and was repeated one time beginning on day 40. Pharmacology studies were performed on day 1 of the first cycle for each patient. Patients began radiation therapy after day 4 of the IdUrd infusion. IdUrd was initially dissolved in 5 ml water and diluted to a final volume of 25 to 39 ml with normal saline solution. The drug solution was transferred into 30 or 50 ml syringes that fit onto a portable pump. The IdUrd infusion was given through a venous catheter placed in the subclavian vein. During each day of the cycle the patient received 12 hours of drug infusion followed by 12 hours without therapy.

At least three patients were treated at each of the dose levels of 250, 500, 850, 1000, and 1200 mg/m^2. The first four dose levels were used to determine plasma pharmacokinetics during the infusion. The final dose level was used to determine plasma kinetics after the end of infusion. Blood samples were drawn into heparinized tubes from a catheter located in a radial artery. Samples were drawn from each patient who received <1200 mg/m^2 on day 1 of chemotherapy just before chemotherapy and 1, 4, 8, and 12 hours after the start of the infusion. Blood from the patients who received 1200 mg/m^2 was sampled at 10, 11, and 12 hours after dosing to determine the steady-state concentration of IdUrd. The kinetics of IUra disappearance from plasma were studied by sampling the blood of patients who received 1200 mg/m^2 0.25, 0.5, 1, 3, 5, 7, 9, and 11 hours after the end of the IdUrd infusion.

Blood samples were immediately stored on ice and centrifuged promptly (<1 hour after collection) at 2,000 rpm for 10 minutes to avoid metabolism of IdUrd in whole blood. After centrifugation the plasma samples were separated, transferred to 4 ml soda lime glass vials, and frozen at $-20°$ C until analyzed. Analytic procedures are described in the Appendix.

In vitro bone marrow toxicity. The relative toxicities of IdUrd and IUra were determined in a semisolid agar CFU-GM assay.[17] Normal human marrow was aspirated from the posterior iliac crest. Human placental conditioned medium was produced and used as the source of colony-stimulating factor.[4] After separation by Ficoll-Hypaque centrifugation, approximately 2×10^6 mononuclear marrow cells were incubated for 24 hours in RPMI 1640 medium with 10% heat-inactivated fetal calf serum and either IdUrd (0.5 to 50 μmol/L) or IUra (5 to 500 μmol/L). Each sample was washed three times with cold phosphate-buffered saline solution and finally resuspended in McCoy's 5A enriched media with 15% fetal calf serum to a final concentration of 2×10^5 cells per well. Samples were incubated at 37° C for 10 to 14 days and the total number of colonies (>35 cells per group) in each sample were counted with an inverted microscope. The dose-response curves were studied in three marrow samples and each drug concentration was measured in triplicate.

Calculations. The disappearance of IUra from plasma after the end of the IdUrd infusion could be described by the Michaelis-Menten expression: $dC/dt = V_{max}C/(Km + C)$, where C is the plasma concentration of IUra, V_{max} is the maximum IUra elimination rate, and Km is the IUra concentration at which the elimination rate is half maximal. V_{max} and Km were determined by nonlinear regression.[14]

RESULTS

Iodouracil verification by gas chromatography-mass spectrometry. The pooled collection from the HPLC peaks presumed to correspond to IUra and an equivalent amount of pure IUra were silylated and gave identical retention times for the gas chromatographic separation. Electron impact and chemical ionization mass spectra of the chromatographed isolate and reference derivatives were similar.

Purity of IdUrd pharmaceutical preparation. An aliquot from the dose solution from one patient was $>99.7\%$ pure. One of the contaminants had the same retention and absorption characteristics as IUra and was estimated as 6×10^{-5} gm IUra per gram IdUrd. Another peak had the same retention time as thymine but had a slightly different 254 nm/280 nm absorbance ratio. If the peak was 100% thymine, then estimated contamination would be 1×10^{-4} gm thymine per gram IdUrd. No significant effect on the plasma concentration of any pyrimidine would be induced by the impurities in the parent solution.

IdUrd and IUra pharmacology and effect on endogenous pyrimidines. Fig. 1 shows the concentration-time profile of endogenous and exogenous pyrimidines

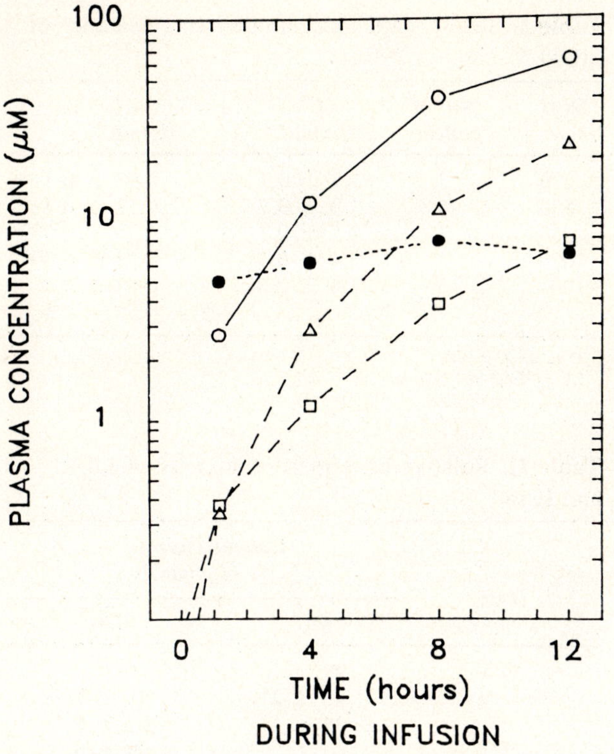

Fig. 1. Plasma concentrations during a 12-hour infusion of 1000 mg/m² IdUrd (●). ○ = IUra; △ = uracil; □ = thymine.

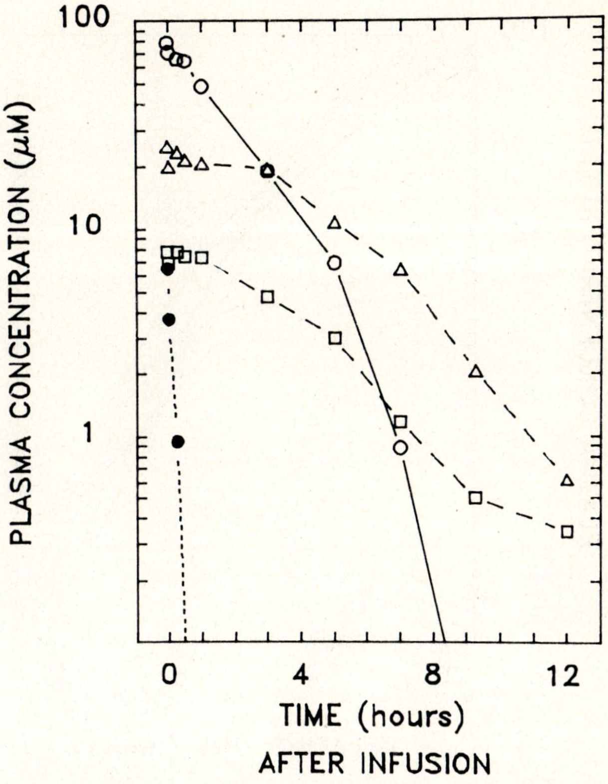

Fig. 2. Plasma disappearance of IdUrd (●), IUra (○), uracil (△), and thymine (□) after the end of a 1200 mg/m² IdUrd infusion. IdUrd was not measurable 30 minutes after the infusion and IUra was not measurable 9 hours after the infusion.

in a patient who received 1000 mg/m². The concentration of IdUrd in plasma reached steady state within 1 hour of the start of the infusion. The steady-state concentration (C^{ss}) of IdUrd was linear over the dose range investigated (Table I). Interpatient variation was remarkably small, as shown by the standard deviations listed in Table I. The disappearance of IdUrd from plasma after the end of the IdUrd infusion was extremely rapid, with a $t_{1/2}$ of <5 minutes (Fig. 2). IdUrd was not measurable (<0.3 μmol/L) 30 minutes after the end of the infusion.

The plasma IUra concentration approached but did not appear to reach steady state during the 12 hours of IdUrd infusion (Fig. 1). The concentration of IUra at the end of the infusion for patients receiving 1000 and 1200 mg/m² was about 10 times the IdUrd concentration (Figs. 1 and 2). Fig. 3 shows the disappearance of plasma IUra in three patients who received 1200 mg/m². The kinetic pattern is typical of a saturable enzymatic system. The Km and V_{max} of IUra were found to be 30 μmol/L and 22 μmol/L/hr, respectively.

The plasma pools of uracil and thymine were substantially altered as a result of the IdUrd infusion (Figs. 1 and 2). At the end of the 1000 and 1200 mg/m² infusions, the concentrations of uracil and thymine were at least 50 to 100 times greater than normal as measured in this laboratory or reported by others.[25] After the infusion, both uracil and thymine concentrations decreased slowly until the concentration of IUra fell below its estimated Km. Subsequently the plasma concentrations of uracil and thymine fell more rapidly (Fig. 3).

We attempted to measure plasma concentrations of the related nucleosides uridine, 2′-deoxyuridine, and thymidine at the end of the infusion. The analysis method for the latter two was not as specific as the methods used for uracil, thymine, IUra, and IdUrd because of ultraviolet-absorbing peaks in the same chromatographic region as 2′-deoxyuridine and thymidine. It was determined, however, that the plasma concentration of 2′-deoxyuridine was always <1 μmol/L and the largest change observed was no greater than a doubling in concentration. Thymidine was below the limit of detection (0.3 μmol/L) before and during IdUrd therapy. The plasma concentration of uridine at the end of the infusion did not change significantly from its normal

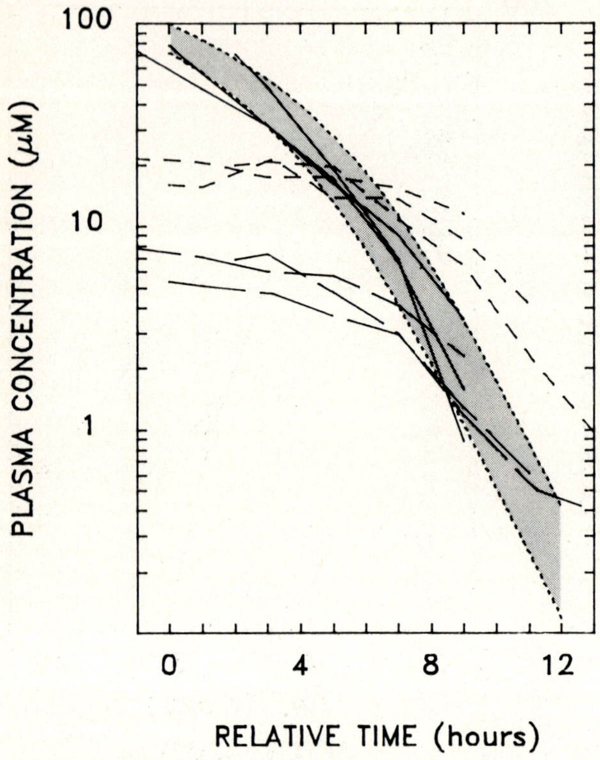

Fig. 3. Overlay of plasma disappearance curves of IUra *(solid line)*, uracil *(short dash)*, and thymine *(long dash)* for three patients who received 1200 mg/m². The zero time sample (last sample during IdUrd infusion) had different plasma IUra values for the three curves shown; therefore, the time scales were shifted for better illustration of the kinetic dependence of uracil and thymine on the plasma disappearance of IUra. The *shaded portion* is the expected plasma concentration of IUra when the zero time sample is between 72 and 100 μmol/L for a Km of 30 μmol/L and a V_{max} of 22 μmol/L/hr.

concentration of about 8 μmol/L as determined in this and other laboratories.[11]

In vitro bone marrow toxicity. Human bone marrow mononuclear cells were incubated with concentrations of IdUrd and IUra that were tenfold greater than those achieved in the plasma of patients receiving 1200 mg/m². IdUrd demonstrated toxicity at 5 μmol/L (Table II). This was analogous to the drug exposure during 1 day of IdUrd therapy for patients receiving 1200 mg/m². On the other hand, IUra did not affect the survival of the marrow cells at a concentration 100-fold greater than that of IdUrd (Table II).

DISCUSSION

The IdUrd total body clearance of 750 ml/min/m² is higher than that of most drugs used in anticancer therapy

Table I. Steady-state concentration and clearance of IdUrd

Dose (mg/m²)	*No. of patients*	C^{ss} *(μmol/L)*	*CL (L/min/m²)*
250	3	1.1 ± 0.1	0.93 ± 0.1
500	4	2.9 ± 0.7	0.71 ± 0.2
850	3	4.5 ± 0.1	0.75 ± 0.02
1000	3	5.6 ± 0.7	0.71 ± 0.09
1200	5	7.4 ± 2.0	0.67 ± 0.2
			Σ = 0.75 ± 0.1

Data are $\overline{X}$ ± SD.
CL = Total body clearance.

Table II. Relative bone marrow toxicity of IdUrd and IUra

Dose (μmol/L)	*Colonies formed (% of control)*	
	IdUrd	*IUra*
0.5	99 ± 7	*
5	48 ± 21	98 ± 7
50	38 ± 17	101 ± 5
500	*	98 ± 6

Data are $\overline{X}$ ± SD of three experiments.
*Concentration not evaluated.

but lower than the rates for other pyrimidine deoxyribosides. The reported total body clearance of bromodeoxyuridine is 1.9 L/min/m²,[23] and values of 15 and 23 L/min/m² can be calculated from data for fluorodeoxyuridine[9] and thymidine.[10] The IdUrd elimination $t_{1/2}$ after the end of the infusion was too short (< 5 minutes) to determine with conventional sampling protocols.

Both the nonlinear kinetics of IUra disappearance from plasma and the large increases in plasma concentration of uracil and thymine can readily be explained by saturation of the enzyme known as dihydrouracil dehydrogenase. In vitro studies with liver homogenates have shown that the catabolism of uracil and thymine is competitively inhibited by each other and by 5-halouracils.[1,3,24] As the plasma concentration of IUra decreased to the range of its K_m, the rate of disappearance of IUra increased, followed by increases in the rates of disappearance of uracil and thymine. This type of competitive interaction in vivo has been demonstrated in clinical studies in which 5-fluorouracil was given simultaneously with thymidine. Thymidine is rapidly catabolized to thymine, which competitively inhibits 5-fluorouracil catabolism by dihydrouracil dehydrogenase.[2] The plasma elimination of 5-fluorouracil decreased about sevenfold during thymidine coadministration. The apparent whole body Km of 30 μmol/L for IUra is similar to the Km value of 15 to 20 μmol/L for 5-fluorouracil.[7]

The presence of IUra in the circulation in amounts tenfold greater than IdUrd raised the question of which was the active species. 5-Fluorouracil, an analog of IUra, is toxic at concentrations of 1 μmol/L during continuous infusion. Because the clinical toxicities of IdUrd therapy include myelosuppression,[6,13] bone marrow was a convenient site at which to address the issue of active species. It would appear that IdUrd is at least 100-fold more potent than IUra and dominates the myelotoxicity. Similar observations were obtained with experimental tumor cells.*

The ultimate effects of pyrimidines (or exogenous pyrimidine analogs) are mediated through nucleotides that are incorporated into or disrupt the synthesis of nucleic acids. Nucleotides cannot be given directly, since phosphorylated forms do not cross cell membranes. Nucleosides can be administered directly, can enter cells, and can be converted to phosphorylated forms by intracellular kinases.[21] With the notable exception of 5-fluorouracil, pyrimidine bases have not been used directly. Both high concentrations of the base and a source of deoxyribose 1-phosphate are required for incorporation into DNA.[8] A lack of sufficient quantities of deoxyribose 1-phosphate may explain the low potency of IUra we noted. On the other hand, 5-fluorouracil is quite cytotoxic because it has both DNA and ribonucleic acid effects.[16]

The observed modulation of endogenous pyrimidine bases opens a new area that could develop into an approach to the manipulation of nucleic acid synthesis. One of the difficulties in the evaluation of the role of pyrimidine bases is a general lack of information concerning their levels in normal states and under the influence of pyrimidine analog therapy. Endogenous nucleosides are not synthesized directly from bases. Increased uracil levels can, however, lead to an enhancement of 5-fluorodeoxyuridine incorporation into DNA.[15] By itself, modulation of pyrimidines is unlikely to alter the course of therapy dramatically. However, it can provide an additional tool for strategies designed to manipulate multiple sites of de novo and salvage metabolic pathways.

We thank Drs. D. Kornhauser at Johns Hopkins University and R. Cysyk and J. Moyer at the National Cancer Institute for stimulating discussions on endogenous pyrimidine alteration.

*Kinsella TJ: Unpublished observations, 1984.

APPENDIX

Analysis of pyrimidines in plasma

Materials. IdUrd was obtained through the Investigational Drug Branch of the National Cancer Institute as a lyophilized powder. The pyrimidine bases, ribosides, and other 5-halogenated analogs were obtained from Sigma Chemical Co. Methanol and acetonitrile were HPLC grade from Burdick & Jackson Laboratories. The ethyl acetate was from MCB Manufacturing Chemists, Inc. and the glacial acetic acid and ammonium acetate were laboratory grade from Fisher Scientific Co. Ammonium acetate solutions were adjusted to pH 6.5 with acetic acid. Water was double distilled in glass.

To measure all the pyrimidine compounds it was necessary to use two different extraction procedures and two HPLC mobile phases. Plasma standards were freshly prepared for each analysis by spiking normal human plasma with pyrimidine solutions. Plasma standards were extracted along with the patient samples. The limits of detection for the analysis procedures were between 0.1 and 1 μmol/L for the pyrimidines measured. There was interference with the peak height measurement of thymine in one patient receiving 1000 mg/m^2, which was probably due to a coadministered drug that extracted and coeluted with thymine.

Extraction procedure I (IdUrd, IUra, 2′-deoxyuridine, and thymidine). Each 0.5 ml of plasma sample or standard received 50 μl internal standard (10^{-4} mol/L) and 50 μl 1 mol/L ammonium acetate. The internal standards used were 5-bromo-2′-deoxyuridine for IdUrd and IUra and 5-fluoro-2′-deoxyuridine for 2′-deoxyuridine and thymidine measurements.

The extractions were performed on C-18 columns (Waters Associates "Sep-pak") conditioned by washing with 4 ml methanol, followed by 4 ml water and finally 4 ml 0.1 mol/L ammonium acetate. The samples were eluted through the extraction columns and the columns were washed with 2 ml 0.1 mol/L ammonium acetate followed by 0.5 ml water. The compounds of interest were eluted and collected from the extraction columns in a 2 ml methanol wash. The methanol was dried under a gentle stream of nitrogen at 40° C in a heated water bath. The residue was dissolved in 150 μl of the HPLC mobile phase and 50 μl was injected onto the HPLC.

Extraction procedure II (uracil and thymine). Each 0.5 ml of sample or standard received 50 μl 5-chlorouracil (10^{-4} mol/L) as internal standard and was gently mixed. A 5 ml aliquot of ethyl acetate was added and each sample was mixed for 20 seconds. The ethyl acetate layer was decanted into a separate tube after freezing the lower (aqueous) layer by shallow insertion of the sample tube into powdered dry ice. The organic phase was evaporated to dryness under a gentle stream of nitrogen at 40° C in a heated water bath. The residue was dissolved in 150 μl of the HPLC mobile phase and passed through a 0.22 μm Gelman Sciences, Inc. filter. Fifty microliters was injected onto the HPLC.

HPLC conditions. The chromatographic separations were obtained with a 5 μm radial-pak C-18 column (Waters Associates). Absorbance was measured at 254 and 280 nm on a Waters 440 fixed-wavelength detector and at 280 or 310 nm on an SF 770 variable wavelength detector (Kratos Inc., Schoeffel Instrument Division). The analytic column was washed with 55% acetonitrile (CH_3CN) for about 30 seconds after each sample run and the column was allowed to equilibrate for 10 minutes before the next sample injection. The mobile phase for analysis of IdUrd and IUra was 25 mmol/L acetic acid with 6% (v/v) CH_3CN at a flow rate of 2 ml/min. For analysis of uracil and thymine, the flow was also 2 ml/min but the mobile phase consisted of 20 mmol/L acetic acid and 1% (v/v) CH_3CN. 2′-Deoxyuridine and thymidine were measured with the same HPLC mobile phase as uracil and thymine, but the flow was increased to 3 ml/min. For analysis of the dose solution of IdUrd, an aliquot was injected directly onto the HPLC with a mobile phase consisting of 3.5% CH_3CN in 22 mmol/L acetic acid at a flow rate of 2 ml/min.

IdUrd was measured at 310 nm even though it had maximum absorbance at 286 nm. At 310 nm IdUrd absorbance was 50% to 70% less than that at 280 nm. However, an endogenous plasma component that had interfered in the detection of IdUrd at 280 nm did not have any absorbance at 310 nm and the loss of sensitivity did not effect the measurability of IdUrd. The other pyrimidines (uracil, thymine, 2′-deoxyuridine, and thymidine) were verified by retention time and peak height ratios at 254 nm/280 nm or 280 nm/310 nm.

Verification of IUra. The 8- and 12-hour plasma samples from three patients receiving 1000 mg/m^2 were pooled for extraction. An aliquot of 1 mol/L ammonium acetate was added in the proportions of 100 μl per milliliter pooled plasma. The C-18 extraction columns were conditioned as before. A volume of 2 ml pooled plasma was added to each column, followed by a water wash of 1.5 ml. A 2 ml methanol wash was collected from each column. All the methanol collections were pooled and dried under a steady stream of nitrogen at 40° C in a water bath. The residue was redissolved in 400 μl of the new HPLC mobile phase, 6% CH_3CN (v/v) in water. The presumed IUra peak was collected from the HPLC after two 200 μl injections of the concentrated pooled sample. The HPLC collection was lyophilized. The residue was derivatized with 50 μl bis-silyltrifluoroacetamide for 10 minutes at 50° C. The derivatized material was identified by gas chromatography-mass spectrometry. Chromatography of IUra was achieved on a 4 ft × 2 mm id glass column packed with 3% OV-17 on chromosorb 100/120 mesh Supelcorp (Supelco). Helium was the carrier gas at a flow rate of 20 ml/min. The injection and interface temperatures were 250° C and the column temperature was 150° C. Electron impact mass spectra at 70 eV and chemical ionization mass spectra with methane at a source pressure of 1 torr were obtained on a Riebermag R-1010-C mass spectrometer (Delsi Instruments-Nermag).

References

1. Agarwal DP, Eickhoff K, Goedde HW: A note on in vitro inhibition of thymine degradation by some pyrimidine analogues and related products. Z Naturforsch **24b:**469-470, 1969.
2. Au JL-S, Rustum YM, Ledesma EJ, Mittelman A, Creaven PJ: Clinical pharmacology studies of concurrent infusion of 5-fluorouracil and thymidine in treatment of colorectal carcinomas. Cancer Res **42:**2930-2937, 1982.
3. Barrett HW, Munavalli SN, Newmark P: Synthetic pyrimidines as inhibitors of uracil and thymine degradation by rat-liver supernatant. Biochim Biophys Acta **91:**199-204, 1964.
4. Burgess AW, Wilson EMA, Metcalf D: Stimulation by human placental conditioned medium of hemopoietic colony formation by human marrow cells. Blood **49:**573-583, 1977.
5. Calabresi P: Regional protection in cancer chemotherapy. I. Infusions of thymidine into external carotid artery of patients receiving systemic 5-iodo-2′-deoxyuridine. J Clin Invest **41:**1484-1491, 1962.
6. Calabresi P, Cardoso SS, Finch SC, Kligerman MM, von Essen CF, Chu MY, Welch AD: Initial clinical studies with 5-iodo-2′-deoxyuridine. Cancer Res **21:**550-559, 1961.
7. Collins JM, Dedrick RL, King FG, Speyer JL, Myers CE: Nonlinear pharmacokinetic models for 5-fluorouracil in man: Intravenous and intraperitoneal routes. Clin Pharmacol Ther **28:**235-246, 1980.
8. Cooper GM, Dunning WF, Greer S: Role of catabolism in pyrimidine utilization for nucleic acid synthesis in vivo. Cancer Res **32:**390-397, 1972.
9. Ensminger WD, Rosowsky A, Raso V, Levin DC, Glode M, Come S, Steele G, Frei E: A clinical-pharmacological evaluation of hepatic arterial infusions of 5-fluoro-2′-deoxyuridine and 5-fluorouracil. Cancer Res **38:**3784-3792, 1978.
10. Howell SB, Ensminger WD, Krishan A, Frei E: Thymidine rescue of high-dose methotrexate in humans. Cancer Res **38:**325-330, 1978.
11. Karle JM, Anderson LW, Dietrick DD, Cysyk RL: Determination of serum and plasma uridine levels in mice, rats, and humans by high-pressure liquid chromatography. Anal Biochem **109:**41-46, 1980.
12. Kim BD, Keenen S, Bodnar JK, Sander EG: Role of enzymatically catalyzed 5-iodo-5,6-dihydrouracil ring hydrolysis on the dehalogenation of 5-iodouracil. J Biol Chem **251:**6909-6914, 1976.
13. Kinsella TJ, Russo A, Collins J, Klecker R, Rowland J, Jenkins J, Glatstein E: Phase I study of intravenous infusions of iododeoxyuridine (IUdR) as a clinical radiosensitizer. Int J Radiat Oncol Biol Phys **10**(suppl 2):130, 1984.
14. Knott GD: MLAB—A mathematical modeling tool. Comput Programs Biomed **10:**271-280, 1979.
15. Kufe DW, Herrick D, Gunner L: Uracil enhancement of 5-fluorodeoxyuridine incorporation into human breast carcinoma deoxyribonucleic acid. Biochem Pharmacol **33:**2331-2333, 1984.

16. Myers CE: The pharmacology of the fluoropyrimidines. Pharmacol Rev **33:**1-15, 1981.
17. Pike BL, Robinson WA: Human bone marrow colony growth in agar-gel. J Cell Physiol **76:**77-84, 1970.
18. Prusoff WH: Synthesis and biological activities of iododeoxyuridine, an analog of thymidine. Biochim Biophys Acta **32:**295-296, 1959.
19. Prusoff WH: Incorporation of iododeoxyuridine into the deoxyribonucleic acid of mouse Ehrlich ascites tumor cells in vivo. Biochim Biophys Acta **39:**327-331, 1960.
20. Prusoff WH, Chen MS, Fischer PH, Lin TS, Shiau GT: 5-Iodo-2′-deoxyuridine. *In* Hahn FE, editor: Antibiotics. New York, 1979, Springer-Verlag.
21. Prusoff WH, Goz B: Halogenated pyrimidine deoxyribonucleosides. *In* Eichler O, Farah A, Herken H, Welch AD, editors: Handbook of experimental pharmacology. New York, 1975, Springer-Verlag.
22. Prusoff WH, Jaffe JJ, Gunther H: Studies in the mouse of the pharmacology of 5-iododeoxyuridine, an analog of thymidine. Biochem Pharmacol **3:**110-121, 1960.
23. Russo A, Gianni L, Kinsella TJ, Klecker RW, Jenkins J, Rowland J, Glatstein E, Mitchell JB, Collins J, Myers C: Pharmacological evaluation of intravenous delivery of 5-bromodeoxyuridine to patients with brain tumors. Cancer Res **44:**1702-1705, 1984.
24. Sebesta K, Bauerova J, Sormova Z: Inhibition of uracil and thymine degradation by some 5-substituted uracil analogues. Biochim Biophys Acta **50:**393-394, 1961.
25. Taylor GA, Dady PJ, Harrap KR: Quantitative high-performance liquid chromatography of nucleosides and bases in human plasma. J Chromatogr **183:**421-431, 1980.

Effect of acute alcohol consumption on lithium kinetics

Lithium carbonate is used in several psychiatric disorders in the context of alcohol abuse. In a randomized, double-blind, crossover study the single-dose kinetics of lithium were followed after alcohol or placebo. Lithium carbonate capsules were taken by mouth by 10 healthy young men with alcohol on one occasion and with placebo on a separate occasion (at least 7 days apart). Lithium concentrations were determined in serum and urine samples for 24 hours after dosing and served as the basis for kinetic analysis. Acute alcohol had no effect on lithium absorption, elimination, distribution, or clearance. Alcohol did, however, increase the peak serum lithium level in nine of 10 subjects, from a mean of 0.62 mEq/L in the placebo condition to 0.70 mEq/L in the alcohol condition. Our data suggest that alcohol has limited effects on lithium carbonate kinetics. The possibility of elevated serum lithium concentrations when lithium is taken with alcohol is suggested. (CLIN PHARMACOL THER 38:52-55, 1985.)

Raymond F. Anton, M.D., Joseph A. Paladino, Pharm.D., Alex Morton, Pharm.D., and Russel W. Thomas, Pharm.D. *Charleston, S. C., and Rochester and Buffalo, N. Y.*

Lithium carbonate is used in the treatment of psychiatric disorders. The clinical response to lithium depends on an adequate serum lithium level, and the absorption and elimination of lithium are two processes that are among the primary determinants of serum levels. Factors that alter these processes may affect the safe, therapeutic use of lithium. One such factor might be alcohol, because it is a common, socially used drug that is frequently abused by patients receiving lithium.[4,10,12,13] Alcohol has effects on intestinal motility and transit times[15,16] that might affect lithium absorption. Alcohol also has an acute diuretic effect through inhibition of vasopressin.[14] Because renal excretion accounts for almost all lithium clearance, any change in this mechanism may alter lithium serum levels. Both acute and chronic alcohol use can increase brain lithium levels, decrease lithium excretion, and induce greater lithium toxicity in rats and mice.[9]

We examined the effect of acute alcohol consumption on lithium absorption and excretion in normal young subjects to elucidate the potential complications of this pharmacologic interaction.

From the Veterans Administration Medical Center and Medical University of South Carolina, Charleston; Rochester General Hospital, Rochester; and Millard Fillmore Hospital, Buffalo.

Supported in part by the Medical University of South Carolina Biomedical Research Support Grant 1982-1983 and by the Veterans Administration.

Received for publication Dec. 17, 1984; accepted March 4, 1985.

Reprint requests to: Raymond F. Anton, M.D., Psychiatry Service, Veterans Administration Medical Center, 109 Bee St., Charleston, SC 29403.

METHODS

Our subjects were ten young men (mean age 24.7 ± 2.8 years) with no psychiatric or physical abnormalities (including gastrointestinal, kidney, and cardiac disease) or abuse of alcohol or drugs. On two separate occasions at least 1 week apart, each subject was admitted to a special studies unit for 12 hours. Each subject was instructed to take no medication for 7 days, no alcohol for 48 hours, and no food or drink for 12 hours before hospitalization. At 8 AM an indwelling venous catheter was placed and blood was drawn for determinations of the blood alcohol concentration (BAC) and serum lithium level as a baseline check for surreptitious ingestion. In a random, double-blind, crossover fashion, each subject took oral lithium carbonate capsules (600 mg) on two occasions, followed within 15 minutes by either 0.5 gm/kg ethyl alcohol (vodka) in a diet lemon drink (120 ml) or a diet lemon drink alone with alcohol mist as a placebo control. Four hours later, a second drink of the same content as the first was drank. Blood was drawn for serum lithium and BAC determinations 0.25, 0.5, 1, 2, 3, 4, 5, 6, 9, 12, and 24 hours after lithium dosing. Urine was collected in two samples (0 to 12 and 12 to 24 hours after dosing) from each subject under both treatment conditions.

Serum and urine lithium levels were measured in

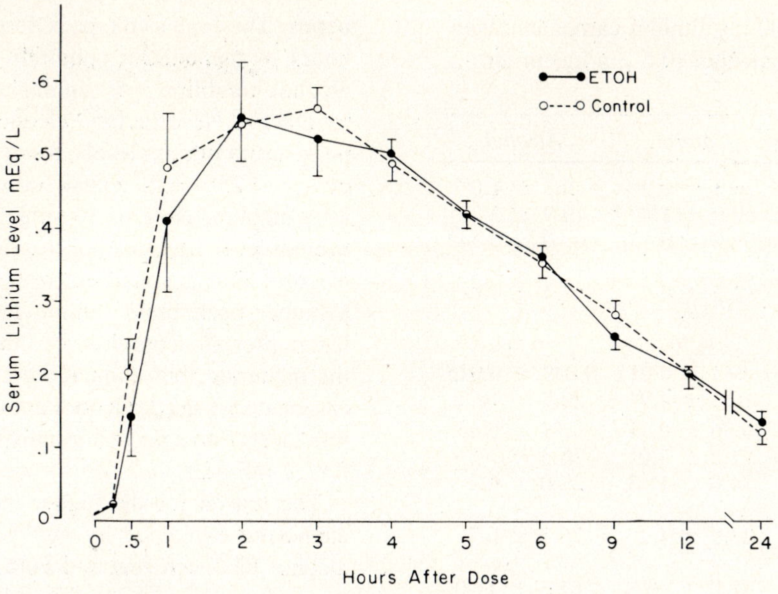

Fig. 1. Serum lithium concentration–time curve for 600 mg lithium carbonate capsules at time 0 with either alcohol (0.5 gm/kg; *ETOH*) or a control nonalcoholic drink. Each *point* represents the $\overline{X}$ ± SE of the same 10 subjects in both conditions.

duplicate by a flame photometric assay with an internal potassium standard. The BAC was measured in duplicate by a spectrophotometric enzymatic assay with alcohol dehydrogenase and the reduction of nicotinamide adenine dinucleotide to dihydronicotinamide adenine dinucleotide with subsequent change in absorbance.

Kinetics for each subject under both conditions were determined (based on standard calculations[5]) from the serum and urine lithium concentrations. The lithium serum AUC over 24 hours (AUC_{0-24}) was calculated by the trapezoidal rule. The total AUC ($AUC_{0-\infty}$) was calculated by adding the 24-hour lithium level divided by the terminal rate constant (k_e) to the AUC_{0-24}. The constant k_e was taken to be the slope of the regression line determined from the semilogarithmetic plot of the serum lithium concentration–time curve over 9 to 24 hours for each subject. These points were chosen because distribution is complete within 6 to 10 hours.[1] The elimination $t_{1/2}$ was calculated by dividing 0.693 by k_e. The apparent volume of distribution (V_z) was calculated from the equation: $V_z = \text{Dose}/AUC_{0-\infty} \cdot k_e$. Plasma clearance ($CL_P$) was determined by dividing the dose by the $AUC_{0-\infty}$. Renal clearance (CL_R) was derived from the equation: [lithium] urine · volume/[lithium] serum midpoint · time. The absorption constant (k_a) was determined from the slope of the residual line, which used mean data points over 1 to 3 hours for the method of residuals.[2] The dose used for all calculations was 16 mEq. The fraction of the dose absorbed was assumed to approximate unity.[8]

Data analysis compared each lithium kinetic parameter under both placebo and alcohol conditions for each subject by repeated-measures ANOVA. Serum lithium levels were also compared at each time point for each subject under both conditions by repeated-measures ANOVA. The k_a for the control condition was compared with that for the alcohol condition by t test to determine the 95% confidence limit around the alcohol condition residual line.

RESULTS

As seen in Fig. 1, the lithium concentration–time curve for both the control and alcohol conditions are similar. When repeated-measures ANOVA was performed for each subject at each time point under both conditions, there was no difference ($F = 0.57$; df = 1,99) in the total curve or at any specific time point.

Table I summarizes the findings. There was no significant difference in the AUC between the conditions. The time to peak serum lithium level was similar and did not differ significantly, but the mean peak serum lithium level was higher in the alcohol group than in the controls. This is not evident in Fig. 1 because different subjects reached peak serum lithium concentra-

Table I. Kinetics of 600 mg lithium carbonate taken with and without ethyl alcohol (0.5 gm/kg) in ten healthy young men

	Control	*Alcohol*
$AUC_{0\text{-}24}$ (mEq/L · hr)	6.3 ± 0.9	6.3 ± 1.0
$AUC_{0\text{-}\infty}$ (mEq/L · hr)	9.9 ± 1.4	10.9 ± 3.2
Observed peak lithium serum level (mEq/L)	0.62 ± 0.15	0.70 ± 0.14*
Time of peak lithium serum level (hr)	2.2 ± 0.9	2.4 ± 1.0
k_a (hr^{-1})	0.79	0.76
k_e (hr^{-1})	0.043 ± 0.011	0.039 ± 0.015
Elimination $t_{1/2}$ (hr)	16.2 ± 4.9	20.7 ± 10.2
V_z (L/kg)	0.56 ± 0.11	0.59 ± 0.13
CL_P (ml/min)	27.5 ± 4.0	26.3 ± 7.2
CL_R, 0 to 12 hr (ml/min)	34.0 ± 11.3	28.0 ± 9.2
CL_R, 12 to 24 hr (ml/min)	22.9 ± 4.1	26.5 ± 6.7
% Dose excreted over 24 hr	71.0 ± 20.8	67.3 ± 11.0

Data are $\overline{X}$ ± SD.
*F = 7.75; df = 1,9; P < 0.02 compared with control value.

tion at different times, which, when averaged, brought the mean for each time under both conditions into the same range. However, when the peak serum lithium level was analyzed irrespective of time, there was a significant difference. There was a mean increase of 16% in the serum lithium concentration in the alcohol group; in nine of 10 subjects the peak serum lithium concentration was higher after alcohol than in the control period.

The values for k_a derived from the slope of the residual line were the same under both conditions. The absorption $t_{1/2}$ was 0.87 hours for the lithium alone condition and 0.90 hours for the alcohol with lithium condition, but these values did not differ significantly. Values for k_e and the elimination $t_{1/2}$ did not differ significantly. The apparent V_z, CL_P, CL_R, and percent dose excreted were all the same under both conditions.

The BAC had two mean peaks. The first occurred between 30 and 60 minutes after the first dose of alcohol and reached a level of 77.5 ± 28.8 mg/dl. The second peak was higher (93.1 ± 27.1 mg/dl) and occurred 1 hour after the second dose of alcohol. At some point after taking alcohol, all subjects reached a BAC of at least 70 mg/dl (the maximum level was 150 mg/dl).

DISCUSSION

The lithium kinetics we report are consistent with reports of others.[1,6,11] It appears that acute alcohol consumption has limited effects on lithium carbonate kinetics. The time to the peak serum lithium level of 2.2 hours in the control condition and 2.4 hours in the alcohol condition was similar to the 2 hours reported by others.[3] Nevertheless, alcohol did elevate the mean peak serum lithium levels; four subjects had an increase of at least 25% in their peak serum lithium concentration after alcohol. Nine of 10 subjects had a higher serum lithium level after alcohol, resulting in a mean increase of 16%. This is consistent with data in the rat showing a higher peak brain lithium level when alcohol was taken after an acute dose of lithium carbonate.[9] Given the moderate, but clinically common, dose of lithium carbonate we used, alcohol did not increase serum lithium levels into a range normally associated with toxicity (>1.2 mEq/L).

The reason for the higher mean peak lithium level cannot be explained by our data. At moderate doses alcohol has been reported both to increase and to decrease gastric emptying time.[7] Because alcohol did not affect the time to peak serum lithium concentration, the lithium absorption constant, or the absorption $t_{1/2}$, a change in gastric emptying seems unlikely to account for the higher observed peak lithium level.

Although alcohol has a reported diuretic effect through inhibition of vasopressin,[14] our data do not support a major influence of alcohol on lithium clearance by the kidney (as reflected in serum lithium levels, CL_P, and CL_R). Our single-dose lithium kinetic data suggest no significant effect of acute alcohol on steady-state lithium levels, but studies of the effects of chronic dosing with both drugs are needed to clarify this issue.

Taken together, our results combined with those in rodents[9] suggest that lithium taken with alcohol might result in higher acute serum and, perhaps, brain levels. However, given a rather homogenous sample of young healthy men, it would seem that there is no gross general effect of acute alcohol consumption on the amount of lithium absorbed or eliminated.

We thank Patricia Reeves, R.N., and Charlene Daniel for their excellent technical assistance. The aid of Dr. Cleatus Wallis in BAC measurement and data analysis is appreciated.

References

1. Amdisen A: Monitoring of lithium treatment through determination of lithium concentration. Danish Med Bull **22**:277-291, 1975.
2. Banker GS, Rhodes CT: Modern pharmaceutics. New York, 1979, Marcel Dekker, Inc.
3. Bone S, Roose SP, Dunner DL, Fieve RR: Bioavailability of lithium carbonate: Single versus multiple daily dosing. J Clin Psychopharmacol **1**:390-391, 1981.

4. Freed EX: Alcoholism and manic-depressive disorders. Quart J Stud Alcohol **31:**62-89, 1970.
5. Gibaldi M, Perrier D: Pharmacokinetics. New York, 1975, Marcel Dekker, Inc.
6. Goode DL, Newton DW, Ueda CT, Wilson JE, Wulf BG, Kafonek D: Effect of antacid on the bioavailability of lithium carbonate. Clin Pharmacol **3:**284-287, 1984.
7. Gottfried EB, Korsten MA, Lieber CS: Gastritis and duodenitis induced by alcohol: An endoscopic and histologic assessment. Gastroenterology **70:**890-898, 1976.
8. Groth U, Prellwitz W, Jahnchen E: Estimation of pharmacokinetic parameters from saliva and urine. CLIN PHARMACOL THER **16:**490-498, 1974.
9. Ho AK, Ho CC: Potentiation of lithium toxicity by ethanol in rats and mice. Alcoholism: Clin Exp Res **2:**386-391, 1978.
10. Kline NS, Wren JC, Cooper TB, Varga E, Canal O: Evaluation of lithium therapy in chronic and periodic alcoholism. Am J Med Sci **268:**15-22, 1974.
11. Mason RW, McQueen EG, Keary PJ, James NM: Pharmacokinetics of lithium: Elimination half-time, renal clearance and apparent volume of distribution in schizophrenia. Clin Pharmacokinet **3:**241-246, 1978.
12. Merry J, Reynolds CM, Bainy J, Copper A: Prophylactic treatment of alcoholism by lithium carbonate. Lancet **2:**481-482, 1976.
13. Morrison JR: Bipolar affective disorder and alcoholism. Am J Psychiatry **131:**1130-1133, 1974.
14. Ogata M: Clinical and experimental studies on water metabolism in alcoholism. Quart J Stud Alcohol **24:**398-411, 1963.
15. Pirola RC, Davis AE: Effects of intravenous alcohol on motility of the duodenum and of the sphincter of Oddi. Aust Ann Med **19:**1-6, 1970.
16. Robles EA, Mezey E, Halsted CH, Schuster MM: Effects of ethanol on the motility of the small intestine. Johns Hopkins Med J **135:**17-24, 1974.

Treatment of recurrent herpes simplex labialis with topical butylated hydroxytoluene

Butylated hydroxytoluene (BHT) is a hydrophobic compound with in vitro activity against many enveloped viruses, including herpes simplex virus. The effect of topical therapy with 15% BHT in mineral oil on the course of recurrent herpes simplex labialis was examined in 30 patients in a double-blind, placebo-controlled pilot study in which treatment was initiated by the physician. Sixteen patients received BHT and 14 received the placebo mineral oil vehicle. The time from lesion onset to dry crust formation was slightly shorter among BHT recipients than among placebo recipients (2.0 and 2.4 days; P = 0.01). Duration of the vesicle-ulcer stages was likewise shorter (1.2 and 2.0 days; P = 0.09), and lesion virus excretion appeared to be less in the subjects who received BHT than in the controls, but these differences were not significant. There was no clinical or laboratory evidence of toxicity. (CLIN PHARMACOL THER 38:56-59, 1985.)

Donna J. Freeman, M.D., Gay Wenerstrom, R.N., and Spotswood L. Spruance, M.D. *Salt Lake City, Utah*

Herpes simplex virus (HSV) is one of several viruses pathogenic for man that is surrounded by a lipid envelope derived from host cell membranes. The envelope mediates viral attachment and entry into the host cell, a potential point of therapeutic intervention. Thus topical agents that affect lipid membranes have been considered as potential antiherpesvirus agents.[1,12] One such agent is butylated hydroxytoluene (BHT), which is used as an antioxidant in foods. BHT is a small, nearly spherical, intensely hydrophobic molecule that has strong perturbing interactions with the hydrocarbon zones of membrane structures.[6] In 1975 Snipes et al.[14] reported that 0.1 to 0.2 mmol/L BHT inactivated HSV and the lipid-containing bacteriophages ø6 and PM2 in vitro. BHT at low concentrations has also been shown to inactivate other enveloped viruses including Newcastle disease virus,[2] human and murine cytomegaloviruses, and Semliki Forest virus.[9] Detailed studies of the effects of BHT on the ø6 bacteriophage have shown that, unlike surfactants, BHT does not remove the virus envelope in conditions in which infectivity is reduced by 99%.[21] Studies with a closely related compound, 1,3-diphenyl-2[5′,5′-dimethyloxazolidinyl-*N*-oxyl]propane, show that a specific structural protein is removed from the viral envelope, with the result that the inactivated virus particles are not able to adsorb to host cells.[5,21]

The in vitro virucidal activity of BHT against enveloped viruses has led to studies of its therapeutic potential in the treatment of HSV infection in animal models. Coohill et al.[3] found milder ocular HSV infections with reduced mortality in rabbits treated with oral BHT. Dietary BHT has also protected chickens exposed to virulent Newcastle disease virus.[2] In a hairless mouse model of experimental cutaneous HSV-1 infection, Keith et al.[8] found that topical BHT was effective in reducing duration of the lesions. In a guinea pig model of genital HSV-2 disease, topical BHT resulted in significant improvement in the healing time of lesions.[11] These results prompted our study of the efficacy and tolerance of topical BHT in recurrent human herpes labialis.

METHODS

Subjects were recruited through the Herpes Study Clinic at the University of Utah. All subjects had a history consistent with recurrent herpes labialis, and 90% had a documented virus culture-positive lesion before the study. Subjects were older than 18 years of

From the Center for Infectious Diseases, Diagnostic Microbiology and Immunology and the Division of Infectious Diseases, Department of Medicine, University of Utah School of Medicine.

Supported in part by a grant from Key Pharmaceuticals, Inc., Miami, Fla.

Received for publication Jan. 22, 1985; accepted March 9, 1985.

Reprint requests to: Dr. Donna Freeman, Division of Infectious Diseases, Department of Medicine, University of Utah School of Medicine, 50 N. Medical Dr., Salt Lake City, UT 84132.

Table I. Pretreatment characteristics of subjects and of the HSL lesions

	Total population (n = 30)		
	BHT *(n = 16)*	*Placebo* *(n = 14)*	*P value**
Percent women	75%	86%	0.47
Age (yr)	31 (25-48)	29 (21-68)	0.37
History of HSL (yr)	20 (7-40)	20 (2-40)	0.95
Historical duration of lesions (days)	10 (5-20)	10 (5-21)	0.95
Lesion age on day 0 (hr)	12 (1-24)	9 (2-21)	0.42
Lesion stage on day 0	3 (2-4)	3 (2-4)	0.28
Lesion area on day 0 (mm^2)	48 (9-192)	88 (35-567)	0.16
Lesion virus titer on day 0 (log_{10} pfu/specimen)	4.6 (0-7.4)	4.1 (0-6.6)	0.88

Data are the median (range).
*Two-tailed Mann-Whitney rank sum test.

Table II. Clinical and virologic measurements of HSL lesions

	Total population (n = 30)		
	BHT *(n = 16)*	*Placebo* *(n = 14)*	*P value**
Clinical			
Time to dry crust (days)	2.0 (1.0-5.3)	2.4 (1.1-9.0)	0.01
Duration of vesicle-ulcer stages (days)	1.2 (1.0-4.9)	2.0 (1.0-8.8)	0.09
Time to total healing (days)	9.9 (1.5-14.0)	11.0 (3.0-16.1)	0.38
Virologic			
Maximum virus titer during therapy (log_{10} pfu/specimen)	4.2 (0-7.0)	5.3 (0-6.8)	0.30
Change in virus titer, days 0 to 1 (log_{10} pfu/specimen)	−0.3 ([−7.4]-7.0)	0.7 ([−2.9]-5.8)	0.38
Change in virus titer, days 0 to 2 (log_{10} pfu/specimen)	−2.2 ([−7.4]-5.4)	−0.1 ([−3.6]-3.8)	0.50
Time to last positive virus culture (days)	2.0 (0-3.0)	2.2 (1.1-3.1)	0.74

Data are median (range).
*Summary Mantel-Haenszel chi-square.

age and had experienced symptoms or signs of herpes labialis for <24 hours before their first clinic visit.

Fifteen percent BHT in mineral oil (w/v) and mineral oil placebo were placed in identical bottles, ordered by a random numbers table, numbered, and dispensed consecutively in a double-blind fashion. Subjects were instructed to apply by their fingertip a drop of the medication sufficient to cover the lesion four times a day for 5 days.

On the initial visit (day 0), a general medical history and history of past episodes of herpes infections were obtained. The current lesion was evaluated for stage, pain, and size. Stages of the lesions were: (1) erythema only, (2) induration or papule (palpable "bump"), (3) vesicle, (4A) ulcer or soft crust, (4B) dry, hard crust, (5) crust shed but still swollen, and (6) completely healed. Pain was scored on a scale of 1 (none) to 4 (severe). Lesion length and width were measured (exclusive of erythema), and the product of these two numbers was considered the lesion area. Subjects were followed on study days 1, 2, 4, and 6 and then every 3 to 4 days until the lesion was completely healed. Lesion onset was defined as the subject's first report of a "bump" (stage 2). Lesion stage, pain, and size were assessed at each visit. To assure the most accurate determination of lesion end points, subjects were questioned about any changes in lesion stage or pain that occurred between visits. Blood and urine specimens were obtained before and after BHT therapy for routine urinalysis, complete blood count, and serum chemistry tests.

Viral cultures were obtained by methods previously described.[15] Specimens were obtained at each visit during lesion stages 1 to 4A. Qualitative assay of infectivity was by inoculating confluent monolayers of mink lung cells[13] with 200 μl aliquots of each specimen. The residual specimen was then frozen at −70° C. Virus-positive samples were subsequently thawed and infectivity was quantitated in triplicate on monolayers of mink lung cells by plaque titration.[16] Cell layers were rinsed twice after virus attachment to remove all traces of drug that might have carried over from the clinical specimen. Lesion virus titers were expressed as $\log_{10}$ plaque forming units (pfu) per specimen.

Differences before dosing between drug- and placebo-treated groups were tested for statistical significance by the two-tailed Mann-Whitney rank sum test. To control for the effect of lesion size at the time of enrollment, a summary Mantel-Haenszel chi-square analysis was used in the analysis of treatment outcome. P values ≤ 0.05 were considered significant.

RESULTS

Thirty-two subjects were enrolled in the study. Two were subsequently unable to comply with the protocol and were not considered in this analysis. Of the remaining 30 subjects, 16 received BHT and 14 received the mineral oil placebo. Pretreatment characteristics of the two groups were generally similar (Table I). The median lesion area before treatment for the group assigned to placebo was 88 mm^2 compared to a median area of 48 mm^2 in the BHT group ($P = 0.16$). Because a larger lesion size correlates with longer healing times and greater virus shedding,[17] statistical probability for the treatment outcome was determined by the summary Mantel-Haenszel chi-square test controlling for day 0 area.

Results of the analysis are shown in Table II. The median time to dry crust formation was slightly shorter in the BHT group than in the controls (2.0 and 2.4 days; $P = 0.01$). Other clinical measures of lesion severity showed a trend in favor of the BHT-treated group, but the differences were not significant. There was no effect of treatment on duration or degree of pain (data not shown).

The maximum lesion virus titer measured during the first 2 days of therapy was lower for the BHT group than for the controls (4.2 and 5.3 $\log_{10}$ pfu), and the drop in virus titer over the 2 days after entry was much greater (−2.2 and −0.1 $\log_{10}$ pfu), but neither of these trends was significant.

Topical therapy with BHT was well tolerated, with no evidence of local or systemic toxicity.

DISCUSSION

The results of our pilot study show that topical BHT is well tolerated and might have a small beneficial effect on the course of herpes labialis. There was statistically significant abbreviation of the interval from the start of therapy to the formation of a dry crust. Clinically, this period of the disease usually involves the greatest discomfort and cosmetic embarrassment. Richards et al.[11] and Keith et al.[8] have found shorter healing times with topical BHT therapy. Because of the small number of subjects in this trial, the suggested clinical benefit we found needs to be confirmed in a much larger study before any definite conclusions about efficacy can be drawn.

Other agents that alter lipid membranes and are active against HSV in vitro have been evaluated in clinical trials as topical antiherpes agents. Ether was found to have no significant effect on the course of labial[7] or genital[4] herpes infections and caused excruciating pain on application to genital lesions. Nonoxynol 9, a nonionic surfactant that inactivates HSV in vitro by breakdown of the viral envelope,[1] was also found to have no effect on the course of genital herpes.[20] Interestingly, chloroform accelerated scab formation in oral lesions,[19] which is similar to our results.

One reason for the generally disappointing results with surfactants may be that, once infection is established, interference with the adherence of viral particles to host cells by destruction of the viral envelope plays a minor role in the prevention of virus propagation. Lodmell et al.[10] suggested that once cell monolayers have been infected, viral spread may occur through intracellular bridges. Rather than destroying the lipid envelope, BHT may become incorporated into the membrane and disturb function by altering the geometry of the lipid bilayer.[5,6,21] The possible effects of this geometric alteration on intracellular viral transfer have not yet been elucidated. The effect of BHT on viral plaque formation in vitro is difficult to assess because of the extreme insolubility of the drug in aqueous media.* Its different mode of action may give BHT an advantage over the envelope-stripping surfactants in vivo.

BHT is an unusual agent possessing virucidal activity

*Freeman DJ, Spruance SL: Unpublished observations, 1984.

at low concentrations and a probable mode of action different from that of the other surfactants or nucleoside analogs. Despite limited in vitro data, BHT has demonstrated moderate in vivo activity in a succession of animal models.[2,3,8,11] There was also a small effect in our study despite delay of treatment until the first clinic visit[18] and the limited number of subjects. Further studies of BHT to examine its possible role in the treatment of herpesvirus infections are warranted.

We thank P. J. Kinzalow for technical assistance with virologic studies and R. Mick for statistical consultation.

References

1. Asculai SS, Weis MT, Rancourt MW, Kupferberg AB: Inactivation of herpes simplex viruses by nonionic surfactants. Antimicrob Agents Chemother **13:**686-690, 1978.
2. Brugh M Jr: Butylated hydroxytoluene protects chickens exposed to Newcastle Disease virus. Science **197:**1291-1292, 1977.
3. Coohill TP, Ferrell BR, Carson D, Elliott LP: Orally administered butylated hydroxytoluene inhibits herpes simplex virus (type 1) infection in rabbits. Presented at the Eighty-third Annual Meeting of the American Society for Microbiology, New Orleans, La., March 6-11, 1983. (Abst. No. S41.)
4. Corey L, Reeves WC, Chiang WT, Vontver LA, Remington M, Winter C, Holmes KK: Ineffectiveness of topical ether for the treatment of genital herpes simplex virus infection. N Engl J Med **299:**237-239, 1978.
5. DeLuca N, Keith A, Snipes W: Studies with a hydrophobic, spin-labeled virucidal agent. Antimicrob Agents Chemother **17:**63-70, 1980.
6. Eletr S, Williams MA, Watkins T, Keith AD: Perturbations of the dynamics of lipid alkyl chains in membrane systems: Effect on the activity of membrane-bound enzymes. Biochim Biophys Acta **339:**190-201, 1974.
7. Guinan ME, MacCalman J, Kern ER, Overall JC Jr, Spruance SL: Topical ether and herpes simplex labialis. JAMA **243:**1059-1061, 1980.
8. Keith AD, Arruda D, Snipes W, Frost P: The antiviral effectiveness of butylated hydroxytoluene on herpes cutaneous infections in hairless mice. Proc Soc Exp Biol Med **170:**237-244, 1982.
9. Kim KS, Moon HM, Sapienza V, Carp RI, Pullarkat R: Inactivation of cytomegalovirus and Semliki Forest virus by butylated hydroxytoluene. J Infect Dis **138:**91-94, 1978.
10. Lodmell DL, Niwa A, Hayashi K, Notkins AL: Prevention of cell-to-cell spread of herpes simplex virus by leucocytes. J Exp Med **137:**706-720, 1973.
11. Richards JT, Katz M, Kern ER: Topical butylated hydroxytoluene treatment of genital herpes simplex virus infections of guinea pigs. Antiviral Res. (In press.)
12. Sabin AB: Misery of recurrent herpes: What to do? N Engl J Med **293:**986-988, 1975.
13. Salmon VC, Stanberry LR, Overall JC Jr: More rapid isolation of herpes simplex virus in a continuous cell line of mink lung cells than in vero or human fibroblast cells. Diagn Micro Infect Dis **2:**317-324, 1984.
14. Snipes W, Person S, Keith A, Cupp J: Butylated hydroxytoluene inactivates lipid-containing viruses. Science **188:**64-65, 1975.
15. Spruance SL, Crumpacker CS, Haines H, Bader C, Mehr K, MacCalman J, Schnipper LE, Klauber MR, Overall JC Jr, the Collaborative Study Group: Ineffectiveness of topical adenine arabinoside 5′-monophosphate in the treatment of recurrent herpes simplex labialis. N Engl J Med **300:**1180-1184, 1979.
16. Spruance SL, McKeough MB, Cardinal JR: Penetration of guinea pig skin by acyclovir in different vehicles and correlation with the efficacy of topical therapy of experimental cutaneous herpes simplex virus infection. Antimicrob Agents Chemother **25:**10-15, 1984.
17. Spruance SL, Overall JC Jr, Kern ER, Krueger GG, Pliam V, Miller W: The natural history of recurrent herpes simplex labialis: Implications for antiviral therapy. N Engl J Med **297:**69-75, 1977.
18. Spruance SL, Schnipper LE, Overall JC Jr, Kern ER, Wester B, Modlin J, Wenerstrom G, Burton C, Arndt KA, Chiu GL, Crumpacker CS: Treatment of herpes simplex labialis with topical acyclovir in polyethylene glycol. J Infect Dis **146:**85-90, 1982.
19. Taylor CA, Hendley O, Greer KE, Gwaltney JM Jr: Topical treatment of herpes labialis with chloroform. Arch Dermatol **113:**1550-1552, 1977.
20. Vontver LA, Reeves WC, Rattray M, Corey L, Remington MA, Tolentino E, Schweid A, Holmes KK: Clinical course and diagnosis of genital herpes simplex virus infection and evaluation of topical surfactant therapy. Am J Obstet Gynecol **133:**548-554, 1979.
21. Wanda P, Cupp J, Snipes W, Keith A, Rucinsky T, Polish L, Sands J: Inactivation of the enveloped bacteriophage ø6 by butylated hydroxytoluene and butylated hydroxyanisole. Antimicrob Agents Chemother **10:**96-101, 1976.

Effects of chronic nitrendipine on casual (office) and 24-hour ambulatory blood pressure

To assess the clinical efficacy of chronic nitrendipine therapy in mild to moderate essential hypertension, we studied blood pressure (BP) and heart rate responses in 22 subjects receiving maintenance nitrendipine therapy. Ten subjects (45%) whose hypertension was controlled with chronic monotherapy had an 11/12 mm Hg decrease in supine BP ($P < 0.05$) with a mean (±SD) dose of 71 ± 15 mg/day. The 12 (55%) subjects whose hypertension was not controlled with monotherapy had a comparatively higher baseline BP than the other 10 (156/105 ± 10/6 compared with 150/98 ± 15/4 mm Hg; $P < 0.05$). Eight of the 10 subjects demonstrating office BP control with chronic nitrendipine monotherapy who also had full-time employment underwent continuous ambulatory BP monitoring before and after maintenance monotherapy. Nitrendipine induced a reduction in the mean 24-hour BP and mean BP at home, but did not reduce the BP during work or while asleep. These data suggest that nitrendipine lowers BP when assessed by casual office methods. The ambulatory BP monitor data demonstrate that the hypotensive response to chronic nitrendipine is modified during work periods, which are generally associated with increased adrenergic activity. Ambulatory BP monitoring may be superior to office (casual) monitoring in the assessment of the overall efficacy of antihypertensive drugs. (CLIN PHARMACOL THER 38:60-64, 1985.)

William B. White, M.D., Vivienne-E. Smith, M.D., Ellen J. McCabe, R.N., and Moideen K. Meeran, M.D. *Farmington, Conn.*

Nitrendipine is a dihydropyridine calcium channel blocker that shares some of the coronary and peripheral vasodilatory properties of nifedipine.[17] Studies of the effects of acute nitrendipine in patients with hypertension have suggested that nitrendipine lowers arterial blood pressure (BP) due to arteriolar dilatation.[1,16] The reduction in BP is associated with a reflex increase in heart rate (HR) and cardiac index.[8,16] Short-term nitrendipine therapy in patients with hypertension has significantly reduced systemic vascular resistance.[3] The alteration in cardiac output and HR varies among individuals, however, and may depend on the dosage used and the degree of venodilation.[3,15]

We investigated the BP and HR responses of patients with hypertension to chronic monotherapy with nitrendipine. We also evaluated the effect of nitrendipine on BP reduction over 24 hours, at work, at home, and during sleep.

From the Divisions of General Internal Medicine (Hypertension Clinic) and Cardiology, Department of Medicine, University of Connecticut School of Medicine.

Supported in part by a grant-in-aid from Miles Laboratories, West Haven, Conn.

Presented in part at the Eastern Section Meeting of the American Federation for Clinical Research, Philadephia, Pa., Oct. 18, 1984.[18]

Reprint requests to: Dr. William B. White, L-2071A, University of Connecticut Health Center, Farmington, CT 06032.

METHODS

Our open study was designed to determine the general safety and efficacy of nitrendipine as monotherapy for hypertension. Our subjects were 22 white patients (19 men and three women; age range 38 to 65 years) with mild to moderate essential hypertension. Patients were enrolled if the untreated supine diastolic BP (Korotkoff phase V sound) in the office setting was 90 to 114 mm Hg.

All subjects underwent 2 weeks of baseline evaluation during which a complete history, physical examination, and baseline laboratory data (12-lead ECG, complete blood count with differential and platelet count, SMA-24, urinalysis, and chest x-ray photography) were obtained. Weekly measurements of supine and erect HR and BP were made during a 2-week "drug washout" period and during a 2-week placebo period. Casual BP and HR were measured after the subject had been supine 10 minutes and after standing 2 minutes. Subjects whose supine diastolic BP fell 10 mm Hg or

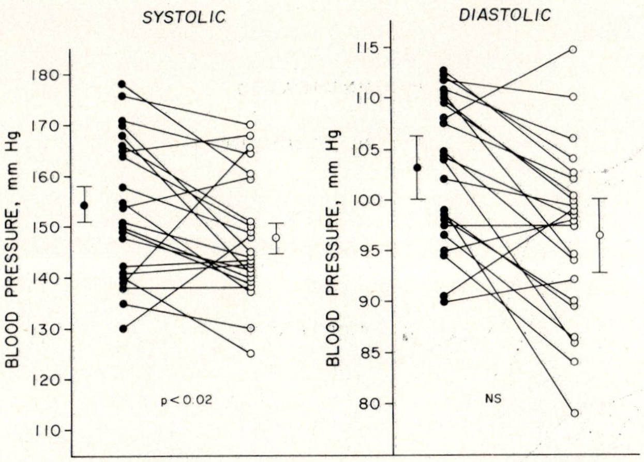

Fig. 1. Individual supine office BPs at the end of placebo phase (●) and after 3 months nitrendipine dosing (○). Mean (± SD) dose was 18 ± 7 mg twice a day. All readings were made 8 to 10 hours after dosing.

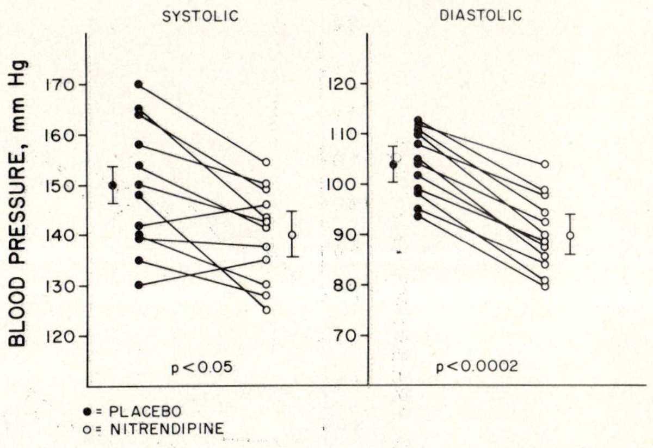

Fig. 2. Individual supine office BPs after higher doses of nitrendipine monotherapy for 1 year (mean [± SD] dose was 36 ± 9 mg twice a day). All readings were made 8 to 10 hours after dosing.

was <90 mm Hg during placebo dosing were dropped from the study.

Afterwards, subjects were seen weekly during a titration period when nitrendipine was given in dosages of 10 to 80 mg/day in two divided doses. The treatment goal was a drop of ≥10 mm Hg in diastolic BP for those subjects entering with a supine diastolic BP between 90 and 99 mm Hg, or a diastolic BP of ≤90 mm Hg in those subjects with an entry supine diastolic BP >100 mm Hg. If these goals were not achieved with the maximally tolerated dose of nitrendipine, a second drug (propranolol or hydrocholorothiazide) could be added to nitrendipine therapy. All subjects were then followed for 1 year at monthly intervals while receiving either nitrendipine monotherapy or combination therapy.

In addition to the general evaluation and routine laboratory studies, eight of 10 subjects whose hypertension was controlled in the office setting by nitrendipine monotherapy and also held full-time employment underwent ambulatory BP measurements after 2 weeks of drug washout and at the end of 1 year of nitrendipine therapy. In general, all these subjects had sedentary types of employment but characterized their jobs as mentally stressful. BP and HR were measured every 15 minutes for the entire 24-hour period with an ambulatory monitoring system. BP values recorded by the monitoring equipment were compared with those measured simultaneously with a standard mercury sphygmomanometer. The correlations between the two systolic and diastolic BP levels obtained at the start of the monitoring were significant (systolic: $r = 0.90$, $P < 0.001$; diastolic: $r = 0.92$, $P < 0.001$), as were those obtained at the end of the monitoring period (systolic: $r = 0.88$, $P < 0.001$; diastolic: $r = 0.86$, $P < 0.001$). Readings that showed an inconsistent increase or decrease in systolic or diastolic BP >25 mm Hg and those with pulse pressures <10 mm Hg were not considered in the analysis. Tracings were analyzed only if ≥80% of the maximal number of 96 readings during the 24-hour period passed the deletion criteria. Diaries were carefully kept by the subjects and data were analyzed for the entire 24-hour period and subanalyzed for the periods of work, home (while awake), and during sleep. Statistical analysis was by a two-tailed paired t test. Data are expressed as $\overline{X}$ ± SD.

RESULTS

The individual supine office BP responses to nitrendipine monotherapy in doses of 10 to 20 mg twice a day are shown in Fig. 1. The average systolic BP was reduced from 154 ± 14 to 148 ± 12 mm Hg ($P < 0.02$) by nitrendipine, while supine diastolic BP fell from 103 ± 7 to 97 ± 9 mm Hg (NS). The supine and erect HR for the group increased by only 3 bpm ($P = 0.06$) after nitrendipine. The effect of the higher dosages (30 to 40 mg twice a day) of nitrendipine on office BP in 12 subjects remaining on chronic monotherapy for 1 year is shown in Fig. 2. Supine systolic BP fell from 150 ± 13 to 140 ± 9 mm Hg ($P < 0.05$) and the average reduction in diastolic BP was from 104 ± 6 to 90 ± 7 mm Hg ($P < 0.0002$). It is noteworthy that the hypertension of two of these 12 subjects was not controlled at the 1-year reading, but that at earlier checks (8 and 10 months) these subjects had a supine diastolic BP <90 mm Hg with nitrendipine

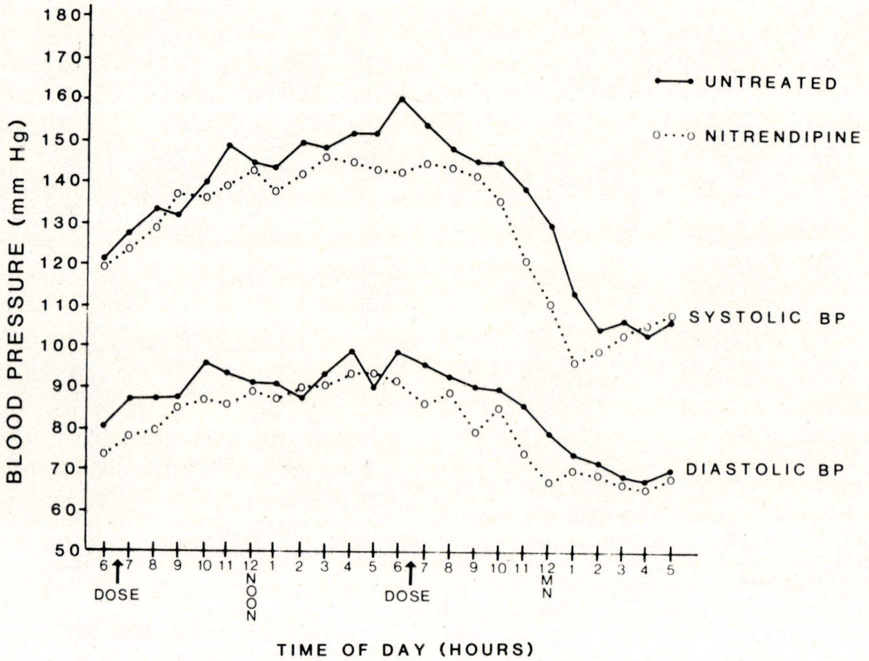

Fig. 3. Twenty-four–hour curves of mean hourly systolic and diastolic BPs before and after 1 year of therapy with higher doses (36 ± 9 mg twice a day) of nitrendipine. *MN* = Midnight.

Table I. Effects of nitrendipine monotherapy on BP and HR

	SBP (mm Hg)	*DBP (mm Hg)*	*HR (bpm)*
Casual readings			
Baseline	148 ± 7	99 ± 9	77 ± 4
Nitrendipine	140 ± 8*	89 ± 6*	78 ± 4
24-hr			
Baseline	136 ± 7	85 ± 9	76 ± 5
Nitrendipine	129 ± 5†	81 ± 4	75 ± 7
Work			
Baseline	145 ± 6	92 ± 11	82 ± 5
Nitrendipine	142 ± 7	90 ± 5	80 ± 5
Home (awake)			
Baseline	149 ± 12	91 ± 13	81 ± 5
Nitrendipine	136 ± 7*	84 ± 4†	84 ± 7
Sleep			
Baseline	109 ± 8	72 ± 7	62 ± 10
Nitrendipine	108 ± 10	68 ± 7	66 ± 12

Data are $\overline{X}$ ± SD.
SBP = Systolic BP; DBP = diastolic BP.
*P < 0.01, †P < 0.05 compared with baseline value.

monotherapy. There was no significant difference in HR after the higher doses of nitrendipine.

The mean 24-hour ambulatory systolic BP was slightly but significantly (P < 0.05) reduced by nitrendipine; however, the reduction in mean 24-hour diastolic BP was only 4 mm Hg (NS; Table I). BP while at home fell by 13/7 mm Hg (P < 0.05 for both systolic and diastolic BPs) with nitrendipine, but BPs during work periods and during sleep were not significantly reduced. In this same group of eight subjects the casual supine BP significantly (P < 0.01) fell from 148/99 ± 7/9 to 140/89 ± 8/6 (Table I).

The pretreatment 24-hour curves showed a circadian pattern similar to that reported previously (Fig. 3).[9] Nitrendipine therapy reduced systolic BP throughout the day and during the awake periods at night. The

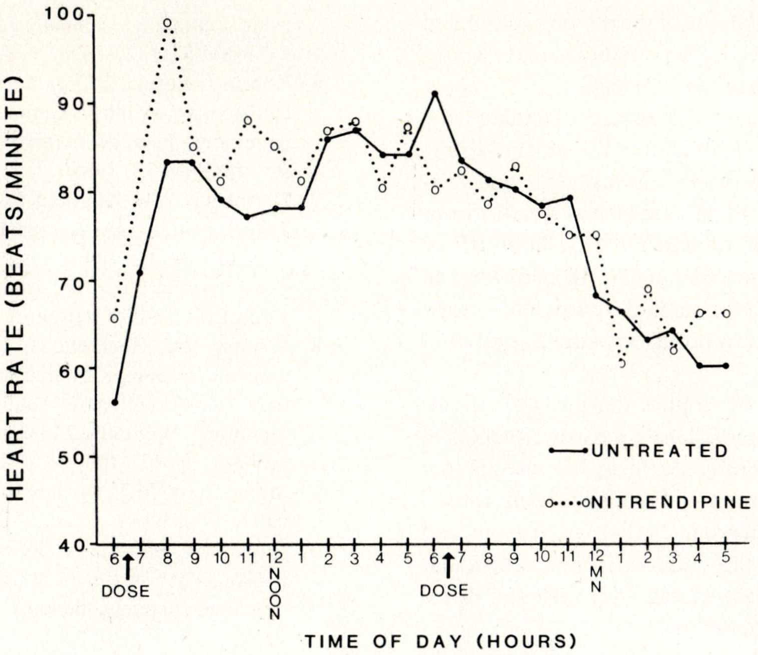

Fig. 4. Twenty-four–hour curve of mean hourly HR before and after therapy with higher doses (36 ± 9 mg twice a day) of nitrendipine. *MN* = Midnight.

diastolic BP was reduced from 6 PM until midnight and may have reflected the evening dose. The mean hourly HR was elevated with nitrendipine during the early morning hours (Fig. 4) and may have reflected the morning dose. Otherwise, there was no difference in the ambulatory HR with nitrendipine.

Three subjects complained of global headaches approximately 1 hour after each dose; this phenomenon spontaneously resolved in all subjects after 2 to 4 weeks of therapy. Two subjects noted ankle edema and received diuretics with good response. There were no persistent abnormalities in the various blood chemistry or hematologic data.

DISCUSSION

Our data demonstrate that chronic therapy with nitrendipine effectively lowers the casual (office) BP without increasing HR. It was apparent in our subjects that a more effective hypotensive response was obtained with doses between 40 and 80 mg/day. However, in the group of patients whose BP was presumably controlled by nitrendipine in the office setting, BP reduction assessed by 24-hour noninvasive ambulatory monitoring was much less.

The beneficial effects of calcium channel blockers in hypertension result from their ability to induce systemic vasodilation.[11] The dihydropyridine calcium channel blockers, including nitrendipine, induce marked peripheral vasodilation and thereby lower peripheral resistance and arterial pressure.[10,14] In the spontaneously hypertensive rat, acute BP reduction is associated with variable changes in HR and cardiac output, but alterations in HR are not significant after chronic therapy.[3,15] In our study we followed subjects for 1 year of nitrendipine therapy. The average HR changes were not significantly affected, although some subjects had persistent and substantial increases in supine-to-erect HR that may have blunted the ambulatory hypotensive effect of nitrendipine.

The 24-hour BP response to nitrendipine was evaluated by noninvasive monitoring to examine the duration of efficacy with the standardized dosing interval. Ambulatory monitoring also allows evaluation of the BP response away from the hospital environment and during daily activities.

In our subjects there was a small reduction in the 24-hour BP with nitrendipine but no significant reduction in the diastolic BP during work. Studies involving intraarterial techniques to examine ambulatory BP with nifedipine[5] and verapamil[4] demonstrated a moderate decrease in awake hourly BP readings, but subanalysis during work compared with home or sleep was not reported. In a 4-week study with use of a patient-automated noninvasive ambulatory monitor,[12] nitrendipine alone or with hydrochlorothiazide lowered the average ambulatory BP by 14/7 mm Hg with a dose of

20 mg twice a day. Limitations of the patient-automated recorder include the lack of automaticity and the inability to assess variations during sleep.

A recent report by Devereux et al.[2] elucidated the importance of measurement of the BP during work. The correlation between the BP during work and posterior left ventricular wall thickness was much closer than was the correlation of either the 24-hour BP or office BP with left ventricular mass. In addition, an association between development of ventricular ectopy and work systolic BP was reported in patients with mild hypertension.[7]

Whether the lack of BP control during work by nitrendipine or other antihypertensives is detrimental in the prevention of hypertensive heart disease is not known. Kobrin et al.[6] reported that nitrendipine caused regression of cardiac mass in both hypertensive and normotensive rats, but the changes in left ventricular mass were not directly associated with systemic or regional hemodynamic alterations.

In our recent experience[13] we have found no association between reduction in BP and regression of left ventricular mass or improvement in left ventricular diastolic filling in patients receiving 6 months of therapy with nitrendipine alone or with propranolol. However, because these studies did not evaluate 24-hour BP during baseline and treatment phases, further investigation is needed to assess fully the relationship between ambulatory control of hypertension, reduction of left ventricular hypertrophy, and improved diastolic performance.

We thank Laura Kearney, R.N., for excellent technical assistance throughout the study and Arnold M. Katz, M.D., for valuable review of the manuscript.

References

1. Burris JF, Notargiacomo AV, Papademetriou V, Freis ED: Acute and short-term effects of a new calcium antagonist in hypertension. Hypertension **4:**(suppl II):32-35, 1982.
2. Devereaux RB, Pickering TG, Harshfield GA, et al: Left ventricular hypertrophy in patients with hypertension: Importance of blood pressure response to regularly recurring stress. Circulation **68:**470-476, 1983.
3. Fouad FM, Aboul-Khair M, Tarazi RC: Heterogeneity of systemic hemodynamic response to a new calcium entry blocker, nitrendipine. J Cardiovasc Pharmacol **4:**S383-S386, 1982.
4. Gould BA, Mann S, Kieso H, Subramanian VB, Raftery EB: The 24-hour ambulatory blood pressure profile with verapamil. Circulation **65:**22-27, 1982.
5. Hornung RS, Gould BA, Jones RI, Sonecha TN, Raftery EB: Nifedipine tablets for systemic hypertension: A study using continuous ambulatory intraarterial recording. Am J Cardiol **51:**1323-1327, 1983.
6. Kobrin I, Sesoka S, Pegram BL, Frolich ED: Reduced cardiac mass by nitrendipine is dissociated from systemic or regional haemodynamic changes in rats. Cardiovasc Res **18:**158-162, 1984.
7. Kornienko WA, Kligfield P, Devereaux RB, Pickering TG, Harshfield GA, Laragh JH: Ventricular arrhythmias in mild essential hypertension: Association with workplace systolic blood pressure and left ventricular mass. J Am Coll Cardiol. (In press.)
8. Lehman HV, Hochrein H, Witt E, Mies HW: Hemodynamic responses of nitrendipine in hypertensive patients. *In* Scriabine A, Vanov S, Deck K, editors: Nitrendipine. Baltimore-Munich, 1984, Urban and Schwarzenberg, pp 491-499.
9. Millar-Craig MW, Bishop CN, Raftery EB: Circadian variation of blood pressure. Lancet **1:**795-798, 1978.
10. Olivari MT, Bartorelli C, Polese A, Fiorentini C, Maruzzi P, Guazzi M: Treatment of hypertension with nifedipine, a calcium channel antagonist. Circulation **59:**1056-1062, 1979.
11. Packer M, Frishman WH: Calcium-channel antagonists in perspective. *In* Packer M, Frishman WH, editors: Calcium-channel antagonists in cardiovascular disease. Norwalk, Conn, 1984, Appleton-Century-Crofts, Inc, pp 17-21.
12. Ram CVS, Carnegie AL, Kaplan NM: Effect of nitrendipine therapy on ambulatory blood pressures. *In* Scriabine A, Vanov S, Deck K, editors: Nitrendipine. Baltimore-Munich, 1984, Urban and Schwarzenberg, pp 501-507.
13. Smith VE, White WB, Karimeddini MK, Meeran M, Schulman P: Improved left ventricular filling accompanies reduced left ventricular mass during therapy of essential hypertension. Circulation **70:**(II):377, 1984. (Abst.)
14. Smith VE, White WB, Meeran M: Nitrendipine in mild to moderate hypertension. Clin Res **32:**338A, 1984. (Abst.)
15. Tarazi RC, Aboul-Khair M, Kobayashi K: Cardiac and hemodynamic effects of nitrendipine in normotensive and hypertensive rats. *In* Scriabine A, Vanov S, Deck K, editors: Nitrendipine. Baltimore-Munich, 1984, Urban and Schwarzenberg, pp 251-270.
16. Ventura HO, Messerli FH, Oigman W, Dunn FG, Reisin E, Frolich ED: Immediate hemodynamic effects of a new calcium-channel blocking agent (nitrendipine) in essential hypertension. Am J Cardiol **51:**783-786, 1983.
17. Warltier DC, Lamping KA, Zyvoloski MG, Gross GJ, Brooks HL: The slow-channel calcium blocking agent, nitrendipine, and coronary blood flow. J Cardiovasc Pharmacol **5:**272-277, 1983.
18. White WB, Smith VE: Comparison of office versus ambulatory blood pressure response to chronic nitrendipine monotherapy. Clin Res **32:**688A, 1984. (Abst.)

Nonsteroidal anti-inflammatory effect of sulindac sulfoxide and sulfide on gastric mucosa

Gastric injury resulting from nonsteroidal anti-inflammatory drugs is thought to require direct contact of the drug with the gastric mucosa. An inactive form of a drug (as a prodrug) should protect against mucosal damage. Because sulindac sulfoxide has little effect on prostaglandin synthesis until it is reduced to sulindac sulfide after absorption, we performed a double-blind, crossover endoscopic study in 15 normal subjects to compare the prodrug sulindac sulfoxide (200 mg b.i.d.), the active sulfide metabolite sulindac sulfide (100 mg b.i.d., which yields similar sulfide blood concentrations), a positive control (aspirin, 650 mg q.i.d.), and a negative control (placebo). Each drug was taken for 1 week and gastric mucosa were endoscopically assessed before and after 2, 5, and 7 days of dosing. Aspirin predictably damaged the gastric mucosa, whereas the effects of sulindac sulfoxide and sulindac sulfide could not be distinguished from those of the placebo. We conclude that sulindac sulfoxide as a prodrug is not directly responsible for the reduced severity of gastric mucosal lesions. Both sulindac sulfoxide and sulindac sulfide are poorly soluble in acid gastric contents and the reduced damage may relate to the inability of high concentrations of the drug to enter gastric mucosal cells. (CLIN PHARMACOL THER 38:65-70, 1985.)

David Y. Graham, M.D., J. Lacey Smith, M.D., Geoffrey I. Holmes, B.A., and Richard O. Davies, M.D., Ph.D. *Houston, Tex., and West Point, Pa.*

Aspirin and other nonsteroidal anti-inflammatory drugs (NSAIDs) may be associated with acute damage to the gastric mucosa. The gastric mucosal changes associated with NSAIDs include submucosal hemorrhages, superficial erosions, and, on occasion, acute ulcers.[6,13,15] Most new NSAIDs have been evaluated (usually compared with aspirin and placebo) for their ability to damage gastric mucosa by endoscopic studies in normal volunteers.[11] When sulindac sulfoxide was evaluated by this technique, it had only minimal adverse effects on the gastric mucosa.[12] Sulindac sulfoxide has little effect on prostaglandin synthesis, but after absorption it undergoes a major reversible biotransformation (reduction) to sulindac sulfide (the moiety containing the prostaglandin synthetase inhibitor activity) and an irreversible oxidation to the inactive sulfone metabolite.[3,10] Thus as administered, sulindac is a prodrug.

From the Digestive Disease Section, Veterans Administration Medical Center, Baylor College of Medicine, Houston, and Merck Sharp & Dohme Research Laboratories, West Point.

Received for publication Dec. 23, 1984; accepted March 14, 1985.

Reprint requests to: David Y. Graham, M.D. (111D), Veterans Administration Medical Center, 2002 Holcombe Blvd., Houston, TX 77211.

Investigators have suggested that the gastric damage associated with NSAIDs is directly related to the ability to inhibit prostaglandin synthesis, and concurrent dosing with prostaglandins is associated with reduced macroscopic gastric mucosal damage.[5] Mucosal damage is thought also to require direct contact between the NSAID and the gastric mucosa, since intravenous aspirin does not damage the gastric mucosa in man.[1,10,13] Our study compared the effects of sulindac sulfoxide and its active metabolite, sulindac sulfide, on the gastric mucosa in normal healthy subjects to determine if the low severity of damage associated with sulindac is related to its use as a prodrug.

METHODS

Our study was a double-blind, randomized, crossover gastroscopic study in healthy men. The drugs and dosages tested were: sulindac sulfoxide, 200 mg; sulindac sulfide, 100 mg (shown to yield blood concentrations of the biologically active sulfide metabolite similar to doses of 200 mg sulindac sulfoxide); aspirin, 650 mg (a positive control); or placebo (a negative control). Drug dosing was by a double-placebo design in which each subject received drugs at 6-hour intervals (sulindac sulfoxide or sulfide at 1 AM and 1 PM, placebo at 7 AM

Table I. Endoscopic grading scale (modified scale of Lanza)

Score	*Description*
0	Normal
1	One area of submucosal hemorrhage
2	>1 area of submucosal hemorrhage/erosion but not numerous or widespread
3	Numerous (>3) areas of submucosal hemorrhage/erosion
4	Widespread involvement of the stomach with submucosal hemorrhage/erosion

and 7 PM, and aspirin four times a day). Our subjects were 15 healthy men 23 to 44 years old ($\bar{X} \pm SD = 31 \pm 7$ years; average weight 174 ± 32 lb). Subjects took no alcohol or any other drugs during the study. The study was of a randomized, crossover design consisting of 1 week of drug dosing and a minimum washout of 3 weeks between drug dosing. An endoscopic score assessment of no damage was required before each treatment week.

Gastroscopy was performed with a Pentax 34F endoscope before the first dose of each regimen, on days 2 and 5 (immediately before the morning dose), and on day 7 (6 hours after the final dose). Gastric mucosa were also evaluated 2 weeks after the end of each drug protocol. Blood samples for drug analysis were drawn after 1, 4, and 7 days of dosing. Each subject kept a diary of side effects.

The gastric mucosa were evaluated endoscopically by two different scales: the modified scale of Lanza (Table I) and a new scale that attempted to quantitate the degree of injury and the area of the stomach involved (Table II; Fig. 1). Endoscopic grading scales fall into two groups: those that simply count lesions without respect to lesion location,[15] and modifications of the Lanza scale that take both number and distribution into account. All such gastroscopic grading scales are nonlinear (categoric) scoring systems, and the grades 0 to 4 could have been labeled A, B, C, D, and E without changing the interpretation. Although grade 1 is not clinically distinguishable from grade 0, we consider grades 1 and 2 as mild damage and grades 3 and 4 as severe damage.

Because the scales are not linear, statistical analysis was by nonparametric ranking methods (principally Friedman's test)[8] in which each subject is considered as a block receiving the four different dosing regimens. The four regimens are ranked according to their relative damage compared with the other treatments for each subject. For example, if placebo resulted in less damage than any other regimen, it would receive the lowest rank (grade 0); if aspirin caused the most damage, it would receive the highest rank (grade 3). A tie in the amount of damage would result in an even split of two or more ranks. For each drug this rank of relative severity is then added for all 15 subjects to yield a total sum of ranks, which yields an estimate of the relative damage of each regimen compared with the others. Statistical testing is then used to determine if the difference in ranks represents a significant difference in damage. The sum of ranks provides an overall estimate of the relative damage, i.e., a sum of 0 represents an ideal "best" drug and the maximum score of 45 represents the ideal "worst" drug.

Sulindac sulfoxide, sulfone, and sulfide levels were determined in plasma by HPLC.[14]

Table II. New system for endoscopic scoring

A. Definition of severity and area of mucosal injury

Subscore	*Severity*	*Area**
0	Normal	Normal
1	Submucosal hemorrhages (≤3-5/area)	1 area only
2	Many submucosal hemorrhages/area, erosions	2 to 4 discrete areas: a. Antrum only b. Body only c. Mixed
3	Confluent erosions, ulcerations	Widespread involvement

B. Scoring system

Final score	*Severity*	*Area**
1	1	1
2	1	2
	2	1
3	1	3
	2	2
	2	3
4	3	1
	3	2
5	3	3

*See Fig. 1 for description of areas.

RESULTS

The two endoscopic rating scales gave essentially identical results, and therefore the simpler scale modified from Lanza[6] was used. Our attempt to increase precision with a new, more complicated rating scale

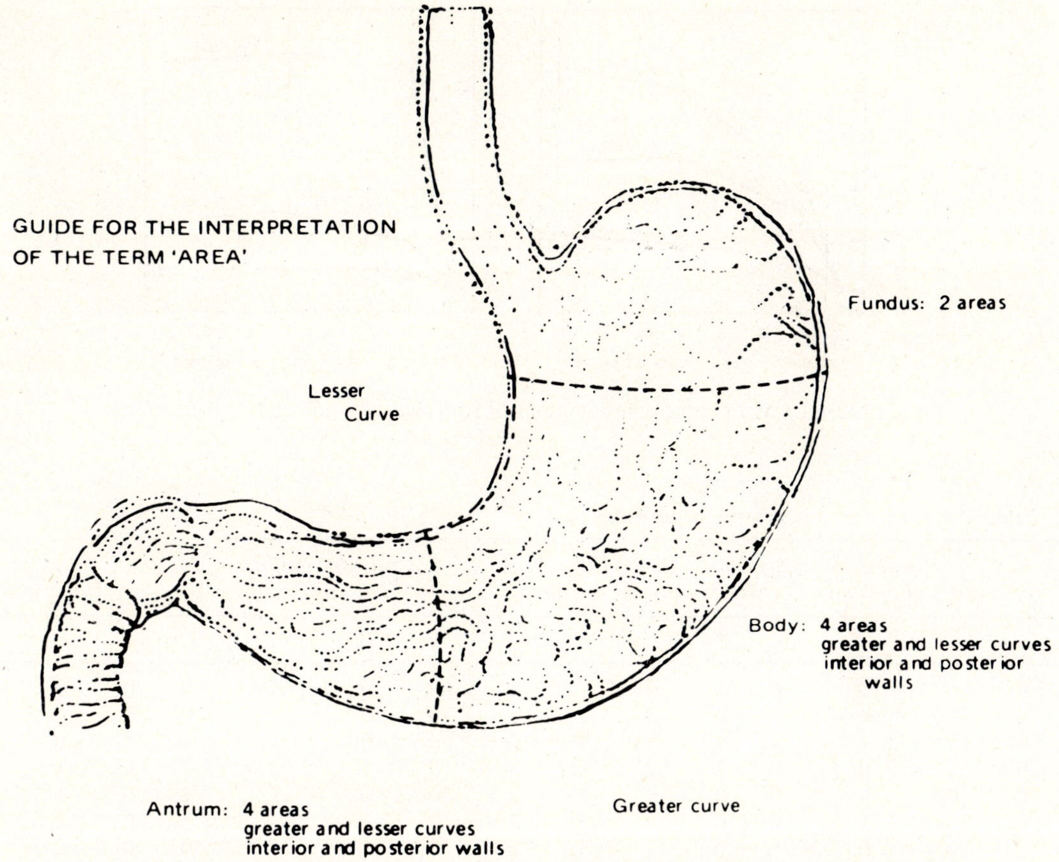

Fig. 1. Guide for interpretation of the term "area" in new endoscopic scoring system.

was judged a failure, emphasizing the value of the previously used rating scale.

Aspirin predictably induced severe gastric mucosal damage; the median endoscopic score was 3 after 1, 4, or 7 days of therapy (Table III). In contrast, the median score for placebo was 0, while sulindac sulfoxide and sulindac sulfide had a median score of 1. There was significantly more damage ($P < 0.01$) with aspirin than with any of the other regimens, but there was no significant difference between placebo and either of the sulindac compounds (Table III). The sum of ranks for aspirin was between 41 and 42.5 for all 3 days of evaluation, whereas the sums of ranks for placebo (12.5 to 14), sulindac sulfoxide (16.5 to 18), and sulindac sulfide (18 to 19.5) were virtually identical.

Fig. 2 shows the mean plasma concentrations for sulindac sulfoxide and its metabolites. The plasma concentration of sulindac sulfide reached steady state sooner after sulindac sulfide than after sulindac sulfoxide ($P < 0.01$). The difference in plasma concentration after 1 day was no longer evident after 4 days of dosing, and drug levels were essentially identical after 7 days. No correlations could be found between the endoscopic score and the plasma concentrations of sulindac sulfide.

Six subjects reported 14 side effects ranging from epigastric fullness, indigestion, and heartburn to diarrhea. Sulindac sulfoxide was associated with six episodes of side effects, the sulfide metabolite with four, placebo with two, and aspirin with two; there were no significant differences between symptoms associated with the four regimens. Multichannel serum chemistry profile results showed no significant abnormalities associated with any of drugs, although there was a slight, statistically significant increase in both BUN and urine-specific gravity associated with aspirin, sulindac sulfoxide, and sulindac sulfide compared with placebo or the prestudy examinations: the BUN during prestudy and placebo was 12.8 ± 3, and 12.6 ± 3 mg/dl ($\overline{X} \pm SD$), respectively, whereas with sulindac sulfoxide, sulindac sulfide, and aspirin the values were 15.6 ± 3, 15.7 ± 3, and 14.7 ± 3 mg/dl. This minor

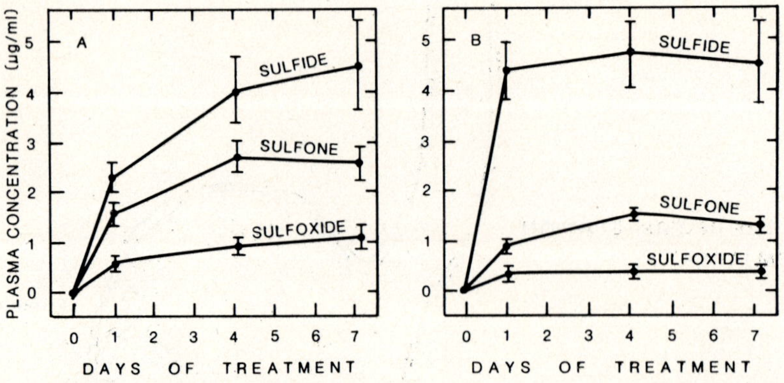

Fig. 2. Mean (±SE) plasma concentrations of sulindac sulfoxide and its metabolites.

Table III. Endoscopic scores for treatment periods

Subject No.	*Placebo (days of therapy)*				*Aspirin (days of therapy)*				*Sulindac sulfoxide (days of therapy)*				*Sulindac sulfide (days of therapy)*			
	0	*1*	*4*	*7*	*0*	*1*	*4*	*7*	*0*	*1*	*4*	*7*	*0*	*1*	*4*	*7*
1	0	0	0	0	0	3	3	2	0	0	0	0	0	0	0	0
2	0	0	0	0	0	3	2	3	0	0	1	0	0	0	1	1
3	0	1	1	1	0	3	3	3	0	0	1	1	0	0	2	0
4	0	1	0	0	0	2	4	3	0	1	2	3	0	1	2	1
5	0	0	0	0	0	4	3	3	0	0	2	2	0	1	1	2
6	0	0	1	0	0	4	3	3	0	0	1	1	0	0	2	1
7	0	0	0	0	0	3	3	2	0	1	1	0	0	2	2	2
8	0	0	1	1	0	1	3	3	0	0	0	0	0	2	2	1
9	0	0	0	0	0	1	0	3	0	0	0	0	0	0	0	0
10	0	1	2	3	0	0	3	1	0	0	0	0	0	0	0	0
11	0	1	2	2	0	3	2	4	0	2	2	1	0	2	2	1
12	0	0	2	1	0	2	3	2	0	1	2	2	0	1	1	1
13	0	2	2	3	0	4	4	4	0	4	2	2	0	1	1	1
14	0	0	0	0	0	3	4	3	0	1	1	2	0	0	0	0
15	0	0	0	0	0	3	3	3	0	0	0	2	0	0	0	0
Median	0	0	0	0	0	3	3	3		0	1	1		0	1	1
Sum of ranks*	0	13.5	12.5	14	0	41	42	42.5	0	16.5	17.5	18	0	19	18	19.5

*For each subject each day, damage caused by a drug is ranked against damage by other drugs (0 = least damage; 3 = most damage). For each drug, all ranks from each subject are summed to represent a damage grade relative to the other drugs, with ideal ''least damage'' sum of ranks = 0, ''maximum damage'' = 45.

difference may be related to prostaglandin inhibition of renal function. There were no changes in urinary sediment.

DISCUSSION

In normal subjects who take oral sulindac, endoscopic evaluation of the gastric mucosa has shown that the drug has a very low propensity to induce mucosal damage; i.e., damage occurs in only a few subjects and is usually slight.[12] The low frequency of gastric mucosal damage in acute endoscopic studies in normal subjects and in long-term studies in patients with arthritis has been thought to be related to sulindac's action as a prodrug. In other words, sulindac in its inactive form (sulfoxide) circumvents a direct action of the drug on gastric prostaglandin synthesis.

The metabolism of sulindac is complicated and includes a reversible reaction between the active sulfide and the inactive sulfoxide forms. There is also a nonreversible oxidation pathway to sulindac sulfone. Although the active sulindac sulfide has negligible renal and low biliary clearance, sulindac sulfide might enter the stomach after sulindac sulfoxide dosing because sulindac and its metabolite undergo enterohepatic circulation.[4,9] If reflux of duodenal contents into the stomach occurs, sulindac sulfide could reflux into the stomach. However, this seems unlikely to be a cause of gastric mucosal damage, because most of the drug in the enterohepatic circulation is in the form of inactive sulfoxide or sulfone derivatives. The low biliary clearance of sulindac sulfide results in an average biliary clearance ratio of 1:12:12 for sulindac sulfide, sulfoxide, and sulfone, respectively.

We used both the active sulindac sulfide and the inactive sulindac sulfoxide and found that both were well tolerated and induced very little damage. The damage induced could not be endoscopically distinguished from the effects of placebo. Studies of aspirin in man have suggested that direct contact with the gastric mucosa is necessary for injury, because there is no change in the gastric mucosal potential difference after intravenous aspirin[10] and because aspirin in the enteric-coated form or with a large quantity of soluble buffer (in which the aspirin remains ionized) is rarely associated with visible gastric injury.[7,13,15,16] Our data suggest that sulindac may not have access to the gastric mucosal cells. The solubility of sulindac is directly related to the pH of the solution, and it is poorly soluble at low pH; for example, the solubility of sulindac sulfide at pH 7 is <0.03 mg/ml and it is <0.002 mg/ml at pH 3 or less, whereas sulindac sulfoxide solubility is 3.0 mg/ml at pH 7 and falls to <0.05 mg/ml at pH 4.8.* This suggests that the lack of injury may be related to insolubility and subsequent poor local absorption.

Available NSAIDs are weak organic acids and are sparingly soluble in water at acid pH.[1,2,17] They are lipid soluble and are not thought to be transported actively; thus the maximum gastric epithelial or interstitial drug concentration will be less than the gastric luminal concentration at acid pH (less than the pKa of the drug) even if there is a neutral pH layer at the epithelial surface. NSAIDs can be ranked by potency (e.g., the concentrations necessary for blocking prostaglandin synthesis), although these rankings fail to correlate with the potential to damage gastric mucosa. For instance, aspirin is less than one-hundredth as effective (on a weight-concentration basis) at inhibiting prostaglandin production as indomethacin,[1] yet aspirin induces more mucosal damage. At pH 7 the solubility of aspirin (pKa 3.5) is approximately 3 mg/ml, well above the range in which it inhibits prostaglandin synthesis. Indomethacin (pKa 4.5), however, is "practically insoluble" at pH 7[2] and even less soluble at acid pH. Other drugs, such as naproxen, tolmetin, and ibuprofen, have weight-concentration potencies 10 to 30 times greater than that of aspirin, but are all less soluble than aspirin. It is tempting to speculate that there is a direct relationship between the potential to induce acute gastric mucosal injury and solubility at acid pH; if so, a scale might be constructed to rank the various NSAIDs as to their potential to damage the gastric mucosa.

*Dobrinska MR: Personal communication, 1984.

References

1. Carty TJ, Eskra JD, Lombardino JG, Hoffman WW: Piroxicam, a potent inhibitor of prostaglandin production in cell culture. Structure-activity study. Prostaglandins **19:**51-59, 1980.
2. Chowhan ZT: pH-solubility profiles of organic carboxylic acids and their salts. J Pharm Sci **67:**1257-1260, 1978.
3. Duggan DE, Hooke KF, Noll RM, Hucker HB, Van-Arman CG: Comparative disposition of sulindac and metabolites in five species. Biochem Pharmacol **27:**2311-2320, 1978.
4. Dujovne CA, Pitterman A, Vincek WC, et al: Enterohepatic circulation of sulindac and metabolites. CLIN PHARMACOL THER **33:**172-177, 1983.
5. Gilbert DA, Surawicz CM, Silverstein FE, et al: Prevention of acute aspirin-induced gastric mucosal injury by 15-R-15 methyl prostaglandin E_2: An endoscopic study. Gastroenterology **86:**339-345, 1984.
6. Graham DY, Smith JL, Dobbs SM: Gastric adaptation occurs with aspirin administration in man. Dig Dis Sci **28:**1-6, 1983.
7. Heftiezer JW, Silvoso GR, Burks M, Ivey KJ: Comparison of the effects of regular and enteric-coated aspirin on gastroduodenal mucosa of man. Lancet **2:**609-612, 1980.
8. Hollander M, Wolfe DA: Nonparametric statistical methods. New York, 1973, John Wiley & Sons.
9. Hucker HB, Stauffer SC, White SD, et al: Physiological disposition and metabolic fate of a new anti-inflammatory agent, cis-5-fluoro-2-methyl-1-[1-p(methyl-sulfinyl)-benzylidenyl]indene-3-acetic acid in rat, dog, monkey and man. Drug Metab Dispos **1:**721-736, 1973.
10. Ivey KJ, Paone DB, Krause WJ: Acute effect of systemic aspirin on gastric mucosa in man. Dig Dis Sci **25:**97-99, 1980.
11. Lanza FL: Endoscopic studies of gastric and duodenal injury after the use of ibuprofen, aspirin, and other nonsteroidal anti-inflammatory agents. Am J Med **77:**19-24, 1984.
12. Lanza FL, Nelson RS, Rack MF: A controlled endoscopic study comparing the toxic effects of sulindac, naproxen, aspirin, and placebo on the gastric mucosa of healthy volunteers. J Clin Pharmacol **24:**89-95, 1984.
13. Lanza FL, Royer GL Jr, Nelson RS: Endoscopic evaluation of the effects of aspirin, buffered aspirin, and

enteric-coated aspirin on gastric and duodenal mucosa. N Engl J Med **303:**136-138, 1980.

14. Musson DM, Vincek WC, Constanzer ML, Detty TE: Analytical methods for the determination of sulindac in metabolites in plasma, urine, bile, and gastric fluid by HPLC using ultraviolet detection. J Pharm Sci **73:**1270, 1984.
15. O'Laughlin JC, Hoftiezer JW, Ivey KJ: Effect of aspirin on the human stomach in normals: Endoscopic comparison of damage produced one hour, 24 hours, and 2 weeks after administration. Scand J Gastroenterol **16:**211-214, 1981.
16. Thorsen WB, Western D, Tanaka Y, Morrissey JF: Aspirin injury to the gastric mucosa. Gastrocamera observations of the effect of pH. Arch Intern Med **121:**499-506, 1968.
17. Windholz M, editor: The Merck index, ed 9. Rahway, N.J., 1976, Merck & Co., Inc.

Effects of d,l-verapamil on atrioventricular conduction in relation to its stereoselective first-pass metabolism

After the oral administration of 160 mg pseudoracemic verapamil (80 mg dideuterodextro *(d)* isomer and 80 mg levo *(l)* isomer), the prolongation of the PR interval was assessed in relation to *d*- and *l*-verapamil plasma concentrations. Concentration-effect curves were analyzed with the sigmoidal E_{max} model. Because of stereoselective first-pass metabolism, the mean plasma *d*- to *l*-verapamil concentration ratio of 4.5 ± 1.2 was substantially greater than that of 2.1 ± 0.3 after intravenous dosing. Compared with the concentration after intravenous injection, the total verapamil concentration after oral dosing consisted of a substantially smaller proportion of the more potent *l*-isomer. These differences in isomer composition of the total verapamil plasma concentration as a result of the route of administration explain the diminished negative dromotropic potency of racemic verapamil after oral dosing. The concentration required to reach 50% of the maximum effect (EC_{50}) for total verapamil concentration was 129.0 ± 22.9 ng/ml, which was more than three times higher than that after intravenous injection. To assess the relative contributions of the *d*- and *l*-isomers to overall dromotropic potency, changes in the PR interval were measured after separate oral dosing with 250 mg *d*-verapamil and 100 mg *l*-verapamil. The EC_{50} showed an 11-fold difference between the *l*- (36.9 ± 14.7 ng/ml) and *d*- (363.1 ± 64.2 ng/ml) isomers. The EC_{50} for the *l*-isomer concentration after oral pseudoracemic verapamil (20.2 ± 6.3 ng/ml) did not differ significantly from that after *l*-verapamil alone (36.9 ± 14.7 ng/ml). We conclude that the *l*-isomer determines the negative dromotropic effects of verapamil and that the *d*-isomer is of minor importance. (Clin Pharmacol Ther 38:71-76, 1985.)

Hirotoshi Echizen, M.D.,* Barbara Vogelgesang, M.PSc., and Michel Eichelbaum, M.D. *Bonn, West Germany*

Verapamil is a calcium antagonist with antiarrhythmic, antianginal, and antihypertensive properties.[5] Because of its negative dromotropic effects on atrioventricular (AV) conduction,[6] verapamil has been successful in the treatment of paroxysmal supraventricular tachycardia, atrial fibrillation, and atrial flutter.[12-14,22] Its negative dromotropic effects on AV nodal conduction, which are considered to be responsible for its efficacy in this type of arrhythmia, can be assessed in the surface ECG as a prolongation of the PR interval. Thus verapamil offers the opportunity to investigate by noninvasive methods its antiarrhythmic effects in relation to its plasma concentrations. Studies in healthy subjects have established a close relationship between the verapamil plasma concentration and PR interval prolongation after intravenous and oral dosing.[2,15,19] These studies have shown, however, that at equivalent plasma concentrations, an oral dose is one half to one third as potent as the intravenous dose. The drug preparation used clinically is a racemic mixture of equal amounts of the optical isomers dextro- and levo-verapamil. Studies in dogs[7,11,18,20] have shown that the *l*-isomer is six to 10 times more potent with respect to negative dromotropic effects on AV conduction. It has been proposed that the differences in negative dromotropic potency in relation to route of administration result from stereoselective first-pass metabolism during which the more potent *l*-isomer is preferentially metabolized.[2] As a consequence of stereoselective first-pass metabolism, the total verapamil plasma concentration would consist of a substantially smaller proportion of the more active *l*-isomer after oral dosing than after intravenous injection. If the concentration-effect curve is based on the total verapamil concentration, the curve thus shifts to the right. It would therefore appear that the drug is less potent after oral dosing.

From the Department of Medicine, University of Bonn.

Supported by grants from the Landesamt für Forschung des Landes Nordrhein-Westfalen (4 B 5 FA 886), the Sandoz-Stiftung für Therapeutische Forschung, Dr. Robert PflegerStiftung, and Knoll AG, Ludwigshafen.

Received for publication Jan. 7, 1985; accepted March 15, 1985.

Reprint requests to: Michel Eichelbaum, M.D., Department of Medicine, University of Bonn, Sigmund-Freud-Straβe 25, D-5300 Bonn, West Germany.

*Alexander von Humboldt Fellow.

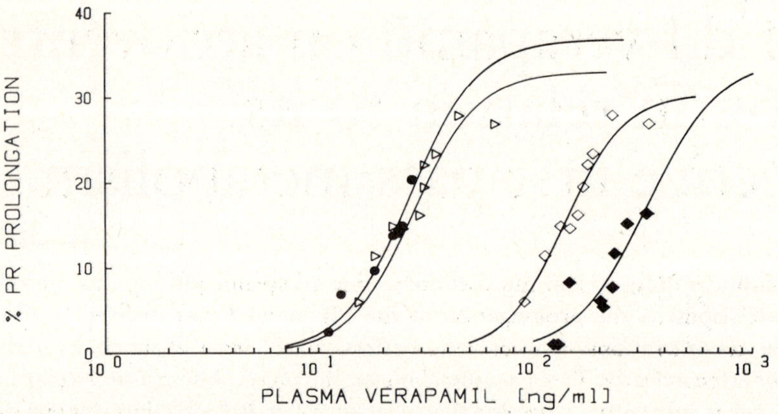

Fig. 1. Relationship between plasma verapamil concentration and percent PR prolongation after oral dosing with 250 mg *d*- (◆), 100 mg *l*- (●), and 160 mg pseudoracemic (◇) verapamil. The curve with the *open triangles* was calculated from *l*-isomer plasma concentrations after pseudoracemic verapamil. (Data from subject 1 in Table I.)

In support of this contention, we recently demonstrated that verapamil exhibits stereoselective first-pass metabolism during which the more potent *l*-isomer is preferentially eliminated.[24] To assess if the stereoselective first-pass metabolism of *d,l*-verapamil could account for the discrepancies in the apparent dromotropic potency according to the route of administration, the changes in the PR interval in relation to *l*- and *d,l*-verapamil concentrations were studied in five healthy subjects after oral dosing with 160 mg pseudoracemic verapamil containing 80 mg of the dideuterated *d*-isomer and 80 mg unlabeled *l*-verapamil. With this stable isotope technique it is possible to measure both isomers after racemic verapamil dosing. In addition, the relative contributions of the *d*- and *l*-isomers to the overall negative dromotropic effects of racemic verapamil were assessed in four subjects who received 250 mg *d*- and 100 mg *l*-verapamil by mouth on separate occasions.

METHODS

Our subjects were five healthy men aged 23 to 27 years weighing 68 to 91 kg. All subjects had normal liver and renal function as assessed by physical examination and appropriate laboratory tests. A standard 12-lead ECG revealed no signs of conduction abnormalities. None of the subjects regularly took any drugs. Two were smokers, but they refrained from smoking for 12 hours before and throughout the study. Beverages containing alcohol or caffeine were prohibited before and throughout the study.

After an overnight fast, subjects received the following verapamil preparations on separate days in random order at least 3 days apart: 160 mg pseudoracemic verapamil, 250 mg *d*-verapamil, and 100 mg *l*-verapamil. The drugs were dissolved in 100 ml carbonated water and were swallowed. Pseudoracemic verapamil was a 1:1 mixture of unlabeled *l*- and dideuterated *d*-verapamil. Two hours after drug dosing subjects ate a normal hospital breakfast. Dideuterated *d*- and unlabeled *l*-verapamil was synthesized in our laboratory according to a recently reported method.[24] Dideuterated *d*-verapamil was 99.8% isotopically pure. Optical purity of *d*- and *l*-verapamil was 99% and 95%. Blood samples were drawn through an indwelling cannula into glass tubes at the following times: 0.25, 0.5, 0.75, 1.0, 1.5, 1.75, 2.0, 3.0, 4.0, 5.0, 6.0, 7.0, 9.0, 11.0, 12.0, 15.0, and 24 hours after dosing. Blood samples were immediately centrifuged at 3000 × g for 10 minutes and separated plasma was stored at −20° C until analyzed.

Plasma verapamil concentrations were analyzed by mass fragmentography with d_7-verapamil as internal standard, as described previously[21] with a recent modification.[3] Unlabeled *l*- and dideuterated *d*-isomers were separately measured at each sampling time after pseudoracemic verapamil dosing. The racemate concentration was calculated as the sum of the isomer concentrations.

Subjects rested at least 30 minutes before baseline ECG measurements and drug dosing. A standard lead II ECG was recorded at a paper speed of 100 mm/sec at each blood sampling. PR intervals were measured by hand and averaged for at least 10 consecutive heart beats. PR interval changes are expressed as percent changes from predose values. The change in PR interval was plotted against the concomitantly measured ver-

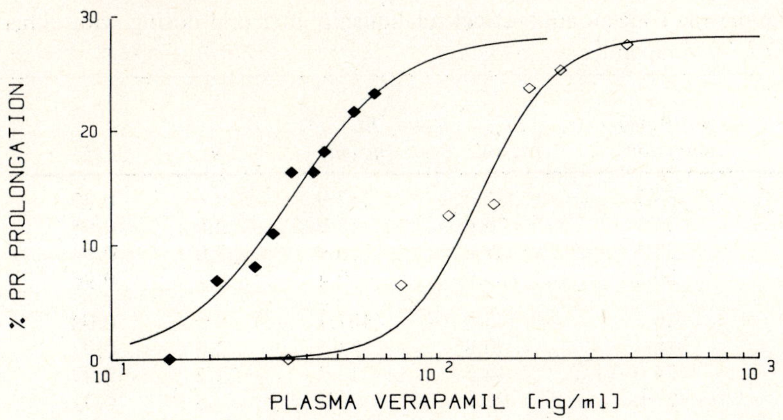

Fig. 2. Relationship between plasma verapamil concentration and percent PR prolongation after 10 mg intravenous (◆) and 160 mg oral (◇) racemic verapamil. E_{max} was identical (intravenous, 28.4%; oral, 28.3%), whereas EC_{50} showed a threefold difference (intravenous, 35.9 ng/ml; oral, 135.9 ng/ml).

apamil plasma concentration to assess the presence or absence of hysteresis. When a hysteresis effect was present, the data points on the slope of the offset part of the curve were used to analyze the plasma concentration-effect relationship.

The plasma verapamil concentration-effect relationship was analyzed by the sigmoidal E_{max} model: $E = (E_{max} \cdot C^N)/(EC_{50}^N \cdot C^N)$, where E is the intensity of pharmacologic effect, C is the plasma drug concentration, E_{max} is the maximum drug effect attributable to the drug, EC_{50} is the drug concentration producing 50% E_{max}, and N is a parameter affecting the shape of the curve. If $N > 1$, then the curve becomes more sigmoidal.[9] Parameters for the E_{max} model were calculated with the nonlinear least-squares regression method.[17] To compare the concentration-effect curves after oral dosing with those after intravenous injection, we used data from a previous study in which all of our present subjects had participated.[1] After oral dosing with racemic verapamil, drug effects were correlated with the total racemate concentration as well as the *l*-isomer concentration.

Data were analyzed by ANOVA. Multiple comparisons among means were by the Student-Newman-Keuls test. A P value <0.05 was considered significant.

RESULTS

The concentration-effect curves of *d*-, *l*-, and racemic verapamil in a representative subject are shown in Fig. 1. Data for all subjects are listed in Table I. There were no significant differences in E_{max} between *d*-, *l*-, and racemic verapamil. Values for EC_{50}, however, differed significantly. Based on the EC_{50}, *l*-verapamil is 3.3 times more potent than racemic verapamil and 11 times more potent than *d*-verapamil. If the concentration-effect curves after oral dosing with pseudoracemic verapamil are calculated only for *l*-verapamil plasma concentrations, these curves are very similar to those obtained after oral *l*-verapamil (Fig. 1; Table I). Thus after oral racemic verapamil, most of the negative dromotropic effect on AV conduction can be attributed to *l*-verapamil.

Fig. 2 shows the concentration-effect curves in subject 5, who received racemic verapamil, 10 mg iv (data from ref. 1) and 160 mg by mouth. Whereas E_{max} was almost identical, there was a 3.7-fold difference in EC_{50} between intravenous and oral dosing. These differences in apparent negative dromotropic potency of the total verapamil plasma concentration can be explained by the different *d*- to *l*-isomer plasma concentration ratios of verapamil after intravenous and oral dosing (Table I). After intravenous dosing the *d*- to *l*-verapamil plasma concentration ratio in this subject was 1.8, whereas after oral dosing this ratio was 6.5. There were similar differences in the *d*- to *l*-verapamil plasma concentration ratio in relation to route of administration in all subjects (data from ref. 1). After intravenous injection the *d*- to *l*-isomer plasma concentration ratio was 1.85, whereas after oral dosing this ratio averaged 4.5. Thus the more potent *l*-isomer was preferentially metabolized after oral racemic verapamil. Because of stereoselective first-pass metabolism, the percentage of the more potent *l*-isomer in the total verapamil plasma concentration was substantially less after oral than after intravenous dosing. The 2.5-fold difference in the *d*- to *l*-isomer plasma concentration ratio was very similar

Table I. Analysis of the plasma concentration-effect relationship after oral dosing with either 250 mg *d*-, 100 mg *l*-, or 160 mg racemic *(d,l-)* verapamil

Subject	Drug form	E_{max} (% PR prolongation)	EC_{50} (ng/ml)	EC_{10} (ng/ml)	N	r^2	d-/l- isomer ratio iv	d-/l- isomer ratio po
1	*d*	34.7	336.4	237.9	2.6	0.80		
	l	36.9	26.6	18.9	2.8	0.95		
	$l_{d,l}$	33.1	27.6	20.9	3.0	0.94		
	d,l	30.5	139.0	110.4	3.1	0.96	1.83	4.2
2	*d*	26.1	445.0	407.1	5.3	0.98		
	l	25.4	40.3	34.5	2.8	0.93		
	$l_{d,l}$	24.0	14.3	12.9	3.2	0.99		
	d,l	27.0	91.9	74.5	2.6	0.91	2.10	3.3
3	*d*	33.9	294.1	204.6	2.4	0.98		
	l	56.3	56.3	33.8	3.0	0.96		
	$l_{d,l}$	76.9	26.4	17.3	4.5	0.96		
	d,l	58.6	137.7	96.5	4.4	0.99	1.37	4.3
4	*d*	36.7	377.0	236.2	2.1	0.98		
	l	46.9	24.5	16.3	3.2	0.96		
	$l_{d,l}$	50.4	16.7	12.7	4.9	0.83		
	d,l	45.6	100.1	89.8	6.1	0.94	2.07	4.3
5	$l_{d,l}$	29.6	16.0	12.1	2.3	0.93		
	d,l	30.4	135.8	102.1	2.5	0.96	1.85	6.5
$\bar{X} \pm SD$	*d*	32.9 ±4.7	363.1 ±64.2	271.5 ±91.7	3.10 ±1.48			
	l	41.4 ±13.2	36.9 ±14.7	25.9 ±9.6	2.95 ±0.19			
	$l_{d,l}$	42.8 ±21.5	20.2 ±6.3	15.1 ±3.8	3.58 ±1.08			
	d,l	38.4 ±13.4	120.9 ±22.9	94.7 ±13.6	3.74 ±1.51		1.84 ±0.29	4.52 ±1.18
	d,l_{iv}	39.9 ±23.6	40.2 ±25.0	21.9 ±8.7	2.80 ±1.11			
	l_{iv}	28.5 ±12.4	15.4 ±10.6	12.5 ±8.1				

(Brackets marked * in the EC_{50} column join *d* vs. *l*, *l* vs. $l_{d,l}$, and *d,l* vs. d,l_{iv}.)

EC_{10} = Drug concentration required to elicit 10% PR interval prolongation; N = parameter affecting shape of curve; r^2 = correlation coefficient; iv = intravenous; po = oral; $l_{d,l}$ = results based on *l*-verapamil concentrations after racemic verapamil; *d,l* and d,l_{iv} refer to data from ref. 1 after intravenous racemic and *l*-verapamil.
*$P < 0.05$.

to the more than 3.7-fold difference in EC_{50} between intravenous and oral racemic verapamil.

DISCUSSION

Our data demonstrate that after oral dosing with racemic verapamil, the *d*- to *l*-isomer plasma concentration ratio is quite different from that after intravenous injection because of stereoselective first-pass metabolism. Furthermore, this study confirms our initial observations and those of other authors that much higher verapamil plasma concentrations are required after oral racemic verapamil to elicit the same prolongation in the PR interval that occurs after intravenous injection.[3,9,19] To assess the relative contribution of the two isomers to the overall negative dromotropic effect of *d,l*-verapamil, the subjects received the *l*- and *d*-isomers on separate occasions. In accord with a recent study from our laboratory in which the effects of *d*-, *l*-, and *d,l*-verapamil on AV conduction in man were studied after intravenous injection, there were similar differences in the negative dromotropic potency between *l*- and *d*-verapamil in our study.[1] No significant differences in E_{max}, EC_{50}, and the shape of the concentration-effect curve were observed for *l*- and *d*-verapamil, irrespective of route of administration. Thus it is rather unlikely that differences in tissue distribution of verapamil according to the route of administration can explain the differences in negative dromotropic potency of racemic verapamil after intravenous and oral dosing, as has been suggested.[10] Our data strongly support the hypothesis that the differences in apparent dromotropic potency of racemic verapamil in relation to route of administration are a result of stereoselective first-pass metabolism, during which the more potent *l*-isomer is preferentially metabolized. In support of this contention are the recent findings that the bioavailability of *l*-verapamil is only 20% compared with 50% for *d*-verapamil.[24] Because of these differences in bioavailability of the *l*- and *d*-isomers, the total verapamil plasma concentration consists of a substantially smaller proportion of *l*-verapamil after oral dosing with racemic verapamil than after intravenous injection. Differences in the apparent dromotropic potency of the total verapamil plasma concentration can be accounted for by differences in isomer composition, because *l*-verapamil is mainly responsible for the effects on AV conduction. Thus after oral dosing the concentration-effect curve is shifted to the right, and it appears that the drug is less potent than after intravenous injection even though the total plasma concentrations of verapamil are identical.

Based on our results, it is unlikely that verapamil metabolites contribute greatly to the negative dromotropic effect of verapamil.[16] Although the fraction of the dose converted to metabolites is the same after intravenous and oral dosing, the concentration-time profile of the metabolites differs because of first-pass metabolism. Because of presystemic elimination, oral doses greatly exceeding the intravenous dose must be given to achieve comparable plasma levels of the parent drug. If active metabolites are being formed during first-pass metabolism, their plasma concentrations will be much higher. Depending on the pharmacologic activity, the metabolites could substantially contribute to the therapeutic effects. If under these circumstances the concentration-effect curves are calculated only with unchanged drug concentrations, the curve is shifted to the left and it would appear that the drug is more potent after oral dosing. Because there were no significant differences in E_{max} and EC_{50} after intravenous and oral *l*- and *d*-verapamil, the contribution of verapamil metabolites to the overall drug effect seems to be of negligible or minor importance.

Verapamil has been extensively used in the treatment of paroxysmal supraventricular tachycardia, atrial fibrillation, and atrial flutter.[12,13,22] The efficacy of verapamil in the treatment of these arrhythmias has been assessed in several studies during long-term dosing.[8,13,23,25] Some investigators have attempted to establish the effective plasma concentration range for the acute termination and for the prophylaxis of supraventricular tachyarrhythmias.[13,22] Our study has demonstrated, however, that the apparent dromotropic potency of verapamil is not related to total plasma concentration but to the *l*-isomer concentration, especially after oral dosing. It has also been shown that there are substantial intra- and interindividual variations in the bioavailability of verapamil during chronic dosing.[4] To date it is not possible to determine *l*- and *d*-verapamil after the dosing of racemic verapamil except by a stable isotope technique. Therefore, plasma level monitoring with conventional analytic methods seems to be of little value in establishing therapeutic plasma concentrations during multiple oral dosing.

We thank Miss J. Casper, Mrs. M. Geisler, and Mrs. R. Korneli for their skillful technical assistance.

References

1. Echizen H, Brecht T, Niedergesäß S, Vogelgesang B, Eichelbaum M: The effect of dextro-, levo- and racemic-verapamil on atrioventricular conduction in man. Am Heart J **109**:210-217, 1985.
2. Eichelbaum M, Birkel P, Grube E, Gutgemann U, Somogyi A: Effects of verapamil on P-R intervals in relation to verapamil plasma levels following single i.v. and oral administration and during chronic treatment. Klin Wochenschr **58**:919-925, 1980.
3. Eichelbaum M, Mikus G, Vogelgesang B: Pharmacokinetics of dextro, levo and racemic verapamil after intravenous administration. Br J Clin Pharmacol **17**:453-458, 1984.
4. Eichelbaum M, Somogyi A: Inter- and intra-subject variation in the first-pass elimination of highly cleared drugs during chronic dosing. Studies with deuterated verapamil. Eur J Clin Pharmacol **26**:47-53, 1984.
5. Ellrodt G, Chew CYC, Singh BN: Therapeutic implications of slow-channel blockade in cardiovasculatory disorders. Circulation **62**:669-679, 1980.
6. Fleckenstein A: Influence of calcium antagonists on normal calcium dependent pacemaker activity. *In* Fleckenstein A, editor: Calcium antagonism in heart and smooth muscle. New York, 1983, John Wiley & Sons, Inc.
7. Gloor HO, Urthalen F: Differential effect of verapamil isomers on sinus node and AV functional region. Am J Physiol **244**:H80-88, 1983.
8. Gonzalez R, Scheinmann MM: Treatment of supraventricular arrhythmias with intravenous and oral verapamil. Chest **80**:465-470, 1981.
9. Holford NHG, Scheiner LB: Understanding the dose-effect relationship: Clinical application of pharmacokinetic and pharmacodynamic models. Clin Pharmacokinet **6**:429-453, 1981.
10. Hamman SR, Todd GD, McAllister RG: The pharmacology of verapamil. V. Tissue distribution of verapamil and norverapamil in rat and dog. Pharmacology **27**:1-8, 1983.
11. Kaumann A, Serur JR: Optical isomers of verapamil on canine heart. Prevention of ventricular fibrillation in-

duced by coronary artery occlusion, impaired atrioventricular conduction and negative inotropic and chronotropic effects. Naunyn Schmeidebergs Arch Pharmacol **292:**21-27, 1976.

12. Klein GJ, Gulamhussein S, Prystowsky EV: Comparison of the electrophysiological effects of intravenous and oral verapamil in patients with paroxysmal supraventricular tachycardia. Am J Cardiol **49:**117-124, 1981.
13. Klein HO, Panzar H, Segni ED, David D, Kaplinsky E: The beneficial effects of verapamil in chronic atrial fibrillation. Arch Intern Med **139:**747-749, 1979.
14. Lang R, Klein HO, Weiss E, David D, Sareli P, Levy A, Guerrero J, Di Segni E, Kaplinsky E: Superiority of oral verapamil therapy to digoxin in treatment of chronic atrial fibrillation. Chest **83:**491-499, 1983.
15. McAllister RG, Kirsten E: The pharmacology of verapamil. IV. Kinetics and dynamic effects after single intravenous and oral doses. CLIN PHARMACOL THER **31:**418-426, 1982.
16. Neugebauer G: Comparative cardiovascular action of verapamil and its major metabolites in the anesthetized dog. Cardiovasc Res **12:**247-254, 1978.
17. Nichols AI, Peck CC: General weighted least squares nonlinear regression program, version 1.0. Bethesda, 1981, Uniformed Service University for the Health Sciences.
18. Raschack M: Relationship of antiarrhythmic to inotropic activity and antiarrhythmic qualities of the optical isomers of verapamil. Naunyn Schmeidebergs Arch Pharmacol **294:**285-291, 1976.
19. Reiter MJ, Shand DG, Pritchett EJC: Comparison of intravenous and oral verapamil dosing. CLIN PHARMACOL THER **32:**711-720, 1982.
20. Satoh K, Yanagisawa T, Taira N: Effects on atrioventricular conduction and blood flow of enantiomers of verapamil and the tetrodotoxin injected into the posterior and the anterior septal artery of atrioventricular node preparation of the dog. Naunyn Schmiedebergs Arch Pharmacol **308:**89-98, 1979.
21. Spiegelhalder B, Eichelbaum M: Determination of verapamil in human plasma by mass fragmentography using stable-labelled verapamil as an internal standard. Arzneimittelforsch **27:**94-97, 1977.
22. Sung RJ, Elsner B, McAllister RG: Intravenous verapamil for termination of re-entrant supraventricular tachycardia. Ann Intern Med **93:**682-689, 1980.
23. Tonkin AM, Aylward PE, Joe SE: Verapamil in prophylaxis of paroxysmal atrioventricular nodal re-entrant tachycardia. J Cardiovasc Pharmacol **2:**473-480, 1980.
24. Vogelgesang B, Echizen H, Schmidt E, Eichelbaum M: Stereoselective first-pass metabolism of highly cleared drugs: Studies of the bioavailability of l- and d-verapamil examined with a stable isotope technique. Br J Clin Pharmacol **18:**733-740, 1984.
25. Waxman HL, Myerburg RJ, Appel R, Sung RJ: Verapamil for control of ventricular rate in paroxysmal supraventricular tachycardia and atrial fibrillation of flutter. Ann Intern Med **94:**1-6, 1981.

Food-induced changes in theophylline absorption from controlled-release formulations. Part I. Substantial increased and decreased absorption with Uniphyl tablets and Theo-Dur Sprinkle

Food-induced changes in absorption from two controlled-release formulations of theophylline (Uniphyl tablets [Purdue Frederick Co.] and Theo-Dur Sprinkle [Key Pharmaceuticals, Inc.]) were studied in healthy male nonsmokers. Although the two forms exhibited a theophylline in vitro dissolution rate that was independent of changes in pH from 1 to 8, they showed substantial but opposite food-induced absorption changes. In a 12-subject, three-way, single-dose, randomized, crossover study the bioavailability of theophylline relative to immediate-release aminophylline tablets increased from 53% ± 23% ($\bar{X}$ ± SD) to 96% ± 46% when Uniphyl (two 400 mg tablets) was taken under fasting and nonfasting (high fat content meal) conditions, respectively. On the other hand, in a separate six-subject, two-way, randomized, crossover study, food reduced the bioavailability of theophylline from Theo-Dur Sprinkle: Theophylline bioavailability in the nonfasting state was only 53% ± 9% that in the fasting state. (CLIN PHARMACOL THER 38:77-83, 1985.)

Aziz Karim, Ph.D., Thomas Burns, M.S., Lorraine Wearley, B.S., Janice Streicher, B.S., and Michael Palmer, M.S. *Skokie, Ill.*

Theophylline has a variable and relatively short elimination $t_{1/2}$ averaging 4 hours in children and 8 hours in adult nonsmokers.[4,13] Therapy with immediate-release dosage forms requires repeated 4- to 6-hour dosing to maintain therapeutic serum concentrations. Because multiple daily dosing regimens often result in poor compliance, controlled-release theophylline formulations have become the products of choice for maintenance therapy. Food-induced absorption changes such as decreases in the rate[7,9,11,16] or extent,[12] increases in the rate and extent,[3,6,20] and more erratic[12] or variable theophylline absorption have been reported with controlled-release theophylline.

Recently, Vaughan et al.[20] reported that a meal with a high fat content increased the rate and extent of theophylline absorption from an ultraslow absorbing formulation (Theo-24; G. D. Searle & Co.) with a pH-dependent in vitro dissolution rate. Our objective was to assess food-induced absorption changes with formulations having pH-independent in vitro dissolution rates under conditions similar to those of Vaughan et al.[20]

From Searle Research & Development, a Division of G. D. Searle & Co.

Received for publication Jan. 26, 1985; accepted March 15, 1985.

Reprint requests to: Aziz Karim, Ph.D., Searle Research & Development, Division of G. D. Searle & Co., 4901 Searle Pkwy., Skokie, IL 60077.

METHODS

Dosage forms. The following commercially available drug forms were used: Uniphyl, 400 mg tablets (Purdue Frederick Co.); Aminophyllin, 200 mg tablets (Searle & Co.); and Theo-Dur Sprinkle, 50 and 200 mg capsules (Key Pharmaceuticals, Inc.)

The time course of theophylline in vitro dissolution from the Uniphyl (n = 15) and Theo-Dur Sprinkle (n = 12) forms was determined by the USP basket method in 1000 ml 0.05 mol/L phosphate buffer at pH 6.6 at 37° C and 100 rpm. Additional in vitro dissolution studies at 37° C and 100 rpm were also conducted at a pH between 1 and 8.

Subjects. Twelve healthy male nonsmokers participated in the Uniphyl study and six additional subjects

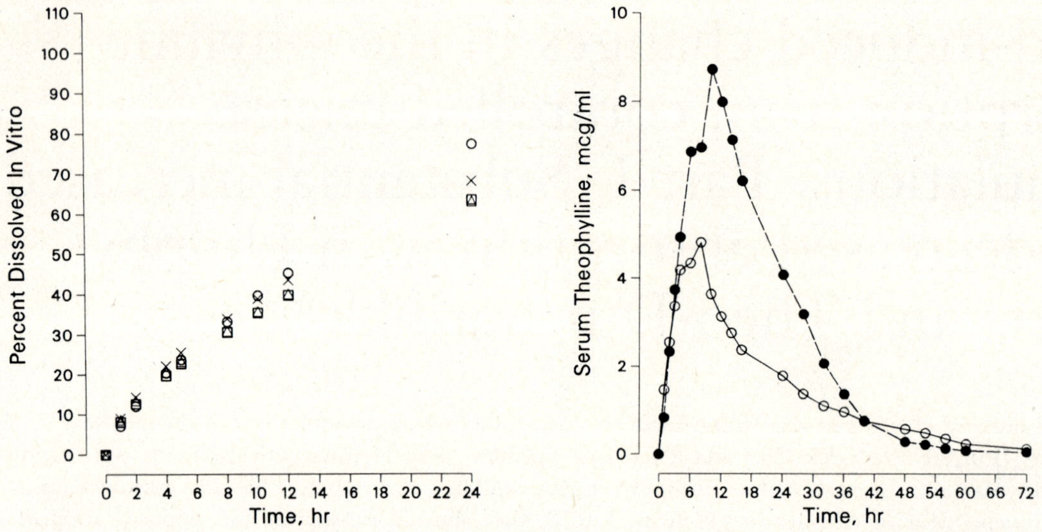

Fig. 1. Left panel, Mean percent theophylline dissolved in vitro from 400 mg Uniphyl tablets (lot 09W) at pH 1.2 (○; n = 3), 6.6 (□; n = 15), 7.5 (△; n = 3), and 8.0 (X; n = 3). **Right panel,** Mean theophylline serum concentration-time curves in 12 healthy male nonsmokers who received 800 mg Uniphyl (two 400 mg tablets) during fasting conditions (○) and immediately after a high-fat breakfast (●).

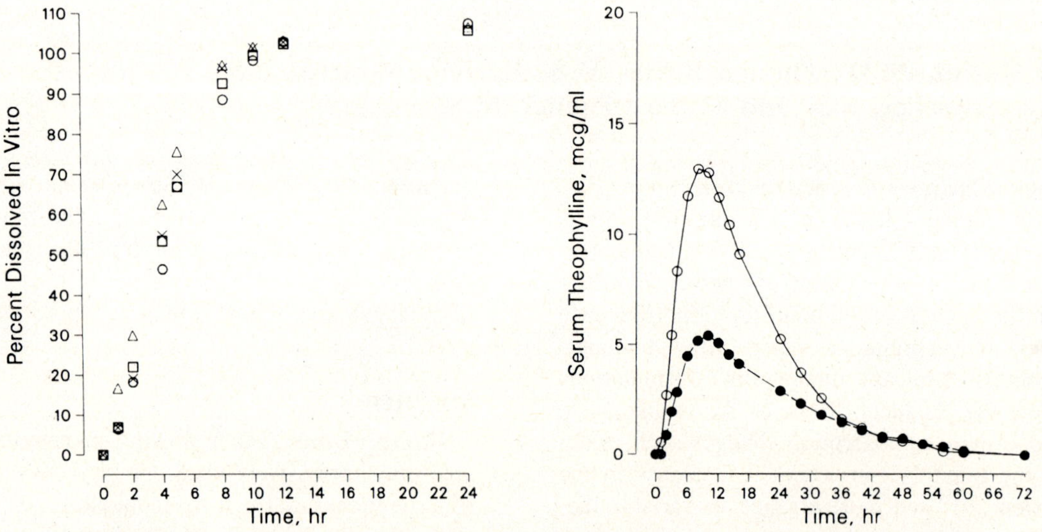

Fig. 2. Left panel, Mean percent theophylline dissolved in vitro from 125 mg Theo-Dur Sprinkle capsules (lot 385841) at pH 1.2 (○; n = 3), 6.6 (□; n = 3), 7.5 (△; n = 3), and 8.0 (X; n = 3). **Right panel,** Mean theophylline serum concentration-time curves in six healthy male nonsmokers who received 900 mg Theo-Dur Sprinkle (four 200 mg [lot 304501] and two 50 mg [lot 265201] capsules mixed with 1 tablespoon applesauce) during fasting conditions (○) and immediately after a high-fat breakfast (●).

participated in the Theo-Dur Sprinkle study. Subjects were judged healthy on the basis of history, physical examination, routine laboratory data, standard ECG, and blood pressure; all subjects weighed within ±10% of the ideal body weight for age and height.

Study design. Ingestion of alcohol- and xanthine-containing food or beverages was prohibited for 48 hours before, during, and 72 hours after each drug dosing. No drug except theophylline was taken by the subjects for 1 week before and throughout each study.

Table I. Theophylline in vitro dissolution characteristics of Uniphyl tablets and Theo-Dur Sprinkle

	Percent labeled dose released		
	Uniphyl 400 mg tablets	*Theo-Dur Sprinkle (N = 12)*	
Time (hr)	*(n = 15)*	*200 mg capsules*	*50 mg capsules*
1	8.1 ± 0.2	6.1 ± 0.4	6.7 ± 0.9
2	12.7 ± 9.3	18.7 ± 1.0	21.4 ± 2.0
4	19.7 ± 0.6	47.2 ± 1.8	51.8 ± 3.6
8	30.6 ± 1.0	89.2 ± 1.9	92.0 ± 3.3
10	35.4 ± 1.4	98.2 ± 1.9	100.5 ± 2.4
12	39.8 ± 1.5	103.1 ± 1.9	104.1 ± 2.4
24	63.7 ± 2.3	—	—

Data are $\overline{X}$ ± SD.

The Uniphyl study was a three-way, randomized, balanced, crossover (7-day washout) study in which each of the 12 subjects received: (a) three 200 mg Aminophyllin tablets (total theophylline dose 480 mg) under fasting conditions, (b) two 400 mg Uniphyl tablets (total theophylline dose 800 mg) under fasting conditions, and (c) the same Uniphyl dose under nonfasting conditions.

Under fasting conditions, subjects fasted overnight for at least 10 hours and for an additional 4 hours after drug dosing and then received the standardized high-fat breakfast.* Under nonfasting conditions the drug was taken immediately after the high-fat breakfast. All doses were taken with 120 ml water. Dosing was done under observation at the clinical facility and standardized diet and activity were observed during the subjects' confinement.

Blood samples for determination of theophylline serum levels were drawn into heparinized Vacutainer tubes (Becton-Dickinson) at 0 (immediately before dosing), 1, 2, 3, 4, 6, 8, 10, 12, 14, 16, 24, 28, 32, 36, 40, 48, 52, 56, 60, and 72 hours after the Uniphyl tablets and at the same times up to 48 hours after Aminophyllin dosing.

The Theo-Dur Sprinkle study was a two-way, randomized, balanced, crossover (7-day washout) study in which each of a separate group of six subjects received a 900 mg dose (the contents of four 200 mg and two 50 mg capsules mixed with 1 tablespoon applesauce) under fasting and nonfasting conditions similar to the Uniphyl study.

Analytic techniques. Serum theophylline concentrations were determined by an enzyme immunoassay system (EMIT; Syva Co.). Between-day coefficients of variation ranged from 3% to 14% at serum concentrations of 0.6 to 20 μg/ml. Concentrations below the 0.6 μg/ml detection limit were considered as zero in all calculations.

Pharmacokinetic and statistical data analyses. Theophylline serum clearance (CL_s) was derived from Eq. 1 from the concentration-time data after a single dose of aminophylline immediate-release tablets:

$$CL_s = \frac{F \cdot D}{AUC_{0\text{-}\infty}} \qquad (1)$$

where F is the fraction of the dose (D) absorbed (F = 1 for aminophylline tablets[17]) and $AUC_{0\text{-}\infty}$ is the serum AUC from time zero to infinity calculated from Eq. 2:

$$AUC_{0\text{-}\infty} = AUC_{0\text{-}t} + \frac{C_t}{k_e} \qquad (2)$$

where $AUC_{0\text{-}t}$ is the serum AUC from time zero to the last measurable data point (derived from the trapezoidal rule) and k_e is the elimination rate constant (derived from regression analysis of the semilogarithmic serum concentration-time curve in the postabsorptive phase). The elimination $t_{1/2}$ was calculated from Eq. 3 as:

$$t_{1/2} = \frac{0.693}{k_e} \qquad (3)$$

The rate and extent of theophylline absorption from Uniphyl tablets were assessed from Eq. 4, a modification[24] of the Wagner-Nelson method[22]:

$$F_t = \frac{(X_A)_t}{(X_A)_T} = \frac{C_t/k_e + AUC_{0\text{-}t}}{AUC_{0\text{-}\infty}} \qquad (4)$$

where F_t is the fraction of the administered dose absorbed at each time t, $(X_A)_t$ is the amount absorbed up to time t, and $(X_A)_T$ is the total amount of drug available for absorption (i.e., the dose given).

*The breakfast consisted of two slices of toasted white bread with butter, two eggs fried in butter, two slices of bacon, 2 oz hash-browned potatoes, and 8 oz whole milk (approximately 33 gm protein, 55 gm fat, and 58 gm carbohydrate; 850 calories).

Table II. Subject characteristics of and theophylline disposition in 12 subjects in the Uniphyl fasting and nonfasting studies

Subject characteristics							*Theophylline disposition (dose 480 mg theophylline as IR product)*					
Number	*Age (yr)*	*Weight (kg)*	*Height (cm)*	*Randomization schedule**			C_{max} (μg/ml)	t_{max} (hr)	AUC_{0-t} (μg · hr/ml)	CL_s (ml/min/kg)	k_e (hr^{-1})	$t_{1/2}$ (hr)
1	26	69.1	164	U-F	IR	U-NF	14.6	2.0	192	0.60	0.104	6.66
2	25	74.8	162	U-NF	IR	U-F	12.3	2.0	115	0.93	0.128	5.41
3	33	67.5	177	U-NF	U-F	IR	14.0	2.0	101	1.17	0.204	3.40
4	23	70.5	170	IR	U-NF	U-F	13.5	1.0	89	1.28	0.188	3.69
5	31	65.2	161	IR	U-F	U-NF	8.6	4.0	80	1.53	0.178	3.89
6	29	65.9	184	U-NF	U-F	IR	16.7	1.0	91	1.33	0.200	3.47
7	31	70.8	162	IR	U-F	U-NF	12.6	1.0	90	1.26	0.180	3.85
8	40	82.0	187	U-F	IR	U-NF	9.4	3.0	107	0.91	0.128	5.41
9	32	71.4	171	U-NF	IR	U-F	11.8	1.0	87	1.29	0.178	3.89
10	25	78.7	177	IR	U-NF	U-F	11.3	3.0	133	0.76	0.103	6.73
11	35	74.5	174	U-F	U-NF	IR	12.4	3.0	168	0.64	0.113	6.13
12	36	79.6	175	U-F	U-NF	IR	12.9	2.0	158	0.64	0.099	7.00
$\bar{X}$	31	72.5	172	—	—	—	12.5	2.1	118	1.03	0.150	4.96
SD	5	5.5	9	—	—	—	2.2	1.0	37	0.32	0.041	1.41

*IR = Three 200 mg Aminophyllin immediate-release tablets (total dose 480 mg theophylline) under fasting conditions; U-F = two 400 mg Uniphyl tablets (total dose 800 mg theophylline) under fasting conditions; U-NF = two 400 mg Uniphyl tablets (total dose 800 mg theophylline) immediately after a high-fat breakfast.

Table III. Cumulative fraction of the dose absorbed after single 800 mg dose of Uniphyl (two 400 mg tablets) under fasting (F) and nonfasting (NF) conditions

	Fraction of dose absorbed		
Time (hr)	*F (n = 12)*	*NF (n = 12)*	*NF* (n = 11)*
2	0.11 ± 0.03	0.10 ± 0.04	0.09 ± 0.03
4	0.20 ± 0.04	0.23 ± 0.09	0.22 ± 0.07
8	0.29 ± 0.07	0.45 ± 0.19	0.41 ± 0.12
12	0.34 ± 0.09	0.66 ± 0.26	0.59 ± 0.12
16	0.37 ± 0.12	0.75 ± 0.34	0.66 ± 0.14
24	0.44 ± 0.17	0.89 ± 0.44	0.77 ± 0.13
48	0.52 ± 0.22	0.96 ± 0.46	0.83 ± 0.12
72	0.53 ± 0.23	0.96 ± 0.46	0.83 ± 0.12

Data are $\bar{X}$ ± SD.
*One of the subjects (no. 5) had an artifactually high fraction of the dose absorbed (2.38). Absorption data for this subject have been deleted in computing the values in this column.

Statistical comparisons of the model-independent pharmacokinetic parameters peak concentration (C_{max}), time to C_{max} (t_{max}), and AUC for the Uniphyl study were by univariate repeated-measures ANOVA. The ANOVA model included terms for individual subjects, treatment, sequence of treatment, period of treatment, and treatment by period interaction. The fraction absorbed was compared for Uniphyl under fasting and nonfasting conditions by the paired t test. For the Theo-Dur Sprinkle study, C_{max}, t_{max}, and AUC were analyzed with an ANOVA model consisting of terms for individual subjects, treatment, sequence of treatment, and period of treatment.

RESULTS

In vitro dissolution profiles. Theophylline dissolution from 400 mg Uniphyl tablets was extremely slow (Table I) and amounted to 39.8% ± 1.5% ($\bar{X}$ ± SD) and 63.7% ± 2.3% at 12 and 24 hours, respectively. For Theo-Dur Sprinkle the dissolution rate was more rapid and at 12 hours amounted to 104.1% ± 2.4% from the 50 mg capsules and 103.1% ± 1.9% from the 200 mg capsules. These dissolution rates did not change substantially between pH 1 and 8 for both Uniphyl and Theo-Dur Sprinkle (Figs. 1 and 2).

Effect of food and bioavailability with Uniphyl. Subjects participating in the Uniphyl study had mean theophylline elimination $t_{1/2}$ and CL_s values of 4.96 hours (range 3.40 to 7.00 hours) and 1.03 ml/min/kg (range 0.60 to 1.53 ml/min/kg; Table II). The time course of the fraction of the theophylline dose absorbed under fasting and nonfasting conditions is listed in Table III. Marked enhancement of theophylline absorption from 53% ± 23% to 96% ± 46% occurred when the conditions were changed from fasting to nonfasting, respectively. Almost 100% differences occurred in C_{max}, t_{max}, and AUC_{0-72} values (Table IV).

Effect of food with Theo-Dur Sprinkle. The food

Table IV. Model-independent theophylline pharmacokinetics in 12 healthy male nonsmokers after a single 800 mg dose of Uniphyl (two 400 mg tablets) in the fasting state (F) and immediately after a high-fat breakfast (NF)

Subject No.	C_{max} (μg/ml) F	C_{max} NF	C_{max} NF/F	t_{max} (hr) F	t_{max} NF	t_{max} NF/F	AUC_{0-72} (μg · hr/ml) F	AUC_{0-72} NF	AUC_{0-72} NF/F	Fraction absorbed* F	Fraction absorbed* NF
1	5.8	11.4	1.97	6.0	12.0	2.00	219	286	1.31	0.73	0.91
2	3.7	7.5	2.03	4.0	12.0	3.00	112	172	1.54	0.58	0.90
3	5.3	8.9	1.68	4.0	10.0	2.50	74	145	1.96	0.44	0.87
4	4.2	4.9	1.17	6.0	12.0	2.00	80	132	1.65	0.54	0.90
5	4.9	14.3	2.92	8.0	12.0	1.50	133	315	2.38	1.00	2.38†
6	5.6	4.2	0.75	8.0	24.0	3.00	75	106	1.41	0.49	0.70
7	4.7	8.2	1.74	4.0	8.0	2.00	64	99	1.55	0.43	0.67
8	2.5	9.1	3.64	4.0	12.0	3.00	57	172	3.04	0.32	0.97
9	3.8	8.1	2.13	4.0	12.0	3.00	107	132	1.23	0.74	0.91
10	4.4	7.0	1.59	4.0	10.0	2.50	56	198	3.55	0.25	0.89
11	4.1	10.6	2.59	6.0	10.0	1.67	56	171	3.04	0.20	0.61
12	5.0	9.2	1.84	8.0	10.0	1.25	163	221	1.36	0.62	0.84
$\overline{X}$	4.50	8.62	2.00	5.50	12.00	2.29	100	179	2.00	0.53	0.96
SD	0.92	2.73	0.77	1.73	4.00	0.64	51	67	0.80	0.23	0.46
P value	<0.05			<0.001			<0.001			<0.05	

*Over 72 hours (Eq. 4).
†This outlier contributed to the high standard deviation (see Table II for values without this outlier).

Table V. Subject characteristics, randomization schedule, and model-independent pharmacokinetics of theophylline in six healthy male nonsmokers after a single 900 mg dose of Theo-Dur Sprinkle in the fasting state (F) and immediately after a high-fat breakfast (NF)

Number	Age (yr)	Weight (kg)	Height (cm)	Randomization schedule*		C_{max} (μg/ml) F	C_{max} NF	C_{max} NF/F	t_{max} (hr) F	t_{max} NF	t_{max} NF/F	AUC_{0-72} (μg · hr/ml) F	AUC_{0-72} NF	AUC_{0-72} NF/F
13	23	81.3	178	NF	F	14.9	4.2	0.28	10.0	10.0	1.00	381	155	0.41
14	34	90.6	168	F	NF	15.9	6.6	0.42	8.0	12.0	1.50	335	162	0.48
15	19	78.3	176	F	NF	16.4	9.2	0.56	10.0	10.0	1.00	336	186	0.55
16	29	80.2	182	NF	F	10.4	3.4	0.33	8.0	10.0	1.25	151	94	0.62
17	25	73.0	164	NF	F	8.4	3.6	0.43	8.0	8.0	1.00	141	91	0.65
18	20	64.6	174	F	NF	12.9	5.9	0.46	8.0	8.0	1.00	231	106	0.46
$\overline{X}$	25	78.0	174	—	—	13.2	5.5	0.41	8.7	9.7	1.13	263	132	0.53
SD	6	8.7	7	—	—	3.2	2.2	0.10	1.0	1.5	0.21	103	41	0.09
P value						<0.05			NS			<0.05		

NS = Not significant.
*F = Contents of four 200 mg and two 50 mg capsules mixed with one tablespoon applesauce; total dose 900 mg theophylline administered fasting; NF = contents of four 200 mg and two 50 mg capsules mixed with one tablespoon applesauce; total dose 900 mg theophylline administered immediately after a high-fat breakfast.

effect with Theo-Dur Sprinkle was opposite to that with Uniphyl. There was a marked food-induced decrease in theophylline absorption (Fig. 2; Table V): the decrease averaged 59% for C_{max} and 47% for AUC_{0-72}, while the t_{max} remained essentially unchanged. These findings are similar to those of Pedersen and Møller-Petersen.[12]

DISCUSSION

Theo-Dur Sprinkle is a beaded multiple-unit and Uniphyl a cellulose matrix single-unit controlled-release formulation of theophylline. Although both have pH-independent in vitro dissolution rates, both showed substantial and opposite food-induced absorption changes. Relative to the fasting condition, Uniphyl tablets showed almost a 100% increase while Theo-Dur Sprinkle showed about a 50% decrease in theophylline absorption when taken with a high-fat meal. The mechanism of these absorption changes remains unknown. Because a high-fat meal delays gastric emptying and increases secretion of bile, pancreatic fluid, digestive enzymes, and gastric hormones, one or a combination of these factors may be responsible for the absorption changes. It is apparent from our data that pH dependency in dissolution rate does not alone predict food-induced absorption changes. Innovative in vitro systems that simulate high-fat meal–related in vivo conditions are needed to predict better the food-induced absorption changes from test formulations.

We assessed the rate and extent of theophylline absorption from Uniphyl by the modified[24] Wagner-Nelson method in which the time course of the fraction of the dose absorbed was evaluated with the use of k_e derived from a fully bioavailable immediate-release product. Limitations of this modified method have been discussed by Wagner[21] in view of the great intrasubject variability in theophylline CL_s and k_e reported by Upton et al.[18,19] However, great intrasubject variability was not found in children with asthma.[2] In any case, accurate determination of k_e from an ultraslow absorbing formulation such as Uniphyl cannot be made from the terminal phase of the log concentration-time curve in a single-dose study, even though blood is sampled for 2 to 3 days. With such formulations there is the possibility of a "flip-flop" pharmacokinetic model and/or continued "trickle" absorption. In the assessment of rate and extent of absorption by the modified Wagner-Nelson method, it is assumed that the kinetics of orally administered theophylline follow a single-compartment model and that there is neither dose-dependent nor time-variable pharmacokinetics. Dose-dependent theophylline kinetics have been reported,[8,10,14,15,23] but this can be minimized by adjusting doses of the controlled-release and immediate-release products to give similar ranges of serum concentrations.

The 53% ± 23% ($\overline{X}$ ± SD) theophylline bioavailability from Uniphyl during the fasting state appears to be unusually low. This value may have been slightly underestimated because of prolonged "trickle" absorption beyond a point at which low theophylline serum concentrations could not be assayed (levels <0.6 μg/ml). A more accurate and clinically meaningful value for the extent of absorption is obtained from a multiple-dose study under steady-state conditions in which blood samples are drawn throughout a 24-hour period rather than over one dosing interval; this is to avoid a potential confounding effect from circadian fluctuation in absorption after dosing every 12 hours.[1,3,5] Nevertheless, a single-dose study does provide a simple and convenient method of ascertaining major absorption changes from formulations dosed under fasting and nonfasting conditions.

Because we found pronounced food-induced absorption changes, patients taking Uniphyl tablets or Theo-Dur Sprinkle should be instructed to take these preparations under consistent conditions of fasting or nonfasting states to assure reproducible absorption or clinical response. It is also recommended that further studies with these formulations be done to examine the effect of meal composition and dosing time relative to meal intake on the rate and extent of theophylline absorption.

Clinical phases of the Uniphyl tablet and Theo-Dur Sprinkle studies were conducted at Quincy Research Center, Kansas City, Mo., with John D. Arnold, M.D., as principal investigator. Theophylline serum levels were determined in the Bioanalytical Department of G. D. Searle & Co., under the direction of Charles L. Jeuell, Ph.D.

References

1. Bauer LA, Gibaldi M, Vestal RE: Influence of pharmacokinetic diurnal variation on bioavailability estimates. Clin Pharmacokinet **9**:184-187, 1984.
2. Ginchansky E, Weinberger M: Relationship of theophylline clearance to oral dosage in children in chronic asthma. J Pediatr **91**:655-660, 1977.
3. Hendeles L, Iafrate RP, Weinberger M: A clinical and pharmacokinetic basis for the selection and use of slow release theophylline products. Clin Pharmacokinet **9**:95-135, 1984.
4. Jusko WJ, Schentag JJ, Clark JH, Gardner M, Yurchak AM: Enhanced biotransformation of theophylline in marihuana and tobacco smokers. CLIN PHARMACOL THER **24**:406-410, 1978.
5. Karim A: Commentary on the paper by Weinberger MM: Theophylline QID, TID, BID and now QD? A report on 24-hour dosing with slow-release theophylline formulations with emphasis on analyses of data used to obtain Food and Drug Administration approval for Theo-24. Pharmacotherapy **4**:192-198, 1984.
6. Lagas M, Jonkman JHG: Greatly enhanced bioavailability of theophylline on postprandial administration of a sustained release tablet. Eur J Clin Pharmacol **24**:761-767, 1983.
7. Leeds NH, Gal P, Purohit AA, Walter JB: Effect of food on the bioavailability and pattern of release of a sustained-release theophylline tablet. J Clin Pharmacol **22**:196-200, 1982.
8. Milavetz G, Weinberger M, Vaughan L: Dose dependency for absorption and elimination rates of theophylline. Implications for studies of bioavailability. Pharmacotherapy **4**:216-220, 1984.

9. Osman MA, Patel RB, Irwin DS, Welling PG: Absorption of theophylline from enteric coated and sustained release formulations in fasted and non-fasted subjects. Biopharm Drug Dispos **4**:63-72, 1983.
10. Pancorbo S, Benson J, Goetz D, Moore K, Vaida A, Johnson D: Evaluation of the effect of nonlinear kinetics on dosage adjustments of theophylline. Ther Drug Monitor **5**:173-177, 1983.
11. Pedersen S: Delay in the absorption rate of theophylline from a sustained release theophylline preparation caused by food. Br J Clin Pharmacol **12**:904-905, 1981.
12. Pedersen S, Møller-Petersen J: Erratic absorption of a slow-release theophylline sprinkle product. Pediatrics **74**:534-538, 1984.
13. Penna PM: *In* Herfindal ET, Hirschman JL, editors: Clinical pharmacy and therapeutics. Baltimore, 1979, Williams & Wilkins Co.
14. Sarrazin E, Hendeles L, Weinberger M, Muir K, Riegelman S: Dose-dependent kinetics for theophylline: Observations among ambulatory asthmatic children. J Pediatr **97**:825-828, 1980.
15. Tang-Liu DD, Williams RL, Riegelman S: Nonlinear theophylline elimination. CLIN PHARMACOL THER **31**: 358-369, 1982.
16. Thompson PJ, Kemp MW, McAllister WAC, Turner-Warwick M: Slow-release theophylline in patients with airways obstruction with particular reference to the effects of food upon serum levels. Br J Dis Chest **77**:293-298, 1983.
17. Upton RA, Sansom L, Guentert TW, Powell JR, Thiercelin J-F, Shah VP, Coates PE, Riegelman S: Evaluation of the absorption from 15 commercial theophylline products indicating deficiencies in currently applied bioavailability criteria. J Pharmacokinet Biopharm **8**:229-242, 1980.
18. Upton RA, Thiercelin J-F, Guentert TW, Wallace SM, Powell JR, Sansom L, Riegelman S: Intraindividual variability in theophylline pharmacokinetics: Statistical verification in 39 of 60 healthy young adults. J Pharmacokinet Biopharm **10**:123-134, 1982.
19. Upton RA, Thiercelin J-F, Moore JK, Riegelman S: A method for estimating within-individual variability in clearance and in volume of distribution from standard bioavailability studies. J Pharmacokinet Biopharm **10**: 135-146, 1982.
20. Vaughan L, Milavetz G, Hill M, Weinberger M, Hendeles L: Food-induced dose-dumping of Theo-24, a "once-daily" slow-release theophylline product. Drug Intell Clin Pharm **18**:510, 1984.
21. Wagner JG: Effect of using an incorrect elimination rate constant in application of the Wagner-Nelson method to theophylline data in cases of zero order absorption. Biopharm Drug Dispos **5**:75-83, 1984.
22. Wagner JG, Nelson E: Per cent absorbed time plots derived from blood level and/or urinary excretion data. J Pharm Sci **52**:610-611, 1963.
23. Weinberger M, Ginchansky E: Dose-dependent kinetics of theophylline disposition in asthmatic children. J Pediatr **91**:820-824, 1977.
24. Weinberger M, Hendeles L, Bighley L: The relation of product formulation to absorption of oral theophylline. N Engl J Med **299**:852-857, 1978.

Hemodynamic and respiratory effects of dezocine, ciramadol, and morphine

The hemodynamic and respiratory effects of dezocine and ciramadol, two agonist-antagonist analgesics, were compared with those of morphine in 30 patients undergoing diagnostic cardiac catheterization. Each subject received a single intravenous dose of dezocine (0.125 mg/kg), ciramadol (0.6 mg/kg), or morphine (0.125 mg/kg) in a double-blind fashion. Hemodynamic and respiratory parameters were measured at baseline and 5, 10, and 20 minutes after dosing. Dezocine increased the cardiac index (CI; 2.67 to 2.92 L/min/m^2), stroke volume index (SVI; 43.6 to 47.6 ml/beat/m^2), left ventricular stroke work index (LVSWI; 57.4 to 64.7 gm-m/m^2), and pulmonary vascular resistance (PVR; 105.6 to 154.0 dynes · sec/cm^5). Ciramadol increased the CI (2.78 to 3.22 L/min/m^2), SVI (40.9 to 48.2 ml/beat/m^2), LVSWI (51.1 to 57.9 gm-m/m^2), and mean pulmonary arterial pressure (PA; 14.7 to 18.9 mm Hg). Morphine had no effect on CI, SVI, LVSWI, PA, or PVR, but it significantly lowered systolic and diastolic blood pressures. There were no appreciable changes in heart rate, left ventricular end-diastolic pressure, mean arterial pressure, or mean pulmonary capillary wedge pressure after any of the drugs. All three drugs significantly decreased systemic vascular resistance. There were no clinically significant changes in respiratory parameters. We conclude that dezocine, ciramadol, and morphine have no clinically important adverse effects on cardiac performance. (CLIN PHARMACOL THER 38:84-88, 1985.)

Robert L. Rothbard, M.D., Bernard F. Schreiner, M.D., and Paul N. Yu, M.D.
Rochester, N. Y.

Patients with acute myocardial infarction and coronary artery disease are predisposed to some degree of pulmonary congestion, arterial hypoxemia, a fall in CO, and metabolic acidosis.[7] An analgesic used in such patients should be free of adverse cardiopulmonary effects that could augment the already decompensated cardiac status of the patient. For many years morphine has been the most commonly used analgesic in the treatment of severe pain associated with myocardial ischemia. The adverse effects of morphine such as hypotension and respiratory depression have stimulated research into the use of agonist-antagonist analgesics in cardiac patients.[1,7-9,12,14]

Dezocine, a bridge aminotetralin,[2] is a potent analgesic with opioid agonist and antagonist activity.[11] In man it is at least as potent as morphine (on a milligram basis), with a similar duration of analgesic activity.[5,13,18] Ciramadol, a synthetic benzylamine,[19] is another agonist-antagonist analgesic. It is suggested that 30 to 60 mg ciramadol induces analgesia of the order of that induced by 10 mg morphine.[15] The effects of dezocine and ciramadol on the cardiovascular system have not been evaluated in man, but results of preclinical studies indicate that both may have advantages over morphine, including fewer hemodynamic effects.[10]

Our double-blind parallel study was designed to compare the hemodynamic and respiratory effects of dezocine, ciramadol, and morphine in patients under-

Abbreviations

CI	Cardiac index
CO	Cardiac output
HR	Heart rate
LVEDP	Left ventricular end-diastolic pressure
LVSWI	Left ventricular stroke work index
PA	Mean pulmonary arterial pressure
P_{CO_2}	Arterial carbon dioxide pressure
PCW	Mean pulmonary capillary wedge pressure
P_{O_2}	Arterial oxygen pressure
PVR	Pulmonary vascular resistance
RR	Respiratory rate
SA	Mean systemic arterial pressure
SVI	Stroke volume index
SVR	Systemic vascular resistance
TRP	Total pulmonary resistance

From the Cardiology Unit, Department of Medicine, University of Rochester School of Medicine and Dentistry and Strong Memorial Hospital.
Supported by a grant from Wyeth Laboratories, Philadelphia, Pa.
Received for publication Nov. 28, 1984; accepted March 18, 1985.
Reprint requests to: Robert L. Rothbard, M.D., Cardiology Unit, University of Rochester School of Medicine and Dentistry, 601 Elmwood Ave., Rochester, NY 14642.

going cardiac catheterization for evaluation of chest pain.

METHODS

Our subjects were 30 patients undergoing diagnostic cardiac catheterization for evaluation of chest pain. They were 35 to 69 years old, weighed between 50 and 103 kg, and had not had a myocardial infarction within the preceding 6 months. Patients with evidence of unstable angina pectoris, valvular heart disease, congestive heart failure, or pulmonary, hepatic, or renal disease were excluded. All subjects had an extensive prestudy clinical evaluation that included physical examination, a complete blood count, urinalysis, serum electrolyte determinations, a 12-lead ECG, an echocardiogram, and, when feasible, a treadmill exercise test.

All subjects fasted before the study and had received no premedication. The left brachial artery was cannulated percutaneously for measuring arterial pressure and for drawing arterial blood samples. A 7-F Swan-Ganz catheter (Edwards Labs) was inserted into the right antecubital vein and advanced to the pulmonary artery under fluoroscopic guidance. With the use of the Seldinger technique, a 7-F pigtail catheter was inserted into the right femoral artery and was advanced to the left ventricle. A thermistor was taped beneath the nostril to measure RR. After a 20-minute equilibration period, each subject received a single intravenous injection of dezocine (0.125 mg/kg), ciramadol (0.60 mg/kg), or morphine (0.125 mg/kg) over 15 seconds. Hemodynamic and respiratory performance was assessed before dosing and 5, 10, and 20 minutes thereafter.

The hemodynamic parameters (CO [by the indicator dye dilution technique], HR, PA, PCW, LVEDP, and SA) were measured at each assessment time. The RR, Po_2, Pco_2, and pH were also measured. Standard methods[1,4] were used to calculate the CI, SVI, LVSWI, SVR, TPR, and PVR. Any adverse effects reported by the subject or observed by the investigator were recorded.

Demographic characteristics and baseline hemodynamic and respiratory parameter values were compared among groups by ANOVA and the chi-square test, as appropriate. Within-group changes from baseline in the hemodynamic and respiratory parameters were analyzed by the paired t test; comparisons among the groups were based on one-way ANCOVA with baseline levels as the covariates.

RESULTS

Ten subjects were randomly assigned to each of the three drug groups. There were no significant differences among the groups in demographic characteristics or baseline hemodynamic or respiratory performance. All subjects had had a precatheterization diagnosis of chest pain, coronary artery disease, or stable angina pectoris.

In one subject no data were collected beyond the baseline period, because after receiving dezocine this subject experienced light-headedness, flushing, and arm numbness along with a decreased HR and blood pressure. In the past he had experienced a number of vasovagal episodes that were associated with medical procedures such as starting intravenous infusion, and may have thus experienced a vasovagal reaction. This subject was dropped from the study.

Mean ($\pm$SE) values for all hemodynamic parameters are listed in Table I. At 10 minutes after dosing PA was significantly elevated from baseline (+4.2 mm Hg) in the ciramadol group, but there were no changes in the dezocine or morphine groups. Other recorded pressures (PCW, LVEDP, and SA) did not change significantly in any group. When systolic and diastolic systemic arterial pressures were evaluated separately, however, there were significant decreases in the morphine group. Five minutes after morphine injection the mean systolic blood pressure fell from 146.6 to 140.0 mm Hg, and 20 minutes after morphine the mean diastolic blood pressure fell from 81.0 to 76.4 mm Hg. There were decreases in systolic blood pressure $\geq$10 mm Hg in five of the 10 subjects in the morphine group. There were no decreases in systolic and diastolic blood pressures after dezocine or ciramadol.

The SVR fell from baseline levels 10 and 20 minutes after dezocine injection, 20 minutes after ciramadol, and 10 minutes after morphine. The only significant change in PVR occurred 10 minutes after dosing in the dezocine group (+48.4 dynes · sec/cm^5). There were no significant changes in TPR in any of the drug groups.

There were significant increases from baseline values in the mean CI at 10 minutes (+0.24 L/min/m^2) and 20 minutes (+0.25 L/min/m^2) in the dezocine group and at 20 minutes (+0.44 L/min/m^2) in the ciramadol group. The CI also rose in the morphine group, but the change was not significant. The changes in CO were similar. There were no significant changes from baseline HR in any group. There were significant increases from baseline values in SVI 10 and 20 minutes after dosing in both the dezocine and ciramadol groups. There were also significant increases in LVSWI in the dezocine group at 5 and 10 minutes (+5.1 and +7.4 gm-m/m^2, respectively) and in the ciramadol group at 10 and 20 minutes (+3.7 and +6.8 gm-m/m^2, respectively). Although SVI and LVSWI tended to rise after morphine, the changes were not significant.

Table II shows the effect of the drugs on the respi-

Table I. Hemodynamic effects of dezocine, ciramadol, and morphine

Group	*HR (bpm)*	*PA (mm Hg)*	*SA (mm Hg)*	*LVEDP (mm Hg)*	*PCW (mm Hg)*
Dezocine					
Baseline	61.7 ± 2.8	16.7 ± 1.3	109.7 ± 4.9	18.0 ± 2.0	10.25 ± 0.86
5 min	62.8 ± 3.3	18.2 ± 1.6	112.7 ± 4.3	16.6 ± 1.6	9.63 ± 1.28
10 min	62.6 ± 3.0	20.4 ± 2.0	110.9 ± 4.6	17.1 ± 2.0	10.00 ± 1.21
20 min	63.2 ± 3.1	18.4 ± 1.7	107.6 ± 4.8	15.9 ± 2.1	9.89 ± 1.20
Ciramadol					
Baseline	69.5 ± 3.4	14.7 ± 0.9	99.6 ± 3.0	13.7 ± 2.6	8.10 ± 1.47
5 min	68.9 ± 3.5	17.6 ± 2.3	99.1 ± 3.0	13.9 ± 2.9	8.50 ± 1.70
10 min	68.9 ± 3.5	18.9 ± 2.5*	98.9 ± 2.8	14.4 ± 2.9	8.90 ± 1.88
20 min	68.2 ± 4.4	17.6 ± 2.1	98.0 ± 4.0	14.6 ± 3.0	9.00 ± 1.47
Morphine					
Baseline	66.2 ± 4.2	14.6 ± 1.7	105.0 ± 3.9	14.7 ± 1.9	8.50 ± 1.58
5 min	62.5 ± 3.0	14.3 ± 1.7	102.8 ± 4.2	13.0 ± 1.7	7.40 ± 1.27
10 min	64.9 ± 3.8	14.7 ± 1.4	100.0 ± 5.8	12.7 ± 1.5	7.90 ± 1.20
20 min	65.7 ± 4.2	15.3 ± 1.3	102.5 ± 4.3	13.8 ± 1.6	8.50 ± 1.28

Data are $\bar{X} \pm SE$.
*$P < 0.05$, †$P < 0.01$ compared with baseline.

ratory variables. The mean RR decreased significantly from baseline at 5 and 10 minutes (−2.4 and −3.4 breaths/min, respectively) in the dezocine group and at 5 minutes (−2.0 breaths/min) in the ciramadol group. By 20 minutes after dosing the RR did not differ significantly from baseline in either group. Morphine had no effect on the RR. Although the mean values for pH never fell below 7.41, there were decreases from baseline values at every assessment point for all three groups. Changes in Po_2 and Pco_2 were minimal and not clinically important.

Except for one subject (discussed earlier), all adverse effects were mild and did not necessitate withdrawal from the study. In the dezocine and ciramadol groups, dizziness (three and four subjects, respectively) and sedation (three subjects in each group) were the most commonly reported adverse effects. Vasomotor symptoms, including flushing and feeling warm, were the most commonly reported adverse effects in the morphine group (three subjects). There were no significant differences among the groups in frequency of any adverse effect.

DISCUSSION

Our data show that in the doses used, there are differences in the hemodynamic effects of dezocine, ciramadol, and morphine. While the direction of change was generally the same, the magnitude of change differed for each drug. At the doses used, all three drugs had a tendency to induce respiratory depression of a similar degree (indicated by a rise in Pco_2 and falls in Po_2 and pH). The results of others[3,16] who evaluated the respiratory effects of dezocine and morphine in a more comprehensive fashion indicate that after larger doses, the respiratory effects of dezocine differ from those of morphine. While morphine induced dose-related increases in respiratory depression, dezocine has a respiratory depressant ceiling at doses of 20 to 30 mg per 70 kg body weight.[3,16] A similar effect has been reported for nalbuphine[4] and butorphanol,[6] but it is not yet clear if a respiratory ceiling is a general characteristic of the agonist-antagonist analgesics.

In our study the mean PVR increased during the first 10 minutes after dezocine injection and tended to increase after ciramadol injection. These increases in PVR were accompanied by significant increases in PA after 10 minutes in the ciramadol group. There have been similar increases in PA after pentazocine[1,8] and butorphanol.[14] Unlike pentazocine, however, ciramadol did not induce a sustained effect on PA, which remained within the normal range (10 to 20 mm Hg). Mean TPR also increased during the first 10 minutes after dosing in the dezocine and ciramadol groups, although the increases were not significant in either group and were not sustained. It thus appears that at the doses used, the changes in pulmonary hemodynamics after dezocine or ciramadol are not long lasting and are not clinically important. Pulmonary hemodynamics were relatively unchanged in the morphine group.

Systolic and diastolic arterial blood pressures were significantly decreased by morphine. In 50% of the subjects who received morphine there was a fall in systolic arterial blood pressure, which is consistent with literature reports.[1,17] Systolic and diastolic blood pressures were not affected by dezocine or ciramadol.

We found no change in CI or LVSWI after morphine.

CI (L/min/m²)	SVI (ml/beat/m²)	LVSWI (gm-m/m²)	SVR (dynes · sec/cm⁵)	TPR (dynes · sec/cm⁵)	PVR (dynes · sec/cm⁵)
2.67 ± 0.17	43.6 ± 3.1	57.4 ± 5.3	1765 ± 118	274.9 ± 34.6	105.6 ± 16.5
2.81 ± 0.18	45.1 ± 3.2	62.5 ± 6.2*	1715 ± 98	283.6 ± 35.4	119.7 ± 14.2
2.90 ± 0.19†	47.6 ± 3.5†	64.7 ± 7.1*	1640 ± 89*	305.8 ± 36.6	154.0 ± 18.5*
2.92 ± 0.20*	47.3 ± 3.9*	62.9 ± 7.5	1595 ± 112*	276.8 ± 34.6	125.2 ± 17.6
2.78 ± 0.24	40.9 ± 3.5	51.1 ± 4.7	1661 ± 284	262.3 ± 70.3	94.9 ± 11.3
2.93 ± 0.22	43.3 ± 3.4	53.0 ± 4.2	1528 ± 225	299.9 ± 98.8	144.5 ± 34.4
3.03 ± 0.25	45.1 ± 3.8*	54.8 ± 4.5*	1494 ± 218	319.7 ± 107.5	158.0 ± 36.9
3.22 ± 0.29*	48.2 ± 3.9†	57.9 ± 5.1†	1401 ± 214*	277.6 ± 89.4	124.7 ± 32.1
2.53 ± 0.20	38.2 ± 2.1	49.6 ± 3.4	1882 ± 264	259.3 ± 43.5	101.9 ± 16.6
2.48 ± 0.20	39.5 ± 1.8	51.0 ± 3.1	1858 ± 253	252.1 ± 39.6	119.1 ± 20.7
2.57 ± 0.20	39.9 ± 2.2	50.6 ± 4.6	1734 ± 239*	253.7 ± 37.6	113.1 ± 16.7
2.77 ± 0.30	42.0 ± 2.6	53.6 ± 4.1	1715 ± 255	254.1 ± 37.8	105.6 ± 16.5

Table II. Effects of dezocine, ciramadol, and morphine on respiration

Group	RR (breaths/min)	P_{O_2} (mm Hg)	P_{CO_2} (mm Hg)	pH
Dezocine				
Baseline	14.6 ± 1.3	73.3 ± 3.1	36.1 ± 2.2	7.46 ± 0.1
5 min	12.1 ± 0.8*	63.4 ± 5.1	38.1 ± 2.8	7.43 ± 0.01*
10 min	11.1 ± 0.8*	66.0 ± 2.5*	38.6 ± 1.7	7.42 ± 0.01†
20 min	11.7 ± 0.8	68.0 ± 2.3	39.6 ± 1.5	7.41 ± 0.01‡
Ciramadol				
Baseline	16.7 ± 1.0	73.7 ± 3.6	34.1 ± 0.8	7.47 ± 0.01
5 min	14.7 ± 1.1*	68.7 ± 2.0	35.6 ± 1.3	7.44 ± 0.01*
10 min	15.0 ± 1.0	70.8 ± 2.7	35.7 ± 1.0*	7.43 ± 0.01‡
20 min	15.1 ± 1.3	74.1 ± 2.2	36.7 ± 1.3*	7.42 ± 0.01†
Morphine				
Baseline	16.1 ± 1.0	75.3 ± 2.3	34.0 ± 0.9	7.46 ± 0.01
5 min	14.9 ± 1.2	71.5 ± 2.4†	34.8 ± 0.9	7.45 ± 0.01†
10 min	16.1 ± 1.4	73.4 ± 3.7	34.7 ± 1.1	7.44 ± 0.01*
20 min	15.4 ± 1.5	72.0 ± 2.2	35.5 ± 1.1	7.44 ± 0.1†

Data are $\bar{X}$ ± SE.
*P < 0.05, †P < 0.01, ‡P < 0.001 compared with baseline.

Reported morphine effects on CI and LVSWI have been inconsistent.[1,8,9,14] Dezocine and ciramadol induced a clinically significant and progressive rise in CI, most likely because of decreased afterload (SVR fell significantly after both drugs). There is little evidence that the increases in CI were the result of changes in preload, as LVEDP and PCW did not change.

Our data indicate that relatively low doses of dezocine, ciramadol, and morphine have no major adverse effects on hemodynamic and respiratory performance in stable cardiac patients. Whether the differences in hemodynamic effects between these drugs increase after larger doses is not known. Because dezocine and ciramadol did not reduce systolic and diastolic blood pressures, these drugs may be preferable to morphine in patients with arterial hypotension.

We thank G. S. Littman, Ph.D., and his colleagues for the statistical analyses and M. A. Messick, Pharm.D., for technical assistance.

References

1. Alderman EL, Barry WH, Graham AF, Harrison DC: Hemodynamic effects of morphine and pentazocine differ in cardiac patients. N Engl J Med **287**:623-627, 1972.
2. Freed ME, Potoski JR, Freed EH, Gluckman MI, Malis JL: Bridged aminotetralins. Adv Biochem Psychopharmacol **8**:137-144, 1974.
3. Gal TJ, DiFazio CA: Ventilatory and analgesic effects of dezocine in humans. Anesthesiology **61**:716-722, 1984.

4. Gal TJ, DiFazio CA, Moscicki J: Analgesic and respiratory depressant activity of nalbuphine: A comparison with morphine. Anesthesiology **57:**367-374, 1982.
5. Gravenstein JS: Dezocine for postoperative wound pain. Int J Clin Pharmacol Ther Toxicol **22:**502-505, 1984.
6. Kallos T, Caruso F: Respiratory effects of butorphanol. Clin Pharmacol Ther **21:**A107, 1977.
7. Lal S, Savidge RS, Chhabra GP: Cardiovascular and respiratory effects of morphine and pentazocine in patients with myocardial infarction. Lancet **1:**379-381, 1969.
8. Lee G, Demaria AN, Amsterdam EA, Realyvasquez F, Angel J, Morrison S, Mason DT: Comparative effects of morphine, meperidine and pentazocine on cardiocirculatory dynamics in patients with acute myocardial infarction. Am J Med **60:**949-955, 1976.
9. Lee G, Low RI, Amsterdam EA, DeMaria AN, Huber PW, Mason DT: Hemodynamic effects of morphine and nalbuphine in acute myocardial infarction. Clin Pharmacol Ther **29:**576-581, 1981.
10. Lewis AJ, Kirchner T: A comparison of cardiorespiratory effects of ciramadol, dezocine, morphine and pentazocine in the anesthetized dog. Arch Int Pharmacodyn **250:**73-83, 1981.
11. Malis JL, Rosenthale ME, Gluckman MI: Animal pharmacology of Wy-16,225, a new analgesic agent. J Pharmacol Exp Ther **194:**488-494, 1975.
12. Nagashima H, Karamanian A, Malovany R, Radnay P, Ang M, Koerner S, Foldes FF: Respiratory and circulatory effects of intravenous butorphanol and morphine. Clin Pharmacol Ther **19:**738-745, 1976.
13. Pandit UA, Kothary SP, Kunz N, Pandit SK: Intravenous dezocine (WY-16,225) for postoperative pain relief. Anesthesiology **61:**3A, 1984.
14. Popio KA, Jackson DH, Ross AM, Schreiner BF, Yu PN: Hemodynamic and respiratory effects of morphine and butorphanol. Clin Pharmacol Ther **23:**281-287, 1978.
15. Powell WF: A double-blind comparison of multiple intramuscular doses of ciramadol, morphine, and placebo for the treatment of postoperative pain. Anesth Analg [Cleve]. (In press.)
16. Romagnoli A, Keats AS: Ceiling respiratory depression by dezocine. Clin Pharmacol Ther **35:**367-373, 1984.
17. Thomas M, Malmcrona R, Fillmore S, Shillingford J: Hemodynamic effects of morphine in patients with myocardial infarction. Br Heart J **27:**863-875, 1965.
18. Vinik HR, McFarland L, Wright D, Baker W: Double-blind postoperative study comparing multiple doses of dezocine (WY-16,225) with morphine and placebo. Anesthesiology **57:**A189, 1982.
19. Yardley JP, Fletcher H, Russell PB: A potent benzylamine analgesic: (−)cis-2(a-methylamino-m-hydroxybenzyl)cyclohexanol. Experientia **34:**1124-1125, 1979.

Temporal variation in the disposition of theophylline and its metabolites

The temporal aspects of theophylline disposition are of interest, as there are predictable time-dependent fluctuations in the pulmonary function of patients with asthma and theophylline serum concentrations may vary throughout a 24-hour period. We studied the extent to which there are significant temporal changes in theophylline kinetics and the relative contribution of distribution, metabolism, and excretion to this phenomenon. Eight healthy men received an intravenous dose (6 mg/kg) of theophylline at 8 AM and 8 PM at 1-week intervals. Serum and urine were analyzed for theophylline and its three major metabolites by HPLC. Distribution volumes and total body and nonrenal clearances showed no differences between morning and evening dosing. The elimination rate was 12% greater after morning dosing. Renal clearance was 24% greater after morning dosing and was accompanied by an increased excretion fraction of unchanged theophylline. Based on total urinary metabolite excretion and the metabolite serum AUCs, there was no evidence of time-dependent variation in theophylline biotransformation. Although theophylline renal clearance is greater after morning dosing, it is only a small fraction of the overall drug elimination and does not change the total body clearance after morning or evening dosing. (CLIN PHARMACOL THER 38:89-95, 1985.)

Marie V. St-Pierre, M.Sc.Phm., Michael Spino, Pharm.D., Alan F. Isles, M.B., M.Sc.,* A. Tesoro, and Stuart M. MacLeod, M.D., Ph.D.
Toronto, Ontario, Canada

With the increasing awareness of circadian rhythms in physiologic and pathologic processes, time-dependent variation in drug disposition is of concern.[1,9,20] Such daily cyclic variations might be expected to modify the intended response to and handling of some drugs. Many diseases are associated with temporal variation in the severity and manifestation of symptoms.[4,19,32,38] Several investigators have studied the temporal characteristics of symptom variation in respiratory distress secondary to bronchial asthma,[10,23,26,30] because patients with asthma commonly experience exacerbation of symptoms nocturnally or during the early morning hours.[10] Investigators measured dyspnea and peak expiratory flow rate (PEF) throughout 24-hour periods and found the former to be greatest upon awakening (7 AM) and least in the mid-afternoon.[26] The change in the latter followed a corresponding pattern, with a minimum at 7 AM and a maximum at 3 PM. The clinical observations of increased airway reactivity at predictable times of the day, coupled with observations of variation in theophylline serum concentrations,[14,16,29] form the basis for continued interest in the chronopharmacokinetics of theophylline.

Previous chronokinetic studies of theophylline have used various methodologies, with either intravenous or oral theophylline dosing to patients with asthma or to healthy subjects.[7,8,12,22,25,35] Most studies involving oral dosing concur in the conclusion that the absorptive process is responsible, at least in part, for the different theophylline concentration-time profile after daytime and nighttime dosing.[7,11,22,25,29,35] Investigations involving intravenous dosing are fewer[8,11,12,35] but they disagree about the role of systemic clearance as a determinant of diurnal variation in theophylline serum concentrations.

About 85% of theophylline total body clearance (CL) is attributed to drug biotransformation.[34] The major metabolites of theophylline in man are 1,3-dimethyluric acid (1,3-DU), 3-methylxanthine (3-MX), and 1-methyluric acid (1-MU).[5] The oxidation and demethylation processes that form 1,3-DU and 3-MX are mediated by

From the Faculties of Pharmacy and Medicine, Departments of Pediatrics and Pharmacology, University of Toronto and Division of Clinical Pharmacology, Research Institute, The Hospital for Sick Children.

Supported in part by Medical Research Council of Canada Grant No. MA 8066 and a grant-in-aid from Astra Pharmaceuticals, Canada.

Received for publication Nov. 23, 1984; accepted March 19, 1985.

Reprint requests to: Michael Spino, Pharm.D., Faculty of Pharmacy, University of Toronto, 19 Russell St., Toronto, Ontario M5S 1A1, Canada.

*Present address: Royal Children's Hospital, Herston Road, Brisbane, Australia.

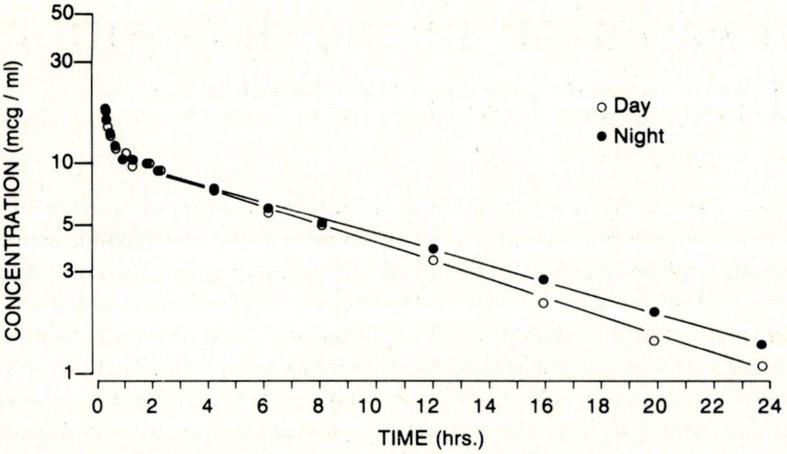

Fig. 1. Mean serum theophylline concentrations after two single intravenous doses (6 mg/kg) at 8 AM and 8 PM in eight normal subjects.

the hepatic microsomal mixed-function oxidase system.[17] An intermediary metabolite, 1-methylxanthine, is oxidized by xanthine oxidase to form 1-MU.[3] In view of the circadian variations in hepatic drug metabolizing enzyme activity in animals,[13,24,36] the possibility of temporal variation in theophylline metabolism should be considered. Renal clearance accounts for the remaining 10% to 15% of CL and is believed to depend on urine flow.[33] Because urine flow varies according to the state of hydration, food and fluid intake, and posture and activity, it may also be subject to underlying circadian influences.[4] Therefore, both renal (CL_R) and nonrenal (CL_{NR}) clearance of theophylline and its metabolites must be considered in assessing the temporal variation in theophylline disposition. Our study was designed to investigate the influence of time of dosing on the kinetics and metabolism of single oral and intravenous doses of theophylline in healthy subjects.

METHODS

Our subjects were 8 healthy nonsmoking men 18 to 25 years old (mean [±SD] weight 70.6 ± 7.0 kg). Subjects were screened by physical examination and baseline laboratory tests. Each subject received four doses of theophylline in random order at 7-day intervals. On two occasions a theophylline dose of 6 mg/kg (aminophylline) was infused intravenously over 15 minutes at 8 AM and 8 PM. On two other occasions the subjects were randomized to receive either 6 mg/kg of a conventional-release tablet (Theolair; Riker Canada, Inc.) or 10 mg/kg of a sustained-release preparation (Theo-Dur; Astra Pharmaceutical Canada Ltd.). The oral studies were part of a larger study reported elsewhere.[27]

An overnight fast preceded the 8 AM doses, while an unsupervised light meal was permitted 3 hours before the evening doses, thus approximating normal dietary patterns. Xanthine-containing foods and beverages were restricted for 48 hours before and 48 hours after each study. During the study day meals were standardized and eaten at 10 AM, noon, and 5 and 10 PM. Subjects were recumbent from midnight to 7 AM and remained seated as much as possible during the day. Blood samples (2 ml) were drawn from the arm contralateral to the injection site immediately before and 5, 10, 15, 25, 45, 60, and 90 minutes and 2, 3, 4, 6, 8, 12, 16, 20, and 24 hours after the infusion. The need for total urine collection was stressed and urine was collected before and at timed intervals for 48 hours after drug dosing. Urine and serum samples were assayed for theophylline and its major metabolites 1-MU, 3-MX, and 1,3-DU by HPLC methods developed in our laboratory.[28]

A two-compartment open model with elimination from the central compartment was fit by computer to the data with a weighting of $1/y^2$ and the nonlinear least-squares regression program ADAPT.[6] CL and CL_R were determined from the model-independent equations: $CL = Dose/AUC_{0-\infty}$ and $CL_R = \Sigma Ae_{0-\infty}/AUC_{0-\infty}$, where $\Sigma Ae_{0-\infty}$ is the amount of theophylline excreted unchanged in the urine up to infinity (48 hours). The fraction excreted unchanged (f_e) was determined as: $f_e = \Sigma Ae_{0-48}/dose_{iv}$, where ΣAe_{0-48} is the total amount of theophylline excreted unchanged within 48 hours and $dose_{iv}$ is the intravenous dose infused.

Table I. A comparison of mean (±SE) theophylline kinetics after 6 mg/kg iv (n = 8) at 8 AM and 8 PM

	8 AM dosing	*8 PM dosing*
β (hr^{-1})	0.112 ± 0.115	0.098 ± 0.011*
V_c (L)	11.2 ± 2.7	14.0 ± 2.0
V_z (L)	31.7 ± 0.9	33.2 ± 1.9
V_{ss} (L)	29.9 ± 0.8	32.3 ± 1.8
$k_{12} \cdot V_c$ (L/hr)	74.7 ± 27.6	40.2 ± 5.4
$k_{21} \cdot V_p$ (L/hr)	49.1 ± 11.1	41.3 ± 5.5
CL (L/hr)	3.58 ± 0.35	3.32 ± 0.38
AUC (μg/ml · hr)	116.4 ± 15.0	127.6 ± 16.1

V_c = Volume of distribution of the central compartment; V_z = volume of distribution of the area; V_{ss} = volume of distribution at steady state; k_{12} and k_{21} = intercompartmental transfer rate constants; V_p = volume of distribution of the peripheral compartment.
P = 0.07 (paired t test).

The CL_R of each metabolite ($CL_{R(mi)}$) was determined from individual concentrations in serum and urine as: $CL_{R(mi)} = Mu_{0-24}/AUC_{(mi)0-24}$, where Mu_{0-24} is the cumulative amount of the metabolite excreted in the urine from time zero to 24 hours and $AUC_{(mi)0-24}$ is the individual metabolite serum AUC after intravenous theophylline.

Student's t test for paired data, Wilcoxon's signed-rank test, and ANOVA were used in statistical analysis of the data.[31] Unless otherwise indicated, data are expressed as $\overline{X}$ ± SE.

RESULTS

Mean theophylline serum concentration-time data plotted on log-linear axes showed a biexponential decline, with a rapid distribution phase and a slower elimination phase (Fig. 1). The computer-fit curves were much the same after both dosing times, but the terminal elimination rate constant (β) was 12% slower after the 8 PM dose (P = 0.07). The CL of the morning dose (51 ml/hr/kg) was similar to that after the evening doses (47 ml/hr/kg), as reflected in the similar AUCs (Table I). The remaining rate constants (α, k_{10}, k_{21}, k_{12}) did not differ significantly, nor did the mean volume terms and mean intercompartmental clearances (Table I).

Concentrations of unchanged drug and major metabolites excreted in the urine were compared after morning and evening dosing. The mean percentage of the dose recovered in the urine after 48 hours (Table II) was not significantly different after morning and evening dosing (97.3% ± 6.6% and 93.5% ± 3.5%), but the mean theophylline f_e was 0.165 ± 0.018 after morning and 0.134 ± 0.012 after evening dosing. Similarly, mean CL_R was higher after morning than after evening dosing (9.6 ± 1.6 and 7.2 ± 0.7 ml/min; Table III).

Table II. Mean (±SE; n = 7) urinary recovery of theophylline and metabolites*

	8 AM dosing	*8 PM dosing*
Theophylline	16.5 ± 1.8	13.4 ± 1.2†
1-MU	20.6 ± 1.5	22.3 ± 2.2
3-MX	14.0 ± 1.7	13.7 ± 1.2
1,3-DU	46.1 ± 3.0	44.2 ± 1.5
Total	97.3 ± 6.6	93.5 ± 3.5

*Values are expressed on a molar basis and represent the amount excreted in 48 hours as percentage of theophylline dose.
†P < 0.05 (Wilcoxon's signed-rank test).

Mean CL_{NR} was similar after morning and evening dosing (49.05 ± 5.76 and 49.97 ± 6.66 ml/min). The mean fraction metabolized (f_m), which is an estimate of the extent of biotransformation, was the same after morning and evening dosing (0.83 ± 0.02 and 0.87 ± 0.01), as was the recovery pattern for metabolites in the urine (Tables II and III). Values for $CL_{R(mi)}$ did not differ significantly for the two dosing times (Table IV). Values for $CL_{R(mi)}$ averaged over both morning and evening theophylline doses were 346 ml/min for 1-MU, 188 ml/min for 3-MX, and 412 ml/min for 1,3-DU.

Individual metabolite serum concentration-time profiles after the intravenous theophylline doses were compared by measurement of the AUC_{mi} from time 0 to 24 hours after dosing. There were no significant differences among any of the three metabolites after morning or evening dosing (Table IV). The mean metabolite serum concentration-time profiles after both dosing times had similar patterns of formation and decay (Figs. 2 and 3). 1,3-DU reached the highest concentrations and appeared to decline in a log-linear fashion after a brief initial plateau. 1-MU serum concentrations appeared to reach a maximum concentration rapidly, maintaining this level for approximately 8 hours. The 3-MX serum concentrations peaked more slowly, with a plateau period for 12 hours or more (Figs. 2 and 3).

DISCUSSION

Preliminary information from our laboratory on theophylline kinetics in five children with asthma[29] suggested that increased theophylline clearance occurred in the evening, contributing to lower serum concentrations. However, interpretation of that study was marred because the subjects had received a maintenance dose of sustained-release theophylline 12 hours before the intravenous study dose and some continued drug absorption might have occurred. The design of our study allowed evaluation of the temporal variation in theoph-

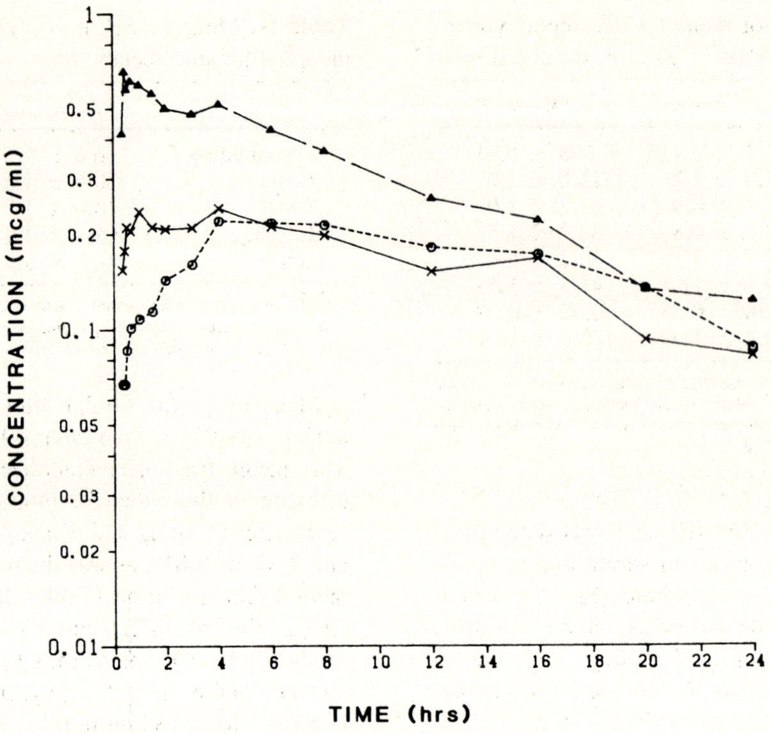

Fig. 2. Mean serum concentrations of 1,3-DU (▲), 3-MX (○), and 1-MU (X) after a single intravenous dose of theophylline (6 mg/kg) at 8 AM in eight normal subjects.

Table III. Mean (±SE; n = 7) theophylline CL_R and CL_{NR} and estimate of fraction metabolized

	8 AM dosing	*8 PM dosing*
CL_R (ml/min)	9.64 ± 1.59	7.20 ± 0.67*
CL_{NR} (ml/min)	49.05 ± 5.76	49.47 ± 6.66
f_m	0.83 ± 0.02	0.87 ± 0.01

*P < 0.05 (Wilcoxon's signed-rank test).

ylline disposition. Our results reveal no significant differences in the CL or volume of distribution of theophylline after intravenous dosing in the morning or evening. The elimination rate constant β was 12% greater after morning dosing but the difference was not significant. Other chronokinetic studies involving theophylline have reported no change in CL[35] as well as altered CL[8] after intravenous dosing. The latter study reported a 17% decrease in CL (P = 0.05) with a 15% increase in the terminal $t_{1/2}$ after nighttime dosing.

The lack of a significant difference in the values for β we report does not rule out the possibility that elimination may, in fact, be marginally greater after morning dosing. It is therefore imperative that the power of the statistical test be considered to assess the risk of committing a type II error. For example, with a power of 0.80 and an α of 0.05, our study would have required a sample of 16 subjects to be able to establish a 12% difference as significant.[31] Because mean CL was slightly greater and the mean volume of distribution tended to be slightly lower after morning dosing, there is a pharmacokinetic rationale for expecting a steeper elimination slope after morning dosing. Results of an additional eight subjects are currently being analyzed to determine whether β may be significantly greater after morning dosing.

We found an increased theophylline CL_R of approximately 24% after morning dosing, accompanied by an increased theophylline f_e. Giacona et al.[8] reported a similarly elevated CL_R during the same time period after intravenous infusion (18% change; P = 0.04). While results of these two studies agreed with respect to the magnitude of the change in CL_R, the lack of a parallel increase in CL in our study was at variance with the earlier report. Giacona et al. suggested that the 18% increase in daytime CL_R was responsible for the 17% increase in CL, but such an increase in CL_R, which

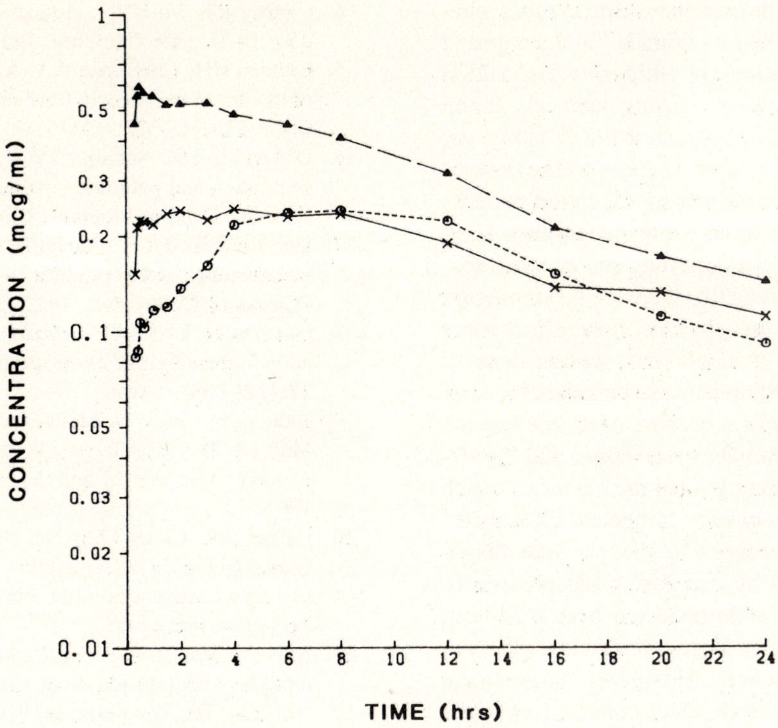

Fig. 3. Mean serum concentrations of 1,3-DU (▲), 3-MX (○), and 1-MU (X) after a single intravenous dose of theophylline (6 mg/kg) at 8 PM in eight normal subjects.

accounts for approximately 15% of CL, combined with constant CL_{NR} such as we found, would be expected to induce only a 3% change in CL. Other factors must therefore have accounted for the increased CL demonstrated by Giacona et al. The 24% increase in CL_R we found theoretically predicts a 4% increase in CL, which is very close to the observed 7.3% mean increase in CL after morning dosing.

The reason for this temporal effect of dosing time on CL_R is not known. Since theophylline CL_R may depend on urine flow,[33] it can be postulated that the increased CL_R is associated with the greater urine volume and, consequently, the enhanced urine flow rate during the day. Urine flow is a variable parameter whose daily maximum and minimum values are closely associated with the excretion of electrolytes such as sodium and chloride.[4] The excretion rate of these solutes declines nocturnally, with lower values from approximately 10 PM to 8 AM.[15] The mean (± SD) urine volume excreted by our subjects from 8 AM to 8 PM was 1510 ± 300 ml and decreased by 20% during the 8 PM to 8 AM period to 1212 ± 189 ml (P = 0.07). If these values are representative of diurnal and nocturnal urine production, the difference in CL_R, which was of a similar magnitude (24%), could be related to circadian variation in urine flow and volume. Another explanation of altered CL_R may be found in the diuretic response to theophylline,[18] which may be less pronounced after evening dosing, thus resulting in proportionately lower urine volume and flow rate. Such a time-dependent alteration in renal mechanisms has been suggested to account for the difference in saliuresis after recumbency, which was less marked at 4 AM than at 7 PM.[21]

Temporal fluctuations in the serum concentrations of a drug subject to microsomal biotransformation might

Table IV. Mean (±SE; n = 8) $CL_{R(mi)}$ and $AUC_{(mi)0\rightarrow24}$

	8 AM dosing	*8 PM dosing*
$CL_{R(mi)}$ (ml/min)		
1-MU	340.7 ± 15.9	351.3 ± 47.3
3-MX	188.2 ± 22.8	188.2 ± 15.7
1,3-DU	431.1 ± 40.6	393.7 ± 40.6
$AUC_{(mi)0\text{-}24}$ (μg/ml · min)		
1-MU	179.7 ± 25.5	193.2 ± 31.2
3-MX	223.7 ± 22.3	232.8 ± 18.6
1,3-DU	419.7 ± 41.2	464.2 ± 46.9

indicate rhythmicity in drug metabolism. Such a phenomenon has been reported in animals[24] and suggested in man to explain variations in antipyrine disposition when data from two separate dosing intervals (noon and midnight) were used to estimate the $t_{1/2}$.[37] However, this possibility does not appear to apply to the case of theophylline. The metabolite urinary excretion patterns and serum AUC_{mi} of the three major metabolites (1,3-DU, 3-MX, and 1-MU) after morning and evening dosing did not differ, suggesting that there are no significant circadian differences in theophylline metabolism when the drug is infused as a single intravenous dose to healthy adults. Theophylline may not be subject to temporal variation in metabolism because of its low hepatic extraction. Studies in animals have shown that the extraction ratio of a drug may govern the extent to which it is subject to time dependency in hepatic clearance.[2]

Time-dependent differences in theophylline disposition were investigated by comparing the pharmacokinetics calculated from data collected over a 24-hour period, which would have been subject to both nocturnal and diurnal influences. However, reassessment of parameters generated from data collected over the first 12-hour period after each dosing did not reveal any differences from findings based on the 24-hour period and did not alter the results of the original morning and evening comparison.

Both earlier studies and our chronokinetic study provide sufficient data to warrant continued research until the extent and therapeutic implications of temporal variation in theophylline disposition are defined. On the basis of our finding of a constant CL in healthy subjects, and in light of the reports of differences in serum theophylline concentrations after daytime and nighttime dosing with oral doses,[7,12,22,28,35] it appears reasonable to conclude that the absorption process rather than metabolism is subject to variation.

We thank J. Correia, R.N., and J. Tanner, R.N., for assistance in the clinical aspects of the study and all the volunteers who participated in the study.

References

1. Aschoff J: Desynchronization and resynchronization of human circadian rhythms. Aerospace Med **40:**844-849, 1969.
2. Belanger PM, Labrecque G, Dore F: Rate limiting steps in the temporal variations in the metabolism of selected drugs. Int J Chronobiol **7:**208, 1981.
3. Birkett DJ, Miners JD, Attwood J: Secondary metabolism of theophylline biotransformation products in man—Route of formation of 1-methyluric acid. Br J Clin Pharmacol **15:**117-119, 1983.
4. Conroy RT, Mills JN: Human circadian rhythms. London, 1970, J&A Churchill, Ltd.
5. Cornish HH, Christman AA: A study of the metabolism of theobromine, theophylline and caffeine in man. J Biol Chem **228:**315-323, 1957.
6. D'Argenio DZ, Schumitzky A: A program package for simulation and parameter estimation in pharmacokinetic systems. Comput Programs Biomed **9:**115-134, 1979.
7. Decourt S, Fodor F, Flouvat B, Pradalier A, Dry J: Pharmacokinetics of theophylline in night workers. Br J Clin Pharmacol **13:**567-569, 1982.
8. Giacona N, Elvin AT, Seligsohn R, et al: Diurnal variation in theophylline elimination. Drug Intell Clin Pharm **17:**452, 1983. (Abst.)
9. Halberg F, Frank G, Matthews J, Aaker H, Gravem H, Melby J: The adrenal cycle in men on different schedules of motor and mental activity. Experientia **17:**282-284, 1961.
10. Hetzel MR, Clark TJH: The clinical importance of circadian factors in severe asthma. *In* Reinberg A, Halberg F, editors: Advances in the biosciences. Toronto, 1979, Pergamon Press Ltd.
11. Isles A, MacLeod S, Levinson H: Theophylline: New thoughts about an old drug. Chest **82:**495-545, 1982.
12. Jonkman JH, VanderBoon W: Nocturnal theophylline plasma concentrations. Lancet **1:**1278, 1983.
13. Jori A, DiSalle E, Santini V: Daily rhythmic variation and liver drug metabolism in rats. Biochem Pharmacol **20:**2965-2969, 1971.
14. Kyle GM, Smolensky MH, Thorne LG, McGovern JP: Indirect monitoring of theophylline blood levels utilizing saliva: A practical noninvasive approach to verifying dosage and understanding temporal variability in pharmacokinetics. *In* Smolensky MH, Reinberg A, McGovern JP, editors: Recent advances in chronobiology of allergy and immunology. Oxford, 1980, Pergamon Press Ltd.
15. Lakatua DJ, Blomquist CH, Haus E, Sackett-Lundeen L, Berg H, Swoyer J: Circadian rhythmic urinary *n*-acetyl-β-glucosaminidase of clinically healthy subjects. Am J Clin Pathol **78:**69-77, 1982.
16. Lesko LJ, Brousseau D, Canada AT, Eastwood G: Temporal variations in trough serum theophylline concentrations at steady-state. J Pharm Sci **69:**358-359, 1980.
17. Lohmann SM, Miech RP: Theophylline metabolism by the rat liver microsomal system. J Pharmacol Exp Ther **196:**213-224, 1976.
18. Maren TH: The additive renal effect of oral aminophylline and trichlormethiazide in man. Clin Res **9:**57, 1961.
19. Millar-Craig MW, Bishop CN, Raftery EB: Circadian variation of blood pressure. Lancet **1:**795-797, 1978.
20. Mills JN, Minors DS, Waterhouse JM: The circadian rhythms of human subjects without timepieces or indication of the alternation of day and night. J Physiol **240:**567-594, 1974.
21. Minors DS, Waterhouse JM: Circadian rhythms of uri-

nary excretion: The relationship between the amount excreted and the circadian changes. J Physiol **321**:39-51, 1982.
22. Primrose WR: Asthma at night. Lancet **1**:927, 1983.
23. Rachiele A, Molo JL, Cartier A, Pineau L, Ghezzo H, Martin RR: Circadian variations of airway response to histamine in asthmatic subjects. Physiology **19**:465-469, 1983.
24. Radzialowski RM, Bousquet WF: Daily rhythmic variation in hepatic drug metabolism in the rat and mouse. J Pharmacol Exp Ther **163**:229-238, 1968.
25. Reed RC, Schwartz HJ: Circadian variation in trough theophylline concentrations. Drug Intell Clin Pharm **17**:444, 1983. (Abst.)
26. Reinberg A, Guillet P, Gervais P, Ghata J, Vignaud D, Albuker C: One month chronocorticotherapy (Dutimelan® 8-15 Mite). Control of the asthmatic condition without adrenal suppression and circadian rhythm alteration. Chronobiologia **4**:295-312, 1977.
27. St-Pierre M, Leeder S, Spino M, Isles A, MacLeod S: Circadian variation in theophylline absorption. Ann Rev Chronopharmacol **1**:81-84, 1984.
28. St-Pierre MV, Tesoro A, Spino M, MacLeod SM: An HPLC method for the determination of theophylline and its metabolites in serum and urine. J Liquid Chromatogr **7**:1593-1606, 1984.
29. Scott PH, Tabachnik E, MacLeod SM, Correia J, Newth C, Levison H: Sustained-release theophylline for childhood asthma: Evidence for circadian variation of theophylline pharmacokinetics. J Pediatr **99**:476-479, 1981.
30. Smolensky M, Harris R, Scott P, MacLeod S, Newth C, Levinson H, Reinberg A: A chronobiological evaluation of a sustained release theophylline compound. *In* Takahashi R, Halberg F, editors: Towards chronopharmacology. Oxford, 1982, Pergamon Press Ltd.
31. Snedecor W, Cochran WG: Statistical methods. Ames, 1980, The Iowa State University Press.
32. Sowers JR, Stern N, Nyby MD, Jasberg KA: Dopaminergic regulation of circadian rhythms of blood pressure, renin and aldosterone in essential hypertension. Cardiovasc Res **16**:317-323, 1982.
33. Tang-Liu DDS, Tozer TN, Riegelman S: Urine flow dependence of theophylline renal clearance in man. J Pharmacokinet Biopharm **10**:351-364, 1982.
34. Tang-Liu DDS, Williams RL, Riegelman S: Nonlinear theophylline elimination. CLIN PHARMACOL THER **31**: 358-369, 1982.
35. Taylor DR, Duffin D, Kinney CD, McDevitt DG: Investigation of diurnal changes in the disposition of theophylline. Br J Clin Pharmacol **16**:413-416, 1983.
36. Tredger JM, Chhabra RS: Circadian variation in microsomal drug metabolising enzyme activities in rat and rabbit tissues. Xenobiotica **7**:481-489, 1977.
37. Vesell ES, Shively CA, Passananti GT: Temporal variations in antipyrine half-life in man. CLIN PHARMACOL THER **22**:843-852, 1977.
38. Wehr TA, Sack D, Rosenthal N, Duncan W, Gillin JG: Circadian rhythm disturbance in manic-depressive illness. Fed Proc **42**:2809-2814, 1983.

Effects of the calcium antagonist tiapamil on pulmonary gas exchange in patients with chronic obstructive pulmonary disease who receive salbutamol

Patients with chronic obstructive pulmonary disease (COPD) and cardiovascular diseases are frequently given combination therapy with a β_2-agonist and a calcium antagonist. Each drug is known to increase ventilation-perfusion inequalities. It was our aim to define the effects of their combination on lung function and on pulmonary gas exchange in eight subjects with COPD but partially reversible airway obstruction. Sixty minutes after placebo or 450 mg tiapamil, subjects inhaled 0.2 mg salbutamol. There was no significant effect of tiapamil on specific airway conductance and the forced expiratory volume in 1 second before or after the inhalation of salbutamol. Blood was drawn 30, 55, 80, and 100 minutes after placebo or tiapamil dosing. After placebo the mean (±SD) arterial oxygen tension (Pa_{O_2}) fell from 67.1 ± 7.3 to 64.4 ± 5.5 mm Hg and the mean alveolar-arterial oxygen tension difference (AaD_{O_2}) rose from 34.6 ± 8.4 to 40.5 ± 6.8 mm Hg. After tiapamil the mean Pa_{O_2} fell from 68.7 ± 7.3 to 66.4 ± 5.8 mm Hg and the mean AaD_{O_2} rose from 35.1 ± 6.8 to 38.7 ± 7.4 mm Hg. The changes in Pa_{O_2} were not significant. The increase in AaD_{O_2} after placebo was significant, but that after tiapamil was not. We conclude that the combination of the calcium antagonist tiapamil and the bronchodilator salbutamol is safe with respect to lung function in COPD. There is no evidence that tiapamil increases β_2-agonist–induced impairment in pulmonary gas exchange. (Clin Pharmacol Ther 38:96-100, 1985.)

Matthias Gugger, M.D., A. Marco Crivelli, M.D., Renato L. Galeazzi, M.D., and Hans Bachofen, M.D. *Berne, Switzerland*

Chronic obstructive pulmonary disease (COPD) is often associated with coronary heart disease and hypertension, which usually requires combined therapy with bronchodilators and cardiovascular drugs. The choice of these drugs deserves careful consideration: Benefits of cardiovascular drugs may be outweighed by adverse effects on pulmonary function, and vice versa. Recent experience suggests that a combination of a calcium antagonist with inhalations of a β_2-agonist may improve hemodynamic performance as well as airway obstruction with a favorable risk-benefit ratio.[7,10,11,14] However, little attention has been paid to the potential risks of this combination. Calcium antagonists and β_2-agonists induce arterial hypoxemia by increasing ven-

From the Department of Medicine, University of Berne.

Supported in part by Hoffmann-La Roche Pharmaceuticals, Basel, Switzerland.

Presented in part at the Third Congress of the European Society of Pneumology, Basel, Switzerland, Sept. 16-22, 1984.

Received for publication Nov. 29, 1984; accepted March 25, 1985.

Reprint requests to: Dr. Matthias Gugger, University of Berne, Department of Medicine, Inselspital, CH-3010 Berne, Switzerland.

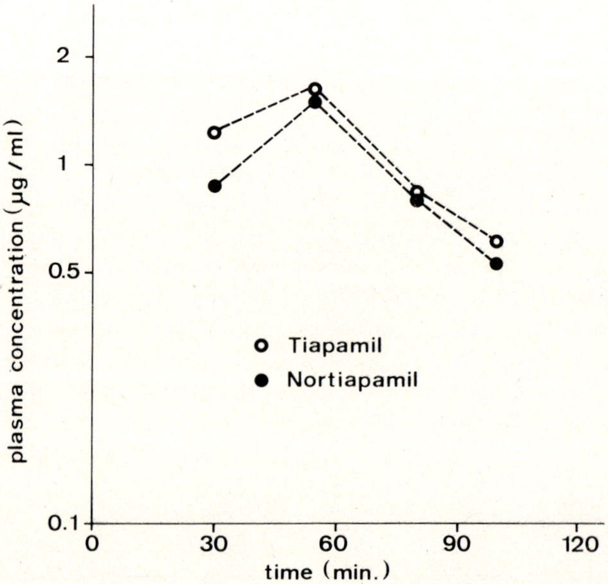

Fig. 1. Average plasma concentrations of tiapamil and its main metabolite nortiapamil during 100 minutes after tiapamil, 450 mg by mouth.

Table I. Subject characteristics before orciprenalin inhalation

Subject No.	*Age (yr)*	*Sex*	*VC (% Pred)*	*RV (% Pred)*	*TLC (% Pred)*	*FEV_1 (% VC)*	*Pa_{O_2} (mm Hg)*	*Pa_{CO_2} (mm Hg)*
1	65	F	73	141	98	56	54	36.8
2	56	M	76	165	102	50	66.5	42.7
3	65	M	68	198	111	49	58	40.7
4	56	M	85	198	118	40	73.5	40.6
5	62	M	70	192	108	33	66.5	43.3
6	42	M	96	122	102	55	65.5	38.9
7	52	M	106	161	121	53	76.5	37
8	56	M	106	145	117	60	73.5	35.8

Pred = Predicted; RV = residual volume; TLC = total lung capacity; F = female; M = male.

tilation perfusion inequalities ($\dot{V}_A/\dot{Q}$) in patients with COPD.[13,15,22,23] Thus an additive effect of both drugs might transiently decrease pulmonary gas exchange and reduce oxygen delivery to sensitive organs. In a randomized, placebo-controlled, double-blind crossover study we examined the combined effect of tiapamil, a calcium antagonist,[24] and standard inhalations of salbutamol on pulmonary gas exchange in eight patients with COPD but partially reversible airway obstruction.

METHODS

Our subjects were eight outpatients with COPD selected by the following criteria: (1) The airway disease was relatively stable; (2) airway obstruction was partially reversible as assessed by a short inhalation of 1.5 mg orciprenaline (increase in forced expiratory volume in 1 second [FEV_1] of >10%); (3) subjects were not receiving steroids and had discontinued all medications and all methylxanthine-containing foods at least 12 hours before the study. Only subject 1 continued regular inhalations every 4 hours; (4) the upper age limit was 65 years; and (5) patients with congestive heart failure, arrhythmias, or liver or renal failure were excluded.

Age, sex, and the results of lung function studies of all subjects before the experiment are shown in Table I. Each subject was studied on 2 consecutive days during the same hours starting at 8 AM. The following parameters were repeatedly determined: FEV_1, specific airway conductance (SGaw), vital capacity (VC), pulse rate, blood pressure, arterial oxygen tension (Pa_{O_2}), arterial carbon dioxide tension (Pa_{CO_2}), pH, and plasma concentrations of tiapamil. VC and FEV_1 were recorded with a water-sealed spirometer. A modified volume-displacement plethysmograph was used to determine SGaw.[6] Arterial blood gases were measured with a blood gas analyzer. An HPLC method on C-18 phase with ultraviolet detection at 278 nm was used to determine tiapamil plasma concentration.[12] The calculation of alveolar-arterial oxygen tension differences (AaD_{O_2}) was based on the "ideal" alveolar air concept, assuming a respiratory exchange ratio of 0.85.[1] For the double-blind, placebo-controlled, crossover study the subjects were randomly assigned to 450 mg tiapamil in a single oral dose or placebo on the first day and the alternate regimen on the second day. Sixty minutes after the subject took tiapamil or placebo, he or she inhaled two puffs of salbutamol (0.2 mg) from a metered-dose aerosol. Arterial blood was drawn through a needle inserted into a brachial artery for gas analyses and for determinations of plasma tiapamil concentrations 30, 55, 80, and 100 minutes after tiapamil or placebo. At the onset of the experiment and 45, 75, 95, 125, and 185 minutes later, values for FEV_1, SGaw, VC, blood pressure, and pulse rate were determined.

RESULTS

The average plasma concentrations of tiapamil and nortiapamil (the main metabolite) are shown in Fig. 1. Thirty, 55, 80, and 100 minutes after 450 mg tiapamil, mean (±SE) tiapamil plasma concentrations were 1.24 ± 0.45, 1.63 ± 0.30, 0.84 ± 0.20, and 0.62 ± 0.19 μg/ml and corresponding mean nortiapamil plasma concentrations were 0.88 ± 0.38, 1.54 ± 0.21, 0.80 ± 0.19, and 0.52 ± 0.07 μg/ml. The time course of plasma concentrations corresponds with reports of other authors.[28] Concentrations before salbutamol inhalation and during the observation period were in the recommended therapeutic range.[28] A carryover effect could be excluded, in that no tiapamil could be detected in the plasma of patients who received placebo.

Figs. 2 and 3 illustrate the effects of the combination on lung function. There was no significant difference in FEV_1 between tiapamil and placebo dosing at any time. Tiapamil did not significantly influence SGaw before or after the salbutamol inhalation; i.e., no modification of bronchodilatory effects of salbutamol was evident. Fig. 3, *A* shows the changes in the arterial

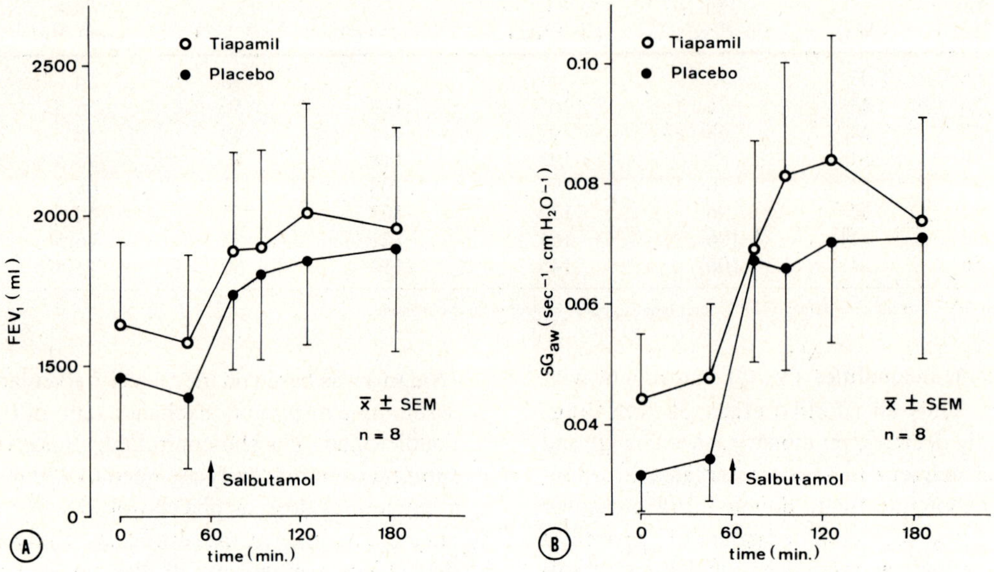

Fig. 2. FEV_1 **(A)** and SGaw **(B)** during 180 minutes after tiapamil, 450 mg by mouth, or placebo. Salbutamol, 0.2 mg, was inhaled 60 minutes after tiapamil or placebo, after the measurement at t = 0.

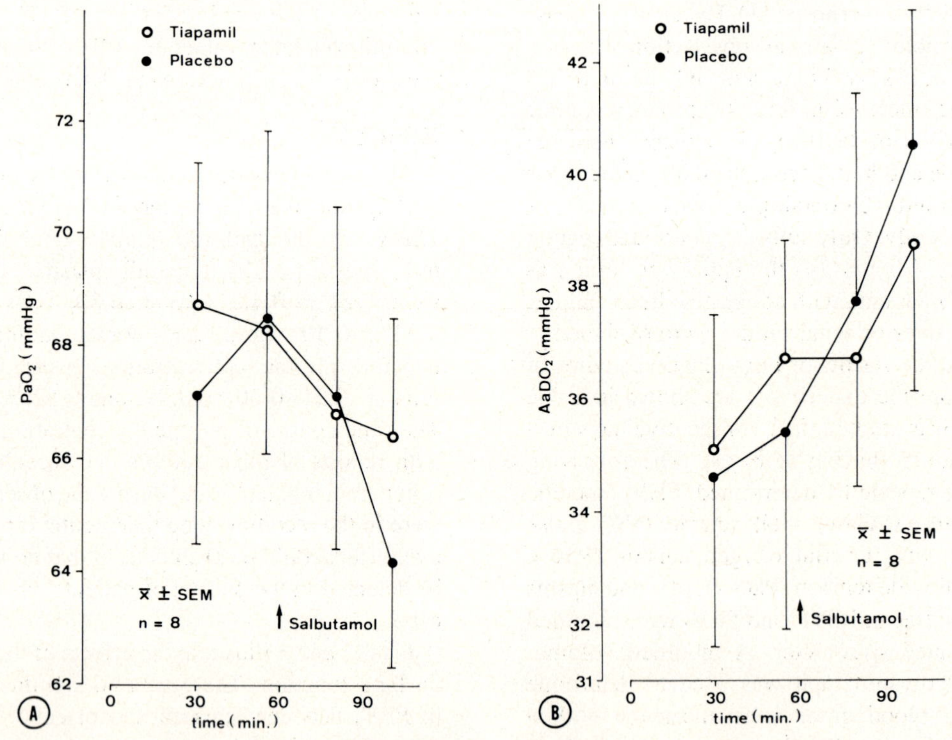

Fig. 3. Pa_{O_2} **(A)** and AaD_{O_2} **(B)** during 100 minutes after tiapamil, 450 mg by mouth, or placebo. Salbutamol, 0.2 mg, was inhaled 60 minutes after tiapamil or placebo, after the measurement at t = 0.

oxygen tensions. There was mild aggravation of the preexisting arterial hypoxemia after bronchodilation, but it appears that the calcium antagonist attenuated rather than accentuated the increased arterial oxygen deficit. Fig. 3, *B* shows that the decrease in Pa_{O_2} predominantly reflects an increase in AaD_{O_2}. The AaD_{O_2} after placebo is significantly increased ($P < 0.05$), but this was not the case after tiapamil.

Although plasma tiapamil concentrations were in the therapeutic range, there were no significant changes in blood pressure and pulse rate in our normotensive subjects, none of whom had heart failure.

DISCUSSION

Possible deterioration of airway obstruction precludes the use of β-antagonists in patients with COPD. Calcium antagonists may be a safe alternative, but it has been shown that calcium antagonists also act on tracheobronchial[8,19,26,27] and pulmonary vascular smooth[15,18,25] muscles. Such effects are rather unpredictable and appear to depend on the preexisting state of the lung, the particular calcium antagonist, and its dose.[3,5,9,17] Information about the combined effects of β-agonists and calcium antagonists on respiratory function in patients with COPD is scarce.

Our short-term study indicates that the calcium antagonist tiapamil does not affect lung mechanics and pulmonary gas exchange, nor does it significantly modify the action of salbutamol. The apparent inefficacy of tiapamil on airway caliber is not surprising. Other evaluations of calcium antagonists indicate that these drugs barely change the resting bronchial tone[4,20] and that, if an adequate dose of β_2-agonists is used, they do not potentiate the bronchodilatory effect of inhalations.[26,27] They seem to prolong the bronchodilatory effect of salbutamol,[16] but it cannot be excluded that tiapamil taken for longer periods might have the same beneficial effect on airway hyperreactivity as nifedipine.[7,10,19]

Tiapamil did not impair pulmonary gas exchange in our subjects with COPD who received salbutamol, but it attenuated a well-known side effect of the β_2-agonists, i.e., the increase of ventilation-perfusion mismatching and the ensuing arterial hypoxemia.[13,22] There is no unequivocal explanation of this finding. It is conceivable that tiapamil has a weaker vasodilatory effect on the pulmonary vessels than other calcium antagonists. Indeed, there is some evidence that different calcium antagonists affect pulmonary vascular tone differently.[5] This result may also well be explained by a tiapamil-induced increase in cardiac output[2] and a corresponding increase in mixed venous oxygen tension as occurs after nifedipine.[23] This clinically important problem might be solved by detailed analysis of the $\dot{V}_A/\dot{Q}$ distribution pattern with a multiple inert gas elimination technique. Our study does not indicate if tiapamil acts differently on pulmonary gas exchange in patients with both COPD and cardiovascular disorders, but there is sufficient evidence that calcium antagonists increase rather than decrease cardiac output in patients with hypertension and angina pectoris.[4,21] It can therefore be reasonably concluded that the drugs improve rather than impair pulmonary gas exchange and oxygen delivery to organs.[15,23]

We thank Dr. M. Eckert, Hoffmann-La Roche Pharmaceuticals, Basel, Switzerland, for the determinations of tiapamil plasma concentrations.

References

1. Bachofen H, Hobi HJ, Scherrer M: Alveolar-arterial N2 gradients at rest and during exercise in healthy men of different ages. J Appl Physiol **34:**137-142, 1973.
2. Bopp P, Mérier G, Scheidegger D, Gabathuler J, Rutishauser W: Acute hemodynamic effects of intravenous tiapamil in patients with coronary artery disease. Cardiology **69**(Suppl 1):91-98, 1982.
3. Brown SE, Linden GS, King RR, Blair GP, Stansbury DW, Light R: Effects of verapamil on pulmonary haemodynamics during hypoxaemia, at rest, and during exercise in patients with chronic obstructive pulmonary disease. Thorax **38:**840-844, 1983.
4. Cerrina J, Denjean A, Alexandre G, Lockhart A, Duroux P: Inhibition of exercise-induced asthma by a calcium antagonist, nifedipine. Am Rev Respir Dis **123:**156-160, 1981.
5. Crevey BJ, Dantzker DR, Bower JS, Popat KD, Walker SD: Hemodynamic and gas exchange effects of intravenous diltiazem in patients with pulmonary hypertension. Am J Cardiol **49:**578-583, 1982.
6. Derron M, Bachofen H: A simple method for computing airway resistance and specific airway conductance from scalar plethysmographic recordings. Respiration **38:**327-331, 1979.
7. Eliraz A, Wishnitzer R, Fink A: Exacerbation of asthmatic symptoms after cessation of nifedipine therapy. Ann Allergy **52:**125-127, 1984.
8. Fanta CH, Drazen JM: Calcium blockers and bronchoconstriction. Am Rev Respir Dis **127:**673-674, 1983.
9. Farber HW, Karlinsky JB, Faling LJ: Fatal outcome following nifedipine for pulmonary hypertension. Chest **83:**708-709, 1983.
10. Gonzalez JM, Morice RC, Bloom K, Akers S, Raizner AE, Stevens PM: Inhibition of airway reactivity by nifedipine in patients with coronary artery disease. Am Rev Respir Dis **127:**155-157, 1983.
11. Griessel HJ, Offermeier J: Investigation of the efficacy of bronchodilator combinations. S Afr J Sci **77:**280-281, 1981.

12. Heizmann P: The determination of tiapamil and nortiapamil in plasma and urine. Roche Research Report No. B-104'657. Basel, 1984, Hoffmann-La Roche Pharmaceuticals.
13. Ishikawa S, Linzmayer I, Segal MS: Gas exchange and arterial blood gas tensions to terbutaline sulfate in older patients with reversible airway obstruction. Ann Allergy **39:**303-305, 1977.
14. Jaiprakash SS, Sahay JN, Chatterjee SS, MacDonald G: Efficacy of nifedipine in the treatment of angina pectoris and chronic airway obstruction. Postgrad Med J **56:**624-628, 1980.
15. Kennedy TP, Michael JR, Huang C, Kallmann CH, Zahka K, Schlott W, Summer W: Nifedipine inhibits hypoxic pulmonary vasoconstriction during rest and exercise in patients with chronic obstructive pulmonary disease. Am Rev Respir Dis **129:**544-551, 1984.
16. Lever AML, Corris PA, Gibson GJ: Nifedipine enhances the bronchodilator effect of salbutamol. Thorax **39:**576-578, 1984.
17. Melot C, Hallemans R, Naeije R, Mols P, Lejeune P: Deleterious effect of nifedipine on pulmonary gas exchange in chronic obstructive pulmonary disease. Am Rev Respir Dis **130:**612-616, 1984.
18. Olivari M-T, Levine TB, Weir EK, Cohn JN: Hemodynamic effects of nifedipine at rest and during exercise in primary pulmonary hypertension. Chest **86:**14-19, 1984.
19. Patakas D, Vlachoianni E, Tsara V, Louridas G, Argiropoulou P: Nifedipine in bronchial asthma. J Allergy Clin Immunol **72:**269-273, 1983.
20. Patel KR: Calcium antagonists in exercise induced asthma. Br Med J **282:**932-933, 1981.
21. Pozenel H: Hemodynamic effects of calcium antagonists in cardiac patients. Cardiology **69**(suppl 1):85-90, 1982.
22. Scherrer M, Bachofen H: Vorteile der Salbutamol-Tacholiquin-gegenüber der Orciprenalin-Tacholiquin-Inhalation bei Bronchialasthma. Schweiz Med Wochenschr **102:**1911-1914, 1972.
23. Simonneau G, Escourrou P, Duroux P, Lockhart A: Inhibition of hypoxic pulmonary vasoconstriction by nifedipine. N Engl J Med **304:**1582-1585, 1981.
24. Singh BN: Use of calcium antagonists in cardiology: Proceedings of the first symposium on tiapamil. Cardiology **69**(suppl 1):1-241, 1982.
25. Sturani C, Bassein L, Schiavina M, Gunella G: Oral nifedipine in chronic cor pulmonale secondary to severe chronic obstructive pulmonary disease. Short- and long-term hemodynamic effects. Chest **84:**135-142, 1983.
26. Svedmyr K, Löfdahl CG, Svedmyr N: Nifedipine—a calcium channel blocker—in asthmatic patients. Allergy **31:**17-22, 1984.
27. Tomioka S, Arai M, Fueki R, Inazawa M, Fueki R, Kobayashi S: The effect of calcium antagonist on bronchoconstriction in asthmatics. Arerugi **31:**1215-1221, 1982.
28. Wendt G: Pharmacokinetics and metabolism of tiapamil. Cardiology **69**(suppl 1):68-78, 1982.

Myocardial ischemia induced by prostacyclin and iloprost

Vasodilators of resistive vessels may induce ischemia in patients with coronary artery disease. To evaluate this possibility during prostacyclin (PGI_2; scalar doses up to 10 ng/kg/min) and prostacyclin analog (iloprost; scalar doses up to 6 ng/kg/min) infusions, we studied 33 patients with angina pectoris and proved coronary artery disease. Patients were also submitted to dipyridamole (0.15 mg/kg/min for 4 minutes) and exercise stress testing (starting at 25 W and increasing 25 W every 2 minutes). In a preliminary study the hemodynamic and side effects of iloprost were studied in seven healthy subjects. At an iloprost dose of 4 to 6 ng/kg/min, these subjects had a significant decrease in mean arterial pressure and total peripheral and pulmonary vascular resistances. Side effects were limited to facial flushing and slight headache and were readily reversible. PGI_2 induced typical chest pain and significant ST segment depression in six patients with severe coronary artery disease (three with left main and three with triple vessel disease) and poor exercise tolerance ($\bar{X} \pm SD = 362 \pm 99$ seconds). All six patients had had angina during the dipyridamole infusion. Similar findings were observed after iloprost infusion in four of these. Aminophylline (125 mg iv) completely relieved chest pain. Although the rate-pressure products occasionally rose during PGI_2 and iloprost infusions, there were no significant changes between ischemic (11.3 ± 2.3 and $10.6 \pm 1.4 \times 10^{-3}$ U) and preischemic (10.8 ± 1.5 and $10.7 \pm 1.4 \times 10^{-3}$ U) rates of infusion. Our data indicate that PGI_2 and iloprost may induce ischemia independently of changes in oxygen demand, and suggest that these drugs dilate small coronary vessels. This may result in decreased subendocardial perfusion pressure and/or "coronary steal." (CLIN PHARMACOL THER 38:101-108, 1985.)

Raffaele Bugiardini, M.D., Marcello Galvani, M.D., Donatella Ferrini, M.D., Claudio Gridelli, M.D., Daniela Tollemeto, M.D., Lucio Mari, M.D., Paolo Puddu, M.D., and Sergio Lenzi, M.D. *Bologna, Italy*

Prostacyclin (PGI_2), a biologic substance produced from arachidonic acid, is under investigation for the treatment of stable and unstable angina pectoris because of its powerful vasodilatory and antiplatelet effects in man.[13,21,30,34] The antiplatelet activity could prevent coronary spasm[31] and intravascular thrombosis.[2,22] The vasodilation may benefit coronary hemodynamics by decreasing left ventricular diastolic pressure[24] and modulating coronary arterial tone.[19] However, drugs that dilate mainly small coronary vessels, such as dipyridamole, may have adverse effects on the distribution of myocardial blood in patients with critical coronary narrowing and, presumably, low poststenotic perfusion pressure.[20,25] Further reductions in coronary pressure distal to the stenosis may account for redistribution of blood away from the subendocardium[4] or diversion of the coronary blood supply from ischemic to nonischemic regions,[5] which may lead to myocardial ischemia.

Although the overall exposure of man to PGI_2 has been broad,[6,7,12,15,17,27,29] there has been no systematic approach to determine its potential adverse effects in patients with coronary artery disease. We assessed the role of PGI_2 in inducing myocardial ischemia in patients with angina pectoris and coronary artery disease. Results were compared with those after an infusion of iloprost, a chemically stable drug with PGI_2-mimetic activities.[3,14,28] The hemodynamics and possible side effects of iloprost were also evaluated in a preliminary study of seven healthy subjects.

METHODS

Preliminary study. Our subjects were three healthy women 40 to 55 years old and four healthy men 45 to 52 years old. All had undergone cardiac catheterization because of atypical chest pain 1 to 2 months earlier and

From Clinica Medica II, Università di Bologna.

Received for publication Nov. 14, 1984; accepted March 27, 1985.

Reprint requests to: Dr. R. Bugiardini, Clinica Medica II, Ospedale Sant'Orsola, Via Massarenti, 9, 40138 Bologna, Italy.

Table I. Changes in heart rate, mean arterial pressure, cardiac index, and mean pulmonary arterial pressure during iloprost infusion (2, 4, or 6 ng/kg/min) in healthy subjects

Subject No.	Age (yr)	HR (bpm) 0	HR 2	HR 4	HR 6	MAP (mm Hg) 0	MAP 2	MAP 4	MAP 6	CI (L/min/m²) 0	CI 2	CI 4	CI 6	MPAP (mm Hg) 0	MPAP 2	MPAP 4	MPAP 6
1	43	74	77	83	86	135	126	125	119	3.85	3.96	4.74	5.03	14	13	14	12
2	55	61	60	59	60	96	87	88	81	4.65	4.30	4.58	4.72	16	17	15	15
3	46	56	60	64	65	107	102	100	96	2.93	3.05	3.92	4.07	10	11	9	9
4	40	58	61	63	71	115	106	107	104	3.54	3.59	4.31	4.93	14	12	12	11
5	45	65	66	74	75	126	123	121	120	3.34	3.12	4.35	4.62	19	16	16	17
6	52	60	59	59	58	100	91	92	87	4.98	4.65	4.89	4.97	15	15	16	16
7	49	70	73	75	78	97	92	89	86	3.18	3.78	4.56	4.61	18	19	17	18
$\overline{X}$	47	63	65	68	70	111	104	103	99	3.78	3.78	4.48	4.71	15	15	14	14
±SD		6	7	9	10	15	16	15	16	0.8	0.6	0.3	0.3	3	3	3	3

HR = Heart rate; MAP = mean arterial pressure; CI = cardiac index; MPAP = mean pulmonary arterial pressure.

Table II. Changes in pulmonary capillary wedge pressure, right atrial pressure, total peripheral resistance, and pulmonary vascular resistance during iloprost infusion (2, 4, or 6 μg/kg/min) in healthy subjects

Subject No.	PCWP (mm Hg) 0	PCWP 2	PCWP 4	PCWP 6	RAP (mm Hg) 0	RAP 2	RAP 4	RAP 6	TPR (dyne · sec/cm⁻⁵) 0	TPR 2	TPR 4	TPR 6	PVR (dyne · sec/cm⁻⁵) 0	PVR 2	PVR 4	PVR 6
1	9	8	8	8	1	2	0	2	1497	1348	1134	1001	156	141	127	103
2	11	9	10	10	3	3	3	2	959	936	889	802	165	189	157	152
3	6	7	8	8	2	1	2	3	1419	1312	990	905	135	143	91	88
4	7	7	6	6	3	2	2	2	1653	1515	1275	1082	207	175	146	117
5	10	9	9	9	2	3	1	2	1642	1699	1220	1129	252	226	163	163
6	9	8	8	8	2	2	3	3	808	785	747	693	124	132	134	132
7	10	8	9	9	4	3	4	4	1314	1058	837	800	254	226	167	176
$\overline{X}$	9	8	8	8	2	2	2	3	1327	1266	1013	935	185	176	136	126
±SD	2	1	1	1	1	1	1	1	328	346	202	168	53	40	26	29

PCWP = Pulmonary capillary wedge pressure; RAP = right atrial pressure; TPR = total peripheral resistance; PVR = peripheral vascular resistance.

at that time showed no evidence of coronary or myocardial abnormalities. No subject had ischemic ECG changes during exercise and ergonovine testing.

A 7F Swan-Ganz thermodilution catheter (Edwards Labs) was placed in the pulmonary artery under fluoroscopy and was continuously perfused with normal saline solution. Arterial blood pressure was continuously recorded through an 18-gauge Teflon cannula inserted into the left brachial artery. The catheter and cannula were connected to a Statham P 23 Db pressure transducer (Statham Instruments, Inc.) and an 863 amplifier for a Mingograf 82 recorder (Siemens Inc.). Cardiac output was measured by the thermodilution technique and was calculated as the mean of three consecutive measurements.

Iloprost was obtained in 1 ml vials (pH 8.3) containing sterile, pyrogen-free solution for injection, Tris buffer, hydrochloric acid, sodium chloride, and ethanol, 96 vol%. The infusion was started at a rate of 2 ng/kg/min and was increased, first to 4 ng/kg/min and then to 6 ng/kg/min. Heart rate, the pulmonary wedge, pulmonary artery, atrial, and arterial blood pressures, and cardiac output were recorded during control and iloprost infusions. The cardiac index and total peripheral and pulmonary vascular resistances were calculated by standard formulas.[33]

Main study. Patients were chosen from a pool referred for exercise stress testing to determine the cause of their chest pain. Only those with interpretable resting ECGs and significant (≥0.1 mV) ST segment depression during exercise testing were included. Patients included 12 with only effort angina, two with rest angina, and 19 with both. The mean age of the subjects (31 men and two women) was 57 years (range 44 to 70 years). None had clinical evidence of heart failure but 13 had a history of myocardial infarction. Coronary arteriography (Judkins technique) revealed significant coronary artery disease in all patients (≥50% reduction in luminal diameter of left main coronary artery, and/or ≥75% reduction in left anterior descending, circumflex, or right coronary artery).

All patients were studied 7 to 14 days after coronary

arteriography. They abstained from caffeinated drinks and alcohol for 12 hours before the study. Long-acting nitrates, calcium antagonists, and β-blockers were discontinued 12 hours, 24 hours, and 1 week, respectively, before the study. Patients underwent an upright cycle ergometer exercise test starting at 25 W, with 25 W increments every 2 minutes. A 12-lead ECG was recorded at rest, peak exercise, and immediately after exercise; three leads (V_1, V_5, and aVF) were continuously monitored by a "CASE" recorder (Marquette Inc.), which provided signal-averaged complexes for accurate computation of the ST segment shifts 0.08 seconds after the J point during the entire stress test. Cuff blood pressures were recorded at 1-minute intervals throughout exercise testing. Testing continued until the onset of severe chest pain, 0.3 mV ST segment depression, or exhaustion.

Patients underwent pharmacologic testing on the days after the exercise test. In the first daily session, dipyridamole was injected intravenously (0.15 mg/kg/min for 4 minutes). On the following morning patients received a PGI_2 infusion; the sodium salt of PGI_2 was dissolved in a glycine buffer at pH 10 and injected at 2° C. In each patient the rate of infusion was progressively increased by 2 ng/kg/min every 5 minutes to a maximum of 10 ng/kg/min or until the occurrence of chest pain. In the last daily session the patients received iloprost. The infusion was begun with 1 ng/kg/min and the dose was increased every 5 minutes in a stepwise fashion to 2, 3, 4, and 6 ng/kg/min.

The ECG was monitored during all the pharmacologic interventions. Cuff blood pressures were recorded at regular intervals. Results of exercise tests and interventions were considered positive if they caused at least 0.1 mV horizontal or downsloping ST segment depression or 0.1 mV ST segment elevation for three consecutive beats or in the average complexes of the "CASE" system. Sixteen patients had chest pain during one or more of the infusions. Pain-relieving drugs were given to patients whose pain continued for >3 minutes. Pain relief was generally provided by 125 mg aminophylline injected over 30 seconds. In five patients, dipyridamole induced severe chest pain; relief was achieved with aminophylline followed by 5 mg sublingual isosorbide dinitrate.

Statistical significance was determined by paired and unpaired Student's t tests. Results are presented as $\overline{X} \pm SD$.

RESULTS

Preliminary study. The hemodynamic effects of iloprost during the preliminary study are listed in Tables I and II. Compared with control values, iloprost infusion at 4 and 6 ng/kg/min reduced mean arterial pressure (from 111 ± 15 to 103 ± 15 and 99 ± 16 mm Hg, respectively) and total peripheral resistance (from 1327 ± 328 to 1013 ± 202 and 935 ± 168 dyne · sec/cm^5). The heart rate and cardiac index progressively increased during the infusion and reached maximum at a dose of 6 ng/kg/min (from 63 ± 6 to 70 ± 10 bpm and from 3.8 ± 0.8 to 4.7 ± 0.3 L/min/m^2). There were no consistent changes in right atrial, mean pulmonary arterial, and pulmonary wedge pressures at any of the infusion rates. Side effects were limited to facial flushing and slight headache and were readily reversible.

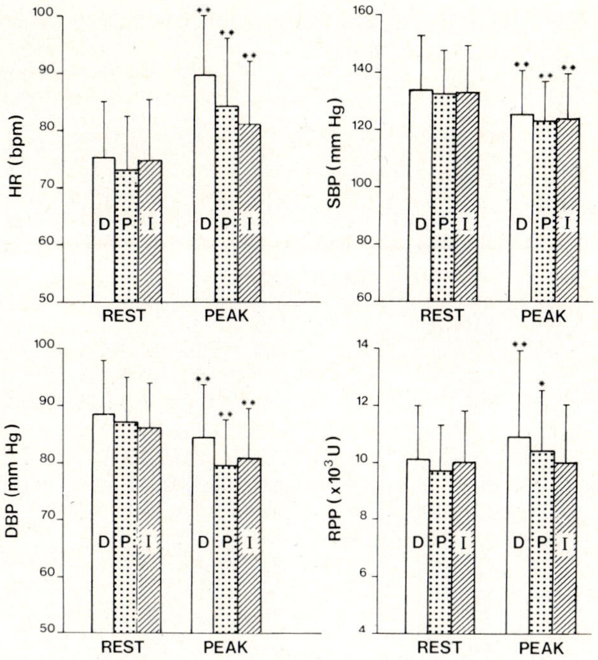

Fig. 1. Peak hemodynamic changes during the infusion of dipyridamole *(D)*, PGI_2 *(P)*, and iloprost *(I)* in 33 patients with coronary artery disease. Dipyridamole and PGI_2 decreased significantly (*P < 0.005; **P < 0.001; paired t test) systolic *(SBP)* and diastolic *(DBP)* blood pressure and consistently increased heart rate *(HR)* and the rate-pressure product *(RPP)*. Iloprost had less of an effect on heart rate; hence the rate-pressure product was unchanged from control.

Main study. Results of coronary arteriography and exercise stress and pharmacologic tests for each of the 33 patients are listed in Table III. All exercise test results were positive, and the mean maximum ST segment depression was 0.18 ± 0.06 mV. This occurred at a mean maximum work capacity of 516 ± 133 seconds and at a maximum rate-pressure product of $23.9 \pm 5.5 \times 10^{-3}$ U.

Dipyridamole induced significant ST segment de-

Table III. Clinical and angiographic findings in patients with coronary artery disease: Results of exercise stress and pharmacologic tests

				Exercise				*Vasodilator-induced ischemia*		
Patient No.	*Symptoms*	*PMI*	*Angiography (% narrowing)*	*Peak RPP* ($\times 10^3 U$)	*Duration (sec)*	*ST depression (mV)*	*Lead*	*DIP*	*PGI_2*	*Iloprost*
1	EF	−	LMCA 95	23.5	324	0.23	V_5	+	+	+
2	EF	−	LMCA 75	19.9	414	0.25	V_5	+	+	+
3	EF+R	−	LMCA 75	14.7	294	0.20	V_5	+	+	+
4	EF+R	+	LAD 75, CX 90, RCA 90	30.1	540	0.26	aVF	+	+	+
5	EF+R	−	LAD 75, CX 90, RCA 95	18.1	276	0.15	aVF	+	+	−
6	EF	+	LAD 100, CX 75, RCA 95	20.2	325	0.16	V_5	+	+	−
7	EF	−	CX 95, RCA 100	21.7	456	0.14	aVF	+	−	−
8	EF+R	+	LAD 75, RCA 100	36.2	492	0.30	V_5	+	−	−
9	EF	+	LAD 100, RCA 100	18.0	438	0.12	V_5	+	−	−
10	EF+R	−	CX 90, RCA 100	21.6	738	0.19	aVF	+	−	−
11	EF	+	LAD 95, CX 90, RCA 100	18.9	480	0.14	V_5	+	−	−
12	EF+R	+	LAD 90, RCA 95	18.0	438	0.12	V_5	+	−	−
13	EF+R	+	LAD 100, CX 90	25.0	534	0.14	V_5	+	−	−
14	EF	−	LMCA 50, RCA 90	16.1	204	0.10	aVF	+	−	−
15	EF+R	−	LAD 75, CX 95, RCA 95	17.5	528	0.15	V_5	+	−	−
16	EF+R	−	LAD 90, CX 90,	22.3	600	0.25	V_5	+	−	−
17	EF	−	LAD 90	26.2	600	0.10	V_5	−	−	−
18	EF+R	+	CX 95, RCA 75	26.9	552	0.29	V_5	−	−	−
19	EF	−	LAD 90	31.0	690	0.20	V_5	−	−	−
20	R	−	RCA 75	25.0	636	0.18	V_5	−	−	−
21	EF	−	LAD 75, RCA 75	29.8	516	0.15	aVF	−	−	−
22	EF+R	+	LAD 90	25.1	522	0.16	V_5	−	−	−
23	EF+R	+	CX 75, RCA 95	24.6	642	0.31	V_5	−	−	−
24	EF+R	−	CX 90	24.4	498	0.18	V_5	−	−	−
25	EF	−	LAD 75, CX 90, RCA 100	20.2	600	0.19	aVF	−	−	−
26	R	+	RCA 100	24.6	522	0.12	V_5	−	−	−
27	EF+R	−	LAD 95	21.9	396	0.14	V_5	−	−	−
28	EF+R	−	CX 75	25.9	556	0.10	aVF	−	−	−
29	EF+R	+	LAD 90	32.2	588	0.30	aVF	−	−	−
30	EF	+	LAD 100, RCA 95	21.1	654	0.15	V_5	−	−	−
31	EF+R	−	RCA 90	30.4	612	0.29	aVF	−	−	−
32	EF+R	−	RCA 100	21.1	556	0.14	aVF	−	−	−
33	EF+R		RCA 75	36.4	798	0.17	aVF	−	−	−
$\bar{X}$				23.9	515.7	0.18				
±SD				5.5	133.4	0.06				

PMI = Previous myocardial infarction; RPP = rate-pressure product; DIP = dipyridamole; EF = effort angina; − = no; LMCA = left main coronary artery; + = yes; R = rest angina; LAD = left anterior descending artery; CX = circumflex coronary artery; RCA = right coronary artery.

pression in 16 patients. Slight to severe chest pain occurred in all patients with ST segment depression. Two patients with no ECG changes complained of some degree of chest discomfort. ECG changes and chest pain appeared simultaneously 2 to 3 minutes after the end of the infusion. Aminophylline completely relieved the symptoms in 13 of the 18 patients; relief in the other five was achieved with aminophylline and 5 mg sublingual isosorbide dinitrate. There were hemodynamic changes consistent with marked arterial dilation during and after dipyridamole injection (Fig. 1). Systolic blood pressure fell from 134 ± 19 to 125 ± 16 mm Hg and heart rate rose from 75 ± 10 to 90 ± 12 bpm. The rate-pressure product rose at the time of the maximal hemodynamic change (from 10.1 ± 1.9 to 10.9 ± 3 × 10^{-3} U).

PGI_2 infusion induced flushing in all 33 patients, moderate headache in seven, and chest pain in six. The six who had chest pain also had significant ST segment depression (≥0.1 mV). The ST segment depression

Table IV. Hemodynamic changes during PGI_2 infusion in patients with drug-induced ischemia

Patient No.		*PGI_2 infusion (ng/kg/min)*					
		0	*2*	*4*	*6*	*8*	*10*
1	HR	76	76	78	81	84	85
	SBP	140	140	140	135	130	150
	DBP	90	90	90	90	85	95
2	HR	88	92	98	101	—	—
	SBP	135	130	120	140	—	—
	DBP	85	85	80	90	—	—
3	HR	63	66	81	—	—	—
	SBP	155	150	140	—	—	—
	DBP	90	90	85	—	—	—
4	HR	74	87	88	88	95	100
	SBP	140	140	145	130	130	120
	DBP	90	90	90	90	80	75
5	HR	77	78	74	71	70	68
	SBP	130	130	130	120	80	80
	DBP	90	90	85	80	80	80
6	HR	84	87	89	90	92	94
	SBP	125	120	120	115	110	110
	DBP	80	80	80	80	75	70
$\overline{X} \pm SD$	HR	77 ± 9	81 ± 10	85 ± 9	86 ± 11	85 ± 11	87 ± 14
	SBP	138 ± 10	135 ± 11	133 ± 11	128 ± 10	123 ± 10	123 ± 19
	DBP	88 ± 4	88 ± 4	85 ± 4	86 ± 5	80 ± 4	80 ± 11

HR = Heart rate (bpm); SBP = systolic blood pressure (mm Hg); DBP = diastolic blood pressure (mm Hg).

occurred in one patient (no. 3) when PGI_2 was infused at 4 ng/kg/min, in another (no. 2) at 6 ng/kg/min, and in four at 10 ng/kg/min (Table IV). Prolonged chest pain (≥3 minutes) occurred in all six patients and was relieved by intravenous injection of 125 mg aminophylline (Fig. 2). Six to ten minutes after the end of the PGI_2 infusion, all nonanginal adverse reactions disappeared.

The hemodynamic effects at peak PGI_2 infusion are shown in Fig. 1. PGI_2 increased heart rate (from 73 ± 9 to 84 ± 12 bpm) and the rate-pressure product (from 9.7 ± 1.6 to 10.4 ± 2.1 × 10^{-3} U) and decreased systolic (from 133 ± 15 to 123 ± 14 mm Hg) and diastolic (from 87 ± 8 to 79 ± 8 mm Hg) blood pressures. The results were similar considering only patients with drug-induced angina (Table IV), even though patients 1 and 2, who had severe chest pain, had a slight increase in arterial blood pressure consistent with a generalized increase in sympathetic nervous system activity. No differences in the rate-pressure product and diastolic blood pressure were found between ischemic or preischemic rates of infusion in all six patients with PGI_2-induced angina (from 11.0 ± 3.0 to 10.1 ± 2.4 × 10^{-3} U and from 83 ± 9 to 82 ± 5 mm Hg). Preischemic rates of infusion were defined as the last tolerated dose of PGI_2 without significant (≥0.1 mV) ST segment depression or chest pain.

After iloprost infusion, all patients had facial flushing accompanied by a sensation of warmth. The flushing in some patients was apparent at 2 ng/kg/min and in all at 6 ng/kg/min. Chest pain and ST segment depression developed in four patients who had similar signs during PGI_2 infusion. In the latter there was significant ST segment depression when the infusion rate reached 6 ng/kg/min. In all patients the pain lasted >3 minutes and was relieved by 125 mg aminophylline.

Hemodynamic changes during iloprost infusion are shown in Fig. 1. At peak infusion, heart rate increased by approximately 8%, diastolic and systolic blood pressures decreased, and the rate-pressure product remained essentially unchanged (9.9 ± 1.8 and 10.0 ± 2.9 × 10^{-3} U). The results were much the same in patients with drug-induced ischemia. The rate-pressure products and diastolic blood pressures during preischemic rates of infusion did not differ from those during ischemia (10.7 ± 1.4 and 10.8 ± 1.5 × 10^{-3} U and 79 ± 9 and 78 ± 10 mm Hg).

No patient with a negative dipyridamole response had a positive response to PGI_2 or iloprost. Dipyridamole induced myocardial ischemia in 64% and 83% of patients with two- and three-vessel disease, respectively, and in all patients with ≥50% reduction of left main diameter. PGI_2 induced ischemia in 50% of patients with triple vessel disease and in 75% with left main

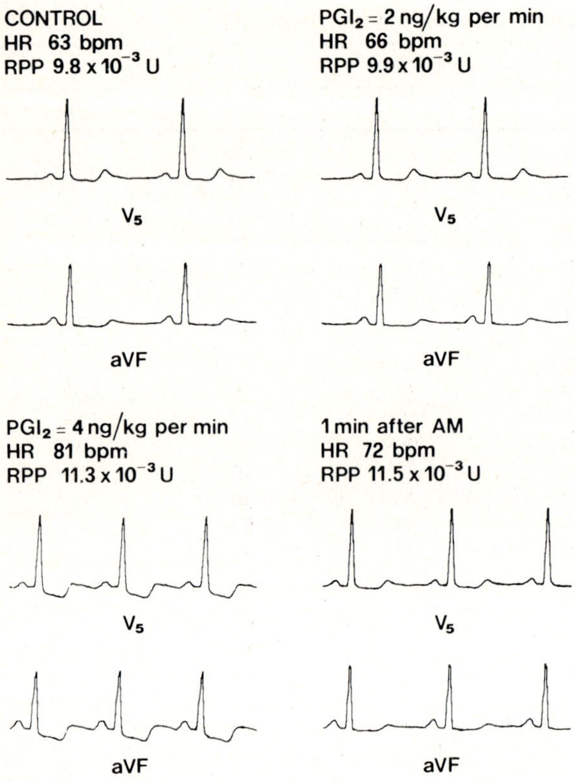

Fig. 2. Response to PGI_2 infusion in patient no. 3 with drug-induced ischemia. PGI_2 induced dose-dependent changes in heart rate *(HR)* and blood pressure. There was chest pain and significant ST segment depression at a PGI_2 infusion rate of 4 ng/kg/min. Three minutes after the end of the infusion, 125 mg aminophylline *(AM)* was injected. Despite a slight rise in the rate-pressure product *(RPP)*, chest pain and ST segment depression were promptly relieved.

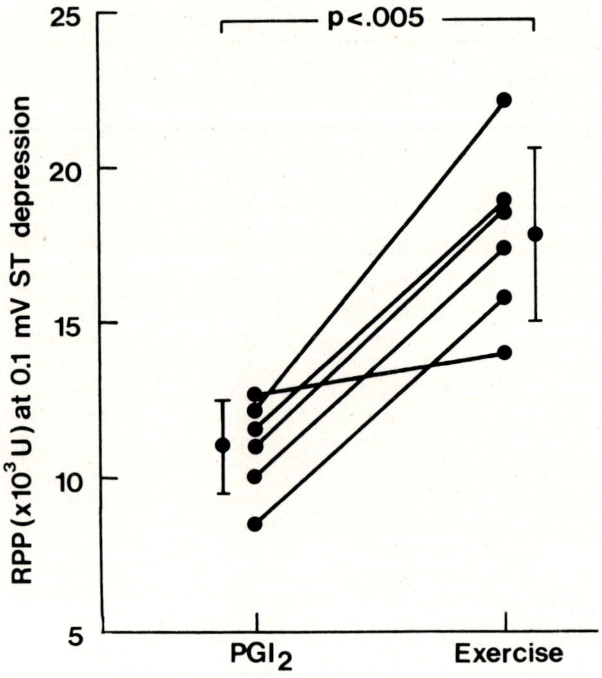

Fig. 3. The rate-pressure product *(RPP)* during PGI_2 infusion and exercise stress testing with reference to 0.1 mV ST segment depression. Ischemia during PGI_2 infusion developed at a rate-pressure product significantly lower than that during exercise stress testing.

narrowings. In most of these the ischemia was also induced by iloprost infusion (Table III). PGI_2 responders had a lower exercise duration than nonresponders (362 ± 99 and 550 ± 116 seconds).

In patients with PGI_2-induced subendocardial ischemia, the rate-pressure products calculated at 0.1 mV ST segment depression were lower under infusion than during exercise (11.0 ± 1.5 and 17.8 ± 2.8 × 10^{-3} U; Fig. 3).

DISCUSSION

Powerful dilators of resistive vessels, such as dipyridamole, have been shown to affect coronary perfusion adversely and to induce myocardial ischemia in patients with coronary artery disease.[11,20,32] PGI_2 has also been shown to decrease systemic, pulmonary, and coronary resistances.[16] We noted similar hemodynamics in our study during the iloprost infusion; vascular resistances fell by 32% and total peripheral resistances fell by 34%.

In keeping with other sporadic observations and suggestions, PGI_2 and its analog iloprost were expected to induce ischemia when infused in patients with fairly severe coronary narrowing.[8,16] In our study of 33 patients with coronary artery disease, intravenous PGI_2 acted as an arteriolar dilator, reducing blood pressure slightly, increasing heart rate, and inducing slight headache and facial flushing. In six patients it induced typical chest pain and ST segment depression; the results were similar in four patients during iloprost infusion. Thus the cause of ischemia cannot be attributed to the PGI_2 vehicle and pH of the solution.

Pain relief after the end of PGI_2 or iloprost infusion was prompt and complete after the administration of aminophylline, a virtually instantaneous antagonist of dipyridamole.[1]

Specific binding of PGI_2 to a variety of cells or tissues has been correlated with the accumulation of cyclic adenosine monophosphate.[9,23] This could account for part of its vasodilating effect, in that the enzymatic hydrolysis of the cyclic compound may generate adenosine, which dilates arterioles and precapillary vessels.

This is in keeping with experiments in isolated heart preparations[10] showing that prostacyclin increases adenosine release in a dose-dependent manner and with the observation that aminophylline, a selective antagonist of adenosine receptors,[1] reduces the increase in coronary perfusion after PGI_2. Because aminophylline has been shown to relieve ischemia caused by dipyridamole (which actually increases adenosine levels and adversely affects coronary perfusion), it was conceivable that the same could apply to PGI_2-induced ischemia.

Our data confirm this working hypothesis and suggest that the effect of PGI_2 on the coronary system is at least partially developed through an adenosine-mediated mechanism. This is also supported by the observation that PGI_2 induced ischemia only in patients who had had angina during dipyridamole infusion.

PGI_2-induced myocardial ischemia may result from several mechanisms. These can be divided into actions on the systemic circulation, which may influence the balance between myocardial oxygen consumption and fixed supply, and actions on coronary perfusion pressure. Increased cardiac work does not seem to play a major role because there was a 0.1 mV ST segment depression during PGI_2 infusion at levels of rate-pressure products below those usually tolerated during exercise, without signs or symptoms of myocardial ischemia.

When maximum poststenotic vasodilation is reached and compensatory autoregulation is almost completely abolished, small decreases in diastolic blood pressure may adversely affect coronary perfusion.[26] However, two patients (nos. 1 and 2) had severe chest pain and significant ST segment depression during PGI_2 infusion accompanied by a slight increase in diastolic blood pressure, consistent with sympathetic reflex stimulation. Also, there were no differences in diastolic blood pressure and rate-pressure products between ischemic and preischemic rates of infusion.

Because adenosine, which could be increased by PGI_2, may induce myocardial ischemia through reduced poststenotic coronary pressure and "coronary steal,"[18] a similar mechanism may be involved in patients with PGI_2- and iloprost-induced angina. The term "steal" is not specific and refers to a spectrum of pressure-flow changes occurring distally to a critical coronary stenosis. There are two hemodynamic conditions in which the term "steal" has been applied. The first refers to an absolute reduction in coronary flow distal to a severe stenosis,[5] and the second concerns a diversion of flow from the subendocardial to the subepicardial layers, which occurs despite increased total coronary blood flow.[4]

Our results do not distinguish the mechanisms responsible for ischemia during PGI_2 infusion, but the induction of ischemia only in patients with severe coronary narrowings and poor exercise tolerance, and the occurrence of ST segment depression indicative of subendocardial injury, suggest that PGI_2 may induce ischemia by lowering the poststenotic coronary pressure. Moreover, because aminophylline, a specific antagonist of the dipyridamole effect at the level of coronary vascular resistance, promptly relieved myocardial ischemia both after PGI_2 and iloprost infusions, these drugs may induce ischemia by a dipyridamole-like maldistribution of flow.

Our data do not rule out the therapeutic potential of PGI_2 and iloprost in patients with angina pectoris. Accordingly, PGI_2 infusion has been shown to prolong the pacing time to angina in patients with coronary artery disease[7] and, occasionally, to reduce the number of episodes of myocardial ischemia due to coronary spasm.[12,31] However, extreme care must be taken in patients with severe coronary narrowings and poor exercise tolerance because PGI_2 and its analogs may induce myocardial ischemia.

We thank Dr. T. Krais and Dr. S. Del Mastro, Schering AG, West Germany, for the iloprost and Prof. C. Patrono, Catholic University School of Medicine, Rome, Italy, for the PGI_2. The technical assistance of Nicodemo Macri, B.S., is greatly appreciated.

References

1. Afonso S: Inhibition of coronary vasodilating action of dipyridamole and adenosine by aminophylline in the dog. Circ Res **26:**743-752, 1970.
2. Aiken JW, Gorman RR, Shebuski RJ: Prevention of blockage of partially obstructed coronary arteries with prostacyclin correlates with inhibition of platelet aggregation. Prostaglandins **17:**483-495, 1979.
3. Aiken JW, Shebuski RJ: Comparison in anesthetized dogs of the anti-aggregatory and hemodynamic effects of prostacyclin and a chemically stable prostacyclin analog, 6a-CARBA-PGI_2 (Carbacyclin). Prostaglandins **19:**629-643, 1980.
4. Bache RJ, Schwartz JS: Effect of perfusion pressure distal to a coronary stenosis on transmural myocardial blood flow. Circulation **65:**928-935, 1982.
5. Becker LC: Conditions for vasodilator-induced coronary steal in experimental myocardial ischemia. Circulation **57:**1103-1110, 1978.
6. Belch JJF, Newman P, Drury JK, McKenzie F, Capell H, Leiberman P, Forbes CD, Prentice CRM: Intermittent epoprostenol (prostacyclin) infusion in patients with Raynaud's syndrome. A double-blind controlled trial. Lancet **1:**313-315, 1983.
7. Bergman G, Daly K, Atkinson L, Rothman M, Richardson PJ, Jackson G, Jewitt DE: Prostacyclin: Hae-

modynamic and metabolic effects in patients with coronary artery disease. Lancet **1:**569-572, 1981.

8. Bergman G, Kiff PS, Atkinson L, Jewitt DE: Failure of intravenous prostacyclin to influence the initial progress of patients with unstable angina. Circulation **68**(suppl III):397, 1983. (Abst.)
9. Best LC, Martin T, Russel RG, Preston F: Prostacyclin increases cyclic AMP levels and adenylate cyclase activity in platelets. Nature **267:**850-852, 1977.
10. Blass KE, Föster W, Zehl U: Coronary vasodilation: Interactions between prostacyclin and adenosine. Br J Pharmacol **69:**555-559, 1980.
11. Brown BG, Josephson MA, Petersen RB, Pierce CD, Wong M, Hecht HS, Bolson E, Dodge HT: Intravenous dipyridamole combined with isometric handgrip for near maximal acute increase in coronary flow in patients with coronary artery disease. Am J Cardiol **48:**1077-1085, 1981.
12. Chierchia S, Patrono C, Crea F, Ciabattoni G, De Caterina R, Cinotti GA, Distante A, Maseri A: Effects of intravenous prostacyclin in variant angina. Circulation **65:**470-477, 1982.
13. Data JL, Molony BA, Meinzinger MM, Gorman RR: Intravenous infusion of prostacyclin sodium in man: Clinical effects and influence on platelet adenosine diphosphate sensitivity and adenosine 3′:5′-cyclic monophosphate levels. Circulation **64:**4-11, 1981.
14. Darius H, Matzky R: The action of ZK 36374, a chemically stable carbacyclin derivative, on platelet aggregation and vascular tone in vitro. Arch Pharmacol **316**(suppl R):29-32, 1981.
15. Edhag O, Henriksson P, Wennmalm Å: Prostacyclin infusion in patients with acute myocardial infarction (preliminary report). N Engl J Med **308:**1032-1033, 1983.
16. Firth BG, Winniford MD, Campbell WB, Hillis LD: Hemodynamic effects of intravenous prostacyclin in stable angina pectoris. Am J Cardiol **52:**439-443, 1983.
17. FitzGerald GA, Roberts LJ II, Maas D, Brash AR, Oates JA: Intravenous prostacyclin in thrombotic thrombocytopenic purpura. *In* Lewis PJ, O'Grady J, editors: Clinical pharmacology of prostacyclin. New York, 1981, Raven Press.
18. Gallagher KP, Folts JD, Shebuski RJ, Rankin JHG, Rowe GG: Subepicardial vasodilator reserve in the presence of critical coronary stenosis in dogs. Am J Cardiol **46:**67-73, 1980.
19. Ginsburg R, Bristow MR, Harrison DC, Stinson EB: Studies with isolated human coronary arteries. Some general observations, potential mediators of spasm, role of calcium antagonists. Chest **78**(suppl 1):180-186, 1980.
20. Gould KL, Westcott RJ, Albro PC, Hamilton GW: Noninvasive assessment of coronary stenoses by myocardial imaging during pharmacologic coronary vasodilation. II. Clinical methodology and feasibility. Am J Cardiol **41:**279-287, 1978.
21. Gryglewski RJ, Szczeklik A, Nizankowski R: Antiplatelet action of intravenous infusion of prostacyclin in man. Thromb Res **13:**153-163, 1978.
22. Higgs EA, Higgs GA, Moncada S, Vane J: Prostacyclin (PGI_2) inhibits the formation of platelet thrombi in arterioles and venules of the hamster cheek pouch. Br J Pharmacol **63:**535-539, 1978.
23. Ito T, Ogawa K, Enomoto I, Hashimoto H, Kai I, Satake T: Comparison of the effects of PGI_2 and PGE_1 on coronary and systemic hemodynamics and coronary arterial cyclic nucleotide levels in dogs. *In* Samuelson B, Ramwell P, Paoletti R, editors: Advances in prostaglandin and thromboxane research. New York, 1980, Raven Press, vol 7.
24. Mehta J, Nichols WW, Mehta P, Pepine C, Conti CR: Effects of prostacyclin on systemic and coronary hemodynamics in the dog. Am Heart J **102:**835-840, 1981.
25. Opherk D, Zebe H, Schwarz F, Manthey J, Baller D, Kübler W: Intravenous carbochromen: A potent and effective drug for estimation of coronary dilatory capacity. J Am Coll Cardiol **1:**694, 1983. (Abst.)
26. Rouleau J, Boerboom LE, Surjadhana A, Hoffman JIE: The role of autoregulation and tissue diastolic pressures in the transmural distribution of left ventricular blood flow in anesthetized dogs. Circ Res **45:**804-815, 1979.
27. Rubin LJ, Groves BM, Reeves JT, Frosolono M, Handel F, Cato AE: Prostacyclin-induced acute pulmonary vasodilation in primary pulmonary hypertension. Circulation **66:**334-338, 1982.
28. Schrör K, Darius H, Matzky R, Ohlendorf R: The antiplatelet and cardiovascular action of a new carbacyclin derivative (ZK 36374)—Equipotent to PGI_2 in vitro. Naunyn Schmiedebergs Arch Pharmacol **316:**252-255, 1981.
29. Szczeklik A, Nizankowski R, Skawinski S, Szczeklik J, Gluszko P, Gryglewski RJ: Successful therapy of advanced arteriosclerosis obliterans with prostacyclin. Lancet **1:**1111-1114, 1979.
30. Szczeklik J, Szczeklik A, Nizankowski R: Haemodynamic changes induced by prostacyclin in man. Br Heart J **44:**254-258, 1980.
31. Szczeklik A, Szczeklik J, Nizankowski R, Gluszko P: Prostacyclin for acute coronary insufficiency. Artery **8:**7-11, 1980.
32. Tavazzi L, Previtali M, Salerno JA, Chimienti M, Ray M, Medici A, Specchia G, Bobba P: Dipyridamole test in angina pectoris: Diagnostic value and pathophysiological implications. Cardiology **69:**34-41, 1982.
33. Yang SS, Bentivoglio LG, Maranhão V, Goldberg H: From cardiac catheterization data to hemodynamic parameters. Philadelphia, 1978, F. A. Davis Company.
34. Warrington SJ, Smith PR, O'Grady J: Noninvasive assessment of the cardiovascular effects of prostacyclin (PGI_2) in man. Eur J Cardiol **12:**73-80, 1980.

Effects of smoke deprivation interval on puff topography

Our purpose in this series of three studies was to determine the effects of deprivation interval on smoking topography. In experiment 1, subjects were allowed to smoke ad libitum for 1 hour after 3, 30, and 300 minutes of tobacco smoke deprivation. An increased latency to the first cigarette developed after 3 minutes deprivation and an increase in the number of cigarettes smoked occurred after 300 minutes of deprivation. In experiment 2, puff number and spacing were held constant to determine if smokers would compensate for long deprivation intervals by more intense smoking, i.e., increased puff volume. Puff volumes and carbon monoxide (CO) boosts did not differ across smoking bouts preceded by either 30, 100, or 300 minutes of tobacco smoke deprivation. In experiment 3, average puff volumes and CO boosts were examined during smoking periods with short (3, 10, and 30 minutes) deprivation intervals. Subjects smoked less intensely (lower puff volumes and CO boosts) when smoking was spaced by 3 than by 30 minutes. We conclude that smokers do not increase puff volume after long deprivation intervals up to 300 minutes, but they may decrease puff volumes after short (3 minutes) deprivation intervals when puff number and spacing cannot be used as compensatory mechanisms. (CLIN PHARMACOL THER 38:109-115, 1985.)

James P. Zacny, Ph.D., and Maxine L. Stitzer, Ph.D. *Baltimore, Md.*

Puff volume is the amount of smoky air drawn through the cigarette rod into the mouth with each puff. Puff volume is an important measure in smoking research because it correlates with biologic exposure as measured by expired air carbon monoxide (CO)[9,12] and plasma nicotine[13] levels. Recent research has shown that puff volume is responsive to a number of smoking parameter alterations. Puff volume can be altered by puff size instructions[22] and nicotine yield variations,[3,9,12,16,20,21] and is sensitive to the draw characteristics of a cigarette.[4] Cigarette availability, on the other hand, has not been shown to influence puff volume. In one study of smokers enrolled in a smoking cessation program that included gradual reduction in the number of cigarettes smoked per day, puff volumes did not change as cigarette consumption declined.[6] However, the effects of decreased cigarette consumption rates on puff volume were confounded with the motivational set of the subjects (i.e., desire to quit smoking).

From the Department of Psychiatry, Francis Scott Key Medical Center and The Johns Hopkins University School of Medicine.

Supported by National Cancer Institute Grant No. 1 RO1 CA 37736-01 and United States Public Health Service Grant No. T 32 DA 07209.

Received for publication Dec. 24, 1984; accepted April 8, 1985.

Reprint requests to: James P. Zacny, Behavioral Pharmacology Research Unit, D-5-West, Francis Scott Key Medical Center, 4940 Eastern Ave., Baltimore, MD 21224.

In another study in which the cigarette presentation rate was doubled and quadrupled, the number of puffs on each of the presented cigarettes decreased, while puff volume did not change.[8] It is possible, however, that smokers would use puff volume to compensate for changes in availability, especially if other avenues of compensation such as puff frequency were blocked.

We explored a range of cigarette availability parameters and procedures to determine if there are conditions under which puff volume is sensitive to altered cigarette availability. In experiment 1, effects of 3, 30, and 300 minutes of tobacco smoke deprivation were assessed on a number of smoking parameters, including puff number and puff volume. In the next experiment, number and spacing of puffs was held constant after deprivation periods up to 300 minutes. Under these conditions, subjects could compensate for reduced cigarette availability by varying puff volume but not by varying number or spacing of puffs. The third and last experiment explored the effects on puff volume of presenting consecutive smoking opportunities much more frequently than usual when number and spacing of puffs were again not available as compensatory mechanisms.

METHODS

Subjects. Our subjects were nine cigarette smokers (mean age, 32.7 years [range 25 to 47 years]; mean

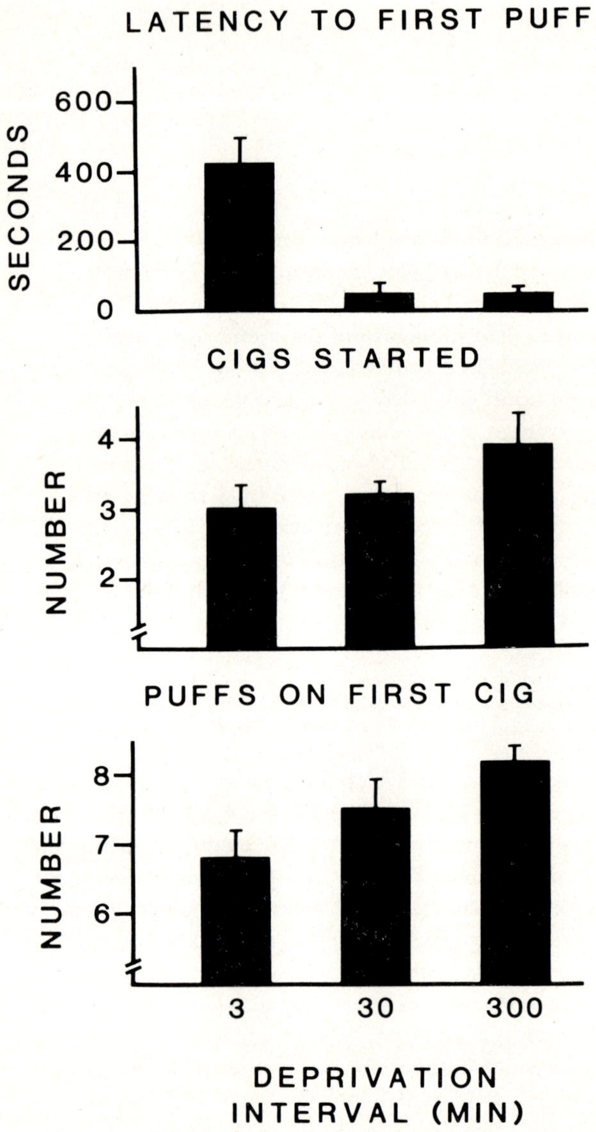

Fig. 1. Experiment 1, the effect of tobacco smoke deprivation on latency to the first puff *(top panel),* number of cigarettes started *(middle panel),* and number of puffs on the first cigarette *(bottom panel),* averaged across subjects. *Brackets* indicate standard error of the mean.

years smoking, 15.2 years [range 11 to 30 years]; mean number of cigarettes smoked per day, 38.9 [range 20 to 60]). All subjects smoked their usual brand of cigarettes, which delivered medium to high levels of nicotine and tar (Federal Trade Commission levels: mean nicotine, 1.1 mg per cigarette; mean tar, 16.7 mg per cigarette). Five subjects (L. W., S. B., E. M., C. W., L. H.) were women and four (B. C., B. E., W. C., C. B.) were men. Four subjects (L. W., S. B., E. M., C. B.), three subjects (E. M., B. E., W. L.), and six subjects (E. M., B. C., C. W., B. E., L. H., C. B.) participated in experiments 1, 2, and 3, respectively.

Puff measurement apparatus. Puff number was measured by a pressure-sensitive switch attached to a needle that protruded through a plastic cigarette holder. The system used to measure puff volume has been described in detail elsewhere[10] and has the pneumotachograph as its principal component. The pneumotachograph, situated distal to the cigarette rod, was attached by rubber tubing and a rubber stopper to a glass cylinder. Before each puff the smoker attached the glass cylinder to another rubber stopper that contained the cigarette holder and lighted cigarette. When the smoker took a puff from the cigarette holder, pressure changes measured by the pneumotachograph were converted into an electric signal by a differential pressure transducer. The signal was conditioned by a polygraph, fed into an analog-to-digital converter, and then entered into a microcomputer, which mathematically converted pressure changes to flow rates. The relationship between pressure change and flow rate is linear over the normal range of puffing rates of 0 to 100 ml/sec; the integration of flow rates over the duration of the puff provides the puff volume measure. The puff volume measurement system was periodically calibrated by sending flow rates of known amounts (zero to 2500 ml/min) into the pneumotachograph.

General procedures. At the start of each experimental session, subjects were seated in a room housing the smoking measurement equipment. Subjects smoked their usual cigarette brand during all three experiments, with puffs taken through the cigarette holder and tube to obtain puff volume measures. A CO boost measure was obtained by comparing expired air CO before and 90 seconds after smoking. Subjects exhaled residual air from their lungs into the atmosphere before taking and holding for 20 seconds a deep breath. They then exhaled a small amount of air into the atmosphere before expiring another 1 L into a CO sample collection bag. A portable CO measurement device was used to measure expired air CO. In each experiment there were three cigarette deprivation conditions. Order of exposure to conditions was determined by a randomized block and subjects were exposed to each cigarette deprivation condition three times. In experiments 1 and 2, subjects were exposed to one condition each day during 9-day experiments; in experiment 3, subjects were exposed to all three conditions within a single day during the 3-day experiment.

Experiment 1: Effects of tobacco smoke deprivation interval on ad libitum smoking. The purpose of this study was to identify smoking parameters that change in response to altered cigarette deprivation conditions. Parameters examined included puff frequency and spacing as well as puff volume. At the start of each session, subjects gave a breath sample for CO analysis, then smoked a cigarette; 90 seconds after the last puff they gave another breath sample. The experimental deprivation interval, timed from the last puff of this baseline cigarette, was either 3, 30, or 300 minutes. This was followed by a third breath sample and a 1-hour smoking period, during which subjects smoked ad libitum using the cylinder and holder. The experimenter was present in the smoking room at this time to record when subjects lit and put out their cigarettes and to adjust the equipment when necessary. A final breath sample for CO analysis was collected after this 1-hour free smoking period.

The following smoking topography variables were measured during the free smoking period: latency to the light-up puff of the first cigarette, number of cigarettes started in a session, puff number per cigarette, average puff volume, and pre- and postsmoking period CO level. The light-up puff was not counted as an actual puff because it bears no resemblance to subsequent puffs in terms of volume and duration, and is often not inhaled by the smoker. CO boost, which is the amount of CO absorbed as a result of smoking, was obtained by subtracting the presmoking period CO level from the postsmoking period CO level. All these measures were analyzed by repeated-measures ANOVA, with three individual replications from each subject at each deprivation condition. Tukey post hoc comparison tests were used, when appropriate.

Experiment 2: Effects of long deprivation intervals on puff volume. The purpose of experiment 2 was to determine if puff volume is used as a compensatory mechanism after long deprivation intervals if distribution and number of puffs are not available as compensatory mechanisms. Subjects started each session by smoking one of their cigarettes. Either 30, 100, or 300 minutes later, subjects took four puffs, spaced 40 seconds apart, from the cigarette. The experimenter lit the cigarette for the subject and indicated when puffs should occur. Breath CO samples were obtained before the first puff and after the last puff. Subjects were not allowed to smoke for 30 minutes after the four-puff smoking bout to ensure that puffing immediately after deprivation would not be influenced by subsequent opportunity to smoke.

Each subject contributed 12 puff volumes (four puff volumes/bout × three replications) and three CO boosts (one CO boost/bout × three replications) from

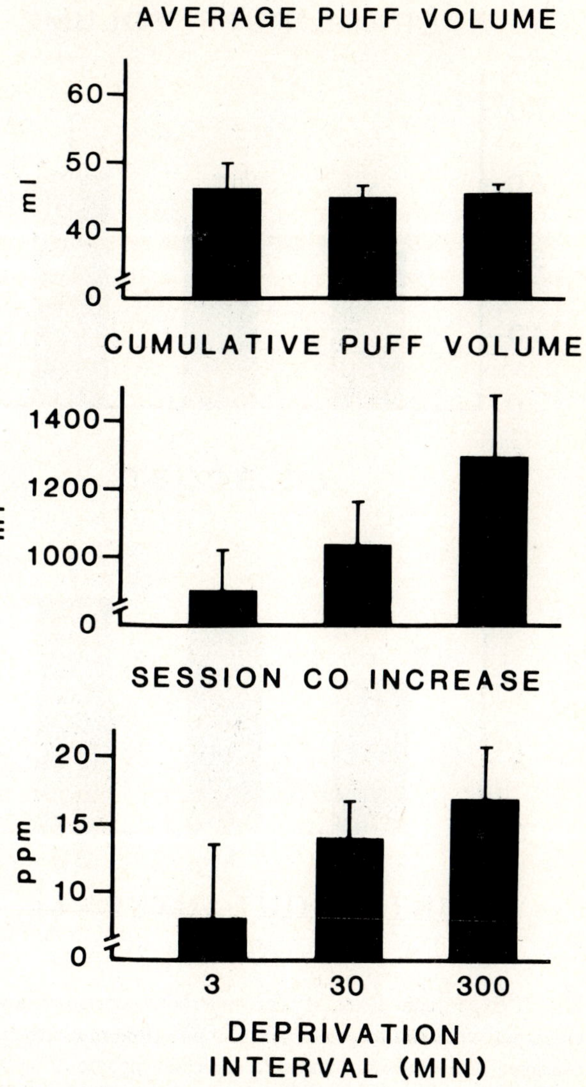

Fig. 2. Experiment 1, the effect of tobacco smoke deprivation on average puff volume *(top panel),* cumulative puff volume *(middle panel),* and session CO increase *(bottom panel),* averaged across subjects. *Brackets* indicate standard error of the mean.

each deprivation interval condition to repeated-measures ANOVA. Factors analyzed in the puff volume ANOVA were deprivation interval, replications, and trials (four puff volumes/bout); factors analyzed in the CO boost ANOVA were deprivation interval and replications.

Experiment 3. Effects of short deprivation intervals on puff volume. In experiment 3 we determined whether puff volume is used as a compensatory mechanism after short deprivation intervals if distribution and number of puffs are not available as compensatory mechanisms. Each daily session consisted of three ex-

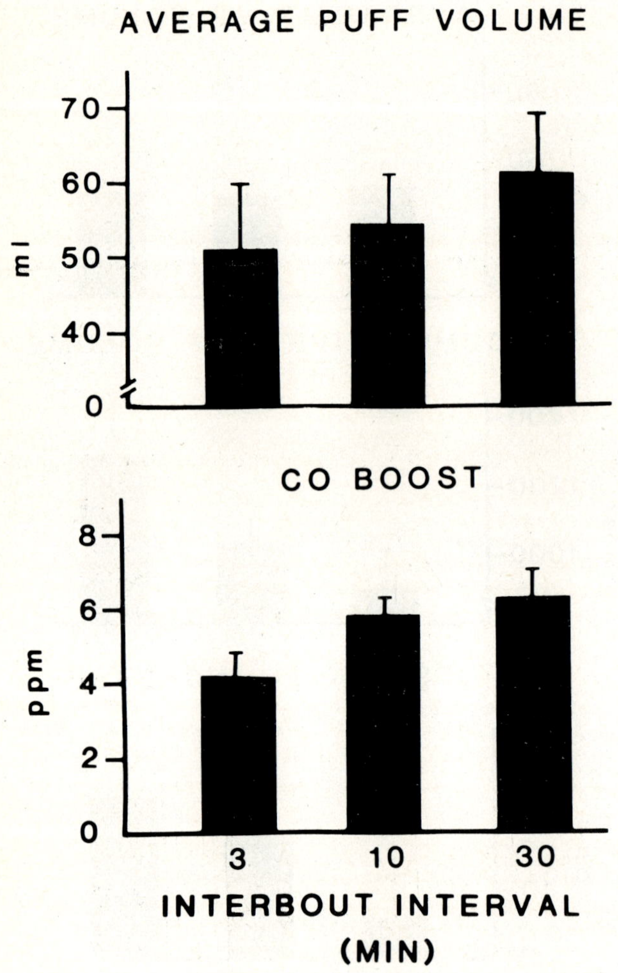

Fig. 3. Experiment 3, the effect of interbout interval on average puff volume *(top panel)* and CO boost *(bottom panel)*, averaged across subjects. *Brackets* indicate standard error of the mean.

perimental smoking periods separated by approximately 45 minutes. During each experimental smoking period, subjects took 20 puffs from their cigarettes: five bouts of four puffs each were separated by 3, 10, or 30 minutes. Within each bout, puffs were spaced 40 seconds apart. During the 45 minutes that separated one experimental period from another, subjects could smoke as they pleased. This procedure was designed to reduce interactions between experimental smoking periods. Breath CO samples were obtained before and 90 seconds after each four-puff bout, except in the 3-minute deprivation interval condition, when the postbout breath CO sample also served as the prebout breath CO sample for the next bout.

Data from the first bout of each experimental smoking period were excluded from analysis because this first bout was not separated from prior smoking by an appropriate experimental interval. Puff volumes and CO boost from each of the subsequent four bouts of each experimental smoking period were included in the data analysis. Each subject contributed 48 puff volume values (four bouts/condition/day × four puffs/bout × three replications across days) and 12 CO boost values (four bouts/condition/day × one CO boost/bout × three replications across days) from each experimental condition to the data analysis. Effects of deprivation interval, bout order, and replications on both puff volume and CO boost, and effects of puff order on puff volume were analyzed with repeated-measures ANOVA. Tukey post-hoc comparison tests were used, when appropriate.

RESULTS

Experiment 1. Deprivation interval influenced latency from the start of the smoking period to the light-up puff of the first free smoking period cigarette. Fig. 1, *top,* shows that mean latencies to the light-up puff were 406.2, 52.9, and 53.4 seconds, respectively, after 3, 30, and 300 minutes of deprivation ($F(2,6) = 21.0$; $P < 0.01$). Post-hoc tests revealed that mean latency was significantly longer in the 3-minute deprivation interval condition than in the other two conditions. Smoking deprivation also influenced several frequency measures. First, as shown in the *middle panel* of Fig. 1, the mean number of cigarettes started during the smoking period was 3.0, 3.2, and 3.9 after 3, 30, and 300 minutes of deprivation ($F(2,6) = 18.2$; $P < 0.01$). Post-hoc tests indicated that subjects started more cigarettes after the 300-minute deprivation interval than after the other two deprivation intervals. When comparing number of cigarettes started after 3 and 300 minutes of deprivation, an extra cigarette was smoked in the latter condition on 10 of 12 occasions. As expected from the increased number of cigarettes started, total number of puffs in the smoking period varied as a function of the previous deprivation interval. Mean number of puffs per session was 20.3, 22.3, and 28.3 after 3, 30, and 300 minutes of deprivation ($F(2,6) = 15.4$; $P < 0.01$). Post-hoc tests revealed that subjects took significantly more puffs after the 300-minute deprivation interval than after the other two deprivation intervals.

Analysis of the average number of puffs taken on a cigarette during the smoking period as a function of deprivation interval revealed no overall significant differences between the three conditions. To determine whether there was a transient effect of deprivation on puffs per cigarette, this parameter was examined separately for the first and second cigarettes of the free smoking period. As shown in the *bottom panel* of Fig. 1, mean puff numbers for the first cigarette were 6.8, 7.5, and 8.2 after 3, 30, and 300 minutes of deprivation ($F(2,6) = 6.26$; $P < 0.05$). Post-hoc tests revealed that subjects took significantly more puffs on their first cigarette after the 300-minute deprivation interval than after the 3-minute deprivation interval. No difference in puff number was apparent as a function of the preceding deprivation interval for the second cigarette of the smoking period.

The *top panel* of Fig. 2 indicates that there was no significant difference in average puff volume as a function of the previous deprivation interval. Mean puff volumes were 45.8, 45.2, and 46.3 ml after 3, 30, and 300 minutes of deprivation. To determine if deprivation interval had a transient effect on puff volume, an analysis was done with the first cigarette of the smoking period. Again, there were no differences in puff volume as a function of previous deprivation. The *middle panel* of Fig. 2 shows that cumulative puff volume changed as a function of deprivation interval. Mean cumulative puff volumes were 903.7, 1040.8, and 1304.4 ml after 3, 30, and 300 minutes of deprivation ($F(2,6) = 6.71$; $P < 0.01$). Post-hoc tests revealed that cumulative puff volumes were significantly larger after 300 minutes of deprivation than after 3 minutes of deprivation. These differences in cumulative puff volume are primarily due to the extra cigarette smoked after the longer deprivation interval. Changes in cumulative puff volume were reflected in the biologic exposure measure. The *bottom panel* of Fig. 1 depicts the pre- to postsession CO increase as a function of the previous deprivation interval. CO boost changed in an orderly fashion in response to deprivation interval alterations. Mean increases in CO from pre- to postsession were 8.1, 14.0, and 17.0 ppm after 3, 30, and 300 minutes of deprivation ($F(2,6) = 5.10$; $P < 0.05$). Post-hoc tests revealed that CO increased significantly more after the smoking period that was preceded by the 300-minute deprivation condition than after the smoking period preceded by the 3-minute deprivation condition.

Experiment 2. Mean (±SE) puff volumes for the four-puff smoking bouts after 30, 100, and 300 minutes of deprivation, respectively, were 57.3 ± 8.5, 60.6 ± 5.5, and 61.1 ± 6.9 ml; these differences are not significant. Puff volume also did not differ as a function of order within the four-puff bout (trials factor) or session order (replications factor). Average prebout CO levels were affected by the previous deprivation period. CO levels were 40.2, 33.7, and 24.4 ppm after 30, 100, and 300 minutes of deprivation. There were no significant differences, however, in CO boost as a function of deprivation interval. Mean CO boosts were 6.0, 2.4, and 4.9 ppm after 30, 100, and 300 minutes of deprivation. CO boost did not differ as a function of session order.

Experiment 3. As shown in the *top panel* of Fig. 3, mean puff volumes were 60.7, 54.1, and 51.0 ml after 30, 10, and 3 minutes of deprivation ($F(2,10) = 6.46$; $P < 0.05$). Post-hoc tests revealed that the average puff volume for the 3-minute deprivation interval was smaller than that for the 30-minute deprivation interval. Examination of individual subject data revealed that three of the six subjects had an average puff volume in the 3-minute deprivation interval condition that was at least 10 ml smaller than the average puff volume in the 30-minute deprivation interval condition. Two of the six subjects had puff volumes in the 3- and 30-minute deprivation conditions that differed by no more than 3 ml.

Puff volume decreased as a function of order within the four-puff bout ($F(3,15) = 10.6$; $P < 0.001$), but average puff volume did not differ across replications. Although there was no main effect of bout order on puff volume, an interaction between bout order and deprivation interval approached significance, ($F(6,30) = 2.34$; $P < 0.06$). Unlike the other two conditions, the 3-minute deprivation interval condition showed progressive changes in puff volume as a function of successive puff bouts. Mean puff volumes for sequential bouts were 55.2, 51.5, 49.5, and 47.7 ml.

The *bottom panel* of Fig. 3 shows the relationship between mean CO boost and deprivation interval. As the interval shortened, CO boost decreased. The mean CO boosts were 6.3, 5.8, and 4.2 ppm after 30, 10, and 3 minutes of deprivation ($F(2,10) = 5.70$; $P < 0.05$). Post-hoc tests revealed that mean CO was larger for the 30-minute deprivation interval condition than for the 3-minute deprivation interval condition. Neither replications nor bout order had an impact on CO boost.

DISCUSSION

Experiment 1 showed that the tobacco smoke deprivation interval had an impact on subsequent puff number and spacing. When given the opportunity to smoke after 3 minutes of deprivation, subjects did not immediately light a cigarette but waited an average of 6 minutes. When given the opportunity to smoke after 30 minutes without smoking, subjects lit a cigarette within 1 minute of being allowed to do so, but took a similar number of puffs during the free smoking period as after 3 minutes of deprivation. After 300 minutes of deprivation, subjects lit their first cigarette quickly, took more puffs on the first cigarette, and smoked an additional cigarette during the 1-hour smoking period (relative to the 3-minute smoking deprivation condition).

The results of experiment 1 are for the most part consistent with other experiments that have varied smoking bout spacing. In one such study[11] subjects started to smoke sooner after 1 or 3 hours of cigarette deprivation than after 2 minutes of cigarette unavailability; also, two of the three subjects increased puff number in a free smoking session as a function of the previous deprivation interval. In another smoking availability study,[7] as the interval between smoking bouts increased, subjects took more puffs during the bouts. Neither in our study nor in a study of smokers who were motivated to quit smoking[6] did puff volume increase as a function of cigarette deprivation.

In experiment 2 we examined the effects of deprivation on puff volume when puff number and spacing were not available as compensatory mechanisms. Puff volumes after 100 and 300 minutes of tobacco smoke deprivation did not differ from that after 30 minutes of smoke deprivation. Because we did not measure normal intervals between cigarettes in our subjects, it is possible that 30 minutes of no smoking was a deprivation condition for our subjects and that all the puff volumes observed in this study were larger than normal. We were able to compare puff volumes after experimental deprivation periods with those obtained from the baseline cigarettes that immediately preceded the deprivation periods. Subjects had been smoking ad libitum before this, so there is strong reason to believe subjects were not deprived of cigarettes to any great extent. Average puff volume for the first four puffs of the baseline cigarettes was 56.7 ± 4 ml, compared with an average puff volume of 59.7 ± 3.4 ml for all the puff bouts that followed the experimental deprivation conditions (a difference of only 3 ml). This suggests that the puff volumes obtained after experimental periods of deprivation were similar to the normal puff volumes of these subjects. Why volume is not used as a compensatory mechanism after smoke deprivation is not clear. One possibility is that smokers are unable to take larger-than-normal puffs. Another possibility is that larger-than-normal puff volumes create nicotine toxicity and/or irritation of the airway passages, and are therefore avoided even after long smoke deprivation periods.

In a previous experiment in which smokers were presented with cigarettes at two and four times their normal smoking rate, they compensated by taking fewer puffs on the presented cigarettes.[8] Puff volume was not used as a compensatory mechanism. In experiment 3 we wanted to determine if puff volume is used as a compensatory mechanism during relatively short deprivation intervals under conditions in which puff number and puff distribution do not change. In this experiment, most subjects had lower puff volumes when four-puff bouts were spaced by 3-minute intervals than when 30 minutes elapsed between bouts. In lowering puff volume, subjects also lowered their exposure to CO. The average CO boost was significantly lower in the 3-minute than in the 30-minute bout spacing condition, but the magnitude of the differences in puff volume and CO exposure was small and not entirely consistent across subjects.

Previous studies and ours involving cigarette spacing alterations suggest that smokers do not use puff volume as a compensatory mechanism when puff number and puff spacing are also available as compensatory mechanisms. When puff number and spacing are not available as compensatory mechanisms, puff volume can decrease in response to short deprivation intervals, but does not readily increase in response to long deprivation intervals.

Currently there are two controlled smoking strategies available for smokers who are unable or unwilling to abstain completely from smoking but who wish to decrease health risks of smoking: Smokers can reduce the nicotine yield of their cigarettes or they can reduce their smoking rate. There is mixed evidence about the efficacy of reducing nicotine yield. Many studies have demonstrated either no relationship between nicotine yield and biologic exposure levels[2,5,14] or increased smoking intensity in response to nicotine yield reduction.[1,9,13,15,20] However, several studies involving smokers who were motivated to reduce have shown that nicotine fading can reduce biologic exposure levels, as reflected in thiocyanate and CO levels.[17-19] Our data suggest that cigarette restriction may be a viable strategy for health risk reduction, because smokers who reduce cigarette intake will probably not increase their puff volumes. However, if the number of puffs taken from each cigarette increases when cigarette access becomes limited, biologic exposure levels may not be reduced. Further research is needed to determine the relative efficacy of the cigarette and yield reduction strategy for lowering health risks of smoking.

We thank Fran Brown for assistance in conducting the studies.

References

1. Ashton H, Watson DW: Puffing frequency and nicotine intake in cigarette smokers. Br Med J **3**:679-681, 1970.
2. Benowitz NL, Hall SM, Herning RI, Jacob PJ, Jones RT, Osman AL: Smokers of low yield cigarettes do not consume less nicotine. N Engl J Med **309**:139-142, 1983.
3. Creighton DE, Lewis PH: The effect of different cigarettes on human smoking patterns. *In* Thornton RE, editor: Smoking behavior—Physiological and psychological influences. London, 1978, Churchill-Livingstone, pp 289-300.
4. Dunn PJ: The effects of a reduced draw resistance cigarette on human smoking parameters and alveolar carbon monoxide levels. *In* Thornton RE, editor: Smoking behavior—Physiological and psychological influences. London, 1978, Churchill-Livingstone, pp 203-207.
5. Ebert RV, McNabb ME, McCusker KT, Snow SL: Amount of nicotine and carbon monoxide inhaled by smokers of low tar, low nicotine cigarettes. JAMA **250**:2840-2842, 1983.
6. Epstein LH, Ossip PJ, Coleman P, Hughes JW, Wiist W: Measurement of smoking topography during withdrawal or deprivation. Behav Ther **12**:507-519, 1981.
7. Griffiths RR, Henningfield JE, Bigelow GE: Human cigarette smoking: Manipulation of number of puffs per bout, interbout interval, and nicotine dose. J Pharmacol Exp Ther **220**:256-265, 1982.
8. Gritz ER, Rose JE, Jarvik ME: Regulation of tobacco smoke intake with paced cigarette presentation. Pharmacol Biochem Behav **18**:457-462, 1983.
9. Gust SW, Pickens RW: Does cigarette nicotine yield affect puff volume? Clin Pharmacol Ther **32**:418-422, 1982.
10. Gust SW, Pickens RW, Pechacek TF: Recording puff volume in smoking. Behav Res Methods Instrumentation **15**:341-343, 1983.
11. Henningfield JE, Griffiths RR: A preparation for the experimental analysis of human cigarette smoking behavior. Behav Res Methods Instrumentation **11**:538-544, 1979.
12. Herning RI, Jones RT, Bachman JB, Mines AH: Puff volume increases when low nicotine cigarettes are smoked. Br Med J **283**:1-7, 1981.
13. Herning RI, Jones RT, Benowitz NL, Mines AH: How a cigarette is smoked determines blood nicotine levels. Clin Pharmacol Ther **33**:84-90, 1983.
14. Hill PK, Haley NJ, Wynder EL: Cigarette smoking: Carboxyhemoglobin, plasma nicotine, cotinine, and thiocyanate vs self-reported smoking data and cardiovascular disease. J Chronic Dis **36**:439-449, 1983.
15. Jarvik ME, Popek P, Schneider NG, Baer-Weiss V, Gritz ER: Can cigarette size and nicotine content influence smoking and puffing rates? Psychopharmacology **58**:303-306, 1978.
16. Kumar R, Cooke EL, Lader MH, Russell MAH: Is tobacco smoking a form of nicotine dependence? *In* Thornton RE, editor: Smoking behavior—Physiological and psychological influences. London, 1978, Churchill-Livingstone, pp 244-258.
17. Martin JE, Prue DM, Collins FC, Thames CJ: The effects of graduated filters on smoking exposure: Risk reduction or compensation? Addict Behav **6**:161-176, 1981.
18. Prue DM, Krapfl JE, Martin JE: Biochemical exposure following changes in low tar and nicotine cigarettes. Behav Res Ther **21**:400-416, 1983.
19. Prue DM, Scott RR, Martin JE, Lomax BD: Carbon monoxide levels and rates of consumption after changing to low tar and nicotine cigarettes. Behav Res Ther **21**:201-207, 1983.
20. Rawbone RG, Martin K, Tate SJ: The analysis of smoking parameters, inhalation and absorption of tobacco smoke in studies of human smoking behavior. *In* Thornton RE, editor: Smoking behavior—Physiological and psychological influences. London, 1978, Churchill-Livingstone, pp 171-194.
21. Tobin MJ, Sackner MA: Monitoring smoking patterns of low and high tar cigarettes with inductive plethysmography. Am Rev Respir Dis **126**:258-264, 1982.
22. Zacny JP, Stitzer ML: Effect of puff size instructions on puff volume. Addict Behav. (In press.)

Notes of the American Society for Clinical Pharmacology and Therapeutics

Notice of workshop

The Academy of Pharmaceutical Sciences, the ASCPT, the Drug Information Association, and the Food and Drug Administration will sponsor a workshop entitled "Controlled Release Dosage Forms: Issues and Controversies," in Washington, D.C., on Sept. 29-Oct. 2, 1985. Co-Chairmen will be Leslie Z. Benet, Ph.D., President, Academy of Pharmaceutical Sciences; David T. Lowenthal, M.D., President, ASCPT; and Jerome P. Skelly, Ph.D., Acting Director, Division of Biopharmaceutics, Food and Drug Administration. Major topics to be covered at the workshop include: pharmacokinetic considerations, biopharmaceutic considerations, clinical/pharmacodynamic considerations, regulatory considerations for therapeutic equivalence, and an open forum on biopharmaceutic concerns in controlled-release dosage forms.

Due to limited space, early registration is requested.

More detailed information, including program and registration materials, can be obtained from: Drug Information Association, P.O. Box 113, Maple Glen, PA 19002. Telephone: (215) 628-2288.

David T. Lowenthal, M.D.
President, ASCPT

Future meeting dates and sites of the ASCPT

March 20-22, 1986	Sheraton Washington Hotel, Washington, D.C.
March 25-28, 1987	Marriott Orlando World Center, Walt Disney World, Fla.
March 9-11, 1988	Town and Country Hotel, San Diego, Calif.

Call for scientific program abstracts forms for 1986 meeting in Washington, D.C., March 20-22, are included in this issue of the JOURNAL and will also appear in the June and August issues. Additional forms are available on request to Elaine Galasso, 1718 Gallagher Rd., Norristown, PA 19401; (215) 825-3838.

USAN Council

List No. 262

New Names

The following nonproprietary names for the compounds described have been adopted by the United States Adopted Names (USAN) Council, which is sponsored by the American Medical Association, the American Pharmaceutical Association, and the US Pharmacopeial Convention, Inc., in cooperation with the respective pharmaceutical manufacturers. The designation USAN (United States Adopted Name) distinguishes these formally adopted nonproprietary names from other names. The information given under the category Therapeutic Claim is based on the manufacturer's claims at the time of publication. Adoption of USAN does not imply endorsement of the claims or products by the AMA, the US Pharmacopeia, or the APhA.

In some instances, the drugs listed are available only from the manufacturer to properly qualified investigators for clinical study.

USAN — AMFILCON A

Pronunciation — ăm′ fĭl″ kŏn

Ingredient function — contact lens material (hydrophilic)

Chemical names

(1) 2-hydroxyethyl 2-methyl-2-propenoate polymer with 2-methyl-2-propenoic acid and 1,2-ethanediyl bis(2-methyl-2-propenoate)

(2) 2-hydroxyethyl methacrylate polymer with methacrylic acid and ethylene dimethacrylate

Structural formula

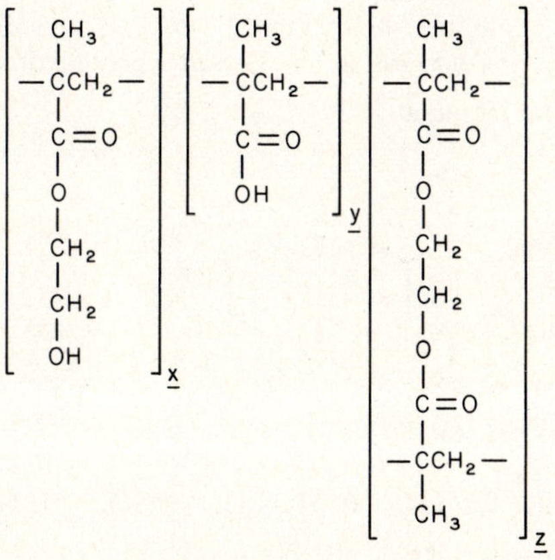

Molecular formula — $(C_6H_{10}O_3)x(C_4H_6O_2)y(C_{10}H_{14}O_4)z$

Manufacturer — Applied Optics

CAS registry No. — 33410-59-2

USAN — CETIRIZINE HYDROCHLORIDE

Pronunciation — sĕ tĭ′ rĭ zēn

Therapeutic claim — antihistamine

Chemical names

(1) (±)-[2-[4-[(4-chlorophenyl)phenylmethyl]-1-piperazinyl]ethoxy]acetic acid, dihydrochloride

(2) (±)-[2-[4-(*p*-chloro-α-phenylbenzyl)-1-piperazinyl]ethoxy]acetic acid, dihydrochloride

Structural formula

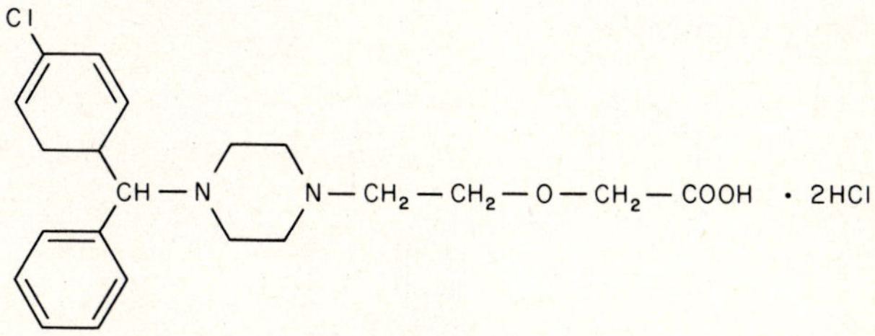

Molecular formula — $C_{21}H_{25}ClN_2O_3 \cdot 2HCl$

Molecular weight — 461.8

Manufacturer — Pfizer Inc.

Code designation — P 071

CAS registry No. — 83881-52-1

USAN — REMOXIPRIDE

Pronunciation — rĕ mŏks′ ĭ prīd″

Therapeutic claim — antipsychotic

Chemical names

(1) (*S*)-3-bromo-*N*-[(1-ethyl-2-pyrrolidinyl)methyl]-2,6-dimethoxybenzamide

(2) (−)-(*S*)-3-bromo-*N*-[(1-ethyl-2-pyrrolidinyl)methyl]-2,6-dimethoxybenzamide

Structural formula

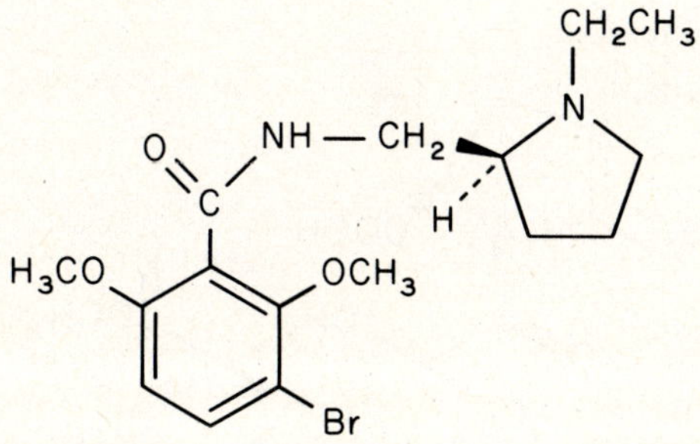

Molecular formula — $C_{16}H_{23}BrN_2O_3$

Molecular weight — 371.27

Manufacturer — Aktiebolaget Astra (Sweden)

Code designations — A 33547; FLA 731

CAS registry No. — 80125-14-0

USAN PELRINONE HYDROCHLORIDE

Pronunciation pĕl′ rĭ nōn

Therapeutic claim cardiotonic

Chemical names

(1) 1,4-dihydro-2-methyl-4-oxo-6-[(3-pyridinylmethyl)amino]-5-pyrimidinecarbonitrile monohydrochloride

(2) 1,4-dihydro-2-methyl-4-oxo-6-[(3-pyridylmethyl)amino]-5-pyrimidinecarbonitrile monohydrochloride

Structural formula

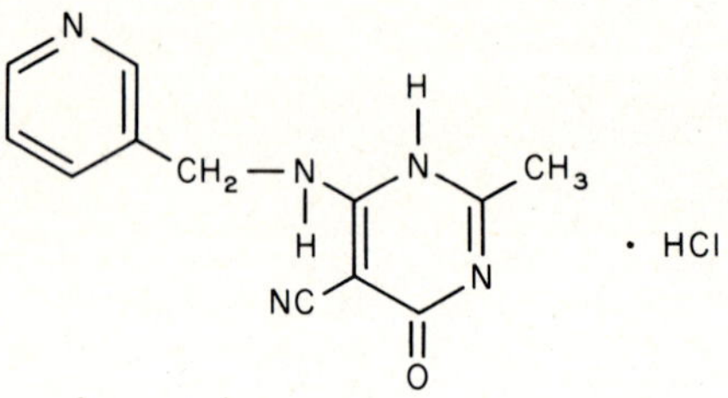

Molecular formula $C_{12}H_{11}N_5O \cdot HCl$

Molecular weight 277.5

Manufacturer Ayerst Laboratories

Code designation AY-28,768

CAS registry No. 89232-84-8

USAN PENTOPRIL

Pronunciation pĕn′ tō prĭl

Therapeutic claim antihypertensive (ACE inhibitor)

Chemical names

(1) ethyl [2*S*-[1(α*S**,γ*S**),2*R**]]-2-carboxy-2,3-dihydro-α,γ-dimethyl-δ-oxo-1*H*-indole-1-pentanoate

(2) ethyl (α*R*,γ*R*,2*S*)-2-carboxy-α,γ-dimethyl-δ-oxo-1-indolinevalerate

Structural formula

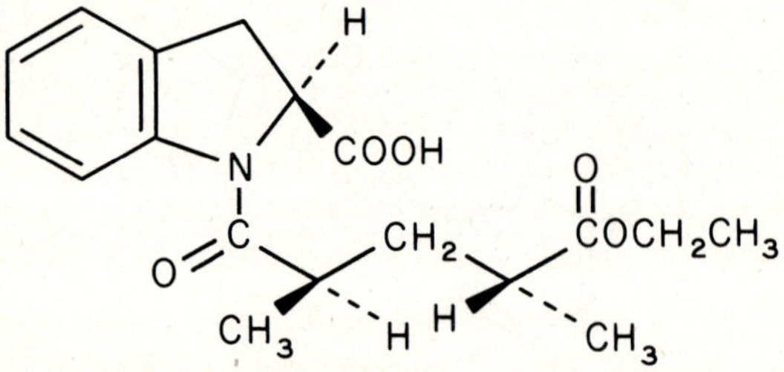

Molecular formula $C_{18}H_{23}NO_5$

Molecular weight 333.37

Manufacturer Ciba-Geigy Corporation

Code designation CGS 13945

CAS registry No. 82924-03-6

USAN FLESTOLOL SULFATE

Pronunciation flĕs′ tō lōl

Therapeutic claim antiadrenergic (β-receptor)

Chemical names

(1) (±)-3-[[2-[(aminocarbonyl)amino]-1,1-dimethylethyl]amino]-2-hydroxypropyl 2-fluorobenzoate, sulfate (1:1) (salt)

(2) *o*-fluorobenzoic acid, 3-ester with (±)-[2-[(2,3-dihydroxypropyl)amino]-2-methylpropyl]urea, sulfate (1:1) (salt)

Structural formula

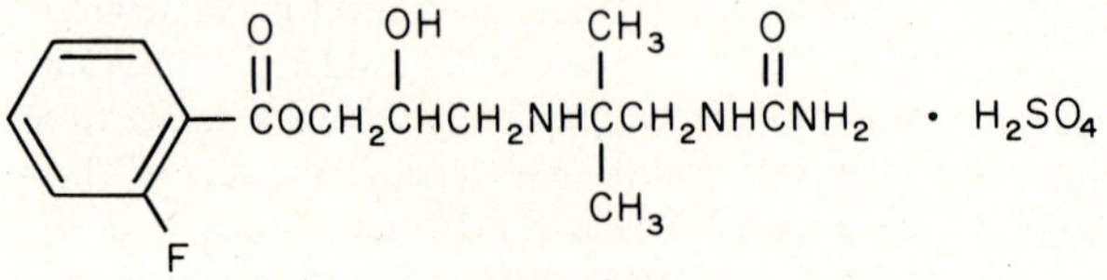

Molecular formula $C_{15}H_{22}FN_3O_4 \cdot H_2SO_4$

Molecular weight 425.43

Manufacturer American Critical Care

Code designation ACC-9089

CAS registry No. 88844-73-9

USAN TROSPECTOMYCIN SULFATE

Pronunciation trō′ spĕk tō mī″ sĭn

Therapeutic claim antibiotic

Chemical names

(1) [2*R*-(2α,4aβ,5aβ,6β,7β,8β,9α,9aα,10aβ)]-2-butyldecahydro-4a,7,9-trihydroxy-6,8-bis(methylamino)-4*H*-pyrano[2,3-*b*][1,4]benzodioxin-4-one sulfate (1:1), pentahydrate

(2) (2*R*,4a*R*,5a*R*,6*S*,7*S*,8*R*,9*S*,9a*R*,10a*S*)-2-butyldecadro-4a,7,9-trihydroxy-6,8-bis(methylamino)-4*H*-pyrano[2,3-*b*][1,4]benzodioxin-4-one sulfate (1:1) (salt), pentahydrate

Structural formula

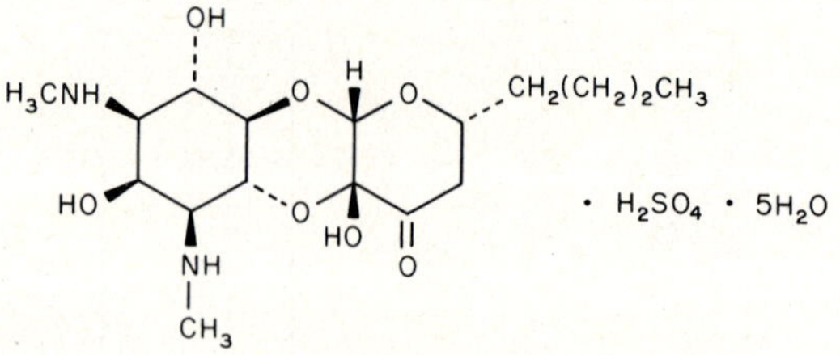

Molecular formula $C_{17}H_{30}N_2O_7 \cdot H_2SO_4 \cdot 5H_2O$

Molecular weight 562.60

Manufacturer The Upjohn Company

Code designation U-63,366F

CAS registry No. 88851-61-0

CLINICAL PHARMACOLOGY & THERAPEUTICS
VOLUME 38 NUMBER 2 AUGUST 1985

ORIGINAL ARTICLES

Effect of probenecid on the formation and elimination of acyl glucuronides: Studies with zomepirac

When 100 mg oral zomepirac was taken with 500 mg b.i.d. oral probenecid by six healthy subjects, the disposition of zomepirac was markedly altered. Probenecid decreased total plasma clearance of zomepirac by 64%, which resulted in an increase in bioavailability from 0.55 without probenecid to 0.84 when given concurrently. The apparent metabolic clearance of zomepirac to form zomepirac acyl glucuronide was reduced 71% and zomepirac renal clearance, a minor elimination route, was reduced by 79%. When assayed by a method that prevents degradation of the labile acyl glucuronide, zomepirac glucuronide concentrations in plasma were comparable to those of zomepirac. Probenecid decreased the renal clearance of zomepirac glucuronide by 72%, which, together with the increased zomepirac levels, resulted in a 2.8-fold increase in the AUC of the conjugate. Urinary excretion of zomepirac glucuronide was reduced from 72% to 58% of the dose, but the excretion of free zomepirac was unchanged at 5% of the dose. The ratio of the total clearance/bioavailability of zomepirac in control subjects was 682 ± 246 ml/min, which is double the value reported in previous studies of zomepirac disposition. We believe that this difference is

Philip C. Smith, Ph.D.,* Pim N. J. Langendijk, M.S.,**
John A. Bosso, Pharm.D.,* and Leslie Z. Benet, Ph.D.** *San Francisco, Calif.*

From the Department of Pharmacy, University of California, San Francisco.

Supported in part by a grant from McNeil Pharmaceutical, Spring House, Pa., and by National Institutes of Health Grant No. GM26691.

Received for publication Jan. 15, 1985; accepted April 18, 1985.

Reprint requests to: Dr. Leslie Z. Benet, Department of Pharmacy, University of California, San Francisco, CA 94143.

*Merck Fellow of the American Foundation for Pharmaceutical Education.

**Present address: National Poison Control Centre, National Institute of Health and Environmental Hygiene, P.O. Box 1, 3720 BA Bilthoven, The Netherlands.

***Present address: Department of Pharmacy Practice, College of Pharmacy, University of Utah, Salt Lake City, UT 84112.

due to degradation of the unstable zomepirac acyl glucuronide in the previous analytic methodologies used. Qualitatively, the effects of probenecid on zomepirac disposition are similar to those previously reported for other drugs of this class that are metabolized to acyl glucuronides. However, zomepirac appears unusual in that significant levels of its acyl glucuronide metabolite are found in vivo. (CLIN PHARMACOL THER 38:121-127, 1985.)

Zomepirac (5-(4-chlorobenzoyl)-1,4-dimethyl-1*H*-pyrrole-2-acetic acid) is a nonsteroidal anti-inflammatory drug (NSAID)[2] previously marketed as the dihydrate of the sodium salt in the United States under the tradename Zomax (McNeil Pharmaceutical). It was voluntarily withdrawn from distribution in the United States because of unexplained anaphylactic reactions that in some cases resulted in death.[14,17] In man, zomepirac is primarily eliminated by metabolic conjugation to the acyl glucuronide, which is subsequently excreted in the urine.[6,10,11,20] A minor oxidative metabolite, hydroxyzomepirac, has also been reported in man and this, too, is excreted in the urine.[6,11]

Probenecid (4-[dipropylaminosulfonyl]benzoic acid) is often used with NSAIDs for the treatment of gout.[4] Because probenecid can alter the renal excretion of acids,[4] it was of interest to determine whether it would affect the disposition of zomepirac in man. Probenecid interacts to varying degrees with all of the NSAIDs of the aryl-alkanoic acid class that have been examined for such a possible interaction. These include indomethacin,[1,3,5] naproxen,[13] ketoprofen,[16] and carprofen,[21] all of which are metabolized to acyl glucuronides to a significant extent. The mechanism for the effect of probenecid on the disposition of NSAIDs and other acidic compounds that are eliminated by formation of acyl glucuronides as well as by renal elimination has not been resolved. Probenecid may competitively inhibit formation of the glucuronide or it may block renal excretion of the conjugate, with subsequent chemical or enzymatic hydrolysis of the labile conjugate in vivo. We describe the effect of probenecid on zomepirac and zomepirac glucuronide disposition and discuss the possible basis for this interaction.

METHODS

Six men took 100 mg zomepirac as a tablet (Zomax) by mouth on two separate occasions. On one occasion, zomepirac was given at 8 AM without concurrent probenecid. The other zomepirac dose was given after previous oral dosing with 500 mg b.i.d. probenecid (Benemid; Merck, Sharpe & Dohme) for 3 days before zomepirac dosing and dosing continued throughout the blood sampling period. On the day of zomepirac dosing, the morning probenecid dose was taken 30 minutes before zomepirac dosing. The two experiments were separated by 7 to 10 days and subjects were randomly assigned to a particular dosing regimen.

All the subjects were healthy men between the ages of 21 and 30 years who weighed from 68 to 84 kg. Studies were conducted in September 1982, before the discontinuation of Zomax distribution in the United States. Before and after the study the subjects were determined to be healthy by physical examination, blood analysis, and urinalysis. Creatinine, bilirubin, and liver transaminase levels were normal for all subjects both before and after the study. None of the subjects smoked. Other drugs and alcohol were excluded for 14 days before and during the study. Subjects fasted from 10 PM the day before each study. At 8 AM, a 100 mg tablet of zomepirac was taken by mouth with 180 ml water. A light liquid lunch was served after blood sampling 4 hours after dosing and dinner was eaten as desired after the blood sampling 10 hours after dosing. Water and cranberry juice were taken ad libitum throughout the study. Cranberry juice was provided to acidify the urine, and subjects were instructed to avoid foods that might increase the urine pH, such as cabbage, bananas, cantaloupe, and large amounts of vegetables.[12] Subjects were ambulatory during the study, but were instructed not to engage in strenuous exercise.

An indwelling catheter with a heparin lock was inserted into the forearm of each subject to allow for blood sampling during the part of the study when samples were taken frequently. Between samples the catheter was flushed with a solution of heparin, 10 U/ml, in normal saline solution. The heparin was discarded before blood was sampled. Once drawn, blood samples were immediately placed in a tube cooled on ice containing 143 U heparin, then mixed. Within 15 minutes the cooled blood was centrifuged for 10 minutes at 0° to 4° C to separate plasma, then the plasma (about 2.5 ml) was transferred to a vial containing 25 μl 86% phosphoric acid, which decreased the pH to between pH 2 and 4. This rapid handling of blood and plasma at reduced temperatures minimized the loss of zomepirac glucuronide by hydrolysis and acyl migration, which is appreciable at room temperature and physiologic pH.[7,15] Under this procedure, zomepirac glucuronide loss was kept to <4% when control spiked blood samples were analyzed.[15] Plasma once buffered to a pH between 2 and 4 was frozen at −20° C until analyzed by HPLC within several weeks. Blood was drawn before zomepirac dosing and 10, 20, 30, 40, 60, and 90 minutes and 3, 4, 5, 6, 8, 10, 12, and 24 hours thereafter. When probenecid was given concurrently, additional blood samples were drawn at 28, 32, 34, 36, and 48 hours.

Precautions for ensuring zomepirac glucuronide stability in urine were also implemented through use of the best possible methods short of urinary bladder catheterization. Because the stability of zomepirac glucuronide improves quite dramatically with a decrease of pH from 7.4 to 5.0,[7] diet was modified as described above to maintain urine pH <6, if possible. For the short intervals of urine collection between 0 and 8 hours after dosing, the pH and volume were recorded and a 15 ml aliquot was saved for analysis. Urine was processed upon collection to minimize artifactual zomepirac glucuronide loss. The urine for analysis was added to a vial containing 75 μl 86% phosphoric acid, which reduced the pH to between pH 2 and 4. Urine was then frozen at −20° C before analysis for zomepirac and zomepirac glucuronide (within 1 month). Over long collection intervals that necessitated voiding during the interval, urine was collected in a container with 1 ml 86% phosphoric acid and then kept refrigerated until the end of the collection interval. The combined urine sample for an interval was adjusted to a pH between 2 and 4 with 86% phosphoric acid before volume measurement and a 15 ml aliquot was frozen at −20° C. Urine collection intervals were 0 to 1, 1 to 2, 2 to 3, 3 to 4, 4 to 6, 6 to 8, 8 to 12, 12 to 24, and 24 to 48 hours after dosing. When probenecid was given concurrently, additional urine collections were made from 24 to 36, 36 to 48, and 48 to 72 hours after dosing.

Plasma and urine were assayed for zomepirac, zomepirac glucuronide (directly), and probenecid by an HPLC method developed in our laboratory.[8] This method minimizes zomepirac glucuronide loss, which may be a significant problem with previous assays for zomepirac.

Kinetic analysis was by model-independent equations. Zomepirac absorption was assumed to be complete, as has been reported.[10,11] The AUC was calculated by the linear trapezoidal method from time zero to the time of the last peak observed, after which the log-linear trapezoidal method was used. The terminal AUC was estimated as the last concentration measured divided by β, where β was determined by the last two or three points that appeared to be log linear. Kinetic parameters were calculated with methods previously used for zomepirac.[11] These kinetic equations assume complete absorption of an oral zomepirac dose and that all metabolism of zomepirac occurs in the liver,[11] as there have been no reports of the renal metabolism of zomepirac. Under these assumptions, $CL_z/F_z = Dose_z/AUC_z = CL_{int,\,z}$,[19] where CL_z is the total body clearance of zomepirac, F_z is its bioavailability, and $CL_{int,\,z}$ is the intrinsic clearance of zomepirac. Values for hepatic blood flow and the blood/plasma ratio for zomepirac were those used by O'Neill et al.,[11] 1450 ml/min and 0.52, respectively. Four additional equations were used for estimating metabolic and renal clearances:

$$CL_{z \rightarrow zg} = Ae_{zg}(0 - \infty) \cdot CL_{P,z}/dose_z \quad (1)$$

$$CL_{R,z} = Ae_z(0 - \infty)/\ AUC_z \quad (2)$$

$$CL_{z \rightarrow other} = CL_{P,z} - CL_{z \rightarrow zg} - CL_{R,z} \quad (3)$$

$$CL_{R,zg} = Ae_{zg}(t_n - t_{n-1})/AUC_{zg}(t_n - t_{n-1}) \quad (4)$$

where $CL_{z \rightarrow zg}$ is the apparent metabolic clearance to form zomepirac glucuronide, Ae_{zg} and Ae_z are the amounts of zomepirac glucuronide and zomepirac excreted in the urine, $CL_{P,z}$ is the plasma clearance of zomepirac, $CL_{R,z}$ and $CL_{R,zg}$ are the renal clearances of zomepirac and zomepirac glucuronide, and t is time. As mentioned above, absorption is assumed to be complete both in the presence and absence of probenecid, and "other" refers to metabolic clearance not accounted for by that of zomepirac glucuronide. In Eq. 4, $CL_{R,zg}$ is calculated as the amount of metabolite excreted during a particular time interval $(t_n - t_{n-1})$ divided by the AUC for the metabolite during that time interval.

It is assumed that once formed, all zomepirac glucuronide is excreted in the urine, as a previous study indicated that >90% of an oral ^{14}C-labeled dose is excreted in the urine.[11] The possible hydrolysis of zomepirac glucuronide in vivo is not accounted for in Eq. 1; this clearance term reflects net elimination of zomepirac by metabolism to zomepirac glucuronide.

Statistical analysis was by a two-tailed paired Student's t test comparing control and probenecid treatments for each subject. A P value ≤0.05 was considered significant.

RESULTS

Analysis of the plasma samples revealed that zomepirac glucuronide levels were higher than expected based on a previous report.[11] The concentration of zomepirac glucuronide in plasma approached and at some times exceeded zomepirac levels even when expressed

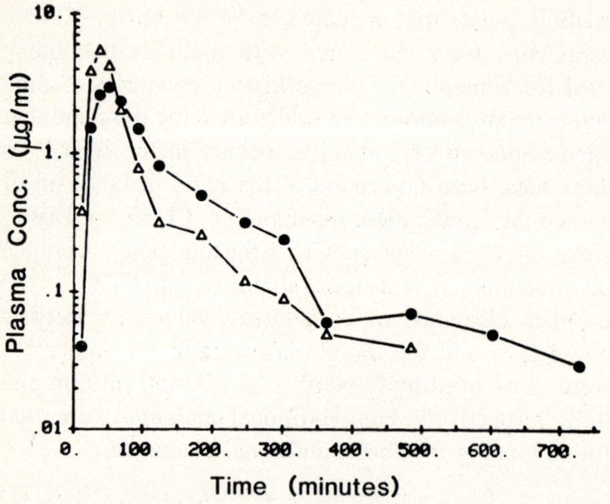

Fig. 1. Representative plasma concentration profile of zomepirac (△) and zomepirac glucuronide (●; reported as zomepirac equivalents) after a single 100 mg oral dose of zomepirac.

in molar units and when no probenecid was present. In the control experiments, the mean AUC_{zg} was slightly higher than the AUC_z. When probenecid was added the mean AUC_z increased by 4.3-fold, while AUC_{zg} increased by a lesser amount (2.8-fold). Fig. 1 shows a representative plasma concentration profile. The irregular shape of the profile with the existence of secondary peaks and shoulders may be indicative of enterohepatic recycling, which has been observed in animals.[6] Absorption also seemed irregular, with late peak times for several of the subjects, as reflected in the wide variance of the peak times (Table I). As a result, time to peak and peak concentration were not significantly different between controls and subjects who received probenecid (Table I). As mentioned in Methods, zomepirac glucuronide can hydrolyze to form zomepirac or rearrange to form isomeric conjugates in blood and plasma,[15] but the sample handling procedure minimized this loss to ≤4%.[8,15] As shown in Fig. 2, many of the HPLC chromatograms contained isomeric conjugate peaks representing >4% total conjugates. This indicates that acyl migration is occurring in vivo, although the extent of this rearrangement was not fully evaluated because of the limited resolution of this HPLC method. In the analysis used here, zomepirac glucuronide and its isomeric conjugates were combined and are referred to simply as zomepirac glucuronide. In most subjects the concentration-time profile of zomepirac glucuronide was nearly parallel to zomepirac levels, which indicates that the zomepirac glucuronide $t_{1/2}$ was probably controlled by its rate of formation from zomepirac.

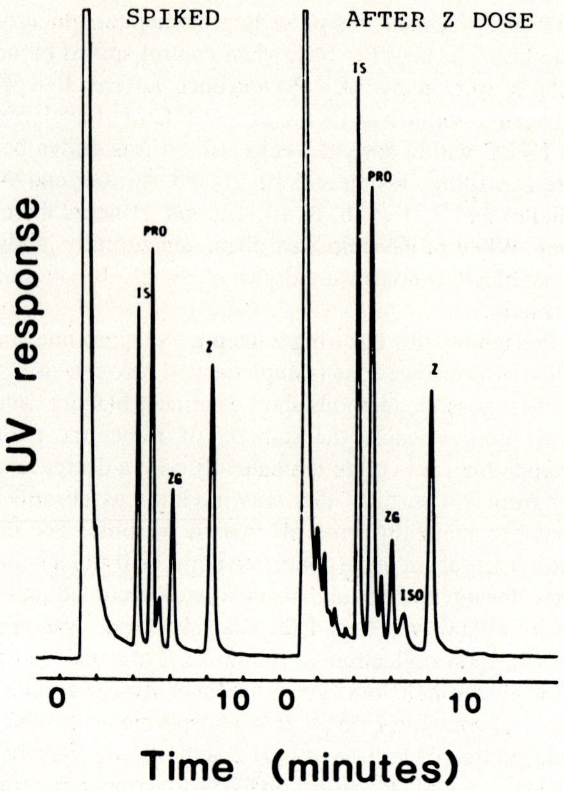

Fig. 2. Chromatograms of plasma spiked with internal standard *(IS)* and 1 μg/ml of zomepirac *(Z)* and zomepirac glucuronide *(ZG)* with probenecid *(PRO)* and plasma 1 hour after a 100 mg oral dose of zomepirac from a subject pretreated with probenecid. *ISO* = Isomeric conjugates of zomepirac glucuronide.

Clearance parameters for zomepirac and zomepirac glucuronide were altered significantly by probenecid (Table I). Mean CL_z/F_z was reduced from 682 to 155 ml/min. When analyzed further, this decline was due to a reduction in clearance and a decrease in the extent of first-pass metabolism. The primary clearance mechanism for zomepirac, $CL_{z \rightarrow zg}$, decreased 71%, from 252 to 74 ml/min. $CL_{R,z}$ was much less than metabolic clearance, but it too was decreased 79% by probenecid, from 36 to 8 ml/min. However, zomepirac clearance by all other routes was unchanged at 60 and 45 ml/min, respectively. When combined, $CL_{P,z}$ was reduced from 348 to 127 ml/min by probenecid. Adding the effects of an increased availability from 0.55 to 0.84, the resultant CL_z/F shows an even greater change of 77%, from 682 to 155 ml/min. Finally, $CL_{R,zg}$ was reduced by probenecid from 406 to 115 ml/min.

When combined, Ae_z and Ae_{zg} accounted for 78% and 63% of the total dose in the controls and subjects

Table I. Summary of the kinetic analysis of a 100 mg oral dose of zomepirac with and without concurrent probenecid dosing

	Zomepirac alone	*Zomepirac and probenecid*	*Ratio of treatments, probenecid/control*
$C_{max,z}$ (μg/ml)	1.60 ± 1.74	3.54 ± 1.58	2.21
$t_{max,z}$ (min)	145 ± 126	101 ± 87	0.70
$C_{max,zg}$ (μg/ml)	1.09 ± 0.42	1.70 ± 0.72	1.62
$t_{max,zg}$ (min)	138 ± 110	139 ± 78	1.01
CL_z/F_z (ml/min)	682 ± 246	155 ± 58	0.23*
$CL_{P,z}$ (ml/min)	348 ± 71	127 ± 40	0.36*
$CL_{z\rightarrow zg}$ (ml/min)	252 ± 60	74 ± 27	0.29*
$CL_{R,z}$ (ml/min)	36 ± 10	7.7 ± 2.6	0.21*
$CL_{z\rightarrow other}$ (ml/min)	60 ± 16	45 ± 14	0.75
$CL_{R,zg}$ (ml/min)	406 ± 110	115 ± 32	0.28*
Extraction $ratio_z$	0.45 ± 0.10	0.16 ± 0.078	0.36*
Ae_z (0-∞) (mg)	5.5 ± 0.98	5.1 ± 0.58	0.93
Ae_{zg} (0-∞) (mg)	72 ± 5.9	58 ± 5.1	0.81*
Ae_{total} (0-∞) (mg)	78 ± 5.2	63 ± 5.3	0.81*
AUC_z (μg · min/ml)	165 ± 64	708 ± 308	4.29*
AUC_{zg} (μg · min/ml)	180 ± 57	499 ± 134	2.77*

Data are $\bar{X}$ ± SD. All concentrations and amounts are in zomepirac equivalents.
C_{max} = Maximum concentration; t_{max} = time to C_{max}.
*$P < 0.05$ (paired t test; n = 6).

who received probenecid, respectively. Almost all the zomepirac eliminated in the urine was as zomepirac glucuronide, with only about 5% of the total dose eliminated in the urine as unmetabolized zomepirac in both controls and subjects receiving probenecid. Even with the precautions taken to maintain zomepirac glucuronide stability in urine, the value of unchanged drug in the urine may be overestimated, as was noted for acyl glucuronide conjugates by Upton et al.[16] Urinary recovery of zomepirac glucuronide was significantly decreased from 72% to 58% by concurrent probenecid dosing (Table I).

Probenecid concentrations in plasma were usually in the range of 20 to 100 μg/ml during the studies when probenecid was dosed concurrently. These levels are about twentyfold higher molar concentrations than those observed for zomepirac. Urine pH was always ≤6.5 when measured, with most urine samples at pH 5.5.

DISCUSSION

The effect of probenecid on the disposition of zomepirac is qualitatively similar to that of the other NSAIDs tested for this interaction. Our results of zomepirac disposition in control experiments, however, differ from reports in the literature that did not control for zomepirac glucuronide instability in blood or plasma. The CL_z/F_z values obtained by other investigators for zomepirac in healthy subjects were, when normalized to a 70 kg man, calculated by us to be 297,[6] 200,[10] 259,[20] and 254 ml/min,[11] whereas our value was 682 ml/min (Table I). We believe that all of the previous estimates of zomepirac clearance are artifactually low because of the problem of zomepirac glucuronide hydrolysis during sample handling and analysis. A comparison of our analytic method with that used by O'Neill et al.[11] has shown[15] that zomepirac glucuronide degrades entirely to zomepirac and isomeric conjugates when no precautions are taken to maintain the stability of the labile acyl glucuronide, zomepirac glucuronide.

Urinary excretion data from our study are in better agreement with published work. In control experiments almost all zomepirac is eliminated in the urine as zomepirac glucuronide,[6,10,11,20] and our results show that only about 5% of the dose was excreted unchanged. Although zomepirac glucuronide loss does occur at a urine pH of 5 to 7, it is slow and results primarily in the formation of isomeric conjugates[7] that are cleaved by base hydrolysis. The high $CL_{R,zg}$ in control subjects of 406 ml/min is much higher than the glomerular filtration rate, indicating extensive active secretion of zomepirac glucuronide. This secretion is dramatically decreased by probenecid, a compound known to competitively block active secretion of organic acids.[4]

Peak plasma concentrations of zomepirac and the time to reach the peak were quite variable. This variability resulted in no significant difference being noted when probenecid was added even though AUC_z increased more than fourfold. Multiple peaks were observed for many of the plasma concentration-time profiles, which may be indicative of either enterohepatic recycling, as occurs in rats,[6] or perhaps of variable and unpredictable absorption. The irregular shape of the concentration-time profile was evident in a recent report on zomepirac disposition in man.[20] Likewise, O'Neill et al.[11] stated that their data were not appropriate for individual fitting to traditional kinetic models.

A direct comparison of our results with previous studies of the probenecid/NSAID interaction yields the same conclusion that Upton et al.[16] stated earlier—that the mechanism of the interaction differs more quantitatively than qualitatively when NSAIDs are compared. Naproxen, indomethacin, carprofen, ketoprofen, and zomepirac are eliminated primarily by conjugation with glucuronic acid, with varying degrees of phase 1 metabolism. Once formed, the glucuronides are then primarily excreted in the urine. Probenecid appears to affect the glucuronidation and renal clearance of zomepirac, but has no discernable effect on other metabolic clearance processes. Probenecid, which is given in larger doses, has much higher plasma concentration than zomepirac. A major route of elimination for probenecid is conjugation with glucuronic acid,[4] which may competitively decrease zomepirac glucuronide formation, as shown by a reduction in $CL_{z \rightarrow zg}$ of 71%. However, this is not easily distinguished from inhibition of renal secretion of the conjugate with subsequent hydrolysis of the labile acyl glucuronide in vivo. This alternative mechanism was discussed by Upton et al.,[16] and Verbeeck et al.[18] suggest that this is the favored explanation for the decrease in ketoprofen clearance in the elderly. More recently, Meffin et al.[9] have shown by dosing intravenous clofibric acid glucuronide to rabbits that the conjugate is cleaved very rapidly in vivo. Preliminary studies in our laboratory have shown that zomepirac glucuronide is also quickly hydrolyzed in vivo when it is given intravenously to rabbits or guinea pigs. Nonetheless, the net effect is that probenecid dramatically reduces the apparent clearance of zomepirac through conjugation with glucuronic acid. Metabolic clearance by other routes could also be affected by probenecid. Because urinary recoveries of zomepirac and zomepirac glucuronide did not account for the total dose administered, the term $CL_{z \rightarrow other}$ need not represent hydroxyzomepirac, which was not measured by our assay. Although $CL_{z \rightarrow other}$ did not change, the AUC_z increased 4.3-fold and the apparent $CL_{z \rightarrow zg}$ fell even further, which may result in an increased fraction of the total dose undergoing phase 1 metabolism, as was observed for naproxen when probenecid was given concurrently.[13] This may explain the decrease in Ae_{zg} when probenecid was coadministered.

Probenecid depressed $CL_{R,z}$, which is expected. However, as with the previous studies of the probenecid/NSAID interaction, this contributes little to the mechanism of the interaction, because renal clearance is only a small fraction of the total clearance.

Two previous studies with indomethacin[1] and ketoprofen[16] that attempted to measure glucuronide conjugates in plasma reported very little conjugate relative to parent drug. However, in neither of the studies was sample handling or HPLC analysis controlled to prevent the possible degradation of the labile glucuronide. Measurement of low concentrations of the conjugate by the difference in the parent drug found after hydrolysis with β-glucuronidase or addition of base is often inaccurate. Also, the isomeric conjugates formed by acyl migration are not susceptible to cleavage by β-glucuronidase.[7] Zomepirac may be unusual in that zomepirac glucuronide levels in vivo approximate those of zomepirac, but until proper procedures are developed for the analysis of labile acyl glucuronides, the interpretation of other studies with NSAIDs may be questioned. To provide unambiguous answers to resolve the mechanism by which probenecid alters the disposition of NSAIDs, animal studies must be done to characterize the disposition of the glucuronide metabolite.

References

1. Baber N, Halliday L, Sibeon R, Littler T, Orme MLE: The interaction between indomethacin and probenecid. Clin Pharmacol Ther **24**:298-307, 1978.
2. Baird WM, Turek D: Comparison of zomepirac, APC with codeine, codeine and placebo in the treatment of moderate and severe post operative pain. J Clin Pharmacol **20**:243-249, 1980.
3. Brooks PM, Bell MA, Sturrock RD, Famaey JP, Dick WC: The clinical significance of indomethacin-probenecid interaction. Br J Clin Pharmacol **1**:287-290, 1974.
4. Cunningham RF, Israili ZH, Dayton PG: Clinical pharmacokinetics of probenecid. Clin Pharmacokinet **6**:135-151, 1981.
5. Duggan DE, Hooke KF, White SD, Noll RM, Stevenson CR: The effects of probenecid upon the individual components of indomethacin elimination. J Pharmacol Exp Ther **201**:463-470, 1977.
6. Grindel JM, O'Neill PJ, Yorgey KA, Schwartz MH, McKown LA, Migdalof BH, Wu WN: Metabolism of zomepirac sodium. I. Disposition in laboratory animals and man. Drug Metab Dispos **8**:343-348, 1980.

7. Hasegawa J, Smith PC, Benet LZ: Apparent intramolecular acyl migration of zomepirac glucuronide. Drug Metab Dispos **10:**469-473, 1982.
8. Langendijk PNJ, Smith PC, Hasegawa J, Benet LZ: Simultaneous determination of zomepirac and its major metabolite zomepirac glucuronide in human plasma and urine. J Chromatogr **307:**371-379, 1984.
9. Meffin PJ, Zilm DM, Veenendaal JR: Reduced clofibric acid clearance in renal dysfunction is due to a futile cycle. J Pharmacol Exp Ther **227:**732-738, 1983.
10. Nayak RK, Ng KT, Gottlieb S, Plostnieks J: Zomepirac kinetics in healthy males. CLIN PHARMACOL THER **27:**395-401, 1980.
11. O'Neill PJ, Yorgey KA, Renzi NL, Williams RL, Benet LZ: Disposition of zomepirac sodium in healthy subjects. J Clin Pharmacol **22:**470-476, 1982.
12. Pemberton CM, Gastinea CF: Mayo clinic diet manual. Philadelphia, 1981, WB Saunders Co.
13. Runkel R, Mroszczak E, Chaplin M, Sevelius H, Segre E: Naproxen-probenecid interaction. CLIN PHARMACOL THER **24:**706-713, 1978.
14. Samuel SA: Apparent anaphylactic reaction to zomepirac (Zomax). N Engl J Med **304:**978, 1981.
15. Smith PC, Hasegawa J, Langendijk PNJ, Benet LZ: Stability of acyl glucuronides in biological fluids: Studies with zomepirac. Drug Metab Dispos **13:**110-112, 1985.
16. Upton RA, Williams RL, Buskin JN, Jones RM: Effects of probenecid on ketoprofen kinetics. CLIN PHARMACOL THER **31:**705-712, 1982.
17. US Congress, Committee on Government Operations, Intergovernment Relations and Human Resources: FDA's regulation of Zomax[R]. Washington, DC, 1982, Proceedings of the Ninety-eighth Congress.
18. Verbeeck RK, Wallace SM, Loewen GR: Reduced elimination of ketoprofen in the elderly is not necessarily due to impaired glucuronidation. Br J Clin Pharmacol **17:**783-784, 1984.
19. Wilkinson GR, Shand DG: A physiological approach to hepatic drug clearance. CLIN PHARMACOL THER **18:**277-390, 1975.
20. Witassek F, Bircher J, Huguenin P, Preisig R: Abnormal glucuronidation in patients with cirrhosis of the liver. Hepatology **3:**415-422, 1983.
21. Yu TF, Perel J: Pharmacokinetic and clinical studies of carprofen in gout. J Clin Pharmacol **20:**347-351, 1980.

Future meeting dates and sites of the ASCPT

March 20-22, 1986	Sheraton Washington Hotel, Washington, D.C.
March 25-28, 1987	Marriott Orlando World Center, Walt Disney World, Fla.
March 9-11, 1988	Town and Country Hotel, San Diego, Calif.

Call for scientific program abstracts forms for 1986 meeting in Washington, D.C., March 20-22, are included in this issue of the JOURNAL and also appeared in the June and July issues. Additional forms are available on request to Elaine Galasso, 1718 Gallagher Rd., Norristown, PA 19401; (215) 825-3838.

Metabolism of methoxyphenamine in extensive and poor metabolizers of debrisoquin

Urine and plasma concentrations of methoxyphenamine (MP) and three of its metabolites were determined after a single oral 60.3 mg dose of MP hydrochloride to healthy subjects of known debrisoquin (D) phenotype. Urine was collected from five extensive (EM) and five poor (PM) metabolizers of D for 12 hours and analyzed after treatment with β-glucuronidase/sulfatase. There were marked interphenotype differences in the total urinary excretion of *O*-demethylmethoxyphenamine (ODMP) and 5-hydroxymethoxyphenamine (5HMP), as well as in MP/ODMP and MP/5HMP ratios. In contrast, the urinary output of *N*-demethylmethoxyphenamine (NDMP) or MP/NDMP ratios showed no interphenotype differences. Plasma data from two EMs and two PMs showed that the mean values for maximum concentration, $t_{1/2}$, and total AUC for MP were two-, three-, and sixfold greater, respectively, in PMs than in EMs. The plasma levels of ODMP and 5HMP were higher in EMs than in PMs, whereas the converse was true for NDMP. Thus, *O*-demethylation and aromatic 5-hydroxylation of MP are defective in PMs of D, resulting in increased MP and NDMP plasma levels. The form of cytochrome P-450 involved in the *N*-demethylation of MP is different from that responsible for *O*-demethylation and aromatic 5-hydroxylation. (Clin Pharmacol Ther 38:128-133, 1985.)

Samir D. Roy, B.Pharm., Edward M. Hawes, Ph.D., Gordon McKay, Ph.D., Elarien D. Korchinski, M.D., and Kamal K. Midha, Ph.D.
Saskatoon, Saskatchewan, Canada

Genetic defects in some people have been observed for several oxidative metabolic reactions, including alicyclic hydroxylation of D,[9] aromatic hydroxylation of phenformin,[13] *O*-dealkylation of encainide,[17] and supposed *N*-oxidation of sparteine.[5] There is evidence that these oxidation reactions are mediated by the same form of cytochrome P-450. The *N*-demethylations of amitriptyline[11] and antipyrine[4] have been reported to be mediated through a different cytochrome P-450 isozyme, because no correlation has been found between *N*-demethylations of these drugs and the oxidation reactions of D and sparteine.

MP, a β_2-adrenergic stimulant, is metabolized in man by three distinctly different oxidative metabolic pathways: *N*-demethylation, *O*-demethylation, and hydroxylation at the 5-position of the benzene ring, to yield NDMP, ODMP, and 5HMP, respectively (Fig. 1).[10,12] A study with single oral doses of MP in Lewis and Dark Agouti rats, which are respective models for human EMs and PMs of D, indicated that ODMP and 5HMP are metabolized by the same form of cytochrome P-450 involved in the 4-hydroxylation of D. In contrast, *N*-demethylation of MP appeared to be mediated by a different cytochrome P-450 isozyme.[14] Because many drugs are similar to MP in that they are metabolized in

Abbreviations

D	Debrisoquin
EM	Extensive metabolizer
4HD	4-Hydroxydebrisoquin
5HMP	5-Hydroxymethoxyphenamine
MP	Methoxyphenamine
NDMP	*N*-Demethylmethoxyphenamine
ODMP	*O*-Demethylmethoxyphenamine
PM	Poor metabolizer

From the Colleges of Pharmacy and Medicine, University of Saskatchewan.

Supported by Grant No. MA-8673 from the Medical Research Council of Canada, Ottawa.

Received for publication Jan. 15, 1985; accepted April 9, 1985.

Reprint requests to: Dr. Kamal K. Midha, College of Pharmacy, University of Saskatchewan, Saskatoon, Saskatchewan, S7N 0W0 Canada.

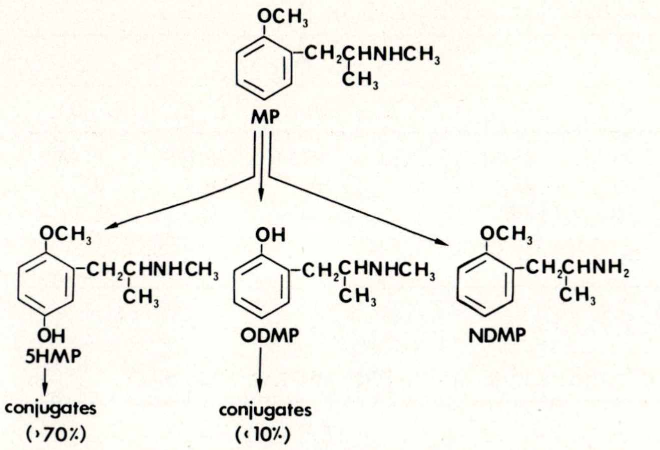

Fig. 1. Known routes of MP metabolism in man.

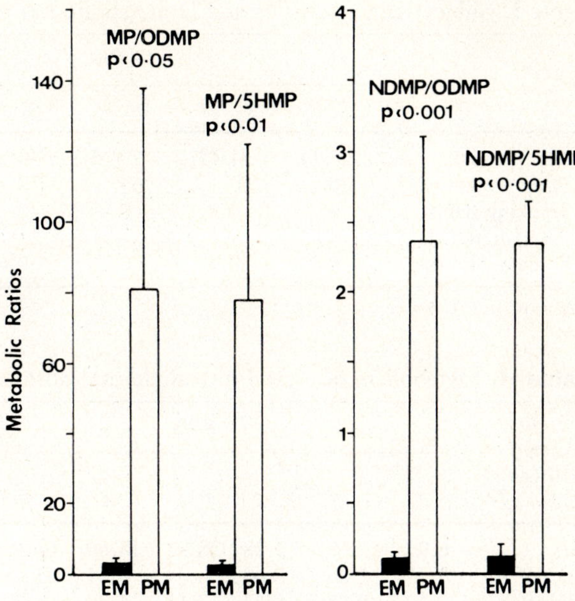

Fig. 2. Mean metabolic ratios in 0-to-12–hour urine samples of five EMs and five PMs after a 60.3 mg oral dose of MP hydrochloride.

man by different routes often involving different forms of cytochrome P-450, MP was examined in two groups of healthy subjects previously phenotyped as EMs or PMs of D. A single dose of MP was taken by mouth and urine and plasma concentrations of MP and the three metabolites were measured. This allowed us to study the effect on an alternative metabolic pathway when one or more genetically determined oxidations are impaired in a drug metabolized by multiple routes.

METHODS

Ten healthy subjects were selected according to their ability to hydroxylate D. A 10 mg oral dose of D was taken after an overnight fast. Aliquots of the 0 to 8–hour urine sample were analyzed for D and 4HD according to the method of Lennard et al.[8] Five subjects were EMs with metabolic ratios in the range of 0.13 to 0.65, and the other five were PMs with ratios in the range of 10.8 to 108. Clinical details are listed in Table I. The two groups were similar in age and body weight. No other medications were allowed at the time of the study.

At least 2 weeks after the D dose, subjects were each given a single oral 60.3 mg dose of MP hydrochloride. The drug was taken after an overnight fast as an extemporaneously prepared capsule with 250 ml water. Food was allowed after 2 hours. Urine was collected for 12 hours and the pH was immediately determined. Portions of the pooled 0 to 12–hour urine sample were stored at $-20°$ C until analysis. Venous blood samples (10 ml) were drawn from selected EMs ($n = 2$) and PMs ($n = 2$) at 12 different times over 27 hours for the PMs and over 32 hours for the EMs after drug dosing. After centrifugation the plasma was collected and stored at $-20°$ C.

Urine concentrations of MP and its three metabolites were determined by modification of the gas chromatographic assay described by Inoue et al.[7] for MP, NDMP, and ODMP. In the modified procedure[15] in which 5HMP was also analyzed, 2 ml urine samples were hydrolyzed with sulfatase enzyme (also containing β-glucuronidase activity) at pH 5.2 for 16 hours. The parent drug, its three metabolites, and the internal standard 3,4-dimethoxyphenethylamine were extracted with ethyl acetate from urine adjusted to pH 9.2 and derivatized with trifluoroacetic anhydride to form mono *N*-acyl derivatives. The chromatographic conditions and other experimental details were the same as those described by Inoue et al.[7] The measured concentrations of MP and its three metabolites were in all cases well above the quantitation limits of the assays.

Plasma concentrations of MP and its three metabolites were measured by gas chromatography, with a nitrogen-selective detector for MP and an electron capture detector for the metabolites.[16] Concentrations were determined as the unconjugated form, as there was no enzymatic treatment of the plasma samples. Quantitation limits (coefficients of variation $<10\%$) were 1.6, 2.2, 3.1, and 3.8 ng/ml for NDMP, 5HMP, ODMP, and MP, respectively.

From the urine data the metabolic ratio for each metabolite in the 0 to 12–hour bulked sample was calculated as the ratio: excretion of MP/excretion of metabolite. The correlation between log MP/metabolite for

Table I. Subject characteristics and D metabolic ratios of the five PMs and five EMs of D

	EMs					PMs				
	S. R.	*G. M.*	*K. R.*	*T. I.*	*B. C.*	*P. H.*	*D. L.*	*R. H.*	*G. C.*	*G. Mc.*
Age (yr)/sex	26/M	31/M	29/M	44/M	25/M	25/M	23/M	36/M	38/F	23/M
Body weight (kg)	70	80	65	70	65	75	70	68	60	70
Smoking habits (cigarettes/day)	0	0	0	0	10	20	0	0	0	0
D metabolic ratio	0.2	0.4	0.1	0.6	0.6	10.8	52.0	84.4	93.3	108

M = Male; F = female.

Table II. Metabolism of a 60.3 mg single oral dose of MP hydrochloride in five PMs and five EMs of D

% Dose excreted in 0-12-hr urine as:	EMs						PMs					
	S. R.	*G. M.*	*K. R.*	*T. I.*	*B. C.*	*X̄ ± SD*	*P. H.*	*D. L.*	*R. H.*	*G. C.*	*G. Mc.*	*X̄ ± SD*
MP	6.93	13.68	13.28	18.92	18.59	14.28 ± 4.89	39.04	25.05	36.10	30.22	22.07	30.50 ± 7.16*
NDMP	0.25	1.26	0.60	0.84	0.31	0.65 ± 0.41	2.22	0.52	1.09	1.11	0.63	1.11 ± 0.67
ODMP	4.17	8.41	5.24	7.14	5.35	6.06 ± 1.69	1.12	0.14	0.56	0.79	0.25	0.57 ± 0.40†
5HMP	4.95	4.80	4.72	5.12	9.52	5.82 ± 2.07	0.98	0.20	0.50	0.55	0.23	0.49 ± 0.31†
Total	16.30	28.15	23.84	32.02	33.77	26.82 ± 7.01	43.36	25.91	38.25	32.67	23.18	32.67 ± 8.38

*$P < 0.01$; †$P < 0.001$.

each metabolite and log D/4HD was assessed by Spearman's rank correlation (r_s), and the significance of each correlation was evaluated by a two-tailed t test. A log plasma concentration-time curve was plotted for each subject. The decline over time in the MP concentration after oral dosing was monoexponential. The plasma AUC was calculated by the linear trapezoidal rule to the last measured calibration time point, and in the case of MP was extrapolated to infinity by adding the MP concentration at the last measured time divided by the first-order rate constant.

RESULTS

The urinary excretion of MP, ODMP, NDMP, 5HMP, and their sum, expressed as the percentage of the 60.3 mg dose found in the 12-hour collection sample, is listed in Table II for each of the subjects. These values were determined from the analysis of extracts obtained after the hydrolysis of urine samples with sulfatase/β-glucuronidase and, therefore, represent totals of free plus conjugated compounds. There was no significant interphenotype difference in the mean urinary pH, but there were significant differences in the mean excretion of MP, ODMP, and 5HMP between EMs and PMs of D. However, between these phenotypes there were no significant differences in the mean urinary excretions of NDMP and the total excretions of MP and the three metabolites.

To allow more detailed analysis of the data in Table II, the mean (±SD) metabolic ratios of MP/5HMP, MP/ODMP, NDMP/ODMP, and NDMP/5HMP for each phenotype are shown in Fig. 2. There were statistically significant differences between PMs and EMs in the means of all these ratios. There is a strong positive correlation ($r_s = 0.87$; $P < 0.01$) between the log MP/ODMP and log D/4HD ratios, as well as between log MP/5HMP and log D/4HD ratios ($r_s = 0.79$; $P < 0.01$; Fig. 3). In contrast, Fig. 3 also shows that there is a weak correlation ($r_s = 0.45$; NS) between log MP/NDMP and log D/4HD ratios. However, a strong positive correlation (Fig. 3; $r_s = 0.90$; $P < 0.001$) between log MP/ODMP and log MP/5HMP ratios indicates that both *O*-demethylation and aromatic 5-hydroxylation are mediated through a closely related isozyme.

Individual plasma concentration-time curves of MP and its three metabolites for two EMs and two PMs are shown in Fig. 4. MP plasma concentrations in samples taken at 24 hours had to be estimated in EMs, while in PMs the concentrations of MP in the samples at the last time point (27 hours) were well above the quantitation limit. Similarly, NDMP plasma concentrations could be followed up to 27 hours in PMs, whereas in all plasma samples from EMs these concentrations were below the quantitation limit of the assay for NDMP. Conversely for the two other metabolites, 5HMP and ODMP, concentrations could be determined up to 12 and 32 hours, respectively, in plasma samples from both

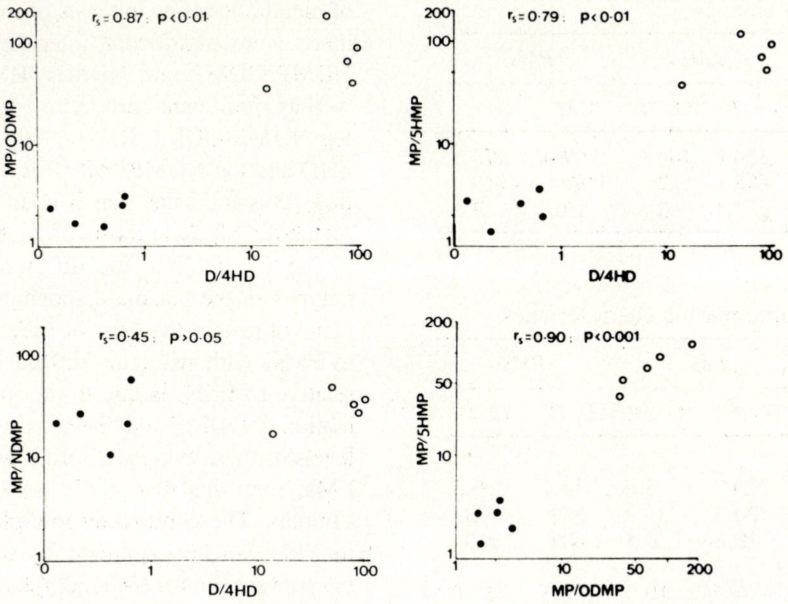

Fig. 3. Relationships between log metabolic ratios in urine in five EMs (●) and five PMs (○).

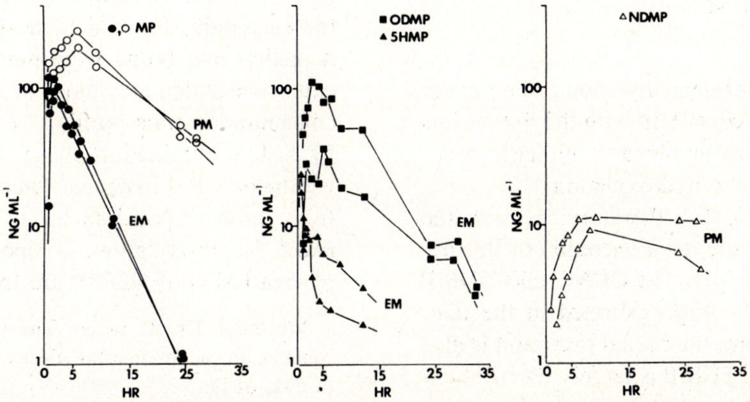

Fig. 4. Plasma concentration-time profiles of MP, ODMP, 5HMP, and NDMP in two EMs *(closed symbols)* and two PMs *(open symbols)* after a 60.3 mg oral dose of MP hydrochloride. Metabolite profiles are not shown for those subjects in whom 5HMP, NDMP, and ODMP plasma concentrations could only be occasionally quantitated.

EMs, while for both PMs these metabolites could not be quantitated in most of the collected plasma samples. Table III details the MP plasma kinetics for all subjects, while values for the three metabolites are listed for all subjects in Table IV. In the case of MP, the maximum concentration, $t_{1/2}$, and total AUC were about two-, three-, and sixfold higher, respectively, in the two PMs than in the two EMs.

DISCUSSION

Our results (Table II; Figs. 2 and 3) indicate that two of the primary routes of metabolism of MP, separately involving *O*-demethylation and aromatic 5-hydroxylation, are probably under the control of the same genetic mechanisms as D. Only for bufuralol[3] and D[19] has more than one route of metabolism of a compound been shown to be likely coinherited with genetically determined D hydroxylation deficiency. However, the third route of metabolism of MP, involving *N*-demethylation, did not correlate with *D*-hydroxylation (Fig. 3). Neither did this *N*-demethylation correlate with the *O*-demethylation (r_s = 0.60; NS) or the aromatic 5-hydroxylation (r_s = 0.28; NS) of MP, when log MP/NDMP ratios were compared with log MP/ODMP and log MP/5HMP ratios, respectively. Thus the form of cytochrome P-450 involved in the *N*-demethylation of MP is different

Table III. MP plasma kinetics

	EMs		*PMs*	
	S. R.	*G. M.*	*P. H.*	*G. C.*
C_{max} (ng/ml)	124.6	100.9	199.0	273.2
Total AUC (ng · hr/ml)	698	582	3489	4049
$t_{1/2}$ (hr)	3.1	3.3	10.5	7.9

C_{max} = Maximum concentration.

Table IV. MP metabolite plasma characteristics

	EMs		*PMs*	
	S. R.	*G. M.*	*P. H.*	*G. C.*
C_{max} (ng/ml)				
NDMP	ND	5.6	14.7	9.3
ODMP	120.2	37.9	ND	ND
5HMP (free)	18.6	6.5	ND	ND
AUC_{0-24} (ng · hr/ml)				
NDMP	—	10.3	194.5	163.6
ODMP	1168	396.3	—	—
5HMP*	46.3	48.9	—	—

C_{max} = Maximum concentration; ND = not determined.
*AUC_{0-12}.

from that responsible for *O*-demethylation and aromatic 5-hydroxylation. This is consistent with the hypothesis that different isozymes are involved in aliphatic *N*-demethylation and D alicyclic hydroxylation.[4,11]

The pKa of MP is 10.45[18]; therefore, as with the related amphetamines,[1,2] the renal excretion of this basic drug depends on urine pH. The ODMP and NDMP metabolites are largely (>90%) excreted in the nonconjugated form; therefore, their renal excretion is also pH dependent. However, 5HMP is largely (>70%) excreted in the urine as glucuronide and/or sulfate conjugates, and its renal excretion is independent of urinary pH. This implies that a metabolic ratio expressed in terms of MP and 5HMP is affected by urine pH. Thus the MP/ODMP ratio is a more reliable indicator of carbon hydroxylation phenotype status.[14] Nevertheless, although we did not control for the urine pH, the correlations between log D/4HD and either log MP/ODMP or log MP/5HMP were similar.

Because the D metabolic ratio is invariably expressed in terms of parent drug values divided by values of the metabolite,[9] analogous ratios for other drugs exhibiting D-type polymorphism are usually similarly defined. However, as in the case of MP, the renal excretion of the parent drug often depends on phenotype, and the appropriateness of expressing metabolic ratios in terms of the parent drug has been questioned.[6] Because we measured NDMP, we could investigate the expression of metabolic ratios in terms of two metabolites. In fact, there were significant interphenotype differences in NDMP/ODMP and NDMP/5HMP ratios (Fig. 2), as well as significant correlations between log D/4HD and log NDMP/ODMP (r_s = 0.79; $P < 0.01$) and log D/4HD and log NDMP/5HMP (r_s = 0.74; $P < 0.02$) ratios. This indicates that it is as appropriate to express metabolic ratios in terms of NDMP as in terms of MP.

There were dramatic differences between the phenotypes in the plasma disposition of MP and the three metabolites. In the case of MP, the high plasma levels in PMs, with resultant sixfold increase in total AUC relative to EMs, is due to the impaired ability for formation of ODMP and 5HMP. Consequently, the plasma levels of these two metabolites were lower in PMs than EMs, such that they could not be quantitated in most samples. The contrasting low plasma levels of NDMP in EMs can be explained by the low activity of the enzyme system for *N*-demethylation relative to the other competing metabolic pathways. The comparatively high plasma levels of MP in PMs allowed more NDMP to be formed. A similar situation has been described for encainide, for which the plasma levels of the *N*-demethyl metabolite were higher in the poor than the extensive *O*-demethylators of encainide.[17] The plasma concentration-time profile of NDMP was characterized by a slow elimination phase. Even though *N*-demethylation of MP is likely carried out by isozymes different from those responsible for *O*-demethylation and aromatic 5-hydroxylation, compensatory increases in the plasma levels of NDMP are found in PMs.

We thank Dr. T. Inaba, The University of Toronto, Toronto, Canada for helpful discussions and providing access to PMs of D.

References

1. Beckett AH, Rowland M: Urinary excretion kinetics of methylamphetamine in man. J Pharm Pharmacol **17:** 109S-114S, 1965.
2. Beckett AH, Rowland M: Urinary excretion kinetics of amphetamine in man. J Pharm Pharmacol **17:**628-639, 1965.
3. Dayer P, Leemann T, Kupfer A, Francis R, Meyer UA: Debrisoquin-type polymorphism: Aliphatic and aromatic bufuralol oxidation are under the same genetic control but display opposite stereoselectivity. Presented at the Sixth International Symposium on Microsomes and Drug Oxidations, Brighton, England, Aug. 9-10, 1984. (Abst. p 4/17).
4. Eichelbaum M, Bertilsson L, Säwe J: Antipyrine metabolism in relation to polymorphic oxidations of sparteine and debrisoquine. Br J Clin Pharmacol **15:**317-321, 1983.

5. Eichelbaum M, Spannbrucker N, Steincke B, Dengler HJ: Defective N-oxidation of sparteine in man: A new pharmacogenetic defect. Eur J Clin Pharmacol **16:**183-187, 1979.
6. Inaba T, Otton SV, Kalow W: Debrisoquine hydroxylation capacity: Problems of assessment in two populations. CLIN PHARMACOL THER **29:**218-223, 1981,
7. Inoue T, Niwaguchi T, Emoto M: Studies on metabolism of methamphetamine analogs. III. Urinary excretion of methoxyphenamine and its metabolites. Kagaku Keisatsu Kenkyusho Hokoku, Hokagaku Hen **33:**89-93, 1980.
8. Lennard MS, Silas JH, Smith AJ, Tucker GT: Determination of debrisoquine and its 4-hydroxy metabolites in biological fluids by gas chromatography with flame ionization and nitrogen selective detection. J Chromatogr **133:**161-166, 1977.
9. Mahgoub A, Idle JR, Dring LG, Lancaster R, Smith RL: Polymorphic hydroxylation of debrisoquine in man. Lancet **2:**584-586, 1977.
10. McKay G, Cooper JK, Hawes EM, Roy SD, Midha KK: Identification of new secondary metabolites of methoxyphenamine in man. Xenobiotica **13:**257-264, 1983.
11. Mellström B, Bertilsson L, Lou Y-C, Säwe J, Sjöqvist F: Amitriptyline metabolism: Relationship to polymorphic debrisoquine hydroxylation. CLIN PHARMACOL THER **34:**516-520, 1983.
12. Midha KK, Cooper JK, McGilveray IJ, Coutts RT, Dawe R: Metabolism of methoxyphenamine in man and in monkey. Drug Metab Dispos **4:**568-576, 1976.
13. Oates NS, Shah RR, Idle JR, Smith RL: Genetic polymorphism of phenformin 4-hydroxylation in man. CLIN PHARMACOL THER **32:**81-89, 1982.
14. Roy SD, Hawes EM, Hubbard JW, McKay G, Midha KK: Methoxyphenamine and dextromethorphan as safe probes for debrisoquine hydroxylation polymorphism. Lancet **2:**1393, 1984.
15. Roy SD, Hawes EM, Midha KK: Methoxyphenamine metabolism in rat models of human debrisoquine phenotypes. Can J Phys Pharmacol. (In press.)
16. Roy SD, McKay G, Hawes EM, Midha KK: Gas chromatographic quantitation of methoxyphenamine and three of its metabolites in plasma. J Chromatogr Biomed Appl **310:**307-317, 1984.
17. Wang T, Roden DM, Wolfenden HT, Woosley RL, Wood AJJ, Wilkinson GR: Influence of genetic polymorphism on the metabolism and disposition of encainide in man. J Pharmacol Exp Ther **228:**605-611, 1984.
18. Warren RJ, Begosh PP, Zarembo JE: Identification of amphetamines and related sympathomimetic amines. J Assoc Off Anal Chem **54:**1179-1191, 1971.
19. Woolhouse NM, Andoh B, Mahgoub A, Sloan TP, Idle JR, Smith RL: Debrisoquine hydroxylation polymorphism among Ghanaians and Caucasians. CLIN PHARMACOL THER **26:**584-591, 1979.

Clinical pharmacology of timentin (ticarcillin and clavulanic acid)

Ticarcillin (4 gm) and clavulanic acid (0.1 gm) were simultaneously administered as timentin to patients with cancer as therapy for infections. The pharmacokinetics of both ticarcillin and clavulanic acid were studied in 15 patients after 30-minute and 2-hour intravenous infusions. The mean (±SD) ticarcillin plasma peak concentrations after the two infusions were 341 ± 76 and 210 ± 60 μg/ml. The plasma terminal $t_{1/2}$ values of ticarcillin were 80 ± 32 and 56 ± 12 minutes. The AUCs were 631 ± 189 and 601 ± 230 mg/L · hr. The volumes of distribution of the area were 15 ± 5 and 21 ± 7 L and total clearances were 115 ± 36 and 127 ± 54 ml/min. The corresponding values for clavulanic acid after the infusions are as follows: mean peak concentrations, 5 ± 1 and 4 ± 1 μg/ml; plasma terminal $t_{1/2}$ values, 84 ± 24 and 74 ± 36 minutes; AUCs, 11 ± 3 and 11 ± 6 mg/L · hr; volumes of distribution of the area, 22 ± 3 and 32 ± 6 L; and total clearances, 170 ± 58 and 175 ± 68 ml/min. (Clin Pharmacol Ther 37:134-139, 1985.)

Gerald P. Bodey, M.D., Edna Yeo, M.D., Dah Hsi Ho, Ph.D., Kenneth Rolston, M.D., and Barbara LeBlanc, B.S. *Houston, Tex.*

Pseudomonas aeruginosa has emerged as a major cause of nosocomial infection in most tertiary hospital centers. Until the introduction of the antipseudomonal penicillins, therapy was frequently unsatisfactory. Ticarcillin (α-carboxyl-3-thienylmethyl penicillin; see structure) is a semisynthetic penicillin used extensively in the treatment of *Pseudomonas* infections.[3,16] Because ticarcillin is susceptible to inactivation by many β-lactamases, it is ineffective against some important pathogens such as *Klebsiella pneumoniae* and *Staphylococcus aureus*.[2,3,11]

Clavulanic acid (BRL 14151; see structure), isolated from *Streptomycin clavuligerus* ATCC 27064, is a β-lactam derivative.[8] Although it has relatively weak intrinsic antibacterial activity, clavulanic acid is a potent irreversible inhibitor of β-lactamases.[4,12,14] When used with ticarcillin, clavulanic acid not only enhances the antimicrobial spectrum of ticarcillin,[7,11,13] but it is also synergistic with ticarcillin against many β-lactamase–producing organisms, including *Escherichia coli, K. pneumoniae* and *Staphlococcus aureus*.[9,13]

The pharmacokinetics of clavulanic acid and ticarcillin have been studied in children with cystic fibrosis and in healthy subjects.[6,10,17,20] We studied the kinetics of timentin (ticarcillin and clavulanic acid) in patients with cancer and compared the kinetics of both drugs after 30-minute and 2-hour intravenous infusions.

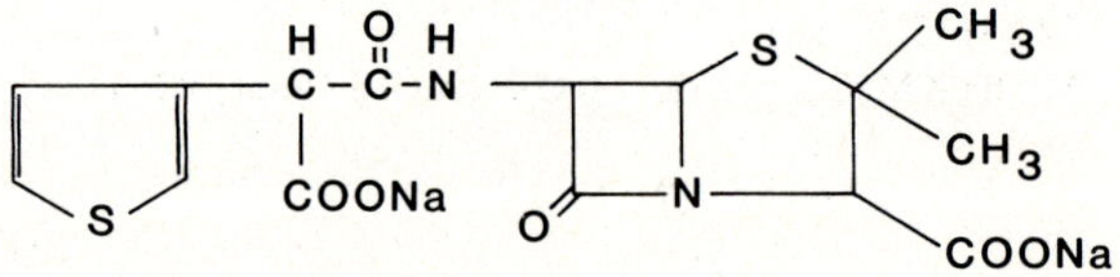

Ticarcillin Disodium

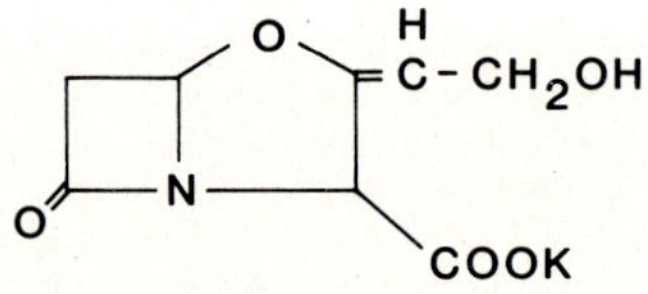

Potassium Clavulanate

Ticarcillin disodium and potassium clavulanate

METHODS

Seventeen studies in 15 female patients with metastatic cancer were conducted during therapy with timentin for presumed or proven infection. Mean (±SD) age was 55 ± 11 years (range 34 to 67 years). All

From the Division of Medicine, The University of Texas M. D. Anderson Hospital.

Supported in part by a grant-in-aid from Beecham Laboratories, Bristol, Tenn.

Received for publication Jan. 15, 1985; accepted March 15, 1985.

Reprint requests to: D. H. Ho, Ph.D., Division of Medicine, M. D. Anderson Hospital, 6723 Bertner Ave., Houston, TX 77030.

patients had normal renal and hepatic function and no known severe hypersensitivity to either of the study drugs or to other β-lactams. The dosage schedule was 4 gm ticarcillin disodium plus 0.1 gm potassium clavulanate given as timentin every 4 hours. Timentin was mixed in 180 ml 0.9% NaCl and infused with an infusion pump. The infusion rate was constant (360 and 90 ml/hr for the 30-minute and 2-hour infusions) and the error in infusion time was <1 minute.

The 2-hour infusion studies were performed on day 2 of therapy in eight patients. Blood samples were drawn at 0, 0.5, 1, and 2 hours during the infusion and at 0.5, 1, and 2 hours after the infusion. The 30-minute infusion studies were carried out in seven patients approximately 18 to 24 hours after the last therapeutic dose of timentin. Heparinized blood samples were drawn before and at the end of infusion and 0.5, 1, 2, 2.5, 3.5, and 5.5 hours thereafter. Peak concentrations were defined as samples taken immediately after infusion for both infusion studies, and trough concentrations were defined as the level 4 hours after the start of therapy. All samples were kept on ice before a brief centrifugation period. Plasma was removed and frozen at −70° C in two portions to avoid frequent freezing and thawing.

Plasma concentrations of ticarcillin and clavulanic acid were determined by agar disk assays. *P. aeruginosa* (ATCC 29336) was used to determine the concentrations of ticarcillin and *K. pneumoniae* (ATCC 29665) was used to determine the concentrations of clavulanic acid. Assay organisms were incubated in trypticase soy broth overnight at 35° C. The broth was then diluted with saline solution to give 50% transmittance at 550 nm on a spectrometer. For ticarcillin assays, 0.125 ml of the *P. aeruginosa* suspension was added to 100 ml 1.5% antibiotic medium A (BBL 10943) to prepare the seed agar. For clavulanic acid assays, 0.125 ml of the *K. pneumoniae* suspension was added to 100 ml 1.5% nutrient agar (BBL 11476) containing 60 μg benzyl penicillin per milliliter.

Assay plates were prepared as follows: For ticarcillin assays, a base agar of 30 ml 1.5% antibiotic medium E (BBL 10943) was prepared and 15 ml seed agar was added. For clavulanic acid assays, a base agar of 30 ml 1.5% nutrient agar (BBL 11476) was prepared and 15 ml seed agar was added.

Ticarcillin standards were prepared in pooled human plasma to provide concentrations ranging from 4 to 200 μg/ml. Clavulanic acid standards were prepared in pooled human plasma providing concentrations of 0.1 to 1.6 μg/ml. Thirty milliliters of the standard or unknowns was pipetted onto the disks, which were then placed onto the agar plates. The plates were incubated at 35° C for 18 hours and zone sizes were measured. Three disks were used for each standard and six disks were used for each unknown. Assay variation ranged from 1% to 7% between operators, from 2% to 5% between experiments performed by the same operator, and from 2% to 6% with triplicate determinations.

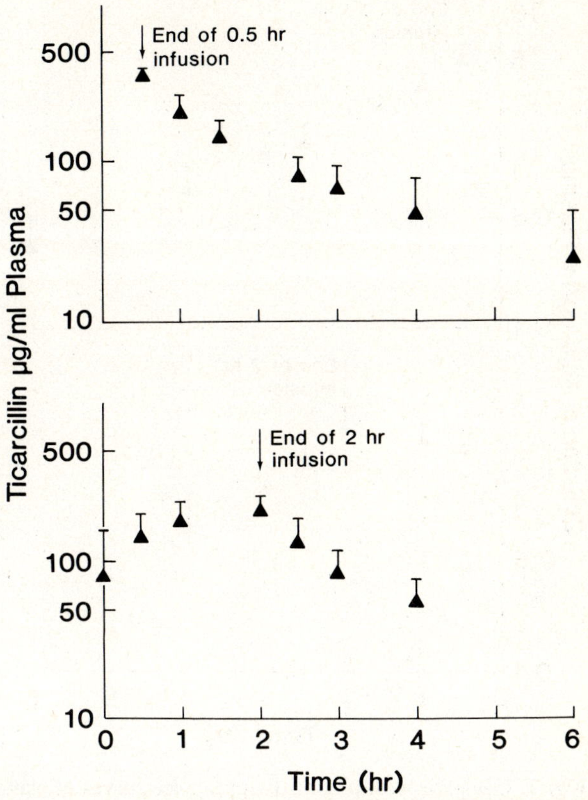

Fig. 1. Comparison of plasma disappearance curves of ticarcillin after 30-minute (eight studies) and 2-hour (nine studies) infusions of timentin (data are $\overline{X}$ ± SD).

The blood AUC was determined by the trapezoidal rule and pharmacokinetic parameters (plasma $t_{1/2}$, volume of distribution of the area [V_z], and total clearance [CL]) were calculated by the method of Ritschel.[15] The Mann-Whitney test[19] was used for statistical analyses.

RESULTS

Fig. 1 shows the plasma disappearance curve of ticarcillin for the 30-minute and 2-hour infusions of timentin. The mean peak concentration at the end of the 30-minute infusion was 341 ± 76 μg/ml, which fell to 37 ± 22 μg/ml 4 hours after the start of timentin. The mean peak concentration at the end of the 2-hour infusion was 210 ± 60 μg/ml and the mean trough concentration was 42 ± 19 μg/ml. The peak clavulanic acid concentrations after the 30-minute and 2-hour timentin infusions were 5.1 ± 1.2 and 3.6 ± 1.3 μg/

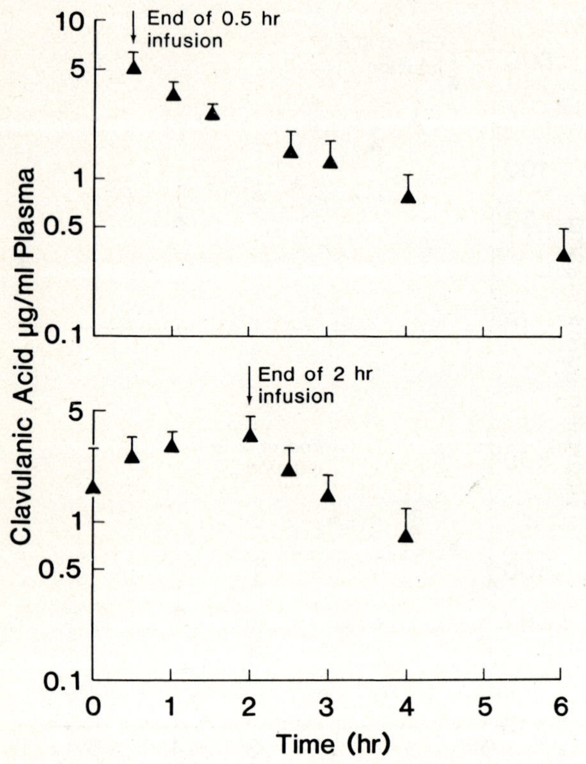

Fig. 2. Comparison of plasma disappearance curves of clavulanic acid after 30-minute (eight studies) and 2-hour (nine studies) infusions of timentin (data are $\overline{X}$ ± SD).

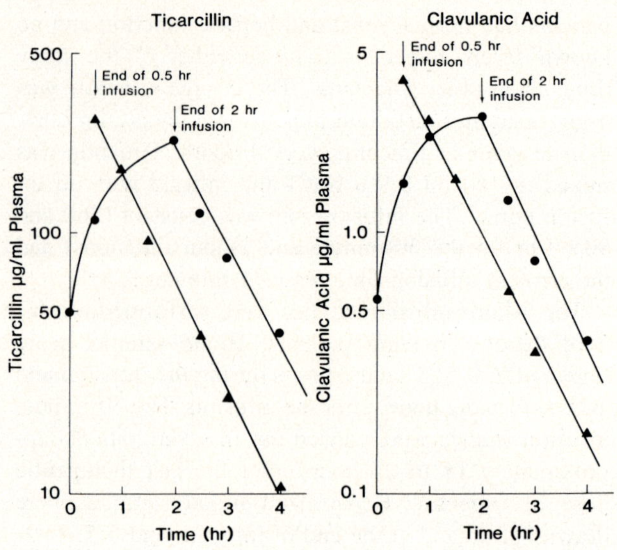

Fig. 3. Plasma disappearance curves of ticarcillin and clavulanic acid. The 30-minute and 2-hour infusion studies were performed in the same patient.

ml, respectively (Fig. 2). At 4 hours the mean concentrations were the same (8.0 ± 0.4 µg/ml) with both infusions. Because the 30-minute infusion studies were performed 18 to 24 hours after the last therapeutic treatment of 2-hour infusions, plasma ticarcillin and clavulanic acid levels were monitored to ascertain that no drug was measurable before the 30-minute infusion study began.

In one patient it was possible to conduct both 30-minute and 2-hour infusion studies (Fig. 3). At the end of the 30-minute infusion, the peak plasma concentrations of ticarcillin and clavulanic acid in this patient were higher than those after the 2-hour infusion, as expected. However, after one hour the plasma concentrations remained higher when timentin was given by the 2-hour infusion. One hour after the start of both regimens the levels of the 2-hour infusion were higher and remained higher for the rest of the study.

Pharmacokinetic parameters of all 17 studies are presented in Tables I and II for ticarcillin and clavulanic acid; mean values are listed in Table III. Except for the peak and trough plasma concentrations, the kinetics were similar with both dosage schedules.

The mean peak concentration ratio of ticarcillin to clavulanic acid after the 30-minute infusion was 68 ± 14, which does not differ significantly from the mean ratio of 60 ± 15 after the 2-hour infusion. The mean trough ratios were also similar for the 30-minute (61 ± 26) and 2-hour (56 ± 26) infusions. The mean ratios of the two drugs remained relatively constant during the study.

None of the patients developed any adverse side effects while receiving timentin.

DISCUSSION

The ability to inhibit β-lactamase activity represents a novel approach to antibiotic therapy. Clavulanic acid is the first of these inhibitors to undergo clinical investigation. It binds irreversibly to many of the common β-lactamases, including the class III TEM β-lactamase that is widespread among *Enterobacteriaceae, Pseudomonadaceae, Hemophilus influenzae,* and *Neisseria gonorrhoeae*. It also inhibits the β-lactamases of *Staphlococcus aureus, Klebsiella ssp, Proteus ssp,* and *Bacteroides fragilis.*[18] Ticarcillin is generally inactive against strains of *K. pneumoniae* because of their production of β-lactamases. Hence the addition of clavulanic acid has expanded the spectrum of ticarcillin to include *K. pneumoniae*. Unfortunately, the strains of *P. aeruginosa* that have developed resistance to ticarcillin are not affected by clavulanic acid. Studies in animals indicate that clavulanic acid reaches sites of infection and protects ticarcillin from inactivation by the β-lactamases of infecting organisms.[1]

In the United States, timentin is supplied as 3 gm

Table I. Ticarcillin pharmacokinetics

Study No.	*Timentin infusion (hr)*	*Plasma concentration (μg/ml)*		$t_{1/2\beta}$ *(min)*	$AUC_{0\rightarrow\infty}$ *(mg/L · hr)*	V_z *(L)*	*CL (ml/min)*
		Peak	*Trough*				
1	0.5	414	67	119	831	16.1	80
2	0.5	276	10	44	361	14.7	185
3	0.5	359	52	97	717	15.2	93
4	0.5	303	21	50	535	10.5	125
5	0.5	332	21	58	478	14.3	139
6	0.5	474	65	79	936	9.4	71
7	0.5	333	24	64	615	11.7	109
8	0.5	235	33	130	576	24.5	116
9	2	93	23	58	266	37.2	251
10	2	221	39	52	557	20.0	120
11	2	247	72	74	791	16.8	84
12	2	188	30	46	472	21.2	141
13	2	208	41	53	561	19.3	119
14	2	213	32	55	707	17.3	94
15	2	322	77	76	1070	13.1	62
16	2	198	33	42	493	19.5	135
17	2	200	34	50	495	20.3	135

$t_{1/2\beta}$ = Terminal $t_{1/2}$.

Table II. Clavulanic acid pharmacokinetics

Study No.	*Timentin infusion (hr)*	*Plasma concentration (μg/ml)*		$t_{1/2\beta}$ *(min)*	$AUC_{0\rightarrow\infty}$ *(mg/L · hr)*	V_z *(L)*	*CL (ml/min)*
		Peak	*Trough*				
1	0.5	4.5	1.2	103	11.9	23.6	140
2	0.5	3.9	0.2	53	5.7	27.3	295
3	0.5	4.6	0.4	72	8.6	23.6	194
4	0.5	5.2	0.4	63	9.1	19.8	184
5	0.5	4.0	0.6	77	9.7	21.5	171
6	0.5	6.8	1.2	101	15.6	18.0	107
7	0.5	7.2	0.9	76	11.7	18.7	142
8	0.5	4.4	1.1	126	13.0	26.0	128
9	2	3.0	0.8	76	9.5	31.6	175
10	2	2.8	0.3	43	6.6	40.5	253
11	2	3.9	1.4	79	13.3	25.7	126
12	2	3.0	0.7	60	9.4	33.6	177
13	2	3.3	1.0	76	10.7	29.8	155
14	2	4.6	1.1	76	15.3	23.9	109
15	2	6.6	1.2	160	23.0	26.8	73
16	2	2.6	0.4	46	6.9	38.7	241
17	2	2.7	0.4	47	6.2	39.9	269

$t_{1/2\beta}$ = Terminal $t_{1/2}$.

ticarcillin with 0.1 gm clavulanic acid. We added an additional 1 gm of ticarcillin because our usual dose of ticarcillin for treating serious *Pseudomonas* infections has been 4 gm every 4 hours.[16] Pharmacokinetic studies were conducted with a rapid infusion (30 minutes) schedule and our usual 2-hour schedule of infusion. This schedule was chosen to ensure continuous optimum serum concentrations in patients with neutropenia who lack adequate host defense mechanisms. Animal studies have confirmed the importance of achieving this objective.[18]

As might be expected, the more rapid infusion sched-

Table III. Mean (±SD) ticarcillin and clavulanic acid pharmacokinetics

	No. of studies	Timentin infusion (hr)	Plasma concentration (μg/ml) Peak	Trough	$t_{1/2\beta}$ (min)	$AUC_{0\rightarrow\infty}$ (mg/L · hr)	V_z (L)	CL (ml/min)
Ticarcillin	8	0.5	341 ± 76*	37 ± 22	80 ± 32	631 ± 189	14.6 ± 4.7	115 ± 36
	9	2	210 ± 60	42 ± 19	56 ± 12	601 ± 230	20.5 ± 6.7	127 ± 54
Clavulanic acid	8	0.5	5.1 ± 1.3*	0.8 ± 0.4	84 ± 24	11 ± 3	22.3 ± 3.2	170 ± 58
	9	2	3.6 ± 1.3	0.8 ± 0.4	74 ± 36	11 ± 6	32.3 ± 6.3	175 ± 68

$t_{1/2\beta}$ = Terminal $t_{1/2}$.
*Significantly different ($P < 0.01$) from value at the end of the 2-hour infusion.

ule produced a higher mean peak plasma concentration of both drugs, whereas the longer infusion maintained somewhat higher plasma concentrations. The kinetics were similar with both schedules. Infusion time did not affect the terminal plasma $t_{1/2}$ values of either ticarcillin or clavulanic acid, as expected for linear kinetics.

It is difficult to compare the results of this study with those of other studies because of differences in doses and schedules. In other studies, 3 gm ticarcillin was given with 0.1 or 0.2 gm clavulanic acid.[1,5,9,15] The mean peak plasma levels of ticarcillin reported were 226 to 600 μg/ml. The $t_{1/2}$ and AUC were 1.1 to 1.6 hours and about 600 μg/ml · hr. The corresponding values for clavulanic acid were: plasma peak level, 3.6 to 16 μg/ml; t½, about 1 hour; and AUC, 7 to 14 μg/ml · hr. Our results were comparable with the above findings when dosage and schedule of administration are considered.

We thank Beecham Laboratories for the supply of timentin.

References

1. Bennett S, Wise R, Weston D, Dent J: Pharmacokinetics and tissue penetration of ticarcillin combined with clavulanic acid. Antimicrob Agents Chemother **23:**831-834, 1983.
2. Bodey GP, Deerhake B: *In vitro* studies of α-carboxyl-3-thienyl methyl penicillin, a new semi synthetic penicillin. Appl Microbiol **21:**61-65, 1971.
3. Brogden RN, Heel RC, Speight TM, Avery GS: Ticarcillin: A review of its pharmacological properties and therapeutic efficacy. Drugs **20:**325-352, 1980.
4. Cole M: Biochemistry and action of clavulanic acid. Scott Med J**27:**510-516, 1982.
5. Davis BE, Humphrey MJ, Langley PF, Lees L, Legg B, Wadds GA: Pharmacokinetics of ticarcillin in man. Eur J Clin Pharmacol **23:**167-172, 1982.
6. Ferslew KE, Daigneault EA, Aten EM, Roseman JM: Pharmacokinetics and urinary excretion of clavulanic acid after oral administration of amoxicillin and potassium clavulanate. J Clin Pharmacol **24:**452-456, 1984.
7. Fuchs PC, Barry AL, Thornsberry C, Jones RN: *In vitro* activity of ticarcillin plus clavulanic acid against 632 clinical isolates. Antimicrob Agents Chemother **25:**392-394, 1984.
8. Howarth TT, Brown AG, King TJ: Clavulanic acid, a novel beta-lactam isolated from streptomyces clavuligerus; X-ray crystal structure analysis. J Chem Soc Chem Commun **1976:**226-267, 1976.
9. Hunter PA, Coleman K, Fisher J, Taylor D: *In vitro* synergistic properties of clavulanic acid, with ampicillin, amoxycillin and ticarcillin. J Antimicrob Chemother **6:**455-470, 1980.
10. Jacobs R, Warren R, Kluza R, Trang J, Underwood F, Brown A, Dorman D: Single dose pharmacokinetics of timenten (ticarcillin/clavulanic acid) in children with cystic fibrosis. Proceedings of the American Society of Microbiology, Las Vegas, March 6-11, 1983. (Abst. No. 844.)
11. Neu HC: The role of beta-lactamases in the resistance of gram-negative bacteria to penicillin and cephalosporin derivatives. Infect Dis Rev **11:**133-149, 1974.
12. Neu HC, Fu KP: Clavulanic acid a novel inhibitor of β-lactamase. Antimicrob Agents Chemother **14:**650-655, 1978.
13. Paisley JW, Washington JA II: Combined activity of clavulanic acid and ticarcillin against ticarcillin-resistant, gram-negative bacilli. Antimicrob Agents Chemother **14:**224-227, 1978.
14. Reading C, Cole M: Clavulanic acid: A beta-lactamase–inhibiting beta-lactam from *Streptomyces clavuligerus*. Antimicrob Agents Chemother **11:**852-857, 1977.
15. Ritschel WA: Handbook of basic pharmacokinetics. Hamilton, Ill., 1976, Drug Intelligence Publications Inc.
16. Rodriguez V, Bodey GP, Horikoshi N, Inagaki J, McCredie KB: Ticarcillin therapy of infections. Antimicrob Agents Chemother **4:**427-431, 1973.
17. Scully BE, Neu HC: The normal human pharmacokinetics of clavulanic acid and ticarcillin combined. Pro-

ceedings of the American Society of Microbiology, Las Vegas, March 6-11, 1983. (Abst. No. 843.)
18. Slocombe B, Beale AS, Boon RJ, Griffin KE, Masters PJ, Sutherland R, White AR: Antibacterial activity *in vitro* and *in vivo* of amoxicillin in the presence of clavulanic acid. Postgrad Med **76**(suppl):29-49, 1984.
19. Sokal RR, Rohlf FJ: Assumption of analysis of statistics in biological research. San Francisco, 1969, WH Freeman.
20. Staniforth DH, Jackson D, Horton R: Pharmacokinetics of parenteral ticarcillin and clavulanic acid. Proceedings of the American Society of Microbiology, Chicago, Nov. 4-6, 1981. (Abst. No. 443.)

Isosorbide dinitrate bioavailability, kinetics, and metabolism

We studied the kinetics of isosorbide dinitrate (ISDN) after a dose of 5 mg iv and the bioavailability of a sublingual and an oral preparation of ISDN. Plasma levels of isosorbide 5-mononitrate (IS-5-MN), isosorbide 2-mononitrate (IS-2-MN), and ISDN were determined by GLC. After intravenous and sublingual dosing, ISDN plasma levels declined biexponentially and could adequately be described by an open two-compartment body model. Distribution was rapid; the $t_{1/2}$ was 4.7 minutes after intravenous injection and 8.7 minutes after sublingual dosing. The volume of distribution at steady state was 90 L. The terminal disappearance $t_{1/2}$ was 54.7 minutes after intravenous injection, 48.8 minutes after sublingual dosing, and 47.7 minutes after oral dosing. Total plasma clearance was 136 L/hr, exceeding normal liver plasma flow and indicating extrahepatic metabolism of ISDN. ISDN bioavailability after oral (10 mg) or sublingual dosing (10 mg) was similar (about 29%), indicating that the first-pass effect cannot be avoided by sublingual ISDN dosing. After intravenous ISDN, mononitrate plasma levels could be adequately described by another two-compartment body model. The terminal $t_{1/2}$ was 4.33 hours for IS-5-MN and 1.83 hours for IS-2-MN. Noncompartmental calculations of the mononitrate levels revealed 100% systemic availability after oral and sublingual ISDN. We assume that ISDN was completely absorbed from the gastrointestinal tract, but 70% was metabolized during the first pass through the liver. After 5 mg iv ISDN, 16 μmol IS-5-MN and 5.3 μmol IS-2-MN reached systemic circulation. The entire dose of ISDN was converted to its two metabolites in a ratio of 3:1 (i.e., 75% IS-5-MN and 25% IS-2-MN). (Clin Pharmacol Ther 38:140-149, 1985.)

Peter Straehl, Pharm.D., and Renato L. Galeazzi, M.D. *Berne, Switzerland*

Isosorbide dinitrate (ISDN) has long been in clinical use. It is taken orally,[17,33] sublingually,[19] intravenously,[5] and transdermally in the treatment and prophylaxis of angina pectoris, vasospastic angina,[5] and congestive heart failure.[8] Despite extensive clinical experience with ISDN, investigators have only recently studied its kinetics[2,9,10,18,19,22,31] because of the development of suitable analytic methods for the determination of low ISDN concentrations in plasma.[16,23] However, reports of ISDN kinetics are still somewhat controversial.[8,31,32] Several studies have shown that oral ISDN provided sustained hemodynamic and antianginal effects,[3,17] but the relationships between the ISDN dose, route of administration, and plasma drug concentrations have not been clearly defined.

A large proportion of ISDN is metabolized to the main metabolites isosorbide 2-mononitrate (IS-2-MN) and isosorbide 5-mononitrate (IS-5-MN).[7,15] Both mononitrates are pharmacologically active in animals[4] and man.[27] Our goal was to examine the kinetics of ISDN and its metabolites and the formation rates of these metabolites in young healthy subjects after intravenous, sublingual, and oral dosing.

METHODS

Our subjects were five healthy young men 22 to 34 years old weighing 55 to 80 kg. They received intravenous, sublingual, and oral doses of ISDN (Table I). In the intravenous studies, 5 ml of a commercial ISDN solution (1 mg/ml NaCl 0.9%; Sorbidilat; Globopharm AG) was slowly injected over 5 minutes into an arm vein. Venous blood samples were drawn from the opposite arm at appropriate intervals and immediately centrifuged, and the plasma was kept frozen (−20° C) until analyzed. In the sublingual studies, ISDN tablets (2 × 5 mg) were kept under the tongue until completely disintegrated (after about 3 minutes). In the oral studies, the 10 mg tablets were swallowed with 100 ml water. All subjects received all three preparations. They rested in a supine position during the first 2 hours of each study. They fasted for 12 hours before and until

From the Department of Medicine, University of Berne.
Supported by a grant from The Swiss National Science Foundation and a grant-in-aid from Globopharm AG, Küsnacht, Switzerland.
Received for publication Oct. 9, 1984; accepted March 22, 1985.
Reprint requests to: R. L. Galeazzi, M.D., Department of Medicine, University of Berne, Inselspital, CH-3010 Berne, Switzerland.

Table I. Subject characteristics

Subject	*Age (yr)*	*Body weight (kg)*	*Height (cm)*
P. S.	34	55	171
K. S.	24	80	186
D. T.	23	78	179
D. R.	23	70	183
G. Z.	22	65	184

2 hours after the start of the study, when a light standard breakfast was eaten.

One milliliter of plasma was assayed for ISDN, IS-5-MN, and IS-2-MN by two separate GLC methods. Quantification of unchanged ISDN was by a modification of the method of Laufen et al.[16] Extraction was performed with pentane and 20 ng isomannide dinitrate was added as internal standard. The ISDN detection limit was about 0.5 ng/ml. Within-day coefficients of variation were 6.3% at a concentration of 1 ng/ml and 3.8% at a concentration of 20 ng/ml (n = 5). Day-to-day variability was 4.6% for 25 ng/ml assayed over a period of 3 months (n = 48). Total recoveries of ISDN and the internal standard throughout the analytic procedures were 70% to 75% over the total concentration range. Detection limits for IS-5-MN and IS-2-MN were 0.5 and 1 ng/ml, respectively. Extraction was with ether after alkalinization of the plasma and addition of 50 ng isomannide dinitrate as internal standard.[28]

We use a 16 mm long capillary column coated with SE 54 (Supelco) and cross-linked. Linear calibration curves based on peak height ratios were obtained up to 100 ng/ml for the mononitrates and up to 50 ng/ml for ISDN. After regular use the column was rinsed every month and reconditioned.

Both noncompartmental and compartmental methods were used to estimate the most relevant kinetic parameters. The plasma AUC and the area under the moment curve (AUMC) were calculated by fitting a spline function to the individual data and integrating the results. Values were extrapolated to infinity according to Benet and Galeazzi.[1] The curve used is the natural spline.

Compartmental-independent plasma clearance (CL) was calculated as originally derived by Dost[6] as: CL = Dose/AUC. The volume of distribution at steady state (V_{ss}) and the mean disposition residence time (i.e., mean residence time after intravenous bolus) are calculated according to Benet and Galeazzi.[1] For the extrapolation of the areas, an individual λ value was calculated by log-linear regression of the last few concentrations, which lay on a straight line when plotted semilogarithmically (determined by visual inspection). Absolute bioavailability (F_{abs}) was calculated by dividing the dose-corrected AUC. For ISDN the formula was: $F_{abs} = (AUC_{non\text{-}iv}/dose_{non\text{-}iv})/AUC_{iv}/dose_{iv})$. Values for the metabolites after ISDN dosing were calculated as: $F_{abs\text{-}met} = (AUC_{met\ non\text{-}iv}/dose_{ISDN\ non\text{-}iv})/(AUC_{met\text{-}iv}/dose_{ISDN\ iv})$.

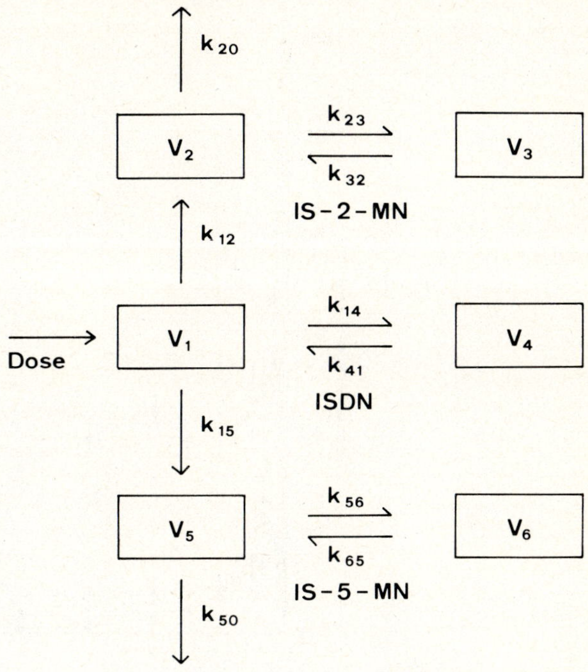

Fig. 1. Schematic representation of the three two-compartment body models used to describe the disposition of ISDN and its mononitrate metabolites.

For compartmental analysis a two-compartment body model with zero-order input was necessary and sufficient to describe plasma ISDN concentrations after intravenous and sublingual dosing (Fig. 1). After oral dosing the two-compartment body model was necessary for only two subjects. Data of the other three subjects were analyzed by a one-compartment body model with first-order absorption. Nonlinear parameters were estimated by the method of extended least squares[25] with the computer program ELSFIT.[24] In this method, which adds a variance model, weights for the dependent variable are found by estimating additional weighting parameters along with the kinetic parameters from the data.[21] In each case a variance model with variances proportional to some power of the predicted value of the dependent variable are chosen. The formation and disposition of the mononitrates after intravenous ISDN are best described by additional two-compartment body models (Fig. 1).[12] The time course of IS-5-MN plasma concentrations was calculated as shown in Eq. 1:

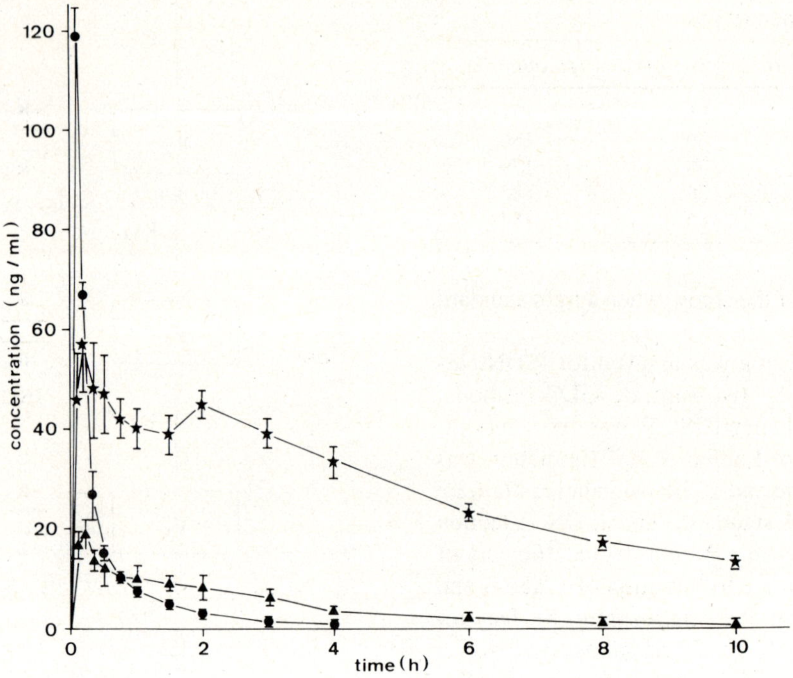

Fig. 2. Mean (±SE; n = 5) plasma levels of ISDN (●), IS-5-MN (★), and IS-2-MN (▲) after ISDN, 5 mg iv.

$$C_{5MN} = \frac{k_{15} \cdot \text{dose ISDN} \cdot (k_{41} - \lambda_1) \cdot (k_{65} - \lambda_1)}{(\lambda_4 - \lambda_1) \cdot (\lambda_5 - \lambda_1) \cdot (\lambda_6 - \lambda_1) \cdot V_5} e^{-\lambda_1 \cdot t} + \frac{k_{15} \cdot \text{dose ISDN} \cdot (k_{41} - \lambda_4) \cdot (k_{65} - \lambda_4)}{(\lambda_1 - \lambda_4) \cdot (\lambda_5 - \lambda_4) \cdot (\lambda_6 - \lambda_4) \cdot V_5} e^{-\lambda_4 \cdot t} + \frac{k_{15} \cdot \text{dose ISDN} \cdot (k_{41} - \lambda_5) \cdot (k_{65} - \lambda_5)}{(\lambda_1 - \lambda_5) \cdot (\lambda_4 - \lambda_5) \cdot (\lambda_6 - \lambda_5) \cdot V_5} e^{-\lambda_5 \cdot t} + \frac{k_{15} \cdot \text{dose ISDN} \cdot (k_{41} - \lambda_6) \cdot (k_{65} - \lambda_6)}{(\lambda_1 - \lambda_6) \cdot (\lambda_4 - \lambda_6) \cdot (\lambda_5 - \lambda_6) \cdot V_5} e^{-\lambda_6 \cdot t} \quad (1)$$

where λ_1 and λ_4 are the hybrid disposition rate constants for ISDN and λ_5 and λ_6 for those for IS-5-MN and V is the volume term. For IS-2-MN the equation was changed to give λ_2 and λ_3 as hybrid rate constants for IS-2-MN.

RESULTS

Intravenous studies. Mean plasma concentrations of ISDN, IS-5-MN, and IS-2-MN in five subjects after intravenous injection of 5 mg ISDN over 5 minutes are shown in Fig. 2. ISDN levels could be fit to a two-compartment body model (Fig. 3) with a mean $t_{1/2}$ of 4.7 minutes for the λ_1 phase (distribution $t_{1/2}$) and 54.7 minutes for the λ_4 phase (terminal $t_{1/2}$; Table II). For ISDN the kinetic parameters of CL and V_{ss} were calculated by compartmental-dependent and -independent evaluations. CL values were in good agreement between the two-compartment (135.1 ± 5.7 L/hr [$\overline{X}$ ± SD]) and noncompartmental (134.6 ± 4.1 L/hr) models. For V_{ss} the respective values are 89.4 ± 12.2 and 97.1 ± 11.8 L. The resulting $t_{1/2}$ values in the log terminal phase are 0.912 hours (54.7 minutes) for the compartmental model and 0.964 hours (57.8 minutes) for the noncompartmental model.

Plasma concentrations of the mononitrates could also be fit to a two-compartment body model (Figs. 1 and 4). Assuming a CL for IS-5-MN of 8.3 L/hr from a previous study,[29] a rate constant of formation (k_{15}) of 2.58 hours^{-1} could be calculated (Table III). Assuming a CL for IS-2-MN of 23.05 L/hr from the previous study,[29] a rate constant of formation (k_{12}) of 0.92 hours^{-1} could be calculated (Table IV).

Sublingual studies. Mean plasma concentrations of ISDN, IS-5-MN, and IS-2-MN after sublingual dosing are shown in Fig. 5. The best fit generated from these values by nonlinear least-squares analysis gave the following values: absorption rate constant (k_a), 26.8 ± 4.93 hours^{-1} ($\overline{X}$ ± SE), or 1.55 minutes; distribution rate constant (λ_1), 4.76 ± 1.3 hours^{-1}, or 8.7 minutes; and terminal rate constant (λ_4), 0.851 ± 0.131 hours^{-1}, or 48.8 minutes (Table V; Fig. 6).

IS-5-MN levels peaked after 2 hours and declined

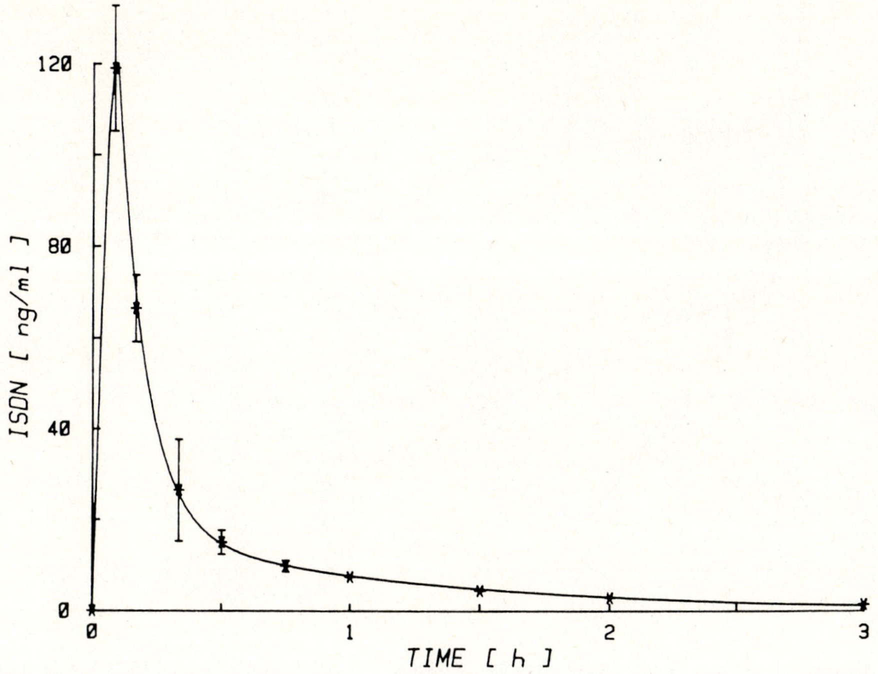

Fig. 3. Mean (±SD; n = 5) plasma levels of ISDN after a 5 mg iv dose. *Line* represents best fit of a two-compartment body model.

Table II. ISDN kinetics after intravenous injection

	Two-compartment body model				*Noncompartmental*	
Subject	λ_1 *(hr^{-1})*	λ_4 *(hr^{-1})*	V_{ss} *(L)*	*CL (L/hr)*	V_{ss} *(L)*	*CL (L/hr)*
P. S.	7.47	0.675	102.4	130.2	92.5	132.8
G. Z.	11.82	0.727	100.0	139.8	116.0	135.7
D. R.	13.23	0.762	90.8	132.7	98.0	139.2
D. T.	4.60	0.542	79.2	130.4	83.9	128.6
K. S.	6.94	1.130	74.9	142.6	95.2	137.0
$\overline{X}$	8.81	0.760	89.4	135.1	97.1	134.6
±SE	1.60	0.098	5.4	2.5	5.2	1.8
$t_{1/2}$ (min)	4.7	54.7				

with a terminal $t_{1/2}$ of 4.6 ± 0.80 hours. The IS-2-MN levels peaked after 60 minutes and declined with a $t_{1/2}$ of 2.01 ± 0.40 hours.

Oral studies. Mean plasma concentrations of ISDN, IS-5-MN, and IS-2-MN after oral dosing with 10 mg ISDN are shown in Fig. 7. Thirty minutes after dosing there was a mean peak ISDN concentration of 14.5 ng/ml. Thereafter the plasma levels in three subjects declined monoexponentially and levels of the other two subjects could best be fit by a two-compartment body model. In three subjects absorption was delayed, necessitating the addition of a lag time factor. The mean lag time in three subjects (two with a two-compartmental model and one with a noncompartmental model) was 13.5 minutes. Data of the other two subjects were best fit by a one-compartment body model with a lag time factor. Because of this variability the estimation of the absorption rate constant k_a was not very precise (6.45 ± 2.54 hours^{-1}, or 6.4 minutes). A mean distribution constant of 3.73 ± 0.08 hours^{-1} was calculated from only two subjects and the distribution time of 11.14 minutes was not representative because of the limited number of subjects. The mean terminal $t_{1/2}$ (n = 5) was 47.5 minutes. Mean data were tentatively

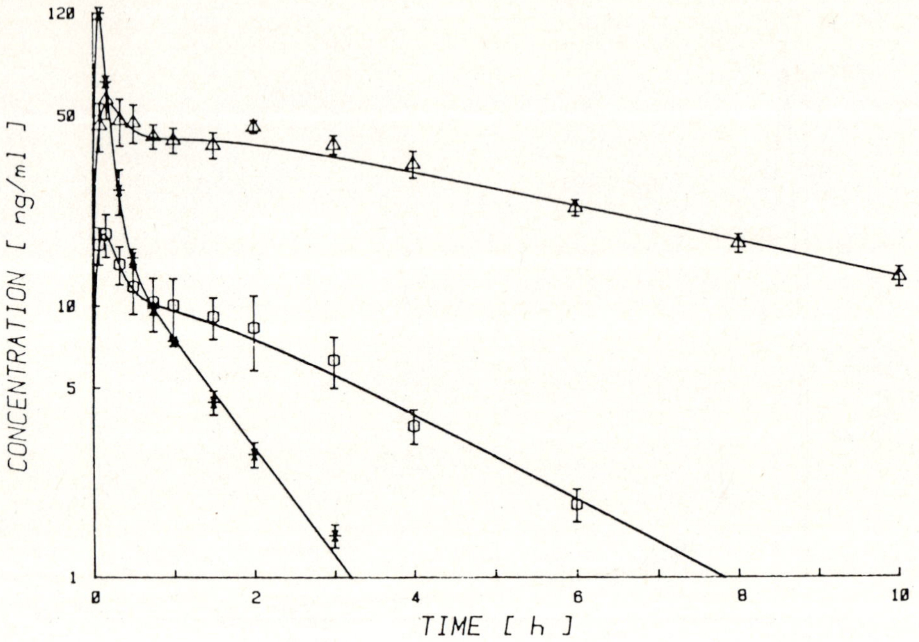

Fig. 4. Mean (±SE; n = 5) plasma levels of ISDN (*), IS-5-MN (△) and IS-2-MN (○) after ISDN, 5 mg iv. *Lines* represent best fit of a combination of three two-compartment body models.

Table III. Compartmental analysis of IS-5-MN kinetics after ISDN, 5 mg iv

Subject	λ_5 *(hr⁻¹)*	λ_6 *(hr⁻¹)*	k_{65} *(hr⁻¹)*	k_{50} *(hr⁻¹)**	V_5 *(ml)†*	k_{15} *(hr⁻¹)†*
P. S.	6.67	0.156	1.32	0.788	8248	2.44
G. Z.	12.44	0.187	3.54	0.657	12633	3.30
D. R.	9.56	0.159	3.10	0.490	16938	3.35
D. T.	7.10	0.162	2.45	0.469	17697	1.78
K. S.	4.39	0.140	1.36	0.451	18403	2.04
$\overline{X}$	8.03	0.160	2.35	0.571	14783	2.58
±SE	1.37	0.007	0.448	0.065	1917	0.321
$t_{1/2}$	5.17 min	4.33 hr				

*Calculated as: $(\lambda_5 \cdot \lambda_6)/k_{65} = k_{50}$.
†Calculated from the estimated parameter (k_{15}/V_5) by use of an IS-5-MN CL value from a previous study.[29]

fit to a one-compartment body model with a lag time factor (Fig. 6; Table VI).

Mean IS-5-MN levels peaked 2 hours after dosing. After 12 hours the mean levels were still 20 ng/ml. For IS-2-MN the peak was reached after 45 minutes and 12 hours later there was a level of 0.6 ng/ml in all subjects.

Amounts of ISDN, IS-5-MN, and IS-2-MN. As shown in Table VII, the bioavailability of ISDN calculated as the ratio of dose-corrected AUCs (compared with intravenous injection) was in the same range for the 5 mg sublingual tablet (29.6%) and the 10 mg oral dose (29.0%). The standard deviation varied much more after oral dosing (±13.9% after oral dosing and 3.6% after sublingual dosing).

To approximate amounts of the mononitrates generated by ISDN metabolism after intravenous, sublingual, and oral ISDN, the AUCs for the metabolites were followed up to 10 hours after intravenous injection and up to 12 hours after sublingual and oral dosing. While IS-2-MN levels were low at the sampling points, the IS-5-MN levels were fairly high and the experimental areas had to be extrapolated to infinity. As can be seen in Table VIII, the mean AUC for IS-5-MN after ISDN, 5 mg iv, was 370.3 ng/ml · hr and after oral ISDN, 10 mg, the mean AUC was 789.0 ng/ml · hr, which gives an F value of 106.5%. For IS-2-MN the corresponding AUC values of 44.1 and 88.8 ng/ml · hr indicated an F value of 100.7%. With the CL values of these metabolites determined in another study[29] in a similar

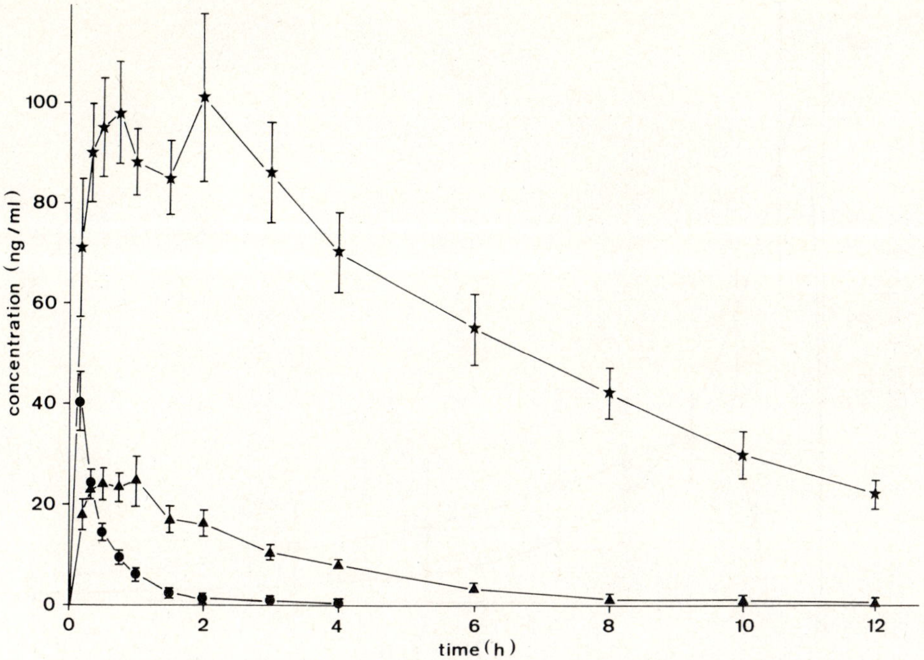

Fig. 5. Mean (±SE; n = 5) plasma levels of ISDN (●), IS-5-MN (★), and IS-2-MN (▲) after ISDN, 10 mg sublingually.

Table IV. Compartmental analysis of IS-2-MN kinetics after ISDN, 5 mg iv

Subject	λ_2 (hr^{-1})	λ_3 (hr^{-1})	k_{32} (hr^{-1})	k_{20} (hr^{-1})*	V_2 (ml)†	k_{12} (hr^{-1})†
P. S.	7.04	0.241	0.492	3.44	7877	0.642
G. Z.	9.00	0.404	1.54	2.36	9745	0.984
D. R.	3.28	0.383	1.37	0.916	25109	1.094
D. T.	12.99	0.475	4.62	1.33	17293	0.734
K. S.	11.04	0.398	2.33	1.88	12344	1.16
$\overline{X}$	8.67	0.380	2.07	1.98	14473	0.922
±SE	1.67	0.038	0.701	0.438	3094	0.100
$t_{1/2}$	4.79 min	1.82 hr				

*Calculated as: $(\lambda_2 \cdot \lambda_3)/k_{32} = k_{20}$.
†Calculated from the estimated parameter (k_{12}/V_2) by use of an IS-2-MN CL value from previous study.[29]

group of subjects, the amounts of mononitrates generated after ISDN dosing could be calculated. For IS-5-MN the CL value was 8.30 L/hr and the calculated dose was 3.07 mg after ISDN, 5 mg iv; 6.54 mg after ISDN, 10 mg by mouth; and 6.96 mg after ISDN, 10 mg sublingual. Corresponding values for IS-2-MN were as follows: CL, 23.05 L/hr; 1.01 mg after intravenous ISDN; 2.04 mg after oral ISDN; and 1.9 mg after sublingual ISDN. After ISDN, 5 mg iv (a dose corresponding to 21.18 μmol), there was 16.07 μmol IS-5-MN (3.07 mg) and 5.28 μmol IS-2-MN (1.01 mg), indicating that the total amount of ISDN was converted into the metabolites with a ratio of 3:1 (i.e., 75% was converted to IS-5-MN and 25% was converted to IS-2-MN). After oral and sublingual dosing the total ISDN dose (42.36 μmol) was metabolized to the mononitrates in about the same 3:1 ratio.

DISCUSSION

We analyzed the kinetics of ISDN by both compartmental and noncompartmental methods to check for consistency of results. Because the mean CL and V_{ss} values between the two methods do not differ, we conclude that a two-compartment body model is adequate to describe the time course of ISDN plasma concentrations after intravenous injection. There was also biexponential decay of the ISDN plasma levels after sublingual dosing, but coefficients of variation were considerably smaller for intravenous than for sublingual data. For oral data it was more difficult to find the best

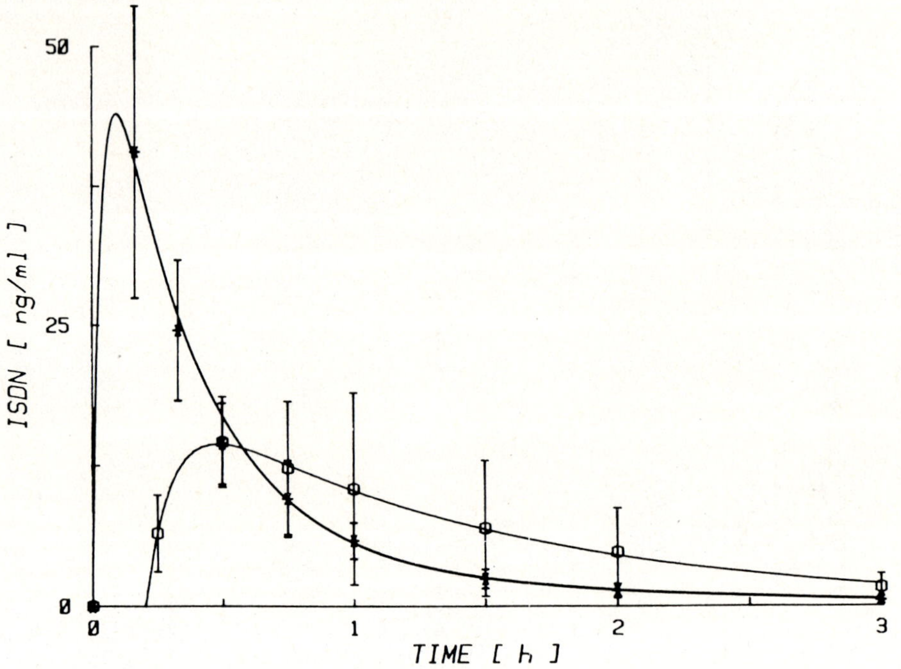

Fig. 6. Mean (±SD; n = 5) plasma levels of ISDN after a 10 mg sublingual (*) and a 10 mg oral (○) dose. *Lines* represent best fit of a two-compartment body model for the sublingual dose and a one-compartment body model with lag time for the oral dose.

Table V. ISDN kinetics after sublingual dosing

Subject	λ_1 (hr^{-1})	λ_4 (hr^{-1})	k_a (hr^{-1})
P. S.	9.07	1.11	17.4
G. Z.	3.17	0.596	26.0
D. R.	1.88	1.07	15.5
D. T.	6.50	1.01	41.8
K. S.	3.21	0.471	33.5
$\overline{X}$	4.76	0.851	26.8
±SE	1.31	0.13	4.93
$t_{1/2}$ (min)	8.7	48.8	1.55

model, because the data of two subjects were best analyzed by a two-compartmental body model and the data of the other three subjects were best fit by a one-compartment body model.

Compared with the terminal λ_4 phase, the λ_1 distribution phase was very short (4.7 and 54.7 minutes after intravenous dosing and 8.7 and 48.8 minutes after sublingual dosing). Values for the terminal elimination rate after intravenous dosing were in close agreement with the oral $t_{1/2}$ (47.7 minutes) but differ mainly due to interindividual variations. A prolonged elimination phase as described by others[11] was not detected in our normal healthy subjects.

Since a study[26] showed that ISDN levels in the whole blood and in plasma are in the same range and that ISDN is not concentrated in erythrocytes, it is therefore valid to compare plasma clearance to organ plasma flow rates. The CL of 135.6 L/hr exceeded hepatic plasma flow (assumed to be about 90 L/hr). Since ISDN is completely metabolized it can be assumed that there is considerable extrahepatic metabolism. It has been demonstrated that ISDN is denitrated when incubated in vitro with blood vessel homogenates.[30] Glutathione sulfotransferases, the enzymes responsible for ISDN metabolism, have been found in all tissues examined in rats[13] and in man.[14] It therefore seems plausible to assume that organs other than the liver contribute to the elimination of ISDN in man. Our V_{ss} of about 90 L corresponds closely to published data.[18,19,22] The systemic availability of ISDN after sublingual and oral tablets was in the same range (about 29%). The plasma levels of the metabolites after 10 mg sublingual and 10 mg oral doses (Figs. 5 and 7) and the AUCs of these metabolites (Table VIII) are of the same order. It can thus be concluded that after sublingual ISDN, not more unchanged ISDN reaches systemic circulation than after normal oral dosing. The only advantage of sublingual dosing seems to be the rapid disintegration and dissolution of the tablet: ISDN is probably swallowed and promptly absorbed. We did not find any suggestion of

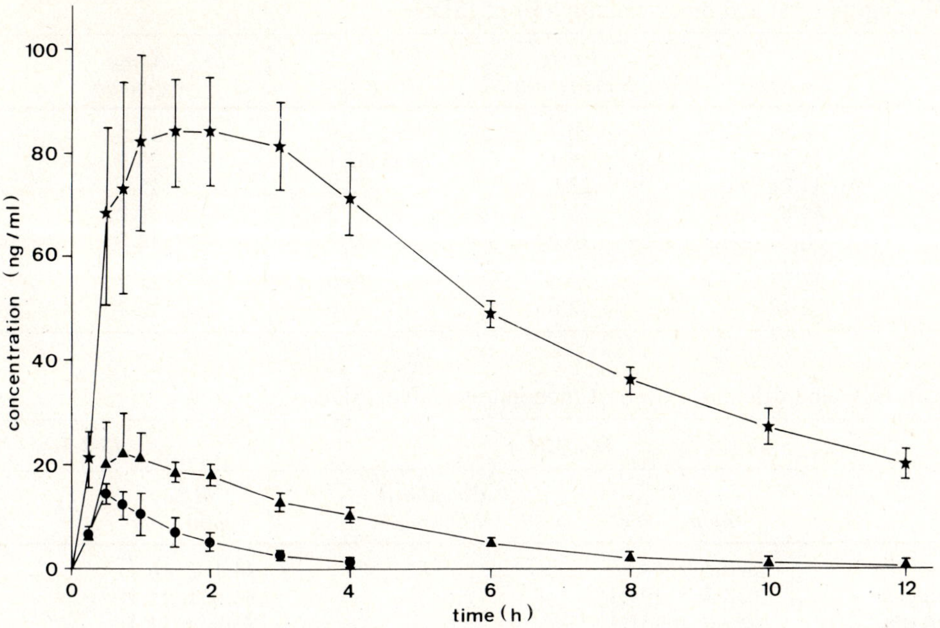

Fig. 7. Mean (±SE; n = 5) plasma levels of ISDN (●), IS-5-MN (★), and IS-2-MN (▲) after ISDN, 10 mg by mouth (normal tablet).

Table VI. ISDN kinetics after oral dosing

	Two-compartment body model			One-compartment body model		
Subject	λ_1 *(hr⁻¹)*	λ_4 *(hr⁻¹)*	k_a *(hr⁻¹)*	k_a *(hr⁻¹)*	λ_4 *(hr⁻¹)*	*Lag time (hr)*
P. S.	3.65	0.456	15.00			0.229
K. S.	3.81	0.655	9.05			0.240
G. Z.				1.44	1.15	
D. R.				5.09	0.632	0.210
D. T.				1.71	1.49	
$\overline{X}$		0.876	6.45			0.226
±SE		0.191	2.54			0.006
$t_{1/2}$ (min)		47.5	6.4			

avoidance of first-pass effect through the liver, as was suggested by Needlemann.[20]

Plasma levels of IS-2-MN and IS-5-MN after intravenous, sublingual, and oral doses of ISDN are shown in Figs. 2, 4, 5, 6, and 7. Peak plasma IS-5-MN concentrations were 3.1 times higher than those of IS-2-MN after intravenous dosing and 3.8 times higher after the oral doses. This ratio is much higher for IS-5-MN during chronic dosing because IS-5-MN accumulates in the body due to its much slower CL.[29] Compartmental analysis of the formation and disposition of the two mononitrates after intravenous ISDN revealed terminal rate constants (λ_6 and λ_3 for IS-5-MN and IS-2-MN, respectively) that were in good agreement with the terminal $t_{1/2}$ after the intravenous injection of the mononitrates in a similar group of subjects; namely, 4.33 hours and 1.83 hours for IS-5-MN and IS-2-MN in our current study and 4.15 and 1.93 in our previous study.[29] After 4 hours the disposition of ISDN no longer contributes to the plasma concentrations of the mononitrate, and their plasma time course seems to be log linear.

Mean AUCs (Table VIII) show a good dose relationship for IS-2-MN after ISDN, 5 mg iv (44.1 ng/ml · hr), and the sublingual and oral values. There was a similar relationship for IS-5-MN. This indicates that the bioavailability of the mononitrates after ISDN dosing is complete (i.e., 100%). Systemic availability of the mononitrates given as the metabolite was also 100%.[29] If the bioavailability of the mononitrate metabolites is 100% and if the bioavailability of the mother

Table VII. AUCs (ng/ml · hr) and bioavailability (F) of ISDN

Subject	*5 mg iv*	*10 mg sublingually*	*F (%)*	*10 mg by mouth*	*F (%)*
P. S.	38.88	20.1	25.9	11.0	14.2
G. Z.	36.82	24.1	32.1	23.1	31.2
D. R.	35.91	23.6	32.8	25.3	35.2
D. T.	38.8	24.2	31.2	37.2	47.9
K. S.	36.48	18.6	25.5	12.0	16.5
$\bar{X}$	37.39	22.1	29.6	21.7	29.0
±SD	1.38	2.6	3.6	10.8	13.9

Table VIII. Mean AUC and calculated dose of mononitrates after ISDN

	IS-5-MN		*IS-2-MN*	
ISDN	*AUC (ng/ml · hr)*	*Calculated dose (mg)**	*AUC (ng/ml · hr)*	*Calculated dose (mg)**
5 mg iv	370.3 ± 64.3	3.07	44.1 ± 16.2	1.01
10 mg sublingual	838.7 ± 194.2	6.96	82.6 ± 15.1	1.90
10 mg by mouth	789.0 ± 131.1	6.54	88.8 ± 14.4	2.04

Data are $\bar{X}$ ± SD.
*From CL values from another mononitrate study[29] for IS-5-MN of 8.3 L/hr and for IS-2-MN of 23.05 L/hr.

substance ISDN is 29%, then ISDN given orally or sublingually is completely absorbed and 70% of ISDN is metabolized during the first pass through the liver.

Because a similar group of subjects was investigated in a recent study,[29] it was possible to calculate the doses of IS-2-MN and IS-5-MN generated after ISDN dosing. Accordingly, the Cl of IS-2-MN was 8.3 L/hr and that of IS-5-MN was 23.05 L/hr. For intravenous ISDN the dose of the mononitrates produced by denitration of ISDN was calculated as: Dose = CL · AUC. Since the sum of the results (3.07 mg, or 16.07 μmol for IS-5-MN and 1.01 mg, or 5.28 μmol for IS-2-MN) is identical to the applied dose of ISDN (5 mg, or 21.18 μmol), we conclude that all the ISDN was metabolized to the two mononitrate metabolites in a ratio of about 3:1. The same metabolization rate was found after oral and sublingual dosing of ISDN. These results correspond to a conversion of 75% and 25% of the ISDN dose into IS-5-MN and IS-2-MN, respectively. With the compartmental analysis of the mononitrates after intravenous ISDN (Eq. 1), the ratio of k_{15} to k_{12} (the formation rates of the mononitrates) is also about 3:1.

We thank Mrs. L. Luethi for the excellent technical assistance and Pharma Schwartz GmbH, West Germany, for the supply of isomannide dinitrate.

References

1. Benet LZ, Galeazzi RL: Non-compartmental determination of the steady state volume of distribution. J Pharm Sci **68:**1071-1074, 1979.
2. Chasseaud LF, Darragh A, Doyle E, Lambe RF, Taylor T: Isosorbide dinitrate plasma concentrations and bioavailability in human subjects after administration of standard oral and sublingual formulations. J Pharm Sci **73:**699-701, 1984.
3. Danahy DT, Burwell DT, Aronow WS: Sustained hemodynamic and antianginal effect of high dose oral isosorbide dinitrate. Circulation **55:**381-387, 1977.
4. Dietmann K, Sponer G, Voss E: Pharmakodynamik, Pharmakokinetik und Metabolismus der Nitrate des Isosorbids am wachen Hund. Med Welt **32:**481-491, 1981.
5. Distante A, Maseri A, Severi S: Management of vasospastic angina at rest with continuous infusion of isosorbide dinitrate. Am J Cardiol **44:**533-539, 1979.
6. Dost FH: Grundlagen der Pharmakokinetik. Stuttgart, 1976, Georg Thieme.
7. Down WH, Chasseaud LF, Grundy RK: Biotransformation of isosorbide dinitrate in humans. J Pharm Sci **63:**1147-1149, 1974.
8. Franciosa JA, Cohn JN: Hemodynamic responsiveness to short- and long-acting vasodilators in left ventricular failure. Am J Med **65:**126-131, 1978.
9. Frydmann A, Levenson J, Simon A, Safar M, Bieder A, Bertharion J, Gaillot J: Pharmacocinétique du dinitrate d'isosorbide. Nouv Presse Med **27:**2049-2056, 1982.
10. Fung HL, McNiff EF, Ruggirello D, Darke A, Thadani U, Parker JO: Kinetics of isosorbide dinitrate and relationships to pharmacological effects. Br J Clin Pharmacol **11:**579-590, 1981.
11. Fung HL, Parker JO: Prolonged plasma half life after oral isosorbide dinitrate in patients with angina pectoris. Br J Clin Pharmacol **15:**746-748, 1983.

12. Gibaldi M, Perrier D: Pharmacokinetics. New York, 1975, Marcel Dekker Inc.
13. Kaplowitz N, Clifton G, Kuhlenkamp J, Wallin JD: Comparison of renal and hepatic glutathione-s-transferases of the rat. Biochem J **158:**243-248, 1976.
14. Kaplowitz N, Spina C, Graham M, Kuhlenkamp J: Glutathione-s-transferases in human lymphoid cell lines and fractionated peripheral leucocytes. Biochem J **169:**465-470, 1978.
15. Laufen H, Aumann M, Leitold M: Oral absorption and disposition of isosorbide dinitrate and isosorbide mononitrates in man. Drug Res **33:**980-984, 1983.
16. Laufen H, Scharpf F, Bartsch G: Improved method for the rapid determination of isosorbide dinitrate in human plasma and its application in pharmacokinetic studies. J Chromatogr **146:**457-464, 1978.
17. Markis JE, Gorlin R, Mills RM, Williams RA, Schwitzer P, Ransil BJ: Sustained effect of orally administered isosorbide dinitrate on exercise performance of patients with angina pectoris. Am J Cardiol **43:**265-271, 1979.
18. Morrison RA, Fung HL, Hoehmann D, Meinertz T, Jaehnchen E: Isosorbide dinitrate: Pharmacokinetics after intravenous administration. J Pharm Sci **71:**721-723, 1982.
19. Morrison RA, Weigand UW, Jaehnchen E, Hoehmann D, Berchtold H, Meinertz T, Fung HL: Isosorbide dinitrate kinetics and dynamics after intravenous, sublingual and percutaneous dosing in angina. CLIN PHARMACOL THER **33:**747-756, 1983.
20. Needlemann P: Organic nitrate metabolism. Ann Rev Pharmacol Toxicol **16:**81-93, 1976.
21. Peck CC, Sheiner LB, Nichols AI: The problem of choosing weights in nonlinear regression analysis of pharmacokinetic data. Drug Metab Rev **15:**133-148, 1984.
22. Platzer R, Reutemann G, Galeazzi RL: Pharmacokinetics of intravenous isosorbide dinitrate. J Pharmacokinet Biopharm **10:**575-585, 1982.
23. Rosseel MT, Bogaert MG: Simultaneous determination of isosorbide dinitrate and its mononitrates in human plasma by capillary column GLC. J Pharm Sci **68:**659-660, 1979.
24. Sheiner LB: ELSFIT. A program for the extended least squares fit to individual pharmacokinetic data. University of San Francisco, 1980, Division of Clinical Pharmacology.
25. Sheiner LB, Beal S: Evaluation of methods for estimating population pharmacokinetics parameters I. J Pharmacokinet Biopharm **8:**553-571, 1980.
26. Sisewine SF, Ruelius HW: Plasma concentrations and urinary excretion of isosorbide dinitrate and its metabolites in dog. J Pharmacol Exp Ther **176:**296-301, 1970.
27. Stauch M, Grewe N: Die Wirkung von Isosorbid-Dinitrat, Isosorbid-2- und 5-Mononitrat auf das Belastungs-EKG und auf die Haemodynamik während Vorhofsstimulation bei Patienten mit Angina pectoris. Z Kardiol **68:**687-693, 1979.
28. Straehl P, Galeazzi RL: Determination of isosorbide 5-mononitrate in human plasma by capillary column gas liquid chromatography. J Pharm Sci **73:**1317-1319, 1984.
29. Straehl P, Galeazzi RL, Soliva M: Isosorbide 5-mononitrate and isosorbide 2-mononitrate kinetics after intravenous and oral dosing. CLIN PHARMACOL THER **36:**485-493, 1984.
30. Sutton SC, Fung HL: Metabolism of isosorbide dinitrate by rat blood vessels and other tissues. Acad Pharm Sci **12:**68, 1982. (Abst.)
31. Taylor T, Chasseaud LF, Doyle E, Bonn R, Darragh A, Lambe RF: Isosorbide dinitrate pharmacokinetics. Drug Res **32:**1329-1533, 1982.
32. Taylor T, Chasseaud LF, Doyle E, Darragh A, O'Kelley DA, Fitzgerald D: Pharmacokinetics of isosorbide dinitrate after intravenous infusion in human subjects. Biopharm Drug Dispos **1:**149-156, 1980.
33. Thadani U, Darke AC, Fung HL, Parker JO: Dose response and duration of action of oral isosorbide dinitrate (ISDN) during sustained therapy in angina pectoris. Am J Cardiol **45:**478-487, 1980.

Moxalactam epimer disposition in patients undergoing continuous ambulatory peritoneal dialysis

The kinetics of the epimers of moxalactam (*R*-MOX, *S*-MOX) were investigated in patients without infections who were receiving continuous ambulatory peritoneal dialysis after both intravenous and intraperitoneal injections of moxalactam. *R*-MOX and *S*-MOX were well absorbed from the peritoneal cavity, with mean systemic availability of 0.71 ± 0.18 and 0.79 ± 0.18, respectively. After intravenous MOX, serum clearance was 10.2 ± 3.4 (*R*-MOX) and 10.9 ± 3.2 (*S*-MOX) ml/hr/kg. Net time-averaged peritoneal dialysis clearance of both epimers was minimal, about 10% of serum clearance. Serum and dialysate MOX concentrations were above the minimum inhibitory concentrations for susceptible bacteria for 24 hours after a 2.0 or 1.0 gm intravenous or intraperitoneal dose. Gastrointestinal side effects occurred after a 2.0 gm dose (both intravenous and intraperitoneal) but not after a 1.0 gm dose. There were no significant differences in the kinetics of *R*-MOX and *S*-MOX. A single 1.0 gm ip dose leads to serum and dialysate MOX concentrations above the minimum inhibitory concentration for susceptible pathogens for 24 hours. (CLIN PHARMACOL THER 38:150-156, 1985.)

Gene Morse, Pharm.D., David Janicke, Pharm.D., Robert Cafarell, Pharm.D., Katherine Piontek, B.S., Michael Apicella, M.D., William J. Jusko, Ph.D., and John Walshe, M.D. *Buffalo, N. Y.*

Continuous ambulatory peritoneal dialysis (CAPD) has become an accepted alternative to hemodialysis for many patients with end-stage renal disease (ESRD).[14,16] The development of bacterial peritonitis, primarily caused by staphylococci and aerobic gram-negative bacilli, is a major complication of CAPD.[6,18] Initial antibiotic therapy is primarily empiric and usually includes a first-generation cephalosporin or vancomycin, with or without an aminoglycoside.[6] Moxalactam (MOX), with its broad spectrum of activity, may be an acceptable alternative in the treatment of CAPD peritonitis caused by susceptible bacteria.[5] This antibiotic exists as a pair of stereoisomers (*R*-MOX and *S*-MOX), which have different antimicrobial activity[22,23] and kinetics.[22,23] These epimers are primarily excreted by glomerular filtration, and differences in renal clearance have been noted in patients with normal renal function.[11,22,24] Varying degrees of plasma protein binding[24] may explain the higher renal clearance of the *R* epimer.

We examined the disposition of the epimers of MOX after intravenous and intraperitoneal dosing in patients with CAPD who were free of infection.

METHODS

Our subjects were five adult patients (four men and one woman) with ESRD. Patients with a history of recent infection, a history of penicillin or cephalosporin allergy, abnormal coagulation parameters, or a hematocrit <20% or who had received antibiotic therapy within 2 weeks before the study were excluded. All subjects were functionally anephric (creatinine clearance <3 ml/min).

A crossover design was used whereby each subject received both an intravenous and an intraperitoneal dose of MOX with a 1 to 2 week washout between doses. Subjects were studied in the CAPD unit for the first 24 hours and then on an ambulatory basis for the remaining studies. Before MOX dosing, a complete blood count was performed and serum electrolyte, creatinine, glucose, and BUN levels and prothrombin time were determined.

After a 10-minute gravity-fed infusion of 2 L dialysis

From the Departments of Pharmacy and Medicine, State University of New York at Buffalo, Erie County Medical Center.
Supported by a grant-in-aid from Eli Lilly and Company.
Received for publication Nov. 30, 1984; accepted April 5, 1985.
Reprint requests to: John Walshe, M.D., Assistant Professor of Medicine, Renal Division, State University of New York at Buffalo, Erie County Medical Center, 462 Grider St., Buffalo, NY 14215.

fluid (Dianeal 137 [Travenol Laboratories, Inc.] with 1.5% dextrose) into the peritoneum, a single 1.0 or 2.0 gm iv dose of MOX (50:50 *R/S* mixture) was injected over 2 to 4 minutes through an indwelling venous catheter. During the study period, dialysis fluid exchanges were made approximately every 6 hours. Blood samples (5 ml) were collected in nonheparinized Vacutainer tubes (Becton-Dickinson) from an indwelling venous catheter in the arm contralateral to the infusion site at 0, 0.08, 0.25, 0.5, 0.75, 1, 2, 4, 6 (end of first dialysis cycle), 7, 9, 12 (end of second dialysis cycle), 24, and 48 hours after drug dosing. Peritoneal dialysis fluid samples (5 ml) were drawn after discarding the first 7 ml (peritoneal catheter volume) at 0, 0.25, 0.5, 0.75, 1, 2, 4, 6, 7, 9, and 12 hours after dosing. Dialysis fluid exchanges continued every 4 to 8 hours, with the volume of each exchange recorded and an aliquot taken at each exchange.

For the intraperitoneal study, a single 1.0 or 2.0 gm dose of MOX was mixed with 2,000 ml dialysis fluid and was infused into the peritoneal cavity by gravity infusion over 10 minutes. Blood and dialysis fluid samples were collected as described after intravenous dosing.

Blood was allowed to clot at room temperature and serum was obtained by centrifugation. Serum and dialysate samples were placed on dry ice within 1 hour of collection and were then stored at −70° C until assayed. Dialysate samples collected on an ambulatory basis were stored at room temperature for up to 12 hours before freezing. The concentration of *R*-MOX and *S*-MOX in serum and dialysate was determined by HPLC. The mobile phase consisted of 9% methanol/91% 0.1 mol/L phosphate buffer at pH 7.0. Separation was achieved on a Whatman Instruments RAC ODS column at a flow rate of 3.0 ml/min. The epimers of MOX were detected by ultraviolet absorption at 280 nm. The analytic standard of MOX used was a 50:50 mixture of the epimers. Serum standards were prepared in blank pooled plasma, and the dialysate standards were prepared in 0.1 mol/L phosphate buffer at pH 7.0. Standards (1.56 to 100 μg/ml) were run in duplicate, and chromatographic peak areas were determined by integration. Standard curves were linear over the range 1.56 to 100 μg/ml and typically had correlation coefficients >0.99 for both epimers. If necessary, samples were diluted with pooled plasma or dialysate to concentrations within the range of the standard curve.

MOX was extracted from serum and dialysate by a modification of the method of Ziemniak et al.[25] To 500 μl sample (serum or dialysate), 500 μl 0.07 mol/L KCl-HCl buffer (pH 1.0) and 200 μl concentrated HCl were added, the mixture was vortexed for 60 seconds, and then shaken for 5 minutes. Three milliliters of ethyl acetate containing cephacetrile as the internal standard were added to the mixture, which was then vortexed for 60 seconds, shaken for 5 minutes, and centrifuged at 1,200 × g for 5 minutes. The ethyl acetate phase was decanted, and 500 μl 0.1 mol/L phosphate buffer (pH 8.0) was added, after which the mixture was vortexed, shaken, and centrifuged as above. The ethyl acetate phase was aspirated and the remaining aqueous phase was partially evaporated under nitrogen (28° C for 20 minutes) and injected onto the column. The internal standard eluted after the epimers.

Intraday relative standard deviations were 1.9% (n = 6) for the 50 μg/ml *R*-MOX and *S*-MOX plasma standards. Corresponding intraday values for the 6.25 μg/ml concentration were 1.8% (n = 6) and 3.2% (n = 6). The interday relative standard deviation of the *R*-MOX and *S*-MOX plasma standards was 5.1% (n = 6) for the 50 μg/ml and 6.4% (n = 6) for the 6.25 μg/ml standards. Measured recovery of the *R* and *S* epimers from plasma was 59.8% ± 2.0% and 66.2% ± 2.1% for the 50 μg/ml (n = 4) plasma standard and 59.1% ± 5.4% and 67.1% ± 7.2% for the 6.25 μg/ml (n = 4) plasma standard.

Noncompartmental analysis was used to calculate the time-averaged disposition kinetics of *R*-MOX and *S*-MOX.[9] The apparent serum clearance (CL_s), an estimated net time-averaged peritoneal dialysis clearance ($\overline{CL_D}$), nonperitoneal clearance (CL_{NP}), and steady-state volume of distribution (V_{ss}) were determined for each epimer by the following equations:

$$CL_s = D/AUC \qquad (1)$$

$$\overline{CL_D} = X_D(t_1 - t_2)/AUC(t_t - t_2) \qquad (2)$$

$$CL_{NR} = CL_s - \overline{CL_D} \qquad (3)$$

$$V_{ss} = (AUMC/AUC) \cdot Cl \qquad (4)$$

where X_D ($t_1 - t_2$) is the amount of drug recovered in the dialysis fluid from t_1 to t_2 (intraperitoneal dose: t_1 = 6 hours, t_2 = 24 hours; intravenous dose: t_1 = 0 hour, t_2 = 24 hours), D is the amount of each epimer administered, and AUMC is the area under the (time × concentration) vs. time curve. CL_s and V_{ss} were determined only after intravenous infusion, and $\overline{CL_D}$ reflects net clearance from the peritoneal cavity. AUC and AUMC were calculated by LaGrange polynomial interpolation and integration.[17]

The fraction of MOX systemically absorbed after intraperitoneal infusion (f_{ip}) was calculated as the ratio of AUC after intraperitoneal and intravenous dosing,

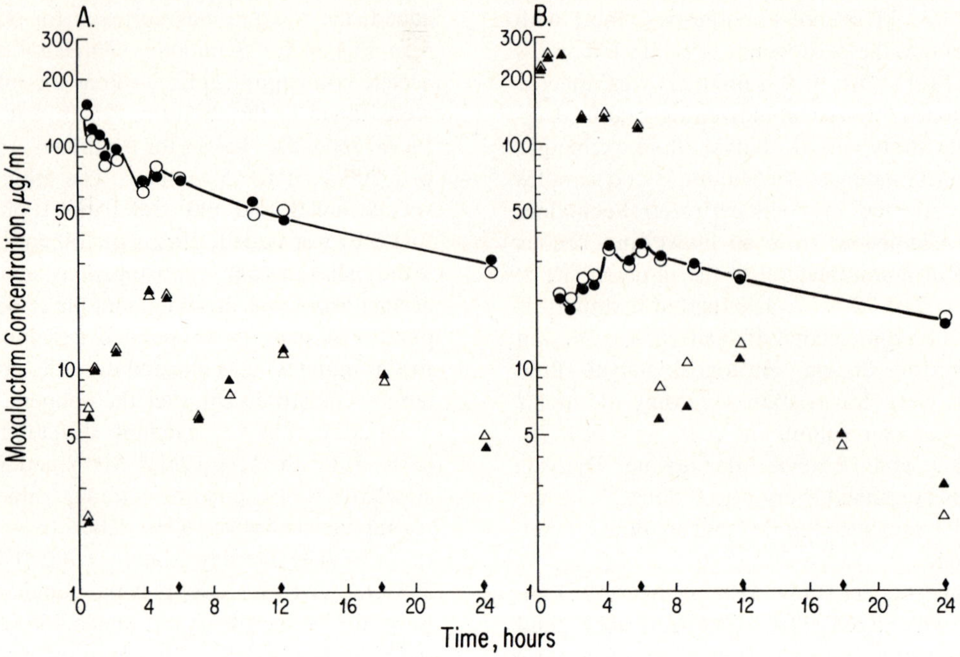

Fig. 1. Serum *(circles)* and dialysate *(triangles)* concentration-time profile of *R*-MOX *(solid symbols)* and *S*-MOX *(open symbols)* for subject 1 after 2.0 gm intravenous **(A)** and intraperitoneal **(B)** doses of MOX. *Diamonds* along the abscissa indicate dialysis exchange time.

with the assumption that CL, remained constant between each part of the study:

$$f_{ip} = AUC_{ip}/AUC_{iv} \quad (5)$$

f_{ip} was also calculated based on the amount of drug recovered in the dialysate after intraperitoneal infusion:

$$f_{ip} = (D_{ip} - X_D)/D_{ip} \quad (6)$$

where X_D is the drug recovered in the dialysate after the initial 6-hour dialysis cycle. The t½ was determined from the terminal slope calculated by linear least-squares regression analysis.

A paired t test was used to assess statistical differences between the kinetics of *R* and *S* epimers.

RESULTS

Physical and laboratory examinations of the subjects at the time of entry into each study revealed no clinical or microbiologic (culture-negative dialysate, <100 white blood cells/mm³) evidence of bacterial peritonitis. All laboratory findings were within expected limits for patients with ESRD. None of the subjects had clinically evident bleeding episodes or prolongation of the prothrombin time.

Two subjects (1 and 2) developed diarrhea approximately 24 hours after a 2.0 gm dose of MOX after both routes. The diarrhea was not associated with abdominal discomfort and lasted <24 hours. Subject 3 withdrew from the study when he developed diarrhea 24 hours after a single 2.0 gm intravenous dose. Subjects 4 and 5 successfully completed both phases of study after 1.0 gm doses without adverse effects.

Representative serum and dialysate concentration-time profiles of *R*-MOX and *S*-MOX after 2.0 and 1.0 gm iv doses are shown in Fig. 1, *A* and Fig. 2, *A*. The serum concentration of *R*-MOX and *S*-MOX declined biexponentially with time after intravenous dosing, and peak dialysate concentrations were achieved at the end of each dialysis period. The mean peak (0.08 hour) MOX serum concentration was 278 ± 41 µg/ml after 2.0 gm iv and 72.6 ± 23 µg/ml after 1.0 gm iv. In all subjects the *R*-MOX and *S*-MOX serum concentrations remained >5 µg/ml for 48 hours. The mean serum concentration ratio of *R*-MOX to *S*-MOX after an intravenous dose was close to unity (1.4 ± 0.04).

Mean dialysate MOX concentration at the end of the initial 6-hour dialysis period was 66 ± 28 µg/ml after 2.0 gm iv and 20 ± 14 µg/ml after 1.0 gm iv. Dialysate concentrations of *R*-MOX and *S*-MOX at the end of subsequent dialysis periods remained >2 µg/ml for 48 hours after 2.0 gm iv and 44 hours after 1.0 gm iv. The mean dialysate concentration ratio of *R*-MOX to *S*-MOX after intravenous dosing was 0.89 ± 0.08 (Tables I and II).

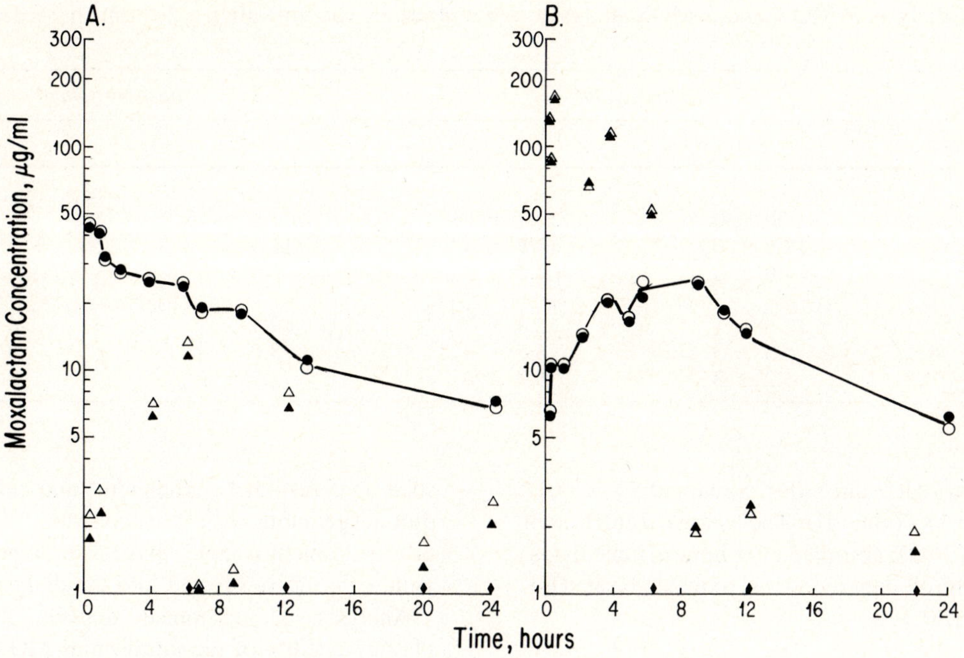

Fig. 2. Serum *(circles)* and dialysate *(triangles)* concentration-time profile of *R*-MOX *(solid symbols)* and *S*-MOX *(open symbols)* for subject 1 after 1.0 gm intravenous **(A)** and intraperitoneal **(B)** doses of MOX. *Diamonds* along the abscissa indicate dialysis exchange time.

Table I. *R*-MOX and *S*-MOX serum concentrations (μg/ml) after a 2.0 gm (n = 3) or 1.0 gm (n = 2) dose

	2.0 gm		*1.0 gm*	
Route	*1 hr*	*24 hr*	*1 hr*	*24 hr*
Intravenous				
R	75.5 ± 24	30.0 ± 10	24.1 ± 10	7.91 ± 0.6
S	70.4 ± 24	27.3 ± 5.0	23.2 ± 11	6.79 ± 0.1
Intraperitoneal				
R	24.8 ± 7.0	17.6 ± 4.0	10.5 ± 0.4	12.1 ± 8.6
S	25.1 ± 7.0	17.8 ± 4.0	11.0 ± 1.0	10.2 ± 6.5

The mean CL_s of *R*-MOX and *S*-MOX was of the same order, 13.0 ± 5.5 ml/hr/kg for *S*-MOX and 12.9 ± 6.9 ml/hr/kg for *R*-MOX (Table III). The $\overline{CL_D}$ of *R*-MOX and *S*-MOX was low and of the same order (1.36 ± 0.64 ml/hr/kg for *S*-MOX and 1.57 ± 0.59 ml/hr/kg for *R*-MOX), approximately 10% of CL_s. The mean V_{ss} of *R*-MOX and *S*-MOX was 0.29 ± 0.13 and 0.33 ± 0.16 L/kg. The mean $t_{1/2}$ values of the *R* and *S* epimers after intravenous dosing were 16.6 ± 3.4 and 17.0 ± 3.3 hours. Overall, there were no significant differences between the kinetics of the *R* and *S* epimers (Table III).

Representative serum and dialysate concentration-time profiles after 2.0 and 1.0 gm ip doses of MOX are shown in Fig. 1, *B* and Fig. 2, *B*. *R*-MOX and *S*-MOX appeared rapidly in the serum and achieved peak concentrations at the end of the initial dialysis period. The mean dialysate MOX concentration was 361 ± 89 μg/ml at 0.5 hour after a 2.0 gm ip dose. At the end of the first 6-hour dialysis cycle, the mean peak serum MOX concentration was 96.7 ± 35 μg/ml after 2.0 gm ip and 44.8 ± 4.9 μg/ml after 1.0 gm ip. Serum concentations of *R*-MOX and *S*-MOX remained >4 μg/ml for 48 hours after both the 1.0 and 2.0 gm ip doses. Serum t½s of both epimers were similar, with a mean of 18.2 ± 3.5 hours for *R*-MOX and 18.2 ± 3.7 hours for *S*-MOX. The $\overline{CL_D}$ was also small after intraperitoneal dosing (1.36 ± 0.6 ml/hr/kg for *R*-MOX and 1.57 ± 0.6 ml/hr/kg for *S*-MOX; Table III).

The mean systemic availabilities of *R*-MOX and *S*-

Table II. End-dialysis *R*-MOX and *S*-MOX dialysate concentrations (μg/ml) after a 2.0 gm (n = 3) or 1.0 gm (n = 2) dose

	Intravenous		Intraperitoneal	
Route	*R*	*S*	*R*	*S*
1.0 gm				
6 hr	30 ± 0	30.7 ± 15	73.1 ± 55	76.6 ± 56
12 hr	18.6 ± 6	17.9 ± 5	11.3 ± 3	13.9 ± 4
24 hr	4.0 ± 2	4.2 ± 2	2.5 ± 0	2.7 ± 1
2.0 gm				
6 hr	12.6 ± 1	15.4 ± 2	69.1 ± 5	76.1 ± 6
12 hr	6.5 ± 3	6.3 ± 4	8.0 ± 4	8.0 ± 6
24 hr	5.2 ± 3	6.7 ± 4	2.8 ± 2	3.1 ± 2

MOX based on AUC values (Eq. 5) were 0.71 ± 0.18 and 0.79 ± 0.18 (Table III). The estimated fraction of *R*-MOX and *S*-MOX absorbed after intraperitoneal dosing based on the amount recovered in the dialysate (Eq. 6) was 0.83 ± 0.12.

DISCUSSION

MOX exists as a pair of stereoisomers of which the *R* epimer has the greater antimicrobial activity.[22,23] In healthy adults, *R* and *S* epimers have been shown to differ in plasma protein binding (*R* = 53%, *S* = 67%), and the *R* epimer has been reported to have a larger V_{ss} than the *S* epimer.[13] The clearance of *R*-MOX has been reported to be somewhat greater than that of *S*-MOX in healthy adults and in children with infections.[12,21]

In patients with normal renal function, the *R/S* serum concentration ratio ranges from 0.5 to 0.8.[11,23] We found the *R/S* serum concentration ratio to be close to unity, with little difference between *R* and *S* kinetics (Table III). Wise et al.[23] reported similar *R/S* ratios in patients with uremia.

Estimates of the net $\overline{CL_D}$ (Eq. 2) revealed similar values for both epimers (*R*, 1.10 ± 0.60 ml/hr/kg; *S*, 1.27 ± 0.62 ml/hr/kg) that were approximately 10% of the mean CL_s values. $\overline{CL_D}$ reflects the relationship between the net amount of drug recovered in the dialysate over a particular sampling time interval ($t_1 - t_2$) and the corresponding cumulative serum concentration-time profile of the drug ($AUC(t_1 - t_2)$). This value is a time-dependent hybrid term that incorporates the distributional clearance across the peritoneum and is influenced by the particular peritoneal dialysis method used.[10] The ease of its estimated calculation (Eq. 2) probably accounts for its common use in CAPD studies. The low $\overline{CL_D}$ values are comparable with those in a previous report describing MOX in patients with CAPD[19] as well as with those involving other β-lactams such as cefazolin,[4] cephalexin,[4] and cefoxitin.[7] In addition, gentamicin,[15,20] vancomycin,[2,3] and trimethoprim-sulfamethoxazole[12] have also demonstrated a low yield of drug transferred into the dialysate.

Analysis of peritoneal dialysis fluid indicated 11.9% ± 2.6% of the intravenous MOX dose was recovered during the study period compared with the 30% to 50% recovery during a 4- to 6-hour hemodialysis period.[1,21] The lower total dialyzing membrane, pore area, lower effective blood flow, and greater resistances to diffusion entailed in peritoneal dialysis may account for these differences.

The amount of antibiotic systemically absorbed after intraperitoneal dosing may be influenced by the volume of dialysis fluid, duration of dwell period, protein concentration in the peritoneal fluid, and permeability characteristics of the peritoneal membrane, the latter of which may be affected by peritoneal infection or inflammation. Studies reporting high bioavailability values have usually involved patients without infections who presumably have minimal protein in their dialysate. Thus after intraperitoneal dosing the peritoneal surface is exposed to high concentrations of "free drug" over prolonged dwell periods, which provides an appreciable driving force for movement of the drug across the mesothelial and endothelial membranes. It is therefore likely that significant systemic absorption occurs. Upon entry into the vascular space, antibiotics bind to serum proteins in varying degrees based on individual physicochemical properties unique to each drug molecule.[8] The serum concentration of unbound antibiotic becomes the driving force for drug distribution from the vasculature into peripheral body compartments. The volume of drug distribution throughout the body is therefore a function of individual drug characteristics, and along with extraperitoneal clearance mechanisms will determine the serum concentrations achieved after an intraperitoneal dose of an antibiotic.

Table III. Kinetics of *R*-MOX and *S*-MOX in patients undergoing CAPD

			CL_s† (ml/hr/kg)		$\overline{CL_D}$ (ml/hr/kg)		CL_{NP}† (ml/hr/kg)		V_{ss}† (L/kg)		$t_{1/2}$ (hr)	
Patient	*Route*	*Dose**	*R*	*S*	*R*	*S*	*R*	*S*	*R*	*S*	*R*	*S*
1	iv	2.0	6.57	7.20	0.80	0.94	5.77	6.26	0.15	0.14	15.3	13.7
	ip	2.0	—	—	0.81	0.96	—	—	—	—	16.6	14.3
2	iv	2.0	7.94	9.20	0.67	1.31	7.27	7.89	0.20	0.25	17.7	18.7
	ip	2.0	—	—	0.50	0.50	—	—	—	—	19.5	20.1
3	iv	2.0	13.2	13.0	1.33	1.38	11.9	11.6	0.26	0.27	13.0	14.0
	ip	—	—	—	—	—	—	—	—	—	—	—
4	iv	1.0	12.9	14.0	1.85	2.50	11.1	11.1	0.44	0.53	22.0	21.6
	ip	1.0	—	—	0.73	0.83	—	—	—	—	22.5	21.7
5	iv	1.0	24.1	21.6	2.14	1.73	22.0	19.9	0.41	0.48	15.0	16.8
	ip	1.0	—	—	—	—	—	—	—	—	14.3	20.7
		$\overline{X}$	12.9	13.0	1.10	1.27	11.6	11.4	0.29	0.33	17.3	18.0
		±SD	6.9	5.5	0.60	0.62	6.3	5.3	0.13	0.16	3.4	3.3

iv = Intravenous; ip = intraperitoneal.
*Total dose of moxalactam (50:50, *R/S* mixture) administered.
†Calculated only from intravenous data.

The combined effect of antibiotic distribution and serum protein binding tends to decrease the diffusion gradient for drug transfer back into the peritoneal cavity.

Many studies of patients with CAPD who are free of infection have yielded dosing recommendations for the treatment of bacterial peritonitis. In doing so it is assumed that the kinetic characteristics of the peritoneum are not significantly altered during infection. Somani et al.[20] demonstrated f_{ip} values for gentamicin in two patients with CAPD and peritonitis equivalent to those seen in patients without infections. Although antibiotics appear to be well absorbed from the noninfected peritoneum,[4,20] there are insufficient data to characterize fully the effects of bacterial infection on this absorption process.

Our data can be used to suggest preliminary dosing guidelines (1.0 gm ip every 24 hours) for use of MOX in the treatment of bacterial peritonitis in patients with CAPD. This recommendation is based on the adverse gastrointestinal effects noted after a 2.0 gm dose and the serum and dialysate concentrations reached after a 1.0 gm dose, which exceed the minimum inhibitory concentrations for pathogens susceptible to MOX. Further study in the patient with CAPD and peritonitis is needed to define precisely the efficacy of this dosing approach.

We thank the nurses in the CAPD unit for their help.

References

1. Aronoff G, Sloan R, Mong S, Luft F, Kleit S: Moxalactam pharmacokinetics during hemodialysis. Antimicrob Agents Chemother **19**:575-577, 1981.
2. Bleuins RD, Halstenson CE, Salem NG, Matzke GI: Pharmacokinetics of vancomycin during continuous ambulatory peritoneal dialysis. Antimicrob Agents Chemother **25**:603-606, 1984.
3. Bunke CM, Aronoff G, Breier ME, Sloan RS, Luft FC: Pharmacokinetics of vancomycin during continuous ambulatory peritoneal dialysis. CLIN PHARMACOL THER **34**: 631-637, 1983.
4. Bunke CM, Aronoff G, Breier ME, Sloan RS, Luft FC: Cefazolin and cephalexin kinetics in continuous ambulatory peritoneal dialysis. CLIN PHARMACOL THER **33**:66-72, 1983.
5. Fitzpatrick BJ, Stardiford HC: A comparative evaluation of moxalactam: Antimicrobial activity, pharmacokinetics, adverse reactions and clinical efficacy. Pharmacotherapy **2**:197-212, 1982.
6. Gokal R: Peritonitis in continuous ambulatory peritoneal dialysis. J Antimicrob Chemother **9**:417-422, 1982.
7. Greaves WL, Krect JH, Ogilvie R, Richards GK: Cefoxitin disposition during peritoneal dialysis. Antimicrob Agents Chemother **19**:253-255, 1981.
8. Gwilt PR, Perrier D: Plasma protein binding and distribution characteristics of drugs as indices of their hemodialyzability. CLIN PHARMACOL THER **24**:154-161, 1978.
9. Jusko WJ: Guidelines for collection and pharmacokinetic analysis of drug disposition data. *In* Evans WE, Schentag JJ, Jusko WJ, editors: Applied pharmacokinetics. San Francisco, 1980, Applied Therapeutics, Inc, pp 639-676.
10. Jusko WJ, Baliah T, Kim KH, Gerbracht LM, Yaffe SJ: Pharmacokinetics of gentamicin during peritoneal dialysis in children. Kidney Int **9**:430-438, 1976.
11. Luthy R, Blaser J, Bonetti A, Simmen H, Wiser R, Siegenthaler R: Comparative multiple-dose pharmacokinetics of cefotaxime, moxalactam, and ceftazidime. Antimicrob Agents Chemother **20**:567-575, 1981.

12. Matzke GR, Halstenson CE, Blevins RB, Salem NG: Trimethoprim-sulfamethoxazole pharmacokinetics during continuous ambulatory peritoneal dialysis. CLIN PHARMACOL THER **33:**235, 1983. (Abst.)
13. Nahata MC, Durell DE, Barson WJ: Moxalactam epimer kinetics in children. CLIN PHARMACOL THER **31:**528-532, 1982.
14. Oreopoulos DG: Chronic peritoneal dialysis. Clin Nephrol **9:**165-173, 1978.
15. Pancorbo S, Comty C: Pharmacokinetics of gentamicin in patients undergoing continuous ambulatory peritoneal dialysis. Antimicrob Agents Chemother **19:**605-607, 1981.
16. Popovich RP, Moncrief JW, Nolph KD, Ghods AJ, Twardowski ZJ, Pyle WK: Continuous ambulatory peritoneal dialysis. Ann Intern Med **88:**449-456, 1978.
17. Rocci ML, Jusko WJ: LAGRAN program for area and moments in pharmacokinetic analysis. Comput Programs Biomed **16:**203-216, 1983.
18. Rubin J, Rogers WA, Taylor HM, Everett ED, Prowant BF, Fruto LV, Nolph KD: Peritonitis during continuous ambulatory peritoneal dialysis. Ann Intern Med **92:**7-13, 1980.
19. Singlas E, Boutron HF, Merdjan H, Brocard JF, Poucheville M, Fries D: Moxalactam kinetics during chronic ambulatory peritoneal dialysis. CLIN PHARMACOL THER **34:**403-407, 1983.
20. Somani P, Shapiro RS, Stockard H, Higgins TT: Unidirectional absorption of gentamicin from the peritoneum during continuous ambulatory peritoneal dialysis. CLIN PHARMACOL THER **32:**113-121, 1982.
21. Srinivasan S, Neu HC: Pharmacokinetics of moxalactam in patients with renal failure and during hemodialysis. Antimicrob Agents Chemother **20:**398-400, 1981.
22. Wise R, Wills PJ, Bedford KA: Epimers of moxalactam: In vitro comparison of activity and stability. Antimicrob Agents Chemother **20:**30-32, 1981.
23. Wise R, Wright N, Wills PJ: Activity, stability, and pharmacology of the epimers of moxalactam. Rev Infect Dis **4:**S564-S568, 1982.
24. Yamada H, Ichihashi T, Hirano K, Kinoshita H: Plasma protein binding and urinary excretion of R- and S-epimers of an arylmalonylamino 1-oxacephem in humans. J Pharm Sci **70:**112-113, 1981.
25. Ziemniak JA, Chiarmonte DA, Miner DJ, Schentag JJ: HPLC determination of D and L moxalactam in human serum and urine. J Pharm Sci **71:**399-402, 1982.

The effects of several weeks of ethanol consumption on ethanol kinetics in normal men and women

We examined in normal men and women the effects of chronic ethanol consumption and the coadministration of cimetidine and ranitidine on the kinetics of ethanol. We found that the consumption of 45 gm ethanol per day for 3 weeks increased the apparent volume of distribution of ethanol in men from 732 to 884 ml/kg ($P < 0.01$) but had no such effect in women (697 ml/kg before ethanol and 746 ml/kg after chronic ethanol consumption). This combined therapy had no effect on the rate of ethanol disappearance in either sex. In men the rate of disappearance was 165 mg/L/hr before and 168 mg/L/hr after chronic consumption, while in women the respective values were 209 and 203 mg/L/hr. The addition of either cimetidine or ranitidine had no effect on either parameter compared with values observed on day 22 of the study. In view of the known inhibitory effects of cimetidine on cytochrome P-450–dependent enzymes, our data suggest that this enzyme system does not metabolize a significant fraction of ingested ethanol in subjects who have consumed moderate doses of alcohol for several weeks. (Clin Pharmacol Ther 38:157-163, 1985.)

Jordan L. Holtzman, M.D., Ph.D., Roger L. Gebhard M.D., John H. Eckfeldt, M.D., Ph.D., Linda R. Mottonen, B.S., Denise K. Finley, R.N., and Fred N. Eshelman, Pharm.D. *Minneapolis, Minn., and Research Triangle Park, N. C.*

It has long been believed that ethanol is more rapidly metabolized in the chronic alcoholic than in naive subjects. A number of controlled studies in man and animals has supported this impression, but others have suggested that alcoholism has no effect on ethanol metabolism (for a review of studies to 1973 see Table of Pieper and Skeen[1]). A major problem in such studies, especially in man, is that it is difficult to control important variables such as the nutritional status of the subjects and to determine both the length of time and the quantity of alcohol the subject has been consuming. Hence it is difficult to compare results observed in different studies.

Both Pieper and Skeen[1] and Lieber's groups[2-4] have sought to avoid these problems by examining this question in nonhuman primates. They used a liquid diet containing up to 50% of the total calories provided by ethanol[5] and have found that in this model there appears to be a significant increase in the rate of ethanol disappearance per unit body weight in the ethanol-treated animals when compared with the pair-fed controls.

A number of mechanisms have been proposed to explain this increased disappearance. Several proposals have been based on the generally accepted concept that ethanol metabolism is catalyzed primarily by the hepatic alcohol dehydrogenases. If so, the limiting factor in ethanol metabolism is the rate of reoxidation of the NADH formed when alcohol is metabolized through this pathway. In support of this general concept, uncouplers of oxidative phosphorylation significantly increase the rate of ethanol metabolism in control but not alcohol-treated rats. These data suggest that the increased metabolism could be due to an increase in mitochondrial metabolism of NADH.[6] Furthermore, Domschke et al.[7] observed that the chronic administration of ethanol decreases the effect of its acute administration on the NAD^+/NADH ratio. A number of biochemical mechanisms might account for these changes in this ratio.[8-26]

Lieber and DiCarli[27] have suggested an alternative

From the Veterans Administration Medical Center and the Departments of Medicine, Pharmacology, and Laboratory Medicine and Pathology, University of Minnesota, Minneapolis, and Glaxo Inc., Research Triangle Park.

Supported in part by a grant from Glaxo Inc.

Received for publication Jan. 18, 1985; accepted April 9, 1985.

Reprint requests to: Jordan L. Holtzman, M.D., Ph.D., Chief, Clinical Pharmacology, Veterans Administration Medical Center, 4801 E. 54th St., Minneapolis, MN 55417.

mechanism for the increased metabolism of ethanol. They and Orme-Johnson and Ziegler[28] observed that the hepatic microsomes contain a mixed-function oxidation system that appears to be able to metabolize alcohols. Lieber and DiCarli have referred to this activity as the microsomal ethanol oxidizing system (MEOS). A number of studies have suggested that this metabolic pathway is associated with the hepatic, microsomal, cytochrome P-450–dependent mixed-function oxidases.[29-35] Lieber and others have found that this system is significantly induced by the chronic consumption of ethanol.[16,27,29,30,33,35-37] However, Cunningham et al.[26] reported that there was no increase in the MEOS after chronic alcohol ingestion in the monkey Macaca fascicularis. Induction of isozymes of cytochrome P-450 by other agents has shown inconsistent results in increasing ethanol metabolism,[34,38-43] suggesting that the oxidation of ethanol is catalyzed by a specific isozyme of cytochrome P-450 that is induced by the chronic administration of alcohol.

A major question that still remains is if there is a true increase in the metabolism of ethanol in alcohol-treated animals. In the most complete study of this question reported to date, Nomura et al.[4] found that, while liver weights were the same in control and the ethanol-fed animals, the body weights were significantly lower in the ethanol-treated animals. Because the treated animals had a higher liver/body weight ratio, they would also have had more enzymatic activity per unit body weight. Hence the observation of increased metabolism of ethanol in the alcoholic could be merely an artifact of the higher liver-to-body weight ratios in the alcohol-treated animals.

These investigators have suggested that, although the overall rate of disappearance of ethanol is the same in the control and treated animals, there may be a significant change in the relative importance of the dehydrogenase and MEOS pathways.[4] They suggest that after chronic alcohol treatment the MEOS may become an important pathway in the metabolism of alcohol. In particular, they point out that with the observed decrease in the activity of the mitochondrial electron chains after chronic alcohol treatment, there would be accumulation of NADH and a corresponding decrease in the activity of the dehydrogenase pathway. Hence the increase in the microsomal oxidation of ethanol may assume increased importance in the metabolism of ethanol and serve to keep the total body metabolism of ethanol at a level comparable to that observed in the control animal.

If the MEOS does represent a major pathway in the metabolism of ethanol, one would anticipate that various inhibitors of the cytochrome P-450–dependent enzyme systems should reduce the metabolism of ethanol, particularly in the alcohol-induced subject. One such well-known inhibitor of the cytochrome P-450 mixed-function oxidases is cimetidine.[44-51] However, Feely and Wood[52] found that this agent had no effect on alcohol disappearance in naive subjects. Similarly, Dobrilla et al.[53] found that neither cimetidine nor ranitidine had any effect in subjects consuming 20 gm ethanol per day. These data would suggest that either the MEOS is not inhibited by cimetidine or that it is not an important pathway in the metabolism of ethanol in uninduced human subjects.

Despite the failure of cimetidine to affect the disappearance of ethanol in control subjects, previous studies in ethanol-treated animals suggest that after higher doses of ethanol, the MEOS might assume greater importance in the metabolism of alcohol. Thus one would predict that the concurrent administration of cimetidine should inhibit the disappearance of alcohol in ethanol-treated subjects. A problem in such studies is that cimetidine has a number of pharmacologic properties in addition to its inhibition of the cytochrome P-450 system. Cimetidine has been reported to decrease hepatic blood flow,[54] although other studies have suggested that these changes do not occur.[55-57] To control for these and other effects of H_2-blockers, it is important to compare the effects of cimetidine with those of an alternative H_2-blocker, such as ranitidine, which does not affect the cytochrome P-450–dependent reactions.[50]

In the current study we examined the effect of moderate doses of alcohol on the disappearance of ethanol in normal men and women. We also investigated whether cimetidine or ranitidine affect ethanol disappearance in these subjects. Our results suggest that in men, the daily consumption of moderate doses of ethanol increases its apparent volume of distribution without affecting its rate of disappearance. On the other hand, we found in women that the chronic consumption of alcohol had no effect on either metabolic parameter. Neither cimetidine nor ranitidine had any effect on ethanol disappearance in either sex when compared with the rates after chronic ethanol consumption. Our results suggest that the moderate consumption of ethanol does not affect its disappearance and that the MEOS probably does not represent a major pathway for ethanol metabolism in human subjects receiving approximately 15% of their calories as ethanol for several weeks.

METHODS

Our subjects were seven normal men and five normal women aged 21 to 42 years old. All subjects had abstained from the consumption of alcoholic beverages for at least 30 days before the study. No subject was taking any other medications, including oral contraceptives, or any drug of abuse. Each subject had normal physical examination and routine laboratory test results including complete blood count with differential and platelet counts, urinalysis, and levels of serum electrolytes, alkaline phosphatase, SGOT, lactate dehydrogenase, bilirubin, and creatinine. All subjects were within 20% of their ideal weights.

After an overnight fast, the subjects were admitted to the Special Diagnostic and Treatment Unit at the Veterans Administration Medical Center, Minneapolis, on days 1, 21, 23, and 33 of the study and received 45 gm ethanol by mouth at 8 AM. The subjects fasted until noon of the study day. Venous blood samples were drawn through a heparin lock 0, 0.5, 1, 2, 3, 4, 5, 6, 8 and 10 hours after dosing. Blood samples were collected in fluoride-oxalate tubes, which were centrifuged and the plasma stored at 4° C until analysis. On all other study days the subjects consumed 45 gm ethanol at bedtime. On study days 22 to 24 and 32 to 34 the subjects received either cimetidine, 300 mg four times a day, or ranitidine, 150 mg twice a day, in a double-blind fashion, such that each subject received drug and placebo at each period. The order of dosing of cimetidine and ranitidine was determined by a random numbers table.

Plasma (100 μl) was mixed with 3.4% $HClO_4$ (2.4 ml). The mixture was centrifuged and the ethanol concentration in the supernatant was determined by an alcohol dehydrogenase method on an automated centrifugal analyzer. The method is sensitive to 100 mg/L and has a reproducibility of >5%.

The rates of metabolism and the zero-time intercepts were determined by least-squares analysis of the linear portion of the concentration-time curves. After the initial peak, all concentration-time curves were linear throughout the study, suggesting that the metabolism of ethanol was zero order to the lowest blood ethanol concentration observed in these subjects. Parameters for each subject were compared within each sex by paired and two-sample t tests as appropriate for the data. On nonstudy days the ethanol dose was consumed at bedtime and in all but two subjects the zero-hour ethanol concentration was zero. Two of the subjects had consumed their last dose of ethanol a few hours before the start of the study and had significant zero-time ethanol levels only during the H_2-blocker portions of the studies. These levels were subtracted from the intercept values and the volume of distribution determined from the difference. The inclusion of these values had no effect on either the overall averages or the significance of the changes in the mean differences.

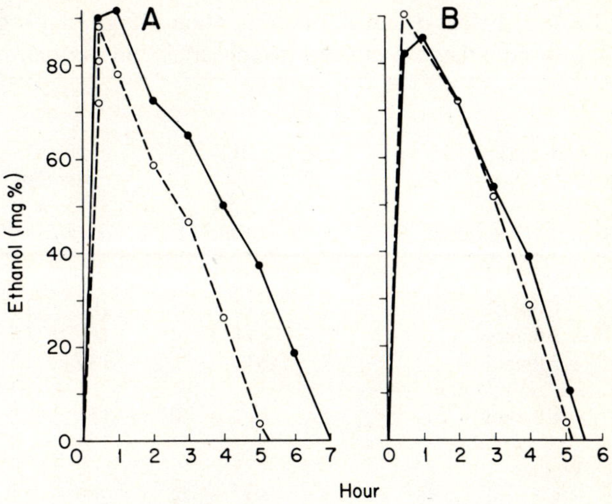

Fig. 1. Ethanol kinetics in a representative male **(A)** and female **(B)** subject before (——) and after (- - - -) 45 gm ethanol per day for 3 weeks.

RESULTS

In male subjects the administration of ethanol for 3 weeks led to a significant increase in the apparent volume of distribution, from 732 ± 36 to 884 ± 44 ml/kg ($P < 0.01$), but had no effect on its rate of disappearance (Fig. 1, *A*; Table I). The addition of either cimetidine or ranitidine did not significantly affect these parameters when compared with values observed after 3 weeks of ethanol.

In female subjects none of the treatments had any effect on either the ethanol volume of distribution or rate of disappearance (Fig. 1, *B*; Table I). It is of interest that, despite the small numbers of subjects, the greater rate of disappearance in women than in men approached statistical significance. Such a result may represent a statistical outlier, since other investigators have not observed any such sex difference in the rate of ethanol disappearance.[58,59]

During the study there were no significant changes in weight, physical examination results, or any of the laboratory values in any of the subjects.

DISCUSSION

Our data suggest that in the normal subject receiving 45 gm ethanol per day, there is no significant increase in its rate of disappearance. It would therefore appear that individuals who are consuming moderate doses of ethanol representing approximately 10% to 15% of their total calories do not show the increased disappearance

Table I. Effect of ethanol consumption (45 gm/day), cimetidine (300 mg four times a day), and ranitidine (150 mg twice a day) on ethanol disappearance in normal men and women

				Change from			
				Day 1*		Day 22	
Treatment	*n*	V_z *(ml/kg)*	*Metabolism (mg/L/hr)*	V_z *(ml/kg)*	*Metabolism (mg/L/hr)*	V_z *(ml/kg)*	*Metabolism (mg/L/hr)*
Men							
Control	7	732 ± 36	165 ± 14†	—	—	—	—
Ethanol	7	884 ± 44	168 ± 15	152 ± 30‡	1 ± 8	—	—
Ethanol + cimetidine	7	840 ± 32	187 ± 17	108 ± 46§	22 ± 15	−44 ± 53	19 ± 11
Ethanol + ranitidine	6	912 ± 70¶	166 ± 21	158 ± 57§	−6 ± 9	12 ± 4	1 ± 12
Women							
Control	5	697 ± 44	209 ± 13	—	—	—	—
Ethanol	5	746 ± 15	203 ± 14	49 ± 47	6 ± 16	—	—
Ethanol + cimetidine	5	686 ± 29	208 ± 9	10 ± 47	−1 ± 14	−59 ± 35	6 ± 16
Ethanol + ranitidine	5	711 ± 40	205 ± 13	14 ± 32	−3 ± 22	−35 ± 37	3 ± 11

Data are $\bar{X}$ ± SE.
*Paired differences for each subject.
†0.1 < P < 0.05, ‡P < 0.01, §P < 0.05 compared with values in women.
¶The discrepancy between the difference of the mean and the average of the difference is due to a lost set of samples, and there were thus data from only six subjects.

reported for human and animal subjects consuming a much higher percentage of their calories as ethanol.

Although we did not observe any change in the rate of ethanol disappearance, there was a significant increase in the apparent volume of distribution of ethanol in men but not in women. It is possible that this change in men was due to an increase in body fat during the study, but this seems unlikely because none of the subjects had a significant weight change. To show such a marked change in the volume of distribution, the subjects would have had to gain 10% or more of their initial body weight, a change that would have been readily observable.

It is possible that the increase in the apparent volume of distribution resulted from either a decrease in the percentage of ethanol absorbed from the gastrointestinal tract or from changes in motility, which would have delayed absorption and indicated an apparent decrease in total absorption. There are several reasons to believe that neither is the case. First, ethanol is readily absorbed from the gut. In fact, it is believed that a significant fraction of the alcohol is passively absorbed from the stomach, so that a significant decrease in the percentage of the ethanol absorbed is unlikely. Second, there were no consistent changes in the times to peak levels. This would suggest that there was no change in intestinal motility, since these times are often used as an index of changes in intestinal motility.

A final consideration is related to the observation that the disappearance of ethanol was consistently zero order; that is, a fixed mass, rather than a fixed fraction, of the total ethanol in the body was metabolized per unit time. As a result, if the changes in the ethanol apparent volume of distribution in the men were due to changes in intestinal motility, then after the drug was totally absorbed the ethanol concentration should be the same before and after chronic ethanol consumption. Yet, at every time point after the peak concentration the concentration in male subjects was lower after chronic ethanol dosing than before (Fig. 1, *A*). These data indicate that the greater apparent volume of distribution after chronic ethanol consumption is not an artifact of the method of statistical analysis.

A more likely explanation for the change in the apparent volume of distribution is that there was a significant increase in the presystemic metabolism of ethanol in men but not in women. It seems unlikely that presystemic metabolism occurs in the liver, because there was no change in the rate of disappearance in the postabsorptive phase. More likely the presystemic metabolism occurs within the gut, in accord with the observations of Carter and Isselbacher[60] and Lamboeuf et al.,[61] who have reported ethanol metabolism in the gastrointestinal tract of the rat. Furthermore, the latter investigators have also observed that this metabolism was increased in alcohol-treated animals.

The failure of cimetidine to affect the disappearance of ethanol would suggest that, irrespective of where the metabolism of ethanol occurs, the MEOS system does not catalyze a significant fraction of this metabolism. Although it is possible that cimetidine may not inhibit the MEOS, this seems unlikely, because cimetidine has been shown to inhibit all the cytochrome P-450–dependent mixed-function oxidases that have been examined. The isozyme of cytochrome P-450, which is induced in human subjects by ethanol, may not be inhibited by the concentrations of cimetidine achieved by usual therapeutic dosages. This hypothesis can only be fully tested when this cytochrome is purified from the human liver. Similarly, the failure of either H_2-blocker to affect ethanol kinetics suggests that the disappearance of ethanol is not affected by changes in such factors as gastric acidity.

In conclusion, our current results indicate that there is a profound sex difference in the disappearance of ethanol after the consumption of moderate amounts of ethanol for 3 to 5 weeks. There may be significant presystemic ethanol metabolism in men, but not in women that is inducible by chronic ethanol consumption. Finally, the inhibition of cytochrome P-450 enzymes does not appear to have a significant effect on ethanol metabolism during its chronic consumption in moderate doses.

References

1. Pieper WA, Skeen MJ: Changes in rate of ethanol elimination associated with chronic administration of ethanol to chimpanzees and Rhesus monkeys. Drug Metab Dispos **1**:634-641, 1973.
2. Salaspuro MP, Lieber CS: Non-uniformity of blood ethanol elimination: Its exaggeration after chronic consumption. Ann Clin Res **10**:294-297, 1978.
3. Pikkarainen PH, Lieber CS: Concentration dependency of ethanol elimination rates in baboons: Effects of chronic alcohol consumption. Alcoholism **4**:40-43, 1980.
4. Nomura F, Pikkarainen H, Jauhonen P, Arai E, Gordon EE, Baraona E, Lieber CS: Effect of ethanol administration on the metabolism of ethanol in baboons. J Pharmacol Exp Ther **227**:78-83, 1983.
5. Lieber CS, DeCarli LM: Animal models of ethanol dependence and liver injury in rats and baboons. Fed Proc **35**:1232-1236, 1976.
6. Videla L, Israel Y: Factors that modify the metabolism of ethanol in rat liver and adaptive changes produced by its chronic administration. Biochem J **118**:275-281, 1970.
7. Domschke D, Domschke W, Lieber CS: Hepatic redox state: Attenuation of the acute effects of ethanol induced by chronic ethanol consumption. Life Sci **15**:1327-1334, 1974.
8. Israel Y, Videla L, Fernandez-Videla V, Bernstein J: Effects of chronic ethanol treatment and thyroxine administration on ethanol metabolism and liver oxidative capacity. J Pharmacol Exp Ther **192**:565-574, 1975.
9. Israel Y, Videla L, Bernstein J: Liver hypermetabolic state after chronic ethanol consumption: Hormonal interrelations and pathogenic implications. Fed Proc **34**:2052-2059, 1975.
10. Bernstein J, Videla L, Israel Y: Metabolic alterations produced in the liver by chronic ethanol administration. Changes related the energetic parameters of the cell. Biochem J **134**:515-521, 1973.
11. Ricci RL, Crawford SS, Miner PB Jr: The effect of ethanol on hepatic sodium plus potassium activated adenosine triphosphatase activity in the rat. Gastroenterology **80**:1445-1450, 1981.
12. Bernstein J, Videla L, Israel Y: Hormonal influences in the development of the hypermetabolic state of the liver produced by chronic administration of ethanol. J Pharmacol Exp Ther **192**:583-591, 1975.
13. Rawat AK, Kuriyama K: Contributions of "substrate shuttles" in the transport of extramitochondrial reducing equivalents by hepatic mitochondria from chronic alcohol-fed mice. Arch Biochem Biophys **152**:44-52, 1972.
14. Spach PI, Parce JW, Cunningham CC: Effect of chronic ethanol administration on energy metabolism and phospholipase A_2 activity in rat liver. Biochem J **178**:23-33, 1979.
15. Cederbaum AI, Lieber CS, Beattie DS, Rubin E: Effect of chronic ethanol ingestion on mitochondrial permeability and the transport of reducing equivalents. Biochem Biophys Res Commun **49**:649-655, 1972.
16. Rubin E, Bacchin P, Gang H, Lieber CS: Induction and inhibition of hepatic microsomal enzymes by ethanol. Lab Invest **22**:569-580, 1970.
17. Rubin E, Beattie DS, Toth A, Lieber CS: Structural and functional effects of ethanol on hepatic mitochondria. Fed Proc **31**:131-140, 1972.
18. Cederbaum AI, Lieber CS, Toth A, Beattie DS, Rubin E: Effects of ethanol and fat on the transport of reducing equivalents into rat liver mitochondria. J Biol Chem **248**:4977-4980, 1973.
19. Gordon ER: Mitochondrial functions in an ethanol-induced fatty liver. J Biol Chem **248**:8271-8280, 1973.
20. Cederbaum AI, Rubin E: Molecular injury to mitochondria produced by ethanol and acetaldehyde. Fed Proc **34**:2045-2051, 1975.

21. Bernstein JD, Penniall R: Effects of chronic ethanol treatment upon rat liver mitochondria. Biochem Pharmacol **27**:2337-2342, 1978.
22. Thayer WS, Rubin E: Effects of chronic ethanol intoxication on oxidative phosphorylation in rat liver submitochondrial particles. J Biol Chem **254**:7717-7723, 1979.
23. Thayer WS, Rubin E: Molecular alterations in the respiratory chain of rat liver after chronic ethanol consumption. J Biol Chem **256**:6090-6097, 1981.
24. Thayer WS, Rubin E: Antimycin inhibition as a probe of mitochondrial function in isolated rat hepatocytes: Effects of chronic ethanol consumption. Biochim Biophys Acta **721**:328-335, 1982.
25. Rubin E, Rottenberg H: Ethanol-induced injury and adaptation in biological membranes. Fed Proc **41**:2465-2471, 1982.
26. Cunningham CC, Bottenus RE, Spach PI, Rudel LL: Ethanol-related changes in liver microsomes and mitochondria from the monkey, Macaca fascicularis. Alcoholism **7**:424-430, 1983.
27. Lieber CS, DeCarli LM: Ethanol oxidation by hepatic microsomes: Adaptive increases after ethanol feeding. Science **162**:917-918, 1968.
28. Orme-Johnson WH, Ziegler DM: Alcohol mixed function oxidase activity of mammalian liver microsomes. Biochem Biophys Res Commun **21**:78-82, 1965.
29. Lieber CS, DeCarli LM: Enhanced nicotinamide-adenine dinucleotide phosphate oxidase: Activity enhanced by ethanol consumption. Science **170**:78-79, 1970.
30. Lieber CS, DeCarli LM: Hepatic microsomal ethanol-oxidizing system: *In vitro* characteristics and adaptive properties *in vivo*. J Biol Chem **245**:2505-2512, 1970.
31. Mezey E, Potter JJ, Reed WD: Ethanol oxidation by a component of liver microsomes rich in cytochrome P-450. J Biol Chem **248**:1183-1187, 1973.
32. Teschke R, Hasumura Y, Lieber CS: Hepatic ethanol metabolism: Respective roles of alcohol dehydrogenase, the microsomal ethanol-oxidizing system and catalase. Arch Biochem Biophys **175**:635-643, 1976.
33. Ohnishi K, Lieber CS: Reconstitution of the microsomal ethanol-oxidizing system: Qualitative and quantitative changes of cytochrome P-450 after chronic ethanol consumption. J Biol Chem **252**:7124-7134, 1977.
34. Miwa GT, Levin W, Thomas PE, Lu AYH: The direct oxidation of ethanol by a catalase- and alcohol dehydrogenase–free reconstituted system containing cytochrome P-450. Arch Biochem Biophys **187**:464-475, 1978.
35. Coon MJ, Koop DR, Morgan ET: Alcohol oxidation by isozyme 3a of liver microsomal cytochrome P-450. Pharmacol Biochem Behav **18**:177-180, 1983.
36. Sinclair JF, Sinclair PR, Smith EL, Bement WJ, Pomeroy J, Bonkowsky H: Ethanol-mediated increase in cytochrome P-450 in cultured hepatocytes. Biochem Pharmacol **30**:2805-2809, 1981.
37. Teschke R, Moreno F, Petrides AS: Hepatic microsomal ethanol oxidizing system (MEOS): Respective roles of ethanol and carbohydrates for the enhanced activity after chronic alcohol consumption. Biochem Pharmacol **30**: 1745-1751, 1981.
38. Klaasen CD: Ethanol metabolism in rats after microsomal metabolizing enzyme induction. Proc Soc Exp Biol Med **132**:1099-1102, 1969.
39. Reinhard JF, Spector E: Effects of phenobarbital, phenylbutazone, 3,4-benzpyrene, or 3-methylcholanthrene on ethanol metabolism in the rat. Toxicol Appli Pharmacol **17**:12-22, 1970.
40. Ugarte G, Pino ME, Pereda T, Iturriaga H: Increased blood ethanol elimination in rats treated with halothane. Pharmacol **9**:275-280, 1973.
41. Mezey E, Robles EA: Effects of phenobarbital administration on rates of ethanol clearance and on ethanol-oxidizing enzymes in man. Gastroenterology **66**:248-253, 1974.
42. Vatsis KP, Coon MJ: On the question of whether cytochrome P-450 catalyzes ethanol oxidation: Studies with purified forms of the cytochrome from rabbit liver microsomes. *In* Thurman R, editor: Alcohol and aldehyde metabolizing systems. New York, 1978, Academic Press, pp 307-322.
43. Moreno F, Petrides AS, Heinen E, Strohmeyer G, Teschke R: Hepatic microsomal ethanol-oxidizing system (MEOS): Increased activity following propylthiouracil administration. Alcoholism **5**:85-91, 1981.
44. Puurunen J, Pelkonen O: Cimetidine inhibits microsomal drug metabolism in the rat. Eur J Pharmacol **55**:335-336, 1979.
45. Klotz U, Reimann I: Delayed clearance of diazepam due to cimetidine. N Engl J Med **302**:1012-1014, 1980.
46. Klotz U, Reimann I: Influence of cimetidine on the pharmacokinetics of desmethyldiazepam and oxazepam. Eur J Clin Pharmacol **18**:517-520, 1980.
47. Desmond PV, Patwardhan RV, Schenker S, Speeg KV: Cimetidine impairs elimination of chlordiazepoxide (Librium) in man. Ann Intern Med **93**:266-268, 1980.
48. Reitberg DP, Bernhard H, Schentag JJ: Alteration of theophylline clearance and half-life by cimetidine in normal volunteers. Ann Intern Med **95**:582-585, 1981.
49. Roberts RK, Grice J, Wood L, Petroff V, McGuffie C: Cimetidine impairs the elimination of theophylline and antipyrine. Gastroenterology **81**:19-21, 1981.
50. Knodell RG, Holtzman JL, Crankshaw DL, Steele NM, Stanley LN: Drumetabolism by rat and human hepatic microsomes in response to interaction with H_2-receptor antagonists. Gastroenterology **82**:84-88, 1982.
51. Abernethy DR, Greenblatt DJ, Divoll M, Ameer B, Shader RI: Differential effect of cimetidine on drug oxidation (antipyrine and diazepam) vs. conjugation (acetaminophen and lorazepam): Prevention of acetaminophen toxicity by cimetidine. J Pharmacol Exp Ther **234**:508-513, 1983.

52. Feely J, Wood AJJ: Effects of cimetidine on the elimination and actions of ethanol. JAMA **247:**2819-2821, 1982.
53. Dobrilla G, de Pretis G, Piazzi L, Chilovi F, Comverlato M, Valentini M, Pastorino A, Vallaperta P: Is ethanol metabolism affected by cimetidine and ranitidine at therapeutic doses? Hepatogastroenterology **31:**35-37, 1984.
54. Feely J, Wilkinson GR, Wood AJJ: Reduction of liver blood flow and propranolol metabolism by cimetidine. N Engl J Med **304:**692-695, 1981.
55. Tyden G, Thulin L, Nyberg B: The effect of cimetidine on liver blood flow in anesthetized man. Acta Chir Scand **149:**303-305, 1983.
56. Henderson JM, Ibrahim SZ, Millikan WJ Jr, Santi M, Warren WD: Cimetidine does not reduce liver blood flow in cirrhosis. Hepatology **3:**919-922, 1983.
57. Daneshmend TK, Ene MD, Parker G, Roberts CJC: Effects of chronic oral cimetidine on apparent liver blood flow and hepatic microsomal enzyme activity in man. Gut **25:**125-128, 1984.
58. Arthur MJP, Lee A, Wright R: Sex differences in the metabolism of ethanol and acetaldehyde in normal subjects. Clin Sci **67:**397-401, 1984.
59. Marshall AW, Kingstone D, Boss M, Morgan MY: Ethanol elimination in males and females: Relationship to menstrual cycle and body composition. Hepatology **3:**701-706, 1983.
60. Carter EA, Isselbacher KJ: The metabolism of ethanol to carbon dioxide by stomach and small intestinal slices. Proc Soc Exp Biol Med **138:**817-819, 1971.
61. Lamboeuf Y, La Droitte P, De Saint-Blanquat G: The gastrointestinal metabolism of ethanol in the rat. Effect of chronic alcoholic intoxication. Arch Int Pharmacodyn Ther **261:**157-169, 1983.

Cigarette smoking as a risk for cardiovascular disease. Part VI. Compensation with nicotine availability as a single variable

In a biochemical investigation of human smoking behavior with filter cigarettes with high draw resistance that varied only in nicotine yield, we attempted to determine which nicotine levels provide desired nicotine intake with a minimum of physiologic and biochemical consequences. Twelve prescreened subjects were divided into two study groups and supplied with cigarettes that varied in nicotine delivery. Both groups were initially monitored while smoking their usual cigarette. At the following visit, smokers in group 1 received incremental increases and smokers in group 2 received incremental decreases in nicotine levels in assigned cigarettes. All subjects were monitored upon first exposure, after 1 week of acclimatization to each experimental cigarette, and upon return to their usual brands. Subjects in both groups were unable to compensate fully for their nicotine uptake from the lowest nicotine cigarette. In subjects in group 1, new nicotine baselines began to develop after 1 week of acclimatization to cigarettes containing 0.9 and 1.3 mg nicotine. New baseline nicotine levels were also noted in subjects receiving decreases in nicotine (group 2) after smoking the cigarette containing 1.3 mg nicotine for 1 week. Carboxyhemoglobin concentrations did not differ from those measured after the usual-brand cigarettes. Plasma cotinine concentrations increased as nicotine content per cigarette increased, except when subjects smoked a 1.3 mg nicotine cigarette. Plasma thiocyanate levels did not vary in either group. Systolic and diastolic blood pressures were generally not different from control values. (CLIN PHARMACOL THER 38:164-170, 1985.)

N. J. Haley, Ph.D., D. W. Sepkovic, Ph.D., D. Hoffmann, Ph.D., and E. L. Wynder, M.D. *Valhalla, N. Y.*

A reduction in nicotine dose and in harmful tobacco smoke constituents should decrease the health risks associated with cigarette smoking. However, previous work from our laboratory[12] and others[1] has demonstrated that most smokers adjust their smoking behavior to maintain a desired nicotine intake. These behavioral changes can result in increased exposure to carbon monoxide (CO) and hydrogen cyanide, as well as to other gas phase and particulate phase constituents of tobacco smoke.[14]

It is well established that individuals alter smoking behavior to compensate for reduced nicotine availability.[7,10,11] Several methods can effectively limit the amount of nicotine a smoker inhales with the mainstream smoke.[16] Martin et al.[9] documented reductions in tobacco smoke constituent exposure through the use of graduated filters. Others have shown that smokers at least partially compensate for a reduction in available nicotine when cigarettes with perforated filter tips are used, and that more cigarettes are smoked when cigarettes of a shorter length than a normal cigarette are used.[3,4,15] In our study, mainstream smoke delivery of particulate and gaseous components in a series of experimental cigarettes was held constant while nicotine levels varied. We attempted to analyze compensatory behavior in response to available nicotine without confounders of smoke yields, pH, or varying air dilution through the use of filters of high draw resistance.

METHODS

Experimental design. Our study consisted of two independent experiments with two distinct study groups. One group was composed of subjects who smoked low-yield cigarettes ($\overline{X} \pm$ SE: 0.73 $\pm$ 0.39 mg nicotine per cigarette) who received gradual increases in nicotine dosage. The second group was com-

From the American Health Foundation, Naylor Dana Institute, Division of Nutrition and Endocrinology.

Received for publication Feb. 18, 1985; accepted April 9, 1985.

Reprint requests to: Dr. D. W. Sepkovic, American Health Foundation, Naylor Dana Institute, Division of Nutrition and Endocrinology, 1 Dana Rd., Valhalla, NY 10595.

Table I. Cigarette component analysis

	Experimental cigarettes (mg nicotine per cigarette)				
	0.06	*0.4*	*0.7*	*0.9*	*1.3*
Cigarette length (mm)	84.0	84.0	84.0	84.0	84.0
Filter length (mm)	21.0	21.0	21.0	21.0	21.0
Diameter (mm)	7.9	7.9	7.9	7.9	7.9
Moisture (%)	12.0	11.0	12.0	12.2	12.2
Effective sample weight (mg)	994.0	981.0	983.0	985.0	996.0
Paper weight (mg)	44.0	45.0	44.0	45.0	44.0
Filter wrapper weight (mg)	163.0	161.0	162.0	162.0	162.0
Cigarette paper permeability	102.9	103.7	103.9	106.4	106.3
Draw resistence (mm H_2O)					
Open vent	141.0	143.0	145.0	149.0	150.0
Closed vent	159.0	161.0	164.0	170.0	175.0
TPM					
Wet (mg)	13.8	15.4	15.1	14.6	15.4
Dry* (mg)	10.6	11.5	11.1	10.9	11.2
Nicotine in smoker (mg)	0.06	0.4	0.7	0.9	1.3
Nicotine transfer (%)	5.2	9.4	9.2	8.0	7.10
CO (vol%)	4.2	4.7	4.7	4.6	4.5
CO (ml)	13.1	13.2	13.4	13.3	12.9
Nicotine in tobacco (%)	0.2	0.8	1.3	1.9	2.9
Nitrate (%)	1.1	1.1	1.1	1.1	1.2
Reducing sugars (%)	11.9	11.8	11.5	11.2	11.4
Total sugars (%)	16.6	16.7	16.3	16.1	16.3
Chloride (%)	0.9	0.9	0.9	0.9	0.9

TPM = Total particulate matter (tar).
*Minus water and nicotine.

posed of subjects who smoked high-nicotine cigarettes (1.03 ± 0.26 mg nicotine per cigarette) who were given gradual reductions in nicotine dosage.

Each clinic visit consisted of two sessions. In session one the subject was monitored smoking the cigarette assigned from the previous week. Subjects were given a supply of these cigarettes and were told to smoke them ad libitum. In session two of each clinic visit, the subject was given a new cigarette assignment and first exposure to that cigarette was monitored according to the procedure outlined below. This experimental design allowed us to measure a variety of both physiologic and biochemical variables simultaneously. Each subject acted as his or her own control. Additionally, all cigarette variables except nicotine were kept constant to avoid the problem of other variables (i.e., "tar") influencing smoker behavior (Table I).

Subjects. Our subjects were six men and six women in good health with no past history of diabetes mellitus, hypertension, or respiratory disorders. Each subject completed a detailed questionnaire about smoking history and related areas including illness and drug use. Subjects were divided into light or moderate smokers according to the number of cigarettes smoked per day, plasma cotinine concentrations, blood carboxyhemoglobin (COHb) levels, and, to a lesser degree, plasma thiocyanate concentrations.[13] No subject had a history of chronic or episodic drug use or alcohol abuse. Diet was not controlled and all subjects had smoked their usual cigarette brand for at least 1 year before the study.

Subjects were prescreened by salivary cotinine analysis to ensure their cigarette smoking behavior was appropriate for our purposes. A minimum salivary cotinine level of 150 ng/ml was considered to reflect adequate nicotine absorption. Subjects in group 1 (n = 6) received graded increases in nicotine availability over the duration of the study. This group smoked cigarettes with approximately 0.75 mg nicotine per cigarette as their usual brands. Group 2 (n = 6) included subjects whose nicotine offering was downtitrated by decreasing the amount of nicotine available over the duration of the study. The cigarettes usually smoked by subjects in group 2 contained an average of 1.0 mg nicotine per cigarette. Subjects came to our clinic at 9 AM once each week to smoke two cigarettes under controlled conditions and to receive a supply of the assigned cigarette for use during the next week.

Procedure. Subjects were monitored upon first exposure to each experimental cigarette and after ad libitum cigarette consumption for 1 week. All subjects

Table II. Self-reported smoking behavior

Subject	*Age (yr)*	*Duration of smoking (yr)*	*Cigarettes/day (usual brand)*	*Experimental cigarettes (cigarettes/day)* 0.06 mg	0.4 mg	0.7 mg	0.9 mg	1.3 mg
Group 1								
A	28	7	18	17	11	9	11	8
B	25	7	15	17	14	14	10	10
C	22	5	22	21	18	18	24	23
D	33	15	15	15	15	15	15	10
E	19	5	17	13	11	11	11	13
F	21	5	30	18	19	19	23	13
$\bar{X}$	24.7	7.33	19.5	16.8	14.7*	14.3*	15.7*	12.8*
±SE	±2.16	±1.6	±2.4	±1.1	±1.4	±1.6	±2.6	±2.2
Group 2								
G	52	30	40	51	43	26	30	25
H	21	5	52	70	73	67	78	75
I	19	5	12	25	12	6	6	6
J	26	9	20	20	40	50	55	6
K	29	8	9	6	5	5	3	3
L	55	20	14	13	12	15	15	21
$\bar{X}$	33.7	12.8	24.5	30.8	30.8	28.2	31.2	22.7
±SE	±6.5	±3.8	±7.2	±10.0	±10.6	±10.3	±12.2	±11.1

*Significantly different ($P < 0.05$; ANOVA) from levels after usual-brand cigarettes.

abstained from smoking for at least 4 hours before reporting to each session. After they were comfortably seated, an indwelling catheter was inserted into the antecubital vein of the right forearm and an automatic blood pressure cuff was placed on the left arm. Catheters were kept open by small infusions of heparin (10 U/ml) and blood samples were drawn through a three-way sterile valve.

Baseline measurements of blood pressure and pulse as well as determinations of COHb, plasma nicotine, cotinine, and thiocyanate levels were taken in duplicate. Subjects then smoked the cigarette assigned the previous week and blood samples and physiologic readings were taken at four puffs, after each cigarette was extinguished, and every 3 minutes thereafter for the next 21 minutes. Saliva samples for cotinine analysis were collected at baseline, immediately after smoking, and 12 and 21 minutes thereafter. After 1 hour, the subjects smoked a second (newly assigned) cigarette while being monitored in the same manner as above. In total, each clinic session provided 20 blood samples and eight saliva samples for analyses. Subjects kept daily records of cigarettes smoked and butts were collected to verify self-reported smoking behavior.

Biochemical analyses. COHb was analyzed in each blood sample, after which the sample was separated and the plasma stored at −20° C for later analysis of nicotine and cotinine. Fresh blood samples were spectophotometrically assayed for total hemoglobin and COHb content. Daily calibration with certified standards guaranteed reproducibility of ±1%. Plasma nicotine and cotinine were quantitated by RIA according to the method of Langone et al.[8] This method uses specific antisera produced by injection into rabbits of *trans*-4-carboxycotinine or *trans*-3-succinylmethylnicotine bound to albumin. The inter- and intra-assay variations are 6%, with a sensitivity of 370 pg/ml for nicotine and cotinine.

Plasma thiocyanate was quantitated by an automated procedure[2] with a coefficient of variation of 1.5%. Subject questionnaires were analyzed by Student's t test and biochemical data were evaluated by univariate ANOVA. Unless otherwise stated, significance was set at the $P < 0.05$ level. Values are expressed as the $\bar{X}$ ± SE.

Cigarettes. The experimental cigarettes were formulated to deliver constant amounts of "tar" (total particulate matter minus water and nicotine) and CO in the mainstream smoke. The cigarettes varied in nicotine content by realistic incremental changes in nicotine per cigarette. Table I describes the physical characteristics of the cigarettes and the data derived from the tobacco and mainstream smoke analyses of machine-smoked cigarettes.

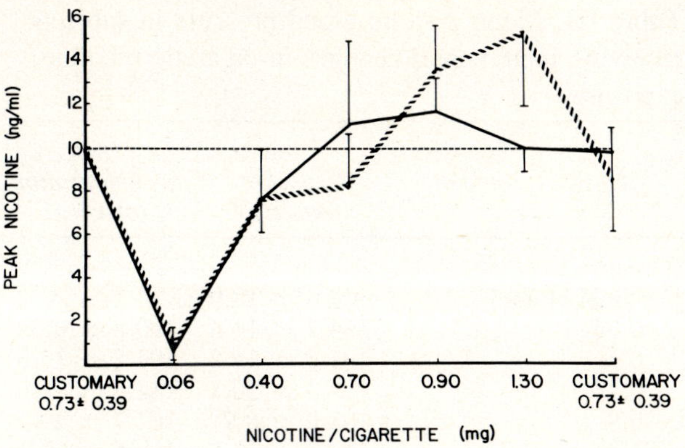

Fig. 1. Mean (±SE) maximum plasma nicotine absorption in smokers who received cigarettes of incrementally increasing nicotine content per cigarette as determined under standard smoking conditions (group 1). The *dashed line* represents maximum plasma nicotine absorption from the smoke of the usual-brand cigarette, the *solid line* represents the first exposure to experimental cigarette, and the *broken line* represents exposure to smoke of the same experimental cigarette after 1 week acclimatization.

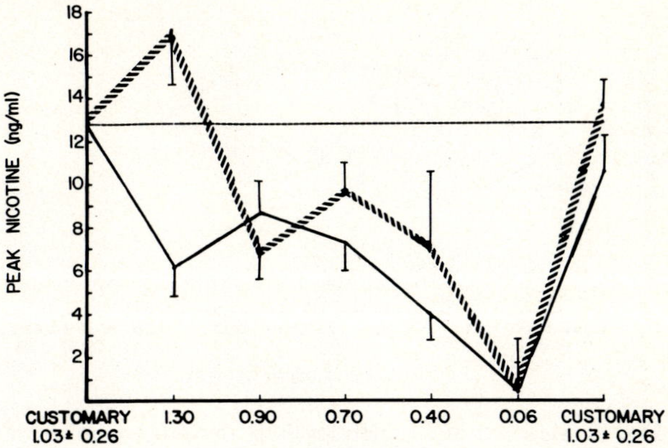

Fig. 2. Mean (±SE) maximum plasma nicotine absorption in smokers who received cigarettes of incrementally decreasing nicotine content as determined under standard smoking conditions (group 2). The *dashed line* represents maximum plasma nicotine absorption from the smoke of the usual-brand cigarette, the *solid line* represents the first exposure to smoke of the experimental cigarette, and the *broken line* represents exposure to smoke of the same experimental cigarette after 1 week acclimatization.

RESULTS

Both groups considered the high-nicotine cigarette (1.3 mg nicotine per cigarette) to be "too strong" relative to their usual brand. This was especially evident in group 1, whose nicotine exposure was increased. For all experimental cigarettes, both groups reported more draw resistance (141 to 150 mm H_2O column) than with their usual brands (<120 mm H_2O column).

Table II lists self-reported data on cigarettes smoked per day. Group 1 had a mean lifetime exposure to cigarette smoking of 7.33 ± 1.6 years and smoked 19.5 ± 2.4 cigarettes per day (usual brand). Subjects in group 2 were generally heavier smokers, with a history of 24.5 ± 7.2 usual-brand cigarettes per day and 12.8 ± 3.8 years of smoking. Significant decreases were noted in the number of cigarettes smoked per day in group 1 as nicotine content per cigarette increased.

Systolic blood pressure did not change in either group when compared with the respective response to the usual brand (Table III), although a positive correlation ($r^2 = 0.81$) between systolic blood pressure and increased nicotine content per cigarette was noted at the first exposure to increased nicotine yield cigarettes in group 1. After 1 week acclimatization, the correlation decreased ($r^2 = 0.34$). A correlation coefficient ($r^2 = 0.45$) was recorded for subjects in group 2 upon their first exposure to decreased nicotine content cigarettes; this did not change after 1 week acclimatization. Mean diastolic blood pressure did not change in either group (Table IV). Hemoglobin levels did not change during each daily session or between sessions.

Fig. 1 shows the maximum plasma nicotine absorption when subjects were exposed to graded increases in nicotine content. Maximum plasma nicotine absorption occurred between 1 and 2 minutes after the subject ceased smoking. Maximum nicotine absorption was determined for each subject by analysis of blood samples, and the group mean was then plotted for each experimental cigarette. When switched from their usual brand to the 0.06 mg nicotine cigarette (group 2), subjects were unable to compensate for such a low level even after ad libitum smoking for 1 week. When exposed to levels of 0.9 or 1.3 mg nicotine per cigarette (group 1), subjects were unable to adjust their nicotine intake and presumably their puff behavior. This resulted in significantly ($P < 0.05$) higher baseline (above that recorded with the usual brand) plasma nicotine concentrations after 1 week. Upon the subject's return to the usual brand (0.75 mg nicotine), plasma nicotine concentrations returned to baseline levels.

Data from subjects who received cigarettes with incrementally higher nicotine levels are shown in Fig. 2. Maximum plasma nicotine absorption for each usual and experimental cigarette are included and plotted

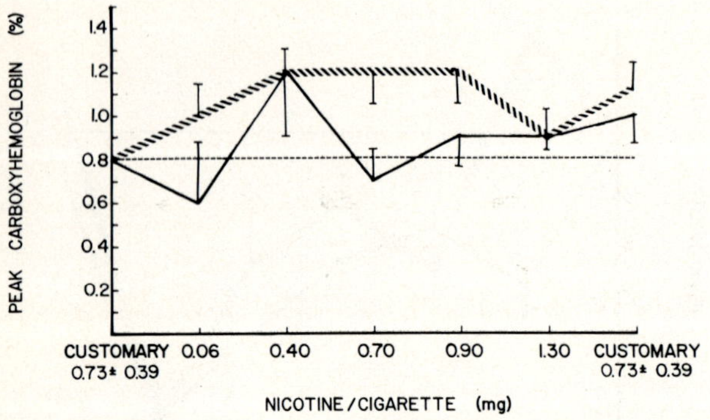

Fig. 3. Mean (±SE) COHb levels at maximum absorption when nicotine content per cigarette is increased (group 1). COHb levels were monitored at first exposure to smoke of the experimental cigarette *(solid line)* and after 1 week ad libitum consumption of the same cigarette *(broken line)*.

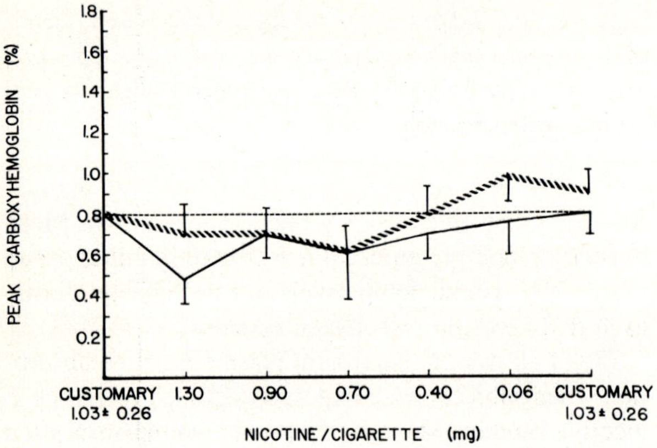

Fig. 4. Mean (±SE) COHb levels at maximum absorption when nicotine content per cigarette is decreased (group 2). COHb levels were monitored at first exposure to smoke of the experimental cigarette *(solid line)* and after 1 week ad libitum consumption of the same cigarette *(broken line)*.

against each weekly session. When subjects were exposed to a cigarette with 1.3 mg nicotine, an unexpected decrease in the plasma nicotine level occurred. However, after 1 week acclimatization to the high draw resistance filter, plasma nicotine absorption rose above that recorded with usual brands. As nicotine exposure was incrementally lowered, subjects appeared unable to compensate for the changing nicotine yield. When nicotine availability became unrealistically low (0.06 mg nicotine per cigarette), subjects were unable to compensate for the lack of a nicotine bolus. Upon return to the usual brand, subjects attempted to return to their former desired nicotine intake. Interestingly, plasma nicotine concentrations were below those observed with

Table III. Mean systolic blood pressure in subjects receiving incremental changes in cigarette nicotine exposure

Nicotine content (mg)	*First exposure (mm Hg)*	*1 wk acclimatization (mm Hg)*
Group 1		
Usual brand	109.6 ± 18.0	—
0.06	104.2 ± 14.4	100.8 ± 8.3
0.4	102.2 ± 15.2	107.8 ± 15.5
0.7	107.3 ± 20.1	112.7 ± 12.6
0.9	108.0 ± 8.9	107.7 ± 19.7
1.3	112.0 ± 13.5	108.6 ± 11.1
Return to usual brand	107.2 ± 11.4	112.0 ± 8.8
Group 2		
Usual brand	117.0 ± 12.2	—
1.3	112.0 ± 12.4	109.2 ± 11.4
0.9	115.2 ± 15.9	110.7 ± 6.5
0.7	113.7 ± 10.6	112.2 ± 10.7
0.4	112.7 ± 10.3	109.3 ± 11.8
0.06	107.0 ± 12.2	114.0 ± 12.5
Return to usual brand	112.2 ± 11.1	110.2 ± 15.4

Data are $\bar{X} \pm$ SE.

usual brands when subjects smoked a 0.9 mg nicotine cigarette, and levels remained depressed until subjects returned to their usual brand.

Fig. 3 shows COHb levels at maximum absorption when nicotine content per cigarette was increased. All experimental cigarettes were designed to deliver constant CO as long as cigarettes were smoked under standardized (i.e., machine smoking) conditions. COHb levels remained relatively constant in smokers in group 1, although a general but not significant increase was noted after 1 week acclimatization to each experimental cigarette.

Fig. 4 shows maximal COHb blood concentrations when subjects smoked the usual and experimental cigarettes. When subjects were assigned the high-nicotine cigarette (1.3 mg nicotine per cigarette), there was an immediate decrease in COHb upon first exposure, at least partially due to the high draw resistance of the filter and the high nicotine delivery per puff. COHb values remained in the range of those noted with usual brands throughout exposure to all experimental cigarettes after the first week of acclimatization.

Fig. 5 shows the change in plasma cotinine levels when subjects smoked the usual and experimental cigarettes. Plasma cotinine concentrations are significantly lower after exposure to a 0.06 mg nicotine cigarette for 1 week (Fig. 5, *A*). As nicotine yield per cigarette increased, there was a corresponding rise in plasma

Table IV. Mean diastolic blood pressure in subjects receiving incremental changes in cigarette nicotine exposure

Nicotine content (mg)	First exposure (mm Hg)	1 wk acclimatization (mm Hg)
Group 1		
Usual brand	63.4 ± 6.4	—
0.06	65.5 ± 9.8	67.3 ± 10.4
0.4	67.2 ± 11.6	65.0 ± 11.3
0.7	70.2 ± 10.6	68.8 ± 11.3
0.9	74.0 ± 7.3	66.0 ± 7.7
1.3	69.8 ± 8.1	69.8 ± 5.9
Return to usual brand	75.5 ± 6.7	69.7 ± 12.5
Group 2		
Usual brand	74.8 ± 5.0	—
1.3	75.7 ± 6.9	72.2 ± 8.9
0.9	71.0 ± 6.6	67.7 ± 4.7
0.7	74.3 ± 7.0	70.2 ± 10.1
0.4	73.2 ± 6.4	62.3 ± 13.3
0.06	68.8 ± 6.2	62.7 ± 9.4
Return to usual brand	68.8 ± 13.2	68.7 ± 7.9

Data are $\bar{X}$ ± SE.

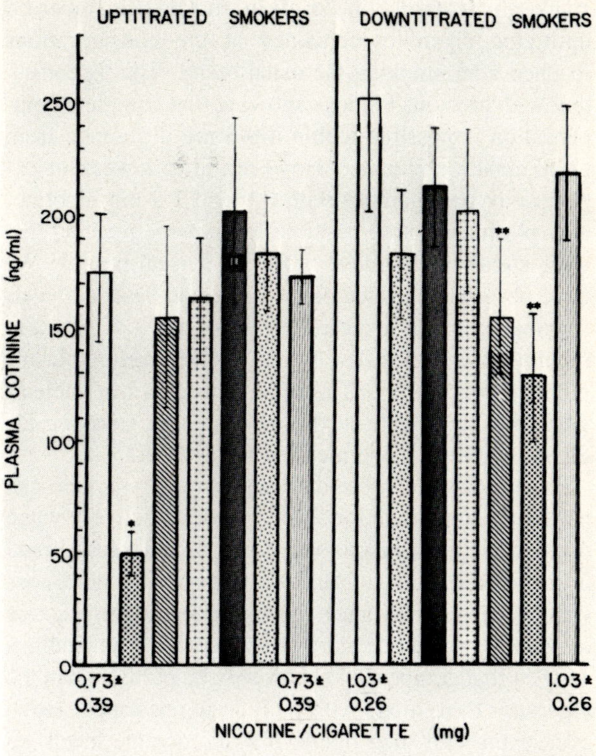

Fig. 5. Mean (± SE) change in plasma cotinine concentrations when subjects smoked the usual or experimental cigarettes for 1 week. □, usual brand; ▩, 0.06 mg nicotine; ▧, 0.40 mg nicotine; ⊞, 0.70 mg nicotine; ■, 0.90 mg nicotine; ▩, 1.30 mg nicotine; ▥, return to usual brand. $^*P < 0.001$; $^{**}P < 0.01$.

cotinine concentrations until subjects smoked the 1.3 mg nicotine cigarette. After 1 week exposure to the cigarette with the highest nicotine yield, plasma cotinine concentrations were no longer rising. These data parallel the plasma nicotine data with the same cigarettes. After subjects smoked their usual brands for 1 week, plasma cotinine levels returned to the levels first recorded after smoking the usual brands.

No change in plasma thiocyanate levels was apparent throughout the study in either group because of the formulation of these cigarettes, which upon smoking provided uniform levels of hydrogen cyanide, the major precursor of thiocyanate.

DISCUSSION

We investigated nicotine tolerance and acute acclimatization in subjects who smoked experimentally prepared cigarettes formulated to deliver constant CO and "tar," but varied nicotine content, under standardized machine-smoking conditions. Each of the experimental cigarettes was prepared with a high draw resistance filter to investigate effects on compensatory behavior. These filters reduced self-titration by limiting inhalation, since nicotine absorption varied with nicotine content per cigarette.

Evidence supporting the diminution of smoker compensation through the use of high draw resistance filters is derived from measuring COHb levels. Percent COHb was statistically unchanged in both groups after 1 week acclimatization to each experimental cigarette. COHb, a good indicator of gas phase absorption by cigarette smokers, has been shown to increase as smokers attempt to titrate nicotine from commercial low-yield products.[14] We observed relatively constant levels of COHb in smokers of the experimental cigarettes formulated with varying nicotine contents.

Plasma thiocyanate formed by detoxification of hydrogen cyanide is an indicator of exposure to both the particulate and the gas phases of tobacco smoke.[5] Thiocyanate levels did not change throughout our study in either group, indicating that the cigarette filters reduced the ability of the smokers to execute behaviorally motivated changes in response to changing nicotine delivery. However, smokers did partially compensate for increased nicotine yield by decreasing cigarette consumption.

As nicotine content per cigarette began to approximate values of the usual-brand cigarettes for each smoker, plasma nicotine levels in smokers who received uptitrated cigarettes remained at the concentrations reached after smoking the usual brand. This is consistent with previous findings showing that complete compensation is possible within a 0.3 mg difference from usual cigarette brands.[14] However, after 1 week of exposure to the cigarettes with 0.9 and 1.3 mg nicotine, new plasma nicotine baseline levels were reached that were significantly above those after usual brands. We have observed elevated plasma nicotine baseline levels in subjects given a cigarette containing 0.4 mg more nicotine than their usual brand.[12] New baseline plasma nicotine concentrations were also observed in subjects who smoked downtitrated cigarettes after smoking the cigarette with 1.3 mg nicotine for 1 week.

Taken together, these data suggest that smokers can partially compensate for altered nicotine delivery when the change from nicotine delivery of the usual brand is not extreme. If CO and tar exposure is held constant, compensatory mechanisms responding to nicotine availability should be more clearly visible. Our findings suggest that compensation can only be partial when the cigarettes have filters with high draw resistance. However, even with such filters, plasma nicotine levels reflect higher exposure than after usual brands when cigarettes formulated for high nicotine delivery are smoked. This reinforces earlier findings demonstrating that smokers cannot completely control increased nicotine availability even by decreasing the number of cigarettes consumed per day.[12] In addition, further work in our laboratories has shown that filter construction can be an important determinant of nicotine and gas phase delivery in mainstream smoke.[6]

Smoker "satisfaction" with respect to nicotine satiation is an important element of any alteration in smoking behavior. More in-depth research is necessary to determine the mechanisms of compensation and the kinetics of nicotine absorption in different categories of cigarette smokers.

We greatly appreciate the valuable technical assistance given by Caryn Axelrad and Kathyrn Tilton.

References

1. Ashton H, Stepney R, Thompson JW: Self-titration by cigarette smokers. Br Med J **2:**357-360, 1979.
2. Butts WC, Kuehneman M, Widdowson GM: Automated method for determining serum thiocyanate to distinguish smokers from non-smokers. Clin Chem **20:**1344, 1974.
3. Chait LD, Griffiths RR: Smoking behavior and tobacco smoke intake: Response of smokers to shortened cigarettes. CLIN PHARMACOL THER **32:**90-97, 1982.
4. Gritz ER, Baer-Weiss V, Jarvik ME: Titration of nicotine intake with full-length and half-length cigarettes. CLIN PHARMACOL THER **20:**552-556, 1976.
5. Haley NJ, Axelrad CM, Tilton KA: Validation of self-reported smoking behavior: Biochemical analyses of cotinine and thiocyanate. Am J Public Health **73:**1204-1207, 1983.
6. Hoffmann DH, Adams JD, Haley NJ: Reported cigarette smoke values: A closer look. Am J Public Health **73:**1050-1053, 1983.
7. Kozlowski LT, Jarvik ME, Gritz ER: Nicotine regulation and cigarette smoking. CLIN PHARMACOL THER **17:**93-97, 1975.
8. Langone JJ, Gjika HB, Van Vunakis H: Nicotine and its metabolites. Radioimmunoassays for nicotine and cotinine. Biochemistry **12:**5025-5030, 1973.
9. Martin JE, Prue DM, Collins FL Jr, Tharnes CJ: The effects of graduated filters on smoking exposure: Risk reduction or compensation. Addict Behav **6:**167-176, 1981.
10. Russell MAH: Realistic goals for smoking and health. Lancet **1:**254-257, 1974.
11. Schachter S: Pharmacological and physiological determinants of smoking. Ann Intern Med **88:**104-114, 1978.
12. Sepkovic DW, Haley NJ, Axelrad CM, Wynder EL: Cigarette smoking as a risk for cardiovascular disease. III. Biochemical effect with higher nicotine yield cigarettes. Addict Behav **8:**59-66, 1983.
13. Sepkovic DW, Haley NJ, Wynder EL: Thyroid activity in cigarette smokers. Arch Intern Med **144:**501-505, 1984.
14. Sepkovic DW, Parker K, Axelrad CM, Haley NJ, Wynder EL: Cigarette smoking as a risk for cardiovascular disease. V. Biochemical parameters with increased and decreased nicotine content cigarettes. Addict Behav **9:**255-263, 1984.
15. Sutton SR, Feyerabend C, Cole PV, Russell MAH: Adjustment of smokers to dilution of tobacco smoke by ventilated cigarette holders. CLIN PHARMACOL THER **24:**395-405, 1978.
16. US Department of Health and Human Services: The changing cigarette. A report of the Surgeon General. D.H.H.S. Publication No. 81-50-156. Washington, DC, 1981, U.S. Government Printing Office.

Pentosane polysulfate: The effect on hemostasis of a continuous 3-day infusion

Pentosane polysulfate (PP) is a sulfated polysaccharide known to exhibit anticoagulant properties that are in part independent of antithrombin III activity. These effects have only been studied in vitro or after single injections in healthy subjects. Our objective was to evaluate the modification of hemostasis induced by a 3-day continuous infusion of PP (4 mg/kg body weight/24 hr) in 10 subjects. No hemorrhagic complication was observed in any patient. Bleeding time was not modified by the infusion, despite a slight decrease in the platelet number. Among the other parameters measured, the automated partial thromboplastin time, prothrombin time, and anti-Xa activity were the most affected by PP. The kinetics of their modifications were quite uniform: clotting times and the anti-Xa effect increased gradually until reaching steady state 24 hours after the start of the infusion. A progressive return to the pretreatment level was then observed during the 6 hours after the end of the infusion. A significant decrease in the factor V concentration was found at day 4. Finally, in contrast with other reported results, no activation of fibrinolysis was induced by PP under the conditions we used, which suggests that discontinuous administration or the route of administration of the drug influences the fibrinolytic effect. In conclusion, we show the excellent tolerance of continuous infusion of PP, detail the modifications in biologic parameters of hemostasis during and after PP infusion, and demonstrate that PP decreases factor V activity. (Clin Pharmacol Ther 38:171-175, 1985.)

Dominique de Prost, M.D., Ph.D., Claude Guérot, M.D., and Florence Karsenty, M.D. *Paris, France*

Pentosane polysulfate (PP), a sulfated polysaccharide, has been shown to exhibit anticoagulant properties. In vitro studies have shown that PP affects coagulation mainly by inhibiting the endogenous activation of factor X and that the mechanism of this inhibition is independent of antithrombin III (AT III) activity.[8] This has led to its use in the prevention of postoperative deep vein thrombosis.[1,2,10] This further suggests that PP could be used in the treatment of patients with AT III deficiency.[7] Very recently it was suggested that PP might potentiate the inactivation of thrombin by plasma through activation of heparin cofactor II.[15]

The effects of PP on the hemostatic system in vivo have been studied mostly after subcutaneous[3,9,13,19] or intramuscular[16] injections. Under these conditions, a more pronounced effect than in vitro was observed, which was associated with the inhibition of factor Xa generation, a direct "anti-Xa" effect, and the release of lipoprotein lipase and plasminogen activator from the vascular endothelial cells.[9,20] To our knowledge, the effects of a continuous intravenous infusion of PP have not yet been studied. They are worth investigating, because this route of administration allows the anticoagulant to be adjusted during administration and is therefore of potential use in postoperative treatment. We measured the effect of a continuous intravenous infusion of the drug over 3 days and analyzed its effects on the components of the hemostatic system and the kinetics of their modification.

METHODS

Our subjects were nine male and one female patients 33 to 77 years old. Subjects were hospitalized in a cardiology unit and were chosen for study because their diseases did not require anticoagulant therapy. They did not receive other drugs that might have interfered with the coagulation data. PP, 4 mg/kg body weight/day, was administered as a continuous infusion for 3 days.

The following tests were performed as described previously[12]: platelet count, automated partial thrombo-

From the Laboratoire d'Immunologie et d'Hématologie and Service de Cardiologie, Centre Hospitalo-Universitaire Xavier Bichat, Université de Paris.

Supported by INSERM Grant No. 842011.

Received for publication Jan. 18, 1985; accepted April 11, 1985.

Reprint requests to: D. de Prost, Laboratoire d'Immunologie et d'Hématologie, Centre Hospitalo-Universitaire Xavier Bichat, 16, rue Henri Huchard, 75018 Paris, France.

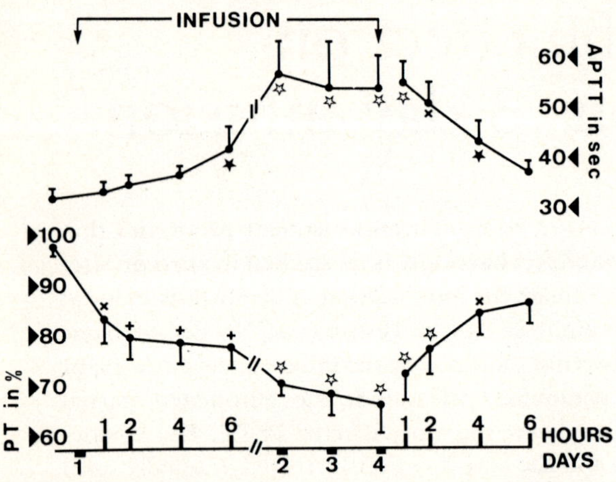

Fig. 1. Mean (±SE) changes in PT and APTT induced by PP infusion. The mean values for APTT and PT are significantly different ($P < 0.001$; ANOVA). The significance of the difference between each value measured after the start of PP infusion and the preinfusion value is indicated by ★ $P < 0.05$, × $P < 0.02$, + $P < 0.01$, ☆ $P < 0.001$. Mean (±SE) preinfusion values are 32.4 ± 1.6 sec for APTT and 97.9% ± 1.3% for PT.

plastin time (APTT), prothrombin time (PT), thrombin time (TT), fibrinogen, euglobulin lysis time, α_2-antiplasmin, and plasmin–α_2-antiplasmin complexes. The prothrombin percentage activity was calculated from a control dilution curve. Bleeding time was determined according to Ivy-Borchgrevink[4]; factors II, V, and VII-X were measured as described by Caen et al.[5] Anti-Xa activity was measured with the synthetic substrate S 2222 (Flow-Kabi) according to the technique of Teien et al.[17] as modified by Soria et al.[16] We adapted this method to the discrete analyzer Isamat (Isa Biologie):265 μl bovine factor Xa (Flow Kabi) diluted in 0.005 mol/L Tris and 0.0075 mol/L Na EDTA at pH 8.4 was added to 33 μl of the plasma sample. The amount of residual protease was evaluated by adding S 2222 to a final concentration of 0.4 mmol/L and measuring the increase in optical density units (Δod/min). A standard curve was obtained by replacing the plasma sample with Tris buffer and using factor Xa at final concentrations of 1.4, 0.7, and 0 nkat/ml. Results are expressed as the percentage of factor Xa neutralized by each plasma sample in the presence of PP. The 100% determination of factor Xa was defined for each subject by determining the residual activity of factor Xa after action of its own plasma without PP.

PP was infused from day 1 at 8:30 AM to day 4 at 8:30 AM. Blood was drawn for coagulation tests at the following times: before treatment; at day 1, 1, 2, 4, and 6 hours after the start of the infusion; in the morning of the 3 following days; and at day 4, 1, 2, 4, and 6 hours after the end of the infusion.

Table I. Percent changes in factor V concentration

Subject No.	*Before PP infusion*	*Day 4*	*Decrease*
4	139	65	−74
5	60	75	+15
6	139	29	−110
8	70	29	−41
9	126	71	−55
10	72	48	−24
$\bar{X}$ ± SE	101 ± 15	53 ± 8*	−48 ± 20

*Significantly different ($P < 0.05$; Student's t test) from value before PP infusion.

Means and standard errors were calculated and followed by ANOVA for each variable. When the means of a test differed, the t test was used to compare assay values obtained before PP infusion with those during or after the infusion. Results are reported as the $\bar{X}$ ± SE.

RESULTS

Neither hemorrhagic complication nor any other adverse effect was observed in any subject. Bleeding time was 3.9 ± 0.4 min before PP infusion and did not change at days 2 and 4 after dosing (data not shown). The platelet number always remained within the normal range (150 to 400,000/μl), although a slight decrease was observed at days 2 and 4. Platelet counts were 288,000 ± 19,090, 254,000 ± 19,650, and 238,000 ± 21,500/μl before PP and at days 2 and 4, respectively.

Fig. 1 shows the APTT and PT values before, during, and after the PP infusion. Before PP the APTT was 32.4 ± 1.6 sec, and 1 hour after the infusion began it had already increased slightly. A maximum effect was reached after 24 hours and persisted throughout the infusion. The difference between this value and the baseline value was still significant 4 hours after the end of the infusion on day 4. Similar kinetics were observed for the PT. Before PP the PT was 98% ± 1.3%. PT was 70% after 24 hours, and 6 hours after the infusion ended it was still 86%.

Factors II and VII-X (baseline values: 98% ± 11% and 94% ± 9%, respectively) were not modified by the infusion (data not shown). Factor V markedly decreased ($P < 0.05$) in five of six subjects studied at day 4 (Table I). In three of them, factor V was <50% on day 4.

Fig. 2 shows the TT and anti-Xa activity level before, during, and after PP infusion. The mean preinfusion

TT was 18.4 ± 0.6 sec. It remained within the normal range, increasing slightly but significantly during the infusion of PP, and returned to the preinfusion level after the end of the infusion. PP also induced a slight increase in anti-Xa activity. A stable and statistically significant inhibitory effect (about 10% less than the baseline value) was observed from day 2 to day 4. This inhibition was of the same order as that induced by 0.05 IU/ml standard heparin.

The preinfusion AT III level was 114% ± 5% and was not modified by PP infusion (data not shown). The fibrinogen level at day 4 (4.85 ± 0.4 gm/L) was slightly higher than the preinfusion value (4.10 ± 0.4 gm/L). The euglobulin lysis time (baseline value >3 hours in all subjects) and the α_2-antiplasmin level (mean preinfusion level 108% ± 3.4%) were not modified. Plasmin–α_2-antiplasmin complexes were measured in seven subjects and were not detected in any.

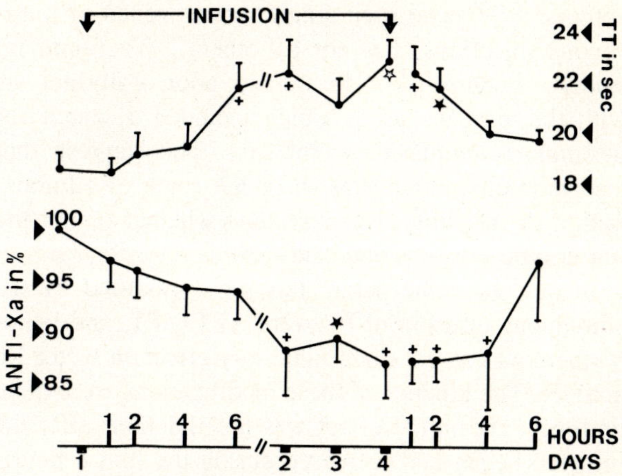

Fig. 2. Mean (±SE) changes in TT and anti-Xa activity induced by PP infusion. The mean values for TT and anti-Xa activity are significantly different ($P < 0.01$ for TT; $P < 0.05$ for anti-Xa activity). The significance of the difference between each value measured after the start of PP infusion and the preinfusion value is indicated by ★ $P < 0.05$, + $P < 0.01$, ☆ $P < 0.001$. Mean (±SE) preinfusion values are 18.4 ± 0.6 sec for TT and 100% for anti-Xa activity.

DISCUSSION

The mechanism of the anticoagulant effect of PP is not yet fully understood, but it is in part independent of AT III. Furthermore, the results of studies in animals and man suggest that PP exerts an antithrombotic effect.[1,2,7,10,18] Our objectives were first, to evaluate how well a continuous infusion of PP would be tolerated and second, to establish the modifications of hemostatic factors during and after such therapy. The drug was infused at a rate of 4 mg/kg/day, as a previous study[16] had shown that the APTT was moderately increased for 8 hours after a single intramuscular injection of 100 mg PP.

The drug was well tolerated; no hemorrhagic complication or other adverse effect was observed in any subject. This information is important, because to our knowledge the effects of continuous intravenous infusion of this drug over several days have not been previously reported.

As already mentioned by other authors who used single subcutaneous injections,[3] the bleeding time was not modified throughout the infusion. However, a slight but statistically significant decrease in the platelet number was observed. This is in accord with the results of Dunn et al.,[6] who showed that PP, like unfractionated heparins, increased the binding of fibrinogen to adenosine diphosphate–treated platelets.

The slight prolongation in TT is also in agreement with a previous study in which PP was administered subcutaneously.[9] Because the effects of PP are usually dose dependent, it is likely that increasing doses would result in greater prolongation of TT. Our study demonstrates that a clear prolongation in APTT is induced by this form of treatment, since the mean APTT values were 56, 54, and 53 sec (mean preinfusion value 32 sec) at days 2, 3, and 4, respectively. Factor Xa activity has been found by most authors to be slightly inhibited when measured by clotting or chromogenic assay,[3,13,16,19] in agreement with our results with a chromogenic assay. Fisher et al.,[9] however, found that subcutaneous injection of PP had a weak anti-Xa effect when measured with a clotting assay and no effect when measured with a chromogenic assay.

The lengthening of PT with a decrease in factor V after 25 to 100 mg intravenous injections has already been mentioned by Sampol et al.[14] Other authors used subcutaneous injections of 50 to 100 mg and found no modifications of PT.[9,19] It is not clear whether this discrepancy is related to the route of administration or to another cause. Although it is tempting to propose a relationship between the decreases in factor V and PT, we cannot draw this conclusion because (1) we have only measured factor V at day 4, and (2) in one subject (no. 5; Table I) the PT decreased from 100% to 72% while factor V increased moderately. We have until now no explanation for the decrease in factor V; however, because factor V is implicated in the activation of factor X, its decrease could be related to the depression of intrinsic factor Xa generation, which has been established by Fisher et al.[9]

The induction by PP of systemic fibrinolytic activity is controversial; it has been found by several authors[9,11,14,20] who used single subcutaneous or intravenous injections, but not by others.[3] We found no evidence in our subjects for the activation of fibrinolysis with the tests we used, which included a search for plasmin–α_2-antiplasmin complexes. This suggests that discontinuous administration or the route of administration of the drug may determine whether or not the fibrinolytic effect is obtained.

In our study the parameters most modified by the continuous infusion of PP were APTT, PT, and factor V; there was also a slight inhibitory effect on factor Xa activity. The kinetics of these modifications were quite uniform. The initial effect was noted 1 hour after the infusion began and increased during the first 6 hours; at 24 hours a steady state was reached, and when the infusion was stopped, there was a progressive return toward normal values that was still incomplete 6 hours later.

The AT III–independent lengthening of APTT could perhaps reflect the inhibition of endogenous factor X activation as described by Fischer et al.[9] Under the conditions we used, the prolongation of APTT was of the same order as that induced by conventional intravenous heparinotherapy. However, the role of PP in preventing the extension of a thrombosis has not yet been defined. If PP does exert such an effect, it could be of great interest especially in patients with AT III deficiency.[7] The potential usefulness of PP merits further studies of its mechanism of action. Of particular interest are the relationship of PP to the factor V decrease and how the route of administration influences this parameter, the activation of fibrinolysis, and the antithrombotic capacities in susceptible patients.

We thank Professors J. Hakim and M. Samama for helpful suggestions and criticisms and Mrs. de Carbonnières, Hôtel Dieu, who dosed the plasmin–α_2-antiplasmin complexes.

References

1. Bergqvist D, Efsing HO, Hallbook T, Lindblad B: Prevention of postoperative thromboembolic complications. Acta Chir Scand **146:**559-568, 1980.
2. Bergqvist D, Ljungner H: A comparative study of dextran 70 and a sulfated polysaccharide in the prevention of postoperative thromboembolic complications. Br J Surg **68:**449-451, 1981.
3. Bergqvist D, Nilsson IM: A sulfated polysaccharide. The effects in vivo and in vitro on the hemostatic system in healthy volunteers. Thromb Res **23:**309-315, 1981.
4. Borchgrevink FA: A method for measuring platelet adhesiveness in vivo. Acta Med Scand **168:**157-164, 1960.
5. Caen JP, Larrieu M-J, Samama M: La coagulation. *In* Caen JP, Larrieu M-J, Samama M, editors: L'hémostase, methodes d'exploration et diagnostic pratique, ed 2. Paris, 1975, Expansion Scientifique, pp 153-162.
6. Dunn F, Soria J, Soria C, Thomaidis A, Tobelem G, Caen JP: Fibrinogen binding on human platelets. Influence of different heparins and of pentosane polysulfate. Thromb Res **29:**141-148, 1983.
7. Fisher AM, Aurousseau MH, Dautzenberg MD, Bentata-Pessayre M, Beguin S: Prevention des thromboses par l'hemoclar. Résultats d'un essai préliminaire chez une malade atteinte de déficit en antithrombine III. Rev Fr Trans Immunohematol **3:**1-8, 1982.
8. Fisher AM, Barrowcliffe TW, Thomas DP: A comparison of pentosan polysulfate (SP54) and heparin. I. Mechanism of action on blood coagulation. Thromb Haemost **47:**104-108, 1982.
9. Fisher AM, Merton RE, Marsh NA, Williams S, Gaffney PJ, Barrowcliffe TW, Thomas DP: A comparison of pentosane polysulphate and heparin. II. Effects of subcutaneous injection. Thromb Haemost **47:**109-113, 1982.
10. Joffe S: Drug prevention of postoperative deep vein thrombosis. A comparative study of calcium heparinate and sodium pentosane polysulfate. Arch Surg **111:**37-40, 1976.
11. Marsh N, Gaffney P: The effect of pentosane polysulfate (SP54) on the fibrinolytic system of man. Nouv Rev Fr Hematol **25:**281, 1983. (Abst.)
12. de Prost D, Guérot C, Laffay N, Horellou MH, Samama M: Intracoronary thrombolysis with streptokinase or lys-plasminogen urokinase in acute myocardial infarction: Effects on recanalization and blood fibrinolysis. Thromb Haemost **50:**792-796, 1983.
13. Ryde M, Eriksson H, Tangen O: Studies on the different mechanisms by which heparin and polysulfated xylan (PZ68) inhibit blood coagulation in man. Thromb Res **23:**435-445, 1981.
14. Sampol J, Angles-Cano E, Benchimol P, Blachére A, Sultan Y: Effet du polysulfate de pentosane (Hemoclar) sur la coagulation et la fibrinolyse après injection intraveineuse de 4 doses différentes chez des volontaires sains. Nouv Rev Fr Hematol **25:**289, 1983. (Abst.)
15. Scully MF, Kakkar VV: Identification of heparin cofactor II as the principal plasma cofactor for the antithrombin activity of pentosane polysulfate (SP54). Thromb Res **36:**187-194, 1984.
16. Soria C, Soria J, Ryckewaert JJ, Holmer E, Caen JP: Anticoagulant activities of a pentosane polysulfate: Comparison with standard heparin and a fraction of low molecular weight heparin. Thromb Res **19:**455-463, 1980.
17. Teien AN, Lie M, Abilgaard U: Evaluation of an amidolytic heparin assay method increased sensitivity by adding purified antithrombin III. Thromb Res **10:**399-410, 1977.
18. Vassiliou I, Wölfl I, Haas S, Stemberger A, Blümel G:

The effect of heparin and polysulfate polysaccharide (SP54) in experimental thrombosis and hemostasis. Presented at the Ninth International Congress on Thrombosis and Hemostasis, Stockholm, July 4-8, 1983.
19. Vinazzer H, Haas S, Stemberger A: Influence on the clotting mechanism of sodium pentosan polysulfate (SP54) in comparison to commercial beef lung sodium heparin. Thromb Res **20**:57-68, 1980.
20. Vinazzer H, Stemberger A, Haas S, Blümel G: Influence of heparin of different heparin fractions and of a low molecular weight heparin-like substance on the mechanism of fibrinolysis. Thromb Res **27**:341-352, 1982.

Oral ciramadol in the treatment of postoperative pain

The efficacy and safety of single oral 15, 30, and 60 mg doses of ciramadol, an investigational agonist/antagonist analgesic, were studied in a postoperative pain model and compared with aspirin, 325 and 650 mg. Two visual analog pain assessment scales were also compared. Results showed that a pain relief score of moderate or better was reported at some time during the 6-hour observation period by 76% of the patients who took 15 mg ciramadol, by 60% of those who took 30 mg ciramadol, by 59% of those who took 60 mg ciramadol, and by 38% and 92% of the patients who took the low and high doses of aspirin, respectively. From 1 to 4 hours after drug dosing, 15 mg ciramadol generally produced higher scores, indicative of greater pain relief, on the three pain intensity efficacy scales used (verbal, linear analog, and curvilinear analog) than did the other two ciramadol doses, but these differences were generally not significant. The differences between 15 mg ciramadol and 650 mg aspirin were generally not significant, although the higher aspirin dose had some advantages over 15 mg ciramadol. The most frequently reported adverse effect was dizziness/vertigo in 22% of patients taking 60 mg ciramadol, in 17% of those taking 30 mg ciramadol, in 13% of those taking 15 mg ciramadol, in 4% of those taking high aspirin doses, and in none of those who received the low aspirin doses. The correlation coefficient for the linear and curvilinear pain analog intensity scales was 0.955, indicating a highly significant correlation ($P < 0.001$). (Clin Pharmacol Ther 38:176-182, 1985.)

Louis Lasagna, M.D., and Jose F. Calimlim, M.D. *Boston, Mass., and Rochester, N. Y.*

Ciramadol, [1*R*-[1α(*R**),2α]]-3-[(dimethylamino)-(2-hydroxycyclohexyl) methyl]phenol hydrochloride, is an investigational analgesic with both narcotic agonist and antagonist properties. In preclinical studies ciramadol has shown analgesic activity in the Eddy hot plate test, phenylbenzoquinone-induced writhing, the rat tail-flick assay, the Randall-Selitto paw pressure test, and monkey shock titration. The narcotic antagonist properties of ciramadol are evident in its ability to inhibit the morphine-induced Straub tail phenomenon, to precipitate jumping in morphine-dependent mice, and to induce withdrawal effects in morphine-dependent monkeys.*

Clinical studies of ciramadol's analgesic efficacy have generated conflicting results. Some investigators, such as Stambaugh et al.[6] and Staquet,[7] have reported positive dose-response curves up to 40, 60, or even 90 mg in trials of oral ciramadol. By contrast, Bloomfield et al.[1] found 30 mg to be better than either 15 or 60 mg by mouth, and Fragen et al.[3] found 30 mg intramuscular ciramadol to be significantly more effective than 60 mg. Furthermore, in the study of Fragen and Caldwell,[2] 20 mg was ''placebo-like'' against moderate pain, and 20 and 40 mg were ''placebo-like'' against severe pain. The most frequently observed side effects have been nausea, vomiting, and dizziness.

Our study was a comparison of ciramadol at three dose levels with the standard drug aspirin at two dose levels in the relief of postoperative pain. As a specific methodologic goal, a comparison was also made of two different visual analog scales.

METHODS

Patients with moderate to severe postsurgical pain of mixed causes were randomly assigned to receive, in double-blind fashion, a single oral dose of either 15 mg ciramadol, 30 mg ciramadol, 60 mg ciramadol, 325 mg aspirin, or 650 mg aspirin. Pregnant women, patients sensitive to narcotics, narcotic antagonists, or aspirin, patients with a history of chronic analgesic or tranquilizer use or known drug dependence, patients taking concomitant interfering or potentially interacting med-

From Tufts University Medical School, Boston, and University of Rochester School of Medicine and Dentistry, Rochester.
Supported in part by Wyeth Laboratories, Philadelphia, Pa.
Received for publication Dec. 10, 1984; accepted April 11, 1985.
Reprint requests to: Louis Lasagna, M.D., Tufts University Medical School, 136 Harrison Ave., Boston, MA 02111.
*Wyeth Laboratories: Personal communication, 1983.

Table I. Mean levels of summary efficacy parameters

Group	No. of patients*	Mean cumulative 6-hr measure: SPID	TOTPAR	Linear SPAID	Curvilinear SPAID	Mean peak relief score
Ciramadol						
15 mg	21	3.3	7.5	75.5	88.6	2.3
30 mg	20	1.8	5.1	49.2	63.1	1.8
60 mg	22	2.4	6.1	62.4	69.2	1.7
Aspirin						
325 mg	24	1.8	4.0	38.9	38.7	1.3
650 mg	24	3.3	8.8	120.4	147.6	2.5

*Cumulative SPID, TOTPAR, and SPAID scores were unavailable for four patients; the SPAID scores on both the linear and the curvilinear scales were unavailable for one patient, while the SPAID score on the curvilinear scale was unavailable for an additional 10 patients.

ications, and any patients who had received an analgesic within 3 hours before the study were excluded.

Four scales were used to record the patients' subjective evaluations of efficacy. Pain intensity was reported on a verbal scale (as "none," "mild," "moderate," or "severe"), a linear analog scale (a 10 cm line, with the ends representing "no pain" and the "worst pain I've ever felt"), and a curvilinear analog scale (a semicircle, divided into 10 equal segments, with the ends representing "no pain" and "severe pain"). Pain relief was noted as "complete," "a lot of," "moderate," "a little," "none," or "worse." Evaluations of pain intensity (all three scales) were made at the time of dosing; subsequent evaluations (all four scales) were scheduled at 30 minutes and 1, 2, 3, 4, 5, and 6 hours thereafter. Patients with unsatisfactory pain relief who requested additional medication could be dropped from the study and given a standard analgesic after the 1-hour observation. For interviews ruled out by such additional medication, patients were assigned scores corresponding to the baseline pain intensity score or to no relief.

At each observation time the degree of sedation ("none," "mild," "moderate," or "marked") was noted and the blood pressure, pulse rate, and respiration rate were recorded (vital signs were not determined at 3 or 5 hours after dosing). Adverse effects were reported, and the investigator noted the likelihood of effect being related to the medication. The patient provided an overall assessment of therapy at the end of the study (as "excellent," "good," "fair," or "poor").

The groups were tested for comparability with respect to age, weight, sex, racial composition, and initial pain intensity (all three scales). The only significant differences detected (at the 0.05 probability level) were in race between the 15 mg ciramadol group (19 whites and five blacks) and each of the 30 mg ciramadol and 325 mg aspirin groups (all whites in both groups). The study population consisted of 62 men (52%) and 57 women (48%), with a racial composition of 110 whites (92%), eight blacks (7%), and one other (1%); the initial pain intensity was moderate for 100 patients (84%) and severe for 19 patients (16%). Age in the study group ranged from 18 to 61 years ($\bar{X}$ = 36 years) and weight ranged from 103 to 232 lb ($\bar{X}$ = 163 lb). Eight of the 119 patients entered were excluded from the efficacy evaluation (six received the test medication within 3 hours of surgery and two were above the protocol weight limit).

The demographic attributes and the baseline efficacy and sedation parameters of the groups were tested for comparability, and assessments were made of efficacy, sedation, the incidence of adverse effects, and changes in vital signs. The demographic and baseline continuous variables were examined by a one-way ANOVA supplemented by the Student-Newman-Keuls test for pairwise comparisons; nominal or categorized variables were analyzed by the chi-square test, with Fisher's exact test used for pairwise comparisons when the variable under consideration was classified into two levels.

The categoric efficacy parameters were analyzed by the generalized Cochran-Mantel-Haenszel procedure with marginal ridit scoring, as discussed by Landis et al.[4,5] The analysis takes the initial pain level as a covariable and provides a test of the average response weighted across the initial pain categories. Comparisons among the groups of the pain-analog scores were by a one-way ANCOVA, with the baseline level as the covariate. To investigate the correlation between the two pain analog scales, consideration was given (across therapy groups) to a scatter diagram comparing the linear with the curvilinear 6-hour sum of the pain analog intensity difference (SPAID) scores, and the Pearson product-moment correlation coefficient was determined for these variables. Vital signs were examined for

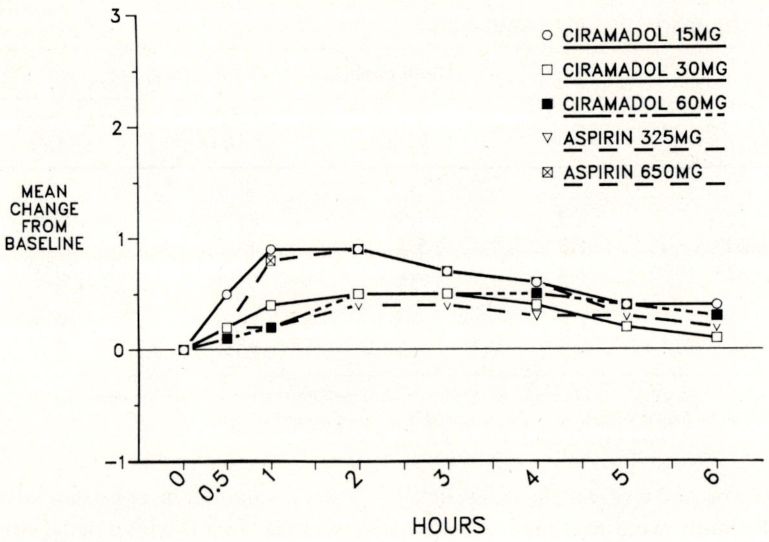

Fig. 1. Mean differences from baseline in pain intensity rating *(PID)* during the 6-hour observation period. Higher scores indicate greater pain relief.

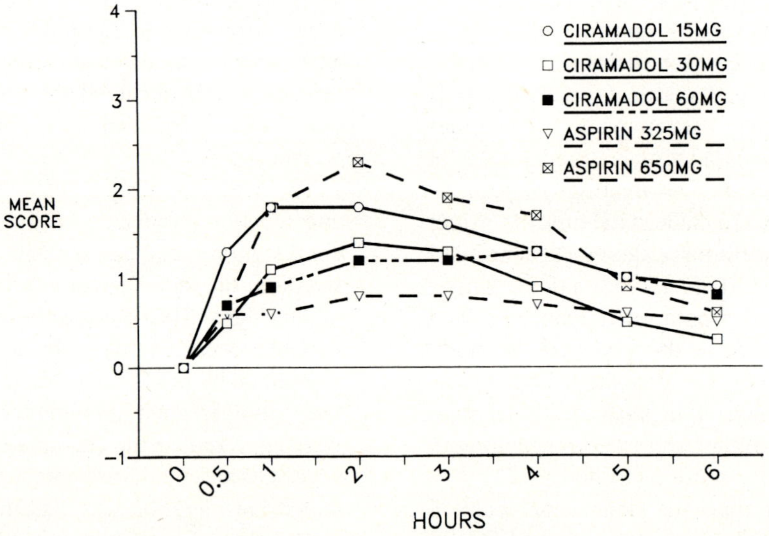

Fig. 2. Mean pain relief scores for the five groups during the 6-hour observation period. Higher scores indicate greater pain relief.

within-group changes from baseline by the paired t test, while comparisons among groups was by a one-way ANCOVA. The frequencies of adverse effects were compared among groups by the chi-square test, supplemented by Fisher's exact test for pairwise comparisons.

RESULTS

The data on pain relief are summarized in Figs. 1 to 5 and Table I. Beginning at 1 hour and persisting through at least 4 hours (depending on the scale), the 650 mg aspirin group showed a consistent and generally significant advantage over the 325 mg aspirin group in the efficacy scores on the four scales. Of the three ciramadol dose groups, the 15 mg group generally had the highest scores on the four efficacy scales, particularly during the first 2 hours; the differences between ciramadol, 30 and 60 mg, were at most times minimal, although at hours 4 through 6 the mean scores in the 60 mg group were somewhat above those in the 30 mg group (and at or only slightly below the levels in the 15 mg group). Differences among the ciramadol dose groups were generally not significant; the only significant differences detected in the efficacy scores were

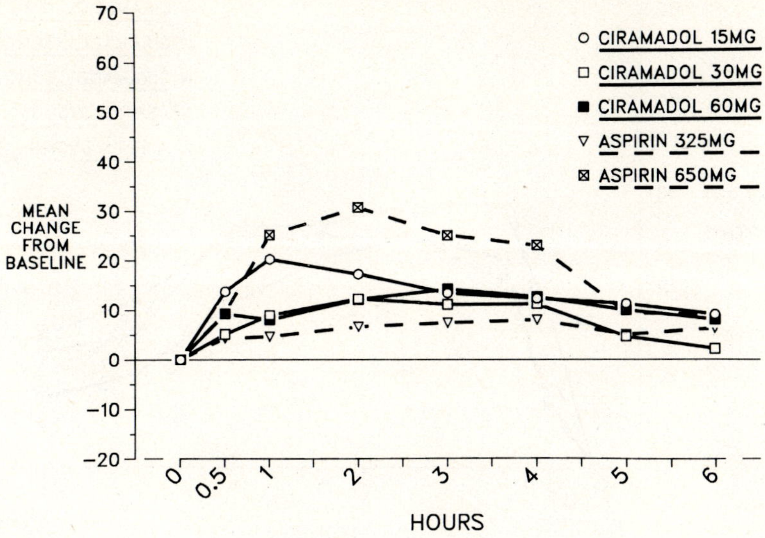

Fig. 3. Mean differences from baseline in pain analog intensity rating *(PAID)* as determined by the linear scale. Higher scores indicate greater pain relief.

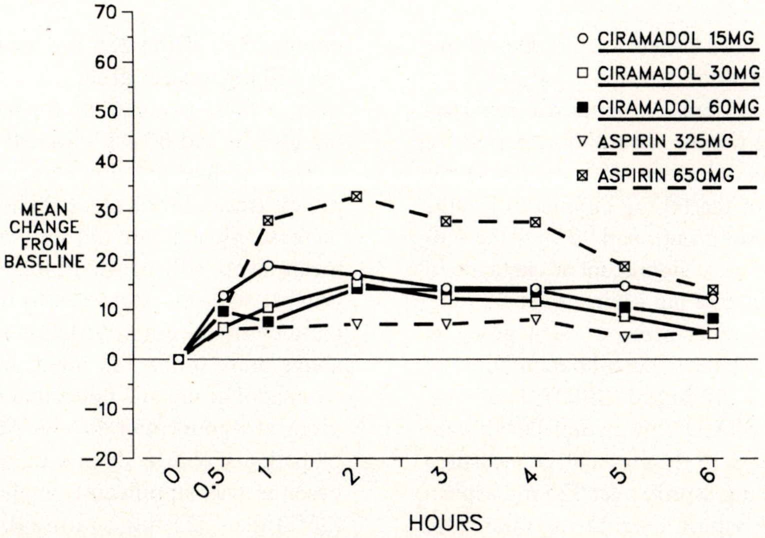

Fig. 4. Mean differences from baseline in pain analog intensity ratings *(PAID)* as determined by the curvilinear scale. Higher scores indicate greater pain relief.

advantages for 15 mg ciramadol over 30 mg ciramadol in the 30-minute relief scores and for 15 mg ciramadol over 60 mg ciramadol in the 30-minute and 1-hour pain intensity difference (PID) scores and the linear 1-hour pain analog intensity difference (PAID) scores.

The differences between 15 mg ciramadol and 650 mg aspirin were generally not significant. The 15 mg ciramadol group had the highest scores at 30 minutes (although the between-group differences were not significant), while the 650 mg aspirin group generally had the highest scores from 2 through 4 hours, showing significant advantages over 15 mg ciramadol in the linear analog scores at 2 hours and in the curvilinear analog scores at 2, 3, and 4 hours; there were no differences between the groups in the mean PID or pain relief scores at these times, however. In most cases, the mean efficacy scores in the 325 mg aspirin group were at or below the levels in the ciramadol 30 and 60 mg groups; there were no significant differences in the pairwise comparisons of the efficacy scores involving these three groups. A number of significant advantages for 15 mg ciramadol over 325 mg aspirin (during the first 3 hours)

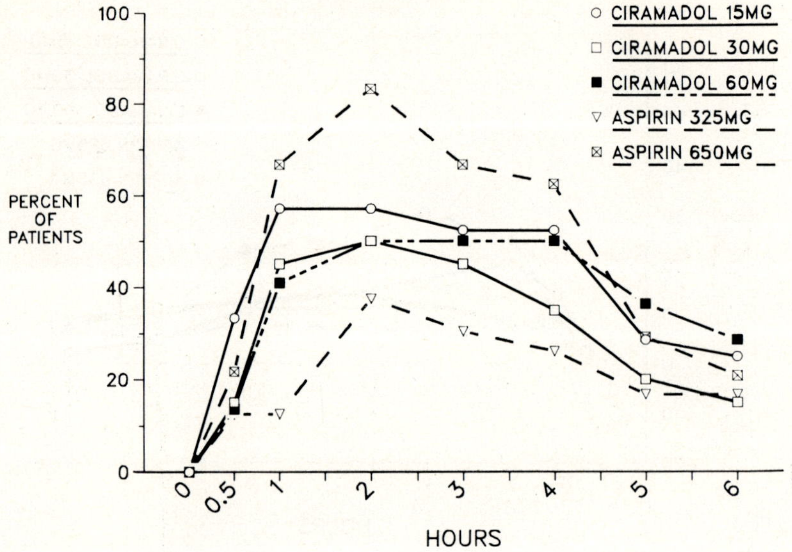

Fig. 5. Percentages of patients in each of the five groups who experienced effective (moderate or better) pain relief during the 6-hour observation period.

and for 650 mg aspirin over ciramadol, 30 and 60 mg (between hours 1 and 4) were detected.

A pain relief score of moderate or better was reported at some time during the 6-hour observation period by 76% of the 15 mg ciramadol group, 60% of the 30 mg ciramadol group, 59% of the 60 mg ciramadol group, 38% of the 325 mg aspirin group, and 92% of the 650 mg aspirin group. There were significant advantages in the peak relief scores for 650 mg aspirin over 325 mg aspirin. The mean peak relief score in each group is listed in Table I, along with the mean 6-hour cumulative sum of the pain intensity difference (SPID), total pain relief (TOTPAR), and SPAID (linear and curvilinear scales) scores. Advantages in the cumulative measures were significant for 650 mg aspirin over 325 mg aspirin (all scales), for 650 mg aspirin over 15 mg ciramadol (SPAID from the curvilinear scale), for 650 mg aspirin over 30 mg ciramadol (SPID and SPAID from both scales), and for 650 mg aspirin over 60 mg ciramadol (SPAID from both scales). It should be noted that although our study was designed as a relative potency assay, formal estimates of relative potency (based on such summary measures as the SPID, TOTPAR, SPAID, and peak relief scores) could not be made because of the lack of a positive dose-response relationship among the ciramadol groups.

Each patient provided an evaluation of the drug response. Overall ratings of either good or excellent were made by 57% of the 15 mg ciramadol group, 60% of the 30 mg ciramadol group, 52% of the 60 mg ciramadol group, 33% of the 325 mg aspirin group, and 83% of the 650 mg aspirin group. A significant advantage was seen in these evaluations for 650 mg aspirin over 325 mg aspirin and 60 mg ciramadol.

The baseline sedation scores were similar in the five groups (mean levels closer to none than to mild). Slight increases in sedation during the observation period (to mean levels still below mild) were noted in all of the groups, with the increases in the aspirin groups being particularly minimal. Sedation scores were significantly above those in the 325 mg aspirin group for the 60 mg ciramadol group at 2 hours and for the 15 mg ciramadol group at 6 hours after dosing. At 2 hours, the proportion of patients with a degree of sedation increased from baseline was significantly higher for 15 mg ciramadol (36%) than 325 mg aspirin (10%).

At least one adverse effect was reported by six of 24 patients taking 15 mg ciramadol (25%), five of 24 patients taking 30 mg ciramadol (21%), five of 23 patients taking 60 mg ciramadol (22%), five of 24 patients taking 325 mg aspirin (21%), and four of 24 patients taking 650 mg aspirin (17%). The most frequently reported adverse effect was dizziness/vertigo, in five patients taking 60 mg ciramadol (22%), four patients taking 30 mg ciramadol (17%), three patients taking 15 mg ciramadol (13%), one patient taking 650 mg aspirin (4%), and none of the patients taking 325 mg aspirin; the difference between the 60 mg ciramadol and 325 mg aspirin groups in this adverse effect was significant.

No statistically significant within-group changes

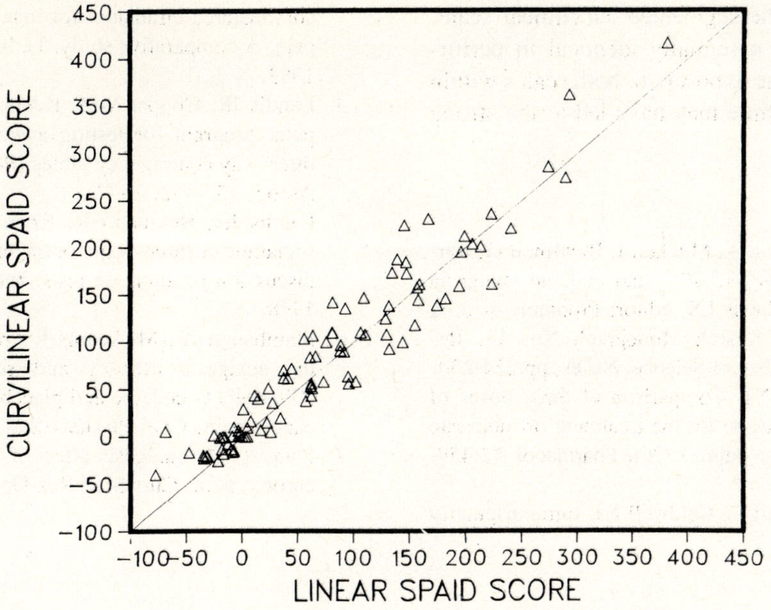

Fig. 6. Individual patient display of 6-hour linear and curvilinear sum of pain analog intensity difference *(SPAID)* scores.

from baseline or between-group differences were detected in pulse rate. The appearance of significant within-group changes in blood pressure (systolic and diastolic) and respiration rate, as well as of between-group differences in these parameters, was generally sporadic in nature. The only consistent significant changes were in the 650 mg aspirin group, in which the diastolic blood pressure was below the baseline (by 3 to 4 mm Hg) at 1, 2, and 4 hours.

There was a high degree of correlation ($P < 0.001$) between the linear and the curvilinear visual analog scales, based on the 6-hour SPAID scores, for the 93 patients with data available on both scales. The correlation coefficient (r) was 0.955 (Fig. 6).

DISCUSSION

Our analgesic data show a clear dose-response relationship for aspirin but not for ciramadol. Indeed, there is an apparent negative relationship for the latter; 15 mg seems more effective than 30 and 60 mg. Because of the greater number of blacks in the 15 mg ciramadol group, we analyzed these responses to see if this would explain the results. It did not; mean scores for blacks and whites were similar. Furthermore, the ciramadol groups did not differ in the percentage of subjects who received narcotics before entry into the study. Because ciramadol has antagonist as well as agonist properties, it is conceivable that at higher doses the former attribute interferes with the latter. In an attempt to analyze for this possibility, we examined the data to see whether ciramadol was more often associated with an increase in pain than was aspirin, since we have seen such "algesic" effects with both nalorphine and naloxone. We found comparable numbers of patients showing increased pain with 60 mg ciramadol and with 325 mg aspirin. Because it seems unlikely that aspirin is "algesic" at this dose, the more parsimonious explanation is that, for whatever reason, ciramadol at the higher doses studied is simply a poorer analgesic.

It has been proposed that ciramadol reaches a plateau in its analgesic efficacy in both animals and man, and that a failure to obtain positive dose-response curves can be thus explained. However, at least in some studies (such as ours), lower doses are not equal to higher ones, but they are superior. In any case, there is considerable variability in the available trials; some show the biphasic curves just described and others show traditional dose-response relationships. There is no clear consensus about the optimal dose, although obviously ciramadol is an analgesic, as predicted from animal data.

The comparison of the two visual analog scales was prompted by previous research from our laboratory on the expressed preferences of subjects for different kinds of scales. The two chosen for comparison were different in two ways: linear vs. curvilinear, and nonsegmented vs. segmented. Despite these differences, which on the basis of our earlier work might have been expected to lead to superiority of the segmented curvilinear scale, the two versions were essentially identical in performance. Conceivably, the exposure to both scales within a very short period of time may have led to the strong correlation.

References

1. Bloomfield SS, Sinkfield A, Mitchell J, Bichlmeir G, Barden TP: Ciramadol (Wy-15,705) and codeine analgesia after episiotomy. *In* Harris LS, editor: Problems of drug dependence. NIDA Research Monograph No. 43. Bethesda, Md., 1983, Office of Science, NIDA, pp 224-230.
2. Fragen RJ, Caldwell NJ: Comparison of three doses of oral ciramadol and placebo for the treatment of moderate to severe postoperative pain. J Clin Pharmacol **22:**459-465, 1982.
3. Fragen RJ, Kouzmanoff C, Caldwell NJ: Intramuscularly administered ciramadol for management of postoperative pain: A comparative study. J Clin Pharmacol **23:**219-226, 1983.
4. Landis JR, Cooper MM, Kennedy T, Koch GG: A computer program for testing average partial association in three-way contingency tables (PARCAT). Proc Am Statist Assoc, 157-162, 1977.
5. Landis JR, Heyman ER, Koch GG: Average partial association in three way contingency tables: A review and discussion of alternate tests. Int Statist Rev **46:**237-254, 1978.
6. Stambaugh JE, McAdams J, Freeland G: Comparison of the analgesic efficacy and safety of oral ciramadol (Ciradol[R]) to codeine and placebo in patients with chronic cancer pain. CLIN PHARMACOL THER **33:**198, 1983.
7. Staquet MJ: Analgesic effect of ciramadol in patients with chronic pain. Curr Med Res Opin **6:**475-477, 1980.

A study of adverse reaction algorithms in a drug surveillance program

To improve agreement among observers, several investigators have recently proposed methods (algorithms) to standardize assessments of causality for presumed adverse drug reactions. We evaluated one such method in the context of an intensive pediatric drug surveillance program. Four observers rated 50 randomly selected case reports drawn from the program, first using only general guidelines and then, several months later, using the strict criteria of the algorithm. Agreement among observers was poor in both study phases. The presence of selected characteristics of adverse events (e.g., major severity) did not improve agreement in either phase of the study. We conclude that routine use of such algorithms in drug surveillance programs is not likely to be of benefit. (Clin Pharmacol Ther 38:183-187, 1985.)

Carol Louik, Sc.D., Peter G. Lacouture, M.S., Allen A. Mitchell, M.D., Ralph Kauffman, M.D., Frederick H. Lovejoy, Jr., M.D., Sumner J. Yaffe, M.D., and Samuel Shapiro, M.B. *Boston, Mass., Detroit, Mich., and Bethesda, Md.*

Adverse drug reactions are a well recognized cause of morbidity, and considerable attention has been devoted to quantifying the extent of this problem. In most cases, however, the determination that a given clinical event is in fact an adverse reaction to a drug has been based on the judgment of a clinical observer. These judgments are almost certainly influenced by both the observer's experience and particular areas of concern, and it is not surprising that low rates of agreement have been documented among different investigators who evaluated selected cases of suspected adverse reactions.[5,6] In response to this problem, several researchers have proposed sets of objective criteria, or "algorithms," to be applied in a systematic manner to suspected drug reactions. These algorithms ask a series of questions, in sequence, the answers to which yield a score intended to measure the probability that the given event was in fact an adverse drug reaction.[4,7,11,12] The algorithms share certain features, and although the precise form of a particular question may differ, there are certain criteria that prove to be crucial in concluding that a clinical event is an adverse drug reaction. These include timing of the event relative to drug exposure, whether the event represents a known reaction to the drug, the possible role of the patient's condition at the time, and the effects of drug withdrawal and, where appropriate, rechallenge.

Such standardized approaches to judging adverse drug reactions are intended to produce greater consistency among evaluators, and enhanced consistency has been demonstrated when such algorithms were tested by their developers.[3,11] However, their potential utility in drug surveillance systems has not been assessed. As part of an intensive pediatric drug surveillance program, we routinely review cases of suspected adverse drug reactions and assess the likelihood that they are due to drugs. In our program, these assessments have been made informally by one observer alone. To determine whether adverse reaction algorithms enhance the consistency and usefulness of these assessments, we studied one such algorithm in the context of the Pediatric Drug Surveillance (PeDS) Program.

METHODS

The PeDS Program is an intensive drug surveillance program established at Children's Hospital in Boston to detect previously unsuspected adverse drug reactions,

From the Division of Clinical Pharmacology and Toxicology, Children's Hospital, Harvard Medical School and the Drug Epidemiology Unit, School of Public Health, Boston University School of Medicine, Boston; Children's Hospital of Michigan, Wayne State University, Detroit; and National Institute of Child Health and Human Development, Bethesda.

Supported by contracts 223-74-3196, 223-75-3036, and 1 UO1 FD 01222 from the Food and Drug Administration, Grant No. GM 24781 from the National Institute of General Medical Sciences, and Grant No. HD 17958 from the National Institute of Child Health and Human Development. The PeDS Program was initiated under a special award from the Burroughs Wellcome Fund. Dr. Louik was supported in part by National Institute of Environmental Health Sciences National Research Service Award 5T32ES07069 from the Harvard School of Public Health.

Received for publication Feb. 10, 1985; accepted April 11, 1985.

Reprint requests to: Dr. Allen A. Mitchell, Pediatric Drug Surveillance Program, Children's Hospital, 300 Longwood Ave., Boston, MA 02115.

quantify known reactions, and identify risk factors for their development. The methods have been described in detail.[9] In brief, nurse monitors are stationed on selected wards where they systematically collect data on patients admitted to these wards. Data are collected in three general areas: patient characteristics, drug exposures, and adverse events. Adverse events include any of a defined set of adverse occurrences (e.g., renal failure, convulsions, rash). Regardless of whether or not such an event is attributed to a drug by a ward observer, the nurse monitor fills out a report form that describes details of the event, date of onset, severity, treatment, duration, and outcome. In addition, reports for events believed to be drug induced include information on the identity of the suspected drug(s), dosage, and an internal assessment by the PeDS Program Director of the likelihood that the event was caused by the implicated drug. The likelihood is rated as definite, probable, possible, or doubtful.

For this investigation we selected a stratified random sample of 50 case reports from among the adverse events reported during the course of routine surveillance of patients. These included 39 "adverse reactions," stratified to include equal numbers of reactions of major, moderate, and minor severity, and 11 events not suspected to be drug induced. For phase I of the study, the 50 case reports were reviewed by three pediatric clinical pharmacologists (R. K., F. H. L., S. J. Y.) who were not directly involved with the PeDS Program and by the PeDS Program Director (A. A. M.), who routinely assesses adverse reaction reports in the Program. To mimic the way assessments are made within the PeDS Program, all reviewers were asked to make an informal judgment as to the probability that each case was an adverse reaction to a suspected drug and to rate each case as "definite," "probable," "possible," "doubtful," or "insufficient information." These terms were deliberately left undefined; we relied on the intuitive understanding of each reviewer to replicate the manner in which these assessments have traditionally been made. The consultant reviewers were told only that we were evaluating our assessments of adverse reactions; at this time no mention was made of algorithms.

Phase II of the study began 3 months after the completion of the first set of reviews. Our consultants were again sent the same 50 case reports, but this time they were asked to assess them using the algorithm proposed by Naranjo et al.[11] This algorithm was chosen because it incorporates the principal features of most others and was judged in our pilot study to be easier to learn and faster to use. This algorithm consists of a set of 10 questions, each of which can be answered "yes," "no," or "do not know," and each of the 10 responses is assigned a score. Our reviewers were asked to answer each question; the scores were tallied and each case report was then categorized according to the established criteria as a "definite," "probable," "possible," or "doubtful" drug-induced event.[11]

In both phases I and II, differences between raters were assessed with the test for marginal homogeneity proposed by Mantel and Byar.[8] This is a generalization of the Mantel-Haenszel test for matched samples. We used Cohen's[1] κ to measure pairwise agreement between all pairs of raters, and then used an approach suggested by Fleiss[2] to measure agreement among more than two raters by taking the average of all pairwise κ values. The statistic κ is a measure of the extent of agreement beyond that expected by chance; it ranges in value from -1 to $+1$. Values >0.75 are generally considered to represent "good" agreement, values between 0.4 and 0.75 to represent "fair" agreement, and values <0.4 to represent "poor" agreement. We also measured agreement with the intraclass correlation coefficient (ρ), a statistic that is essentially equivalent to a weighted κ provided the weights have a particular form.[2] Unlike the unweighted κ, the intraclass correlation coefficient gives partial weighting to partial agreement (e.g., ratings from two reviewers of "definite" and "probable" receive more credit than ratings of "definite" and "doubtful") and would therefore be expected to give slightly higher values than unweighted κ when used to measure agreement in ordered categories.

RESULTS

Table I shows the distribution of ratings for each rater. Because "insufficient information" was used only five times, these ratings were reclassified as "possible" for all analyses. The Mantel-Byar tests for marginal homogeneity indicate that in both phases of the study there were substantial differences in the frequency distributions of ratings for each rater. Thus in the aggregate, some raters were considerably more likely to choose a "definite" or "doubtful" rating. For example, in phase I, rater 2 used "definite" only four times (2%), while rater 1 chose it 15 times (30%). This difference was somewhat less marked in phase II, but still statistically significant.

In Table II, agreement in assignment of ratings to individual cases as measured by both the K statistic and the intraclass correlation coefficient is shown for all pairwise combinations of raters as well as for all four raters considered together. As expected, in all cases the

Table I. Distribution of assessments of 50 adverse events according to rater

	Phase I				Phase II			
Rater	*Definite*	*Probable*	*Possible*	*Doubtful*	*Definite*	*Probable*	*Possible*	*Doubtful*
1	15	10	16	9	0	24	25	1
2	4	20	19	7	5	10	32	3
3	13	12	11	14	1	17	31	1
4	12	13	6	19	7	14	27	2
	X^2 (df = 9; marginal homogeneity) = 35.4 (P < 0.005).				X^2 (df = 9; marginal homogeneity) = 21.7 (P < 0.01).			

Table II. Agreement among raters of 50 adverse events

	Phase I		Phase II	
Sets of raters	K	*r*	K	*r*
1-2	0.12	0.40	0.14	0.30
1-3	0.44	0.74	0.42	0.51
1-4	0.22	0.38	0.31	0.50
2-3	0.21	0.40	0.20	0.38
2-4	0.10	0.28	0.24	0.58
3-4	0.27	0.56	0.36	0.62
All raters	0.24	0.51	0.30	0.48

intraclass correlation coefficient indicates a greater degree of agreement than K. In phase I, when assessments were made without specified guidelines, agreement was poor as measured by either statistic, except for one pair of raters for whom r indicates fairly good agreement (r = 0.74). Application of the algorithm to assess causality in phase II of the study did not improve agreement. Although the overall K indicates slightly better agreement, r is quite similar for the phase I and phase II assessments, and pairwise comparisons show no trend in either direction.

We stratified the events according to characteristics that might affect the level of agreement. Factors selected were severity of the event, whether the event was originally reported as drug attributed, whether treatment was required, and whether blood levels of the suspected drug had been measured (Table III). In general, for a given event characteristic, measures of agreement did not vary substantially in either phase. For example, in phase I, events that were of major severity were no more likely to yield agreement among raters than were events of minor severity; this finding held for phase II as well. However, agreement was better in both phases among the 39 events originally attributed to drugs than among the 11 events that were not.

When results from phase I were compared with those from phase II, there was little evidence that use of the algorithm improved agreement for most of the event characteristics studied, although phase II agreement measures were better for those case reports that included a blood level value of the suspected drug. However, in no category did use of the algorithm raise agreement to "good" levels.

DISCUSSION

For any individual adverse event it is rarely possible to know with absolute certainty whether the event is drug induced. As a first step in approaching truth, one would hope to achieve a consensus among experts. Such consensus is difficult to obtain when judgments are made intuitively and when unspecified criteria are used to make the determination of drug involvement.[5,6] This problem led several investigators to develop methods of standardizing assessments, and reports have suggested that agreement is indeed improved when these methods are used. In particular, Naranjo et al.[11] used a study design similar to ours and demonstrated a change in the intraclass correlation coefficient from 0.49 ("fair") to 0.92 ("good").

Our study is the first to consider the utility of these algorithms in the assessment of adverse events routinely identified as part of an intensive drug surveillance pro-

Table III. Agreement among raters according to selected characteristics of events

	No. of cases	*Phase I* K	*Phase I* *r*	*Phase II* K	*Phase II* *r*
Severity					
Major	14	0.16	0.50	0.26	0.50
Moderate	16	0.21	0.43	0.30	0.53
Minor	20	0.27	0.53	0.31	0.42
Drug attribution					
Yes	39	0.18	0.36	0.24	0.43
No	11	0.05	0.16	−0.20	−0.17
Treatment required					
Yes	24	0.22	0.58	0.34	0.51
No	26	0.24	0.42	0.26	0.48
Blood levels measured					
Yes	12	0.15	0.25	0.28	0.56
No	38	0.24	0.52	0.24	0.29

gram. While levels of agreement before use of the algorithm were similar in both the study of Naranjo et al.[11] ($r = 0.49$) and our own ($r = 0.51$), we were unable to demonstrate that application of the algorithm led to improved agreement among raters.

We believe there are two factors that account for our discordant findings. First, our raters were pediatric clinical pharmacologists who were not experienced in the use of any of the proposed algorithms. This criterion for selection of the raters was intended to assure that their first "informal" assessments would not be influenced by their unconscious application of any standardized set of criteria. If this explanation is correct, it suggests that simple application of these algorithms as they are published will not automatically lead to greater consensus.

Second, our case reports differ from those used in other studies to test algorithms. While we used reports derived from our routine surveillance, Naranjo et al. used published case reports. Unlike reports from intensive surveillance programs, which are necessarily brief and often based on incomplete information, published reports are more complete—in fact, they must contain sufficient evidence of a cause and effect relationship to justify publication. Thus such reports are more likely to include information on many of the important components required by the Naranjo et al. (and other) algorithms. For example, blood levels of the suspected drug would almost certainly be included in published reports, but may only infrequently be available for suspected reactions observed by a surveillance program. It is interesting that in our study, the most marked improvement in agreement with the use of an algorithm occurred for those events for which blood levels were available.

The role of adverse drug reaction algorithms in a drug surveillance program must be kept in perspective. These algorithms are not designed to identify previously unreported adverse drug reactions, and their inclusion in a drug surveillance program would not enhance the capacity to detect such previously unrecognized reactions. That objective is better met by the use of "event surveillance," in which attributions of causality are not relevant.[10] Because event surveillance applies to populations of subjects, it cannot provide useful assessments of causality for individual cases. Algorithms would seem to be an alternative approach to this problem. However, our findings indicate that the use of an algorithm in an intensive drug surveillance program does not improve the uniformity (or validity) of adverse drug reaction assessments.

We thank Jane Sheehan, R.N., Project Coordinator and the nurse monitors of the PeDS Program who collected patient data, and John Farrell and Leonard Gaetano for computer programming assistance.

References

1. Cohen J: A coefficient of agreement for nominal scales. Educ Psychol Meas **20:**37-46, 1960.
2. Fleiss JL: Measuring nominal scale agreement among many raters. Psych Bull **76:**378-382, 1971.
3. Hutchinson TA, Leventhal JM, Kramer MS, Karch FE, Lipman AG, Feinstein AR: An algorithm for the operational assessment of adverse drug reactions. II. Demonstration of reproducibility and validity. JAMA **242:** 633-638, 1979.
4. Karch FE, Lasagna L: Toward the operational identifi-

cation of adverse drug reactions. CLIN PHARMACOL THER **21:**247-254, 1977.

5. Karch FE, Smith CL, Kerzner B, et al: Adverse drug reactions: A matter of opinion. CLIN PHARMACOL THER **19:**489-492, 1976.
6. Koch-Weser J, Sellers EM, Zacest R: The ambiguity of adverse drug reactions. Eur J Clin Pharmacol **1:**75-78, 1977.
7. Kramer MS, Leventhal JM, Hutchinson TA, Feinstein AR: An algorithm for the operational assessment of adverse drug reactions. I. Background, description, and instructions for use. JAMA **242:**623-632, 1979.
8. Mantel N, Byar DP: Marginal homogeneity, symmetry, and independence. Commun Statist Theor Math A7:953-976, 1978.
9. Mitchell AA, Goldman P, Shapiro S, Slone D: Drug utilization and reported adverse reactions in hospitalized children. Am J Epidemiol **110:**196-204, 1979.
10. Mitchell AA, Slone D, Shapiro S, Goldman P: Adverse drug effects and drug surveillance. *In* Yaffe SJ, editor: Pediatric pharmacology: Therapeutic principles in practice. New York, 1980, Grune & Stratton Inc., pp 65-78.
11. Naranjo CA, Busto U, Sellers EM, et al: A method for estimating the probability of adverse drug reactions. CLIN PHARMACOL THER **30:**239-245, 1981.
12. Venulet J, Ciucii A, Berneker GC: Standardized assessment of drug-adverse reaction associations—Rationale and experience. Int J Clin Pharmacol **18:**381-388, 1980.

Treatment of arterial hypertension with ketanserin in mono- and combination therapy

We evaluated the long-term antihypertensive effects of ketanserin, a selective serotonin$_2$-receptor blocker with weak adrenergic receptor blocker properties. Ketanserin was given alone, 40 mg o.d. or b.i.d., for 2 years to 12 patients with essential hypertension. Systolic and diastolic blood pressures (BPs) were significantly reduced 14 days after the start of therapy and remained lowered during the 2-year follow-up period. In a larger group of patients who received ketanserin monotherapy for 2 to 3 months, the response to therapy varied considerably between subjects, with an overall response rate (BP <165/95 mm Hg) of 60% to 75%. During steady-state conditions, the maximum and minimum ketanserin plasma concentrations varied from threefold to fourfold between subjects and did not correlate with individual reductions in BP, but for each individual there was a positive correlation between BP reduction and ketanserin plasma concentration throughout a study day. In combination with β-blockers, ketanserin effectively reduced BP in the supine and standing positions. The plasma concentration profile was not altered as much during combination therapy as when ketanserin was given alone. Side effects were few and tolerable. Ketanserin effectively reduces BP both alone and in combination with β-blockers and may be still another drug useful in the treatment of essential hypertension. (CLIN PHARMACOL THER 38:188-194, 1985.)

Anders Pettersson, M.D., Bengt Persson, M.D., Göran Berglund, M.D., and Thomas Hedner, M.D. *Göteborg, Sweden*

It has been suggested that serotonin (5-hydroxytryptamine [5-HT]) is involved in the regulation of blood pressure (BP) in the periphery[17,22-24] as well as in the central nervous system.[5,12] While the central hypotensive effects of 5-HT have been generally accepted, its role in the control of BP is debated.[10,23-25] Although the vasoconstrictive effects of 5-HT were described early,[17] it did not attract much interest until recently, mainly because 5-HT had variable effects on BP in animals[22] and because early 5-HT antagonists did not lower BP in animals or man.[22] Interest in 5-HT has been renewed because of the recent discovery of vascular 5-HT$_2$ receptors[13,25] and the introduction of selective 5-HT$_2$–receptor blocking drugs such as ketanserin.[6,11,19,25] If the antihypertensive effect of ketanserin is due to 5-HT$_2$–receptor blockade alone,[1,3,4,20] a new principle in the treatment of essential hypertension would be indicated. To explore further the potential usefulness of 5-HT$_2$ antagonism in the long-term management of essential hypertension, we measured BP and ketanserin plasma concentrations after ketanserin alone and in combination with β-blockers.

From the Hypertension Unit, Department of Medicine I and Department of Clinical Pharmacology, Sahlgren's Hospital.
Received for publication Nov. 23, 1984; accepted April 15, 1985.
Reprint requests to: Anders Pettersson, M.D., Department of Clinical Pharmacology, Sahlgren's University Hospital, S-413 45 Göteborg, Sweden.

METHODS

Our subjects were 26 patients (25 men and one woman) with mild to moderate uncomplicated essential hypertension (Table I). Patients who had used antihypertensive drugs were given placebo for 3 to 4 weeks before they were accepted into the study. If their diastolic BP at the end of the placebo washout period was >95 mm Hg, they were included.

The study was carried out in three parts, and active ketanserin was given on a single-blind basis. In the first part of the study, ketanserin was given alone during an 8-to-10–week period in an oral dose of 40 mg once (n = 5) or twice (n = 10) a day. Afterwards, subjects fasted overnight and came to the clinic at 8 AM without having taken their morning tablets. Supine and standing BPs were measured and venous blood (antecubital vein) was drawn for determination of ketanserin plasma con-

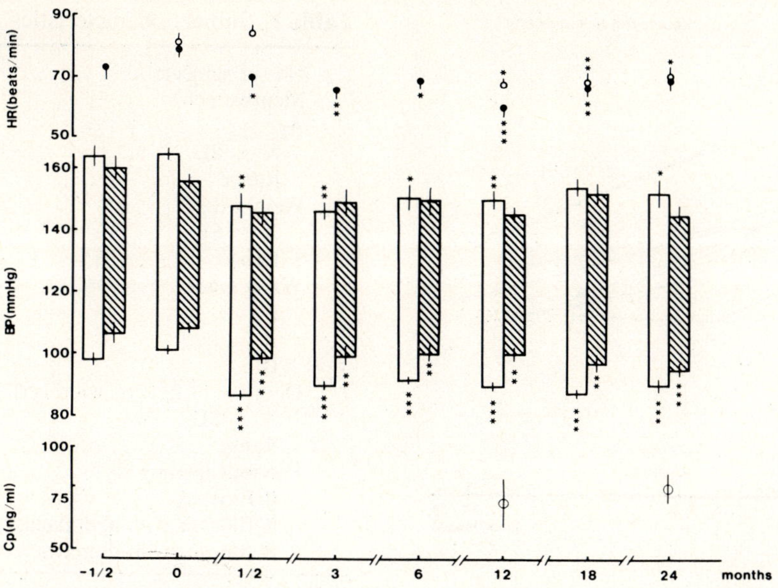

Fig. 1. Effects of 2 years of ketanserin dosing alone (20 mg b.i.d., 40 mg o.d., or 40 mg b.i.d.) in 12 patients with essential hypertension. The mean (±SE) supine *(open bars)* and standing *(hatched bars)* BPs, as well as supine (●) and standing (○) HRs during placebo (times −½ and 0) and ketanserin (times ½ to 24 months) dosing are shown. Mean (±SE) ketanserin plasma concentrations *(Cp)* are shown at 12 and 24 months. *$P < 0.05$, **$P < 0.005$, ***$P < 0.001$ compared with placebo values.

centrations. Assessments preceded dosing and followed at 0.25, 0.5, 1, 2, 4, 6, 12, and 24 hours thereafter. The subjects who took ketanserin twice a day received their second tablet at 8 PM.

In the second part of the study, ketanserin was added to a fixed optimal dose of a β-blocker. After 3 to 4 weeks of a single-blind β-blocker and placebo period, subjects (n = 10) were given ketanserin, 40 mg b.i.d. After 4 weeks, systolic and diastolic BPs, heart rate (HR), and ketanserin plasma concentrations were measured during a 24-hour period. Measurements were made before dosing and at 0.25, 0.5, 1, 2, 4, 6, 12, and 24 hours thereafter. A second tablet was given immediately after the 12-hour assessment.

Finally, 12 patients (some of whom had participated in the first part of the study) participated in a 2-year follow-up. They were given ketanserin, 40 mg once (n = 3) or twice (n = 9) a day for 2 years. Dosage requirements changed only minimally in individuals throughout the 2-year period. The 40 mg dose was chosen based on previous experience.[8,9] Most subjects started a twice-daily regimen. Those subjects who responded (diastolic BP <95 mm Hg) were switched to a once-daily regimen, and if they responded to this regimen it was continued throughout the 2 years. The remaining subjects, both responders and nonresponders, continued therapy with 40 mg b.i.d., as side effects are more common when larger dose increments are used.

Systolic and diastolic BPs and HR were measured in the supine and standing positions on an outpatient basis. Samples for measurements of ketanserin plasma concentrations were drawn at some visits and, with few exceptions, sampling was performed in the morning between 8 and 10 AM, i.e., 1 to 3 hours after dosing. Subjective experiences were recorded after spontaneous reporting.

BP was measured blindly with a semiautomatic manometer.[14] Systolic and diastolic BP readings were made after at least 5 minutes of supine rest and after 2 minutes in the standing position. Korotkoff phase V was taken as the diastolic value. HR was measured automatically over a 30-second interval. Venous blood was sampled and plasma was separated by centrifugation within minutes of collection. Samples were stored at −20° C and later assayed for unchanged ketanserin by HPLC.[15]

Data are presented as the $\overline{X} \pm SE$. Statistical evaluation was by ANOVA with two independent criteria for classification, followed by Student's t test.[2] Regression analysis was by the method of least squares.[2] The relationship between the change in BP and the loga-

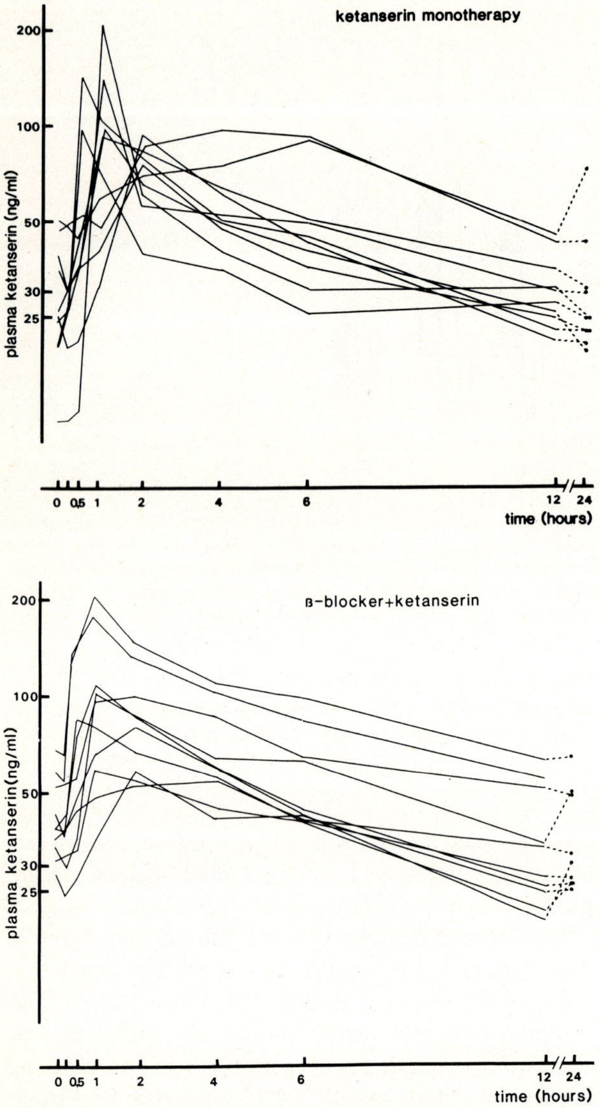

Fig. 2. Individual ketanserin plasma concentrations during 24 hours at steady state after 8 weeks of ketanserin, 40 mg b.i.d. **(top)**, and after 4 weeks of ketanserin, 40 mg b.i.d., in combination with a β-blocker (tablet intake at times 0 and 12) **(bottom)**.

rithms of the ketanserin plasma concentrations was examined by ANOVA. The regression and correlation coefficients between all BP and transformed concentration values (0 to 24 hours) were estimated for each subject. The null hypothesis was that there was no interaction, i.e., equal regression coefficients for each subject. In the case of no interaction, the average within-subject correlations and regression coefficients were estimated from ANOVA and their significance was tested.

Table I. Subject characteristics

No. of subjects	26
Men/women	25:1
Age (yr)	
$\bar{X} \pm$ SE	60 ± 2
Range	41 – 70
Weight (kg)	
$\bar{X} \pm$ SE	85 ± 2
Range	74 – 118
WHO grade	
I	21
II	5
III	0
Duration of hypertension (yr)	
$\bar{X} \pm$ SE	9 ± 1
Range	2 – 21
Previous therapy	
β-Blocker	8
β-Blocker with hydralazine	7
β-Blocker with diuretics	11

RESULTS

Before the start of ketanserin therapy and after a 2-week placebo washout, the supine BP in the group of subjects followed for 2 years was 165 ± 3/101 ± 2 mm Hg. Ketanserin lowered systolic and diastolic BPs in the supine and standing positions after 2 weeks (Fig. 1). This reduction was virtually unchanged during the 2 years of follow-up. After 2 years, seven of 12 subjects had supine BPs <165/95 mm Hg. The response to ketanserin in the supine and standing positions varied markedly between subjects. Thus from the start of therapy to the time of the 2-year follow-up, the reduction in supine diastolic BP varied between 0 and 28 mm Hg and the reduction in standing diastolic BP varied between 7 and 25 mm Hg. HR decreased slightly after ketanserin dosed alone. The BP reaction in the standing position was normal and no orthostatic phenomena were noted at the time of maximal or minimal ketanserin steady-state plasma concentrations (data not shown).

Individual ketanserin plasma concentrations during steady state after 4 to 8 weeks of therapy are shown in Fig. 2. Maximal plasma concentrations generally developed 2 hours after dosing and were 113.5 ± 13 ng/ml for the ketanserin alone group and 102.4 ± 15.6 ng/ml after ketanserin and β-blocker therapy. Minimal plasma concentrations in the two groups were 30.3 ± 3.8 and 41.6 ± 4.2 ng/ml, respectively, and did not differ.

During the 24-hour assessments, maximal BP reductions in both groups coincided with the time of maximal ketanserin plasma concentration (Table II), occurring at 1.9 ± 0.5 and 1.6 ± 0.3 hours after dosing

Table II. BP reduction at steady state after ketanserin alone and in combination with β-blockers

	Placebo	*0 hr*	*Maximal plasma concentration**	*12 hr*
Alone (40 mg b.i.d.)				
Supine BP (mm Hg)				
Systolic	163 ± 3	154 ± 4	144 ± 3†	163 ± 3
Diastolic	102 ± 2	93 ± 3‡	91 ± 2‡	97 ± 2
Standing BP (mm Hg)				
Systolic	156 ± 3	148 ± 5	139 ± 6§	157 ± 5
Diastolic	110 ± 3	102 ± 3§	96 ± 4‡	104 ± 2
Ketanserin, 40 mg b.i.d., with β-blocker				
Supine BP (mm Hg)				
Systolic	166 ± 4	160 ± 5	142 ± 4‡	163 ± 6
Diastolic	107 ± 6	94 ± 3§	87 ± 2†	93 ± 3§
Standing BP (mm Hg)				
Systolic	161 ± 5	152 ± 5	137 ± 5‡	158 ± 6
Diastolic	108 ± 2	99 ± 2§	90 ± 3†	98 ± 2‡

Data are $\overline{X}$ ± SE.
Ketanserin was given 4 to 10 weeks before assessments. Values shown represent BPs at minimal (0 to 12 hours after dosing) and maximal ketanserin plasma concentrations.
*Maximal plasma concentrations occurred at 1.9 ± 0.5 and 1.6 ± 0.3 hours when ketanserin was given alone and in combination with β-blockers, respectively.
†P < 0.001, ‡P < 0.01, §P < 0.05 compared with placebo values.

in the ketanserin alone and in combination with β-blocker groups, respectively. When all individual values between 0 and 24 hours are taken into account (Fig. 3A), there was a positive correlation between plasma concentrations and BP reduction for all individuals, except for the effects on supine diastolic BP when ketanserin was given alone. With the subject in the standing position, ketanserin alone correlated with the lowering of systolic ($r = 0.36$; $P = 0.03$) and diastolic ($r = 0.25$; $P = 0.03$) BPs, and the combination of ketanserin and a β-blocker also correlated significantly with systolic ($r = 0.66$; $P = 0.002$) and diastolic ($r = 0.65$; $P = 0.002$) BP reductions. When the group was taken as a whole, however, there were no significant correlations between minimal or maximal ketanserin plasma concentrations and the BP reduction (Fig. 3B).

During therapy for 1 to 2 months, the most frequent side effect was slight sedation 1 to 2 hours after dosing. This effect was experienced by four of 15 subjects receiving ketanserin alone and by six of 10 subjects receiving ketanserin in combination with a β-blocker. During continuous ketanserin therapy for 2 years, this side effect decreased in frequency. Thus at the end of the follow-up, no subject complained of slight sedation (compared with one subject reporting this effect at the start of the 2-year period). One subject also reported blocked nose and one had dry mouth. Various laboratory parameters as listed previously[6-8] did not change during the 2-year follow-up.

DISCUSSION

Approximately 60% to 70% of the patients responded to chronic oral dosing with ketanserin, 20 to 40 mg b.i.d., which indicates a response rate of the order of that after β-blockers or thiazide diuretics.[9,22] BP was reduced after 2 weeks of ketanserin therapy. During the rest of the 2-year follow-up, supine as well as standing mean BPs remained low and changed little, despite the fixed dosages. Especially in the supine position, HR was reduced during active ketanserin therapy. This has also been reported in double-blind investigations.[3,18] Cardiac output was not decreased, but rather increased slightly because of an increase in stroke volume.[3,16] Thus the most important mechanism by which ketanserin lowers BP is by reducing total peripheral resistance.[3,16] Apart from its 5-HT_2–blocking properties, ketanserin also exerts weak α_1-adrenergic and H_1-histaminergic blockade.

It has been widely questioned whether α_1-adrenergic blockade contributes to the antihypertensive effects of ketanserin. In the spontaneously hypertensive rat, the α_1-blocking property seems to be the single most important factor in the acute effects[3,19]; during chronic dosing, however, there is an antihypertensive effect in this model that is not mediated by α_1-receptors.[20] During chronic oral ketanserin dosing to patients with essential hypertension, the drug slightly alters the dose-response curve to phenylephrine and methoxamine,[3] but unlike the potent α_1-blocker prazosin, ketanserin depresses only the responses to high doses of the α-ag-

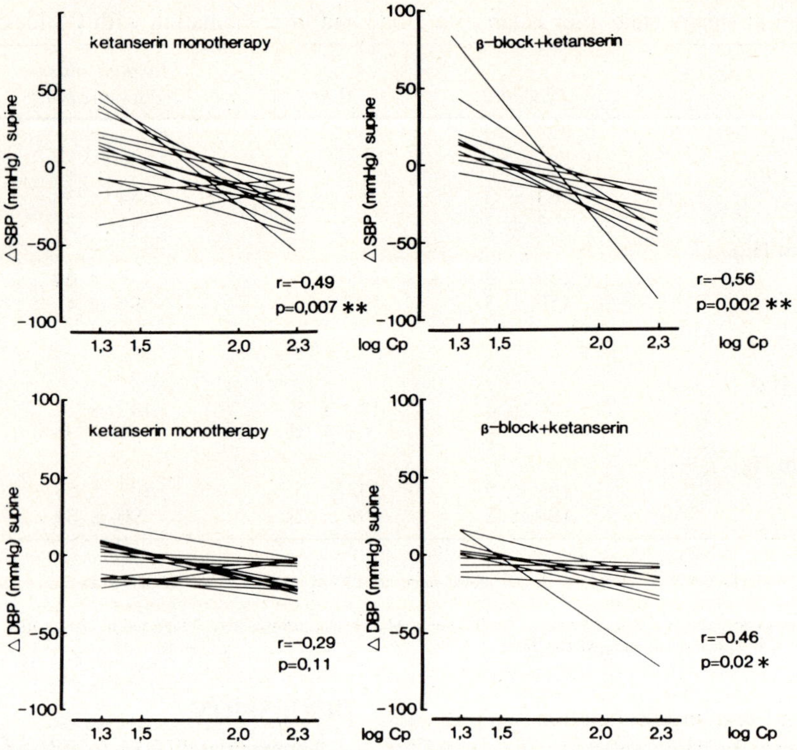

Fig. 3A. Regression lines and average correlation coefficients (r) for the correlation between log ketanserin plasma concentrations *(Cp)* and changes in systolic *(SBP)* and diastolic *(DBP)* BP values in the supine position in patients who received ketanserin alone, 40 mg b.i.d. or o.d. *(left panel)*, or the combination of ketanserin, 40 mg b.i.d., with a β-blocker *(right panel)*.

onists. This matter is still unresolved in its application to chronic therapy,[2,27] but ketanserin seems to lower BP by mechanisms unrelated to α_1-adrenergic blockade. This interpretation may be further substantiated by the fact that no signs of orthostatic hypotension were noted in our subjects during maximal or minimal ketanserin plasma concentrations.

During steady-state conditions, plasma concentrations of unchanged ketanserin (maximal and minimal) varied threefold to fourfold between subjects. There was no correlation between the BP reduction for the different subjects as plotted against the minimal or maximal ketanserin plasma concentrations. In individual subjects, however, BP reduction correlated positively to ketanserin plasma concentrations throughout the study day. The plasma concentration profile did not seem to differ when ketanserin was given alone or in combination with β-blockers. We interpret these data as indicative of individual variable sensitivity to 5-HT–antagonists in patients with essential hypertension and in the potential role of 5-HT in the development and maintenance of high BP. The role of 5-HT may therefore differ between subpopulations of patients with hypertension.

Side effects were mild; the most common was slight sedation. Fewer subjects experienced side effects during long-term therapy. In an on-going international multicenter comparative trial with metoprolol or hydrochlorothiazide, no differences were noted between the regimens.[9,22] The dropout frequency increased markedly after single doses of ⩾60 mg, however, and thus the dose-response curve for the dropout frequency seemed to be steeper than that of the antihypertensive effect.[9] This indicates that the therapeutic dose is 20 to 40 mg twice or possibly once a day.

To establish further the future role of ketanserin in the management of essential hypertension, long-term tolerance studies as well as comparative studies with other antihypertensive drugs need to be performed.

We gratefully acknowledge the technical assistance of Gunnel Dahlén and Gabriella Sahlén.

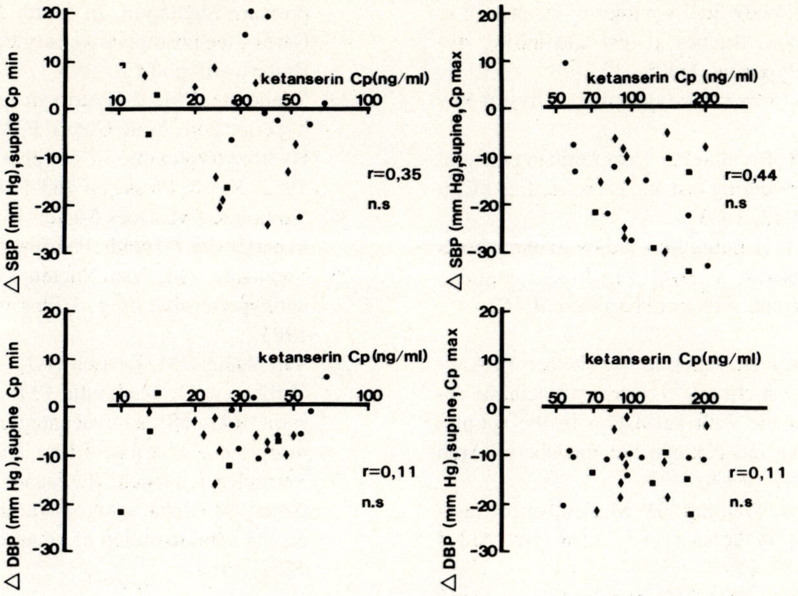

Fig. 3B. Correlations between ketanserin plasma concentrations *(Cp)* and changes in systolic *(SBP)* and diastolic *(DBP)* BP values. Individual values are shown for patients who received ketanserin alone, 40 mg o.d. (■) or b.i.d. (♦) for 8 weeks, or the combination of ketanserin, 40 mg b.i.d., with a β-blocker (●) for 4 weeks. *Cp min* = Minimum plasma concentration; *Cp max* = maximum plasma concentration.

References

1. Ball SG, Zabludowski JR, Robertson JIS: Mechanism of antihypertensive action of ketanserin in man. Br Med J **387:**1065, 1983.
2. Davies OL: Statistical methods in research and production. London, 1949, Oliver and Boyd.
3. Fagard R, Fiocchi R, Lijnen P, Staessen J, Moerman E, De Schaepdryver A, Amery A: Haemodynamic and humoral responses to chronic ketanserin treatment in essential hypertension. Br Heart J **51:**149-156, 1984.
4. Fozard JR: Mechanism of the hypotensive effect of ketanserin. J Cardiovasc Pharmacol **4:**829-838, 1982.
5. Gradin K, Pettersson A, Hjort S, Hedner T, Arvidsson LE, Persson B: Cardiovascular effects in the Sprague-Dawley rat of 8-hydroxy-2 (DI-*N*-propylamino) tetraline (8-OH-DPAT), a selective serotonin receptor agonist. J Pharm Pharmacol **37:**263-265, 1985.
6. Hedner T, Persson B: Ketanserin in combination with β-adrenergic blocking agents in the treatment of essential hypertension. Br J Clin Pharmacol **18:**263-265, 1985.
7. Hedner T, Persson B, Berglund G: Ketanserin, a novel 5-hydroxy-tryptamine antagonist: Monotherapy in essential hypertension. Br J Clin Pharmacol **16:**121-125, 1983.
8. Hedner T, Persson B, Berglund G: Experience with ketanserin, a serotonin (S_2) antagonist, in longterm treatment of esential hypertension. Clin Exp Hypertens **6:**743-751, 1984.
9. Hedner T, Persson B, Berglund G: A comparative and longterm evaluation of ketanserin in essential hypertension. J Cardiovasc Pharmacol. (In press.)
10. Humphrey PPA, Fenuik W, Watts AD: Ketanserin, a novel antihypertensive drug? J Pharm Pharmacol **34:**541, 1982.
11. Janssen PAJ: Paul Janssen replies. Trends Pharmacol Sci **4:**412, 1983.
12. Kuhn DM, Wolf WA, Lovenberg W: Review of the role of the central serotonergic neuronal system in blood pressure regulation. Hypertension **2:**243-245, 1980.
13. Leysen JE, Awouters F, Kenis L, Lauderon J, Vendenberk J, Janssen PAJ: Receptor binding profile of R41468, a novel antagonist of 5-HT_2 receptors. Life Sci **28:**1015-1022, 1981.
14. Nyberg G: Indirect blood pressure and heart rate measured quickly without observer bias using a semiautomatic machine (Auto-Manometer)—Response to isometric exercise in normally healthy males and its modification by β-adrenoreceptor blockade. Br J Clin Pharmacol **4:**275-281, 1977.
15. Okonkwo PO, Riemann I-W, Woesterborgh R, Klotz U: High performance liquid chromatographic assay with fluorimetric detection of ketanserin, a new antihypertensive agent and serotonin (S_2) antagonist in human plasma, blood and urine. J Chromatogr **272:**411-416, 1983.
16. Omvik P, Lund-Johansen P: Long-term effects on central

haemodynamics and body fluid volumes of ketanserin in essential hypertension. Studies at rest and during dynamic exercise. J Hypertens **1**:405-412, 1983.
17. Page IH: Serotonin (5-hydroxytryptamine). Physiol Rev **34**:563-588, 1954.
18. Persson B, Hedner T, Berglund G: Ketanserin in essential hypertension. Effects during rest and exercise. Eur J Clin Pharmacol **25**:307-312, 1983.
19. Persson B, Hedner T, Henning M: Cardiovascular effects in the rat of ketanserin, a novel 5-hydroxytryptamine receptor blocking agent. J Pharm Pharmacol **3**:442-445, 1982.
20. Pettersson A, Persson B, Henning M, Hedner T: Antihypertensive effects of chronic 5-hydroxytryptamine (5-HT_2) receptor blockade with ketanserin in the spontaneously hypertensive rat. Naunyn Schmiedebergs Arch Pharmacol **327**:43-47, 1984.
21. Schalekamp MADH, Wenting GJ: Mechanism of antihypertensive action of ketanserin in man. Br Med J **287**:1300-1301, 1983.
22. Symoens J, Vanhoutte PM: Role of serotonin in blood pressure regulation. *In* Smith JAR, Watkins J, editors: Care of the postoperative surgical patient. London, 1984, Butterworth and Co.
23. Vanhoutte PM: 5-Hydroxytryptamine, vasospasm and hypertension. *In* de Clerck F, Vanhoutte PM, editors: 5-Hydroxytryptamine in peripheral reactions. New York, 1982, Raven Press, pp 163-174.
24. Vanhoutte PM: Does 5-hydroxytryptamine play a role in hypertension? Trends Pharmacol Sci **3**:370-373, 1982.
25. Vanhoutte PM, Van Nueten JM: Ketanserin—A novel antihypertensive drug. J Pharm Pharmacol **35**:339-340, 1983.
26. Van Nueten JM, Janssen PAJ, Van Beek J, Xhonneux R, Verbeuren TJ, Vanhoutte PM: Vascular effect of ketanserin (R41 468), a novel antagonist of 5-HT_2 serotonergic receptors. J Pharmacol Exp Ther **218**:217-230, 1981.
27. Vermylen I, Fiocchi R, Fagard R, Lijnen P, Staessen J, Amery A: $Alpha_1$ antagonistic and antiserotonergic action during administration of ketanserin. Br Med J **287**:1551-1552, 1983.

Losulazine, a new antihypertensive

The efficacy of losulazine was determined in 32 patients with hypertension. Each subject was randomly assigned to receive either losulazine (n = 16) or placebo (n = 16) in a double-blind fashion. Losulazine in the dosage range of 10 to 30 mg b.i.d. effectively lowered the blood pressure. Diastolic blood pressure was lowered to ≤90 mm Hg in over 70% of the subjects receiving losulazine. There was no evidence of an increase in heart rate; to the contrary, there was a tendency for heart rate to decrease. Six subjects dropped out of the study before completion. Four of these were receiving placebo and dropped out because of lack of efficacy. One subject receiving losulazine dropped out for personal reasons during the first week of the study, and the other subject (also taking losulazine) dropped out when a drug-related pruritus (itchy eyes) developed. This event was readily reversed upon discontinuation of the drug. The drug was well tolerated and side effects were minimal, with no evidence of orthostatic effects or sexual dysfunction. There was a suggestion that nasal stuffiness and conjunctival congestion may be drug related. There were no changes in any laboratory values or body weight. (Clin Pharmacol Ther 38:195-198, 1985.)

Randall Gore, M.D., David Musselman, M.D., Edwin Micalizzi, B.A., and Michaline Slomka, M.A. *Portland, Ore., and Kalamazoo, Mich.*

Losulazine hydrochloride (1-((4-fluoropheny)sulfonyl)4-(4-((7-(trifluoromethyl)-4-quinolinyl)amino)benzoyl)piperazine hydrochloride) is being tested as a new antihypertensive in man. Its exact mechanism of action has not been defined, but its hypotensive activity depends on the presence of an intact, functional sympathetic nervous system. Results of animal studies suggest that losulazine exerts its action by modulating sympathetic nerve activity. Hypotensive doses of losulazine in animals reduced norepinephrine levels in the heart and spleen without altering norepinephrine levels in the brain.[5] Orthostatic hypotension was not observed during tilt experiments in conscious monkeys who received losulazine.[5] Additional animal studies showed that losulazine did not block the release of sympathetic neurotransmitters nor the postsynaptic adrenergic receptor sites.[5]

Losulazine has had only limited exposure in man. Initial phase I clinical trials were conducted in normal, healthy men, and it was very well tolerated at doses <100 mg (total daily dose). Our randomized, double-blind, placebo-controlled study is an early efficacy trial of losulazine monotherapy in patients with mild to moderate hypertension.

From the Heart Research Department, Providence Medical Center, Portland, and The Upjohn Company, Kalamazoo.
Received for publication Dec. 10, 1984; accepted April 15, 1985.
Reprint requests to: Edwin Micalizzi, The Upjohn Company, 7000 Portage Rd., Kalamazoo, MI 49001.

METHODS

Our subjects were 22 men and 10 women between 23 and 67 years old. All were white and had hypertension, with initial supine diastolic blood pressures between 96 and 109 mm Hg. Most subjects had been taking medications to control their hypertension.

Each subject was gradually removed from his/her present antihypertensive medication(s) and left untreated for 3 weeks. No placebo was administered during the washout. History, physical examination, chest roentgenogram, ECG, vital signs, and screening laboratory data were obtained just before randomization to either losulazine (n = 16) or placebo (n = 16). Each subject was then started on 5 mg b.i.d. losulazine or placebo and visited the clinic on a weekly basis. Vital signs (average of three readings) were obtained in both the supine (after 5 minutes of rest) and standing (after 5 minutes) positions. Vital signs were determined at each visit and if the supine diastolic blood pressure was >85 mm Hg, the dose was increased by 5 mg b.i.d. increments until a maximum daily dose of 60 mg was reached. When the supine diastolic blood pressure fell <85 mm Hg or the maximum dose was achieved, subjects were maintained on that dose for a total of 4 weeks.

All adverse drug reactions were recorded at each visit. Each subject was asked if he/she had experienced any side effects since the previous visit. All adverse side effects were coded through use of modification of the COSTART National Adverse Drug Reaction Directory.[3] Therefore, similar events were grouped according

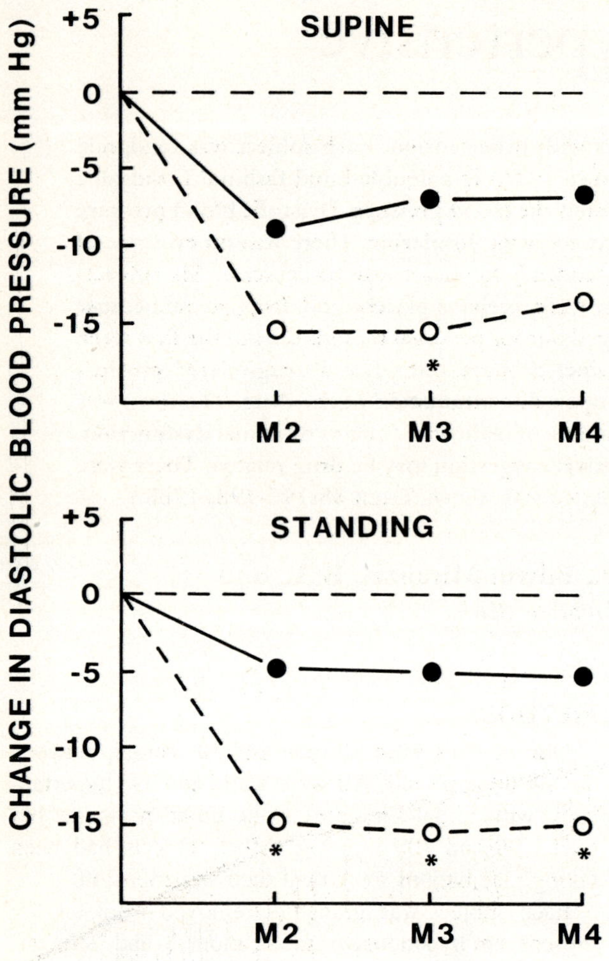

Fig. 1. Change in diastolic blood pressure during losulazine (○) or placebo (●) dosing (n = 12 to 14 subjects). *M2* = After second week; *M3* = after third week, *M4* = after fourth week of maintenance dosing. $^{*}P < 0.01$ compared with value after placebo dosing.

to the COSTART system, and the actual term that was reported may have been changed.

During the study blood chemistry values, electrolyte levels, and enzyme levels were determined at 2-week intervals. At the end of the maintenance phase a chest roentgenogram, ECG, and safety laboratory evaluations were repeated. Subjects stopped taking losulazine or placebo and were switched to conventional antihypertensive medication(s). If a subject dropped out during the washout period, his/her data were not evaluated. If a subject dropped out while receiving losulazine or placebo, his/her data were analyzed to the time of discontinuation.

A standard t test was used to test for differences in means between the two groups, as well as for differences in changes from initial to follow-up determinations between the two groups.

RESULTS

Six subjects dropped out of the study before the end of the maintenance phase. Four subjects taking placebo dropped out because of lack of efficacy, two at the discretion of the investigator (supine diastolic blood pressure >110 mm Hg) and two at the request of the subjects, who were uncomfortable to remain in the study because of their elevated blood pressures (supine diastolic blood pressures >100 mm Hg). Of the two subjects taking losulazine who dropped out, one did so for personal reasons and the other dropped out because of an intolerable adverse drug reaction (itchy eyes).

Four weeks of maintenance losulazine therapy significantly decreased standing diastolic blood pressure (Fig. 1). During the last three visits in the maintenance phase, losulazine reduced the mean supine diastolic blood pressure by 13.5 to 15.5 mm Hg, compared with an average reduction of only 6.8 to 8.9 mm Hg in the placebo group (Table I). During this same interval losulazine also reduced mean standing diastolic blood pressure by 14.6 to 15.3 mm Hg, compared with an average reduction of only 4.7 to 5.3 mm Hg in the placebo group (Table II). Losulazine effectively controlled the supine diastolic blood pressure in 71% to 86% of the subjects, whereas in only 33% to 42% of the subjects taking placebo was the blood pressure controlled. There was no evidence of the development of tolerance.

Losulazine significantly decreased heart rate compared with pretreatment values, but the values were not significantly different from those in the placebo group (Table III). There were no significant changes in body weight. Mean body weight in the placebo group was 179.8 ± 5.24 lb before and 180.6 ± 5.41 lb after dosing and values in the losulazine group were 178.6 ± 10.94 and 178.9 ± 11.04 lb, respectively.

Table IV lists the number of subjects reporting at least one episode of an adverse drug reaction. Nasal stuffiness and conjunctival congestion occurred in more subjects taking losulazine than in those taking placebo. All adverse drug reactions were mild to moderate, except for the severe pruritus (itchy eyes) that resulted in discontinuation of the drug in one subject. All reported effects had disappeared by the end of the study. Chest roentgenograms, ECGs, serum chemistry tests, blood enzyme and electrolyte levels, and urinalysis showed no significant drug-related changes.

Of the subjects receiving losulazine, two (14.3%) took 20 mg/day, one (7.1%) took 30 mg/day, four

Table I. Summary of supine blood pressure after subjects were titrated to an effective (diastolic blood pressure <85 mm Hg) or a maximum (30 mg b.i.d.) dose of losulazine

	Systolic blood pressure (mm Hg)		*Diastolic blood pressure (mm Hg)*	
Visit	*Placebo*	*Losulazine*	*Placebo*	*Losulazine*
Baseline	148.7 ± 3.18	151.4 ± 2.52	99.1 ± 1.08	98.8 ± 0.90
M2	138.8 ± 4.57	137.7 ± 4.13	90.2 ± 2.30	83.3 ± 2.40
M3	143.8 ± 4.34	137.3 ± 5.18	92.2 ± 2.58	83.4 ± 2.35*
M4	144.8 ± 5.26	144.4 ± 4.31	92.3 ± 3.03	85.3 ± 2.50

Data are $\overline{X}$ ± SE.
M2 = After second week, M3 = after third week, M4 = after fourth week of maintenance dosing.
*$P < 0.05$ compared with placebo value.

Table II. Summary of standing blood pressure after subjects were titrated to an effective (diastolic blood pressure <85 mm Hg) or a maximum (30 mg b.i.d.) dose of losulazine

	Systolic blood pressure (mm Hg)		*Diastolic blood pressure (mm Hg)*	
Visit	*Placebo*	*Losulazine*	*Placebo*	*Losulazine*
Baseline	143.3 ± 2.51	147.7 ± 2.50	98.5 ± 0.86	99.6 ± 0.94
M2	138.2 ± 2.18	134.1 ± 3.29	93.8 ± 1.87	85.0 ± 1.94*
M3	134.0 ± 2.69	127.3 ± 3.64	93.5 ± 2.31	84.3 ± 1.94*
M4	137.0 ± 2.44	134.6 ± 4.45	93.2 ± 2.10	84.7 ± 2.34†

Data are $\overline{X}$ ± SE.
M2 = After second week, M3 = after third week, M4 = after fourth week of maintenance dosing.
*$P < 0.05$, †$P < 0.01$ compared with placebo values.

Table III. Summary of supine heart rate after subjects were titrated to an effective (diastolic blood pressure <85 mm Hg) or a maximum (30 mg b.i.d.) dose of losulazine

	Supine heart rate (bpm)		*Standing heart rate (bpm)*	
Visit	*Placebo*	*Losulazine*	*Placebo*	*Losulazine*
Baseline	71.7 ± 1.89	73.9 ± 1.12	77.4 ± 1.87	81.1 ± 1.30
M2	74.0 ± 2.06	70.3 ± 1.37	80.0 ± 2.15	76.7 ± 1.32
M3	70.7 ± 1.62	69.1 ± 1.49	79.3 ± 1.58	76.3 ± 1.78
M4	69.7 ± 1.45	70.4 ± 1.50	75.5 ± 1.64	77.9 ± 1.76

Data are $\overline{X}$ ± SE.
M2 = After second week, M3 = after third week, M4 = after fourth week of maintenance dosing.

(28.6%) took 50 mg/day, and seven (50.0%) took the maximum dose of 60 mg/day. In the placebo group, two (16.7%) took 50 mg/day and 10 (83.3%) took the maximum dose of 60 mg/day.

DISCUSSION

Decreasing the blood pressure of patients with hypertension reduces morbidity and mortality.[1,2,6] This is especially important in the treatment of mild to moderate hypertension, because this tends to be an asymptomatic disease in most patients. Most, if not all, of the present antihypertensive drugs exert side effects[4] or are inconvenient because of their short duration of activity. It is important to find drugs that not only effectively reduce blood pressure but also have few side effects.

Losulazine effectively lowered the blood pressure in patients with hypertension, decreasing mean diastolic blood pressure in the supine and standing positions. The change in diastolic blood pressure from pretreatment levels was much greater (two to three times) in the subjects who received losulazine, and the hypertension in most (71% to 86%) of these subjects was effectively controlled. The reduction in diastolic blood pressure persisted throughout the 4 weeks of the maintenance phase.

Table IV. Number of subjects reporting adverse drug reactions

	Placebo (n = 16)	*Losulazine (n = 16)*
Body as a whole		
Asthenia	1	2
Headache	(2) 1	2
Cardiovascular system		
Flushed		1
Palpitations	(2)	
Digestive system		
Diarrhea		1
Nervous system		
Dizziness	(1)	(1)
Paresthesia	(1)	2
Tremor		1
Respiratory system		
Nasal stuffiness	1	3
Special senses		
Conjunctival congestion		3
Eye pain		1
Pruritus (itchy eyes)		1

Subjects with mild to moderate hypertension were titrated to an effective dose or the maximum of 60 mg/day. Treatment ranged from 5 to 9 weeks. Numbers in parenthesis are side effects reported before the subject received the medication.

Despite a significant decrease in blood pressure, there was no evidence of reflex tachycardia. To the contrary, the heart rate decreased in the subjects who received losulazine. The decrease in heart rate was significant when compared with pretreatment values, but not when compared with the placebo group. The decrease in blood pressure associated with a decrease in heart rate is probably related to the mechanism of action of losulazine. Although this combination of clinical effects can occur with other antihypertensive drugs, it is usually associated with either an increase in peripheral vascular resistance or an effect on the central nervous system. Losulazine appears to modulate the sympathetic nervous system. It decreased arterial blood pressure but did not compromise the ability of the sympathetic nervous system to respond to orthostatic changes, in accord with results in animals.[5] We dosed losulazine twice a day, but substantial evidence from animal studies indicates that a single daily dose may be feasible.

Reported side effects occurred more frequently in the subjects who received losulazine, but most were well tolerated and did not seem to interfere with normal activities. It appears that nasal stuffiness and conjunctival congestion may be drug related, but other side effects occurred with such low frequency that it is difficult to determine which, if any, are drug related. The observation that body weight did not change is encouraging, suggesting that a diuretic may not be needed to control fluid retention. However, the duration of the study was relatively short and longer studies will be needed for confirmation.

New antihypertensive drugs must be effective, convenient, and exert minimal side effects. Losulazine appears to fulfill these requirements, since it possesses efficacy in this patient population without reflex tachycardia or major limiting side effects.

References

1. Hypertension Detection and Follow-up Program Cooperative Group: Five-year findings of the Hypertension Detection and Follow-up Program. JAMA **247:**633, 1982.
2. Kaplan NM: Therapy for mild hypertension. JAMA **249:**365, 1983.
3. National Adverse Drug Reaction Directory: COSTART: Coding Symbols for Thesaurus of Adverse Reaction Terms. Rockville, Md, Food and Drug Administration.
4. Rahn KA: Frequency and significance of side effects of antihypertensive drugs. Cardiovasc Rev Reports **4:**517, 1982.
5. Wendling MG, DuCharme DW, Johnson GA, McCall RB, Pals DT: U-54,669F, A novel hypotensive agent. Fed Proc **42:**162, 1983.
6. W.H.O./I.S.H. Mild Hypertension Liaison Committee: Trials of the treatment of mild hypertension. Lancet **1:**149, 1982.

Enalaprilat, an intravenous angiotensin-converting enzyme inhibitor, in hypertensive crises

The effect of enalaprilat (MK-422), a newly synthesized, intravenous, nonsulfhydryl, angiotensin-converting enzyme inhibitor, was studied in seven patients with either severe or malignant hypertension. All subjects initially received a 1 mg bolus injection of enalaprilat followed in 30 minutes by 10 mg. Five subjects received an additional 40 mg. Mean (±SE) pretreatment blood pressure for the group was 226 ± 9/141 ± 7 mm Hg. Five minutes after the 1 mg enalaprilat dose, blood pressure decreased to 211 ± 10/131 ± 9 mm Hg and further fell to 201 ± 14/123 ± 11 mm Hg at 30 minutes. The maximal reduction in blood pressure to 169 ± 14/112 ± 10 mm Hg occurred 30 minutes after the 10 mg dose. No further blood pressure reduction was observed in those subjects who received the additional 40 mg dose. Within the entire group, five subjects exhibited sustained blood pressure reduction. No adverse side effects or symptomatic hypotension occurred in any subject. (CLIN PHARMACOL THER 38:199-204, 1985.)

Donald J. DiPette, M.D.,* James C. Ferraro, D.O., Robert R. Evans, Pharm.D., and Marcus Martin, M.D. *Pittsburgh, Pa.*

Captopril, an angiotensin-converting enzyme inhibitor, has been successful in reducing blood pressure in several hypertensive settings, including hypertensive emergencies.[3,4,11,26] Captopril can only be administered orally, and has been associated with adverse side effects such as rash, taste disturbances, proteinuria, and leukopenia.[24] It has been postulated that these effects may be related to the sulfhydryl moiety of captopril.[27] Enalapril, a recently developed oral angiotensin-converting enzyme inhibitor that contains no sulfhydryl group, has been shown to be effective in the treatment of hypertension.[13,25] Enalapril is converted to the biologically active diacid enalaprilat (MK-422) in the liver. This active diacid may be parenterally administered. When administered intravenously, enalaprilat has been found to reduce blood pressure in normal subjects.[23] It was our purpose to evaluate the efficacy of acute intravenous enalaprilat administration in patients with severe and malignant hypertension.

From the Department of Medicine, Allegheny-Singer Research Institute and Departments of Medicine, Pharmacy, and Surgery, Allegheny General Hospital.

Received for publication Feb. 7, 1985; accepted April 17, 1985.

Reprint requests to: Dr. Donald J. DiPette, Department of Medicine, Allegheny-Singer Research Institute, Allegheny General Hospital, 320 E. North Ave., Pittsburgh, PA 15212.

*Research activities partially funded by Allegheny-Singer Research Institute and the Pennsylvania Heart Association.

METHODS

Our subjects were seven patients (five blacks and two whites) aged 37 to 74 years with severe hypertension who presented to our Emergency Department. One subject was studied twice, with a 1-month interval between tests. To enter the study, each patient had to have either a supine diastolic blood pressure (BP) $\geq$130 mm Hg or a supine diastolic BP $\geq$110 mm Hg with encephalopathy, retinal hemorrhages or exudates, papilledema, or evidence of congestive heart failure after a rest period of at least 30 minutes in a quiet room (Table I). Patients with a recent (6-month) history of myocardial infarction or a cerebral vascular accident, known bilateral renal artery stenosis, a serum creatinine level $>$3.5 mg/dl, eclampsia, valvular heart disease, suspected pheochromocytoma, aortic dissection, or unstable angina were excluded from study. The following baseline laboratory test values were determined: plasma renin activity, 12-lead ECG, chest x-ray, complete blood count and differential, urinalysis, BUN, serum creatinine, serum electrolytes, blood glucose, serum cholesterol, alkaline phosphatase, SGOT, total bilirubin, serum uric acid, creatinine phosphokinase, and lactate dehydrogenase. Except for the chest x-ray and plasma renin activity, these tests were repeated 24 hours after the start of enalaprilat therapy in all subjects.

After baseline determinations, all subjects received 1 mg enalaprilat by intravenous bolus injection, fol-

Table I. Subject characteristics

Subject No.	*Age (yr)*	*Sex*	*Weight (kg)*	*Race*	*Previous anti-hypertensive therapy*	*Pretreatment serum creatinine (mg/dl)*	*Pretreatment renin activity (ng/ml/hr)*	*Baseline BP (mm Hg)*	*Complications*
1	69	M	84.5	W	DY, MD, PR	1.3	26.3	207/122	Hemorrhages, exudates
2	74	F	74	B	AT, MI, PR, CH	2.1	—	260/111	Encephalopathy, CHF
3	40	M	86	W	—	1.7	60.0	201/151	Encephalopathy, papilledema
4	37	M	91	B	—	1.0	0.3	249/150	None
5a*	42	F	46	B	—	1.7	1.5	244/147	Papilledema
5b*	42	F	46	B	HCT, CL	1.1	12.2	239/175	Papilledema
6	62	M	55	B	PP, ISO	1.1	0.5	193/130	Encephalopathy
7	60	M	66	B	—	1.2	0.3	222/140	None

M = Male; W = white; DY = dyazide; MD = methyldopa; PR = prazosin; F = female; B = black; AT = atenolol; MI = minoxidil; CH = chlorthalidone; CHF = congestive heart failure; HCT = hydrochlorothiazide; CL = clonidine; PP = propranolol; ISO = isosorbide.
*Same subject studied on two separate occasions.

lowed in 30 minutes by 10 mg. Thirty minutes after the 10 mg dose, four subjects received an additional 40 mg. Baseline BP and heart rate were recorded as the average of three readings before the start of enalaprilat dosing, each taken 10 minutes apart. BP and heart rate were determined in the supine position by a third-party observer 5, 10, 15, and 30 minutes after the infusion of each new dosage level of enalaprilat. All BP measurements were taken with a standard mercury sphygmomanometer. After the study, subjects were classified by diastolic BP response to enalaprilat as follows: (1) Complete responders, a diastolic BP of ≤100 mm Hg; (2) partial responders, a sustained decrease of ≥20 mm Hg; (3) nonresponders. Complete responders continued receiving intravenous enalaprilat every 6 to 12 hours for the next 24 to 48 hours, at which time they were converted to oral enalapril, 10 to 20 mg b.i.d. When further BP control was necessary, a diuretic was added.

All data are expressed as the $\overline{X} \pm$ SE. Where indicated, the correlation coefficient was determined by the least-squares method.

RESULTS

The baseline BP for the seven subjects was 226 ± 9/141 ± 7 mm Hg. Within 5 minutes after 1 mg enalaprilat, BP decreased to 211 ± 10/131 ± 9 mm Hg. BP continued to decrease to 194 ± 12/124 ± 9 mm Hg at 15 minutes, but rose to 201 ± 14/123 ± 11 mm Hg at 30 minutes after the 1 mg dose. After 10 mg, BP again decreased within 5 minutes to 194 ± 11/118 ± 10 mm Hg. The maximal reduction in BP (169 ± 14/112 ± 10 mm Hg) occurred 30 minutes after the 10 mg dose. In the five subjects who received an additional 40 mg, no further BP reduction was observed (Fig. 1). Individual BP responses are shown in Table II.

The baseline heart rate for the group was 96 ± 5 bpm. Despite immediate BP reduction in response to enalaprilat injection, no increase in heart rate was observed in the group as a whole or in any individual (Fig. 1).

Three subjects (nos. 1, 2, and 3) achieved a complete response, two (nos. 4 and 5a) had a partial response, and three (nos. 5b, 6, and 7) were nonresponders (Table II). In the complete response group, the average maximal decrease in diastolic BP was 48 mm Hg. This maximal response occurred 30 minutes after the 10 mg dose of enalaprilat. In the partial response group, the maximal decrease in diastolic BP occurred 30 minutes after the 40 mg dose, with an average reduction of 33 mm Hg. In the nonresponder group, there was a maximal decrease of 19 mm Hg in diastolic BP, but this effect was not sustained. In both the partial and nonresponder groups, the 40 mg dose failed to induce further significant BP reduction. The response pattern for systolic BP was similar.

The maximal reduction in both systolic and diastolic BPs correlated with the pretreatment plasma renin activity (r = 0.82, slope = 0.81, intercept = −18.26; and r = 0.87, slope = 0.59, intercept = −18.34, respectively). Although marked reduction in BP occurred in three patients, no adverse reactions or signs or symptoms of hypotension were observed. After 24 to 48 hours of intravenous enalaprilat, the three complete responders were converted to oral enalapril. Two of three remained normotensive with enalapril, 10 mg b.i.d., while the third required oral furosemide, 80 mg

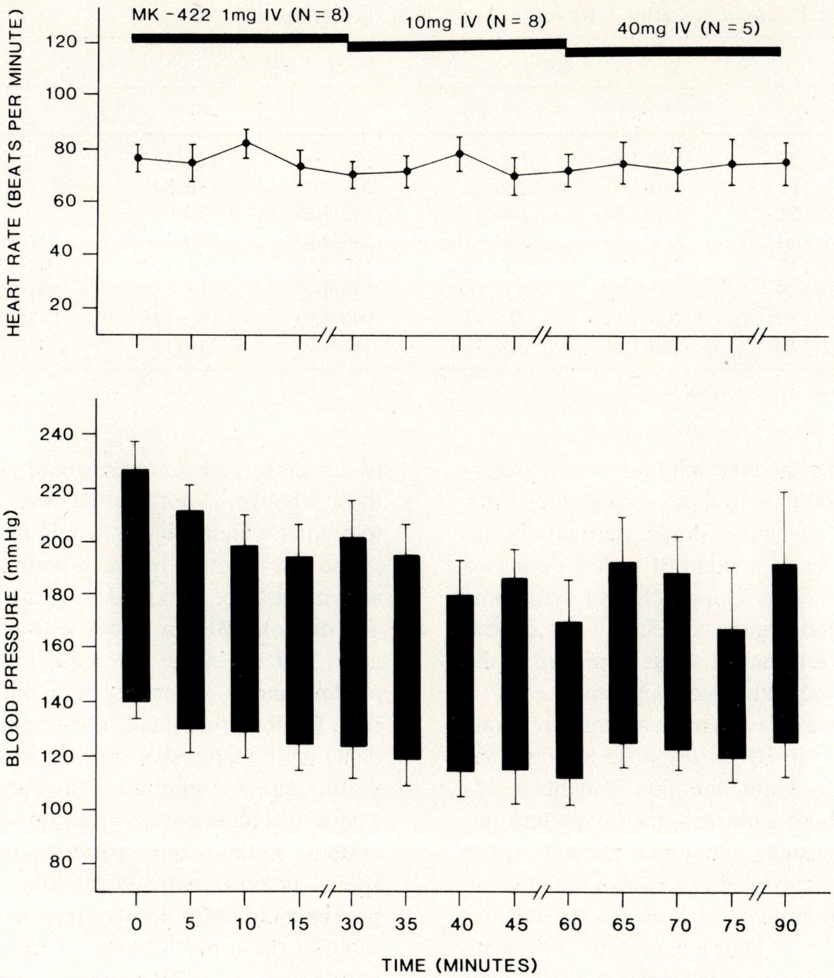

Fig. 1. Average heart rate and systolic and diastolic BP before (time 0) and after enalaprilat *(MK-422)* administration at increasing dosages.

b.i.d., in addition to enalapril, 20 mg b.i.d. The partial and nonresponders received conventional antihypertensive agents after acute enalaprilat dosing.

DISCUSSION

Inhibition of the renin-angiotensin system by blockade of angiotensin-converting enzyme with either parenteral teprotide or oral captopril has been successful in lowering BP both in severe hypertension and in hypertensive crises.[3,6,7,21,22] Our results with enalaprilat, an intravenous nonsulfhydryl angiotensin-converting enzyme inhibitor, further support these observations.

In our study, five of seven subjects with markedly elevated BP (with one being studied on two separate occasions) responded with a reduction in both systolic and diastolic BP within the first hour of enalaprilat. Four of the five subjects who responded had hypertensive encephalopathy or papilledema. Both of these conditions require a rapid reduction in BP, usually by parenteral antihypertensive drugs; however, the rate and extent of BP reduction is still a matter of controversy. One subject (no. 1) returned to normotensive BP levels within minutes after receiving the 1 mg dose. This sudden BP change is disturbing in light of recent reports associating such decreases in BP in patients with malignant hypertension to cerebral ischemia as well as blindness.[9,17] These reports suggest that initial therapy in such patients should aim for a more gradual reduction in BP rather than immediate normalization.

Both enalapril and captopril have been reported to either maintain or improve blood flow to vital organs such as the brain, heart, and kidneys.[1,10,12,18,20] Because

Table II. Individual BP responses after intravenous injection of enalaprilat

Subject No.	Baseline BP (mm Hg)	1 mg		10 mg		40 mg	
		5 min	30 min	5 min	30 min	5 min	30 min
1	207/122	180/100	116/64	132/70	118/73		
2	206/111	250/100	226/92	200/94	186/84		
3	201/151	176/130	160/112	152/100	130/96		
4	249/150	228/130	222/158	234/140	200/120	222/112	210/110
5a*	244/147	214/138	226/136	210/128	198/122	198/126	188/120
5b*	239/175	242/178	222/160	222/162	210/160	204/152	225/170
6	193/130	200/134	210/134	190/120	180/110	172/120	170/118
7	222/140	200/134	224/130	210/130	210/130	204/128	202/130

*Same subject studied on two separate occasions.

angiotensin-converting enzyme inhibitors may preferentially preserve blood flow to these organs, they offer a distinct advantage over other drugs, particularly the direct vasodilators. Despite a rapid BP reduction in two of our subjects, neither developed clinical symptoms referable to these vital organs, especially the central nervous system. In fact, mental status improved in the subjects who presented with encephalopathy.

Patients with elevated plasma renin activity are prone to a marked decrease in BP in response to acute angiotensin-converting enzyme inhibition. Patients in this population include those with malignant hypertension, renovascular hypertension, and those already taking concomitant antihypertensive drugs known to stimulate the renin-angiotensin system, such as direct vasodilators and diuretics.[4,5,11,14,19] Thus angiotensin-converting enzyme inhibitors including enalaprilat must be used with caution in such patients. If a marked BP decrease occurs or symptoms develop, BP may be supported by intravenous saline solution or similar fluid administration. Two of our subjects who had the most pronounced response to enalaprilat were reported to have been receiving previous diuretic therapy.

Recent studies have drawn attention to the use of angiotensin-converting enzyme inhibitors in patients with severe bilateral renal artery stenosis and unilateral stenosis in a solitary kidney. In such patients the use of angiotensin-converting enzyme inhibitors has led to abrupt deterioration in renal function, which is thought to result from inhibition of intrarenal angiotensin-2.[2,15] However, other antihypertensive agents have also been shown to result in rapid renal deterioration in similar patients.[28] Because these patients are rarely known before the start of the emergency antihypertensive procedures, caution is advised when using any antihypertensive agent, including enalaprilat, in this setting.

Since not all of our seven subjects responded to enalaprilat, it would be advantageous to discriminate between those patients who would possibly respond and those who would not. The BP level alone did not appear to predict which subjects would respond. However, we found a correlation between pretreatment plasma renin activity and the maximal decrease in both the systolic and diastolic BPs in response to enalaprilat. This suggests that the acute BP reduction after enalaprilat is predominantly secondary to renin-angiotensin inhibition. On the other hand, non–renin-angiotensin dependent, antihypertensive mechanisms of action for converting enzyme inhibitors have also been suggested.[16] These mechanisms involve the sympathetic nervous system, kinins, and prostaglandins. The partial response noted in two subjects (nos. 4 and 5a) with low pretreatment renin activity may be attributed to one or more of these mechanisms. The two subjects with the most pronounced BP response were white, whereas the remaining subjects were black. It has previously been noted that blacks with hypertension have lower plasma renin activity, particularly if the hypertension is not in an accelerated or malignant phase.[8] Therefore, black patients presenting with just an elevated BP may be less likely to respond to angiotensin-converting enzyme inhibitors.

When used in patients similar to ours, the orally administered angiotensin-converting enzyme inhibitor captopril appears to initiate a BP decrease within 15 minutes, with a maximal decrease occurring 60 to 90 minutes after dosing.[7] In contrast to captopril, intravenous enalaprilat results in a significant BP decrease within minutes. The responding patient can then immediately be discerned and, of greater importance, the nonresponding patient can quickly be changed to alternate therapy. Enalaprilat appears to be extremely potent, as two of our subjects exhibited a marked BP response to 1 mg. On the other hand, 10 mg appeared to be a maximal dose, since the subjects who went on to receive 40 mg had no further BP reduction. Because our initial study was conducted only to determine enalaprilat's effect on BP, further investigations are necessary to determine optimal dosage recommendations. In addition to its rapid onset of action, the parenteral availability of enalaprilat also offers advantages for those patients who present in a lethargic or comatose state or are otherwise unable to take oral medications.

In the responding patients, the effect of enalaprilat on BP administered by intravenous bolus persisted for up to 12 hours. Since enalapril is the parent compound of enalaprilat, the patient can be converted to an oral angiotensin-converting enzyme inhibitor when clinically indicated, as was done in a subset of our subjects. Both enalaprilat and enalapril are nonsulfhydryl-containing compounds. It has been speculated that the sulfhydryl moiety of captopril may be responsible for some of its side effects.[27] Thus the use of enalaprilat and enalapril may not induce similar effects.

In conclusion, enalaprilat given as a bolus injection can rapidly lower BP in patients with severe hypertension without apparent adverse side effects. The mechanism of action by which enalaprilat acutely lowers BP is presumed to be renin-angiotensin inhibition. While patients with the highest plasma renin activity are expected to respond best to enalaprilat, further studies will be necessary to determine the optimal dose.

We thank Debbie Haymaker and Keith Little for illustrations and the Allegheny General Hospital Housestaff for their assistance.

References

1. Bauer JH: Role of angiotensin converting enzyme inhibitors in essential and renal hypertension. Am J Med **77:**43-51, 1984.
2. Bender W, Lafrance N, Walker G: Mechanism of deterioration in renal function in patients with renovascular hypertension treated with enalapril. Hypertension **6**(suppl 1):193-197, 1984.
3. Biollaz J, Waeber B, Brunner HR: Hypertensive crisis treatment with orally administered captopril. Eur J Clin Pharmacol **25:**245-259, 1983.
4. Bravo EL, Tarazi RC: Converting enzyme inhibition with an orally active compound in hypertensive man. Hypertension **1:**39-46, 1979.
5. Case D, Atlas SA, Laragh JH, Sealey JE, Sullivan PA, McKinstry DN: Clinical experience with blockade of the renin-angiotensin-aldosterone system by an oral converting enzyme inhibitor in hypertensive patients. Prog Cardiovasc Dis **21:**195-206, 1978.
6. Case DB, Atlas SA, Laragh JH, Sealey JE, Sullivan PA, McKinstry DN: Clinical experience with blockade of the renin-angiotensin-aldosterone system by an oral converting-enzyme inhibitor (SQ14255, captopril) in hypertensive patients. Prog Cardiovasc Dis **21:**195-206, 1978.
7. Case DB, Atlas SA, Sullivan PA, Laragh JH: Acute and chronic treatment of severe and malignant hypertension with the oral angiotensin-converting enzyme inhibitor captopril. Circulation **64:**765-771, 1981.
8. Chrysant SG, Danisa K, Dem DC, Smith WJ, Dillard BL, Frohlich ED: Racial differences in pressure, volume and renin inter-relationships in essential hypertension. Hypertension **1:**136-141, 1979.
9. Cover DH, Seddon M, Fletcher RF, Dukes DC: Blindness after treatment for malignant hypertension. Br Med J **3:**245-246, 1979.
10. Creager MA, Halperin JL, Bernard DB, Faxon DP, Melidossian CS, Gavras H, Ryan TJ: Acute regional circulatory and renal hemodynamic effects of converting enzyme inhibition in patients with congestive heart failure. Circulation **64:**483-489, 1981.
11. Gavras H, Brunner HR, Turnini GA, Kershaw GR, Tifft CP, Cuttelod S, Gavras I, Vukovich RA, McKinstry DN: Antihypertensive effect of the oral angiotensin converting enzyme inhibitor SQ14255 in man. N Engl J Med **298:**991-995, 1978.
12. Gavras H, Liang CS, Brunner HR: Redistribution of regional blood flow after inhibition of the angiotensin-converting enzyme. Circ Res **43**(suppl 1):I59-62, 1978.
13. Gavras H, Waeber B, Gavras I, Biollaz J, Brunner HR, Davies RO: Antihypertensive effect of the new oral angiotensin converting enzyme inhibitor MK-421. Lancet **2:**543-546, 1981.
14. Havelka J, Vetter H, Studer A, Greminger P, Luscher T, Wollnik S, Siegenthaler N, Vetter W: Acute and chronic effects of the angiotensin converting enzyme inhibitor captopril in severe hypertension. Am J Cardiol **49:**1462-1474, 1982.
15. Hricik DE, Browning PJ, Kopelman R, Goorno WE, Madias NE, Dzau VJ: Captopril-induced functional renal insufficiency in patients with bilateral renal artery stenosis or renal artery stenosis in a solitary kidney. N Engl J Med **308:**373-376, 1983.
16. Johnston CI, Jackson B, Cubela R, Arnolda L: Mechanism for hypotensive action of angiotensin converting enzyme inhibitors. Clin Exp Hypertens [A] **142:**551-561, 1984.
17. Ledingham JG, Rajagopalan B: Cerebral complications in the treatment of accelerated hypertension. Quart J Med **48:**25-41, 1979.
18. Maskin C, Chadwick B, Ocken S, LeJemiel T: Comparative effects of dopamine therapy and angiotensin converting enzyme inhibition with MK-422 on cardiac and renal hemodynamics in heart failure. Circulation **64:**569, 1983.
19. Millar JA, McGrath BP, Matthews PG, Johnston CE: Acute effects of captopril on blood pressure and circulating hormonal levels in salt-replete and depleted normal subjects and essential hypertensive patients. Clin Sci **61:**75-83, 1981.

20. Mimran A, Brunner HR, Turini GA, Waeber B, Brunner DB: Effects of captopril on renal vascular tone in normal subjects and in patients with essential hypertension. Clin Sci **57**(suppl):421-423, 1979.
21. Saragoca MA, Homsi E, Ribeiro A, Filho SR, Ramos O: Hemodynamic mechanism of blood pressure response to captopril in human malignant hypertension. Hypertension **5**(suppl 1):I53-58, 1983.
22. Tifft CP, Gavras H, Kershaw GR, Gavras I, Brunner HR, Liange CS, Chobanian AV: Converting enzyme inhibition in hypertensive emergencies. Ann Intern Med **90:**43-47, 1979.
23. Till AE, Irvin JD, Hichens M, Lee RB, Davies RO, Swanson B, Vlasses PH: Pharmacodynamics and disposition of intravenous MK-422, the diacid metabolite of enalapril maleate. CLIN PHARMACOL THER **31:**275, 1982.
24. Vidt DG, Bravo EL, Fouad FM: Captopril. N Engl J Med **306:**214-219, 1982.
25. Vlasses PH, Rotmensch HH, Swanson BN, Lee RB, Koplin JR, Ferguson RF: Comparative antihypertensive effects of enalapril maleate and hydrochlorothiazide, alone and in combination. J Clin Pharmacol **23:**227-233, 1983.
26. Vlasses PH, Rotmensch HH, Swanson BN, Mojaverian P, Ferguson F: Low-dose captopril: Its use in mild to moderate hypertension unresponsive to diuretic treatment. Arch Intern Med **142:**1098-1101, 1982.
27. Waeber B, Gavras I, Brunner HR, Gavras H: Safety and efficacy of chronic therapy with captopril in hypertensive patients: An update. J Clin Pharmacol **21:**508-516, 1981.
28. Ying CY, Tifft CP, Gavras H, Chobanian AV: Renal revascularization in the azotemic hypertensive patient resistant to therapy. N Engl J Med **311:**1070-1075, 1984.

Felodipine kinetics in healthy men

In a randomized, crossover study, the absorption, distribution, and elimination of intravenous and oral felodipine were investigated in eight healthy men 22 to 31 years old. Felodipine was given as a 2.5 mg iv infusion over 30 minutes and as a 27.5 mg oral solution. Both doses were labeled with 25 μCi ^{14}C-felodipine. Given as an oral solution, felodipine is rapidly (mean time to peak concentration 64 minutes; range 30 to 90 minutes) and completely absorbed. Presystemic elimination reduced the availability to 16% (range 10% to 25%). Felodipine kinetics can be described by a multicompartmental model with three distinct phases. The $t_{1/2}$ for the initial phase was 6.4 minutes (range 1.7 to 10.4 minutes) and felodipine was distributed to a volume of 0.6 L/kg (range 0.4 to 0.9 L/kg), which approximately corresponds to the total body water. The second distribution phase reached pseudoequilibrium with a $t_{1/2}$ of 1.6 hours (range 1.3 to 2.2 hours). The volume of distribution at the end of this phase was 9.7 L/kg (range 6.0 to 18.2 L/kg). The terminal phase had $t_{1/2}$ of 10.2 hours (range 6.7 to 20.7 hours). The contribution of the three phases to the AUC was 15%, 40%, and 45% in the order of increased $t_{1/2}$. Total body clearance of felodipine was 1.2 L/min (range 0.9 to 1.6 L/min). Within 72 hours after drug dosing, 62% to 81% of the felodipine doses were excreted in the urine and feces as metabolites. The rate of excretion by the kidneys had a biphasic pattern, with $t_{1/2}$ values of 4 and 18 hours. Approximately 10% of the doses was excreted in the feces. (Clin Pharmacol Ther 38:205-211, 1985.)

Boo Edgar, B.Sc., C. G. Regårdh, Ph.D., G. Johnsson, M.D., Ph.D., L. Johansson, B.Sc., P. Lundborg, M.D., Ph.D., I. Löfberg, M.Sc., and O. Rönn, M.D., Ph.D. *Mölndal and Göteborg, Sweden*

In recent years calcium antagonists have been increasingly used in essential hypertension.[4,5,13] Felodipine (see structure) is a new dihydropyridine that appears to interfere with intracellular calcium utilization in vascular smooth muscle.[6] In vitro experiments have shown that felodipine has a direct and selective relaxing effect on smooth muscle cells, especially those of resistance vessels.[12] The vasodilating effect of felodipine in healthy subjects decreases systemic vascular resistance and diastolic blood pressure, increases cardiac output, and induces reflex increases in heart rate.[11,15] Felodipine markedly reduces both diastolic and systolic blood pressures in patients with hypertension, both acutely and after long-term use.[1,7,10] Furthermore, it seems to be effective in angina pectoris[8,9] and cardiac failure.[16]

Our objective was to investigate the absorption and disposition characteristics of felodipine in healthy men after acute intravenous and oral administration.

From Research Laboratories, AB Hässle, Mölndal, and Department of Medicine, University of Göteborg, Östra Hospital, Göteborg.
Received for publication Nov. 18, 1984; accepted April 21, 1985.
Reprint requests to: Boo Edgar, B.Sc., Research Laboratories, AB Hässle, Mölndal, Sweden.

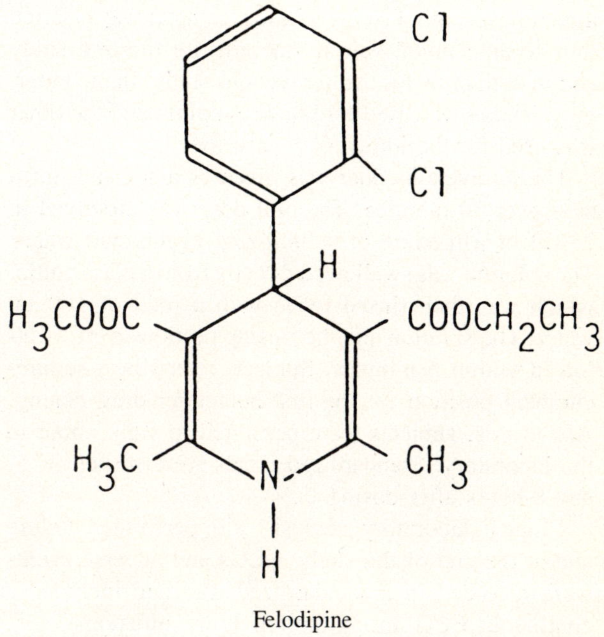

Felodipine

METHODS

Our subjects were eight healthy men between 22 and 31 years old ($\overline{X}$ = 25 years). Mean weight was 74 kg (range 69 to 82 kg) and all subjects were within 10% of their ideal body weight. The experiment was an open,

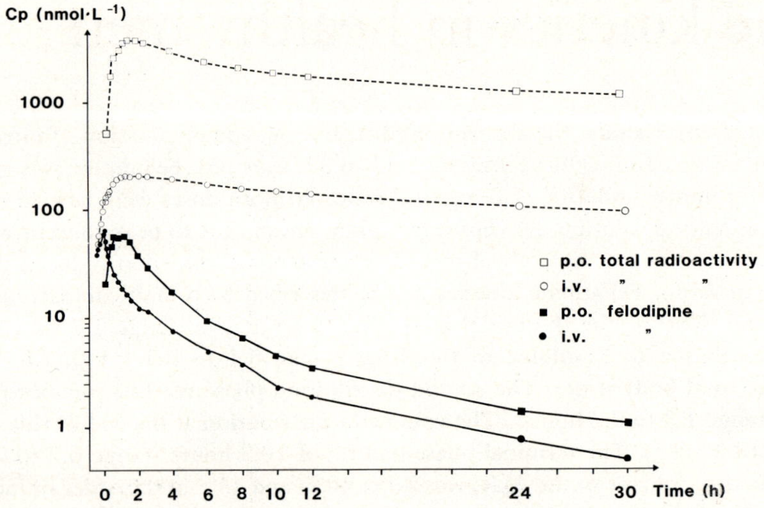

Fig. 1. Mean plasma levels of unchanged felodipine and total radioactivity after 2.5 mg iv ^{14}C-felodipine and 27.5 mg po ^{14}C-felodipine.

randomized, two-way, crossover study in which felodipine was given as a 2.5 mg iv infusion over 30 minutes or as a 27.5 mg oral solution on separate days. Both doses contained 25 μCi ^{14}C-labeled drug. The doses were given on 2 days separated by at least 2 weeks. Subjects arrived at the laboratory about 8 AM after an overnight fast. A veinflow catheter was inserted into an antecubital vein in one arm for the oral study and in both arms for the intravenous study. In the latter, one catheter was used for blood sampling and the other was used for the intravenous infusion.

The intravenous dose was given as a constant infusion over 30 minutes. The oral dose was dissolved in 25 ml of a mixture of solubilizing agents and water. The solution was swallowed directly from a glass bottle, which was then rinsed twice with a total of 100 ml water. The solution and the rinsing portions were swallowed within 5 minutes. Subjects rested in a semirecumbent position for the first hour after drug dosing. Afterwards, subjects were permitted to walk about in the laboratory. Standardized meals were served 3, 5, and 8 hours after dosing.

Clinical laboratory analysis was performed before and at the end of the study. ECGs and adverse events were recorded in a standardized way and included a continuous ECG during the felodipine infusions.

Serial 10 ml blood samples were drawn from an antecubital vein at specified times up to 30 hours after drug dosing. Sampling times were −50, −25, −20, −15, −10, −5, 0, 3, 6, 10, 15, 30, 45, 60, 75, and 90 minutes and 2, 2.5, 4, 6, 8, 10, 12, 24, and 30 hours in the intravenous study and −5, 15, 30, 45, 60, 75, and 90 minutes and 2, 2.5, 4, 6, 8, 10, 12, 24, and 30 hours in the oral study. Zero time is equal to the end of the 30-minute infusion or the intake of the oral dose. After separation of the plasma, samples were kept frozen until analyzed.

Urine was quantitatively collected for 72 hours at the following times: blank, 0 to 4, 4 to 8, 8 to 12, 12 to 24, 24 to 36, 36 to 48, 48 to 60, and 60 to 72 hours. Urine samples were weighed and appropriate volumes (25 ml) were kept frozen until analysis. Feces were collected in 24-hour portions up to 72 hours after drug dosing.

The concentrations of felodipine in plasma and urine were determined by gas chromatography with electron capture detection after extraction with toluene. The method is selective and interference with endogenous plasma substances is low. The within-run reproducibility of spiked samples was 4% to 8% (relative standard deviation) at the 2 nmol/L level. In low concentration samples (0.5 to 2 nmol/L), mean day-to-day reproducibility was ±0.25 nmol/L (standard deviation). The samples can be stored for at least 5 months at −20° C without significant degradation.[2]

Total radioactivity in the plasma and excreta was determined by liquid scintillation counting. Before the measurements, the plasma and urine were diluted twice with water. Ten milliliters Insta-Gel (Packard Instrument Co., Inc.) was added to 1 ml diluted plasma and urine before counting. Each feces sample was diluted with an equal amount of water and homogenized. Of

Table I. Felodipine disposition characteristics after 2.5 mg iv infused over 30 minutes

Subject No.	C_1 *(nmol/L)*	C_2 *(nmol/L)*	C_3 *(nmol/L)*	$t_{1/2\lambda_1}$ *(min)*	$t_{1/2\lambda_2}$ *(hr)*	$t_{1/2\lambda_3}$ *(hr)*	V_c *(L/kg)*	V_z *(L/kg)*	CL_p *(ml/min)*
1	110.0	29.8	4.3	8.5	1.3	8.8	0.55	7.7	811
2	174.0	26.8	6.7	3.5	1.6	7.9	0.39	6.0	709
3	150.0	18.1	1.6	6.5	2.6	20.7	0.51	18.2	780
4	84.6	26.4	4.5	5.9	1.2	8.3	0.76	9.3	960
5	76.3	19.2	4.3	7.9	1.2	8.4	0.94	12.1	1098
6	118.0	26.2	3.6	10.4	2.2	13.3	0.62	9.7	599
7	347.0	36.4	7.0	1.7	1.1	7.6	0.24	7.1	743
8	122.0	21.6	5.1	6.8	1.7	6.7	0.60	7.1	887
$\bar{X}$	147.7	25.56	4.64	6.40	1.61	10.21	0.576	9.65	823.4
SD	86.5	5.97	1.72	2.77	0.54	4.67	0.215	3.96	155.8

the homogenate, 0.1 to 0.2 gm was decolorized by addition of 0.2 ml concentrated $HClO_4$ and 0.2 ml concentrated H_2O_2. The mixture was heated for 30 minutes at 80° C. After the sample cooled to room temperature, 10 ml Insta-Gel was added and the radioactivity was determined by liquid scintillation counting.

The kinetic constants of the three-compartmental model were derived in each subject from the computer-fit triexponential function describing the plasma concentration-time curve after intravenous dosing.[3] Computer fitting was by the least-squares method on a VAX 11/780 computer (Digital Equipment Corp.) with the NONLIN program.[14] Data were weighted by their reciprocals. Total plasma clearance (CL_p) was calculated as: $CL_p = D_{iv}/(C_1/\lambda_1 + C_2/\lambda_2 + C_3\lambda_3)$, in which D is the intravenous dose infused, the denominator represents the AUC after intravenous dosing, and C is the coefficient and λ is the exponent of the computer-fit triexponential function of plasma concentration vs. time. The AUC after oral dosing was determined by the linear trapezoidal method over the interval 0 to 4 hours and by the "lin-log" trapezoidal method[17] between 4 and 30 hours. Extrapolation to infinity was done with use of the term: C_t/λ_3, in which C_t is the concentration in the last blood sample drawn. The felodipine $t_{1/2}$ after oral dosing was determined by regression analysis of individual data in the 4-to-30–hour interval by means of the NONLIN computer program.

Intrinsic hepatic plasma clearance (CL_{int}) was determined from the relationship: $CL_{int} = D_{po}/AUC_{po}$. This equation is valid provided the drug is completely absorbed and eliminated exclusively by metabolism in the liver (these are assumptions that are compatible with the results of our study). Systemic availability of the oral dose (F) was determined as: $F = (AUC_{po} \cdot D_{iv})/(AUC_{iv} \cdot D_{po})$. The fraction of the radioactive dose absorbed from the gastrointestinal tract was calculated from the above equation after replacement of the AUCs of unchanged felodipine by the corresponding AUCs of total radioactivity.

Student's t test for paired observations was used for comparisons between intravenous and oral data. Observed differences were accepted as statistically significant at $P < 0.05$.

RESULTS

The mean plasma concentration-time profile after intravenous dosing is shown in Fig. 1. After the end of the infusion, the felodipine concentration declined triexponentially in all eight subjects, indicating that the disposition might be best described by a three-compartment model. Individual and mean disposition characteristics of felodipine derived from the intravenous study are listed in Table I. The mean contributions of the three individual phases to the overall AUC were 15.1%, 39.5%, and 45.4%, respectively, in the order of increasing $t_{1/2}$.

The mean $t_{1/2}$ of the initial distribution phase ($t_{1/2\lambda_1}$) was 6.4 minutes (range 1.7 to 10.4 minutes) and the drug was initially distributed into a mean body space (V_c) of 0.58 L/kg (0.24 to 0.94 L/kg). The mean $t_{1/2}$ of the second phase ($t_{1/2\lambda_2}$), probably reflecting distribution to slowly equilibrating tissues, was 1.6 hours (range 1.1 to 2.2 hours). The volume of distribution in the terminal phase of the plasma concentration-time curve (V_z) was 9.7 L/kg (range 6.0 to 18.2 L/kg). The felodipine elimination $t_{1/2}$ in the terminal phase of the plasma concentration-time curve ($t_{1/2\lambda_3}$) was 10.2 hours (range 6.7 to 20.7 hours). CL_p as calculated from the intravenous dose was 823 ml/min (range 599 to 1098 ml/min).

The mean plasma concentration-time profile of felo-

Table II. Felodipine absorption and elimination characteristics after an oral dose of 27.5 mg

Subject No.	t_{max} *(min)*	C_{max} *(nmol/L)*	*F (%)*	$t_{1/2}$ *(hr)*	CL_{int} *(L/min)*
1	45	125	24.7	10.0	3.3
2	90	86	25.3	12.7	2.6
3	60	38	11.4	10.6	7.3
4	30	67	12.9	31.6	6.5
5	90	59	14.4	16.8	5.4
6	90	52	11.6	15.9	5.1
7	60	77	19.3	8.6	3.8
8	45	57	10.2	8.9	8.8
$\overline{X}$	63.8	70.1	16.2	14.4	5.3
SD	23.8	26.6	6.2	7.6	2.0

t_{max} = Time to reach maximum concentration; C_{max} = maximum concentration.

Table III. AUCs of the sum of unchanged felodipine and radioactive metabolites over a 30-hour period after intravenous and oral administration of 2.5 and 27.5 mg felodipine, respectively

Subject No.	AUC_{iv} *(μmol · hr/L)*	AUC_{po} *(μmol · hr/L)*	$(AUC_{po} \cdot D_{iv})/(AUC_{iv} \cdot D_{po})$
1	4.80	54.96	1.04
2	4.13	50.32	1.11
3	3.89	45.63	1.07
4	3.91	53.43	1.24
5	5.32	63.89	1.09
6	3.78	47.12	1.13
7	3.68	47.40	1.17
8	4.45	51.33	1.05
$\overline{X}$	4.25	51.70	1.11
SD	0.57	5.86	0.06

dipine after oral dosing is shown in Fig. 1. Individual and mean absorption and elimination characteristics are listed in Table II. Felodipine was rapidly absorbed after oral dosing. The mean time to reach peak plasma concentration was 63.8 minutes (range 30 to 90 minutes). The peak concentration was 70.1 nmol/L, with a threefold variation from 38 to 125 nmol/L. The average fraction of the oral dose available systemically was 16.2% (range 10.2% to 25.3%; Table II).

The concentrations of the total pool of radioactive metabolites in the plasma were substantially higher and declined more slowly than those of the parent drug both after intravenous and oral dosing (Fig. 1). At the end of the infusion, the ratio between the concentrations of radioactive metabolites and felodipine in the plasma was about 3:1. This ratio increased to about 200:1 at the end of the plasma sampling period 30 hours after dosing. For the oral dose the concentrations of the sum of the metabolites exceeded those of the parent drug by a factor 100 to 1000 over the entire period of blood sampling. The mean $t_{1/2}$ of the metabolites over the interval 10 to 30 hours was 28 hours (range 22 to 33 hours) after intravenous dosing; the $t_{1/2}$ over the same period after oral dosing was almost the same. Individual and mean AUC values of the total radioactivity in plasma over 30 hours after intravenous and oral dosing are listed in Table III. The mean ratio between the dose-corrected AUCs was 1.1 (range 1.0 to 1.2).

On average, approximately 70% (range 62.4% to 78.1%) of the intravenous radioactive dose was recovered in the urine during the first 72 hours after dosing. The corresponding urinary recovery after oral dosing was 62% (range 53.6% to 65.4%; Table IV). No unchanged felodipine was detected in any of the individual urine specimens collected in the two studies. The excretion rate of radioactive metabolites by the kidneys declined biexponentially (Fig. 2). Approximately 50% of the recovered radioactivity of the oral dose was excreted with a $t_{1/2}$ of about 4 hours. The $t_{1/2}$ of the remaining fraction was about 18 hours. After intravenous

Table IV. Excretion of total radioactivity (in percent of administered dose) in urine and feces over a 72-hour period after intravenous and oral administration of 2.5 and 27.5 mg ^{14}C-felodipine, respectively

Subject No.	*Urine*		*Feces*		*Urine and feces*	
	iv	*po*	*iv*	*po*	*iv*	*po*
1	62.4	53.6	5.8	8.5	68.2	62.1
2	68.3	62.0	7.9	6.7	76.2	68.7
3	72.9	64.0	11.6	12.9	84.4	76.9
4	70.4	63.9	13.9	11.4	84.4	75.3
5	78.1	63.3	12.3	6.6	90.5	69.9
6	71.2	62.8	13.7	12.3	84.9	75.1
7	69.6	65.4	14.1	11.9	83.7	77.3
8	65.8	61.9	9.8	8.3	75.6	70.2
$\bar{X}$	69.8	62.1	11.1	9.8	81.0	71.9
SD	4.8	3.7	3.1	2.5	7.1	5.1

dosing, the fast excretion phase accounted for about 70% of the amount ultimately recovered in the urine.

During the 3-day period feces were collected, an average fraction of 11% (range 5.8% to 14.1%) of the administered radioactive intravenous dose was excreted in the stools. After oral dosing the mean recovery was 9.8% (range 6.6% to 12.9%) for the same period.

Flushing and headache, both symptoms that might be attributed to the vasodilation induced by felodipine, were observed in or reported by all subjects. In most cases effects were mild and did not lead to withdrawal from the study. All ECGs recorded during the study were considered normal. Some clinical laboratory values were outside the laboratory's normal range, but none were considered to be of clinical significance.

DISCUSSION

Our data after oral dosing show that felodipine is relatively rapidly absorbed from the gastrointestinal tract when given as a solution. The average time to reach peak concentration is about 1 hour. The maximum concentration varied about threefold between subjects, suggesting moderate interindividual variation in drug plasma levels. This is supported by the twofold variation in the systemic availability we found. The reduction in systemic availability to 16% seems primarily to be an effect of presystemic elimination, as the mean ratio between the dose-corrected AUC_{30} of the total radioactivity of the oral and intravenous doses was close to 1.0 (Table III).

It might be argued that the ratio of the AUC_{0-30} values may not give a correct estimate of the systemic availability of the radioactive oral dose due to the considerable rest area beyond 30 hours. However, the ratio between the plasma concentrations of the total radioactivity at 30 hours was almost the same as the ratio between the doses. Furthermore, the $t_{1/2}$ of the total pool of radioactive metabolites was virtually the same in the two studies. The use of AUC_{0-30} instead of AUC will therefore result in approximately the same ratio.

Felodipine is extensively distributed to extravascular sites. The initially available body space (0.58 L/kg, accessible with a $t_{1/2}$ of about 6 minutes) is of the order of the total body water volume. Substantial redistribution occurs during the first few hours after dosing, resulting in an apparent volume of distribution at pseudoequilibrium of about 10 L/kg. This indicates that $<1\%$ of the total amount of the drug in the body is located in the blood during the terminal phase of the plasma concentration-time curve. The $t_{1/2}$ of the second distribution phase is about 1.5 hours.

The absence of felodipine in urine suggests that felodipine is eliminated almost entirely by metabolism. The drug is probably too extensively bound to plasma proteins and too lipophilic to be excreted by the kidneys. The average terminal $t_{1/2}$ is about 10 hours in young healthy subjects and CL_p is about 800 ml/min. Assuming a mean ratio of 0.68 between the concentration of felodipine in blood and plasma (a value derived in a separate study in three healthy subjects), the mean CL would be 1,210 ml/min. If felodipine is eliminated exclusively by the liver, this value is compatible with an extraction ratio of 0.81 based on a mean hepatic blood flow of 1.5 L/min. Almost the same extraction ratio (0.84) was derived from the mean systemic availability of felodipine. This further supports the hypothesis that felodipine is virtually completely taken up from the gastrointestinal tract and that the liver is the major site of presystemic elimination. Provided that felodipine equilibrates momentarily between plasma and the eryth-

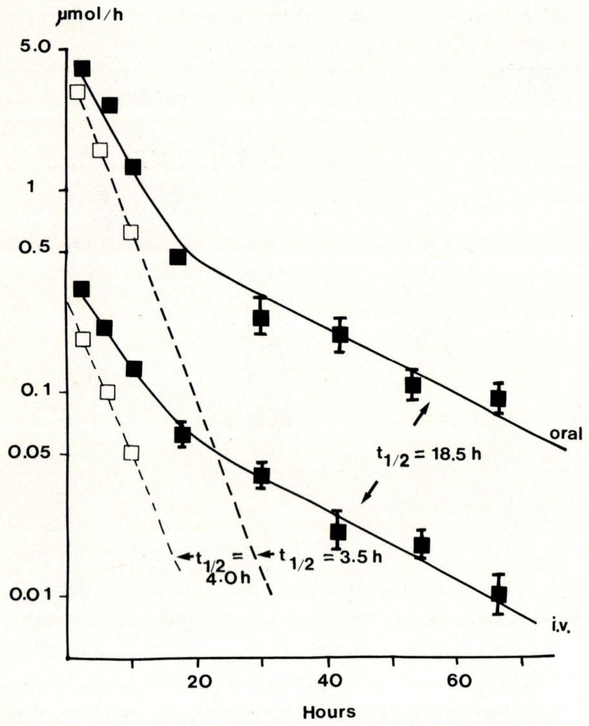

Fig. 2. Mean (± SE) urinary excretion rates of radioactive metabolites over 66 hours after 2.5 mg iv and 27.5 mg po ^{14}C-felodipine. *Open symbols* derived by feathering.

rocytes, the mean CL_{int} of felodipine is about 7.8 L/min (5.3/0.68 L/min), which expresses the liver's maximum capacity to clear felodipine at unlimited blood flow.

The terminal $t_{1/2}$ tended to be longer after oral dosing than after intravenous infusion. One subject eliminated felodipine extremely slowly after oral dosing ($t_{1/2}$ = 31.2 hours). The relatively low plasma levels during the terminal phase of the studies, however, make the determination of $t_{1/2}$ relatively uncertain in some subjects. Because the terminal phase appears at very low plasma concentrations, accumulation of felodipine during long-term therapy will only marginally affect peak concentrations, whereas the trough level might double if the drug is administered every 12 hours and the terminal $t_{1/2}$ is 12 hours. Because the effect of blood pressure is related to the felodipine plasma concentrations,[10] this will presumably lead to a more even effect on blood pressure during a dosing interval with repeated dosing than after a single dose.

The much higher plasma concentrations of radioactive metabolites than of the parent drug is a consequence of extensive metabolism and the much smaller volume of distribution of some of these metabolites than of felodipine. The plasma levels of the metabolites declined biexponentially in both studies, although the two phases were more distinct after oral dosing.

The 72-hour recovery of radioactive metabolites in the urine after intravenous dosing was in good agreement with previously reported urinary excretion of an oral radioactive dose of felodipine.[18] We found 62% of an oral dose in the urine over the same period of time, which is lower than in another study.[18] This might to some extent be due to missed urine collection, as indicated by excretion rate data. It seems unlikely, however, that careless sampling would be the only factor behind the lower recovery of the oral dose. Potentially, a greater fraction of the oral dose than of the intravenous dose was eliminated extrarenally in our subjects.

The biexponentially declining excretion rates of the total pool of metabolites, with mean $t_{1/2}$ values of approximately 4 and 18.5 hours, is compatible with the formation of several metabolites with different excretion or formation rates. After intravenous dosing, about 70% of the total metabolites excreted by the kidneys was eliminated during the rapid phase. The corresponding fraction was 50% after the oral dose. Integration of the equation describing the excretion rate profile gives a total renal excretion of 75% and 66% of the intravenous and oral doses, respectively. In both cases these values are about 5% higher than the observed 72-hour recoveries, indicating that renal excretion of the metabolites continues for >72 hours. The discrepancy between the mean terminal $t_{1/2}$ of the total pool of radioactive metabolites determined from the plasma concentration (28 hours) and renal excretion rates (18.5 hours) is compatible with the formation of some metabolite(s) eliminated by nonrenal mechanisms having lower clearance capacity than the kidneys.

Biliary or gastrointestinal secretion appears to play a moderate role in the elimination of the metabolites, since about 10% of the radioactive doses was recovered in the feces over the 3-day period of the studies. It is probable that the fraction not excreted in the urine (approximately 25%) will be ultimately recovered in the feces; this has been shown in the rat and dog.[18] This assumption is further supported by the good agreement between the cumulative 3-day recovery in the urine and feces, and the $t_{1/2}$ of the metabolites in the plasma. After intravenous dosing, the recovered amount was 80%, and the calculated amount eliminated from the body, assuming a $t_{1/2}$ of 28.0 hours, was 83%.

References

1. Åberg H, Lindsjö M, Mörlin B: Felodipine in comparison with nifedipine. Drugs **29**:S117-123, 1985.

2. Ahnoff M: Determination of felodipine in plasma by gas chromatography with electron capture detection. J Pharm Biomed Anal **2:**519-526, 1984.
3. Allen L, Kimura K, MacKickan J, Ritschel W: Manual of symbols, equations and definitions in pharmacokinetics. J Clin Pharmacol **22:**1S-22S, 1982.
4. Andrén L, Hansson L, Orö L, Ryman T: Experience with nitrendipine—a new calcium antagonist—in hypertension. J Cardiovasc Pharmacol **4:**S387-S391, 1982.
5. Aoki K, Kondo S, Mochizaki A, Yoshida T, Kato S, Kato K, Tahikawa K: Antihypertensive effect of cardiovascular Ca^{24} antagonist in hypertensive patients in the absence and presence of beta-adrenergic blockade. Am Heart J **96:**218-226, 1978.
6. Boström SL, Ljung B, Nordlander M, Johansson B: Action of felodipine in vascular smooth muscle. *In* Hidaka H, Hartshorne D, editors: Calmodulin: Antagonists and cell function. New York, 1984, Academic Press.
7. Collste P, Danielsson M, Elmfeldt D, Felche E, Gelin A, Hedner T, Rydén L: Long term experience of felodipine in combination with β blockade and diuretics in refractory patients. Drugs **29:**S124-130, 1985.
8. Culling W, Sheridan DJ: Acute haemodynamic effects of oral felodipine in β-adrenoceptor blocked patients. Br J Clin Pharmacol **17:**206P-207P, 1984.
9. Detry JM, de Coster PM, Renhin J: Hemodynamic effects of felodipine at rest and during exercise in exertional angina pectoris. Am J Cardiol **52:**453-457, 1983.
10. Elmfeldt D, Hedner T: Felodipine—A new vasodilator, in addition to β-receptor blockade in hypertension. Eur J Clin Pharmacol **25:**571-575, 1983.
11. Johnsson G, Murray G, Tweddel A, Mutton I: Haemodynamic effects of a new vasodilator drug, felodipine, in healthy subjects. Eur J Clin Pharmacol **24:**49-53, 1983.
12. Ljung B, Boström S-L, Hallbäck-Nordlander M: A new dihydropyridine. Blood Vessels **17:**154, 1980.
13. Maeda K, Takasugi T, Tsukemo Y, Tanaka Y, Shiota K: Clinical study on the hypotensive effect of diltiazem hydrochloride. Int J Clin Pharmacol Ther Toxicol **19:**47-55, 1981.
14. Metzler CM, Elfring L, McEven AJ: A users manual for NONLIN and associated programs. Research biostatistics. Kalamazoo, Mich., 1974, The Upjohn Company.
15. Rönn O, Bengtsson B, Edgar B, Raner S: Acute haemodynamic effects of the calcium antagonists felodipine and verapamil in man, singly and with metoprolol. Drugs **29:**S16-25, 1985.
16. Timmis AD, Campbell S, Monaghan MJ, Walker L, Jewitt DE: Acute haemodynamic and metabolic effects of felodipine in congestive heart failure. Br Heart J **51:**445-451, 1984.
17. Yeh KC, Kwan KC: A comparison of numerical algorithms by trapezoidal, Lagrange and spline approximation. J Pharmacokinet Biopharm **6:**79-80, 1970.
18. Weidolf L, Borg KO, Hoffmann K-J: Urinary metabolites of felodipine, a new vasodilator drug in man, dog, rat and mouse. Xenobiotica **14:**S657-666, 1984.

Nitrendipine kinetics in normal and impaired renal function

To test the hypothesis that renal failure alters the absorption and metabolism of nitrendipine and the renal elimination of its metabolites, we gave six normal men and 16 men with various degrees of renal dysfunction a single 20 mg oral dose of nitrendipine. Plasma nitrendipine and nitrendipine pyridine analog metabolite concentrations were measured by HPLC 14 times during 48 hours after dosing. The urinary excretion of four additional metabolites was measured. Standing and supine arterial blood pressure was measured 14 times during the 48 hours after dosing. The mean nitrendipine $t_{1/2}$ was 2.8 ± 2.1 hours and that of the metabolite was 3.4 ± 3.9 hours. No significant effect of decreased renal function on any kinetic parameter was demonstrated. Plasma nitrendipine concentrations correlated with decreased blood pressure, but metabolite concentrations did not. We conclude that renal insufficiency does not alter nitrendipine kinetics in man. (Clin Pharmacol Ther 38:212-218, 1985.)

George R. Aronoff, M.D., and Rebecca S. Sloan, R.N. *Indianapolis, Ind.*

Nitrendipine is a 1,4-dihydropyridine derivative with potent antihypertensive activity.[1,2,7] Chemically related to nifedipine, nitrendipine acts by peripheral vascular smooth muscle relaxation resulting from the inhibition of calcium influx across cellular membranes. As shown in Fig. 1, nitrendipine is metabolized to its inactive pyridine analog (M1) and to more polar metabolites that are excreted in the urine.[5] We examined the influence of decreased renal function on nitrendipine disposition, and determined the effects of uremia on blood pressure response to a single nitrendipine dose. Specifically, we addressed the hypothesis that renal failure would alter the absorption and metabolism of nitrendipine and the renal elimination of its metabolites.

METHODS

Our subjects were 22 adult men. Candidates were excluded if they were allergic to nitrendipine or related drugs or had a history of ischemic heart disease, clinical evidence of heart failure, evidence of major arrhythmia or cardiac conduction defect, or major disorders of any organ system other than the kidneys. For the subjects who passed urine, the creatinine clearance (CL_{CR}) rate was determined by averaging two 12- or 24-hour rates of endogenous CL_{CR} measured during the week before the study. For purposes of analysis, subjects were divided into four groups on the basis of renal function (Table I). Subjects with renal insufficiency had a variety of renal diseases, including glomerulonephritis, glomerulosclerosis, and interstitial nephritis. The anuric subjects were studied during a 48-hour period between hemodialysis treatments. All subjects had a complete physical examination before and after the study. Blood was sampled for a complete blood cell count and the determination of serum levels of sodium, potassium, calcium, phosphorus, bilirubin, SGOT, alkaline phosphatase, BUN, and creatinine. These determinations were performed by an automated method.

Each subject was given a single oral dose of nitrendipine, 20 mg. Blood samples were drawn either by venipuncture or through an indwelling butterfly intermittent infusion set in a forearm vein. Heparin was used to prevent clotting. Samples were drawn before drug dosing and 0.25, 0.5, 0.75, 1, 1.5, 2, 2.5, 3, 4, 6, 8, 12, 24, and 48 hours thereafter. Plasma was separated from blood cells by centrifugation at 2000 × g for 15 minutes at 4° C immediately after collection. All urine was collected from those subjects who passed urine for

From the Nephrology Section, Department of Medicine, Indiana University Medical Center.

Supported by a grant from Miles Laboratories, West Haven, Conn.

Received for publication Dec. 6, 1984; accepted April 22, 1985.

Reprint requests to: George R. Aronoff, M.D., Nephrology Section, Department of Medicine, Indiana University Medical Center, Fesler Hall 108, 1120 South Drive, Indianapolis, IN 46223.

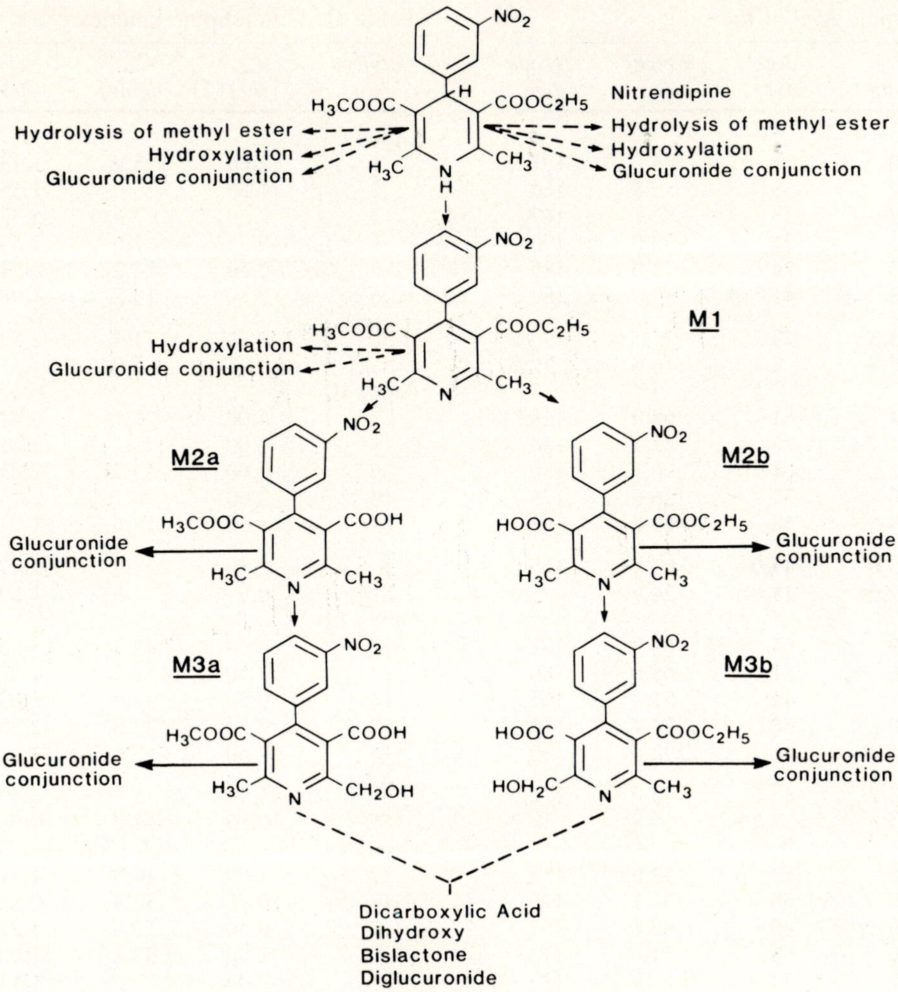

Fig. 1. The metabolic fate of nitrendipine.

48 hours after drug dosing. Plasma and urine samples were frozen at −70° C until assayed for drug and metabolite concentrations. Standing and supine blood pressures were measured each time blood samples were drawn.

Nitrendipine and metabolite concentrations were determined by a modification of an HPLC method.[3] Samples were analyzed on a Spherisorb ODS 15 cm × 4.6 nm column (Applied Science Labs). A Waters Associates M-45 solvent delivery system was used, with sample injection by a Waters autoinjector. Detection was with the aid of a Kratos Model 773 UV detector operated at 238 nm and 0.003 absorbance units full-scale attenuation. The chromatographic solvent consisted of methanol-tetrahydrofuran-water (47:15:38 [v/v/v]). Nimodipine was used as internal standard. Coefficient of variation of the assay was between 1.0% and 3.8%.*

Data for each subject were entered into a computer file. Kinetic analysis was by compartment-independent methods. The maximum plasma nitrendipine and M1 concentrations (C_{max}) and the time to reach the maximum nitrendipine concentration (t_{max}) were determined directly from the data. AUC was determined by the trapezoidal rule. The values reported were extrapolated to infinity with a tail correction by dividing the last measured plasma concentration by β, the slope of the terminal elimination phase of the plasma concentration-time curve determined by least-squares linear regres-

*The assay we used was performed under the direction of George J. Krol, Ph.D., at Miles Laboratories, West Haven, Conn.

Table I. Demographic data of the subjects

Subject No.	*CL_{CR} (ml/min)*	*Age (yr)*	*Weight (kg)*	*Height (cm)*
Group I				
1	140	21	75.0	181
2	124	33	56.8	160
3	117	35	82.1	167
4	115	21	87.0	190
5	110	24	72.0	186
6	83	41	80.0	187
$\overline{X}$	114.8	29.2	75.5	178.5
SD	18.8	8.4	10.6	12.2
Group II				
7	44	51	68.0	168
8	41	43	83.1	180
9	31	61	96.3	180
10	30	32	126.0	178
11	29	58	64.8	177
$\overline{X}$	35.0	49.0	87.6	176.6
SD	7.0	11.8	24.9	5.0
Group III				
12	19	54	69.0	191
13	15	51	65.0	180
14	12	41	51.4	161
15	10	56	72.4	171
16	5	41	92.4	180
$\overline{X}$	12.2	48.6	70.0	176.6
SD	5.3	7.2	14.8	11.2
Group IV				
17	0	63	53.0	158
18	0	56	74.1	170
19	0	46	69.8	168
20	0	68	53.6	173
21	0	53	62.9	173
22	0	60	63.0	165
$\overline{X}$	0	57.7	62.7	167.8
SD	0	7.8	8.5	5.7

Table II. Nitrendipine kinetics

Subject No.	*t_{max} (hr)*	*C_{max} (ng/ml)*	*$t_{1/2}$ (hr)*	*AUC (ng · hr/ml)*
Group I				
1	2.00	5.9	1.13	15.8
2	1.50	15.0	1.35	35.6
3	2.50	7.6	5.37	37.7
4	0.75	7.6	2.59	25.6
5	2.50	14.2	2.71	63.9
6	2.50	18.2	1.98	51.6
$\overline{X}$	1.96	11.4	2.52	38.4
SD	0.71	5.0	1.53	17.4
Group II				
7	4.00	21.1	5.47	203.9
8	2.00	21.3	1.41	64.7
9	2.00	15.2	2.03	48.9
10	2.00	16.1	1.74	50.5
11	1.50	17.6	1.71	46.7
$\overline{X}$	2.30	18.3	2.47	82.9
SD	0.97	2.8	1.69	68.0
Group III				
12	2.50	15.4	3.45	92.0
13	1.50	52.3	4.97	151.7
14	0.50	22.4	3.08	54.4
15	2.50	32.6	2.38	125.4
16	2.50	7.6	3.13	44.3
$\overline{X}$	1.90	26.1	3.40	93.6
SD	0.89	17.3	0.96	45.7
Group IV				
17	1.00	10.9	1.31	30.9
18	0.75	18.4	0.82	33.6
19	0.50	53.4	1.57	83.1
20	2.50	33.8	3.00	136.3
21	2.00	7.5	1.11	17.6
22	2.00	3.6	9.76	29.8
$\overline{X}$	1.46	21.3	2.93	55.2
SD	0.81	19.0	3.43	45.8

sion of the terminal portion of the curve. The $t_{1/2}$ was given by the expression: $t_{1/2} = \ln 2/\beta$. Statistical comparisons were by linear regression analysis with CL_{CR} as the independant variable and ANOVA. The correlation between blood pressures and plasma drug or metabolite concentrations were determined. Where appropriate, t tests were performed to compare mean data. Data are expressed as the $\overline{X} \pm$ SD.

RESULTS

Demographic data for the subjects are listed in Table I. The subjects with decreased renal function were older than the normal subjects in group I, but otherwise the groups were similar. No changes in serial measurements reflecting hematopoietic, renal, or hepatic function were detected, and no adverse effects were reported by any of the subjects.

Mean plasma nitrendipine and M1 concentrations for the four groups are shown in Fig. 2, and kinetic parameters for the drug and its pyridine analog are listed in Tables II and III. Nitrendipine was rapidly absorbed, reaching a C_{max} for all subjects of 19 ± 13.4 ng/ml at 1.9 ± 0.8 hours after dosing. The presence of M1 was also rapidly detected, reaching a mean C_{max} in all subjects of 27.4 ± 13.7 ng/ml at 1.7 ± 0.9 hours after nitrendipine dosing. No significant correlation between

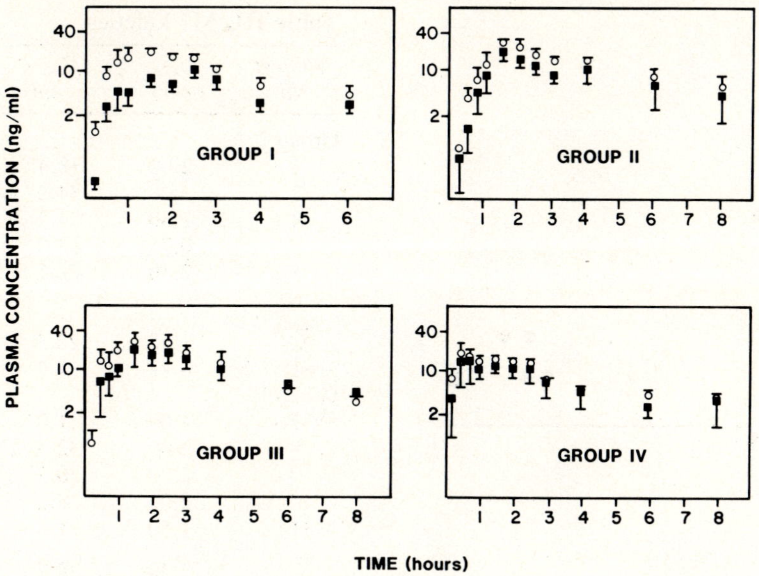

Fig. 2. Mean (±SD) nitrendipine *(closed symbols)* and M1 *(open symbols)* plasma concentrations in the four subject groups.

renal function and the rate or extent of nitrendipine absorption or the formation of M1 could be demonstrated.

The rate of nitrendipine elimination varied, with a $t_{1/2}$ ranging from 0.82 to 9.76 hours ($\overline{X} \pm SD = 2.8 \pm 2.1$ hours). Similar results were found for the pyridine analog. The $t_{1/2}$ of M1 ranged from 0.51 to 16.1 hours ($\overline{X} \pm SD = 3.4 \pm 3.9$ hours). No significant correlation between renal function and the rate of nitrendipine or M1 elimination could be demonstrated. That renal function does not effect the kinetics of nitrendipine and M1 is shown in Fig. 3. There was no significant correlation between CL_{CR} and AUC for nitrendipine or its primary metabolite.

The renal excretion of four additional metabolites was measured in the 16 subjects who passed urine. Overall, these metabolites accounted for 26.2% ± 8.8% of the nitrendipine dose. Metabolite M2a was excreted in the greatest amount, accounting for half the total amount of metabolites recovered in the urine. There was no significant correlation between CL_{CR} and urinary excretion of any of the four measured metabolites. As seen in Table IV, these metabolites accounted for 26.2% ± 4.4% of the nitrendipine dose in subjects with normal renal function and 20% ± 7.9% in subjects with CL_{CR} <20 ml/min.

Nitrendipine plasma concentration correlated with a decrease in both systolic and diastolic blood pressures at all measurements up to 8 hours after dosing ($P < 0.05$). Fig. 4 shows the relationship between nitrendipine plasma concentration and supine systolic and diastolic blood pressures. A similar relationship was found for standing blood pressures up to 8 hours after dosing.

Subjects with impaired renal function had higher systolic and diastolic blood pressures than did subjects with normal renal function. Supine blood pressure in subjects with CL_{CR} >50 ml/min was 105 ± 5/64 ± 7 mm Hg. Supine blood pressure in subjects with CL_{CR} <50 ml/min was 138 ± 25/71 ± 12 mm Hg ($P < 0.05$). Similarly, the decrease in blood pressure after nitrendipine was greater in subjects with CL_{CR} <50 ml/min than in subjects with CL_{CR} >50 ml/min. One hour after dosing the supine systolic blood pressure fell by 19.5 ± 17 mm Hg in the group with less renal function, but by only 4.7 ± 2.2 mm Hg ($P < 0.01$) in the group with normal renal function. The differences in supine and standing systolic and diastolic blood pressure response between these two groups were significant from 0.5 to 3 hours after nitrendipine.

DISCUSSION

Renal failure can lead to abnormalities in hepatic biotransformation.[6] Although Leber and Schutterle[4] demonstrated decreased activity of hepatic mixed-function oxidase in uremic rats, most oxidation reactions

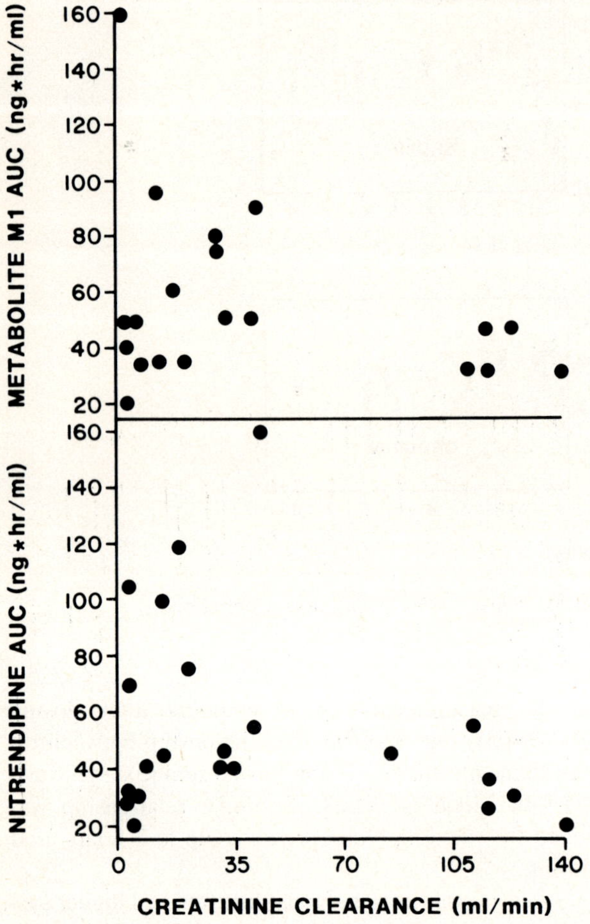

Fig. 3. The relationship between renal function and the plasma AUC for nitrendipine and its M1 metabolite. No significant correlation could be demonstrated.

Table III. M1 kinetics

Subject No.	t_{max} *(hr)*	C_{max} *(ng/ml)*	$t_{1/2}$ *(hr)*	*AUC (ng · hr/ml)*
Group I				
1	2.00	18.4	1.79	51.3
2	1.00	34.2	1.28	79.8
3	1.50	24.7	1.23	50.7
4	0.75	13.0	3.32	80.0
5	2.50	21.1	0.51	50.1
6				
$\overline{X}$	1.55	22.3	1.63	62.4
SD	0.72	7.9	1.05	16.0
Group II				
7	4.00	21.0	5.67	182.0
8	2.00	32.5	1.45	94.2
9	2.00	30.7	1.63	90.7
10	2.00	38.2	4.82	156.6
11	1.50	21.0	11.64	161.1
$\overline{X}$	2.30	28.7	5.04	136.9
SD	0.97	7.5	4.14	41.7
Group III				
12	1.50	10.6	3.22	58.3
13	1.50	56.2	1.79	120.3
14	0.50	34.9	1.11	58.4
15	2.50	51.5	1.62	193.8
16	2.50	22.4	1.93	57.9
$\overline{X}$	1.70	35.1	1.93	97.7
SD	0.84	19.2	0.78	60.1
Group IV				
17	0.75	16.5	6.00	100.0
18	0.50	24.9	16.10	344.1
19	0.50	55.5	2.23	94.2
20	2.50	15.5	0.70	27.1
21	2.00	23.6	1.87	66.4
22	1.50	10.0	0.97	18.9
$\overline{X}$	1.29	24.3	4.64	108.4
SD	0.84	16.2	5.93	120.2

occur at a normal rate in patients with uremia.[4,6] Our data demonstrate that the oxidation of nitrendipine to its inactive pyridine analog M1 occurs quickly and is not altered by renal failure. Similarly, the rate of M1 disappearance from plasma was not altered by renal insufficiency, and there was no difference in the renal excretion of the metabolites. These observations support the notion that the hydrolysis or oxidation of the ester groups on M1 and the hydroxylation of methyl groups on M2a and M2b occur normally in patients with renal failure.

The nitrendipine elimination $t_{1/2}$ we found in subjects with normal and impaired renal function is of the order of that reported by others in normal subjects.[5] However, Hansson et al.[2] reported a much longer $t_{1/2}$ of 8.09 to 11.4 hours in 12 patients with hypertension. To measure nitrendipine plasma concentrations, they used a capillary column gas chromatographic-mass spectrophotometric assay that is 10 times as sensitive than our assay. Nitrendipine terminal elimination from a deep tissue compartment may occur much more slowly than has been presumed, allowing the prolonged presence of low plasma drug levels. Further elucidation of this possibility should be considered in future studies.

We found that nitrendipine lowered blood pressure after a single dose. The effect correlated well with the plasma nitrendipine concentration and lasted for 8 hours after dosing. Subjects with diminished renal function had higher initial blood pressures and a greater decrease

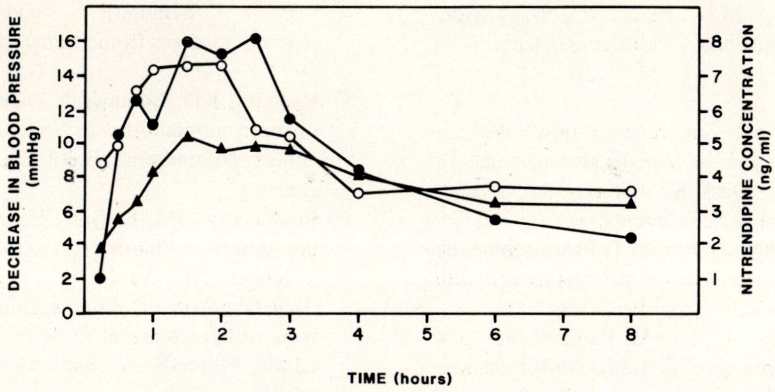

Fig. 4. There was a significant correlation between the mean plasma nitrendipine concentration (●) and the mean decrease in supine systolic (○) and diastolic (▲) blood pressures in all subjects after a single 20 mg oral dose.

Table IV. Urinary excretion of nitrendipine metabolites

Subject No.	*M2a (mg)*	*M2b (mg)*	*M3a (mg)*	*M3b (mg)*	*Total (mg)*	*Total (%)*
Group I						
1	3.96	0.69	0.58	0.94	6.17	30.9
2	2.62	0.66	0.53	0.82	4.63	23.2
3	2.2	1.19	0.17	0.78	4.34	21.7
4	3.15	0.77	0.26	0.57	4.75	23.8
5	3.16	1.77	0.61	0.96	6.5	32.5
6	2.8	1.02	0.46	0.71	4.99	25.0
$\overline{X}$	2.98	1.02	0.44	0.80	5.23	26.2
SD	0.60	0.42	0.18	0.15	0.89	4.4
Group II						
7	2.00	1.48	0.5	0.71	4.69	23.5
8	2.81	1.37	0.54	0.97	5.69	28.5
9	3.08	1.39	0.52	1.11	6.1	30.5
10	2.67	2.00	0.52	1.21	6.4	32.0
11	5.08	1.63	1.26	1.65	9.62	48.1
$\overline{X}$	3.13	1.57	0.67	1.13	6.50	32.5
SD	1.16	0.26	0.33	0.35	1.86	9.3
Group III						
12	1.86	0.72	0.81	0.74	4.13	20.7
13	1.92	1.1	1.02	0.7	4.74	23.7
14	1.52	1.11	0.85	0.64	4.12	20.6
15	2.63	0.95	0.88	1.14	5.6	28.0
16	0.61	0.29	0.28	0.21	1.39	7.0
$\overline{X}$	1.71	0.8	0.8	0.7	4.0	20.0
SD	0.73	0.3	0.3	0.3	1.6	7.9

in blood pressure than did subjects with normal renal function.

We conclude that renal failure does not alter the absorption and metabolism of nitrendipine and that the accumulation of metabolites should not occur in nonoligouric patients. Multiple-dose safety, efficacy, and kinetic studies of nitrendipine in patients with renal insufficiency are warranted.

We thank Svetislav Vanov, M.D., Ph.D., Russell J. Taylor, Ph.D., and George J. Krol, Ph.D., for their assistance.

References

1. Burris JF, Freis ED: Single- and repeated-dose tolerance and activity of nitrendipine in hypertensive patients. *In* Scriabine A, Vanov S, Deck K, editors: Nitrendipine. Baltimore, 1984, Urban & Schwarzenberg.
2. Hansson L, Andren L, Oro L, Ryman T: Pharmacokinetic and pharmacodynamic parameters in patients treated with nitrendipine. Hypertension **5**(suppl II):25-28, 1983.
3. Janis RA, Krol GJ, Noe AJ, Pan M: Radioreceptor and high-performance chromatographic assays for the calcium channel antagonist nitrendipine in serum. J Clin Pharmacol **23:**266-273, 1983.
4. Leber HW, Schutterle E: Oxidative drug metabolism in liver microsomes from uremic rats. Kidney Int **2:**152-158, 1972.
5. Raemsch KD, Sommer J: Pharmacokinetics and metabolism of nitrendipine. *In* Scriabine A, Vanov S, Deck K, editors: Nitrendipine, Baltimore, 1984, Urban & Schwarzenberg.
6. Reidenberg MM, Drayer DE: Drug therapy in renal failure. Ann Rev Pharmacol Toxicol **20:**45-54, 1980.
7. Vlachakis ND, Vanov SK, Taylor RJ, Pun EFC: Controlled comparison of nitrendipine and placebo in the treatment of hypertension. *In* Scriabine A, Vanov S, Deck K, editors: Nitrendipine. Baltimore, 1984, Urban & Schwarzenberg.

Self-administration of clonidine, oxazepam, and hydromorphone by patients undergoing methadone detoxification

The extent to which hydromorphone, clonidine, and oxazepam alleviate the symptoms of opioid withdrawal and the extent and pattern of self-administration of these drugs during methadone detoxification were examined within a residential laboratory in three groups of patients dependent on methadone. Six times over the course of detoxification, acute effects of orally administered placebo and a single active drug (hydromorphone HCl, 3 mg, clonidine HCl, 0.3 mg, or oxazepam, 30 mg, all given twice daily) were tested, followed by an opportunity for subjects to self-administer the drug and dose of their choice. Hydromorphone significantly decreased opioid withdrawal symptoms and was more preferred for self-administration than the placebo. Clonidine and oxazepam did not significantly decrease withdrawal symptoms, nor was either drug self-administered significantly more than placebo. Clonidine, however, did induce side effects. (CLIN PHARMACOL THER 38:219-227, 1985.)

Kenzie L. Preston, Ph.D., George E. Bigelow, Ph.D., and Ira A. Liebson, M.D.
Baltimore, Md.

A common goal in drug addiction therapy is that patients attain drug-free status. Detoxification is the pharmacologic process for the initial achievement of drug-free status, and for many years routine detoxification procedures have involved therapy with methadone and gradual reduction of methadone dose. The opioid withdrawal symptoms that accompany detoxification from methadone, however, present major obstacles for many patients. Efforts have thus been made to alleviate withdrawal symptoms through pharmacologic intervention with adjunctive medications.

Compounds with opioid agonist properties have been shown to decrease opioid withdrawal symptoms.[7,8] Although opioid agonists are effective in alleviating the signs and symptoms of detoxification, the abuse liability and physical dependence–producing properties of these agents necessarily limit their usefulness. More recently, clonidine has been shown to be effective in decreasing the symptoms of abrupt withdrawal from chronic methadone[1,15]; however, its usefulness in gradual methadone detoxification, a procedure more commonly used in outpatient methadone clinics, has yet to be demonstrated. There is some suggestion that clonidine may also possess some potential abuse liability; clonidine has been shown to support intravenous self-administration in both the rat[2] and the rhesus monkey,[17] and the availability of clonidine on the illicit street market and the existence of some degree of drug abuse have been reported.[3] Benzodiazepines and related compounds have been used as adjuncts in the treatment of opioid withdrawal syndrome,[9] but their efficacy as adjuvants in methadone detoxification has not been demonstrated in controlled studies. It is well established that the benzodiazepines possess some degree of abuse potential and will be self-administered by opioid addicts.[14,16] The reinforcing properties of the benzodiazepines may account for their popularity in the treatment of methadone withdrawal symptoms.

The purpose of our investigation was to study the effects of two nonopioid drugs, clonidine and a benzodiazepine, oxazepam, currently used or recommended as adjuncts for treatment of opioid withdrawal symptoms in patients in a methadone maintenance program who are undergoing gradual inpatient detoxification, and to compare their effects with those of an opioid agonist, hydromorphone. The extent to which these drugs alleviated the symptoms of opioid withdrawal and the extent and pattern of self-administration of these drugs during methadone detoxification were examined.

From The Johns Hopkins University School of Medicine and Francis Scott Key Medical Center.

Supported by United States Public Health Service Research Grant No. DA03894, Research Training Grant No. DA07209, and Research Scientist Development Award No. DA00050.

Received for publication Feb. 13, 1985; accepted March 19, 1985.

Reprint requests to: George E. Bigelow, Ph.D., Behavioral Pharmacology Research Unit, Department of Psychiatry, D-5-West, Johns Hopkins/Key Medical Center, Baltimore, MD 21224.

Table I. Demographic characteristics and addiction history of subjects

Subject No.	*Race*	*Age (yr)*	*Yr of opiate abuse*	*Daily methadone dose (mg)*
Clonidine				
1	B	32	12	40
2	B	34	11	30
3	B	27	12	50
4	W	34	11	30
5	B	31	12	40
12	B	40	25	30
Oxazepam				
6	B	41	25	50
7	B	23	3	45
9	W	33	4	30
13	B	31	14	30
15	B	29	14	50
17	B	28	13	50
Hydromorphone				
8	B	27	14	30
10	B	31	10	30
11	B	35	4	60
14	B	33	18	40
16	W	31	13	50
18	B	28	14	35

B = Black; W = white.
Subject number indicates order of participation in the study.

Three groups of patients undergoing gradual methadone detoxification were used; in each group the effects of one active drug (clonidine, oxazepam, or hydromorphone) were compared with those of placebo. The procedures used were the same for all three groups and consisted of two components: (1) to assess efficacy, subjects were exposed to active drug and placebo, and the acute effects of the two agents and their effects on withdrawal symptoms were monitored; and (2) to assess drug preference, after the forced exposure subjects were given the opportunity in self-administration trials to choose between active drug and placebo and to choose the dose they would receive. These preference data gave an indication of patient acceptability of the drug and possibly some measure of abuse liability. The two components were repeated six times over the course of detoxification to assess the relationship between drug efficacy and preference and withdrawal symptoms as symptoms changed over the course of methadone detoxification.

METHODS

Subjects and general procedures. Our subjects were 18 men undergoing methadone maintenance therapy who requested inpatient detoxification from methadone. Demographic and addiction histories are presented in Table I. On the basis of physical examination, history, routine laboratory chemistry test, and chest x-ray results, subjects were found to be without significant medical or psychiatric disturbances other than drug abuse, with the exception of subject 6 whose essential hypertension was controlled with chlorthalidone, 50 mg/day.

Subjects participated while residing in an eight-bed behavioral pharmacology research ward as previously described[5]; typically, two beds were allocated to our subjects. To increase independence of observations between subjects, whenever two subjects were simultaneously participating, their schedules of adjunct medication administration were set out-of-phase, such that one subject had nonchoice trials on the days in which the other subject had choice trials. Occasionally three subjects participated at the same time; when this occurred the third subject's entire daily schedule was shifted 1 hour earlier than that of the other two subjects.

Before admission into the study and independent of the subject selection process, subjects were assigned to either the clonidine (n = 6), oxazepam (n = 6), or hydromorphone (n = 6) group. Group assignment was determined by the order in which patients were admitted onto the ward. The study was run in double-blind fashion such that neither the subjects nor the staff were informed of the methadone detoxification schedule or group assignment. Research protocols started on the third or fourth day after admission onto the research ward.

Methadone detoxification schedule. Methadone HCl (Methadose; Mallinckrodt, Inc.) was administered in a constant volume (60 ml) of cherry syrup solution once daily at 6 PM. Subjects received their maintenance doses for the first 5 to 6 days of the protocol, followed by 5 days at one half the maintenance dose. The methadone dose was then decreased to zero over the next 10 days. The subject continued to receive a constant volume of methadone placebo (cherry syrup) throughout the rest of the study (15 days). No attempt was made to mask the taste of the methadone placebo.

Adjunct medications. Placebo (lactose) and commercially available preparations of oxazepam (Serax; Wyeth Laboratories), clonidine HCl (Catapres; Boehringer Ingelheim), and hydromorphone HCl (Dilaudid; Knoll Pharmaceutical Co.) were orally administered in distinctively colored opaque capsules and given an arbitrary letter code. Letter and color codes varied between subjects but were held constant within each subject's protocol. The adjunct medication schedule began on the first day of methadone dose reduction (50% maintenance dose) and was arranged into six blocks of 5 days. Because of occasional subject dropout prior to completion of the study, some subjects completed fewer

Table II. Visual analog scales

	Hydromorphone, 3 mg b.i.d.		*Clonidine, 0.3 mg b.i.d.*		*Oxazepam, 30 mg b.i.d.*	
	H	*P*	*C*	*P*	*O*	*P*
Drug effect						
Morning	1.82	1.72	4.70*	2.30	1.32	0.67
	(0.55)	(0.50)	(0.70)	(1.00)	(0.70)	(0.45)
Evening	2.40	1.70	6.07*	2.30	1.22	0.75
	(0.53)	(0.51)	(0.77)	(0.97)	(0.77)	(0.56)
Liking						
Morning	2.09	0.68	2.25	1.10	1.07	0.78
	(0.69)	(0.23)	(0.62)	(0.35)	(0.71)	(0.55)
Evening	2.30*	0.90	2.42	0.80	1.05	0.60
	(0.66)	(0.36)	(0.74)	(0.35)	(0.76)	(0.42)
Good effects						
Morning	2.37*	0.68	2.52	1.20	1.18	0.78
	(0.67)	(0.24)	(0.55)	(0.44)	(0.69)	(0.52)
Evening	2.60*	0.90	3.58*	0.97	1.12	0.65
	(0.67)	(0.28)	(0.75)	(0.34)	(0.75)	(0.45)
Bad effects						
Morning	0.92	2.50	3.67	3.02	1.02	0.78
	(0.36)	(0.93)	(0.66)	(1.27)	(0.39)	(0.53)
Evening	1.12	2.82	4.28	2.42	0.85	0.92
	(0.35)	(0.97)	(0.67)	(1.14)	(0.39)	(0.71)

Data are $\overline{X}$ ($\pm$SE) (n = 6).
H = Hydromorphone; C = clonidine; O = oxazepam; P = placebo, 3 capsules twice a day.
*Significantly different ($P < 0.05$; ANOVA) from placebo value.

than six blocks. On day 1 of each block (baseline) no adjunct medications were given. On days 2 and 3 of each block (nonchoice trials), the subjects were given three capsules of placebo or drug (oxazepam, 10 mg/capsule, clonidine HCl, 0.1 mg/capsule, or hydromorphone HCl, 1 mg/capsule) two times a day at 9 AM and 3 PM. The order of placebo or drug dosing was counterbalanced over the six blocks and across subjects. On days 4 and 5 of each block (choice trials), subjects were given the opportunity at each of the scheduled dosings (9 AM and 3 PM) to choose which of the two drugs they would receive and the number of capsules (one, two, or three) they would receive. Subjects were required to take at least one capsule of their choice at each drug dosing. The opportunity to choose the number of capsules to take allowed subjects to titrate the drug effect. The doses of clonidine, oxazepam, and hydromorphone given in the nonchoice trials are within the upper dosage range recommended by the manufacturers.

Subjective measures. Multiple subjective effects measures were recorded throughout the day on four subjective effect questionnaires.

Questionnaire 1. A physical symptoms questionnaire developed in this laboratory to measure opioid withdrawal symptoms experienced over the previous 24 hours was completed at 8:30 AM. The questionnaire contained seven subscales and consisted of 60 items that the subjects rated on a four-point scale from not at all (0) to severe (3). The withdrawal subscale, the results of which are reported below, consisted of 21 items derived from the Himmelsbach system for withdrawal assessment[8] and from other symptoms typical of opioid withdrawal. The items included muscle cramps, sneezing, painful joints, sick to stomach, diarrhea, nausea, runny nose, shaky, goose flesh, yawning, muscle twitches, weak knees, watery eyes, clammy skin, poor appetite, backache, hot and cold flashes, sweating, abdominal cramps, craving for heroin, and craving more methadone.

Questionnaire 2. At 11:30 AM and 5:30 PM (2.5 hours after each adjunct medication dosing), subjects completed a visual analog questionnaire that contained scales for strength of drug effects, drug liking, and "good" and "bad" drug effects. Each scale consisted of a 10 cm line marked at either end with "not at all" and "extremely." Subjects were instructed to indicate on the scale how they would rate the adjunct medication at the time they completed the form.

Questionnaire 3. Also at 11:30 AM and 5:30 PM subjects answered a 49-item true/false questionnaire drawn

Table III. ARCI scales

	Hydromorphone, 3 mg b.i.d.		*Clonidine, 0.3 mg b.i.d.*		*Oxazepam, 30 mg b.i.d.*	
	H	*P*	*C*	*P*	*O*	*P*
AG						
Morning	4.8	4.1	3.0*	3.9	4.9	4.7
	(1.0)	(1.0)	(0.7)	(0.8)	(1.1)	(1.1)
Evening	4.7	4.4	3.4	4.0	4.6	4.4
	(1.0)	(0.9)	(0.8)	(0.9)	(1.1)	(1.1)
BG						
Morning	6.2*	5.4	3.5	5.2	6.6	6.9
	(1.4)	(1.4)	(0.6)	(1.0)	(1.0)	(1.0)
Evening	6.2	5.5	4.1	5.2	6.3	6.5
	(1.2)	(1.2)	(0.8)	(0.8)	(0.7)	(0.9)
MBG						
Morning	6.3	4.7	4.2	4.8	6.6	6.5
	(1.4)	(1.5)	(1.3)	(1.2)	(2.0)	(1.9)
Evening	6.2*	5.0	4.4	5.0	6.4	6.2
	(1.7)	(1.3)	(1.3)	(0.8)	(2.1)	(2.0)
PCAG						
Morning	5.5	5.9	9.2*	6.0	5.6	5.4
	(1.1)	(1.1)	(0.7)	(1.2)	(1.1)	(0.8)
Evening	4.8*	6.4	8.8*	5.7	5.1	5.1
	(1.0)	(1.0)	(0.8)	(1.0)	(0.9)	(0.8)
LSD						
Morning	5.2	5.4	6.2	5.9	4.8	4.3
	(1.4)	(1.3)	(0.9)	(0.8)	(0.6)	(0.5)
Evening	5.4	6.0	6.9	6.0	4.7	4.7
	(1.2)	(1.4)	(0.9)	(0.7)	(0.5)	(0.6)

Data are $\bar{X}$ ($\pm$SE) (n = 6).
H = Hydromorphone; C = clonidine; O = oxazepam; P = placebo, 3 capsules twice a day.
*Significantly different ($P < 0.05$; ANOVA) from placebo value.

from the Addiction Research Center Inventory (ARCI) and containing five major subscales: MBG (a measure of euphoria), PCAG (a measure of sedation), LSD (a measure of dysphoric and psychotomimetic changes), and BG and AG scales (empirically derived amphetamine-sensitive scales.[8,10]

Questionnaire 4. At 5:30 PM subjects also completed the Profile of Mood States (POMS), a questionnaire[12] consisting of a 65-item five-point adjective rating scale on which eight categories were distinguished for scoring purposes: tension-anxiety, anger-hostility, confusion, depression-dejection, fatigue, vigor, friendliness, and total mood disturbance.

Staff-rated withdrawal. At 11:30 AM and 5:30 PM, the nursing staff rated the severity of withdrawal signs and symptoms based on observations made over the previous 2-hour period and at the same time as blood pressure was measured. The items on the withdrawal evaluation questionnaire were derived from the Himmelsbach system for withdrawal assessment[8] and included lacrimation, rhinorrhea, sweating, chills, mydriasis, tremor, yawning, dozing, irritability, restlessness, inactivity, social interaction, and general withdrawal discomfort.

Physiologic and performance measures. At 8:30 AM and 11:30 AM blood pressure was recorded. Psychomotor/cognitive performance was measured by two performance tasks: a computerized Digit Symbol Substitution Test (DSST)[11] at 11:30 AM and 5:30, 8:30, and 10 PM, and the circular lights task, a test of hand-eye coordination, at 8:30 and 11:30 AM and 5:30, 8:30, and 10 PM. In the DSST, randomly selected digits appeared in the center of the video screen. The subject used the numeric key pad to reproduce a geometric pattern associated with the digit by using the digit symbol code presented continuously at the top of the screen. The score was the number of correct responses during the 90-second session. In the circular lights task, during 1-minute sessions subjects earned points by pressing a series of 16 buttons as rapidly as possible in response to the random-sequenced illumination of their associated lights. Score was the number of correct responses during the 1-minute session.

Data analysis. Data are reported that compare the

Table IV. Psychomotor performance

	Hydromorphone, 3 mg b.i.d.		*Clonidine, 0.3 mg b.i.d.*		*Oxazepam, 30 mg b.i.d.*	
	H	*P*	*C*	*P*	*O*	*P*
Circular lights						
8:30 AM	80.4	79.9	83.6	83.0	79.4	82.6
	(2.1)	(2.9)	(2.1)	(2.1)	(1.5)	(2.1)
10:30 PM	84.1*	81.4	80.9*	87.9	84.8	87.3
	(2.5)	(2.1)	(1.7)	(2.0)	(3.0)	(2.7)
5:30 PM	84.4*	81.4	74.9*	90.6	83.5*	86.7
	(2.5)	(2.6)	(2.4)	(2.9)	(3.0)	(2.4)
8:30 PM	84.2	82.8	83.0	89.3	82.8	86.8
	(2.2)	(2.1)	(3.3)	(2.8)	(2.9)	(2.5)
10 PM	79.8	81.0	85.2*	89.6	82.1*	85.6
	(1.6)	(2.1)	(3.0)	(3.4)	(2.9)	(2.0)
DSST						
10:30 AM	39.1	37.8	37.0*	40.8	37.0	37.8
	(2.7)	(2.6)	(5.1)	(5.1)	(0.9)	(0.9)
5:30 PM	38.2	36.9	35.3*	40.2	37.5	38.3
	(2.7)	(2.4)	(5.6)	(4.6)	(1.0)	(0.9)
8:30 PM	37.8	37.3	38.1	41.0	35.5	37.7
	(2.5)	(2.7)	(5.5)	(5.2)	(1.3)	(1.1)
10 PM	36.1	38.2	39.9	41.1	35.2*	37.6
	(6.0)	(3.1)	(5.2)	(5.0)	(1.3)	(1.2)

Data are $\overline{X}$ (±SE) (n = 6).
H = Hydromorphone; C = clonidine; O = oxazepam; P = placebo, 3 capsules twice a day.
*Significantly different (P < 0.05; ANOVA) from placebo value.

effects of active drug with placebo on drug preference and self-administration behavior, withdrawal symptoms and other subjective measures, and psychomotor/cognitive performance. Results of individual measures were averaged across trials for individual subjects to determine an overall score. A one-way repeated-measures ANOVA was then conducted on the individual overall scores for placebo and active drug. Data collected on days 2 and 3 of each block (nonchoice trials) are reported for subjective, physiologic, and performance measures. Self-administration (preference) data reported were collected on days 4 and 5 (choice trials) of each block. Unless otherwise indicated, data are reported as the $\overline{X}$ ± SE.

RESULTS

Subjective effects measures (nonchoice trials). Results of the visual analog subjective effects measures are listed in Table II. Hydromorphone was rated significantly greater than placebo in drug liking in the afternoon ratings ($F(1,5) = 7.50$; $P = 0.04$) and as having significantly more "good" effects than placebo in both morning ($F(1,5) = 8.56$; $P = 0.03$) and afternoon ($F(1,5) = 8.89$; $P = 0.03$) ratings. No significant differences between hydromorphone and placebo were found for the strength of drug effect or on bad effects. Clonidine was rated as having significantly greater drug effects than placebo in both morning ($F(1,5) = 16.06$; $P = 0.01$) and afternoon ($F(1,5) = 18.13$; $P = 0.01$) ratings and as having significantly greater good effects than placebo only in the afternoon ($F(1,5) = 11.50$; $P = 0.02$). No significant differences between clonidine and placebo were found on the drug liking or bad effects rating scales. Oxazepam was not rated significantly different from placebo on any of the visual analog scales.

Results of the ARCI short-form questionnaire are shown in Table III. Hydromorphone significantly increased scores on the BG (amphetamine-sensitive scale) in the morning ($F(1,5) = 7.3$; $P = 0.04$) and on the MBG (euphoria scale) in the afternoon ($F(1,5) = 8.7$; $P = 0.03$) compared with placebo and significantly decreased scores on the PCAG (sedation scale) in the afternoon ($F(1,5) = 13.0$; $P = 0.02$) compared with placebo. Clonidine significantly decreased scores on the AG (amphetamine-sensitive scale) in the morning ($F(1,5) = 13.1$; $P = 0.02$) and significantly increased scores on the PCAG (sedation scale) in both the morning ($F(1,5) = 14.4$; $P = 0.01$) and afternoon ($F(1,5) = 7.5$; $P = 0.04$) compared with placebo. Oxazepam had no significant effect on any of the ARCI scales.

On the POMS questionnaire, hydromorphone sig-

Table V. Withdrawal ratings

	Hydromorphone, 3 mg b.i.d.		*Clonidine, 0.3 mg b.i.d.*		*Oxazepam, 30 mg b.i.d.*	
	H	*P*	*C*	*P*	*O*	*P*
Self-rated withdrawal scale	12.2* (5.0)	14.6 (5.4)	14.8 (3.5)	16.3 (3.8)	7.4 (2.2)	8.1 (2.0)
Staff-rated withdrawal scale						
Morning	18.3 (0.6)	19.1 (0.3)	24.0† (1.1)	18.9 (0.6)	18.9 (0.5)	17.8 (0.6)
Evening	18.7* (1.0)	20.1 (1.3)	24.8† (1.7)	19.4 (1.5)	19.4 (1.1)	19.3 (0.6)

Data are $\overline{X}$ (±SE) (n = 6).
H = Hydromorphone; C = clonidine; O = oxazepam; P = placebo, 3 capsules twice a day.
*Significantly different (P < 0.05; ANOVA) from placebo value.
†n = 2; not tested by ANOVA.

Table VI. Self-administration of hydromorphone, clonidine, and oxazepam

	Hydromorphone		*Clonidine*		*Oxazepam*	
	H	*P*	*C*	*P*	*O*	*P*
Total capsules taken	45.7* (6.3)	14.7 (3.9)	27.7 (8.5)	19.0 (9.0)	38.0 (8.8)	18.5 (8.0)
Total choices	16.0* (2.0)	5.3 (1.4)	11.5 (3.1)	8.5 (3.5)	14.3 (2.8)	8.2 (3.2)

Data are $\overline{X}$ (±SE) (n = 6).
H = Hydromorphone, 1 mg/capsule; C = clonidine, 0.1 mg/capsule; O = oxazepam, 10 mg/capsule; P = placebo.
*Significantly different (P < 0.05; ANOVA) from placebo.

nificantly increased scores on the vigor (9.8 ± 2.0 vs. 7.9 ± 2.5; F(1,5) = 9.00; P = 0.03) and friendly (14.3 ± 2.0 vs. 12.6 ± 2.1; F(1,5) = 6.8; P = 0.047) scales compared with placebo, while clonidine significantly decreased scores on the vigor scale (3.7 ± 1.0 vs. 6.0 ± 0.4; F(1,5) = 7.7; P = 0.04) compared with placebo. Oxazepam effects did not differ significantly from those of placebo on any of the POMS scales.

Physiologic and performance measures (nonchoice trials). As expected from its primary clinical indication, clonidine significantly decreased both systolic (−11.79 ± 2.6 vs. 0.70 ± 1.4 mm Hg; F(1,5) = 12.3; P = 0.018) and diastolic (−9.0 ± 0.8 vs. 0.25 ± 1.8 mm Hg; F(1,5) = 28.5; P = 0.004) blood pressure compared with placebo. Neither hydromorphone nor oxazepam had significant effects on systolic or diastolic blood pressure.

All three drugs had some effect on the two measures of psychomotor performance (Table IV). Hydromorphone significantly improved performance on the hand-eye coordination test compared with placebo for each of the two testing times 1.5 hours after drug dosing (10:30 AM: F(1,5) = 6.9, P = 0.047; 5:30 PM: F(1,5) = 10.3, P = 0.024), but had no significant effect on DSST scores at any test time. Clonidine significantly decreased scores on the hand-eye coordination test compared with placebo throughout the day after the first drug dosing (10:30 AM: F(1,5) = 16.2, P = 0.011; 5:30 PM: F(1,5) = 39.2, P = 0.002; 10:00 PM: F(1,5) = 10.7, P = 0.022) and significantly decreased performance on the DSST at the two testing times 1.5 hours after drug dosing (10:30 AM: F(1,5) = 9.8, P = 0.026; 4:30 AM: F(1,5) = 14.1, P = 0.014). Oxazepam had no significant effects early in the day, but produced significant impairments late in the day on both the hand-eye coordination test (8:30 PM: F(1,5) = 38.8, P = 0.002; 10:00 PM: F(1,5) = 6.9, P = 0.047) and on the DSST (10:00 PM: F(1,5) = 23.5, P = 0.005).

Withdrawal severity measures (nonchoice trials). Results of the overall measures of withdrawal severity are listed in Table V. Of the three drugs studied, only hydromorphone significantly decreased the overall self-reported withdrawal scores (F(1,5) = 8.77; P = 0.031). Hydromorphone also significantly decreased afternoon staff-rated withdrawal scores (F(1,5) = 8.35; P = 0.03). Oxazepam had no significant effect on

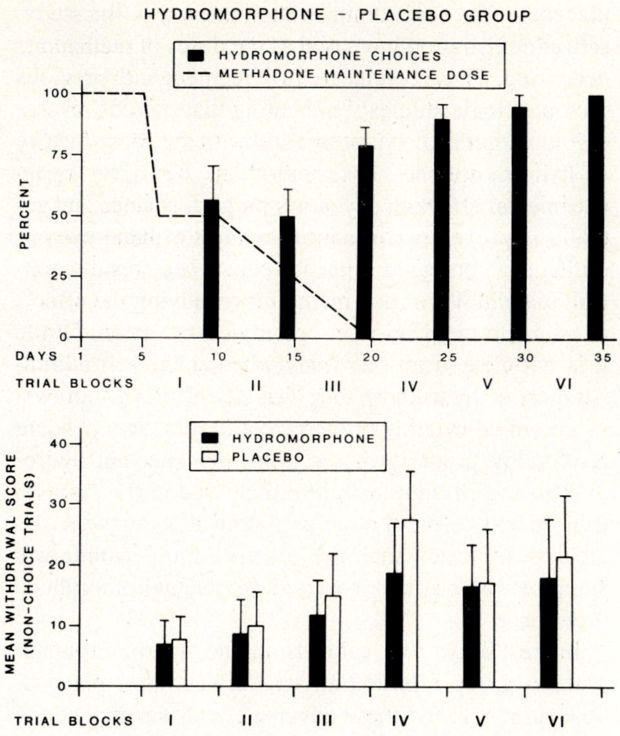

Fig. 1. *Upper graph* shows methadone dose (as percent of entry methadone maintenance dose) over days and mean (±SE) percent of hydromorphone choices over successive trial blocks. *Lower graph* shows mean (±SE) self-rated withdrawal score over successive trial blocks.

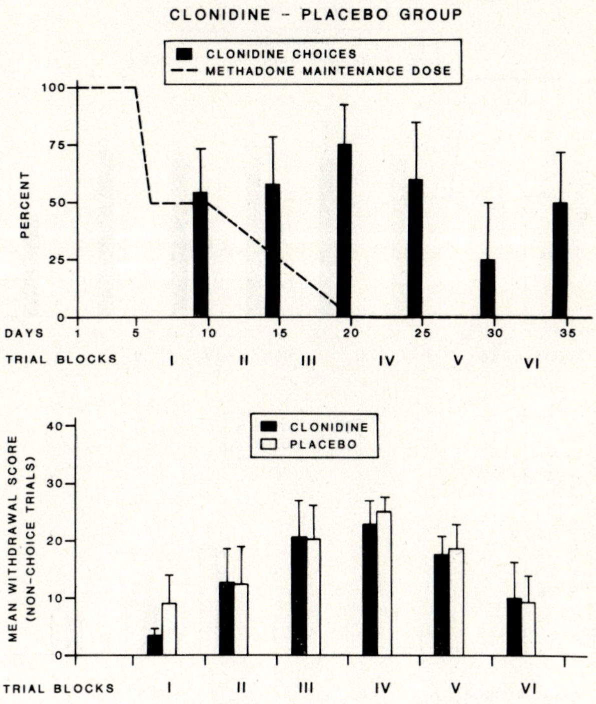

Fig. 2. *Upper graph* shows methadone dose (as percent of entry methadone maintenance dose) over days and mean (±SE) percent of clonidine choices over successive trial blocks. *Lower graph* shows mean (±SE) self-rated withdrawal score over successive trial blocks.

morning or afternoon staff-rated withdrawal scores. In the clonidine/placebo group, staff-rated withdrawal scores were collected for only two of the six subjects. Interestingly, these staff-rated withdrawal scores for both morning and afternoon were greater after clonidine dosing than after placebo dosing, indicating that in these two subjects, at least, clonidine may have increased the discomfort apparent to observers during methadone detoxification.

Self-administration measures (choice trials). Results of the self-administration portion of the study are listed in Table VI. Hydromorphone was chosen in significantly more choice trials than was placebo ($F(1.5) = 10.8$; $P = 0.022$). The total number of hydromorphone capsules taken was also significantly greater than the total number of placebo capsules taken ($F(1.5) = 11.4$; $P = 0.02$). Neither oxazepam nor clonidine was found to differ significantly from placebo either in terms of the numbers of total choices or total capsules ingested, although for both drugs the absolute differences from placebo were in the direction of greater self-administration of the active compound.

Figs. 1, 2, and 3 show the results of the self-administration and the self-reported withdrawal scores during individual trial blocks in relationship to the methadone dose reduction for the three drug groups. Self-reported withdrawal scores increased during methadone dose reduction, peaked during the fourth trial block when the methadone dose was decreased to zero, and then decreased in the final two trial blocks in all three groups. Only the group receiving hydromorphone reported consistently lower withdrawal scores after active drug than after placebo (Fig. 1). Hydromorphone was chosen in approximately 50% of the opportunities in the first two trial blocks. The frequency of choices for hydromorphone then increased over the last four trial blocks as the methadone dose decreased, with hydromorphone chosen in 100% of the opportunities during the last trial block. Clonidine did not consistently decrease withdrawal scores over time compared with placebo (Fig. 2). Clonidine self-administration varied over the six trial blocks, from a mean of 75% to 25% choices for active drug. The pattern of clonidine self-administration did not appear to be related to either methadone dose reduction or self-reported withdrawal scores. Oxaze-

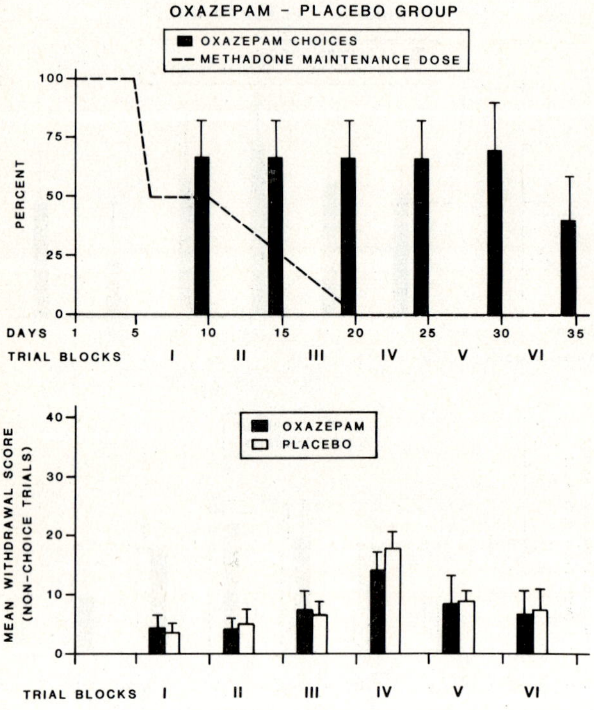

Fig. 3. *Upper graph* shows methadone dose (as percent of entry methadone maintenance dose) over days and mean (±SE) percent of oxazepam choices over successive trial blocks. *Lower graph* shows mean (±SE) self-rated withdrawal score over successive trial blocks.

pam also did not consistently decrease withdrawal scores relative to placebo (Fig. 3). The mean percent choices of oxazepam was constant over the first five trial blocks at approximately 65%. Choices for oxazepam dropped to approximately 40% during the last trial block. There was no apparent relationship between oxazepam self-administration and either the methadone dose reduction or withdrawal scores.

DISCUSSION

Only the opioid agonist hydromorphone, which was included in this study as a positive control drug, suppressed withdrawal signs and symptoms below placebo levels. At the doses tested, neither clonidine nor the short-acting benzodiazepine oxazepam significantly suppressed withdrawal or maintained self-administration. While clonidine did induce some significant effects, they were often in a direction opposite to those induced by hydromorphone and suggestive of drug-induced side effects rather than withdrawal relief.

Results show that hydromorphone was more effective than placebo in decreasing opioid withdrawal both as measured by subjective effect forms and by observer ratings. In addition, hydromorphone was preferred over placebo in the self-administration portion of the study; self-administration increased as the doses of methadone decreased. These results are in agreement with previous pharmacologic studies[7,8] indicating that opioids reverse opioid withdrawal symptoms and with the abuse history of hydromorphone. Hydromorphone had little or no detrimental effect on psychomotor performance and actually improved performance on a test of hand-eye coordination compared with placebo. These results confirm the validity of this method for studying the effects of adjuvant medication in opioid detoxification. While it is not clear from our study whether the self-administration of hydromorphone was due to its withdrawal symptom–alleviating properties or to some independent reinforcing property of the drug, the fact that hydromorphone self-administration increased in the last two trial blocks even though withdrawal symptoms decreased indicates that the alleviation of withdrawal symptoms alone did not account for the hydromorphone preference.

Interestingly, two subjects in the hydromorphone/placebo group reported adverse effects after placebo. One subject found these adverse effects severe enough to consider withdrawing from the study to avoid taking further doses of placebo. This phenomenon may have resulted from the contrast between placebo and hydromorphone or, perhaps, from a conditioned abstinence response to placebo.

Clonidine was not effective in decreasing withdrawal symptoms compared with placebo as measured by a subjective effect questionnaire. For the two subjects for which observer-rated withdrawal scores were made, the staff rated subjects as having more severe symptoms on days in which subjects received clonidine than on days on which placebo had been given. This finding may have been related to the sedative properties of clonidine. Clonidine increased PCAG (sedative) scores on the ARCI questionnaire and significantly decreased the vigor score on the POMS questionnaire compared with placebo. Clonidine was also not self-administered significantly more often than placebo. There was considerable between-subject variability in the free-choice self-administration of clonidine. Two subjects consistently chose placebo over clonidine and complained to the nursing staff of side effects on the days when clonidine was administered in the nonchoice trials. Other subjects, however, consistently chose clonidine over placebo, and clonidine was rated as having significantly greater "drug effect" and "good" effects than placebo on the visual analog scales. Although clonidine was not effective in alleviating withdrawal symptoms at the dose tested, clonidine did induce significant side effects including decreased blood pressure and impaired psychomotor performance. Therefore, although higher doses of clonidine may have provided more alleviation of withdrawal symptoms, it is likely that increased side effects would have offset any beneficial effects.

At the doses tested, oxazepam was not effective in decreasing self-reported or staff-rated withdrawal symptoms compared with placebo, nor was oxazepam self-administered significantly more frequently than placebo. Oxazepam was also not significantly different from placebo on any of the subjective effects measured. Oxazepam, however, did impair performance on both the psychomotor-cognitive tests at the two measurements taken latest in the day. These results might indicate that the oxazepam onset of action was too slow to be detected by the subjects and to have any significant effects on withdrawal symptoms during the daytime hours, or that the dose of oxazepam tested was too low to produce the desired effect. Higher doses may not be recommended, however, since oxazepam 30 mg b.i.d., is at the upper end of the recommended dose range and did impair psychomotor performance.

Throughout the study self-reported withdrawal scores tended to be lower in the oxazepam/placebo group than in either the clonidine or hydromorphine groups. The possibility that this could be a drug effect resulting from carryover of oxazepam effects into placebo days has been considered; however, this is not likely given the schedule and counterbalanced order of dosing. Rather, it seems most likely that this is a coincidental result of variability among the groups in the intensity of their complaints about symptoms; staff-rated withdrawal scores were similar in all three subject groups.

We selected oxazepam as the test benzodiazepine because it is pharmacokinetically short acting, i.e., it does not have long-acting metabolites as diazepam does. However, we have subsequently obtained data indicating that oxazepam has a slow onset of action—with peak effect 6 to 8 hours after oral dosing—and indicating that oxazepam's pharmacodynamic effects may persist longer than those of diazepam.[6] The slow rate of absorption of oxazepam has also been demonstrated in pharmacokinetic studies.[4,13] Thus because of the differences among members of the benzodiazepine class, further testing of other effects of benzodiazepines on opioid detoxification/withdrawal may be warranted.

References

1. Charney DS, Steinberg DE, Kleber HD, Heninger GR, Redmond E: The clinical use of clonidine in abrupt withdrawal from methadone. Arch Gen Psychiatry **38:**1273-1277, 1981.
2. Davis WM, Smith SG: Catecholaminergic mechanisms of reinforcement: Direct assessment by drug self-administration. Life Sci **20:**483-492, 1977.
3. Gold MS, Pottash AC, Sweeney DR, Kleber HD: Opiate withdrawal using clonidine. JAMA **243:**343-346, 1980.
4. Greenblatt SJ, Divoll M, Harmatz JS, Shader RI: Oxazepam kinetics: Effects of age and sex. J Pharmacol Exp Ther **215:**86-91, 1980.
5. Griffiths RR, Bigelow GE, Liebson I, Kaliszak JE: Drug preference in humans: Double-blind choice comparison of pentobarbital, diazepam and placebo. J Pharmacol Exp Ther **215:**649-661, 1980.
6. Griffiths RR, McLeod DR, Bigelow GE, Liebson IA, Roache JD: Relative abuse liability of diazepam and oxazepam: Behavioral and subjective dose effects. Psychopharmacology **84:**147-154, 1984.
7. Himmelsbach CK, Andrews HL: Studies on modification of the morphine abstinence syndrome by drugs. J Pharmacol Exp Ther **77:**17-23, 1943.
8. Jasinski DR: Assessment of the abuse potentiality of morphine like drugs (methods used in man). *In* Martin WR, editor: Drug addiction I. New York, 1977, Springer Verlag.
9. Kleber HD, Gold MS: Use of psychotropic drugs in treatment of methadone maintained narcotic addicts. Ann NY Acad Sci **311:**81-98, 1978.
10. Martin WR, Sloan JW, Sapiro JD, Jasinski DR: Physiologic, subjective, and behavioral effects of amphetamine, methamphetamine, ephedrine, phenmetrazine and methylphenidate in man. CLIN PHARMACOL THER **12:**245-258, 1971.
11. McLeod DR, Griffiths RR, Bigelow GE, Yingling J: An automated version of the digit symbol substitution test (DSST). Behav Res Methods Instrum **14:**463-466, 1982.
12. McNair D, Loor M, Droppleman L: Profile of mood states-(POMS). San Diego, Calif., 1971, Educational and Industrial Testing Services.
13. Salzman C, Shader I, Greenblatt DJ, Harmatz JS: Long and short half-life benzodiazepines in the elderly. Arch Gen Psychiatry **40:**293-297, 1983.
14. Stitzer ML, Griffiths RR, McLellan AT, Grabowski J, Hawthorne JW: Diazepam use among methadone maintenance patients: Patterns and dosages. Drug Alcohol Depend **8:**189-199, 1981.
15. Washton AM, Resnick RB: Clonidine in opiate withdrawal: Review and appraisal of clinical findings. Pharmacotherapy **1:**140-146, 1981.
16. Woody GE, O'Brien CP, Greenstein R: Misuse and abuse of diazepam: An increasingly common medical problem. Int J Addict **10:**843-848, 1975.
17. Woolverton WL, Wessinger WD, Balster RL: Reinforcing properties of clonidine in rhesus monkeys. Psychopharmacology **77:**17-23, 1982.

Effects of age and disease on the pharmacokinetics and pharmacodynamics of sulindac

The disposition and effect on hemostasis of a single 150 mg dose of sulindac was studied in young healthy subjects and in older patients with arthritis. Older patients were restudied after 2 weeks of sulindac, 150 mg b.i.d. The only difference in disposition of the first dose was a reduced plasma sulfone metabolite concentration in the elderly patients with arthritis. Chronic sulindac dosing resulted in accumulation of the drug and its sulfone and sulfide metabolites in plasma to a greater extent than previously reported for young subjects. No differences in renal clearance of sulindac and its sulfone metabolite related to age or chronic drug dosing were observed. No renal excretion of the active sulfide metabolite was detected. Bleeding time in the elderly patients was shorter than in the young healthy subjects before sulindac dosing, but was prolonged in the elderly patients after 2 weeks of dosing to values similar to control data from the young healthy subjects. This change correlated weakly with plasma sulfide metabolite concentrations. Differences in bleeding time were not reflected in changes in platelet aggregation induced by adenosine diphosphate either with respect to age or chronic drug dosing. Our data provide no justification for lowering the recommended dose of sulindac for patients older than 65 years of age. (CLIN PHARMACOL THER 38:228-234, 1985.)

D. S. Sitar, Ph.D., J. A. Owen, Ph.D.,* B. MacDougall, M.D., T. Hunter, M.D., and P. A. Mitenko, M.D. *Winnipeg, Manitoba, Canada*

Sulindac is a nonsteroidal anti-inflammatory drug (NSAID) with analgesic and antipyretic properties introduced for the treatment of rheumatic disorders.[1] It is both oxidized and reduced in the body, and while oxidation to the sulfone metabolite is irreversible, reduction to the sulfide metabolite is reversible. Only unchanged sulindac, the sulfone metabolite, and their glucuronide conjugates are excreted in urine, and about half of the dose is excreted in the feces.[5] The therapeutic activity of this drug has been attributed to its sulfide metabolite.[21] Inhibition of platelet aggregation in vitro also appears to be associated with the sulfide metabolite.[11] Although adverse drug reactions have been reported with the use of sulindac, the mechanism of such actions is not clear.[18] Pharmacokinetic and other studies to date have been performed primarily on healthy younger subjects.[6,7,11,14] Because advanced age and associated disease may affect pharmacokinetics and pharmacodynamics, we conducted this study to assess the potential for effects of age and disease on the use of sulindac in rheumatic diseases.

From the Geriatric Clinical Pharmacology and Rheumatic Disease Units, Departments of Medicine and Pharmacology and Therapeutics, University of Manitoba.

Supported by grants from Merck Frosst Laboratories, Montreal, Quebec; The Royal Canadian Legion, St. James Branch, Winnipeg, Manitoba; and a postdoctoral fellowship to J. A. O. from the Medical Research Council of Canada.

Received for publication Feb. 2, 1985; accepted May 1, 1985.

Reprint requests to: D. S. Sitar, Ph.D., Geriatric Clinical Pharmacology Unit, Department of Pharmacology and Therapeutics, University of Manitoba, 770 Bannatyne Ave., Winnipeg, Manitoba R3E OW3, Canada.

*Present address: Department of Urology, Queen's University, Kingston, Ontario, Canada.

METHODS

Our subjects were 10 young healthy normal subjects and 16 elderly patients with a primary diagnosis of either rheumatoid arthritis (n = 6) or osteoarthritis (n = 10; Table I). All the older patients had arthritis of moderate severity but were otherwise reasonably healthy, and none had any hepatic or renal dysfunction on initial examination. In particular, no subject had creatinine clearance <32 ml/min.

All participants abstained from acetylsalicylic acid for 2 weeks before the first study day, and patients with

Table I. Demographic data for the healthy young subjects and the elderly patients with arthritis

	Subjects	*Patients*
No. of participants	10	16
Sex	6M/4F	4M/12F
Age (yr)	27 ± 2	70 ± 1
Weight (kg)	69.0 ± 3.7	74.1 ± 3.3

Data are $\overline{X}$ ± SE.
M = Male; F = female.

arthritis did not take acetylsalicylic acid during the study. Medications not known to interfere with sulindac disposition or platelet function were allowed and included benzodiazepines, *l*-thyroxine, allopurinol, and a variety of antihypertensive agents. Nine of the 16 patients with arthritis received such therapy during the study. Patients with arthritic disease stopped using NSAIDs 1 week before the study and received sulindac as their only antiarthritic medication for the 2-week duration of the study. These conditions were imposed to prevent changes in platelet function due to any drug other than sulindac. Patients who required supplemental analgesia were given acetaminophen with or without codeine during the prestudy drug withdrawal period and for the duration of the study.

All participants fasted overnight before drug dosing. Sulindac (Clinoril; Merck Sharp & Dohme) was provided as commercially formulated 150 mg tablets (421 μmol). All subjects received their first dose between 7:30 and 8:30 AM. Blood samples (8 ml) were drawn through an indwelling venous cannula kept patent with a heparin in saline solution lock (10 U/ml) and were placed in tubes containing sodium oxalate. Samples were drawn just before dosing and 0.33, 0.67, 1, 2, 3, 4, 6, 8, and 12 hours thereafter. Total urine was also collected in 2-hour aliquots for 12 hours. After this initial study, the patients with arthritis continued to take sulindac, 150 mg every 12 hours, starting the next morning (24 hours after the first dose). On day 8, a blood sample was drawn just before the morning dose for the determination of levels of sulindac and its metabolites. On the morning of day 15, after an overnight fast, patients received a final 150 mg dose of sulindac and the kinetic study described above was repeated.

Concurrent with the kinetic studies, bleeding times were measured in all participants before the morning dose and 6 hours after drug dosing on both study days. In addition, some participants provided blood samples concurrent with the bleeding time studies (9 ml each time) for platelet aggregation determinations with citrated whole blood diluted 50% with normal saline solution and adenosine diphosphate (ADP) as the stimulating agent.[2]

Plasma was separated and frozen until analyzed for sulindac and its sulfone and sulfide metabolites by HPLC.[9] Urine volume was determined and aliquots were frozen for drug and metabolite analyses. All samples were stored at −20° C until the day of analysis. Urine was diluted 25-fold with distilled water. An aliquot (0.5 ml) was mixed with an equal volume of 1 mol/L acetate buffer at pH 4.0 containing the internal standard and extracted with 5 ml ethyl acetate. The ethyl acetate was separated and evaporated under a stream of nitrogen. The residue was dissolved in the running solvent and analyzed for sulindac and its metabolites as described above for plasma.[9] Glucuronide conjugates were hydrolyzed by mixing 1.0 ml diluted urine with 0.2 ml 1N sodium hydroxide solution and allowing the alkalinized urine to stand at room temperature for 1 hour. The solution was then neutralized with 1N hydrochloric acid solution. An aliquot (0.5 ml) was mixed with acetate buffer, extracted with ethyl acetate, and analyzed for sulindac and its metabolites as described for the nonhydrolyzed urine samples.

Noncompartmental methods were used for kinetic analyses. Because the sampling periods after dosing were relatively short, especially for the metabolites, some conventional pharmacokinetic parameters could not be accurately determined. Apparent plasma clearance at steady state was calculated by dividing the dose by the plasma AUC during a dose interval. The AUC was determined by the trapezoidal rule. Statistical analyses were done with ANOVA followed by a multiple range test where appropriate.[8,10,15] All data are presented as the $\overline{X}$ ± SE.

RESULTS

Characteristics of the participants are listed in Table I. Preliminary comparisons of the kinetic data did not reveal differences in sulindac disposition or effect related to the primary diagnosis in elderly patients. Similarly, there were no sex-related differences in disposition. All patients with arthritis are therefore considered as a single group for data presentation and subsequent statistical comparisons.

One of the patients with osteoarthritis, a 75-year-old woman, was withdrawn from the study on day 8 because of anxiety and paranoid ideation. She was assessed clinically and her apprehension was thought to be due to continued participation in the trial and not related to sulindac dosing. She returned to her previous

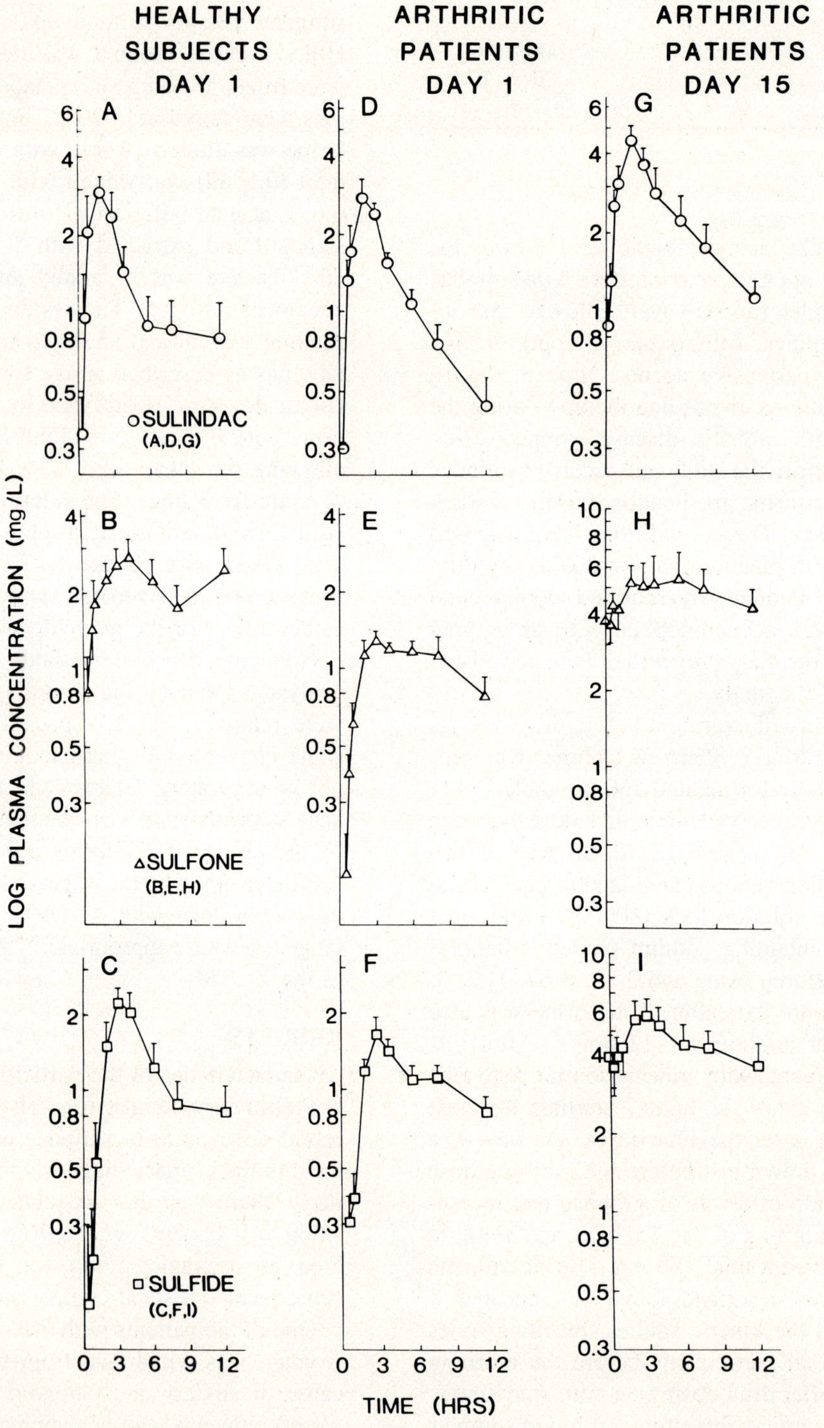

Fig. 1. Mean (±SE) plasma concentrations of sulindac and its sulfone and sulfide metabolites in normal subjects after a single 150 mg dose *(left)* and in patients with arthritis after a single 150 mg dose *(middle)* and after 2 weeks of therapy with 150 mg sulindac every 12 hours *(right)*.

Table II. Kinetic disposition over a dose interval (12 hours) related to plasma analyses for sulindac and its sulfone and sulfide metabolites in normal healthy subjects and in patients with arthritis

	Subjects (day 1)	Patients Day 1	Patients Day 15
Peak concentration (mg/L)			
Sulindac	3.8 ± 0.6*	3.5 ± 0.4*	5.3 ± 0.6
Sulfone	3.2 ± 0.6*	1.6 ± 0.1*†	6.3 ± 1.4
Sulfide	2.6 ± 0.4*	1.9 ± 0.1*	6.4 ± 1.1
AUC (mg/L · hr)			
Sulindac	14.87 ± 2.67*	14.20 ± 1.48*	27.47 ± 4.61
Sulfone	25.14 ± 4.81*	12.06 ± 1.16*†	57.09 ± 12.70
Sulfide	13.82 ± 2.08*	12.74 ± 1.17*	54.27 ± 9.93

Data are $\overline{X}$ ± SE.
*Significantly different ($P < 0.05$) from patients on day 15.
†Significantly different ($P < 0.05$) from healthy subjects on day 1.

Table III. Effects of sulindac on hemostasis in young healthy subjects after a single dose and in older patients with arthritis after a single dose and after 14 days of therapy

	Subjects (Day 1) t = 0 hr	Subjects (Day 1) t = 6 hr	Patients (Day 15) t = 0 hr	Patients (Day 15) t = 6 hr
Bleeding time (min)				
Subjects (n = 10)	5.9 ± 0.9†	6.2 ± 0.4	—	—
Patients (n = 16)*	4.5 ± 0.2	4.9 ± 0.3	5.1 ± 0.4	5.8 ± 0.4†
Platelet aggregation (% full scale)				
Subjects (n = 6)	65 ± 6	61 ± 8	—	—
Patients (n = 9)	49 ± 8	55 ± 9	63 ± 10	62 ± 7
ADP for maximum aggregation (μmol/L)				
Subjects (n = 6)	13 ± 3	13 ± 2	—	—
Patients (n = 9)	12 ± 2	14 ± 3	12 ± 2	13 ± 3

Data are $\overline{X}$ ± SE.
*n = 15 on day 15.
†Significantly different ($P < 0.05$) from patients at t = 0 hours on day 1.

state of health gradually over the next week. All other patients studied had relatively few problems taking the medication, and especially noteworthy was an absence of gastrointestinal symptoms. Although our study was not designed to test the efficacy of the drug, most of the patients achieved good control of their arthritic symptoms while taking sulindac, and 10 of 16 asked to have the sulindac continued at the end of the study.

Plasma concentration-time curves for sulindac and its sulfone and sulfide metabolites are presented in Fig. 1. Peak plasma concentration of sulindac occurred 2 hours after dosing in both young subjects and elderly patients on both study days. Peak plasma concentration of the sulfone and sulfide metabolites occurred 4 hours after dosing and did not vary with the age of subject or the day of drug dosing. The only difference in disposition in patients with arthritis after the first dose was a reduced peak plasma sulfone concentration, which was reflected in a reduced plasma AUC (Table II). Trough plasma concentrations of sulindac and its metabolites in patients on day 8 of the study were similar to those immediately before dosing (t = 0) on day 15. Plasma clearance of sulindac at steady state in the patients was 120 ± 26 ml/kg/hr.

The plasma sulfide concentrations 6 hours after the first dose did not differ in young healthy subjects and older patients with arthritis (1.2 ± 0.3 and 1.1 ± 0.1 mg/L, respectively), nor were they different at t = 0 and t = 6 hours in the patients on day 15 (3.9 ± 1.0 and 4.4 ± 0.9 mg/L, respectively). Bleeding times

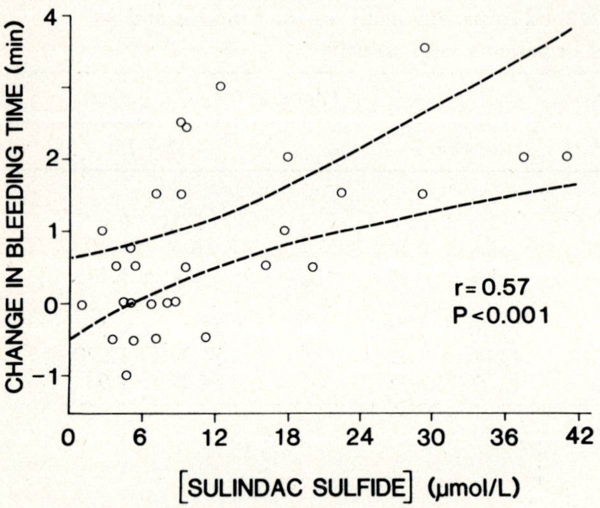

Fig. 2. Change in bleeding time in elderly patients with arthritis (as compared with prestudy control determinations) compared with the sulfide metabolite concentration in plasma just before and 6 hours after a drug dose on day 15 of the study. *Dashed lines* represent the 95% confidence interval for the correlation.

correlated modestly with sulfide metabolite concentration on day 15 compared with prestudy values in the patients (Fig. 2). Although bleeding times showed a lengthening tendency overall, the only significant difference was observed 6 hours after dosing on day 15 compared with prestudy values in the patients. This was not reflected in platelet aggregation induced by ADP either with respect to maximum aggregation or the ADP concentration required to produce maximum aggregation (Table III). These findings occurred with similar and normal platelet concentrations of 241,000 ± 13,000, 254,000 ± 11,000, and 255,000 ± 11,000 cells/mm^3 in the normal subjects and in the patients with arthritis on days 1 and 15 of the study, respectively. Hemoglobin concentrations for these same groups of 144 ± 5, 136 ± 3, and 135 ± 4 gm/L at these times also did not differ.

Urinary excretion data for sulindac and its metabolites are listed in Table IV. There was no difference between elderly patients with arthritis and young healthy subjects, and excretion amounted to 47% of the administered dose at steady state in the patients. Renal clearance of sulindac and its sulfone metabolite (Table V) did not differ after drug dosing. No sulfide metabolite was detected in any of the urine samples analyzed. Creatinine clearance in the patients on day 15 (58 ± 4 ml/min) was less than that on day 1 (64 ± 5 ml/min; P = 0.03). These findings occurred in the presence of unchanged serum creatinine concentrations between days 1 and 15 in the patients (0.09 ± 0.01 mmol/L). BUN values (6.8 ± 0.5 mmol/L on day 1 and 7.4 ± 0.5 mmol/L on day 15) also did not change.

DISCUSSION

Previous reports of sulindac disposition have generally featured young healthy subjects, while the older patients in our study approximated typical users of the drug in terms of age and disease. The younger controls in our study were found to have kinetic parameters similar to those reported.[6,12,17,20] We have some confidence, therefore, in our findings concerning reduced plasma concentrations of the sulfone metabolite (with a corresponding reduction in AUC) on the first day of dosing in our older patients. Because the sulfone metabolite has not been shown to have any biologic effect,[21] this difference is not of particular clinical importance, but it does suggest that sulindac metabolism may change with age.

Of greater interest is the degree of accumulation of sulindac and its metabolites in older people. Swanson et al.[20] found the cumulation factors in young subjects to be 1.23 for sulindac, 2.52 for the sulfide metabolite, and 2.42 for the sulfone metabolite. The dose given was 200 mg b.i.d. and the cumulation factors were calculated by comparing the 12-hour AUCs for the first and seventh day of dosing. The data of Duggan et al.[6] yield similar results for sulindac and the sulfide metabolite. Although the results of Mattila et al.[17] are not as easy to interpret, there appears to be some degree of accumulation of sulindac and the sulfide metabolite but not of the sulfone metabolite. The older patients in our study were found to have corresponding cumulation factors of 1.93 for sulindac, 4.26 for the sulfide metabolite, and 4.73 for the sulfone metabolite after comparing the 12-hour AUCs for days 1 and 15. Because concentrations of sulindac and its metabolites before dosing on day 15 were not different from those on day 8, these values indicate the degree of accumulation of sulindac and its metabolites in older patients at steady state. Although the cumulation factors are substantially higher for our older patients than those reported earlier for younger subjects, the absence of adverse clinical or laboratory effects suggests that this dosage of sulindac for the elderly is not excessive.

Renal excretion of sulindac and its metabolites by older people appears to be qualitatively and quantitatively similar to results found in younger subjects.[6,12,20] We were not able to detect the active sulfide metabolite

Table IV. Urinary excretion of sulindac and metabolites during a dose interval (μmol/12 hours) in young healthy subjects after a single dose and in older patients with arthritis after a single dose and after 14 days of therapy (421 μmol/dose, equivalent to 150 mg sulindac)

	Sulindac	*Sulindac glucuronide*	*Sulfone*	*Sulfone glucuronide*	*Total*
Day 1					
Subjects (n = 10)	18.5 ± 4.1	26.7 ± 4.3	8.0 ± 1.5	29.1 ± 3.9	82 ± 10
Patients (n = 16)	22.1 ± 5.4	21.5 ± 2.4	14.1 ± 2.1	20.2 ± 2.7	78 ± 8
Day 15					
Patients (n = 15)	36.1 ± 9.1	39.2 ± 5.1	39.3 ± 6.4	84.0 ± 9.5	199 ± 17

Data are $\overline{X}$ ± SE.

Table V. Renal clearance of sulindac and its sulfone metabolite (ml/kg/hr) in young healthy subjects after a single dose and in older patients with arthritis after a single dose and after 14 days of therapy

	Sulindac	*Sulfone metabolite*
Subjects (day 1; n = 10)	9.1 ± 2.6	3.1 ± 1.1
Patients (day 1; n = 16)	10.6 ± 2.7	7.5 ± 1.7
Patients (day 15; n = 15)	9.3 ± 2.8	5.6 ± 1.4

in urine, again in agreement with previous studies, and this absence presumably results from the reversible conversion of the sulfide metabolite back to sulindac.[5,6,12] Our use of alkaline hydrolysis for the glucuronide conjugates has been validated.[12]

We do not consider the small change in creatinine clearance observed in our older patients during the 2 weeks of sulindac dosing to be clinically important. This is supported by the unchanged renal clearance of sulindac and its sulfone metabolite over the 2-week period and also by the finding of similar values for serum creatinine and BUN levels. The minimal effect of sulindac on the kidney is supported by earlier studies in younger subjects and is in contrast to the renal effects reported with other NSAIDs.[3,4,19] It should be pointed out, however, that all our older patients had reasonable kidney function for age before sulindac dosing.

Our use of a 6-hour postdose assessment of bleeding time and platelet aggregation is based on the study of Green et al.,[11] who observed maximal inhibition of platelet function and a slightly prolonged bleeding time 6 hours after ingestion of 200 mg sulindac by younger subjects. Our study showed a prolongation of bleeding time in older patients on day 15 only, and a corresponding weak association with the plasma sulfide metabolite concentration (Fig. 2; Table III). The bleeding times for our older patients on day 15 were similar to the day 1 control data in our younger subjects, and our observations on day 1 of a shorter bleeding time in older patients before drug dosing confirm a similar observation by Jorgensen et al.[13] The change in bleeding time in older patients was not reflected by any observable differences in platelet aggregation in our study. Green et al.[11] found such an association, but they used an enriched platelet preparation and an optical assay for their determinations, while we used whole blood and a resistance method to quantify platelet aggregation. Both methods are said to give similar patterns for platelet aggregation,[2] but it may be that the difference in methodology was responsible for the difference in observations.

In conclusion, effects on hemostasis in the elderly are minimal. This dose of sulindac in chronic therapy should be safe in terms of hemorrhagic complications. Coupled with our results concerning sulindac disposition and its effect on renal function, this observation may provide some assurance concerning the use of this drug for older patients. We were not able to separate the effects of age and disease in this study, but since all the older patients were in reasonable health, the differences observed were probably due to age alone. Our study provides no justification for modifying the recommended dose of sulindac for the elderly, but did not address the question of whether larger doses would improve efficacy while maintaining safety.

We thank Mrs. L. Forsyth, R.N., for nursing assistance and Mr. J. Sherwin and Mr. C. Foster for technical assistance in the laboratory. We are also grateful to the patients who agreed to participate. Clinoril was provided by the Frosst Division of Merck Frosst Canada Inc., Montreal, Quebec, Canada.

References

1. Brogden RN, Heel RC, Speight TM, Avery GS: Sulindac: A review of its pharmacological properties and therapeutic efficacy in rheumatic diseases. Drugs **16:**97-114, 1978.
2. Cardinal DC, Flower RJ: The electronic aggregometer: A novel device for assessing platelet behavior in blood. J Pharmacol Methods **3:**135-158, 1980.
3. Ciabattoni G, Cinotti GA, Pierucci A, Simonetti BM, Manzi M, Pugliese F, Barsotti P, Pecci G, Taggi F, Patrono C: Effects of sulindac and ibuprofen in patients with chronic glomerular disease. N Engl J Med **310:**279-283, 1984.
4. Ciabattoni G, Pugliese F, Cinotti GA, Patrono C: Renal effect of anti-inflammatory drugs. Eur J Rheum Inflam **3:**210-221, 1980.
5. Duggan DE: Sulindac: Therapeutic implications of the prodrug/pharmacophore equilibrium. Drug Metab Rev **12:**325-337, 1981.
6. Duggan DE, Hare LE, Ditzler CA, Lei BW, Kwan KC: The disposition of sulindac. CLIN PHARMACOL THER **21:**326-335, 1977.
7. Dujovne CA, Pitterman A, Vincek WC, Dobrinska MR, Davies RO, Duggan DE: Enterohepatic circulation of sulindac and metabolites. CLIN PHARMACOL THER **33:**172-177, 1983.
8. Duncan DB: Multiple range and multiple F tests. Biometrics **11:**1-42, 1955.
9. Dusci LJ, Hackett LP: Determination of sulindac and its metabolites in serum by high-performance liquid chromatography. J Chromatogr **171:**490-493, 1979.
10. Goldstein A: Biostatistics: An introductory text. New York, 1964, Macmillan Company, pp 84-85.
11. Green D, Given KM, Ts'ao C, Whipple JP, Rossi EC: The effect of a new non-steroidal anti-inflammatory agent, sulindac, on platelet function. Thromb Res **10:**283-289, 1977.
12. Hucker HB, Stauffer SC, White SD, Rhodes RE, Arison BH, Umbenhauer ER, Bower RJ, McMahon FG: Physiologic disposition and metabolic fate of a new anti-inflammatory agent, *cis*-5-fluoro-2-methyl-1-(*p*-(methylsulfinyl)-benzylidenyl)-indene-3-acetic acid in the rat, dog, rhesus monkey, and man. Drug Metab Dispos **1:**721-736, 1973.
13. Jorgensen KA, Dyerberg J, Olesen AS, Stoffersen E: Acetylsalicylic acid, bleeding time and age. Thromb Res **19:**799-805, 1980.
14. Juhl RP, Van Thiel DH, Ditlert LW, Albert KS, Smith RB: Ibuprofen and sulindac kinetics in alcoholic liver disease. CLIN PHARMACOL THER **34:**104-109, 1983.
15. Kramer CY: Extension of multiple range tests to group means with unequal numbers of replications. Biometrics **12:**307-310, 1956.
16. Lanza FL, Nelson RS, Rack MF: A controlled endoscopic study comparing the toxic effects of sulindac, naproxen, aspirin and placebo on the gastric mucosa of healthy volunteers. J Clin Pharmacol **24:**89-95, 1984.
17. Mattila J, Mäntylä R, Vuorela A, Lamminsivu U, Männistö P: Pharmacokinetics of graded oral doses of sulindac in man. Arzneimittelforsch **34:**226-229, 1984.
18. Park GD, Spector R, Headstream T, Goldberg M: Serious adverse reactions associated with sulindac. Arch Intern Med **142:**1292-1294, 1982.
19. Sedor JR, Williams SL, Chremos AN, Johnson CL, Dunn MJ: Effects of sulindac and indomethacin on renal prostaglandin synthesis. CLIN PHARMACOL THER **36:**85-91, 1984.
20. Swanson BN, Boppana VK, Vlasses PH, Holmes GI, Monsell K, Ferguson RK: Sulindac disposition when given once and twice daily. CLIN PHARMACOL THER **32:**397-403, 1982.
21. Van Arman CG, Risley EA, Nuss GW, Hucker HB, Duggan DE: Pharmacology of sulindac. *In* Huskisson EC, Franchimont P, editors: Clinoril in the treatment of rheumatic disorders: A new nonsteroidal anti-inflammatory/analgesic agent. Proceedings of the Eighth European Rheumatology Congress, Helsinki, Finland, June 1-7, 1975. New York, 1976, Raven Press, pp 9-36.

Notes of the American Society for Clinical Pharmacology and Therapeutics

A Message from the President

The American Society for Clinical Pharmacology and Therapeutics is the premier organization in the world that represents clinical pharmacology.

The lay public is well aware of the American Heart Association and the American Society of Nephrology or American Kidney Foundation and know that when there are problems related to the heart and kidney, respectively, questions are posed to these organizations and their representatives. To date the ASCPT has not had that type of visibility within the lay public and media. I, as President, feel that it is time that ASCPT has this degree of credibility and visibility. In the past and even now the media have resorted to consulting with Washington-based physician-consumer advocates who generally denigrate both the Food and Drug Administration and the pharmaceutical industry.

I am requesting members of the ASCPT and the readers of CLINICAL PHARMACOLOGY AND THERAPEUTICS to recommend to the media and to the lay public that with regards to controversy and problems related to drugs, that the media or the public be referred to experts within our Society.

By utilizing the Scientific Sections, which include: (1) Analgesia; (2) Epidemiology (adverse drug reactions); (3) Biostatistics and Computer Sciences; (4) Cardiovascular and Pulmonary Drugs; (5) Antihypertensives; (6) Clinical Pathology and Human Toxicology; (7) Clinical Trial Methodology; (8) Dermatologic and Allergic Diseases; (9) Endocrine Drugs; (10) Gastrointestinal and Liver Diseases; (11) Headache; (12) Hematologic and Neoplastic Diseases; (13) Infectious Disease and Antimicrobial Agents; (14) Medico-Legal Matters and Research and Development Administration; (15) Neuropsychopharmacological Drugs; (16) Pediatric Pharmacology; (17) Pharmacokinetics and Drug Metabolism; (18) Pharmacometrics; (19) Renal; and (20) Rheumatology and Immunology, experts from these areas can provide unbiased and accurate information. In addition, the Society has standing committees related to ethics, government affairs, medical education, publications, liaison to the American Medical Association, and the development of the annual scientific program. The annual program is generally in March and is well publicized. Reporters from medical sources generally come to these meetings, but the major newspapers are not always represented.

Any questions from the media or the public can be directed to Elaine Galasso, Executive Secretary, who can then refer whatever question there is to the appropriate individual or individuals. The office address and phone number are: 1718 Gallagher Road, Norristown, PA 19401; (215) 825-3838.

I hope that in the future, ASCPT and its members will be recognized for the accurate dissemination of unbiased information. The knowledge that ASCPT, which has a liaison to both the Food and Drug Administration and the pharmaceutical industry, can be of benefit pro bono publico.

David T. Lowenthal, M.D.
President

Notice of workshop

The Academy of Pharmaceutical Sciences, the ASCPT, the Drug Information Association, and the Food and Drug Administration will sponsor a workshop entitled "Controlled Release Dosage Forms: Issues and Controversies," in Washington, D.C., on Sept. 29-Oct. 2, 1985. Co-Chairmen will be Leslie Z. Benet, Ph.D., President, Academy of Pharmaceutical Sciences; David T. Lowenthal, M.D., President, ASCPT; and Jerome P. Skelly, Ph.D., Acting Director, Division of Biopharmaceutics, Food and Drug Administration. Major topics to be covered at the workshop include: pharmacokinetic considerations, biopharmaceutic considerations, clinical/pharmacodynamic considerations, regulatory considerations for therapeutic equivalence, and an open forum on biopharmaceutic concerns in controlled-release dosage forms.

Due to limited space, early registration is requested.

More detailed information, including program and registration materials, can be obtained from: Drug Information Association, P.O. Box 113, Maple Glen, PA 19002. Telephone: (215) 628-2288.

David T. Lowenthal, M.D.
President, ASCPT

Future meeting dates and sites of the ASCPT

March 20-22, 1986	Sheraton Washington Hotel, Washington, D.C.
March 25-28, 1987	Marriott Orlando World Center, Walt Disney World, Fla.
March 9-11, 1988	Town and Country Hotel, San Diego, Calif.

Call for scientific program abstracts forms for 1986 meeting in Washington, D.C., March 20-22, are included in this issue of the JOURNAL and also appeared in the June and July issues. Additional forms are available on request to Elaine Galasso, 1718 Gallagher Rd., Norristown, PA 19401; (215) 825-3838.

USAN Council

List No. 263

New Names

The following nonproprietary names for the compounds described have been adopted by the United States Adopted Names (USAN) Council, which is sponsored by the American Medical Association, the American Pharmaceutical Association, and the US Pharmacopeial Convention, Inc., in cooperation with the respective pharmaceutical manufacturers. The designation USAN (United States Adopted Name) distinguishes these formally adopted nonproprietary names from other names. The information given under the category Therapeutic Claim is based on the manufacturer's claims at the time of publication. Adoption of USAN does not imply endorsement of the claims or products by the AMA, the US Pharmacopeia, or the APhA.

In some instances, the drugs listed are available only from the manufacturer to properly qualified investigators for clinical study.

USAN: RIFAPENTINE

Pronunciation: rĭf′ ȧ pĕn tēn

Therapeutic claim: antibacterial

Chemical names

(1) 3-[[(4-cyclopentyl-1-piperazinyl)imino]methyl]rifamycin

(2) 3-[*N*-(4-cyclopentyl-1-piperazinyl)formimidoyl]rifamycin

Structural formula

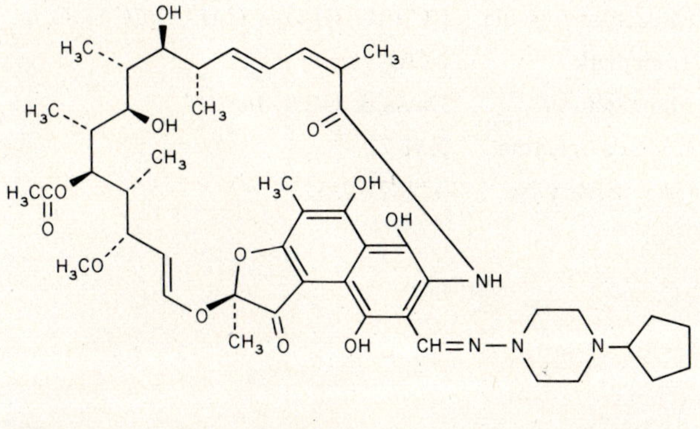

Molecular formula: $C_{47}H_{64}N_4O_{12}$

Molecular weight: 877.04

Manufacturer: Merrell Dow Pharmaceuticals Inc.

Code designation: MDL 473

CAS registry No.: 61379-65-5

USAN: QUINAPRIL HYDROCHLORIDE

Pronunciation: kwĭn′ ȧ prĭl″

Therapeutic claim: antihypertensive (angiotensin-converting enzyme inhibitor)

Chemical names

(1) [3*S*-[2[*R**(*R**)]],3*R**]-2-[2-[[1-(ethoxycarbonyl)-3-phenylpropyl]amino]-1-oxopropyl]-1,2,3,4-tetrahydro-3-isoquinolinecarboxylic acid, monohydrochloride, monohydrate

(2) *(S)*-2-[*(S)*-*N*-[*(S)*-1-carboxy-3-phenylpropyl]alanyl]-1,2,3,4-tetrahydro-3-isoquinolinecarboxylic acid, 1-ethyl ester, monohydrochloride, monohydrate

Structural formula

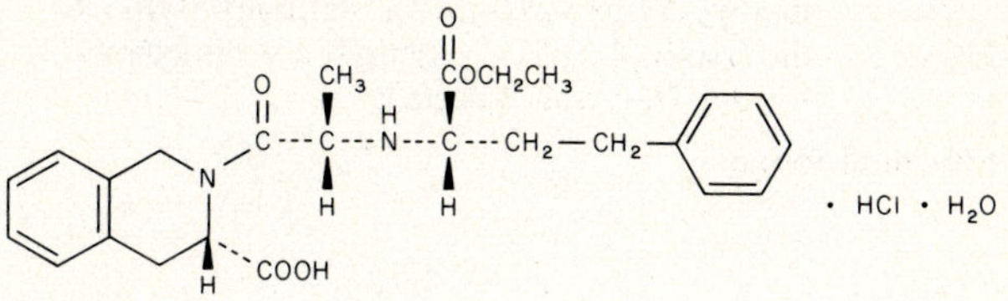

Molecular formula: $C_{25}H_{30}N_2O_5 \cdot HCl \cdot H_2O$

Molecular weight: 493.00

Manufacturer: Parke-Davis

Code designation: CI-906

CAS registry No.: 90243-99-5

USAN: LUPITIDINE HYDROCHLORIDE

Pronunciation: lū pĭ′ tĭ dēn″

Therapeutic claim: histamine H_2-receptor antagonist (veterinary use)

Chemical names

(1) 2-[[2-[[[5-[(dimethylamino)methyl]-2-furanyl]methyl]thio]ethyl]amino]-5-[(6-methyl-3-pyridinyl)methyl]-4(1*H*)-pyrimidinone trihydrochloride

(2) 2-[[2-[[5-[(dimethylamino)methyl]furfuryl]thio]ethyl]amino]-5-[(6-methyl-3-pyridyl)methyl]-4(1*H*)-pyrimidinone trihydrochloride

Structural formula

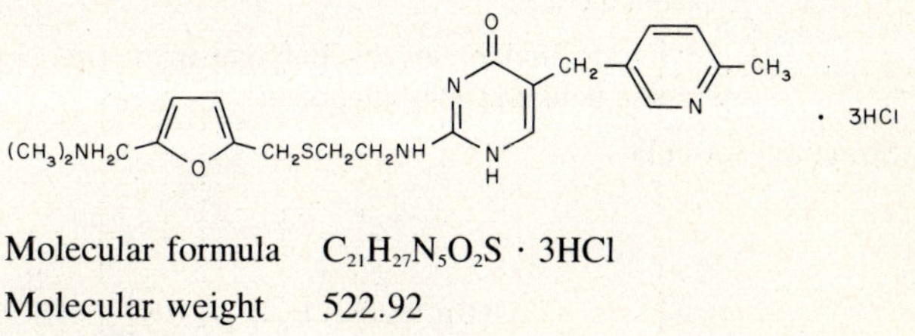

Molecular formula: $C_{21}H_{27}N_5O_2S \cdot 3HCl$

Molecular weight: 522.92

Manufacturer: Smith Kline & French Laboratories

Code designation: SK&F 93479

CAS registry No.: 72716-75-7

USAN	MADURAMICIN
Pronunciation	mă dŭr′ à mī″ sĭn
Therapeutic claim	anticoccidal
Chemical names	

(1) (3*R*,4*S*,5*S*,6*R*,7*S*,22*S*)-23,27-didemethoxy-2,6,22-tridemethyl-11-*O*-demethyl-22-[(2,6-dideoxy-3,4-di-*O*-methyl-β-L-*arabino*-hexopyranosyl)oxy]-6-methoxylonomycin A, monoammonium salt

(2) ammonium (2*R*,3*S*,4*S*,5*R*,6*S*)-tetrahydro-2-hydroxy-6-[(*R*)-1-[(2*S*,5*R*,7*S*,8*R*,9*S*)-9-hydroxy-2,8-dimethyl-2-[(2*S*,2′*R*,3′*S*,5*R*,5′*R*)-octahydro-2-methyl-3′-[[(2*R*,4*S*,5*S*,6*S*)-tetrahydro-4,5-dimethoxy-6-methyl-2*H*-pyran-2-yl]oxy]-5′-[(2*S*,3*S*,5*R*,6*S*)-tetrahydro-6-hydroxy-3,5,6-trimethyl-2*H*-pyran-2-yl][2,2′-bifuran]-5-yl]-1,6-dioxaspiro[4.5]dec-7-yl]ethyl]-4,5-dimethoxy-3-methyl-2*H*-pyran-2-acetate

Structural formula

Molecular formula	($C_{47}H_{83}NO_{17}$)
Molecular weight	934.17
Trademark	Cygro
Manufacturer	American Cyanamid Co.
Code designation	CL 273,703
CAS registry No.	84878-61-5

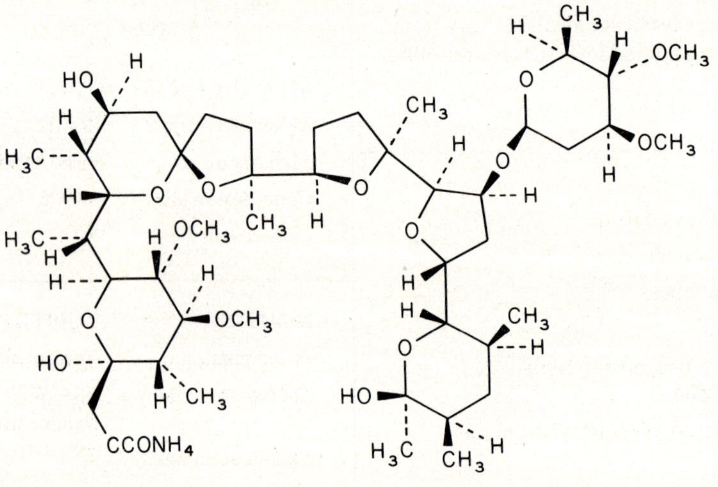

USAN	POLYBUTESTER
Pronunciation	pŏl′ ĭ būt ĕs″ tĕr
Ingredient function	suture (nonabsorbable)
Chemical names	

(1) α-hydro-ω-hydroxypoly(oxy-1,4-butanediyl), polymer with 1,4-benzenedicarboxylic acid and 1,4-butanediol

(2) polytetramethylene glycol, polymer with terephthalic acid and 1,4-butanediol

Structural formula

Molecular formula	$[(C_4H_8O)xH_2O]m(C_8H_6O_4)n(C_4H_{10}O_2)o$
Trademark	NOVAFIL
Manufacturer	Davis & Geck, Inc.
Code designation	XM-72
CAS registry No.	37282-12-5

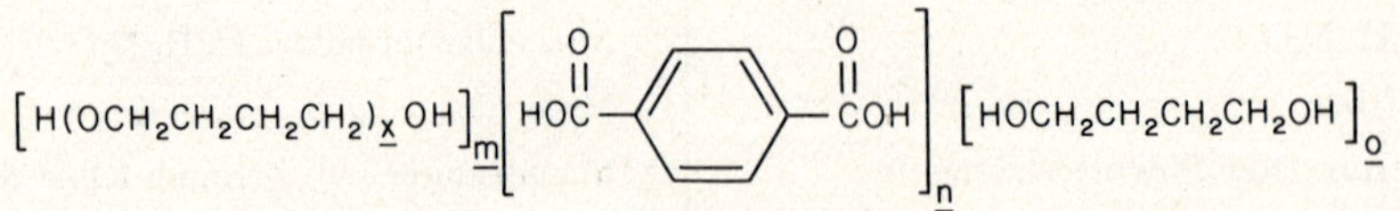

CLINICAL PHARMACOLOGY & THERAPEUTICS
VOLUME 38 NUMBER 3 SEPTEMBER 1985

ORIGINAL ARTICLES

Dose-dependent absorption of amoxycillin and bacampicillin

The relationship between the relative absorption and increasing oral doses of amoxycillin and bacampicillin, a prodrug of ampicillin, was studied testing the hypothesis that a saturable transport system for aminopenicillins exists in the human gut. Each drug was given in four different doses in a randomized order to 12 fasting subjects. One group of subjects was given amoxycillin in single doses of 375, 750, 1500, and 3000 mg, while the other group received bacampicillin in 400, 800, 1600, and 3200 mg doses. The highest dose was four times larger than that normally used in clinical practice. Amoxycillin, and ampicillin generated from bacampicillin, were determined in plasma and urine by modern column liquid chromatographic methods. With increasing doses of the penicillins, there was a saturable increase in peak plasma concentration, plasma AUC, and urinary recovery. The mean (± SD) AUC values after 750, 1500, and 3000 mg amoxycillin were 86% ± 13%, 70% ± 16%, and 55% ± 14% of that expected, when the expected ratio of AUC to dose was that of the 375 mg dose, assuming nonsaturable absorption. The corresponding AUC values after 800, 1600, and 3200 mg bacampicillin were 97% ± 17%, 89% ± 19%, and 76% ± 11% of that expected from the results obtained after the 400 mg dose. The importance of dose of either drug for AUC and urinary recovery was analyzed according to a function implying capacity-limited absorption. The dose-dependency was most pronounced for amoxycillin ($P < 0.001$). Renal drug clearance was stable within subjects throughout the dose range. Our results support the concept of capacity-limited absorption of aminopenicillins, probably by carrier-mediated transport. However, limited solubility of the compounds, especially of bacampicillin, may be a confounding factor. (CLIN PHARMACOL THER 38:241-250, 1985.)

Jan Sjövall, Ph.D., Gunnar Alván, M.D., and Douglas Westerlund, Pharm.D.*
Södertälje and Huddinge, Sweden

From Clinical Pharmacology and The Research and Development Laboratory, Astra Läkemedel AB, Södertälje, and the Department of Clinical Pharmacology, Huddinge Hospital, Huddinge.

Supported by Swedish Medical Research Council Grant No. 3902.

Received for publication Jan. 22, 1985; accepted May 18, 1985.

Reprint requests to: Jan Sjövall, Clinical Pharmacology, Astra Läkemedel AB, S-151 85 Södertälje, Sweden.

*Present address: Department of Analytical Pharmaceutical Chemistry, Uppsala University Biomedical Centre, Uppsala, Sweden.

Amoxycillin and bacampicillin are both well absorbed from the gastrointestinal tract.[19] Bacampicillin, a prodrug of ampicillin, has a relatively high lipophilicity combined with aqueous solubility and would therefore be expected to be absorbed by passive diffusion. Amoxycillin, on the other hand, is virtually completely ionized at the physiologic pH of the intestine. Nevertheless, it is better absorbed than would be anticipated if passive diffusion were the only absorptive process. Animal studies suggest that there is a common specialized and saturable absorption mechanism for amoxycillin and other aminopenicillins.[15,25]

Our aim was to determine if the absorption of amoxycillin and bacampicillin is dose dependent after single oral doses up to 3.2 gm. Dose-dependency would support the hypothesis of capacity-limited absorption. Bacampicillin is rapidly hydrolyzed to ampicillin after absorption, and concentrations of the latter were therefore measured in plasma and urine.

METHODS

Subjects. Two groups of 12 nonobese subjects participated (Table I). All were found to be healthy by routine clinical examinations and laboratory tests performed within 14 days of the study, and none had a history of allergy to penicillins or cephalosporins. Subjects had taken no other drugs for at least 1 week before the study.

Pharmaceutic preparations. The drugs were given in commercially available tablets, namely amoxycillin, 375 mg (Imacillin; Astra Läkemedel, batch no. IB 100), and bacampicillin HCl, 400 mg (Penglobe; Astra Läkemedel, batch no. HI 225). Doses consisted of one to eight tablets. Analysis of the actual mean contents per dosage unit showed $\leq$1.5% deviation from the declared amounts. The in vitro dissolution half-life of the amoxycillin tablet was about 1 minute and that of bacampicillin was 11 minutes, determined at pH 1.2 by the rotating basket method at 100 rpm and in water by the USP paddle apparatus at 150 rpm, respectively. Amoxycillin (molecular weight 365) has a pKa of 2.4 and 7.4, and bacampicillin HCl (molecular weight 502) has a pKa of 6.8.

Experimental design. The study was performed in two separate groups, each consisting of 12 subjects. One group was given amoxycillin in single oral doses of 375, 750, 1500, and 3000 mg. The other group of subjects was given bacampicillin in single doses of 400, 800, 1600, and 3200 mg. The four doses were given in a completely randomized order to each subject with an interval of 1 week between doses. Subjects from both groups participated on each experimental day. Subjects fasted for a minimum of 8 hours (from midnight to drug dosing), with the exception of 250 ml water taken upon rising at least 1 hour before dosing. Tablets were swallowed with 200 ml water. Subjects continued fasting for 3 hours after drug ingestion, except for 150 ml water given after 1 and 2 hours and permitted ad libitum thereafter. A standardized meal was served 3 hours after drug dosing. Subjects were instructed not to engage in any strenuous or athletic activities during the days of drug dosing. Smoking was permitted but snuff was not. The study was reviewed and approved by the local Ethics Committee.

Adverse reactions tended to increase with increasing doses of both drugs. One subject reported symptoms after the lowest dose, one reported symptoms with each of the three highest doses, and another reported adverse reactions with the two highest doses of bacampicillin. Symptoms from the upper or lower gastrointestinal tract were recorded in four subjects after the 3000 mg amoxycillin dose and in seven subjects after the 3200 mg bacampicillin dose.

One subject vomited 2.5 hours after the 3000 mg amoxycillin dose, another had a cold but no fever when given 1500 mg amoxycillin, and a third felt feverish and had signs of an upper respiratory tract infection and vomited 1.3 hours after taking the 3200 mg bacampicillin dose. However, because the plasma concentrations in these subjects were within the same range as in the others, these data have been included in the evaluation of the results.

Sampling. Blood samples (5 ml) for the assay of ampicillin or amoxycillin were drawn just before dosing and 30, 45, 60, and 90 minutes and 2, 2.5, 3, 4, 6, 8, and 10 hours thereafter. All samples were collected from the antecubital vein by direct puncture with evacuated heparinized blood collection tubes. Plasma was quickly separated by centrifugation for 7 minutes at 2500 × g and filtration. The samples were frozen within 20 minutes of collection. Urine was collected before dosing and over the periods of 0 to 1, 1 to 3, 3 to 5, 5 to 7, 7 to 9, and 9 to 11 hours after dosing. The weight of the total volume collected during each interval was recorded and an aliquot was frozen. All samples were stored at −70° C until assayed.

Blood samples (3 ml) for the assay of unchanged bacampicillin were collected in heparinized tubes containing sodium fluoride (5 mg/ml) as an esterase inhibitor just before dosing and 10, 20, 30, 45, 60, and 90 minutes and 2 hours thereafter. Immediately after being drawn, the blood was decanted into a tared and chilled polypropylene tube and was then immediately frozen in ethanol/dry ice.

Chemical assays. Plasma and urine were assayed for ampicillin and amoxycillin by reversed-phase HPLC.

For the determination of ampicillin, plasma was injected into the chromatographic system after precipitation of proteins with trichloroacetic acid and dilution with citrate-phosphate buffer at pH 5.4. Urine was injected after dilution with citrate-phosphate buffer at pH 4.85. For plasma samples, a 3 μm Perkin-Elmer C-18 column (60 × 4 mm id) was used as the support and 30% methanol in phosphate buffer at pH 7.8 was the mobile phase. In the analysis of urine samples, 5 μm Spherisorb RP 18 (100 × 4.6 mm) was used as the support and the mobile phase contained 37.5% ethanol in a phosphate buffer at pH 2.0, with 10^{-2} mol/L sodium lauryl sulphate as counterions to give the required selectivity and an acceptable retention time. A precolumn (5 × 4 mm) loaded with 10 μm Lichrosorb RP 8 was used to increase the life of the analytic columns. After separation, the mercuric mercaptide penicillenic acid was formed postcolumn in an air-segmented stream by the use of aqueous solutions of imidazole (4.85 mol/L) and mercuric chloride (4 × 10^{-3} mol/L) adjusted to pH 7.2 with hydrochloric acid and containing Brij®-35 (0.12%).[26] This reaction is specific for penicillins with an intact ring system. The penicillenic acid mercuric mercaptide was detected by ultraviolet light at 310 nm. With this technique, ampicillin was determined at concentrations of 2 to 3 mg per liter plasma with an intra-assay precision of 0.9% (CV), and in urine at about 40 mg/L with a precision of 1.4% (CV). The detection limits were about 120 ng/ml in plasma and 900 ng/ml in urine.

Amoxycillin was determined by direct injection of a small volume (20 μl) of urine after adjustment to pH 4.9, or of plasma (100 μl) after protein precipitation with perchloric acid and the addition of buffer at pH 5.4, to a reversed-phase system with coupled columns. Two short columns (10 cm) packed with alkyl-bonded silica gel (3 μm Microsphere C-18) were used, preceded by a small (5 × 4 mm id) precolumn (5 μm Spherisorb ODS).[1] Amoxycillin was eluted in the first column by a mobile phase containing 10% methanol in phosphate buffer at pH 7.4 and 10^{-3} mol/L hexylsulphate. In this environment the negatively charged amoxycillin competes with the hydrophobic anion for adsorption sites on the solid phase. The amoxycillin-containing fraction from this column was captured in a large (1 ml) loop. Finally, amoxycillin was chromatographed in the second column as an ion-pair with tetrahexylammonium (10^{-3} mol/L) in phosphate buffer at pH 7.4 containing 30% methanol. The fluorescamine derivative of amoxycillin was formed in a postcolumn packed bed reactor by use of a solution of fluorescamine in acetonitrile and was measured fluorimetrically. The intra-assay precision obtained with 0.35 to 39 mg/L plasma ranged from 5% to 1.3% (CV). The detection limits were about 25 ng/ml in urine and 10 ng/ml in plasma.

Table I. Subject characteristics

Group	*Sex (F/M)*	*Weight (kg)*	*Height (cm)*	*Age (yr)*	*Body surface area (m^2)*
Amoxycillin					
$\bar{X}$	6/6	67.8	176.3	30.4	1.83
SD		11.8	8.3	5.6	0.19
Range		52-84	163-187	22-39	1.60-2.09
Bacampicillin					
$\bar{X}$	6/6	71.8	176.1	31.4	1.88
SD		9.95	11.2	5.2	0.19
Range		60-93	160-200	22-41	1.65-2.30

F = Female; M = male.

Bacampicillin was determined in whole blood after an extraction procedure by reversed-phase HPLC with coupling to a postcolumn derivatization step. The instability of the compound in blood necessitated special care in sampling and storage. Sodium fluoride was added as an enzyme inhibitor. The addition of a large amount of a chemically related compound was necessary to eliminate the adsorption tendencies of the drug. Either a 100-fold excess of a related ester or a 100,000-fold excess of ampicillin was effective. Bacampicillin was extracted into butyl acetate from the frozen blood during thawing after the addition of the internal standard. It was then reextracted into an acidic aqueous buffer at pH 2 and the aqueous phase was extracted with *n*-hexane (for removal of dissolved butyl acetate) before injection into a reversed-phase column. The support was 5 μm Nucleosil C-18 (100 × 2.9 mm id) and acetonitrile/phosphate buffer at pH 7.4 (41/49, v/v) was the mobile phase. To improve the selectivity and sensitivity of the assay, the well-known fluorescamine reaction was used in a postcolumn derivatization system. The detection limit was 2 ng/gm in a 3 gm blood sample, and the intra-assay precision at this level was about 8% (CV).

Because of a breakdown of the freezer over a weekend, the blood samples for the assay of unchanged bacampicillin were stored above −70° C or thawed for some time before being analyzed. A control experiment

Table II. Mean (SD) pharmacokinetics in two groups of 12 subjects receiving either amoxycillin or bacampicillin

	*Dose**								
	mg	*mmol*	C_{max} *(mg/L)*	*AUC (mg · hr/L)*	t_{max}† *(hr)*	*MRT (hr)*	*Urinary recovery (%)*	$t_{1/2}$ *(hr)*	CL_R *(ml/min · 1.73 m²)*
Amoxy-cillin	375	1.03	8.1 (1.8)	19.5 (3.1)	1.0 (0.75-2)	2.3 (0.3)	71.3 (6.4)	1.7 (0.8)	221 (33)
	750	2.05	13.0 (2.3)	33.0 (4.8)	1.5 (0.75-1.5)	2.4 (0.3)	67.0 (7.2)	1.5 (0.3)	245 (39)
	1500	4.11	17.9 (4.7)	53.9 (12.2)	1.75 (1-2)	2.6 (0.4)	51.6 (10.1)	1.6 (0.2)	232 (38)
	3000	8.21	28.7 (7.0)	83.5 (21.5)	2.0 (1-2.5)	2.6 (0.4)	40.1 (8.8)	1.7 (0.4)	232 (38)
Bacampi-cillin	394	0.78	7.1 (1.8)	10.9 (2.3)	0.5 (0.5-1.5)	1.6 (0.2)	60.0 (7.1)	1.1 (0.2)	240 (43)
	787	1.57	11.3 (2.6)	20.9 (3.8)	0.88 (0.5-1.5)	1.8 (0.3)	55.5 (6.7)	1.1 (0.2)	228 (35)
	1575	3.14	17.7 (5.2)	38.8 (8.1)	1.5 (0.5-2)	2.0 (0.1)	54.2 (7.6)	1.3 (0.2)	243 (48)
	3150	6.27	26.2 (5.4)	65.7 (9.8)	1.5 (0.75-2)	2.2 (0.2)	45.3 (5.8)	1.4 (0.3)	236 (33)

*Adjusted for the actual mean content per dosage unit.
†Median (range).

with bacampicillin, 10 and 50 ng/gm in blood, indicated a 60% decrease in bacampicillin concentration during the breakdown period. Relating this to the sensitivity of the assay, the actual detection limit of bacampicillin in the study was still very low, 3 ng/gm in a 3 gm blood sample.

Pharmacokinetic calculations. All pharmacokinetic calculations on the results after bacampicillin were based on its hydrolysis product ampicillin. The plasma AUC was calculated by the linear trapezoidal rule and the logarithmic trapezoidal method in the exponential postabsorption phase.[2] The estimated area from the last sampling time to infinity, the first-order elimination rate constant, and the $t_{1/2}$ were calculated by conventional methods.[7] The mean residence time of a drug in the body (MRT) is defined as:[28]

$$MRT = {}_0\int^{\infty} t\, Cdt / {}_0\int^{\infty} Cdt \qquad (1)$$

where t is time (in hours) and C is the plasma concentration.

Renal clearance (CL_R) was calculated as the amount of unchanged drug excreted in the urine during the sampling period (Ae) divided by the AUC. A fundamental pharmacokinetic equation relates the absorbed fraction (F) of a given dose (D) to the product of plasma clearance (CL) and AUC:

$$CL \cdot AUC = F \cdot D \qquad (2)$$

Assuming first-order kinetics, CL is constant and thus independent of the actual plasma concentration. Let us assume that carrier-mediated absorption occurs with the drug molecules associating with a carrier system of the intestinal mucosa. The complex formed will then dissociate and the systemic delivery of drug per time unit is proportional to the abundance of the complex. This will give a function of the following type, which subsumes the classic Michaelis-Menten equation as a special case[8] and describes the relationship between dose and the amount of drug absorbed:

$$CL \cdot AUC = \frac{A_{max} \cdot D}{K_D + D} \qquad (3)$$

where D is dose, A_{max} is the theoretic maximum amount absorbed at extremely large doses, and K_D the dose at which the amount absorbed is half the theoretic maximum. With the assumption that the intestinal drug concentration can be regarded as proportional to the dose, it is justified to use Eq. 3 in the evaluation of our data. As CL_R was stable within each subject throughout the study, a constant CL was assumed and both sides of Eq. 3 were divided by CL and the resulting A_{max}/CL was exchanged for AUC_{max}:

$$AUC = \frac{AUC_{max} \cdot D}{K_D + D} \qquad (4)$$

Alternatively, Ae can be exchanged for AUC, as CL_R of unchanged aminopenicillin is the main route of elimination. The parameters AUC_{max}, Ae_{max}, and K_D were estimated from the experimental data by linear regression analysis of AUC against AUC/D or Ae against Ae/D from a linear transform of Eq. 4:

$$AUC = AUC_{max} - K_D \cdot \frac{AUC}{D} \qquad (5)$$

This method has been shown to provide the most reliable estimate of the constants regardless of the magnitude of the error in the dependent variable.[4] The degree of saturation was conventionally calculated as AUC/AUC_{max} or Ae/Ae_{max}.

Statistical methods. The relation between pharma-

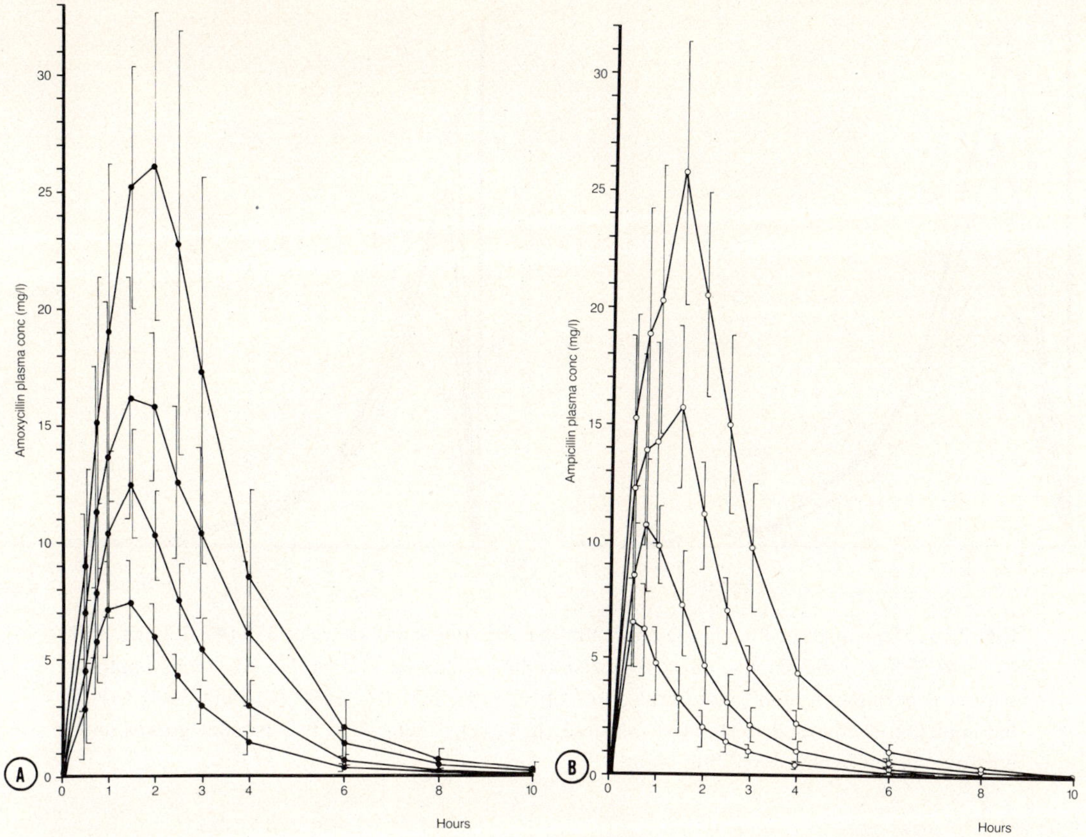

Fig. 1. A, Mean (±SD) amoxycillin plasma concentration after single oral doses of 375, 750, 1500, and 3000 mg amoxycillin (n = 12). **B,** Mean (±SD) ampicillin plasma concentration after single oral doses of 400, 800, 1600, and 3200 mg bacampicillin (n = 12). There were two parallel groups and a crossover design within each drug group.

cokinetic variables and dose was compared with regard to amoxycillin and bacampicillin by ANOVA for repeated measurements.[27] AUC, C_{max}, and Ae were adjusted for differences in dose. ANOVA gives information about differences in mean levels of drugs as well as doses and also about the interaction between drug and dose. The concept of interaction expresses in this context a difference between drugs in the dose course of the variable under analysis. The time to the peak concentration (t_{max}) was analyzed with rank-transformed data. Results were considered as statistically significant for P values <5%. Data are expressed as the $\overline{X}$ ± SD.

RESULTS

Unhydrolyzed bacampicillin was barely detected at 2.6 and 3.4 ng/gm blood in only two samples, taken 60 and 20 minutes after dosing from subjects given the 3200 mg dose of bacampicillin. This analysis was therefore not considered relevant for the samples after the lower doses of bacampicillin. Thus bacampicillin is rapidly and quantitatively converted to ampicillin after absorption and a minimal amount of intact bacampicillin reaches the peripheral blood.

The mean plasma concentrations of amoxycillin and ampicillin after bacampicillin did not increase proportional to the dose (Fig. 1, *A* and *B*). Plots of the plasma concentrations divided by the administered dose could not be superimposed (Fig. 2, *A* and *B*), indicating nonlinear kinetics.

The increase in peak plasma concentration (C_{max}) with dose was also saturable for both drugs (Table II). The C_{max} after 750, 1500, and 3000 mg amoxycillin averaged 77% ± 13%, 53% ± 14%, and 42% ± 10% of that expected, when the expected ratio of C_{max} to dose was that of the 375 mg dose and assuming

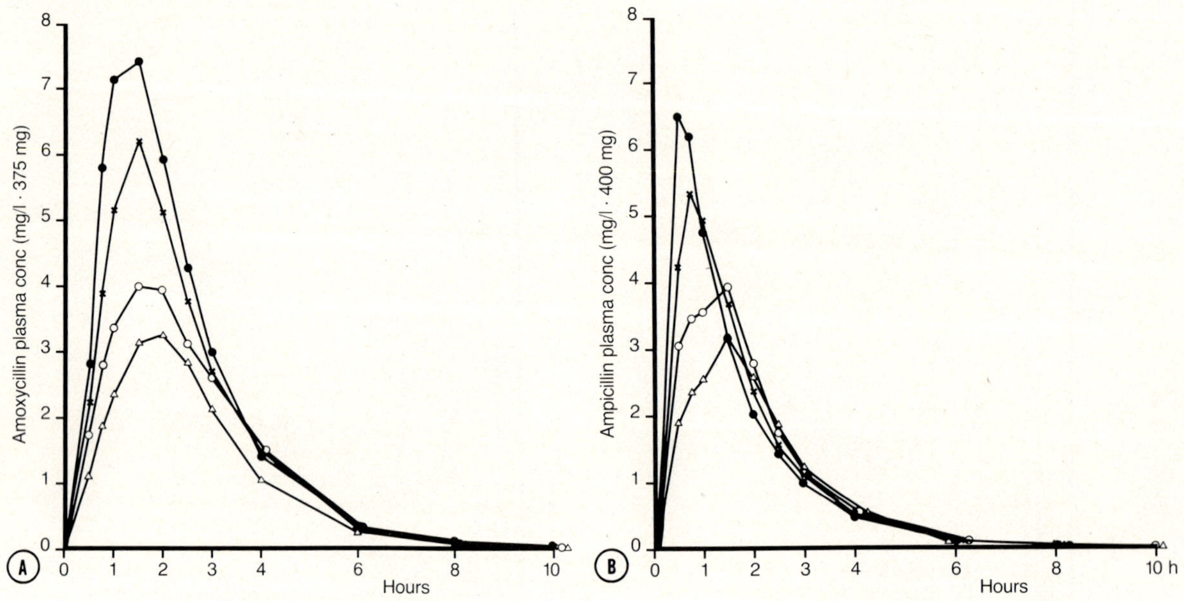

Fig. 2. A, Mean amoxycillin plasma concentration after single oral doses of 375 (●), 750 (x), 1500 (○), and 3000 (△) mg amoxycillin normalized to the 375 mg dose (n = 12). **B,** Mean ampicillin plasma concentration after single oral doses of 400 (●), 800 (x), 1600 (○), and 3200 (△) mg bacampicillin normalized to the 400 mg dose (n = 12). There were two parallel groups and a crossover design within each drug group.

nonsaturable absorption. The corresponding figures after 800, 1600, and 3200 mg bacampicillin were 75% ± 17%, 58% ± 17%, and 43% ± 9% of that expected, when the expected ratio of C_{max} to dose was that of the 400 mg dose.

The t_{max} occurred later with increasing doses for both drugs (Table II), indicating a slower absorption rate at higher doses. However, this difference was not statistically significant. The t_{max} occurred consistently later after amoxycillin and thus reflected a slower absorption of this drug as compared with bacampicillin ($P < 0.01$).

The increase in AUC was also not proportional to dose (Fig. 3), but this saturation was not as pronounced as for C_{max}. The mean AUC values after 750, 1500, and 3000 mg amoxycillin were 86% ± 13%, 70% ± 16%, and 55% ± 14% of that expected, when the expected ratio of AUC to dose was that of the 375 mg dose. The corresponding figures after 800, 1600, and 3200 mg bacampicillin were 97% ± 17%, 89% ± 19%, and 76% ± 11% of that expected, when the expected ratio of AUC to dose was that of the 400 mg dose. This shows a more marked dose-dependency in the absorption of amoxycillin with increasing doses as compared with bacampicillin ($P < 0.001$).

The relationship between AUC and dose with amoxycillin was well described by Eq. 4, with a mean AUC_{max} of 154 ± 68 mg · hr/L and a K_D of 7.11 ± 3.19 mmol (Fig. 3). In the linear regression analysis used to estimate AUC_{max} and K_D by Eq. 5, the coefficient of correlation (r) ranged from 0.79 to 0.98. The relationship between AUC and dose with bacampicillin was also described by Eq. 4, with an AUC_{max} of 157 ± 63 mg · hr/L and a K_D of 9.71 ± 4.32 mmol. The coefficient of correlation in the linear regression was high in seven subjects (r = 0.76 to 0.99) but less remarkable in the other five (r = 0.34 to 0.59). The mean degree of saturation after the highest dose was 58% ± 12% after amoxycillin and 47% ± 16% after bacampicillin.

Urinary excretion was consistent with the results based on plasma concentrations, as the percentage urinary recovery decreased with increasing doses of both drugs ($P < 0.001$; Table II). This effect was also most pronounced with amoxycillin ($P < 0.001$).

Application of Eq. 4 to describe the relationship between Ae and dose of amoxycillin resulted in an Ae_{max} of 2343 ± 980 mg (6.42 ± 2.69 mmol) and a K_D of 7.65 ± 3.49 mmol. The linear regression analysis used to estimate the constants had a high coefficient of correlation for all subjects (r = 0.86 to 1.00). The relationship between Ae and dose with regard to bacampicillin was also well described by Eq. 4, with an Ae_{max}

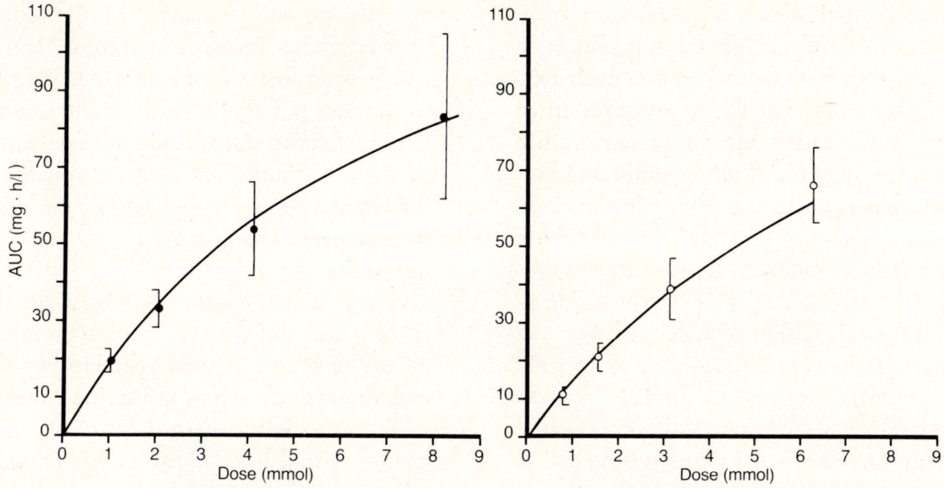

Fig. 3. Mean (±SD) AUC plotted against dose and fitted to Eq. 4 after single oral doses of 375, 750, 1500, and 3000 mg amoxycillin (●; n = 12) and 400, 800, 1600, and 3200 mg bacampicillin (○; n = 12). There were two parallel groups and a crossover design within each drug group.

of 2738 ± 1225 mg (7.84 ± 3.51 mmol) and a K_D of 11.5 ± 5.32 mmol. The coefficient of correlation in the linear regression was high (r = 0.72 to 0.94) in nine subjects and lower (r = 0.31 to 0.47) in the other three. The mean degree of saturation after the highest dose was 56% ± 13% after amoxycillin and 43% ± 18% after bacampicillin based on the amount of drug excreted in the urine.

The mean CL_R was similar after all four doses of both drugs (Table II) and stable within the subjects throughout the dose range. The amoxycillin plasma $t_{1/2}$ was longer than that of ampicillin after bacampicillin dosing ($P < 0.001$). The MRT, which represents the transit time of a drug through the body including dissolution, absorption, and all disposition phases, was longer for amoxycillin than for bacampicillin ($P < 0.001$). There was a prolonged MRT with increasing doses ($P < 0.01$) that was most marked after bacampicillin.

DISCUSSION

Amoxycillin was developed by the introduction of a hydroxy group into the side chain of ampicillin. This minor change of the molecule resulted in only small changes in its physicochemical properties with retained polarity. Still, amoxycillin shows a marked improvement in gastrointestinal absorption, which is contradictory to the classic theory that diffusion of the nonionized lipid-soluble form is a major determinant of absorption. On the other hand, the improved absorption of the ampicillin prodrug bacampicillin has been explained by the markedly increased lipophilicity of the esterified ampicillin.

The successful application of Eq. 4 to describe the relationship of AUC and Ae vs. dose with both drugs indicates a saturable, and thus specialized, transport for both drugs. The mean degree of saturation after the highest dose was about 50% after both drugs. The K_D values calculated from AUC and urinary excretion data were very close, 7.11 and 7.65 mmol, respectively, for amoxycillin and 9.71 and 11.5 mmol, respectively, for bacampicillin.

With regard to bacampicillin, the application of Eq. 4 was less successful in some subjects, as indicated by a low correlation coefficient when estimating AUC_{max} and K_D by linear regression. Eq. 4 also tended to underestimate the results at the highest bacampicillin dose (Fig. 3). Most likely, bacampicillin and other aminopenicillins are absorbed by parallel nonlinear and linear transport processes. In this case, a term proportional to the dose and representing passive diffusion (k · D) should be added to the right-hand side of Eq. 3. The fraction absorbed (F) of a given dose would then be resolved into

$$CL \cdot AUC = \left[\frac{A_{max}}{K_D + D} + k\right] \cdot D \qquad (6)$$

taking both specialized uptake and passive diffusion into account. The relative importance of the linear term increases with higher doses, and the addition of this term may thus improve the estimates for bacampicillin. The addition of a linear term does not seem necessary for amoxycillin. The presence of parallel passive diffusion may have been estimated in a nonlinear regression analysis with AUC_{max}, K_D, and k as parameters.

This approach was not considered, because there were too few observations to estimate the three parameters.

The comparison of the bioavailability after each dose is based on the assumption that CL of amoxycillin or ampicillin is the same in each subject after amoxycillin or bacampicillin. The fraction of amoxycillin and ampicillin excreted unchanged in the urine after intravenous administration amounts to about 80% for both drugs,[20] making renal clearance the main route of elimination. Because CL_R was stable (Table II), this assumption was justified for calculation of AUC and Ae.

The AUC after oral amoxycillin doses of up to 1000 mg has been previously reported to increase proportional to the dose.[21] However, those authors showed a decrease in absorption rate with increasing doses. A proportional increase in AUC with dose has been found after bacampicillin doses up to 800 to 1600 mg in subjects.[11,18] These findings are not inconsistent with our results, as the dose-dependent absorption might be hard to detect in this dose range. At low doses, the dose becomes negligible in comparison with K_D and can be eliminated from the denominator in Eq. 4. Under these conditions, AUC is directly proportional to the dose.

A proportional increase in AUC has been reported after intravenous administration of 250, 500, 1000, 2000, and 5000 mg amoxycillin.[3] These results strongly support our conclusion that the saturation we saw is not due to dose-dependent disposition of amoxycillin.

In some cases, the chemical properties of the drug and the physiology of the gastrointestinal tract have provided explanations for dose-dependent absorption. The dose-dependent absorption of chlorothiazide has been attributed to limited solubility of the drug in the intestinal lumen.[6] The aqueous solubility of both amoxycillin and bacampicillin depends on pH. The solubility curve of amoxycillin is U shaped, with a minimum at pH 5, 5.5 mg/ml at 37° C,[22] and the solubility of bacampicillin markedly decreases with an increase in pH. The aqueous solubility of bacampicillin at 22° C, determined by the intrinsic dissolution rate as described by Nyqvist and Nicklasson,[14] is 400 mg/ml at pH 3.0, 200 mg/ml at pH 4.5, 100 mg/ml at pH 5.0, 20 mg/ml at pH 5.5, 7 mg/ml at pH 6.0, and 2 mg/ml at pH 6.5.* Thus it cannot be ruled out that the dose-dependent absorption of bacampicillin may be due to limited intestinal solubility. The drugs were, however, taken with a large volume of water (200 ml), additional water (150 ml) being given 1 and 2 hours after the dose, and both formulations showed rapid in vitro dissolution at the pH of the stomach. Furthermore, amoxycillin showed more marked saturation than bacampicillin, which is opposite to the expected effect of solubility.

Another possible reason for the saturable absorption with increasing doses could be dose-dependent changes in the distribution of drug within the gut and great differences in absorptive capacity at different parts of the intestine. This hypothesis could not be tested under our study design. However, if the absorption is first order, a linear relationship between the amount absorbed and the dose is expected, even if absorption occurs only in a certain segment of the gut, provided intestinal transit is not affected by dose size.

The quantitative hydrolysis of bacampicillin, shown by the virtual lack of parent compound in blood even after the highest dose, precludes saturation of this step as an explanation for our results.

Another reason for the saturable absorption kinetics may be degradation of the drugs before absorption. If the degradation process is first order, which seems most likely, a constant fraction of each dose would be destroyed. If the process is zero order, the fraction of each dose destroyed would decrease with increasing doses. Thus our results are opposite to those expected from degradation of the drugs before absorption. Impaired gastric emptying and subsequent degradation are also less likely to explain our findings, as the drugs are stable at low pH.

The tendency for a later t_{max} and longer $t_{1/2}$ with increasing doses of bacampicillin (Table II) indicates a slower absorption rate at higher doses. This may be due to hydrolysis of bacampicillin to ampicillin in the epithelial cells. Thus bacampicillin would be efficiently transported into the cells, whereas the intracellularly released and more polar ampicillin would be expected to be transported out of the cell more slowly. This is supported by results with a similar ampicillin ester, pivampicillin, by use of the in situ ligated small intestinal loop technique in rats.[16] ^{14}C-pivampicillin, but not ^{14}C-ampicillin, accumulated rapidly in the intestinal wall in a high concentration and then gradually passed into the blood stream.

The dose-dependent absorption of amoxycillin and bacampicillin supports the concept of a capacity-limited and probably carrier-mediated transport in man. A confounding factor may be limited solubility of the compounds, especially for bacampicillin.

The permeability of the rat small intestine to amoxycillin has been shown to depend on the concentration of the drug in the perfusate within the in situ recirculating perfusion model.[23] Based on the disappearance

*Nyqvist H, Nicklasson M: Personal communication, 1985.

of various β-lactam antibiotics from in situ rat small intestinal loops, carrier-mediated absorption has been suggested to be a common mechanism for the intestinal absorption of amino-β-lactam antibiotics.[15,24,25] Such a process is more likely to be used for endogenous compounds or natural products, as has been shown with dipeptides,[12] riboflavin,[10] folic acid,[9] and ascorbic acid.[13] Penicillin may be regarded as a dipeptide derived from cysteine and valine[5] and thus uses a specialized transport common to the absorption of dipeptides, for which a saturable transport system has been demonstrated in man.[12,17] Substitution of the *N*-terminal amino group of a dipeptide appears to decrease or abolish affinity for transport.[12] Thus the aminopenicillins, all of which have a free amino group in the side chain, may be especially prone to use this transport system.

In relation to the carrier-mediated absorption of aminopenicillins, one could acknowledge their highly specialized transport in another organ. Table II illustrates the well-known fact that tubular secretion is important for renal clearance of the aminopenicillins, as it far exceeds the glomerular filtration rate (125 ml/min).

The mean Ae_{max} values of 2.3 gm for amoxycillin and 2.7 gm for bacampicillin indicate that even if these drugs are given in very high oral doses, 2 to 3 gm of active aminopenicillin is the maximum amount that can be absorbed and excreted in the urine after a single dose. Accordingly, a 50% degree of saturation in relative absorption would need amoxycillin doses in the order of 2.6 and 2.8 gm, calculated from K_D for AUC and Ae, respectively. The corresponding doses for bacampicillin would be in the order of 4.9 and 5.8 gm. A saturable absorption implies that too large a dose may be wasteful and lead to an increased frequency of gastrointestinal reactions and ecologic disturbances of the intestinal microflora.

We are grateful to Bernhard Huitfeldt, Ph.D., for statistical advice and to Erik Vinnars, M.D., for medical supervision of the subjects.

References

1. Carlqvist J, Westerlund D: Automated determination of amoxycillin in biological fluids by column-switching in ion-pair RPLC systems with post-column derivatization. J Chromatogr. (In press.)
2. Chiou WL: Critical evaluation of the potential error in pharmacokinetic studies of using the linear trapezoidal rule method for the calculation of the area under the plasma level time curve. J Pharmacokinet Biopharm **6**:539-546, 1978.
3. Dalhoff A, Koeppe P, von Kobyletzki D: Untersuchungen zur Pharmakokinetik von Amoxicillin nach intravenöser, intramuskulärer und oraler Applikation. Arzneimittelforsch **31**:1148-1157, 1981.
4. Dowd JE, Riggs DS: A comparison of estimates of Michaelis-Menten kinetic constants from various linear transformations. J Biol Chem **240**:863-869, 1965.
5. Doyle FP, Nayler JHC: Penicillins and related structures. *In* Harper NJ, Simmonds AB, editors: Advances in drug research, vol 1. London, 1964, Academic Press, pp 8-13.
6. Dressman JB, Fleisher D, Amidon GL: Physicochemical model for dose-dependent drug absorption. J Pharm Sci **73**:1274-1279, 1984.
7. Gibaldi M, Perrier D: Pharmacokinetics. New York, 1982, Marcel Dekker, Inc.
8. Goldstein A, Aronow L, Kalman SM: Principles of drug action: The basis of pharmacology. New York, 1974, John Wiley & Sons, pp 82-83.
9. Hepner GW, Booth CC, Cowan J, Hoffbrand AV, Mollin DL: Absorption of crystalline folic acid in man. Lancet **2**:302-306, 1968.
10. Levy G, Jusko WJ: Factors affecting the absorption of riboflavin in man. J Pharm Sci **55**:285-289, 1966.
11. Magni L, Sjöberg B, Sjövall J, Wessman J: Clinical pharmacological studies with bacampicillin. *In* Williams JD, Geddes AM, editors: Chemotherapy: Penicillins and cephalosporins, vol 5. New York, 1976, Plenum Press, pp 109-114.
12. Matthews DM: Intestinal absorption of peptides. Biochem Soc Trans **11**:808-810, 1983.
13. Mayersohn M: Ascorbic acid absorption in man—Pharmacokinetic implications. Eur J Pharmacol **19**:140-142, 1972.
14. Nyqvist H, Nicklasson M: Influence of epimer ratio on physicochemical properties of bacampicillin hydrochloride. Acta Pharm Suec. (In press.)
15. Sezaki H, Kimura T: Carrier-mediated transport in drug absorption. *In* Breimer DD, Speiser P, editors: Topics in pharmaceutical sciences. Amsterdam, 1983, Elsevier Science Publishers BV, pp 133-142.
16. Shindo H, Fukuda K, Kawai K, Tanaka K: Studies on intestinal absorption of pivampicillin and species difference in the intestinal esterase activity. J Pharmacobiodyn **1**:310-323, 1978.
17. Silk DBA, Hegarty JE, Fairclough PD, Clark ML: Characterization and nutritional significance of peptide transport in man. Ann Nutr Metab **26**:337-352, 1982.
18. Sjövall J: Dose dependence in human absorption of aminopenicillins. Infection **7**(suppl 5):458-462, 1979.
19. Sjövall J, Magni L, Bergan T: Pharmacokinetics of bacampicillin compared to those of ampicillin, pivampicillin, and amoxycillin. Antimicrob Agents Chemother **13**:90-96, 1978.
20. Sjövall J, Westerlund D, Alván G: Renal excretion of intravenously infused amoxycillin and ampicillin. Br J Clin Pharmacol **19**:191-201, 1985.
21. Spyker DA, Rugloski RJ, Vann RL, O'Brien WM: Phar-

macokinetics of amoxicillin: Dose dependence after intravenous, oral, and intramuscular administration. Antimicrob Agents Chemother **11:**132-141, 1977.

22. Tsuji A, Nakashima E, Hamano S, Yamana T: Physicochemical properties of amphoteric β-lactam antibiotics I: Stability, solubility, and dissolution behavior of aminopenicillins as a function of pH. J Pharm Sci **67:**1059-1066, 1978.
23. Tsuji A, Nakashima E, Kagami I, Honjo N, Yamana T: Effect of dose-concentration on the absorption of amoxicillin and ampicillin from the rat intestine. J Pharm Pharmacol **29:**707-708, 1977.
24. Tsuji A, Nakashima E, Kagami I, Yamana T: Intestinal absorption mechanism of amphoteric β-lactam antibiotics. I. Comparative absorption and evidence for saturable transport of amino-β-lactam antibiotics by in situ rat small intestine. J Pharm Sci **70:**768-772, 1981.
25. Tsuji A, Yamana T: Gastrointestinal absorption of β-lactam antibiotics. *In* Mitsuhashi S, editor: Beta-lactam antibiotics. Tokyo, 1981, Japan Science Society Press, pp 235-258. (Engl.)
26. Westerlund D, Carlqvist J, Theodorsen A: Analysis of penicillins in biological material by reversed phase liquid chromatography and post-column derivatization. Acta Pharm Suec **16:**187-214, 1979.
27. Winer BJ: Statistical principles in experimental design. New York, 1962, McGraw-Hill Book Company.
28. Yamaoka K, Nakagawa T, Uno T: Statistical moments in pharmacokinetics. J Pharmacokinet Biopharm **6:**547-558, 1978.

The pharmacokinetics of baclofen derived from intestinal infusion

The pharmacokinetics of baclofen, a centrally acting muscle relaxant, have been elucidated in man. The pharmacokinetic disposition was determined form plasma concentration-time data and urinary recovery after the administration of rate-limiting intestinal infusions and an oral bolus dose. Based on comparisons between the plasma concentration-time profiles from the intestinal infusions and the oral bolus doses, relative regression parameter assignments were made. The intestinal absorption of baclofen after intestinal infusion was very rapid, such that baclofen disposition was well characterized by an open two-compartment pharmacokinetic model with zero-order input. Intravenous administration of baclofen was precluded from this study because of the potential for severe adverse reactions. The average distribution phase constant (α) was 1.29 hours^{-1} and the average elimination phase constant (β) was 0.191 hours.$^{-1}$ Average volume of the central compartment (V_C/F), volume of the body compartment (V_{area}/F), systemic clearance (CL/F), and renal clearance were 28.8 L, 59.0 L, 180 ml/min, and 103 ml/min, respectively. Pharmacokinetics were dose proportional in the dose range studied. The use of these pharmacokinetic parameters as determined in normal subjects in therapeutic management is particularly relevant, because baclofen is targeted to a patient population subject to renal dysfunction. (CLIN PHARMACOL THER 38:251-257, 1985.)

Gregory M. Kochak, Ph.D., Ashok Rakhit, Ph.D., William E. Wagner, M.D., Frank Honc, M.S., Lorraine Waldes, B.S., and Richard A. Kershaw, Ph.D.
Ardsley, N. Y., and Columbus, Ohio

Baclofen (4-amino-3-(*p*-chlorophenyl)-butanoic acid) is a centrally acting muscle relaxant. It has proved efficacious in the treatment of spasticity resulting from multiple sclerosis, particularly for the relief of flexor spasms and concomitant pain, clonus, and muscle rigidity. Baclofen may also be of some value in patients with spinal cord injuries and other spinal cord diseases. Despite its presence on the United States market for nearly 6 years and previously in Europe, little is known about its pharmacokinetic disposition in man. This may be due in part to baclofen's potential for severe adverse effects resulting in central nervous system, respiratory, and cardiovascular depression, and, therefore, the reluctance to administer the drug intravenously. Ideally, dosage adjustment, particularly in patient populations, is most rationally accomplished based on the pharmacokinetics of a drug.

Riegelman et al.[11] reported that when an oral solution is administered directly into the intestine, the absorption process is extremely fast for some drugs and the plasma concentration-time profile is virtually equivalent to that after an intravenous injection. Because intravenous administration of baclofen has not been reported in man, this study was undertaken to determine the pharma-

Abbreviations

A, B	Infusion preexponential intercepts
A′, B′	Postinfusion preexponential intercepts
α, β, k_a	Exponential terms
C, D	Oral bolus preexponential intercepts
C_C	Plasma concentration in the central compartment
CL	Total systemic clearance
CL_R	Renal clearance
D_{po}	Administered dose by intestinal infusion or oral bolus
F	Absolute bioavailable fraction
T	Infusion duration
t	Time
t′	t-T
t_{lag}	Lag time
V_C	Volume of the central compartment
V_{area}	Volume of the body

From the Pharmaceuticals Division, CIBA-GEIGY Corporation, Ardsley, and Department of Pharmacology, College of Medicine, The Ohio State University, Columbus.
Received for publication Jan. 7, 1985; accepted May 29, 1985.
Reprint requests to: Gregory M. Kochak, Ph.D., Pharmaceuticals Division, CIBA-GEIGY Corporation, Ardsley, NY 10502.

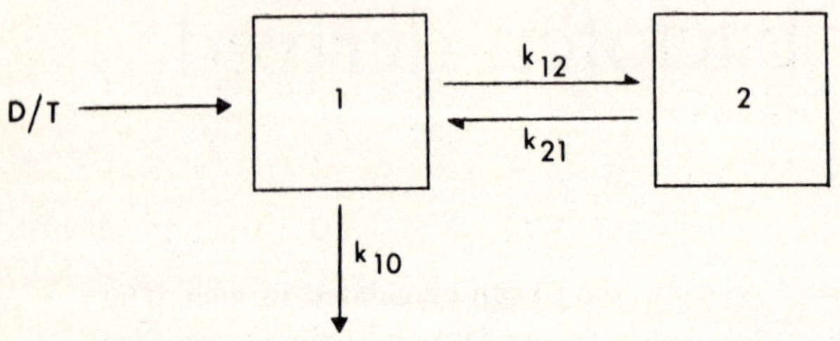

Fig. 1. Schematic representation of a two-compartment pharmacokinetic model with zero-order input.

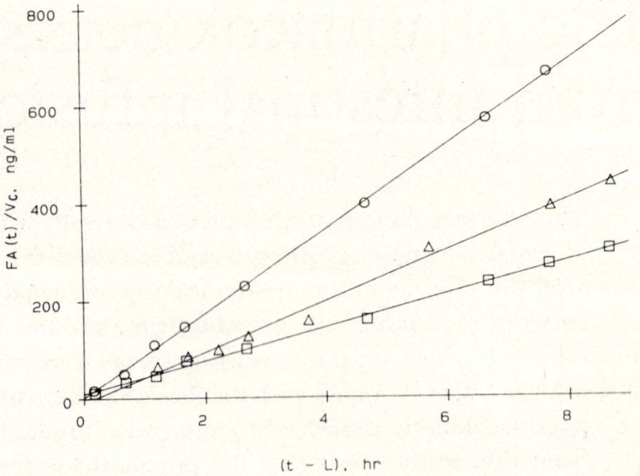

Fig. 2. Loo-Riegelman cumulative absorption profiles for subject 3 showing infusion rate–limited absorption after baclofen administration by three intestinal infusions at rates of 5.86 (○), 2.66 (△), and 1.31 (□) mg/hr. *L*, lag factor (t_{lag}).

cokinetic disposition and dose proportionality at the absorption site of baclofen by direct infusion of baclofen solution into the duodenum over a prolonged infusion interval. Evaluations of the assumption of near instantaneous absorption and appropriateness of treating the data with zero-order input were made.

METHODS

Clinical. Four healthy nonsmoking men 21 to 26 years old were informed of the nature of the experiment and gave written consent to participate. All were within 15% of the standards for body weight,[9] had a history of good health, and denied using prescription drugs, over-the-counter medications, and other drugs during the 7 days before the study. Consumption of alcoholic beverages was prohibited for the 3-day period before any drug study day. A standard physical examination, routine laboratory workup of blood and urine samples, and ECG showed no deviations from accepted values.

Each of the four subjects received an aqueous solution of baclofen over approximately an 8-hour period through a nasogastric tube directly into the duodenum. Intestinal infusions were repeated three times, such that the total delivered doses were approximately 12, 24, and 48 mg. Actual delivered doses were determined as indicated below. In addition to the three infusions, each subject received an oral bolus dose (24 mg) of baclofen in an aqueous solution. The sequence of administration of each preparation followed a four-way Latin squares design balanced for residual effects.

Baclofen was infused by a new portable and disposable infusor unit, the Travenol 24-Hour Infusor (Travenol Laboratories, Inc.). These pumps are designed to deliver 2 ml/hr of 5% dextrose in water injection solution at 30° C with a dynamic viscosity of 0.907 cp. In vitro calibration of the pumps with aqueous solutions of baclofen (density 0.996 gm/ml; viscosity 0.798 cp) at ambient temperature indicated an average (±SD) flow rate of 2.20 ± 0.163 ml/hr (n = 63) over a 9-hour period after allowing dynamic equilibration for the first hour. Stability of the flow rate indicated an average (±SD) decline in the initial rate of 0.03 ± 0.018 ml/hr (n = 7). At intervals of 1 week, the subjects were admitted to the clinical pharmacology unit on the evening before drug dosing. Specially fabricated nasogastric feeding tubes, 43 in long with 8-F end fittings and tungsten weights (Enteriflex feeding tube; Biosearch Medical Products Inc.) were passed through one nostril and fed into the stomach. Enough slack was allowed so that normal peristalsis would carry the tip of the feeding tube into the small bowel overnight. Once the tubes were in place, all subjects, including the nonintubated control, were allowed only 100 ml apple juice and 2 soda crackers per hour to prevent excessive hunger. Three hours after the tube was introduced, a small fluid sample was withdrawn through the nasogastric tube to check for patency. A second sample was taken just before the start of the drug infusion and its pH and color were noted to confirm placement of the tube in the small intestine and to check for patency of the tube.

To prepare the infusion solutions, 66.8, 133.6, and 267.3 mg baclofen was added to 100 ml distilled water. The oral solution was prepared by adding 24 mg drug to 50 ml water. The infusors were loaded with 60 ml of the appropriate infusion solution. Flow was allowed to stabilize for 1 hour before the infusor pumps were capped and weighed. The pumps were then attached to the enteric feeding tubes and the flow rate was approximated by measuring the time needed for the advancing meniscus to traverse a 10 cm distance marked on the tube. The start of the infusion (t_0) was calculated as: t_0 (hr) = t_i + [LG × t]/600, where t_i is the time the infusor pump was attached to the nasogastric tube, LG is the length of the nasogastric tube, and t is time in min for the solution to traverse 10 cm.

The oral baclofen solution was swallowed and followed by three 50 ml washings of the container. At t_0 the three subjects receiving the infusions drank 200 ml water.

Serial 7 ml blood samples were collected by venipuncture in Venoject tubes (Terumo Medical Corp.) containing 143 IU sodium heparin. Blood samples were drawn at 0, 0.5, 1, 1.5, 2, 3, 5, 7, 8, 9, 10, 12, 14, 16, 18, 20, and 24 hours for subjects receiving the drug by infusion. Blood samples after oral bolus dosing were drawn at 0, 0.5, 1, 1.5, 2, 3, 4, 5, 6, 8, 12, 16, and 24 hours. Plasma was separated by centrifugation and stored for analysis. Urine collections were made at 0, 2, 4, 6, 8, 12, 16, 24, and 48 hours. Total volume and pH of the urine collected during each period were measured and a 10 ml portion was retained for analysis.

At the end of the oral infusion, the enteric feeding tube was clamped and removed from each subject. The capped infusion pump was reweighed and the weight of infusion solution delivered was calculated. The actual dose delivered was calculated as: Dose (mg) = [(Net weight delivered (gm)/ρ) − residual volume in the nasogastric tube (ml)] × concentration of baclofen solution (mg/ml), where ρ is the density of baclofen solution (gm/ml).

Sample analysis and storage. All plasma and urine samples were kept frozen at approximately −20° C until analyzed. Plasma and urine concentrations of baclofen were determined by a previously reported GLC method.[5]

Computational. The plasma concentration-time profiles were analyzed by standard nonlinear regression techniques with a weighting factor of 1/C. Initially, the postinfusion curves were fit to an open two-compartment pharmacokinetic model described by the following equation (see Appendix):

$$C_C = A'e^{-\alpha t'} + B'e^{-\beta t'}$$

The cumulative absorption profiles determined by the method of Loo and Riegelman[7] were then generated to determine if the input rates were zero order and limiting. Comparisons were made between the absorption rate normalized for a bioavailable fraction of 1 and the infusion rates determined experimentally in vitro from the net volume of solution delivered and the time interval from attachment of the infusor to the nasogastric tube until removal of the nasogastric tube from the subject.

Subsequently, the entire plasma concentration-time profile was fit to the pharmacokinetic model shown in Fig. 1 when the experimentally determined infusion rate coincided with the absorption rate calculated from in vivo data. The equation used to describe the model in Fig. 1 is as follows:

$$C_C = A(e^{-\alpha(t' - t_{lag})} - e^{-\alpha(t - t_{lag})} + B(e^{-\beta(t' - t_{lag})} - e^{-\beta(t - t_{lag})})$$

where T = t during the infusion and is fixed as a constant after infusion.

The oral bolus dose was fitted to a standard classical two compartment pharmacokinetic model with first-order input. The equation used to describe the model is as follows:

$$C_C = Ce^{-\alpha(t - t_{lag})} + De^{-\beta(t - t_{lag})} - (C + D)e^{-ka(t - t_{lag})}$$

The absorption rate constant was determined directly from regression analysis. Disposition parameter estimates as determined from the intestinal infusions were used as initial estimates in fitting the data after oral bolus dosing. Data are reported as $\overline{X} \pm$ SD.

Table I. Infusion and absorption rates

Subject No.	*Dose (mg)*	*Infusion rate (mg/hr)*	*Absorption rate (mg/hr)**
1	11.8	1.48	1.37
	23.7	2.95	2.86
	41.6	5.21	5.44
2	11.8	1.45	1.41
	23.5	2.93	2.67
	43.3	5.43	6.07
3	11.6	1.45	1.31
	23.1	2.87	2.66
	47.0	5.88	5.86
4	12.1	1.52	1.53
	17.1	2.12	2.03
	44.5	5.59	5.14

*Calculated from in vivo data by the method of Loo and Riegelman and normalized for an F of 1.

RESULTS

Experimental. The cumulative absorption profiles (Fig. 2) for each subject and dose were linear, indicating that the infusion rates were limiting. There is good agreement between the infusion rate and the absorption rate (Table I). Pairwise comparison of the infusion rate and the absorption rate for each subject and dose by the t test found no significant differences ($P \geq 0.05$).

The plasma concentrations of baclofen after the intestinal infusions and oral bolus doses are listed in Table

Table II. Baclofen plasma concentrations (ng/ml) after intestinal infusion and oral bolus

Subject No.	Dose (mg)	t_0 cf (hr)*	Hr after dosing 0.5	1.0	1.5	2.0	3.0	4.0	5.0	6.0	7.0	8.0	9.0
1	11.8	+0.60	15	20	35	54	63		105		115	123	116
	23.7	+0.30	22	55	87	100	195		217		229	204	156
	41.6	−0.34	5	49	61	131	234		352		363	386	331
	24.0†		106	282	293	322	303	176	156	111		70	
2	11.8	+0.38	19	25	29	49	69		75		118	118	85
	23.5	+0.75	23	54	75	119	140		220		248	225	208
	43.3	−0.87		132	171	283	432		697		754	788	444
	24.0†		557	554	462	501	338	247	170	129		102	
3	11.6	+0.86	10	29	36	59	62		75		95	100	99
	23.1	+0.71	62	75	80	90	107		191		194	200	159
	47.0	+0.00	15	43	89	107	141		188		217	233	160
	24.0†		363	610	590	580	260	207	161	108		77	
4	12.1	−0.09	21	44	47	66	73		77		83	81	48
	17.1	+0.41	17	54	71	160	175		264		299	345	253
	44.5	+0.66	39	85	145	169	292		312		427	419	308
	24.0†		330	477	481	405	337	156	122	88		45	

cf = Correction factor; ND = not detectable (<5 ng/ml).
*Positive values are added to the time axis and negative values are subtracted (see text).
†Taken by mouth as a bolus dose.

Table III. Individual regression parameter estimates (by NONLIN) and integrated AUCs

Subject No.	Dose (mg)	A (or C) (ng/ml)	B (or D) (ng/ml)	α (hr^{-1})	β (hr^{-1})	t_{lag} (hr)	k_a (hr^{-1})	$AUC_{0-\infty}$ (ng · hr/ml)
1	11.8	15.1 (31.5)*	150 (27.6)	0.769 (2.23)	0.146 (0.0361)	0.68 (0.32)		1423
	23.7	65.5 (52.4)	210 (48.7)	1.03 (1.27)	0.180 (0.0449)	0.54 (0.18)		2290
	41.6	†	548 (21.6)		0.176 (0.0151)	0.06 (0.14)		4197
	24.0‡	2860 (404000)	278 (167)	0.931 (10.5)	0.150 (0.0480)	0.33 (0.09)	1.09 (11.2)	2044
2	11.8	†	146 (6.96)		0.176 (0.0195)	0.13 (0.21)		1223
	23.5	78.8 (43.6)	205 (37.0)	1.03 (0.927)	0.148 (0.0414)	1.02 (0.15)		2480
	43.3	200 (350)	664 (339)	0.795 (1.29)	0.242 (0.0766)	−0.20 (0.20)		6157
	24.0‡	253 (653)	606 (569)	0.797 (3.75)	0.232 (0.0965)	0.00 (0.18)	3.38 (4.64)	2675
3	11.6	34.8 (9.12)	77.5 (8.59)	1.44 (0.774)	0.177 (0.0247)	1.18 (0.08)		995
	23.1	7.55 (14.9)	237 (17.1)	3.36 (67.9)	0.186 (0.0174)	0.00 (0.00)		2133
	47.0	43.7 (29.0)	227 (28.2)	1.19 (1.15)	0.208 (0.0248)	0.34 (0.08)		2164
	24.0‡	4000 (232000)	544 (373)	1.46 (9.54)	0.256 (0.0908)	0.29 (0.16)	1.83 (11.1)	2388
4	12.1	42.9 (5.27)	76.3 (4.82)	2.43 (1.51)	0.126 (0.0204)	0.17 (0.13)		943
	17.1	61.3 (113)	270 (107)	0.999 (2.06)	0.220 (0.0748)	0.76 (0.14)		2790
	44.5	111 (147)	321 (138)	0.854 (1.28)	0.208 (0.0723)	0.86 (0.19)		3739
	24.0‡	3000 (88900)	342 (345)	1.04 (4.39)	0.220 (0.0986)	0.16 (0.22)	1.38 (5.46)	2021
$\overline{X}$				1.29	0.191	0.462§	1.92	
SD				0.734	0.0377	0.442	1.02	

†Asymptotic parameter standard deviation determined directly by NONLIN.
‡One-compartment model as determined by the Akaike Information Criterion.[13]
‡Taken by mouth as a bolus with 200 ml water.
§Intestinal infusion only.

Hr after dosing						
10.0	*12.0*	*14.0*	*16.0*	*18.0*	*20.0*	*24.0*
85	54	58	30	30	25	15
145	79	57	48	28	25	14
271	228	132	101	77	65	32
	52		35			20
85	62	32	27	18	16	10
131	86	56	51	40	36	25
309	181	108	68	54	53	20
	38		22			10
56	36	24	16	15	11	5
136	81	74	36	27	21	14
140	85	47	37	26	27	7
	39		21			ND
45	32	20	19	14	11	ND
143	93	63	44	35	32	18
233	111	94	56	46	34	25
	32		21			6

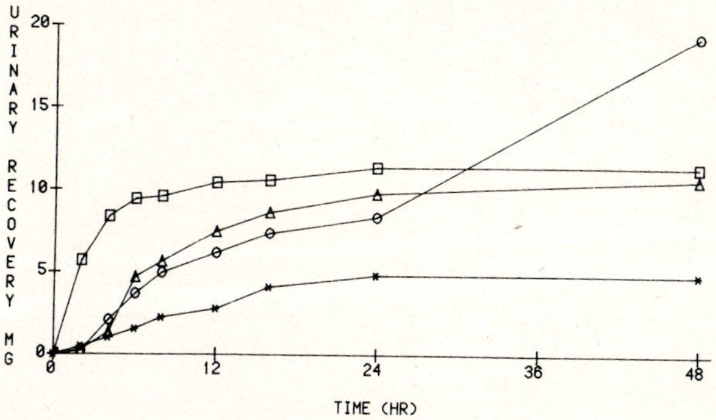

Fig. 3. Cumulative urinary recovery of baclofen after intestinal infusions with doses of 11.6 (*), 23.1 (○), and 47.0 (△) mg and an oral bolus dose of 24.0 mg (□) in subject 3.

II. Because the infusion rates measured by the benchmarks on the nasogastric tubes tended to be variable, possibly due to the initial filling of the nasogastric tube, corrections in t_0 (t_0 cf in Table II) were calculated based on the absorption rate indicated in Table I and the administered dose. Positive values of the correction factor indicate an overestimation of t_0 as measured by the benchmark and negative values as an underestimation of t_0. The duration of the infusion was therefore equivalent to 8 ± (t_0 cf) hours.

The cumulative urinary recovery of baclofen was nearly complete in 24 hours (Fig. 3), with an average of 59% ± 20.0% of the administered dose recovered in 48 hours.

The average relative ratios for the dose-normalized AUC of the three intestinal infusions (I_1, I_2, I_3) compared with the oral bolus dose (O) were 1/1.02/1.20/0.98 ($O/I_1/I_2/I_3$).

Pharmacokinetics. The plasma concentration-time profiles after intestinal infusion were well characterized by an open two-compartment body model with zero-order input (Fig. 4), except for subject 1 when administered a 41.6 mg dose and subject 2 when administered an 11.8 mg dose. In these two subjects the plasma concentration-time profiles collapsed to an open single-compartment body model with zero-order input.

The regression parameter estimates and asymptotic parameter standard deviations determined for each plasma concentration-time profile are presented in Table III, along with the integrated AUCs. The average distribution phase constant α was 1.29 ± 0.734 hours^{-1}, which represents a $t_{1/2\alpha}$ of 0.54 hours. The average elimination phase constant β was 0.191 ± 0.0377 hours^{-1}, which represents a $t_{1/2\beta}$ of 3.63 hours. The t_{lag} after intestinal infusion averaged 0.46 ± 0.442 hours. The absorption rate constant k_a determined from administration of the oral bolus dose averaged 1.92 ± 1.02 hours^{-1}, which represents $t_{1/2a}$ of 0.36 hours.

The pharmacokinetic parameters determined for each dose were averaged for each subject (Table IV). Average volume terms were 28.8 ± 6.68 L for V_c/F and 59.0 ± 8.70 L for V_{area}/F. The V_c/F term was also calculated by dividing the known infusion rate by the slope of the cumulative absorption plot ($F \cdot k_0/V_c$). The average V_c/F term calculated by this method was 33.0 ± 13.05 L and is of the order of that obtained by conventional curve fitting. The average total systemic clearance term (CL/F) and CL_R were 179.6 ± 33.68 and 102.6 ± 7.96 ml/min, respectively.

The pharmacokinetics of baclofen were dose proportional in the range tested as indicated by the constant relative bioavailability (dose-normalized AUC ratios).

DISCUSSION

Ideally, the pharmacokinetic disposition of a drug is best derived from intravenous data. Therapeutic and regulatory considerations for many drugs including baclofen, however, preclude the administration of intravenous doses. Thus one is left with analyzing oral plasma concentration-time data, which can be perplexing.[12] The difficulty in obtaining pharmacokinetic information from orally administered drugs can be re-

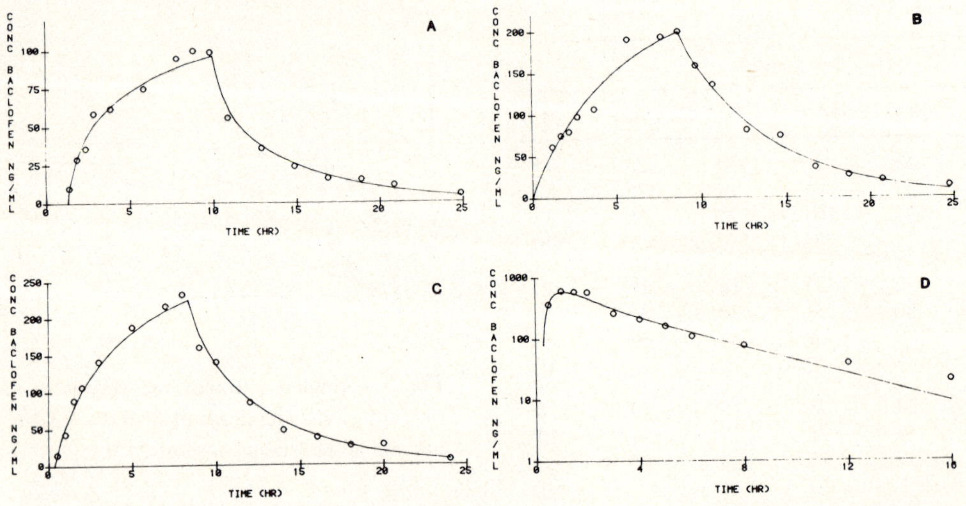

Fig. 4. Plasma concentration-time profiles and associated nonlinear regression best fit after baclofen administration by intestinal infusion with rates of 1.31 **(A)**, 2.66 **(B)**, and 5.86 **(C)** mg/hr and an oral bolus dose of 24.0 mg **(D)** in subject 3.

Table IV. Pharmacokinetic parameter estimates*

Subject No.	*Weight (kg)*	V_C/F *(L)*†	V_{area}/F *(L)*‡	*CL/F (ml/min)*	CL_R *(ml/min)*
1	82.3	34.8	62.2	167.9	96.0
2	69.5	24.9	46.7	146.4	102.1
3	74.1	34.1	67.0	226.1	98.3
4	66.4	21.4	60.2	178.1	113.9
$\overline{X}$	73.1	28.8	59.0	179.6	102.6
SD	6.92	6.68	8.70	33.68	7.96

*Subject average from individual doses.
†Two-compartment model estimates only.
‡Includes both one- and two-compartment model estimates.

solved to a great extent when several formulations or modes of oral administration are given and when intubation directly into the intestine is possible. Both these methods help sort out the relative assignment of α, β, and k_a and in the case of intestinal intubation may result in k_a values so large that the plasma concentration-time profiles are essentially equivalent to those after intravenous administration. Although the absorption process is quite complex, possibly involving first-pass effects, decreased bioavailability, stomach emptying, and other non–first-order absorption processes, it can usually be adequately described by a single rate-limiting process (i.e., first-order input for oral bolus and zero-order input for intestinal infusion under proper infusion rate conditions).

Regression analysis of the postinfusion plasma concentration-time data indicated the necessity of two exponentials in describing the distribution and elimination disposition of baclofen. This was verified after the oral bolus doses resulting in the characteristic "nose" in the plasma concentration-time profile that is commonly associated with a two-compartment pharmacokinetic model and a triexponential equation. Additionally, k_a was computed from the oral bolus doses, resulting in an average value of 1.92 $hours^{-1}$. Most drugs are absorbed more slowly from the stomach than the intestines[10] and in the case of baclofen, with an associated t_{lag} after oral bolus dosing of 0 to 20 minutes, may also be limited by the gastric emptying rate. Because of the amphoteric properties of baclofen, minimal absorption from the stomach would be anticipated. Therefore, the absorption rate after intestinal infusion would be ≥ 1.92 $hours^{-1}$ and the regression exponential constants are defined as $k_a > \alpha > \beta$.

In all but two cases plasma concentration-time profiles after intestinal infusion were adequately described by a two-compartment model with zero-order input. Absorption profiles indicated that the infusion rate was limiting, that the infusion rate determined in vitro and by the absorption plot slope corresponded, and that V_c/F determined from the absorption plot was consistent with the value obtained by conventional curve fitting. Input from the intestines was not instantaneous as indicated by the average t_{lag} of 28 minutes associated with the intestinal infusions. The t_{lag} after intestinal infusion represents any error associated with the determination of t_0 and lag associated with an intestinal compartment. The equations describing the addition of an intestinal compartment connected to the central compartment by a first-order rate constant were also analyzed by nonlinear regression. Comparison of this model with that previously described by the Akaike Information Criterion[13] and the F test[1] indicated the two models were equivalent and the additional compartment redundant. Thus absorption from the intestine was sufficiently rapid so as not to be detected, at least not by the sampling regimen defined in our study. In the two cases in which the two-compartment model collapsed to a single compartment, absorption must have been slowed sufficiently, resulting in a change of the relative values of α, β, k_a, and k_{21} and thereby causing the apparent collapse of the two-compartment model as described by Ronfeld and Benet.[12]

The relatively low ratio of V_{area}/V_C and the slow distribution rate indicates baclofen is distributed primarily in the blood and well-perfused tissues of the central compartment and only slowly penetrates other tissues, even though it is only 30% protein bound.[4] This is consistent with autoradiographic data in rats in which there are high levels of baclofen in the liver and kidneys and relatively low levels in the brain, muscle, and nerve tissues and fat.[3] The bioavailable fraction was reported[2] to be approximately 70% to 80%. Thus the primary route of baclofen elimination is by the kidney, principally by glomerular filtration. This has important therapeutic implications since baclofen is targeted to a patient population that is primarily convalescent and in many cases is subject to renal dysfunction. Although there is little evidence as yet to support a plasma concentration-activity relationship,[6,8] dosage adjustment based on pharmacokinetic evaluation of the patient relative to normal subjects provides the most rational basis for therapeutic management.

We gratefully acknowledge the contributions of Drs. J. R. Lawter and S. Ahuja for their technical assistance in evaluating the in vitro performance of the Travenol 24-Hour Infusors.

APPENDIX

The pharmacokinetic definitions of the preexponential terms A, B, C, and D are as follows:

$$A = \frac{FD_{po}\,(k_{21} - \alpha)}{V_C\,T\alpha\quad(\alpha - \beta)}$$

$$B = \frac{FD_{po}\,(\beta - k_{21})}{V_C\,T\beta\quad(\alpha - \beta)}$$

$$C = \frac{k_a\,FD_{po}\,(k_{21} - \alpha)}{V_C\,(k_a - \alpha)\quad(\beta - \alpha)}$$

$$D = \frac{k_a\,FD_{po}\,(k_{21} - \beta)}{V_C\,(k_a - \beta)\,(\alpha - \beta)}$$

The microscopic constants shown in Fig. 1 can be calculated from the preexponential terms and the following relationships:

$$\alpha + \beta = k_{21} + k_{12} + k_{10}$$
$$\alpha \cdot \beta = k_{21} \cdot k_{10}$$

References

1. Boxenbaum HG, Riegelman S, Elashoff RM: Statistical estimations in pharmacokinetics. J Pharmacokinet Biopharm **2:**123-148, 1974.
2. Faigle JW, Keberle H: The chemistry and kinetics of Lioresal. Postgrad Med J **48:**(suppl):9-13, 1972.
3. Faigle JW, Keberle H: The metabolism and pharmacokinetics of Lioresal. *In* Birkmayer W, editor: Spasticity—A topical survey. Bern, Switzerland, 1972, Verlag-Hans-Huber.
4. Faigle JW, Keberle H, Degan PH: Chemistry and pharmacokinetics of baclofen. *In* Feldman RG, Young RR, Koella WP, editors: Spasticity: Disordered motor control. Miami, Fla, 1980, Symposia Specialists Inc.
5. Kochak G, Honc F: An improved gas-liquid chromatographic method for the determination of baclofen in plasma and urine. J Chromatogr **310:**319-326, 1984.
6. Knutsson E, Lindblom U, Mortensson A: Plasma and cerebrospinal fluid levels of baclofen at optimal therapeutic responses in spastic paresis. J Neurol Sci **23:**473-484, 1974.
7. Loo J, Riegelman S: New method for calculating the intrinsic absorption rate of drugs. J Pharm Sci **57:**918-928, 1968.
8. McLellan DL: Co-contraction and stretch reflexes in spasticity during treatment with baclofen. J Neurol **40:**30-38, 1977.
9. Metropolitan Life Insurance Company: Statistical Bulletin 40. New York, 1959, Metropolitan Life Insurance Company.
10. Nimmo WS: Drugs, diseases, and altered gastric emptying. Clin Pharmacokinet **1:**189-203, 1976.
11. Riegelman J, Collier P: The application of statistical moment theory to the evaluation of in-vivo dissolution time and absorption rate. J Pharmacokinet Biopharm **8:**509-534, 1980.
12. Ronfeld RA, Benet LZ: Interpretation of plasma concentration-time curves after oral dosing. J Pharm Sci **66:**178-180, 1977.
13. Yamaoka K, Nakagawa T, Uno T: Application of Akaike's Information Criterion (AIC) in the evaluation of linear pharmacokinetic equations. J Pharmacokinet Biopharm **6:**165-175, 1978.

Sulindac is not renal sparing in man

We investigated the claimed renal-sparing effect of the cyclooxygenase inhibitor sulindac. Fifteen normal women following a diet of 50 mEq salt a day were randomly assigned to 5 days of either placebo, sulindac, 200 mg b.i.d., or indomethacin, 25 mg q.i.d., after first serving as their own controls. Renal effects were assessed by the excretion rate of prostaglandin (PG) E_2 (an index of renal PG synthesis), sodium balance, plasma renin activity (PRA), and the response to furosemide. Systemic effects were assessed by collagen-induced platelet aggregation and thromboxane B_2 formation and by the urinary excretion of a systemically formed metabolite of $PGF_{2\alpha}$ (PGF-M). Both sulindac and indomethacin resulted in a positive sodium balance and a reduction in 24-hour urinary PGE_2 excretion (range −49% to −86%). Basal PRA was decreased by indomethacin only, but the increases in PRA and in urinary PGE_2 excretion in response to furosemide were inhibited by both sulindac and indomethacin. Sulindac reduced the natriuresis induced by furosemide, and indomethacin reduced the rise in inulin clearance after furosemide. Thus the two nonsteroidal anti-inflammatory drugs had similar effects on the kidney. Indomethacin had a greater effect than sulindac on the inhibition of collagen-induced platelet aggregation and thromboxane synthesis and the two drugs had equivalent effects on the reduction of PGF-M excretion. Peak plasma drug concentrations of indomethacin (1.9 ± 0.4 μg/ml) and sulindac sulfide (7.7 ± 1.9 μg/ml) were those associated with clinical efficacy. We conclude that sulindac has renal effects qualitatively comparable to those of indomethacin. Therefore, caution should continue to be exercised with the use of sulindac, as with other nonsteroidal anti-inflammatory drugs, in clinical situations in which cyclooxygenase inhibitors have been associated with deterioration of renal function. (CLIN PHARMACOL THER 38:258-265, 1985.)

Douglas G. Roberts, M.D.,* John G. Gerber, M.D., John S. Barnes, B.S., Gary O. Zerbe, Ph.D., and Alan S. Nies, M.D.** *Denver, Colo.*

Sulindac (Clinoril; Merck, Sharp & Dohme) is a newer nonsteroidal anti-inflammatory drug (NSAID) reported to differ from other NSAIDs in that it spares renal prostaglandin (PG) synthetase.[5,7,8,30] This would have a potential advantage in some disease states such as severe hepatic dysfunction, in which renal PGs are important in the maintenance of renal blood flow (RBF) and glomerular filtration rate (GFR). However, before clear recommendations can be made about the use of sulindac in disease states, the evidence about its renal sparing properties should be unequivocal. In this report we show that sulindac is not specifically renal sparing; therefore, caution should continue to be exercised with its use in situations in which impairment of renal function with NSAIDs may be expected.

METHODS

Subjects. This study was performed in the Clinical Research Center of the University of Colorado Health Sciences Center after approval by the Human Subjects Committee. Informed consent was obtained from all subjects.

Subjects were 15 normal, nonsmoking women between the ages of 18 and 55 years, within 15% of ideal weight for height,[33] with no active illness or any history of renal disease, and with normal physical examination results. All had normal laboratory screening results including a complete blood count, differential and platelet count, levels of electrolytes, fasting blood sugar, BUN, creatinine, SGOT, alkaline phosphatase, total bilirubin, and total protein, urinalysis, urine culture, and a negative test for pregnancy. They had to be drug free for 2 weeks before the study.

From the Division of Clinical Pharmacology, Departments of Medicine and Pharmacology, and Department of Preventive Medicine and Biometrics, University of Colorado School of Medicine.

Supported in part by Merck, Sharp & Dohme Research Laboratories, West Point, Pa., General Clinical Research Center Program Grant No. M01 RR 00051-22 from the Division of Research Resources, National Institutes of Health (NIH), and Grant No. HL21308 from the Heart, Lung and Blood Institute, NIH.

Received for publication Feb. 20, 1985; accepted June 8, 1985.

Reprint requests to: John G. Gerber, M.D., University of Colorado Health Sciences Center, Box C-237, 4200 E. Ninth Ave., Denver, CO 80262.

*Supported by NIH Training Grant in Clinical Pharmacology No. GM07063-09.

**Established Investigator of the American Heart Association.

Table I. Subject characteristics

	Placebo	*Sulindac*	*Indomethacin*
Age (yr)	33 ± 5	35 ± 2	30 ± 3
Height (cm)	165 ± 1	161 ± 1	165 ± 3
Systolic blood pressure (mm Hg)			
Entry	112 ± 2	106 ± 7	108 ± 5
Day 4	96 ± 4	105 ± 4	103 ± 4
Day 9	99 ± 6	102 ± 3	98 ± 3
Diastolic blood pressure (mm Hg)			
Entry	76 ± 5	72 ± 5	77 ± 3
Day 4	68 ± 1	75 ± 3	75 ± 5
Day 9	71 ± 5	72 ± 4	67 ± 1
Weight (kg)			
Entry	61.6 ± 2.7	54.9 ± 2.3	60.2 ± 3.1
Day 4	59.9 ± 2.5	54.0 ± 2.2	58.8 ± 2.9
Day 9	59.2 ± 2.4	54.3 ± 2.1*	59.1 ± 3.0*

Data are $\overline{X}$ ± SE.
*$P < 0.05$ compared with placebo.

The study lasted 10 days and was timed to begin within 10 days after menstrual onset. Throughout the study, all subjects took individually labeled, identically appearing packets of drug at 7 AM and 1, 7, and 11 PM. The study was divided into two sequential 5-day periods. During the first 5 days (control) all subjects received placebo (single blind), while during the second 5 days (trial) the subjects were randomly assigned (double blind) to placebo, sulindac, 200 mg b.i.d. (7 AM and 7 PM), or indomethacin, 25 mg q.i.d. There were five subjects in each treatment group.

During the study, a 50 mEq sodium and 60 mEq potassium per day diet was provided and vital signs and weight were determined daily. Twenty-four–hour urine samples were collected daily for determination of electrolytes, creatinine, and osmolality. On days 3 and 8, an aliquot was screened for drugs other than sulindac or indomethacin. On days 4 and 9 the excretion rates of PGE_2 and the tetranor metabolite of $PGF_{2\alpha}$ (5α,7α-dihydroxy-11-ketotetranorprostane-1,16-dioic acid; PGF-M) were determined.

The control and trial periods each consisted of 3 days as an outpatient and 2 days as an inpatient. As inpatients, the subjects were required to be flat in bed and fasted from midnight until 1 PM the following day. At 6:30 AM, the subjects were given their morning medication with 200 ml water. A bladder catheter was placed and loading and maintenance intravenous doses of inulin (50 mg/kg; 30 mg/min) and *p*-amino hippurate (PAH; 120 mg; 8 mg/min) were given. After allowing 45 minutes for equilibration, a baseline (control) 45-minute urine collection with a midpoint blood collection was obtained. Furosemide, 40 mg, was then intravenously injected over 5 seconds, and serial urine and blood samples were collected until 1 PM (at 0 to 15, 15 to 30, 30 to 60, 60 to 120, and 120 to 300 minutes after furosemide). Measured water, sodium, and potassium losses were replaced intravenously in the third hour. The urine collection on days 5 and 10 began at 1 PM. Subjects were observed overnight and discharged the next morning.

Baseline measurements included platelet aggregation and thromboxane B_2 generation, plasma drug concentrations, inulin clearance (GFR), PAH clearance (to estimate renal plasma flow), plasma renin activity (PRA), and the excretion rates of PGE_2 and electrolytes. All determinations except drug levels and the platelet studies were repeated at various times after furosemide dosing.

Assays. Sodium and potassium were measured by ion exchange on a Beckman Electrolyte 2 Analyzer (Beckman Instruments Inc.); bilirubin was measured on a Beckman 24 Spectrophotometer; glucose was analyzed with a Beckman Glucose 2 Analyzer; osmolality was determined by freezing-point depression with an Advanced Instruments, Inc. model 3D II; and inulin and PAH were analyzed with an Autoanalyzer I (Technicon Instruments Corp.).[18,23] All other chemistry parameters were measured with a System 203S Analyzer (Gilford Instrument Laboratories Inc.). PRA was determined by standard methods.[34] Urinary PGE_2 was extracted into dichloromethane at pH 3 and measured by RIA with an antibody from Institut Pasteur, Paris.[12,29] Urinary PGF-M was measured by RIA with an antibody.* Standard and tritiated PGF-M were produced

*Obtained from Dr. E. Granstrom.

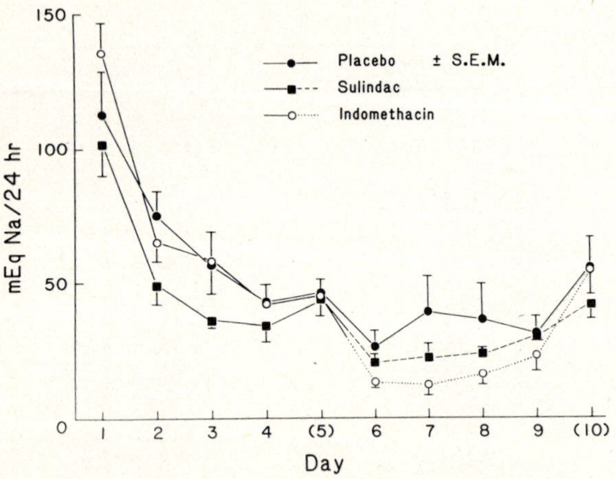

Fig. 1. Daily urinary sodium excretions for groups. All groups started on placebo; drug groups were crossed over on day 6 to either sulindac or indomethacin. Days 5 and 10 are corrected to a 24-hour equivalent (see text).

by a variation of published methods[21,22] from 13,14-dihydro-15-keto-$PGF_{2\alpha}$ (tritiated from Amersham Corp.; cold from Cayman Chemical). Modifications included addition of adenosine diphosphate (ADP), 0.5 mmol/L, and D,L-carnitine, 0.24 mmol/L, to the reaction mixture, extraction of PGF-M at pH 3 into ethyl acetate, and purification of the evaporated residue by reversed-phase HPLC. The presence of PGF-M was confirmed by gas chromatography/mass spectrometry. Platelet aggregation studies were performed with platelet-rich plasma in a Payton aggregometer with collagen and ADP as the proaggregatory agents.[2] The percent aggregation was determined 4 minutes after addition of collagen or ADP. Thromboxane B_2 generated in the platelet-rich plasma was measured by RIA with an antibody from Seragen.

Plasma drug concentrations were measured in duplicate by a modification of current methods.[15,35] Briefly, 200 μl plasma was mixed with 10 μl ethanolic internal standard (indomethacin [Sigma Chemical Co.] for the sulindacs; sulindac sulfoxide [Merck, Sharpe & Dohme] for indomethacin) and 200 μl 750 mmol/L lactic acid buffer at pH 3.0. The mixture was extracted twice with 4 ml CH_2Cl_2, dried under nitrogen at 40° C, and taken up in 100 μl mobile phase. Reversed-phase HPLC was performed with a mobile phase of 40% to 60% acetonitrile in 45 mmol/L aqeuous phosphate buffer at pH 3.0, and a nonlinear gradient (no. 7 setting Waters Model 660 Solvent Programmer, slow upstroke; Waters Associates, Inc.) at a flow rate of 1.5 ml/min over 20 minutes with ultraviolet detection at 327 nm (Waters Model 440 Variable Wavelength UV Spectrophotometer).

Statistics. Data were analyzed by multivariate one-way ANOVA (three levels) appropriate for analysis of repeated measurements over time.[11,32] Intragroup comparisons between trial and control periods and comparisons between groups were determined. The latter allows direct drug-to-drug comparison. Comparisons of drug to placebo are one tailed. Comparisons between drugs or between placebo periods are two tailed. All data are expressed as the $\overline{X} \pm$ SE. A P value <0.05 was considered significant.

RESULTS

The entry profile and the effect of any therapy on weight and blood pressure are listed in Table I. The groups were comparable in age, weight, and blood pressure. Systolic and diastolic sitting blood pressures generally fell over the course of the study, but there were no significant differences between day 9 and day 4 blood pressures in any group. Subjects receiving placebo showed statistically significant weight loss during both control and trial periods of the low-salt diet. Drug groups showed weight loss only for the first (control) half, with no weight loss during drug dosing. Intergroup analysis showed that the absence of continued weight loss while taking sulindac and indomethacin was significantly different from placebo, but the two drugs did not differ from each other.

Fig. 1 shows daily outpatient urinary sodium excretion for each group. The values for inpatient days 5 and 10 do not include the acute study period and are corrected to a 24-hour equivalent. At the start of the control period, sodium excretion differed between groups and probably reflected group differences in the subject's diets. The subjects achieved sodium balance, as sodium excretion equilibrated at about 40 mEq/day by day 4 following the standard diet. For statistical analysis, the nonequilibrium period (days 1 through 3) was excluded. During the trial period, sodium excretion decreased compared with control values for both indomethacin ($P < 0.01$) and sulindac ($P < 0.05$) but not for placebo. There was no significant difference between indomethacin and sulindac. Chloride excretion (data not shown) was similar to sodium excretion. Potassium excretion (data not shown) did not show as marked an initial equilibrium phase, and only the sulindac group showed a significant ($P = 0.01$) decrease, which was relatively small (from 39 ± 4 to 31 ± 2 mEq).

The 24-hour urinary excretion of PGE_2 was compared for day 4 (control) and day 9 (trial period; Table II). The control values between the groups did not differ

Table II. Effects of sulindac and indomethacin on excretion of PGE_2 and PGF-M, urine volume, and on platelet function

	Placebo	*Sulindac*	*Indomethacin*
PGE_2 excretion (ng/gm creatinine)			
Control (day 4)	96 ± 8	91 ± 10	127 ± 28
Drug (day 9; % control)	73 ± 7 (76%)	46 ± 6 (51%)*	28 ± 3 (22%)*†
PGF-M excretion (μg/gm creatinine)			
Control	11.6 ± 1.0	10.5 ± 0.9	16.2 ± 2.8
Drug (% control)	11.1 ± 1.1 (96%)	6.8 ± 0.6 (65%)*	9.2 ± 0.4 (57%)*
24-hr urine volume (L)			
Control	1.89 ± 0.39	2.30 ± 0.64	1.76 ± 0.22
Drug	1.82 ± 0.46	2.45 ± 0.71	1.48 ± 0.19
Platelet aggregation (% maximum)			
Collagen (5 μg/ml)			
Control (day 5)	73 ± 3	76 ± 2	74 ± 3
Drug (day 10; % control)	73 ± 5 (99%)	68 ± 5 (89%)*	34 ± 8 (46%)*†
ADP (10^{-5} mol/L)			
Control	65 ± 4	66 ± 3	60 ± 8
Drug (% control)	62 ± 5 (96%)	56 ± 2 (85%)*	55 ± 2 (90%)
Platelet thromboxane B_2 release (ng/ml)			
Collagen			
Control (day 5)	42 ± 7	41 ± 8	53 ± 10
Drug (day 10; % control)	45 ± 8 (108%)	28 ± 7 (69%)*	2 ± 2 (3%)*†
ADP			
Control	17 ± 10	6 ± 2	11 ± 6
Drug (% control)	13 ± 8 (76%)	0.3 ± 0.3 (5%)*	Below detection (0%)

Data are $\overline{X}$ ± SE.
*P < 0.05 compared with placebo.
†P < 0.05 compared with sulindac.

significantly. During the trial period the placebo group showed a decrease in PGE_2 excretion of 24% (not significant), whereas the indomethacin and sulindac groups showed significantly decreased PGE_2 excretion, by 78% and 49%, respectively. By intergroup comparison, the effect of indomethacin was greater than that of sulindac ($P < 0.05$).

Urinary excretion of PGF-M was examined on days 4 and 9 (Table II). Both indomethacin and sulindac decreased PGF-M excretion as compared with the subjects' own control value ($P < 0.05$), while placebo did not. By intergroup comparison the drugs did not differ from each other.

ADP-stimulated platelet aggregation was minimally affected by sulindac and indomethacin. Collagen-stimulated aggregation was inhibited to a small (11%) but significant extent by sulindac ($P < 0.05$), and to a greater extent (54%) by indomethacin ($P < 0.01$). Intergroup comparison showed that the effect of sulindac on collagen-induced platelet aggregation was significantly less than that of indomethacin ($P < 0.01$). The small amount of thromboxane released from platelets with ADP was suppressed by both sulindac and indomethacin. With collagen-induced platelet aggregation, which causes much greater synthesis of thromboxane B_2, sulindac decreased thromboxane B_2 release by 31% ($P < 0.05$), while indomethacin decreased thromboxane B_2 release by 97% ($P < 0.01$). Intergroup drug comparison revealed that the effect of indomethacin was significantly greater than that of sulindac (Table II).

The response to furosemide is shown in Figs. 2 and 3. Neither sulindac nor indomethacin had great effects on the natriuretic response to furosemide. Compared with the placebo group, sulindac significantly blunted urinary sodium excretion ($P < 0.05$). Indomethacin had a similar effect ($P = 0.07$; Fig. 2). Furosemide induced a large increase in the urinary excretion of PGE_2, which was significantly inhibited by both sulindac and indomethacin (Fig. 2), and the drug effects did not differ. Only indomethacin decreased basal PRA, but 20 minutes after furosemide both sulindac and indomethacin inhibited the rise in PRA, an effect significantly different from placebo (Fig. 3). Although at 60 minutes the rise in PRA continued to be inhibited by both sulindac and indomethacin, the difference from the placebo group was of borderline significance ($P = 0.07$). Neither sulindac nor indomethacin affected PAH clearance during baseline or after furosemide. The GFR before furosemide was not affected by sulindac or indomethacin. However, compared with the

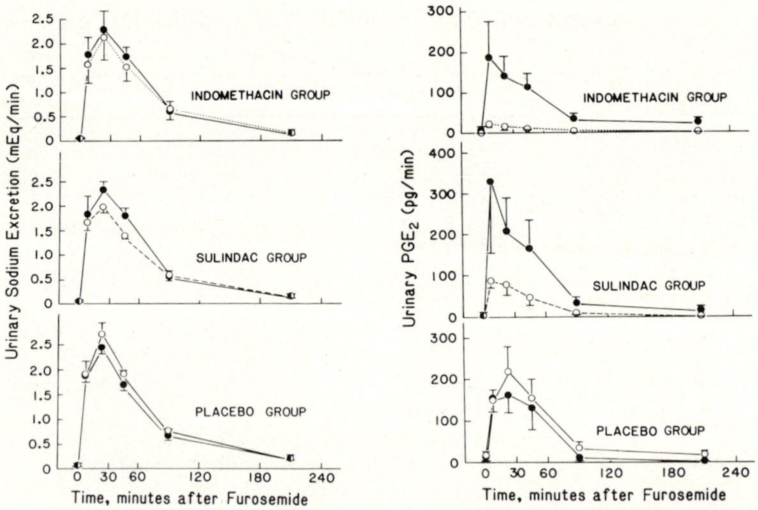

Fig. 2. Left, Timed urinary sodium excretions after furosemide on control day 5 (●) and trial day 10 (○). **Right,** Urinary PGE_2 excretion after furosemide on control day 5 (●) and trial day 10 (○). *Bars* represent standard error of the means. *Solid lines* represent placebo, *dashed lines* represent sulindac, and *dotted lines* represent indomethacin.

placebo group, the furosemide-induced changes in GFR were reduced by indomethacin for the first three collection periods (0 to 15, 15 to 30, and 30 to 60 minutes) and by sulindac at the 15-to-30–minute collection period.

Plasma drug concentrations were as follows: sulindac sulfide (active metabolite), 7.7 ± 1.9 μg/ml; sulindac (inactive parent compound), 6.0 ± 2.4 μg/ml; sulindac sulfone (inactive metabolite), 3.9 ± 0.7 μg/ml; and indomethacin, 1.9 ± 0.4 μg/ml. These peak levels were in the expected range, and all subjects were taking their assigned drugs. Urine drug screening results did not show the presence of salicylates or other drugs.

DISCUSSION

NSAIDs are useful for the relief of fever, pain, and inflammation. Recent evidence has implicated these drugs as causing acute renal failure in clinical conditions that are associated with glomerular disease or circulatory stresses in which both the sympathetic nervous system and the renin-angiotensin system are activated.[1,3,10,36,38] PGs have been demonstrated to modulate the renal effects of these endogenous vasoconstrictors. It is thought that inhibition of PGs by NSAIDs in these settings results in unopposed renal vasoconstriction by angiotensin II and norepinephrine, resulting in acute renal failure.[19]

The development of an NSAID that would spare renal cyclooxygenase would be an important advance in therapeutics. Sulindac has been reported to be renal sparing.[5,7,8,30] Sulindac is a structural analog of indomethacin, but is inactive as dosed and must be reduced to the sulfide form to be active.[14] Experiments in rat and rabbit kidneys have shown that the kidney has the enzymatic machinery to oxidize sulindac sulfide to the inactive forms (the sulfoxide and sulfone).[25] Thus the kidney may be exposed to less of the active form than other organ systems. Consistent with this hypothesis is the finding that little active sulfide is excreted in the urine.[13] On the other hand, the sulfide is present in the circulation and in the renal tissue itself,[25] and thus should be able to affect PG synthesis in the renal vasculature. In addition, infusion of sulindac sulfide into the isolated kidney results in PG inhibition even though no sulfide appears in the venous effluent.[25] Nonetheless, recent clinical reports have suggested that sulindac may indeed be safe in situations in which other NSAIDs have caused a reduction in renal function.[5,7]

Because of the importance of this question of selective cyclooxygenase inhibition, we have compared the effect of sulindac with those of indomethacin and placebo given for 5 days to normal women.[26] The doses of the drugs were those used clinically, and for sulindac the dose used was that reported to have no effect on renal PG synthesis in normal subjects or patients with renal disease. We used collagen-stimulated platelet thromboxane B_2 release as well as the urinary excretion of PGF-M as indices of systemic cyclooxygenase inhibition, and urinary PGE_2 excretion as a measure of renal cyclooxygenase inhibition. In addition, we looked at the effects of these drugs on furosemide-stimulated PGE_2 production and renin release as additional tools to evaluate effects of the drug on renal cyclooxygenase.

Our findings indicate that sulindac does not appear to be renal sparing. The data for this conclusion are several. First, both sulindac and indomethacin induced sodium retention on a moderately sodium-restricted diet and prevented the continued weight loss that occurred in the placebo group. This clinically important effect may reflect either vascular or tubular consequences of inhibiting renal cyclooxygenase. Second, both drugs reduced urinary PGE_2 excretion. Urinary PGE_2 excretion is considered to reflect de novo renal PG synthesis, whereas the urinary excretion of the prostacyclin metabolite, 6-keto-$PGF_{1\alpha}$, may derive from systemic as well as renal sources.[17,28,31] Third, the response to furosemide was similarly altered by the two drugs. Furosemide resulted in a rapid increase in PGE_2 excretion that was inhibited by sulindac and indomethacin. The increase in renin activity after furosemide, which is dependent on PG synthesis, also was inhibited by both sulindac and indomethacin. Finally, sodium excretion after furosemide was decreased to a small extent by sulindac and probably by indomethacin as well.

We have evidence that indomethacin may have had greater effects than sulindac on some indices of renal PG effect (basal PRA, PGE_2 excretion, and GFR). However, the small group size of our study precludes determination of small differences between the drugs. The size of the groups was chosen as the minimum number to confirm the large differences in the drugs that had been reported in the literature. Clearly, such large differences did not exist in our study.

Were the systemic effects of sulindac and indomethacin comparable? The doses used and the blood levels achieved were those associated with clinical anti-inflammatory effects. Compliance was good as judged by these drug concentrations. Effects of the drugs on the renal excretion of PGF-M were comparable. The PGF-M arises from hepatic metabolism of systemically produced $PGF_{2\alpha}$. A reduction in the urinary excretion of PGF-M, therefore, is indicative of a reduction of systemic $PGF_{2\alpha}$ production. Both indomethacin and sulindac had moderate effects on this index of systemic PG synthesis. As another index of systemic effect, collagen- and ADP-induced platelet aggregation and thromboxane production were investigated. ADP has less effect than collagen on the stimulation of platelet aggregation through thromboxane synthesis, and thus to discern differences between cyclooxygenase inhibitors, collagen-induced platelet aggregation may be preferred.[6,20] Indomethacin had a greater effect than sulindac on collagen-induced platelet aggregation and thromboxane production. This implies that either the platelets are spared by sulindac, or that indomethacin had a greater systemic effect than sulindac.

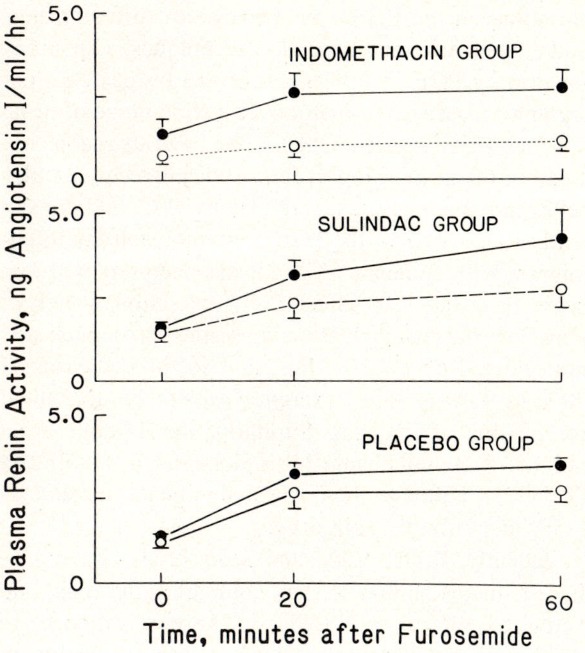

Fig. 3. PRA on control day 5 (●) and trial day 10 (○). *Bars* represent standard error of the means. *Solid lines* represent placebo, *dashed line* represents sulindac, and *dotted line* represents indomethacin.

The literature on the renal effects of sulindac is noteworthy for discrepant results.[4,7,8,16,23,29,30,37] Although study protocols vary, some of the different results remain unexplained. A major question is whether sulindac has systemic effects comparable with those of the other NSAIDs in the various studies. Different methods have been used to evaluate the systemic effects of NSAIDs, but there is no concensus as to their relative meaning or which may be best. We have attempted to assess systemic effect by measuring the excretion of a systemic PG metabolite and by measuring collagen-induced platelet aggregation and thromboxane B_2 production. Others have used ADP-induced platelet aggregation, which is not dependent on cyclooxygenase, or ADP-induced thromboxane B_2 production, and thus is an insensitive measure of cyclooxygenase, since only a small amount of thromboxane is formed. Still others have used thromboxane production by clotted blood, an indirect measure, the meaning of which relative to platelet thromboxane production induced by a standardized stimulus such as collagen is not known.

A final source of differences between studies are

variations in the PG assays because of different antibodies and different extraction techniques. Our assay for urinary PGE_2 has been confirmed by gas chromatography-mass spectrometry over a wide range of urine flow and PGE_2 excretion rates.[27] We have also subjected some of the urine samples from subjects receiving placebo, indomethacin, and sulindac to TLC[9] and consistently found 90% of the PGE_2 immunoreactivity to comigrate with authentic PGE_2. It has been reported that urine flow rate can affect PGE_2 excretion acutely.[27] However, the change in urine flow after furosemide was not affected by the NSAIDs, and so the decreases of 70% to 90% in PGE_2 excretion cannot be accounted for by this mechanism. Similarly, the 24-hour urine volumes were not changed by indomethacin or sulindac (Table II), although there was a significant decrease in PGE_2 excretion by both drugs.

Recently, Brater et al.[4] and Sedor et al.[30] have published studies similar to ours comparing the renal and extrarenal effects of NSAIDs to those of sulindac. In the first study, ibuprofen and naproxen were compared with sulindac after administration of the drugs over a 12-hour period. Differences in terms of the renal and platelet effects were very minor among the three drugs. Brater et al. concluded that sulindac was no more renal sparing than the other two NSAIDs. In the study by Sedor et al., the drug protocol was similar to ours in that sulindac, 200 mg b.i.d., was compared with indomethacin, 25 mg q.i.d. Quantitatively, indomethacin was more potent in inhibiting renal excretion of $PGF_{2\alpha}$, although clearly sulindac had an effect as well. In terms of renal function, neither drug had a major effect in this healthy female population. In terms of platelet effect, sulindac and indomethacin were equivalent in altering ADP-stimulated thromboxane B_2 release in platelet-rich plasma. However, as discussed above, ADP is not a potent stimulator of platelet thromboxane release, and consequently this model may not be the most sensitive method to assess systemic PG inhibition. Another difference between our data and those of Sedor et al. is that in our subjects the peak sulindac sulfide concentration was 7.7 ± 1.9 μg/ml, while Sedor et al. reported a value one third this concentration.

Our data from normal subjects may not apply to subjects with renal disease or those with very high levels of circulating angiotensin II or norepinephrine. We used a modest degree of sodium restriction and furosemide dosing to stimulate renal PG production to simulate the conditions that might exist in disease states. However, the fact that we saw significant effects of sulindac on renal function and cyclooxygenase under these mild conditions cannot be ignored. One would expect patients with renal disease, severe cirrhosis with ascites, dehydration, congestive heart failure, or nephrosis to be at least as sensitive to the effects of sulindac as normal subjects. Caution should therefore be applied with the use of sulindac, as with the use of other NSAIDs, in these conditions.

We thank Dr. Elisabeth Granstrom, Stockholm, for PGF-M antibody; Drs. Bob Strife and Paul Fennessey for gas chromatography/mass spectrometry confirmation of PGF-M; and Dr. Athanassios Chremos and Ms. Mary Ann Tupy-Visich of Merck, Sharp and Dohme Research for administrative assistance.

References

1. Ariz L, Donker AJM, Brentjens JRH, van der Hem GK: The effect of indomethacin on proteinuria and kidney function in the nephrotic syndrome. Acta Med Scand **179:**121-125, 1976.
2. Barnes JS, Dubocovich ML, Nies AS, Gerber JG: Lack of interaction between tricyclic antidepressants and clonidine at the $alpha_2$-adrenoceptor on human platelets. CLIN PHARMACOL THER **32:**744-748, 1982.
3. Boyer TD, Zia P, Reynolds TB: Effect of indomethacin and prostaglandin A, on renal function and plasma renin activity in alcoholic liver disease. Gastroenterology **77:**215-222, 1979.
4. Brater DC, Anderson S, Baird B, Campbell WB: Effects of ibuprofen, naproxen and sulindac on prostaglandins in men. Kidney Int **27:**66-73, 1985.
5. Bunning RD, Barth WF: Sulindac, a potentially renal-sparing non-steroidal anti-inflammatory drug. JAMA **248:**2864-2867, 1982.
6. Charo IF, Feinman RD, Detwiler TC: Interrelations of platelet aggregation and secretion. J Clin Invest **60:**866-873, 1977.
7. Ciabattoni G, Cinotti G, Pierucci A, et al: Effects of sulindac and ibuprofen in patients with chronic glomerular disease. N Engl J Med **310:**279-283, 1984.
8. Ciabattoni G, Pugliese F, Cinotti GA, Patrono C: Renal effects of anti-inflammatory drugs. Eur J Rheum Inflam **3:**210-221, 1980.
9. Ciabattoni G, Pugliese F, Spaldi M, Cinotti GA, Patrono C: Radioimmunoassay measurement of prostaglandin E_2 and $F_{2\alpha}$ in human urine. J Endocrinol Invest **2:**173-182, 1979.
10. Clive DM, Stoff JS: Renal syndromes associated with non-steroidal antiinflammatory drugs. N Engl J Med **310:**563-572, 1984.
11. Cole JWL, Grizzle JE: Applications of multivariate analysis of variance to repeated measurements experiments. Biometrics **22:**810-828, 1966.
12. Dray F, Charbonnel B, Maclouf J: Radioimmunoassay of prostaglandins F_2, E_1 and E_2 in human plasma. Eur J Clin Invest **5:**311-318, 1975.
13. Duggan DE, Hare LE, Ditzler CA, Lei BW, Kwan KC:

Disposition of sulindac. CLIN PHARMACOL THER **21**:326-335, 1977.

14. Duggan DE, Hooke KF, Risley EA, Shen TY, VanArman CG: Identification of the biologically active form of sulindac. J Pharmacol Exp Ther **201**:8-13, 1977.
15. Dusci LJ, Hackett LP: Determination of sulindac and its metabolites in serum by high performance liquid chromatography. J Chromatogr **171**:49-93, 1979.
16. Ferguson RJ, Vlasses PH, Riley LJ, et al: Sulindac and ibuprofen inhibit IV furosemide-stimulated renin release but not natriuresis in sodium-replete men. CLIN PHARMACOL THER **35**:239, 1984. (Abst.)
17. Frolich JC, Wilson TW, Sweetman BJ, et al: Urinary prostaglandins: Identification and origin. J Clin Invest **55**:763-770, 1975.
18. Fuhr F, Kaczmarczyk J, Kruttgen C-D: Eine einfache colorimetrische Methode zur Inulinbestimmung fur Nieren-clearance-untersuchungen bei stoffwechselgesunden und Diabetikern. Klin Wochen **33**:729-730, 1955.
19. Gerber JG, Olson RD, Nies AS: Interrelationship between prostaglandins and renin release. Kidney Int **19**:816-821, 1981.
20. Gerrard JM: Platelet aggregation and the influence of prostaglandins. *In* Lands WEM, Smith WL, editors: Methods in enzymology, vol 86. New York, 1982, Academic Press, pp 642-654.
21. Granstrom E, Kindahl H: Radioimmunoassay of 5α,7α-dihydroxy-11-ketotetranorprostane-1,16-dioic acid, a major prostaglandin F metabolite in blood and urine. *In* Lands WEM, Smith WL, editors: Methods in enzymology, vol 86. New York, 1982, Academic Press, pp 339-356.
22. Hamberg M: Metabolism of prostaglandins in rat liver mitochondria. Eur J Biochem **6**:135-146, 1968.
23. Harvey RB, Brothers AJ: Renal extraction of para-aminohippurate and creatinine measured by continuous *in vivo* sampling of arterial and renal-vein blood. Ann NY Acad Sci **102**:46-54, 1962.
24. Kronborg I, Daskalopoulos D, Katkov W, Zipser RD: Influence of sulindac and indomethacin on renal function and furosemide-induced decreases in patients with cirrhosis and ascites. Clin Res **32**:14A, 1984. (Abst.)
25. Miller MJS, Bednar MM, McGiff JC: Renal metabolism of sulindac: Functional implications. J Pharmacol Exp Ther **231**:449-456, 1984.
26. Patrono C, Wennmalm A, Ciabattoni G, Norvak J, Pugliese F, Cinotti GA: Evidence for extra-renal origin of urinary prostaglandin E_2 in healthy men. Prostaglandins **18**:623-629, 1979.
27. Roberts DG, Strife RJ, Gerber JG, Murphy RC, Nies AS: Effect of urine flow on prostaglandin E_2 excretion in man. Clin Res **31**:440A, 1983. (Abst.)
28. Rosenkranz B, Kitajima W, Frolich JC: Relevance of urinary 6-keto-prostaglandin $F_{1\alpha}$ determination. Kidney Int **19**:755-759, 1979.
29. Ryan JR, Chremos AN, Vargas R, Johnson CL, McMahon FG: The influence of nonsteroidal antiinflammatory drugs (NSAID) [Sulindac (S) and naproxen (N)] in natriuretic, diuretic and renin (PRA) response to furosemide (F). CLIN PHARMACOL THER **34**:271, 1984. (Abst.)
30. Sedor JR, Williams SL, Chremos AN, Johnson CL, Dunn MJ: Effects of sulindac and indomethacin on renal prostaglandin synthesis. CLIN PHARMACOL THER **36**:85-91, 1984.
31. Seyberth HW, Muller H, Solding K, Wille L, Hackenthal E: Urinary excretion rate of 6-keto-prostaglandin $F_{1\alpha}$ as an index of circulating prostacyclin. *In* Samuelsson B, Paoletti R, Ramwell P, editors: Advances in prostaglandin, thromboxane, and leukotriene research, vol 11. New York, 1983, Raven Press, pp 533-538.
32. Starmer CF, Grizzle JE: A computer program for analysis of data by general linear models. Institute of Statistics Mimeograph Series No. 560. Chapel Hill, NC, 1968, University of North Carolina.
33. Statistical Bulletin No. 40, November-December, 1959, Metropolitan Life Insurance Company, New York, NY.
34. Stockigt J, Collins R, Biglieri E: Determination of plasma renin concentration by angiotensin I immunoassay. Diagnostic impact of precise measurement of subnormal renin in hyperaldosteronism. Circ Res **28/29**(suppl II): 175-189, 1971.
35. Swanson BN, Boppana VK: Measurement of sulindac and its metabolites in human plasma and urine by high performance liquid chromatography. J Chromatogr **225**:123-140, 1981.
36. Walshe JJ, Venuto RC: Acute oliguric renal failure induced by indomethacin: Possible mechanism. Ann Intern Med **91**:47-49, 1979.
37. Wong DG, Spence JD, McDonald JWD: Nonsteroidal antiinflammatory drugs (NSAID) vs. placebo in hypertension treated with diuretics and β-blocker. CLIN PHARMACOL THER **35**:284, 1984. (Abst.)
38. Zipser RD, Hoefs JC, Speckart PF, Zia PK, Horton R: Prostaglandins: Modulators of renal function and pressor resistance in chronic liver disease. J Clin Endocrinol Metab **48**:895-900, 1979.

Circulatory effects of intravenous and oral acebutolol in acute myocardial infarction

The hemodynamic dose-response effects of intravenous (25 and 50 mg) and oral (200 and 400 mg) acebutolol were compared in a randomized between-group study in men within 17 hours of an acute uncomplicated myocardial infarction. Six subjects were evaluated in each of the four groups. After a 1-hour control period, hemodynamic variables and plasma drug concentrations were determined at 15 (intravenous therapy only), 30, 60, 90, 120, and 240 minutes after dosing. At the doses studied, hemodynamic dose-response effects were not evident after either intravenous or oral acebutolol. In all groups acebutolol reduced systolic and mean systemic arterial pressure, heart rate, cardiac output, and stroke volume. Pulmonary artery occluded pressure and systemic vascular resistance were transiently increased. Maximum changes developed between 15 and 30 minutes after intravenous dosing and between 1 and 2 hours after oral dosing. However, there were substantial reductions in cardiac output (−0.7 L/min/m²; $P < 0.05$) by 30 minutes after oral dosing. Effects lasted for 2 hours after intravenous dosing and for 4 hours after oral dosing. Our data confirm the hemodynamic safety of acebutolol after acute myocardial infarction. The relevance of the time-dependent hemodynamic differences between intravenous and oral initiation of β-blockade to the overall goal of reducing myocardial oxygen requirements after acute coronary artery occlusion merits closer examination. (Clin Pharmacol Ther 38:266-272, 1985.)

Bernard Silke, M.D., Gregory Nelson, M.B., Satya Prakash Verma, M.D., Janet Clarke, M.B., Ganesh Baliga, M.B., and Stanley H. Taylor, M.D.
Leeds, United Kingdom

Sympathoadrenal activation rapidly follows acute coronary occlusion,[11,30] and the resultant augmentation of myocardial oxygen requirements may extend infarct size[15] and increase the frequency of sinister arrhythmias.[4,10] β-Blocking drugs reduce the major determinants of myocardial oxygen consumption,[17] have limited the extent of experimental myocardial infarction,[13] and in man have reduced the indices of myocardial damage[18,20,22] and the occurrence of dysrhythmias.[28,29] Although the efficacy of β-blockade in reducing long-term mortality after myocardial infarction has been established,[3,19] its role during the acute evolving infarction is still under investigation.[34] It is intriguing, therefore, that the hemodynamic dose-response effects of early β-blockade or comparison of oral and intravenous therapy in this situation do not appear to have been examined.

From the University Departments of Cardiovascular Studies and Medical Cardiology, The General Infirmary.
Supported in part by the Yorkshire Regional Hospital Board, the West Riding Medical Research Trust, and May & Baker, Ltd.
Received for publication May 2, 1984; accepted March 3, 1985.
Reprint requests to: Dr. S. H. Taylor, Department of Medical Cardiology, The General Infirmary, Great George Street, Leeds LS1 3AX, United Kingdom.

Acebutolol is a cardioselective β-adrenoceptor antagonist with intrinsic sympathetic activity[2,12,14] effective in suppressing postinfarction arrhythmias in man.[1] Its hemodynamic safety after stable coronary heart disease has been confirmed.[5,16,21,33] Studies were therefore extended to characterize the hemodynamic dose-response effects of two intravenous and two oral doses of acebutolol in patients with uncomplicated acute myocardial infarction and to examine the influence of route of administration on the time of onset of cardiodynamic action.

METHODS

Our subjects were consecutive male patients admitted to the Coronary Care Unit with a definite transmural myocardial infarction (determined by Q waves). Their average age was 45 years (range 30 to 61 years), and the studies were performed between 3 and 17 hours after the onset of symptoms of acute myocardial infarction. The site of the definite infarction (Minnesota Code Criteria[23]) was equally distributed between anterior and inferior sites. Serum cardiac enzyme levels were substantially elevated in all: creatinine phosphokinase, 611 IU/L (range 86 to 1275 IU/L; normal <60 IU/L), aspartate transaminase, 169 IU/L (range 44 to

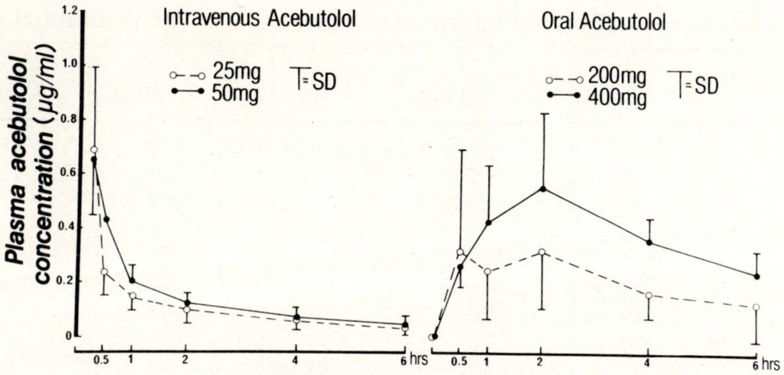

Fig. 1. Plasma acebutolol concentration after intravenous **(left)** or oral **(right)** dosing in acute myocardial infarction.

295 IU/L; normal <22 IU/L), and lactate dehydrogenase, 1542 IU/L (range 545 to 3706 IU/L; normal <480 IU/L). All subjects were in sinus rhythm and had stable systemic arterial pressure (systolic blood pressure >110 mm Hg). Immediately before the study a 6 ft standing posteroanterior chest radiograph was obtained. The average cardiothoracic ratio was 0.42 (range 0.40 to 0.49); no subject had more than grade 1 (upper lobe diversion) changes. Subjects randomized to oral or intravenous therapy were well matched for age, site of infarct, and plasma level of cardiac enzymes as well as baseline hemodynamic variables.

All subjects had received a single dose of diamorphine, 5 mg im or 5 mg iv, 2 hours or more before the start of intravascular monitoring. The serum potassium concentration was increased to >4.5 mmol/L by intravenous therapy in all subjects before intravascular cannulation. Subjects with sinus bradycardia (heart rate <60 bpm), atrioventricular conduction disturbance, insulin-dependent diabetes mellitus, or severe obstructive lung disease were excluded.

Our study was a single-blind, randomized, between-group comparison of the hemodynamic effects of intravenous and oral acebutolol. After intravascular cannulation and confirmation of normal left ventricular function (cardiac output >2.5 L/min/m^2; pulmonary artery occluded pressure [PAOP] <18 mm Hg), subjects were randomized to intravenous or oral acebutolol. Within these categories subjects were allocated to high or low doses according to a predetermined code. The randomized groups were adequately matched for baseline data including age, site of infarction, cardiac enzyme levels, and resting (control) hemodynamic variables. Four hemodynamic measurements were made at 20-minute intervals during the 1-hour control period. The subjects in each group then initially received either intravenous or oral acebutolol according to the following schedule: (1) group 1, acebutolol, 25 mg iv; (2) group 2, acebutolol, 50 mg iv; (3) group 3, acebutolol, 200 mg po; and (4) group 4, acebutolol, 400 mg po. Hemodynamic measurements were then made 15 (intravenous injection only), 30, 60, 120, and 240 minutes after acebutolol dosing. Blood was drawn for the measurement of plasma drug concentrations at each of the above times and at 4, 6, and 8 hours after acebutolol.

Heart rate was measured continuously from the ECG. Pulmonary vascular pressures were measured through a 7-F balloon floatation catheter introduced percutaneously through the median basilic vein and positioned by pressure monitoring. Left ventricular filling pressure was taken to be the PAOP. Systemic arterial pressure was measured through a small brachial cannula (1.2 mm od). Both intravascular pressures were externally transduced, continuously displayed, and recorded. Zero reference was at the mid-chest level. Cardiac output was computed in triplicate by the thermodilution technique with 10 ml 5% dextrose solution in water at 0° C as indicator injected through a gas-operated constant velocity pump.

The plasma concentrations of acebutolol and its metabolite diacetolol were measured by HPLC with fluorometric detection. The assay was specific and linear over the measured range (coefficient of variation 5%), with a lower limit of sensitivity of 0.02 μg/ml for each compound.[8]

Recorded variables were analyzed independently by an observer not involved in data acquisition. Statistical analysis was by standard two-way repeated-measures ANOVA.[6] Fisher's multiple comparison procedure[32] was used to test the difference between doses. The variability of measurements in the control period was determined from the coefficient of variation and expressed as a percentage of the mean.

Table I. Hemodynamic dose-response effects of intravenous acebutolol in acute myocardial infarction

	Dose (mg)	*Control*	*15 min*	*30 min*	*60 min*	*120 min*	*240 min*
Systolic blood pressure (mm Hg)	25	143 ± 6	135 ± 8*	137 ± 8*	139 ± 9	134 ± 9*	131 ± 8*
	50	133 ± 5	125 ± 3*	124 ± 3*	123 ± 4*	124 ± 4*	124 ± 5*
Diastolic blood pressure (mm Hg)	25	80 ± 4	80 ± 3	79 ± 3	81 ± 3	76 ± 3	74 ± 1*
	50	76 ± 4	73 ± 3	75 ± 2	75 ± 3	73 ± 2	71 ± 2*
Mean blood pressure (mm Hg)	25	103 ± 5	100 ± 4	99 ± 4	101 ± 5	98 ± 4	97 ± 4*
	50	100 ± 6	97 ± 4	95 ± 5	97 ± 5	96 ± 4	94 ± 4*
Heart rate (bpm)	25	79 ± 7	74 ± 7*	74 ± 7*	75 ± 8*	74 ± 8*	80 ± 9
	50	79 ± 7	76 ± 6*	77 ± 6	76 ± 5*	75 ± 5*	78 ± 5
PAOP (mm Hg)	25	13 ± 1	15 ± 1*	15 ± 1*	15 ± 1*	14 ± 1	14 ± 1
	50	12 ± 2	14 ± 2*	13 ± 2	13 ± 2	13 ± 2	12 ± 2
Cardiac output (L/min/m^2)	25	3.2 ± 0.2	2.7 ± 0.3*	2.7 ± 0.3*	2.7 ± 0.3*	2.7 ± 0.3*	3.2 ± 0.4
	50	3.9 ± 0.1	3.3 ± 0.1*	3.3 ± 0.1*	3.3 ± 0.1*	3.3 ± 0.1*	3.6 ± 0.1
Stroke volume (ml/m^2)	25	40 ± 2	36 ± 3	36 ± 2	36 ± 2	36 ± 3	40 ± 2
	50	49 ± 3	43 ± 3	43 ± 2	43 ± 2	44 ± 2	46 ± 2
Systemic vascular resistance (dyne · sec · cm^{-5} · m^2)	25	2675 ± 255	3140 ± 300*	3130 ± 275*	3160 ± 360*	3040 ± 340	2625 ± 305
	50	2205 ± 250	2545 ± 270*	2580 ± 310*	2455 ± 270*	2485 ± 255*	2180 ± 210

Data are $\bar{X}$ ± SE.
*$P < 0.05$ compared with control values.

Table II. Hemodynamic dose-response effects of oral acebutalol in acute myocardial infarction

	Dose (mg)	*Control*	*30 min*	*60 min*	*120 min*	*240 min*
Systolic blood pressure (mm Hg)	200	139 ± 4	135 ± 6	135 ± 6	130 ± 6*	130 ± 4*
	400	140 ± 6	140 ± 7	135 ± 9	130 ± 9*	124 ± 7*
Diastolic blood pressure (mm Hg)	200	77 ± 1	77 ± 2	79 ± 2	75 ± 1	77 ± 2
	400	77 ± 4	80 ± 4	80 ± 5	76 ± 5	78 ± 4
Mean blood pressure (mm Hg)	200	103 ± 3	102 ± 2	103 ± 3	100 ± 2	99 ± 3
	400	100 ± 5	102 ± 5	100 ± 6	97 ± 6*	92 ± 5*
Heart rate (bpm)	200	88 ± 4	84 ± 3*	80 ± 3*	79 ± 3*	79 ± 3*
	400	77 ± 7	75 ± 7	71 ± 6*	70 ± 5*	73 ± 5*
PAOP (mm Hg)	200	11 ± 1	11 ± 1	13 ± 1*	13 ± 1*	11 ± 1
	400	12 ± 1	13 ± 1	14 ± 1*	13 ± 1	13 ± 1
Cardiac output (L/min/m^2)	200	4.2 ± 0.2	3.7 ± 0.2*	3.4 ± 0.2*	3.6 ± 0.4*	3.4 ± 0.3*
	400	3.7 ± 0.2	3.3 ± 0.2*	3.0 ± 0.3*	3.0 ± 0.2*	3.1 ± 0.3*
Stroke volume (ml/m^2)	200	48 ± 3	44 ± 2	43 ± 2	46 ± 2	43 ± 3
	400	48 ± 2	44 ± 3	42 ± 2	43 ± 2	42 ± 2
Systemic vascular resistance (dyne · sec · cm^{-5} · m^2)	200	1992 ± 83	2258 ± 164*	2505 ± 232*	2331 ± 272*	2407 ± 229
	400	2216 ± 146	2568 ± 153*	2773 ± 234*	2395 ± 196*	2449 ± 235

Data are $\bar{X}$ ± SE.
*$P < 0.05$ compared with control values.

RESULTS

A total of 24 studies were completed without untoward incident in any subject. No subject developed symptomatic hypotension, bradycardia, or required supportive cardiac therapy or supplementary narcotic analgesia during the study, and all survived to leave the hospital.

The mean plasma AUCs for intravenous and oral acebutolol were: 25 mg iv, 0.95 μg/hr/ml (range 0.72 to 1.6 μg/hr/ml); 50 mg iv, 1.02 μg/hr/ml (range 0.96 to 1.14 μg/hr/ml); 200 mg po, 2.1 μg/hr/ml (range 0.84 to 3.36 μg/hr/ml); and 400 mg po, 3.7 μg/hr/ml (range 2.8 to 4.1 μg/hr/ml). Peak plasma drug concentrations after oral acebutolol occurred 2 hours (0.32 ± 0.23 μg/ml and 0.57 ± 0.30 μg/ml) after the 200 and 400 mg oral doses (Fig. 1). The metabolite diacetolol was detected within 15 minutes of the intravenous injection at each dose level (25 mg iv, 0.09 μg/ml; 50 mg iv, 0.09 μg/ml) and remained constant throughout the study. After oral acebutolol diacetolol

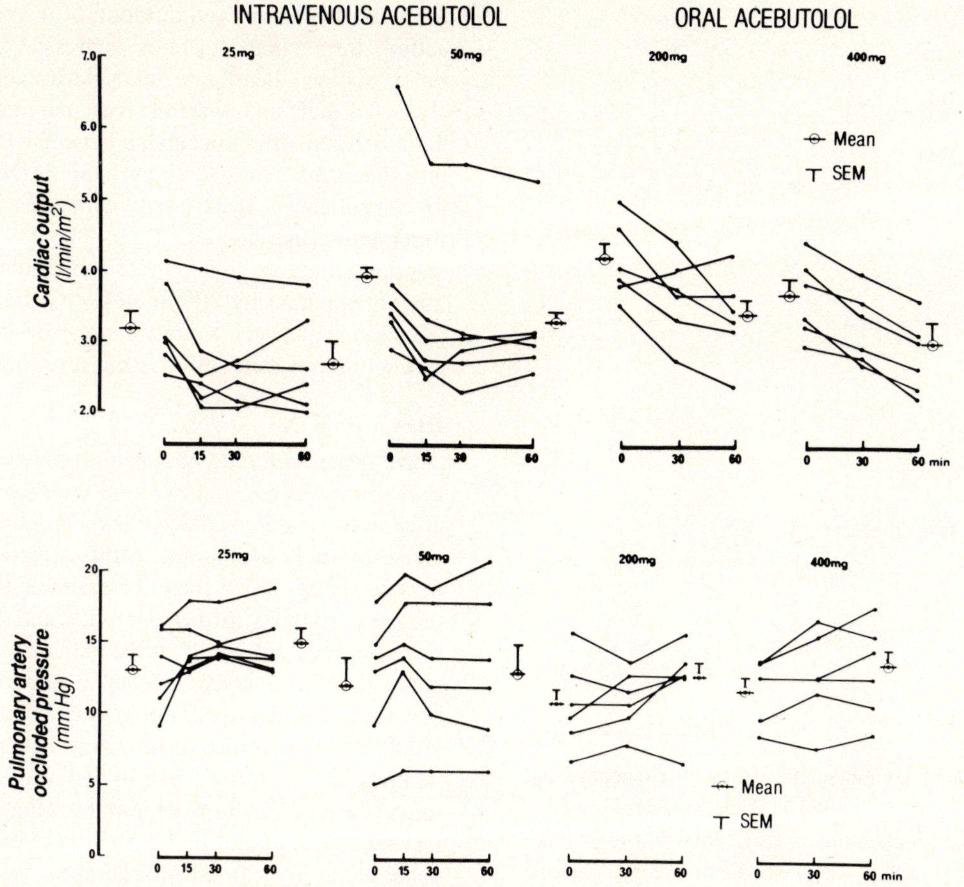

Fig. 2. Effects of intravenous and oral acebutolol on cardiac output **(top)** and PAOP **(bottom).** Data are presented for each subject together with the group mean. Significance levels are indicated in Tables I and II.

was detected within 30 minutes at each dose level and its peak plasma concentration occurred at 2 hours (0.37 ± 0.29 μg/ml) after the 200 mg dose and at 4 hours (0.58 ± 0.27 μg/ml) after the 400 mg dose.

The average coefficients of variation of hemodynamic variables over the control hour were: systolic blood pressure, 3.6% (range 0.8% to 10.2%); diastolic blood pressure, 4.2% (range 1.6% to 12.1%); heart rate, 2.5% (range 0.3% to 10.6%); cardiac output, 6.8% (range 0% to 11.9%); and PAOP, 8.1% (range 2% to 13.5%). There were no between-group differences in the variability or trend to change in any parameter over the 1-hour control period. Accordingly, control data have been averaged from the four determinations taken during this period.

After acebutolol, 25 mg iv (group 1), there was a prompt (15 minutes) and sustained (240 minutes) reduction in systolic arterial pressure ($P < 0.05$; Tables I and II; Figs. 2 and 3); the diastolic and mean component showed a trend to fall over the same time course, becoming significant by 240 minutes. Immediate (15 minutes) reductions in heart rate ($P < 0.05$) and cardiac output ($P < 0.05$) persisted for 120 minutes. Systemic vascular resistance and PAOP were initially increased ($P < 0.05$) over the first 60 minutes, but subsequently returned to control values. After acebutolol, 50 mg iv (group 2), there were reductions in systolic ($P < 0.05$) and mean ($P < 0.05$) systemic arterial pressures, heart rate ($P < 0.05$), and cardiac output ($P < 0.05$), which were similar to those in group 1; transient increases in systemic vascular resistance ($P < 0.05$) and PAOP ($P < 0.05$) were also similar to the changes in the same parameters after acebutolol, 25 mg iv. There were no statistically significant differences in the changes in any hemodynamic parameter between the 25 mg iv and 50 mg iv acebutolol doses over the 4 hours of the study period.

After acebutolol, 200 mg po (group 3), the systolic arterial pressure was reduced within 120 minutes ($P < 0.05$; Tables I and II; Figs. 2 and 3). Diastolic

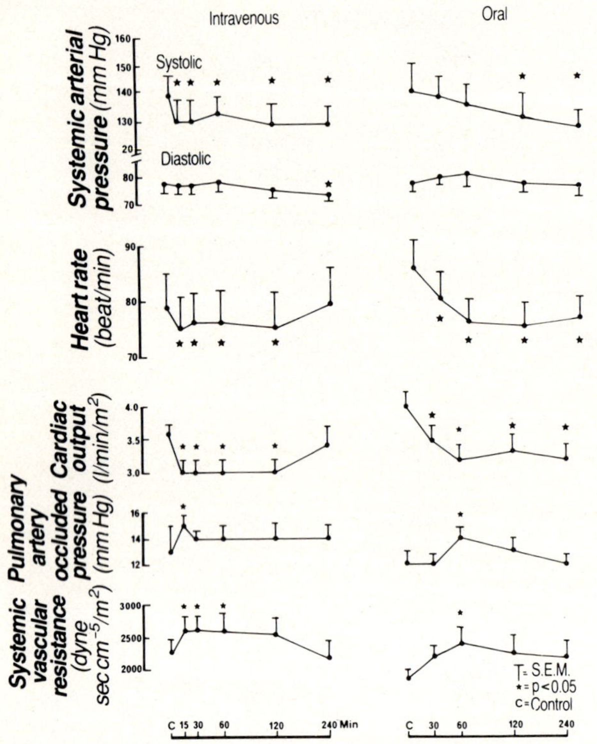

Fig. 3. Comparative hemodynamic effects of intravenous and oral β-blockade with acebutolol in acute myocardial infarction. Data from both the intravenous (25 and 50 mg) and the oral (200 and 400 mg) groups have been combined. Significance levels relate to comparison with control.

and mean systemic arterial pressures remained at control levels. Heart rate ($P < 0.05$) and cardiac output ($P < 0.05$) fell maximally by 60 minutes. Systemic vascular resistance and PAOP were transiently increased. After acebutolol, 400 mg po (group 4), there was a significant fall in systolic and mean systemic arterial pressures ($P < 0.05$) at 120 and 240 minutes without a change in the diastolic component. The reduction in heart rate ($P < 0.05$) and cardiac output ($P < 0.05$) and the increase in systemic vascular resistance ($P < 0.05$) were similar to the changes in the same variables in subjects given the 200 mg po dose. Apart from the greater effect on mean systemic arterial pressure, which was reduced only after the 400 mg po dose, there were no apparent differences in other measured or derived parameters between the two groups.

Because there were no dose-response effects with either mode of administration, we combined groups 1 and 2 (intravenous) and groups 3 and 4 (oral) for comparison of the effects of intravenous and oral therapy (Fig. 3). The major differences between the hemodynamic effects relative to route of administration were in the time of onset and duration of the cardiodynamic action. Intravenous injection depressed systemic arterial pressures, heart rate, and cardiac output and increased PAOP and systemic vascular resistance, with the maximum effect occurring between 15 and 30 minutes; heart rate, cardiac output, and PAOP had returned to control levels by 2 hours. Oral dosing resulted in maximum effect between 1 and 2 hours, although substantial reductions in heart rate and cardiac output were already apparent by 30 minutes. At 4 hours the reductions in mean systemic arterial pressure, heart rate, and cardiac output were still present after oral therapy.

DISCUSSION

We describe the hemodynamic effects of acebutolol at two intravenous and two oral dose levels in patients after an uncomplicated acute myocardial infarction. We chose to study acebutolol in this situation for several reasons. First, it was the only available β-blocker with the properties of cardioselectivity and intrinsic sympathomimetic activity.[12,14] Second, in a dose-response study of its immediate effects in patients with stable coronary heart disease,[25] we found that intravenous acebutolol over a similar dose range had no deleterious hemodynamic effects. Wan et al.[31] have shown maintained cardiac function 30 minutes after 0.5 mg/kg intravenous acebutolol in 15 patients after an uncomplicated acute myocardial infarction.

Before consideration of the results, the validity of the design should be discussed. Valid between-group pharmacodynamic comparisons in relatively small numbers of patients pose considerable difficulties. The comparability of the randomized groups, variability of the measurement techniques, confounding of the analysis by intercurrent therapy, as well as the definition of adequacy of therapeutic effect all influence interpretation of the results. In our study the oral and intravenous groups were well matched for baseline clinical and hemodynamic characteristics. The variability in circulatory changes over the control period was relatively small. Except for a single dose of opiate some hours before the study, alternative cardioactive drugs were excluded. Plasma acebutolol concentrations achieved were within the range associated with a substantial degree of cardiac β-blockade in normal subjects[26]; thus the hemodynamic changes in our study can be taken as representative of the pharmacodynamic-time activity profile of the drug.

Both oral and intravenous acebutolol significantly reduced heart rate and cardiac output and transiently increased left heart filling pressure. Increased systemic vascular resistance was insufficient to offset the falls in systolic and mean systemic arterial pressures. The maximum hemodynamic effects occurred between 15 and 30 minutes after intravenous acebutolol and, except for the fall in systolic arterial pressure, between 60 and 120 minutes of its oral dosing. However, after oral dosing there were already significant falls in cardiac output and heart rate within 30 minutes.

One of our primary aims was to compare the differences between intravenous and oral initiation of β-blockade. Both regimens induced similar directional and quantitative hemodynamic changes but differed in speed of onset and duration of action. The major quantitative differences between these routes of administration were in the falls in systolic and mean systemic arterial pressure, which were maximal within 15 minutes of intravenous acebutolol and at 4 hours after oral dosing. In terms of the speed of onset of hemodynamic effect, intravenous initiation was more efficient, although the magnitude of the changes in heart rate and cardiac output at 30 minutes after oral therapy was similar.

Our findings are in agreement with the small number of reports on the hemodynamic effects of β-adrenoceptor blockade in acute myocardial infarction. Wan et al.[31] examined the effect of a single intravenous acebutolol bolus (0.5 mg/kg). The reductions in cardiac output and the increase in left heart filling pressure were similar to those in our subjects, but the fall in mean systemic arterial pressure (5 mm Hg) calculated from indirect pressure measurements was not significant. How do these findings compare with those from studies in which other β-blocking drugs were used? Studies with practolol[9] and pindolol[7] at approximately equivalent β-blocking doses confirmed falls in cardiac output (-0.3 to -0.5 L/min/m^2) of the order of those in the present study, without change in echocardiographic left ventricular dimension.[7] Changes in arterial pressure were inconsistent. In contrast, however, propranolol, without intrinsic sympathetic activity, appears to induce a proportionately greater fall in cardiac output (-0.6 to -0.9 L/min/m^2) and a consistent fall in systemic arterial pressure.[27] In terms of hemodynamic function of the heart, drugs with intrinsic sympathetic activity may, therefore, induce less overall depression of cardiac function than those without this property. The fall in systolic arterial pressure and cardiac output after both intravenous acebutolol doses in our study did not occur when equivalent doses were given to patients with stable coronary heart disease.[5,16,21,25,33] In states of high sympathetic activity, such as after infarction,[30] the already high systemic vascular resistance[24] may not increase further as cardiac output falls, resulting in a fall in systemic arterial pressure. The absence of any dose-response effect after intravenous or oral acebutolol in our study suggests that doses even smaller than those we used may be adequate to attain β-adrenoceptor blockade in the peri-infarction period.

In conclusion, our data confirm the hemodynamic safety of acebutolol in uncomplicated acute myocardial infarction. Hemodynamic dose-response effects were not seen within the dose range studied. Intravenous initiation of therapy appears to have some hemodynamic advantages over the more convenient oral route of administration, but the extent of superiority was less than anticipated.

We thank Sister S. Winterburn and nurses K. Jefferies and E. Craig for their help and Mrs. A. Richmond, B.Sc., for statistical advice.

References

1. Ahumada GG, Karlsberg RP, Jaffe AS, Dieter AH, Sobel BE, Roberts R: Reduction of early arrhythmias by acebutolol in patients with acute myocardial infarction. Br Heart J **41:**654-659, 1979.
2. Basil B, Jordan D, Loveless AH, Maxwell DR: Beta-adrenoceptor blocking properties and cardioselectivity of M and B 17,803A. Br J Pharmacol **48:**198-211, 1973.
3. Beta-Blocker Heart Attack Trial Research Group: A randomized trial of propranolol in patients with acute myocardial infarction. I. Mortality results. JAMA **247:**1707-1714, 1982.
4. Corr PB, Witkowski FX, Sobel BE: Mechanisms contributing to malignant dysrhythmias induced by ischemia in the cat. J Clin Invest **61:**109-119, 1978.
5. Dalal JJ, Ross K, Wong K, et al: Acute effects of acebutolol on cardiovascular function in man. Br J Clin Pharmacol **11:**265-268, 1981.
6. Dixon WJ, Brown MB, editors: Biomedical computer program—"P" Series. Berkeley, Calif, 1979, University of California Press, pp 540-580.
7. Heikkila J, Nieminen JS: Rapid monitoring of regional myocardial ischaemia with echocardiography and ST segment shifts in man. Acta Med Scand (suppl) **623:**71-95, 1978.
8. Holt JE, Kaye CM, Sankey MG: Use of reverse-phase high pressure liquid chromatography for the assay of acebutolol, practolol and propranolol in plasma. Br J Clin Pharmacol **12:**282P, 1981.
9. Jewitt DE, Burgess PA, Shillingford JP: The circulatory effects of practolol in patients with acute myocardial infarction. Cardiovasc Res **4:**188-193, 1970.
10. Jewitt DE, Mercer CJ, Reid D, Valori C, Thomas M, Shillingford JP: Free noradrenaline and adrenaline excretion in relation to the development of cardiac arrhythmias and heart failure in patients with acute myocardial infarction. Lancet **1:**635-641, 1969.

11. Karlsberg RP, Penkoske PA, Cryer PE, Corr PB, Roberts R: Rapid activation of the sympathetic system following coronary artery occlusion: Relation to infarct size, site and haemodynamic impact. Cardiovasc Res **13:**523-531, 1979.
12. Leary WP: The cardioselectivity of acebutolol (Sectral) in man. Clin Trials **3:**33-35, 1974.
13. Libby P, Maroko PR, Covell JW, Malloch CI, Ross J Jr, Braunwald E: The effects of practolol on left ventricular function and infarct size following acute experimental coronary occlusion. Clin Res **19:**116, 1971.
14. Marmo E, Spaziante G, Pentimalli D, et al: Specific and non-specific activities of acebutolol, atenolol, metoprolol and propranolol; Comparative experimental studies. Int J Clin Pharm Res **11:**41-48, 1982.
15. Maroko PR, Kjekshus JK, Sobel BE, et al: Factors influencing infarct size following experimental coronary artery occlusions. Circulation **43:**67-82, 1971.
16. Mason JW, Specter MJ, Ingels NM, Daughters GT, Ferris AC, Alderman EL: Haemodynamic effects of acebutolol. Br Heart J **40:**29-34, 1978.
17. Mueller H, Ayres SM: Propranolol in acute myocardial infarction in man: Effect on haemodynamics and myocardial oxygenation. Postgrad Med J **52**(suppl 4):141-148, 1976.
18. Norris RM, Clarke ED, Samell NL, Smith WM, Williams B: Protective effect of propranolol in threatened myocardial infarction. Lancet **2:**907-909, 1978.
19. Norwegian Multicentre Study Group: Timolol-induced reduction in mortality and reinfarction in patients surviving acute myocardial infarction. N Engl J Med **304:**801-807, 1981.
20. Pelides LJ, Reid DW, Thomas M, Shillingford JP: Inhibition by beta-blockade of the ST segment elevation after acute myocardial infarction in man. Cardiovasc Res **6:**295-302, 1972.
21. Pfisterer M, Muller-Brand J, Burkart F: Combined acebutolol/nifedipine therapy in patients with chronic coronary artery disease: Additional improvement of ischaemic-induced left ventricular function. Am J Cardiol **49:**1259-1266, 1982.
22. Reid DS, Pelides LJ, Shillingford JP, Thomas M: Electrocardiographic surface mapping of the heart following myocardial infarction and the influence of beta-blockade. Postgrad Med J **52**(suppl 4):135-139, 1976.
23. Rose GA, Blackburn H: Cardiovascular survey methods. WHO monograph series. **56:**137-174, 1968.
24. Seino Y, Takano T, Tanaka K, Hayakawa H: Peripheral circulatory adjustments and the vasodilator intervention in acute myocardial infarction. Proceedings of the Eight Asian Pacific Congress of Cardiology, Taipei, Nov-Dec, 1983, p 154. (Abst.)
25. Silke B, Nelson GIC, Hussain M, Verma SP, Taylor SH: Dose-response effects of cardioselective beta blockade in coronary artery disease. CLIN PHARMACOL THER **36:**40-46, 1984.
26. Silke B, Nelson GIC, Verma SP, et al: Comparative haemodynamic dose-response effects of intravenous propranolol, acebutolol and penbutolol in angina pectoris. Herz **9:**57-64, 1984.
27. Silke B, Nelson GIC, Verma SP, et al: Enhanced haemodynamic effects of propranolol in acute myocardial infarction. Eur Heart J **5:**366-373, 1984.
28. Singh BN, Jewitt DE: Beta-adrenergic receptor blocking drugs in cardiac arrhythmias. Drugs **7:**426-461, 1974.
29. Taylor SH, Burley D: Beta-adrenoceptor drugs in post-myocardial infarction dysrhythmias. Proc R Soc Med **70**(suppl 11):11-16, 1977.
30. Valori C, Thomas M, Shillingford J: Free noradrenaline and adrenaline excretion in relation to clinical syndromes following myocardial infarction. Am J Cardiol **20:**605-617, 1967.
31. Wan SH, Seah CS, Teh LB, Letchmana K: Haemodynamic profile of acebutolol in acute myocardial infarction. Ann Acad Med **9:**440-445, 1980.
32. Winer BJ: Statistical principles in experimental design, ed 2. New York, 1971, McGraw-Hill, pp 197-200.
33. Wollam GL, Cody RJ, Tarazi RC, Bravo EL: Acute hemodynamic effects and cardioselectivity of acebutolol, practolol and propranolol. CLIN PHARMACOL THER **25:**813-820, 1979.
34. Yusuf S, Sleight P, Ross PA, et al: Reduction in infarct size, arrhythmias and chest pain by early intravenous beta-blockade in suspected acute myocardial infarction. Circulation **67**(suppl 1):32-41, 1983.

Prostaglandins and nicotinate-provoked increase in cutaneous blood flow

The mechanism of topically applied methyl nicotinate–induced local cutaneous erythema was studied in normal human subjects. Aqueous methyl nicotinate (0, 0.1, 1.0, 10.0, and 100 mmol/L) was applied to the volar forearms in quadruplicate after oral pretreatments with 25 mg doxepin hydrochloride, 600 mg ibuprofen, 50 mg indomethacin, 975 mg aspirin, and lactose placebo. The cutaneous vascular response was monitored by laser Doppler velocimetry. Although doxepin did not affect the cutaneous vascular response to methyl nicotinate, indomethacin, ibuprofen, and aspirin significantly suppressed the response. Because indomethacin, ibuprofen, and aspirin have different chemical structures, the common property of inhibition of the response to methyl nicotinate may be assigned to their common pharmacologic action, i.e., inhibition of prostaglandin bioformation. (CLIN PHARMACOL THER 38:273-277, 1985.)

Jonathan K. Wilkin, M.D., Glenn Fortner, B.S., Linda A. Reinhardt, M.D., Otero Vogt Flowers, M.D., S. James Kilpatrick, Ph.D., and W. Carson Streeter
Richmond, Va.

Systemic administration of nicotinic acid leads to a generalized cutaneous erythema (flush) mediated at least in part by prostaglandin biosynthesis.[29] Topical applications of nicotinic acid and its esters provoke a local cutaneous erythema.[20] Because prostaglandins are involved in the cutaneous vasodilation provoked by systemic nicotinic acid, we undertook to examine further the mechanism of nicotinate-provoked, local cutaneous vasodilation. Methyl nicotinate was selected because it is readily soluble in water and penetrates rapidly[20] through the interstitial channels, bypassing the keratinized cells.[1]

METHODS

Our subjects were 19 clinically normal human subjects (seven men, 12 women) aged 21 to 33 years. All subjects abstained from prescription and over-the-counter drugs both 10 days before and throughout the study. Patches of coarse porosity, quantitative, ashless grade filter paper (1.23 cm^2) saturated with 0.0, 0.1, 1.0, 10.0, and 100.0 mmol/L aqueous methyl nicotinate were applied to the volar forearm. Each concentration was tested in quadruplicate with randomization of order and location of individual patches. Patches were sequentially applied for 5 minutes, removed for 5 minutes, and then the laser Doppler velocimeter probe was applied for 5 minutes. Preliminary studies* disclosed that the maximal reaction occurred after 5 minutes. Challenges were performed with subjects in the sitting position after oral pretreatment with 25 mg doxepin HCl, 600 mg ibuprofen, 50 mg indomethacin, 975 mg aspirin, and lactose placebo. All subjects were given two capsules before each challenge; one capsule was taken 4 hours before and the other capsule 1 hour before each test. Doxepin or placebo were given 4 hours and ibuprofen, indomethacin, aspirin, or placebo were given 1 hour before topical methyl nicotinate testing. Each of the pretreatment studies was performed on each subject at a minimum interval of 10 days. All oral pretreatments were given in a randomized, double-blind manner in opaque gelatin capsules. During the first half of the study, the unpleasant sedative effect associated with doxepin precluded adequate blinding. The data were then analyzed independent of the investigators directly conducting the study, and doxepin pretreatment was found to have negligible effects. Thus no more

From the Dermatology Section, McGuire Veterans Administration Medical Center and Departments of Pharmacology, Dermatology, and Biostatistics, Medical College of Virginia.

Supported by the A. D. Williams Fund, the National Institutes of Health Student Fellowship Program, and a Veterans Administration Research Grant.

Presented in part at the Annual Meeting of the American Society for Clinical Pharmacology and Therapeutics, Atlanta, Ga., March 13-16, 1984.

Received for publication Feb. 21, 1985; accepted April 4, 1985.

Reprint requests to: Jonathan K. Wilkin, M.D., McGuire Veterans Administration Medical Center, 1201 Broad Rock Blvd., Richmond, VA 23249.

*Wilkin JK, Fortner G: Unpublished observations, 1983.

Table I. Adjusted cutaneous perfusion index (in millivolts)

	Methyl nicotinate levels (mmol/L)				
Pretreatments	*0.1*	*1.0*	*10.0*	*100.0*	*All levels*
Placebo	20.0 ± 7.2	108.0 ± 17.6	232.8 ± 19.2	251.6 ± 18.4	152.0 ± 20.0
Doxepin	16.4 ± 10.0	135.2 ± 24.4	225.2 ± 26.4	226.0 ± 25.6	156.0 ± 26.4
Ibuprofen	6.8 ± 7.2	38.4 ± 17.6	87.6 ± 19.2	118.8 ± 18.4	64.0 ± 20.0
Indomethacin	6.4 ± 7.2	54.0 ± 17.6	64.4 ± 19.2	63.2 ± 18.4	48.0 ± 20.0
Aspirin	5.2 ± 7.2	12.8 ± 17.6	19.2 ± 19.2	17.2 ± 18.4	12.0 ± 20.0
Mean square error (analysis)	24.56	149.76	172.88	162.16	190.4

Data are $\overline{X} \pm$ SE.

doxepin pretreatments were given during the rest of the study.

Vascular response to methyl nicotinate after pharmacologic pretreatment was assessed by laser Doppler velocimetry[3,8,19] (Model LD 5000; MedPacific Inc.). The low-power (5 mW) helium-neon laser source emits light at 632.8 nm, which is delivered to the skin by flexible graded index fiberoptic light guides. A portion of the incident light strikes nonmoving structures and is reflected with no shift in frequency. The portion that strikes moving erythrocytes is reflected with a shift in frequency (Doppler broadening). The reflected light is conducted from the tissue surface through a second fiberoptic light guide, mixed (heterodyned), and analyzed in real time by an analog processor that provides a continuous output of the instantaneous mean Doppler frequency in the photocurrent identified by a square-law detector. The electrical analog of this output (in millivolts) is displayed digitally and on a chart recorder. While not a quantification of skin blood perfusion as volume/weight of tissue per unit time, laser Doppler velocimetry does produce data known to be related to fundamental skin perfusion characteristics, i.e., volume and flow rate,[25] referred to here as the cutaneous perfusion index.

Each of the five pretreatments in each of the 19 subjects were at five methyl nicotinate levels: 0.0, 0.1, 1.0, 10.0, and 100.0 mmol/L. Because subjects differed significantly in baseline responses to water (0.0 mmol/L), each subject's response to water was subtracted from the response to nonzero levels of methyl nicotinate. Except for comments on pretreatment effects on unstimulated cutaneous blood flow, all subsequent results are adjusted values, i.e., flow rate at a specified methyl nicotinate level minus flow rate at 0.0 mmol/L methyl nicotinate.

The methyl nicotinate level was treated as a covariate. To linearize the relationship of flow to methyl nicotinate level, logarithms to the base 10 were taken of the methyl nicotinate levels multiplied by 100. Analyses of each subject's results confirmed that this transformation gave a linear response, indicating that for most subjects the range of methyl nicotinate levels was appropriately scaled.

Global analyses of the data were performed with the general linear model (GLM) of the Statistical Analysis System (SAS) package.[15] This enabled us to treat subjects as a random effect in the model and to test for different slopes of flow (adjusted) vs. log(100 × methyl nicotinate level) for different pretreatments, even though the design was unbalanced in that eight subjects did not receive doxepin. Because of problems of estimation in contrasts involving doxepin, the results that follow are taken either from a global analysis treating levels of methyl nicotinate as a categoric variable or from separate analyses at each level.

RESULTS

In a preliminary analysis of raw data at the control level (0.0 mmol/L), the mean flow for placebo was 83.6 mV. The three prostaglandin synthetase inhibitors gave mean values of 73.5, 73.5, and 60.6 mV for ibuprofen, indomethacin, and aspirin, respectively. Only results with aspirin differ significantly from those with placebo.

Results presented in Table I and Fig. 1 are mean adjusted flow. Over all levels the mean adjusted flow was not significantly different for placebo and doxepin or for ibuprofen and indomethacin. All other differences are significant at the 5% level, allowing for repeated tests of significance. Over the separate levels of methyl nicotinate, there is a gradual trend from no significant differences at the 0.1 mmol/L level to two significantly different but statistically overlapping groups of pretreatments at the 1.0 mmol/L level: for placebo and doxepin and for ibuprofen, indomethacin, and aspirin. At the 10.0 mmol/L level these two groups do not overlap and are quite distinct. The results at the 100.0 mmol/L level are similar to the overall results for all levels combined. At 100.0 mmol/L, placebo and doxepin are not significantly different. However, a significant difference now exists among the three prostaglandin inhibitors, with aspirin having a significantly greater effect than either ibuprofen or indomethacin. Thus aspirin is clearly the most effective inhibitor, with ibuprofen and indomethacin being next effective in suppressing the vascular response. We found no significant differences between placebo and doxepin, results we do not think to be due to the reduced number of subjects taking doxepin. Although no attempt was made to quantify the erythema in response to topical methyl nicotinate, erythema was barely perceptible at low concentrations, especially after ibuprofen, indomethacin, and aspirin, and was most intense at high concentrations, especially after doxepin and placebo.

DISCUSSION

Several aspects of our study deserve special comment. First, not only are the effects of methyl nicotinate on the cutaneous vasculature dose related as assessed by laser Doppler velocimetry, but also the doses of methyl nicotinate used were in the linear portion of the dose-response curve. This is compatible with the conclusions drawn from our unpublished pilot studies that these four doses represent the linear portion of the curve relating dose of methyl nicotinate to laser Doppler velocimetric response. Studies in the linear portion of the dose-response curve are important in detecting pharmacologic effects of antagonists. Second, the use of adjusted data is desirable because it imposes more conservative interpretation of the data. Since pretreatment with prostaglandin synthetase inhibitors was followed by less unstimulated cutaneous blood flow (significant only for aspirin), raw data will include this effect. It is more rigorous to look for a pretreatment effect after subtracting out the effect on baseline cutaneous blood flow.

We have shown that indomethacin, ibuprofen, and aspirin significantly suppressed the cutaneous vascular response to methyl nicotinate. Because these three drugs have different chemical structures, the common property of inhibition of the response to methyl nicotinate may be assigned to their common pharmacologic action, i.e., inhibition of prostaglandin bioformation. Since the systemic cutaneous vascular response to nico-

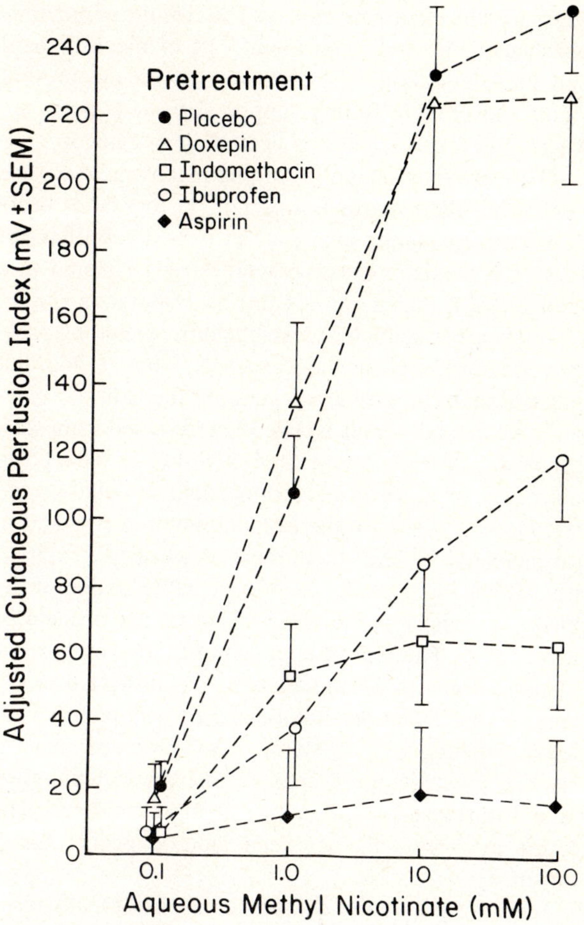

Fig. 1. Cutaneous vascular response to different concentrations of topically applied methyl nicotinate after oral pretreatment with placebo, indomethacin, ibuprofen, aspirin (n = 19 for all), and doxepin (n = 11).

tinic acid and the local cutaneous vascular responses to the methyl ester of nicotinic acid are suppressed by inhibitors of prostaglandin biosynthesis, the effect of the nicotinate moiety on vascular smooth muscle may be mediated by vasodilator prostaglandins.

In contrast, doxepin pretreatment did not affect the measured cutaneous vascular response despite a dosage schedule at which its antihistaminic activity in the cutaneous vasculature is demonstrable.[21] Also, doxepin is an antagonist at both H_1- and H_2-histamine receptors.[16] Thus histamine does not play a major role in methyl nicotinate–provoked local cutaneous erythema.

Because nicotinic acid and its esters (methyl, ethyl, butyl, hexyl, octyl, tetrahydrofurfuryl, and xanthinol) all provoke vasodilation,[5,20,29] it is reasonable to ascribe this pharmacologic activity to the common chemical structure, the nicotinate moiety. Thus results of previous pharmacologic studies on the effects of nicotinic acid and its esters should be compatible with the present study and provide further support for our hypothesis. These data will be adduced according to category.

There are four categories of pharmacologic evidence supporting the role for a mediator, in this case, prostaglandins mediating nicotinate-provoked vasodilation. First, the mediator must be synthesized or stored in a manner such that it can act on the responding tissue. Not only are vasodilator prostaglandins, including prostacyclin, produced in blood vessels,[13] but in addition prostaglandin biosynthesis occurs in the skin.[10,12] Second, the mediator must be liberated (released from storage or immediately synthesized) in response to the pharmacologic agent. In fact, nicotinic acid stimulates prostaglandin synthesis in the isolated rabbit heart[11] and in rat platelets.[26] Third, there must be identity of action, i.e., either the mediator itself or a stable analog of the mediator must reproduce the effect of the pharmacologic agent. The topical application of 16-vinylprostaglandins leads to a similar erythema, restricted to the area of application and not associated with pain, swelling, or itching.[2] The systemic administration of a variety of prostaglandins leads to flushing indistinguishable from that provoked by nicotinic acid.[27,28] The fourth category is the documentation of specific antagonism.

We have previously shown that aspirin blocks nicotinic acid–induced flush.[29] Aspirin also inhibits the vascular response to topically applied tetrahydrofurfuryl nicotinate.[30] Furthermore, indomethacin inhibits nicotinic acid–induced flush in man.[23] However, indomethacin may be a vasoconstrictor as well as an inhibitor of prostaglandin biosynthesis.[4] Thus other prostaglandin synthetase inhibitors should also be studied to discriminate between these two activities. In our study all three chemically dissimilar prostaglandin biosynthesis inhibitors antagonized the nicotinate-provoked vascular response.

Moreover, doxepin, which has potent antihistaminic effects, did not affect the nicotinate vascular response. In previous studies neither the iontophoresis of tripelennamine HCl, an antihistamine, nor the injection of compound 48:80, a mast cell histamine depleting agent, led to inhibition of the erythema provoked by tetrahydrofurfuryl nicotinate.[14,30] Furthermore, should histamine and other mast cell products be involved, one would expect itching and a burning, painful sensation, which do not occur after nicotinates.

The significance of the hypothesis that nicotinate-provoked vasodilation is mediated by prostaglandins includes both basic and clinical aspects. It is important to note that the effect of nicotinates on the blood vessels need not be direct. This could explain the "conduction mechanism" proposed after observing vasodilation in the hamster cheek pouch extending beyond the immediate vasculature in contact with droplets of nicotinate esters.[6] Similarly, although others infer that it is nicotinate that is rapidly transported radially in the dermis,[7] it could be prostaglandins. Certainly, the end point of erythema is insufficient to distinguish between these two possibilities. In fact, since flushing occurs only while the nicotinate concentration in blood is rising and disappears when a constant level of nicotinic acid is maintained,[22] the stimulus for prostaglandin bioformation may be the rate of increase, and not simply the absolute level, of nicotinate. This relationship would invalidate conclusions regarding dermopharmacokinetics,[24] which assume first-order kinetics and a direct relationship between vascular effect and nicotinate presence. Finally, the use of such topical and systemic agents to provoke prostaglandin biosynthesis and vasodilation will be an additional pharmacologic tool in the study of cutaneous and systemic vascular mechanisms and reactivity. Vasodilator prostaglandins may be important in the maintenance of baseline cutaneous blood flow, since we found that unstimulated flow was lower after pretreatment with prostaglandin synthetase inhibitors (significant only after aspirin pretreatment).

The clinical significance of this hypothesis will require further work. Indeed, several directions can be suggested. Topical nicotinate challenge leads to an "atypical" or blanch reaction in atopy,[14,17] psoriasis, rheumatoid arthritis, and dyshidrotic eczema[17] and "nonreactivity" in scleroderma and diabetes mellitus.[14] The diminished reactivity of patients with diabetes might be related to impairment of the vessel wall's ability to manufacture prostacyclin, since this defect has recently been shown in patients with diabetes and vasculopathy.[9,18] The nicotinate reaction must be reevaluated in these various disorders, with an active search for the role of prostaglandin biosynthesis.

In conclusion, previous studies have shown that prostaglandin bioformation occurs in skin and blood vessels; that nicotinates provoke vasodilation; that nicotinates provoke prostaglandin biosynthesis in vitro; and that prostaglandins and stabile prostaglandin analogs provoke a qualitatively identical vascular response to that provoked by nicotinates. We have shown that specific antagonism of prostaglandin biosynthesis inhibits nicotinate-provoked vasodilation in human skin. Thus the nicotinate-provoked vasodilator response is mediated, at least in part, by prostaglandin biosynthesis.

References

1. Albery WJ, Hadgraft J: Percutaneous absorption in vivo experiments. J Pharm Pharmacol **31:**140-147, 1979.
2. Birnbaum JE, Chan PS, Cervoni P: Cutaneous erythema and blood pressure lowering effects of topically applied 16-vinylprostaglandins. Prostaglandins **23:**185-199, 1982.
3. Bonner RF, Chen TR, Bowen PD, Bowman RL: Laser-Doppler continuous real time monitor of pulsatile and mean blood flow in tissue microcirculation. *In* Chen SH, Chu B, Nossal R, editors: Scattering techniques applied to supramolecular and non-equilibrium systems. New York, 1981, Plenum, Publishing Co, pp 685-702.
4. Carlsson I, Wennmalm A: Effect of different prostaglandin synthesis inhibitors on postocclusive blood flow in human forearm. Prostaglandins **26:**241-252, 1983.
5. Davis E, Rozov H: The effects of xanthinol nicotinate on the small vessels. Bibl Anat **11:**334-339, 1973.
6. Fulton GP, Farber EM, Moreci AP: The mechanism of action of rubefacients. J Invest Dermatol **33:**317-325, 1959.
7. Guy RH, Maibach HI: Rapid radial transport of methyl nicotinate in the dermis. Arch Dermatol Res **273:**91-95, 1982.
8. Holloway GA, Watkins DW: Laser Doppler measurement of cutaneous blood flow. J Invest Dermatol **69:**306-309, 1977.
9. Johnson M, Harrison HE, Raftery AT, Elder JB: Vascular prostacyclin may be reduced in diabetes in man. Lancet **1:**325-326, 1979.
10. Johnsson C-E, Anggard E: Biosynthesis and metabolism of prostaglandin E_2 in human skin. Scand J Clin Lab Invest **29:**289-296, 1972.
11. Kaijser L, Wennmalm A: Nicotinic acid stimulates prostaglandin biosynthesis in the rabbit heart without releasing noradrenaline. Acta Physiol Scand **102:**246-247, 1978.
12. Lord JT, Ziboh VA, Poitier J, Legget G, Penneys NS: The effects of photosensitizers and ultraviolet irradiation on the biosynthesis and metabolism of prostaglandins. Br J Dermatol **95:**397-406, 1976.
13. Moncada S, Vane JR: The role of prostacyclin in vascular tissue. Fed Proc **38:**66-71, 1979.
14. Murrell TW Jr, Taylor WM: The cutaneous reaction to nicotinic acid (niacin)-furfuryl. AMA Arch Dermatol **79:** 545-550, 1959.
15. Ray AA, editor: SAS User's Guide: Statistics. Cary, NC, 1982, SAS Institute Inc.
16. Richelson E: Antimuscarinic and other receptor-blocking properties of antidepressants. Mayo Clin Proc **58:**40-46, 1983.
17. Rovensky J, Preis A: The significance of the Trafuril test, with special reference to atopy and rheumatic fever. Ann Paediat **193:**289-303, 1959.
18. Silberbauer K, Schernthauer G, Sinzinger H, Piza-Katzer H, Winter M: Decreased vascular prostacyclin in juvenile-onset diabetes. N Engl J Med **300:**366-376, 1979.
19. Stern MD, Lappe DL, Bowen PD, Chimosky JE, Holloway GA, Keiser HR, Bowman RL: Continuous measurement of tissue blood flow by laser Doppler spectroscopy. Am J Physiol **232:**H441-H448, 1977.
20. Stoughton RB, Clendenning WE, Kruse D: Percutaneous absorption of nicotinic acid and derivatives. J Invest Dermatol **35:**337-341, 1960.
21. Sullivan TJ: Pharmacologic modulation of the whealing response to histamine in human skin: Identification of doxepin as a potent in vivo inhibitor. J Allergy Clin Immunol **69:**260-267, 1982.
22. Svedmyr N, Harthon L, Lundholm L: The relationship between the plasma concentration of free nicotinic acid and some of its pharmacologic effects in man. Clin Pharmacol Ther **10:**559-570, 1969.
23. Svedmyr N, Heggelund A, Aberg G: Influence of indomethacin on flush induced by nicotinic acid in man. Acta Pharmacol Toxicol **41:**397-400, 1977.
24. Tur E, Guy RH, Tur M, Maibach HI: Noninvasive assessment of local nicotinate pharmacodynamics by photoplethysmography. J Invest Dermatol **80:**499-503, 1983.
25. Tur E, Guy RH, Tur M, Maibach HI: Basal perfusion of the cutaneous microcirculation: Measurements as a function of anatomic position. J Invest Dermatol **81:**442-446, 1983.
26. Vincent JE, Zijlstra FJ: Nicotinic acid inhibits thromboxane synthesis in platelets. Prostaglandins **15:**629-636, 1978.
27. Wilkin JK: Flushing reactions: Consequences and mechanisms. Ann Intern Med **95:**468-476, 1981.
28. Wilkin JK: Flushing reactions. *In* Rook AJ, Maibach H, editors: Recent advances in dermatology. vol 6, New York, 1982, Churchill-Livingstone, vol 6, chap 8, pp 157-187.
29. Wilkin JK, Wilkin O, Kapp R, Donachie R, Chernosky ME, Buckner J: Aspirin blocks nicotinic acid-induced flushing. Clin Pharmacol Ther **31:**478-482, 1982.
30. Winkelmann RK, Wilhelmi CM, Horner FA: Experimental studies on dermographism. Arch Dermatol **92:** 436-442, 1965.

Pharmacokinetics of transdermally delivered clonidine

We detail a series of pharmacokinetic investigations to determine the dose linearity, the effect of site of application, the duration of steady-state plasma concentrations, and the effect of chronic application when clonidine is administered transdermally. Dose linearity was assessed in six subjects with normotension after application of increasing sizes of transdermal clonidine systems (3.5, 7.0, and 10.5 cm² size) to the upper outer arm. Of the six subjects studied, five had linear relationships between clonidine plasma concentrations at steady state and system size of >0.975; in the sixth subject the correlation was >0.90. The mean steady-state plasma concentrations with 3.5, 7.0, and 10.5 cm² systems were 0.39, 0.84, and 1.12 ng/ml, respectively. The influence of site and duration of application on the absorption of transdermal clonidine was studied in eight subjects with normotension by use of the 3.5 cm² system. The mean steady-state plasma concentration over the time interval from 3 to 7 days after application to the arm or to the chest did not significantly differ. When a system was left on the chest or arm for a total of 11 days (4 days beyond the recommended time to change systems), the plasma concentrations of seven of eight subjects with application to the arm and of six of eight subjects with application to the chest remained constant through day 11. The influence of consecutive applications of 3.5 cm² transdermal clonidine systems on steady-state plasma clonidine concentrations was also studied in eight subjects with normotension over an 11-day period. Steady-state plasma concentrations were achieved in all eight subjects within 3 days after application of the initial transdermal clonidine system. On days 4 and 7 the previous transdermal system was removed and a new system was applied to the alternate arm. The mean steady-state plasma concentration (3 to 11 days) for the eight subjects was 0.32 ng/ml. There was no apparent difference between the mean plasma concentration at the time the clonidine system was removed and 24 hours after application of a new system. (Clin Pharmacol Ther 38:278-284, 1985.)

Thomas R. MacGregor, M.Sc., Kandace M. Matzek, M.Sc., James J. Keirns, Ph.D., Rudolf G. A. van Wayjen, M.D., Abraham van den Ende, Ph.D., and Rudolf G. L. van Tol, Ph.D. *Ridgefield, Conn., and Amsterdam and Alkmaar, The Netherlands*

Clonidine (Catapres; Boehringer Ingelheim) is an effective drug in the treatment of mild to moderate hypertension when used alone,[6,10] in combination with a diuretic,[5] and as a transdermal delivery system (Catapres-TTS).[7,8,11,12] The transdermal system has been developed to deliver clonidine at a constant rate for 7 days for once-a-week therapy. In cases in which lack of compliance with oral antihypertensive therapy is an obstacle to adequate blood pressure control, a 7-day transdermal system is advantageous in maintaining predictable, therapeutic blood concentrations.

From Boehringer Ingelheim Pharmaceuticals, Inc., Ridgefield; Vereeniging voor Ziekenverpleging and Slotervaart Hospital, Amsterdam; and Boehringer Ingelheim b.v., Alkmaar.

Received for publication Feb. 7, 1985; accepted May 1, 1985.

Reprint requests to: Thomas R. MacGregor, M.Sc., Research and Development, Boehringer Ingelheim, P.O. Box 368, Ridgefield, CT 06877.

Clonidine is a lipid-soluble, relatively potent drug with a high volume of distribution and a therapeutically effective low plasma concentration.[2] These properties permit clonidine to be incorporated into a 7-day transdermal delivery device. The clonidine transdermal delivery system is a tan-colored square unit with rounded edges composed of a flexible system of membranes that adheres to the skin. The development of a specific and sensitive RIA for plasma clonidine determinations[1,3] has facilitated the exploration of the pharmacokinetic properties of the drug.

We describe a series of pharmacokinetic studies undertaken to determine the dose linearity of three different-sized systems, the effect of anatomic site of application, the duration of plasma clonidine steady-state concentrations when the system is not removed after 7 days, and the effect of chronic application of the system on clonidine steady-state plasma concentrations.

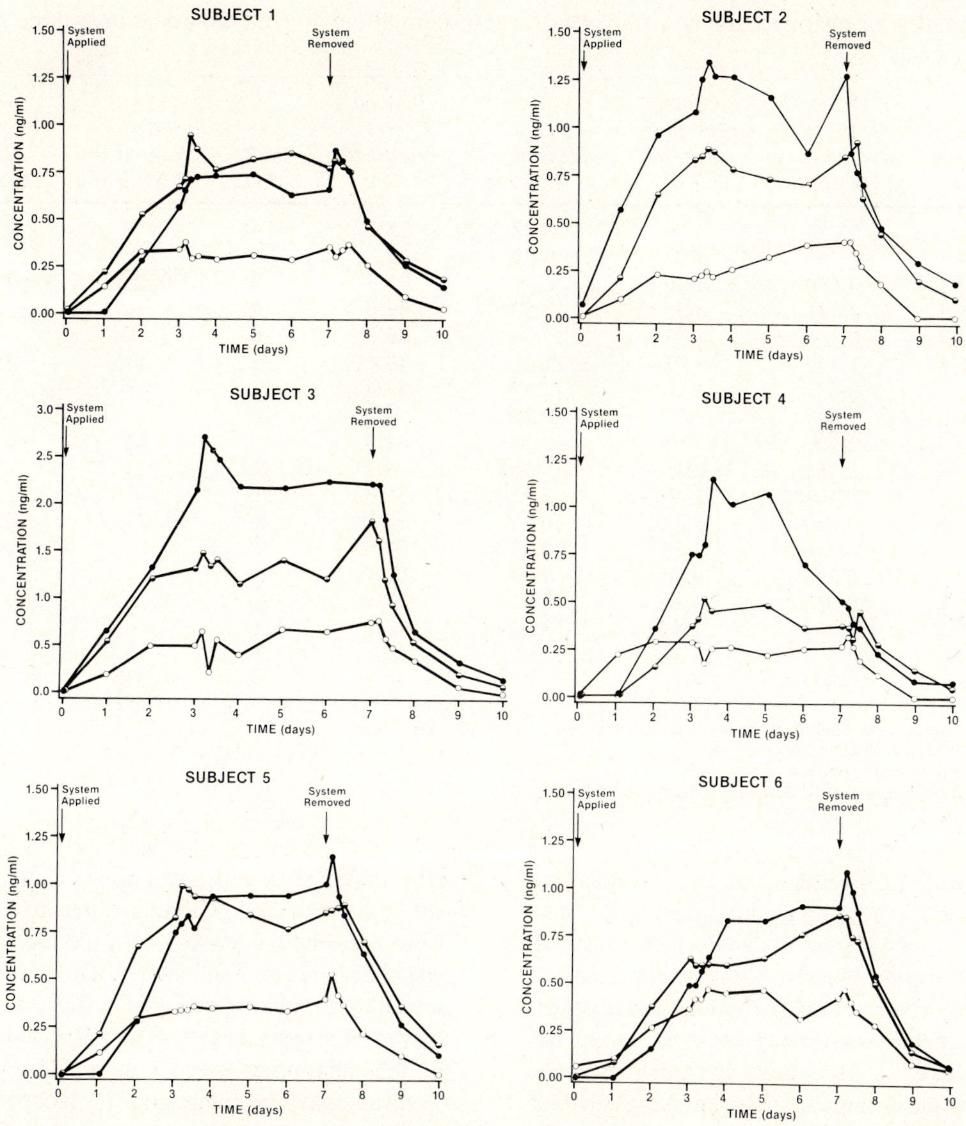

Fig. 1. Clonidine plasma concentrations from the 3.5 (○), 7.0 (◒), and 10.5 (●) cm^2 systems worn over a 7-day period in six subjects. There is a y-axis change in subject 3.

METHODS

Our subjects were men between the ages of 18 and 45 years who had normal weight. All subjects were in good health as documented by history and physical examinations, including chest x-ray, ECG, hematology, clinical chemistry, and urinalysis.

Blood and urine samples for laboratory examination were collected in the morning before the start of and at the end of each study after a 10-hour fast. If laboratory parameters at the end of each study were not within the normal range, laboratory examinations were repeated within 24 hours.

Exclusion criteria were women, recognizable medical problems (cardiovascular, hepatic, renal, hematologic, or other organ abnormality or pathology), skin disease of any type or a history of skin allergies, concomitant medications, blood pressure measured on 2 days (both sitting and standing) of >140/90 mm Hg or <110/70 mm Hg, a resting pulse rate <55 bpm, or suspicion of sinus node dysfunction.

Before application of the transdermal delivery system to a nonhairy area of intact skin, the site of application was cleaned with ethanol. Sites showing any abrasion or irritation were avoided. An overlay adhesive was

Table I. Compilation of pharmacokinetic parameters for transdermally delivered clonidine over three sizes of systems for 7 days of wear

Subject No.	*Size of system (cm^2)*	*C^{ss} (ng/ml)*	*Urine excretion rate (μg/hr)*	*Renal clearance (L/hr)*	*Percent load released* (%)*	*$t_{1/2}$† (hr)*	*β_1‡ (ng/ml/ 3.5 cm^2)*	*β_0‡ (ng/ml)*	*r‡*
1	3.5	0.298	2.60	8.72	25.2	14			
	7.0	0.791	5.07	6.41	48.8	21			
	10.5	0.680	4.36	6.41	40.3	18	0.253	+0.062	0.90
2	3.5	0.341	3.58	10.50	49.6	14			
	7.0	0.766	8.73	10.34	56.2	16			
	10.5	1.145	13.07	11.41	48.1	19	0.386	−0.016	0.99
3	3.5	0.631	4.68	7.42	82.8	15			
	7.0	1.404	8.73	6.22	77.2	17			
	10.5	2.200	17.93	8.15	81.3	17	0.737	−0.047	0.99
4	3.5	0.255	2.13	8.35	48.4	17			
	7.0	0.461	2.40	5.21	38.0	26			
	10.5	0.830	5.22	6.29	30.0	26	0.270	−0.018	0.99
5	3.5	0.366	2.26	6.17	39.6	18			
	7.0	0.858	6.64	7.74	50.4	24			
	10.5	0.965	4.39	4.55	57.3	20	0.339	+0.039	0.98
6	3.5	0.431	1.58	3.67	42.0	20			
	7.0	0.733	1.81	2.47	32.0	20			
	10.5	0.891	1.41	1.58	48.8	18	0.298	+0.068	0.98

C^{ss} = Steady-state plasma concentration; β_1 = slope; β_0 = intercept; r = correlation coefficient.
*Calculated after residual analysis.
†Value is the $t_{1/2}$ of decline after removal of the system.
‡Linear equation and correlation of the steady-state values obtained: $C^{ss} = \beta_1 (n \cdot 3.5 \text{ cm}^2) + \beta_0$.

used. The transdermal system and overlay adhesive were applied and removed by the investigator. Because the clonidine delivery system has an occlusive backing membrane, the overlay adhesive would not be expected to alter either drug delivery or skin hydration properties. There were no dietary restrictions during the study, but subjects were asked to discontinue alcoholic beverages 24 hours before and during the study. Smoking behavior of the subjects was recorded.

At specified times throughout each of the studies (0, 24, 48, 72, 76, 80, 84, 96, 120, 144, 168, 172, 176, 180, 192, 216, and 240 hours for the dose linearity study; additional samples at 264 and 288 hours for the anatomic placement and duration studies; and at 0, 24, 48, 72, 96, 100, 104, 108, 120, 144, 168, 172, 176, 180, 192, 216, 240, 264, 268, and 272 hours for the consecutive application study), venous blood samples (5 ml) were drawn from the median cubital vein in plastic syringes and collected in heparinized tubes. The tubes were inverted twice with foil on top and centrifuged at approximately 300 × g for 3 minutes. The plasma was transferred to plastic tubes that were stored frozen at approximately −20° C until analysis by RIA.

For the dose linearity assessment, a series of three systems were used on the upper outer right arm. Systems of 3.5, 7.0, and 10.5 cm^2 were applied for 7 days and then removed. Clonidine plasma concentrations were measured over a 10-day period with a 14-day washout between applications. Dose linearity was assessed by comparing steady-state plasma concentrations for the three systems 4, 5, 6, and 7 days after application of the appropriate sized system. Linear correlations were assessed by comparing the independent variable of dose (i.e., size of system = 0, 3.5, 7.0, 10.5 cm^2) to the dependent variable of plasma steady-state concentrations (mean of the four 8 AM time points at each dose). Comparisons of linear and quadratic (dose × dose) correlations were by a standard general linear models routine.[9]

For the anatomic site of application assessment, 3.5 cm^2 systems were applied to a nonhairy area of either the arm or the chest. Clonidine plasma concentrations were measured over a 12-day period with a 14-day washout between doses. A paired t test at each sampling point was used to determine a significant difference between sites. The transdermal systems were not removed until 11 days after application, permitting an assessment of the duration of drug release beyond the recommended 7-day application period. Clonidine plasma concentrations on days 4 to 11 for each subject

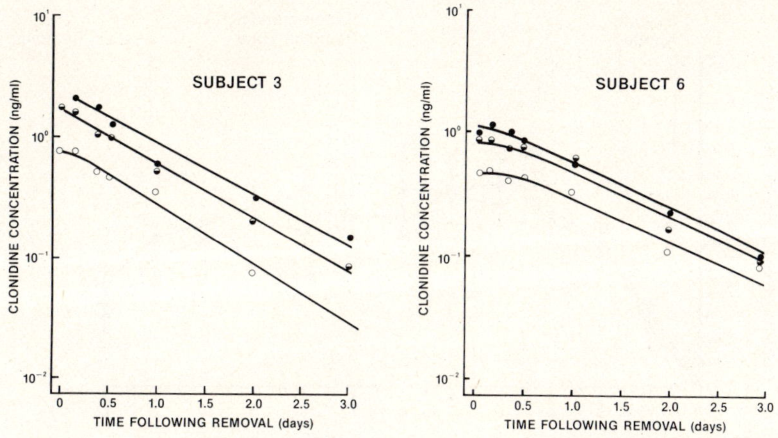

Fig. 2. Representative decline in clonidine plasma concentrations after removal of the 3.5 (○), 7.0 (◒), and 10.5 (●) cm^2 systems in subjects 3 and 6. The limit of detection for the assay is 5×10^{-2} ng/ml.

were analyzed by ANOVA. Trends were also evaluated to determine if the rate of release of clonidine from the transdermal system was lower after the 7-day recommended application period.

The chronic use and replenishment of spent systems on steady-state plasma concentrations was assessed by 3.5 cm^2 systems on alternate arms. Clonidine plasma concentrations were measured in eight subjects over a 12-day period, with used systems replaced with fresh systems on days 4 and 7. Intensive plasma sampling was performed for the 24 hours after replacement to determine if constant plasma concentrations of clonidine were maintained.

Clonidine elimination kinetics after transdermal input were determined from the dose linearity study plasma data points after removal of the delivery systems (i.e., 7, 7.2, 7.3, 7.5, 8, 9, and 10 days after application). Renal clearances were determined by comparing clonidine urinary excretion rates over a 24-hour period at steady state with plasma steady-state concentrations. Total doses administered in each study were calculated by assaying the residual clonidine in the transdermal systems after the exposure period.

RESULTS

Composite curves for the dose linearity study in six subjects are shown in Fig. 1. Kinetic parameters and dose linearity correlations are listed in Table I. Although renal clearance and percent release from the system varied among individuals, subject parameters were internally consistent. Of the six subjects studied for dose linearity, only subject 1 showed a lack of linearity at the larger system size. The $t_{1/2}$ values for all subjects ranged from 14 to 26 hours, with most clustered about 17 to 20 hours. The $t_{1/2}$ values were calculated from the decline in plasma clonidine concentrations after system removal (Fig. 2) and appear to be dose independent. A comparison of anatomic site of application with the 3.5 cm^2 system reveals no significant difference between chest and arm (Fig. 3) over the 7 days recommended for wear. This was consistent with the percent of load delivered (Table II) estimated from residual system analysis after removal on day 11. The 3.5 cm^2 systems were left in place for 4 days past the recommended removal time to determine duration of release. Although there were no significant differences among days 7, 8, 9, 10, and 11, there was a downward trend in mean clonidine plasma concentrations after approximately 9 days of wear. Chronic removal and application of a fresh system was studied at plasma clonidine steady-state concentrations (Fig. 4).

Table II. Comparison of the percent load released after 11 days of wear on chest or arm

Subject No.	*% Released**	
	Arm	*Chest*
1	62.7	64.6
2	54.9	78.0
3	51.9	80.2
4	68.8	64.8
5	51.0	49.4
6	75.6	54.4
7	72.6	83.1
8	81.7	87.5
$\bar{X} \pm SD$	64.9 ± 11.6	70.3 ± 14.0

*Calculated after system residual analysis.

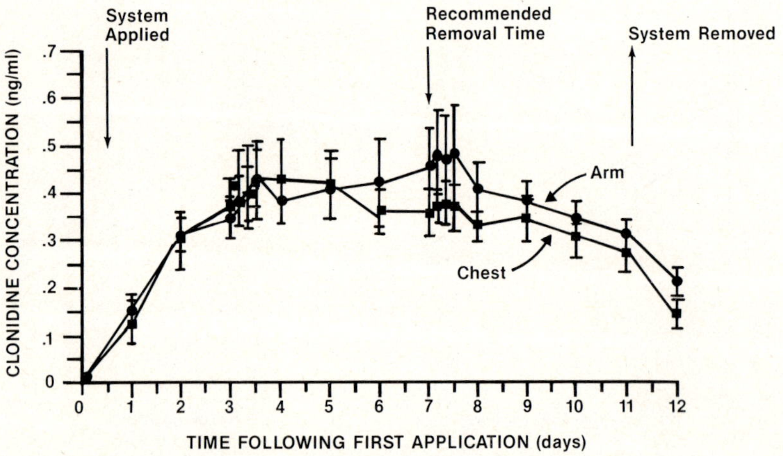

Fig. 3. Time course of mean (±SE) plasma clonidine concentrations in eight subjects receiving 3.5 cm² systems on the arm or the chest for 11 days (4 days past label-recommended removal).

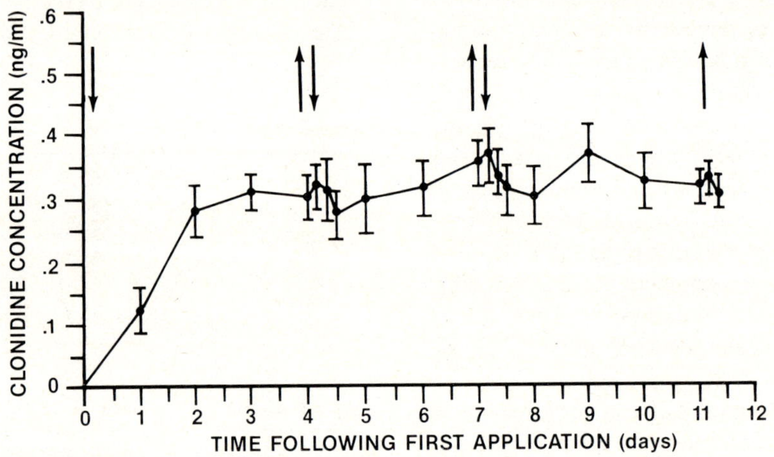

Fig. 4. Time course of mean (±SE) clonidine plasma concentrations in eight subjects receiving consecutive 3.5 cm² systems at 4 and 7 days. ↑ = Removal; ↓ = application.

There was no significant difference between clonidine plasma concentrations at time of replacement and 24 hours later. Most plasma samples assayed for the eight subjects were in the range of 0.3 to 0.4 ng/ml, as desired for a 3.5 cm² transdermal clonidine system.

DISCUSSION

Several factors unique to the pharmacokinetics of a drug are present when input is by transdermal delivery. Factors such as site of application, dose titration, extent of system drug release, and reproducibility of blood concentrations with chronic application must be fully investigated and clearly understood. Our series of studies attempted to evaluate critically transdermally delivered clonidine as a practical therapeutic alternative to oral antihypertensive therapy. Oral clonidine has an effective range in mild to moderate hypertension of 0.3 to 2 ng/ml.[4] Clinical studies have shown transdermal clonidine to be safe and effective in the treatment of hypertension.[7,8,11,12] The dose linearity study gave mean plasma concentrations of 0.39, 0.84, and 1.12 ng/ml for the system sizes of 3.5, 7.0, and 10.5 cm², respectively, thereby covering the therapeutic range reported for oral clonidine.

Dose linearity was established by examining three different-sized systems and correlating surface area of release to the steady-state clonidine plasma concentrations obtained. Within each subject there was approximate linearity, but not all subjects obtained the same plasma steady-state levels. This is primarily due to interindividual variations in the clearance of the drug and in the case of subject 3 to a larger overall dose in all three systems. Therefore, one can surmise that the skin has an influence on the amount of drug released. For therapeutic use the smallest-sized system should be prescribed and eventually titrated up to a larger size if greater blood pressure reduction is desired.

There was a lack of dose dependency in the $t_{1/2}$ and renal clearance, which again emphasizes that the transdermal absorption of clonidine is dose linear. There is no indication from the parameters in Table I of why there is a lack of linearity in subject 1 at the highest dose. This lack of high-dose linearity in this particular subject would not have led to any toxicity problems, as the curve was concave-downward. In a clinical situation this apparent nonlinearity would have been manifested by a lack of increased efficacy when titrating from 7.0 to 10.5 cm^2.

The decline from plasma steady-state levels after system removal is shown for two subjects in Fig. 2. There appears to be a slight increase in plasma clonidine concentrations after system removal in some subjects, as illustrated by subject 6, but this skin depot effect lasted <1 day. The procedure of removing an adhering system from the skin would be expected to increase blood flow to that site and increase drug absorption from the skin. A depot effect can be helpful in system changeover during chronic use if the burst effect of the new system is not enough to compensate for the rate of decline in plasma concentrations from removal of the old system. No perceivable skin depot was seen in subject 3, giving further evidence that in this subject the system membrane was the rate-determining step and the skin had negligible release characteristics.

For chronic therapeutic use in hypertension, various anatomic sites of application are needed to prevent potential skin irritation. This could be accomplished if a patient progressively applies systems from left to right across the arms and chest. In our limited study of eight subjects there were no significant differences in the amounts released from a 3.5 cm^2 system (Table II) or the clonidine plasma steady-state concentrations obtained (Fig. 3).

One major question encountered with dosing every 7 days is what would happen if the patient forgot, for a day or two, to remove the system. In the study depicted in Fig. 3, subjects wore the 3.5 cm^2 system for 11 days and a decline in mean clonidine plasma concentrations was not seen until the tenth day. Of the eight subjects studied, seven had no perceivable decline through all 11 days and one subject (subject 7) declined significantly after day 7. For another subject (subject 8), only the plasma concentrations after application to the chest dropped after 7 days of wear. Thus it can be expected in therapeutic use to be a minor problem if systems are left on for a day or two past the recommended removal date. As is shown in Table II, there is still 20% to 40% of the drug left in the system at 11 days. This much load is needed to drive the drug from the system to the skin at a zero-order rate. Subjects 7 and 8 appeared to have crossed a threshold percent load remaining, and zero-order release was not maintained.

Treatment of hypertension is a chronic multiyear process. It is assumed that once a plasma steady-state level is reached it will be maintained with subsequent application of fresh systems of the same size. This assumption was tested by multiple system changeover at steady state with intensive sampling to evaluate clonidine plasma concentrations for the following 24 hours (Fig. 4). There were no substantial increases or decreases in clonidine plasma concentrations during this 24-hour period, with rises and falls in plasma concentrations of the same magnitude as during studies in which there was no system changeover (Figs. 1 and 3) and intense sampling occurring during the day. Evaluation of the 8 AM time points for each day showed no significant differences and all plasma concentrations were within the range of 0.3 to 0.4 ng/ml, as expected with a 3.5 cm^2 system. Mean residual analysis of systems removed after 4, 3, and 4 days of wear showed 28.3%, 26.1%, and 28.6% of the load released.

Our pharmacokinetic studies were designed to answer many questions indigenous to the labeling of a transdermally delivered drug. We have shown that 3.5, 7.0, and 10.5 cm^2 clonidine systems deliver drug at a rate sufficient to produce plasma concentrations in the established therapeutic range; there are various anatomic sites for placement of the transdermal clonidine system with chronic use; clonidine is delivered at a constant rate for at least 7 days as recommended in the labeling; and during chronic dosing therapeutic clonidine concentrations will be maintained during the 24 hours after system changeover.

We thank Dr. Zacharias for the residual clonidine analysis, Dr. H. Esber, P. Zavorskas, Dr. P. Farina, and C. Homon for the plasma clonidine determinations, and K. O'Connor for helpful technical discussion.

References

1. Arndts D, Stahle H, Förster HJ: Development of a RIA for clonidine and its comparison with the reference methods. J Pharmacol Methods **6**:295-307, 1981.
2. Dollery CR, Davies DS, Draffan GH, Dargie HJ, Dean CR, Reid JL, Clare RA, Murray S: Clinical pharmacology and pharmacokinetics of clonidine. CLIN PHARMACOL THER **19**:11-17, 1976
3. Farina PR, Homon CA, Chow CT, Keirns JJ, Zavorskas

PA, Esber HJ: Solid phase radioimmunoassay for clonidine in human plasma and urine. Ther Drug Monit. (In press.)
4. Frisk-Holmberg M, Paalzow L, Wibell L: Relationship between the cardiovascular effects and steady-state kinetics of clonidine in hypertension. Eur J Clin Pharmacol **26:**309-313, 1984.
5. Grossman S, Gunnels JC: Blood pressure response to a single daily dose of a clonidine-chlorthalidone combination. J Clin Pharmacol **20:**193-196, 1980.
6. Lowenstein J: Clonidine. Ann Intern Med **92:**74-77, 1980.
7. McMahon FG: Some new aspects of modern CATAPRES® therapy in the United States. *In* Bock KD, editor: CATAPRES®(clonidine): Pathways in the development of a pharmaceutical. Aulendorf, FRG, 1983, Editio Cantor, pp 118-125.
8. Mroczek WJ: Preliminary evaluation of transdermal clonidine administration in hypertensive patients receiving a diuretic. *In* Bock KD, editor: CATAPRES® (clonidine): Pathways in the development of a pharmaceutical. Aulendorf, FRG, 1983, Editio Cantor, pp 126-132.
9. SAS Institute Inc: SAS User's Guide: Statistics, 1982 edition. Cary, NC, 1982, SAS Institute Inc, 584.
10. Thananopavarn C, Golub MS, Eggena P, Barrett JD, Sambhi MP: Clonidine, a centrally acting sympathetic inhibitor, as monotherapy for mild to moderate hypertension. Am J Cardiol **49:**153-158, 1982.
11. Weber MA, Drayer JIM: Clinical experience with rate-controlled delivery of antihypertensive therapy by a transdermal system. Am Heart J **108:**231-236, 1984.
12. Weber MA, Drayer JIM, Brewer DD, Lipson JL: Transdermal continuous antihypertensive therapy. Lancet **1:**9-11, 1984.

Pharmacokinetics of intravenous and intraperitoneal cefotaxime in chronic ambulatory peritoneal dialysis

We investigated the kinetics of cefotaxime in eight subjects undergoing continuous ambulatory peritoneal dialysis (CAPD). A single 1 gm iv dose was injected and a 1 gm dose was given intraperitoneally in the CAPD fluid during a 4-hour dwell time. Cefotaxime and desacetylcefotaxime were assayed by HPLC. After intravenous injection the cefotaxime serum kinetic parameters were as follows: plasma t½, 2.31 ± 0.20 hours; volume of distribution, 0.35 ± 0.04 L/kg; total plasma clearance, 118.7 ± 12.3 ml/min; and peritoneal clearance, 6.7 ± 1.3 ml/min. Dialysate cefotaxime concentrations rose rapidly, but only 5% of the dose was eliminated by the peritoneal route. After intraperitoneal instillation, cefotaxime appeared in the serum rapidly and the peak serum concentrations ranged from 9 to 20 μg/ml between 1 and 3 hours. The absorption of cefotaxime from peritoneal space was 58.7% ± 5.4%. Data suggest that cefotaxime has bidirectional exchange characteristics through the peritoneal membrane. Instillation of cefotaxime in CAPD fluid may permit rapid absorption to achieve therapeutic serum concentrations.
(CLIN PHARMACOL THER 38:285-289, 1985.)

H. C. Albin, M.D., F. M. Demotes-Mainard, Ph.D., J. L. Bouchet, M.D., G. A. Vincon, Ph.D., and C. Martin-Dupont, M.D. *Bordeaux, France*

Cefotaxime is a third-generation cephalosporin administered by intravenous or intramuscular injection. It has a broad spectrum of activity against gram-positive and gram-negative aerobic and anaerobic bacteria and is generally more active against gram-negative bacteria than the first- and second-generation cephalosporins. Kinetic studies in normal subjects suggest that the drug is mainly excreted by the kidneys. Cefotaxime pharmacokinetics have also been studied in patients with varying degrees of renal dysfunction.

Continous ambulatory peritoneal dialysis (CAPD) is now widely used as an alternative to hemodialysis in patients with end-stage renal disease. Bacterial peritonitis remains a major complication associated with this kind of dialysis, requiring a suitable, efficient, and well-tolerated antibacterial treatment. Because there is no information on the exchange kinetics of cefotaxime through the peritoneal membrane, we investigated its kinetics after intravenous or intraperitoneal administration in subjects undergoing CAPD.

From the Departments of Clinical Pharmacology and Nephrology, Hôpital Pellegrin.

Supported by a grant from Roussel France.

Received for publication March 22, 1985; accepted May 1, 1985.

Reprint requests to: Dr. H. Albin, Centre de Pharmacologie Clinique, Hôpital Pellegrin, 33076 Bordeaux, France.

METHODS

Our subjects were eight patients (six men and two women) with end-stage renal disease who had been receiving CAPD for 1 to 12 months (Table I). Subjects were clinically stable and were without evidence of peritonitis. None had ever presented signs or symptoms of liver disease. Dialysis was carried out with a Tenckhoff catheter (Bernas Medical) with 1.5% dextrose solution for peritoneal dialysis. Subjects were hospitalized and CAPD was conducted as four 4-hour exchanges and an overnight 8-hour exchange. Each subject received a single 1 gm iv and a single 1 gm ip dose of cefotaxime 8 days apart.

During intravenous dosing, cefotaxime was injected into a forearm vein over 3 minutes. Blood samples (5 ml on dry heparin) were drawn aseptically at 0, 0.08, 0.16, 0.25, 0.33, 0.5, 0.75, 1, 1.5, 2, 3, 4, 5, 6, 8, 10, and 12 hours after cefotaxime injection. Blood was immediately centrifuged and plasma was frozen at −20° C until assayed. Urine samples were collected before injection and at intervals of 0 to 2, 2 to 4, 4 to 6, 6 to 8, 8 to 10, 10 to 12, and 12 to 24 hours after dosing. An aliquot was frozen for analysis. At each change of the dialysis bag the collected volume was determined and an aliquot was kept frozen.

During intraperitoneal dosing, the drug was diluted in 2 L dialysate and the fluid was then instilled over

Table I. Clinical characteristics of subjects undergoing CAPD

Subject No.	*Age (yr)*	*Sex*	*Body weight (kg)*	*Primary diagnosis*	*Duration of CAPD*
1	26	F	39	Chronic glomerulonephritis	5 mo
2	31	M	65	Polycystic kidney disease	11 mo
3	55	F	87	Polycystic kidney disease	9 mo
4	51	M	60	Chronic glomerulonephritis	11 mo
5	72	M	63	Interstitial nephritis	3 mo
6	24	M	64	Diabetic nephropathy	1 mo
7	55	M	58	Nephrosclerosis	3 mo
8	63	M	55	Nephrosclerosis	12 mo

F = Female; M = male.

Table II. Cefotaxime and desacetylcefotaxime kinetics after a single 1 gm iv injection in subjects with renal disease undergoing CAPD

	Cefotaxime	*Desacetyl-cefotaxime*
$t_{1/2}$ (hr)	2.31 ± 0.20	11.4 ± 1.9
β (hr^{-1})	0.318 ± 0.030	0.076 ± 0.016
$AUC_{0\rightarrow\infty}$ (μg · hr/ml)	153.8 ± 20.1	211.4 ± 45.2
V_{area} (L/kg)	0.38 ± 0.05	—
V_{ss} (L/kg)	0.35 ± 0.04	—
CL (ml/min)	118.7 ± 12.3	—
Peritoneal clearance (ml/min)	6.7 ± 1.3	3.6 ± 1.4
CL_R (ml/min)	4.9 ± 1.6	3.5 ± 0.9
Urinary excretion (%)	3.9 ± 0.1	3.3 ± 1.0
Peritoneal excretion (%)	4.9 ± 0.7	2.8 ± 0.6

V_{ss} = Volume of distribution at steady state; CL_R = renal clearance.

15 minutes into the peritoneal cavity. Blood samples (5 ml on dry heparin) were drawn 0, 0.25, 0.5, 0.75, 1, 1.5, 2, 3, 4, 5, 6, 8, 10, and 12 hours after cefotaxime dosing. Urine samples were collected as described above. All samples were stored at −20° C until analysis.

Plasma, dialysate, and urine assays were performed within 48 hours after collection of the samples. Cefotaxime and desacetylcefotaxime were assayed by HPLC. The assay, which required only 100 μl biologic fluid, was performed in the presence of an internal standard, cephaloridine. Separation was carried out by ion-pair chromatography on a radial-pak C-18 column with ultraviolet detection at 270 nm. The minimal detectable limits for cefotaxime and desacetylcefotaxime were 0.5 and 0.25 μg/ml. Details of the method have been published.[4]

The pharmacokinetics were analyzed by an interactive graphic program. The concentration-time data points were fit to a biexponential model by a Gauss-Newton interactive procedure.[7] The AUCs were calculated by the trapezoidal rule with extrapolation to infinity by the terminal slope of the fit curve. Total plasma clearance (CL) was calculated by the formula: $CL = Dose/AUC_{0\rightarrow\infty}$. The apparent volume of distribution (V_{area}) was calculated by the formula: $V_{area} = CL/\beta$, in which β is the terminal phase rate constant. The terminal plasma $t_{1/2}$ was calculated by the equation: $t_{1/2} = 0.693/\beta$. Peritoneal and renal clearances were calculated by the formula of Gibson et al.[6a]: $CL = Q/AUC_{0\rightarrow\infty}$, where Q is the amount of drug removed by peritoneal dialysis or by the kidneys each day. Percent of drug absorbed from the peritoneum was calculated for each subject from the following equation: Percent absorption = (Amount injected − amount recovered)/amount injected × 100.

Results are expressed as the $\overline{X}$ ± SE.

RESULTS

The mean plasma concentrations of cefotaxime and desacetylcefotaxime after intravenous injection are shown in Fig. 1. Data points from all subjects after the intravenous dose suggest an early distribution phase of <30 minutes, followed by linear elimination kinetics. The mean plasma cefotaxime concentrations were 72.2 ± 8.7 μg/ml 0.08 hours and 3.2 ± 1.2 μg/ml 12 hours after dosing. The mean plasma desacetylcefotaxime concentrations were 6.5 ± 1.0 μg/ml 0.08 hours and 5.8 ± 1.5 μg/ml 12 hours after dosing. Kinetic parameters are listed in Table II. The mean plasma $t_{1/2}$ of cefotaxime during peritoneal dialysis was 2.31 ± 0.20 hours. The total amount of drug eliminated through the peritoneal membrane over a single 4-hour dwell time was 28.6 ± 3.4 mg. Peritoneal excretion was low; only 4.9% ± 0.7% of cefotaxime is removed by this route in 24 hours. The mean peritoneal clearance was 6.7 ± 1.4 ml/min (range 2.7 to 12.2 ml/min). Renal excretion of cefotaxime was also low

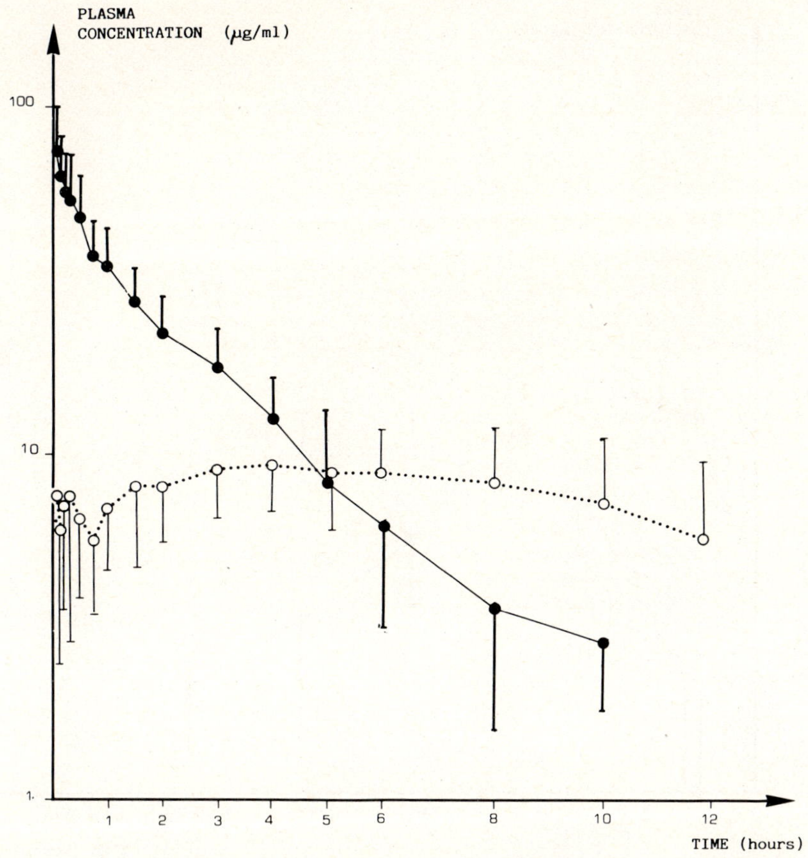

Fig. 1. Mean (±SD) plasma concentrations of cefotaxime and desacetylcefotaxime after intravenous injection of 1 gm (n = 8).

(3.9% ± 0.1% of the dose over 24 hours), but there were wide interindividual variations. The mean renal clearance was 4.9 ± 1.6 ml/min (range 0.09 to 11.4 ml/min). After intravenous administration the mean plasma desacetylcefotaxime $t_{1/2}$ was 11.4 ± 1.9 hours (range 4.6 to 17 hours).

The mean plasma concentrations of cefotaxime and desacetylcefotaxime after intraperitoneal administration are shown in Fig. 2. Serum concentrations of cefotaxime rose rapidly in five subjects after peritoneal instillation: At the end of perfusion the mean plasma cefotaxime concentration was 5.3 ± 1.3 μg/ml. For all subjects, mean plasma cefotaxime concentrations were 6.5 ± 1.2 μg/ml 15 minutes after the end of instillation and 3.1 ± 0.06 μg/ml at 8 hours. Mean plasma desacetylcefotaxime concentrations were 2.2 ± 0.5 μg/ml 1 hour and 3.4 ± 0.8 μg/ml 24 hours after dosing. Because two distinct exponential phases could not be discerned, a one-compartment model was used for the calculation of kinetic parameters (Table III). The mean plasma cefotaxime and desacetylcefotaxime $t_{1/2}$ values were 2.29 ± 0.30 and 13.2 ± 4.3 hours, respectively. Cefotaxime absorption kinetics from the peritoneal compartment were calculated by standard equations for estimating oral drug absorption. Because the drug is

Table III. Cefotaxime and desacetylcefotaxime kinetics after a single 1 gm ip instillation in subjects with renal disease undergoing CAPD

	Cefotaxime	*Desacetyl-cefotaxime*
$AUC_{0\rightarrow\infty}$ (μg · hr/ml)	90.5 ± 12.4	217.3 ± 36.6
C_{max} (μg/ml)	15.0 ± 1.5	9.7 ± 1.4
t_{max} (hr)	2.0 ± 0.3	6.0 ± 1.0
k_e (hr^{-1})	0.334 ± 0.039	0.054 ± 0.013
$t_{1/2}$ (hr)	2.3 ± 0.3	13.2 ± 4.3
k_a (hr^{-1})	0.656 ± 0.121	0.404 ± 0.04
$t_{1/2\alpha}$ (hr)	1.3 ± 0.2	1.8 ± 0.2
Percent absorption	58.7 ± 6.4	—

C_{max} = Maximum plasma concentration; t_{max} = time to reach C_{max}; k_e = elimination rate constant; k_a = absorption rate constant; $t_{1/2\alpha}$ = absorption $t_{1/2}$.

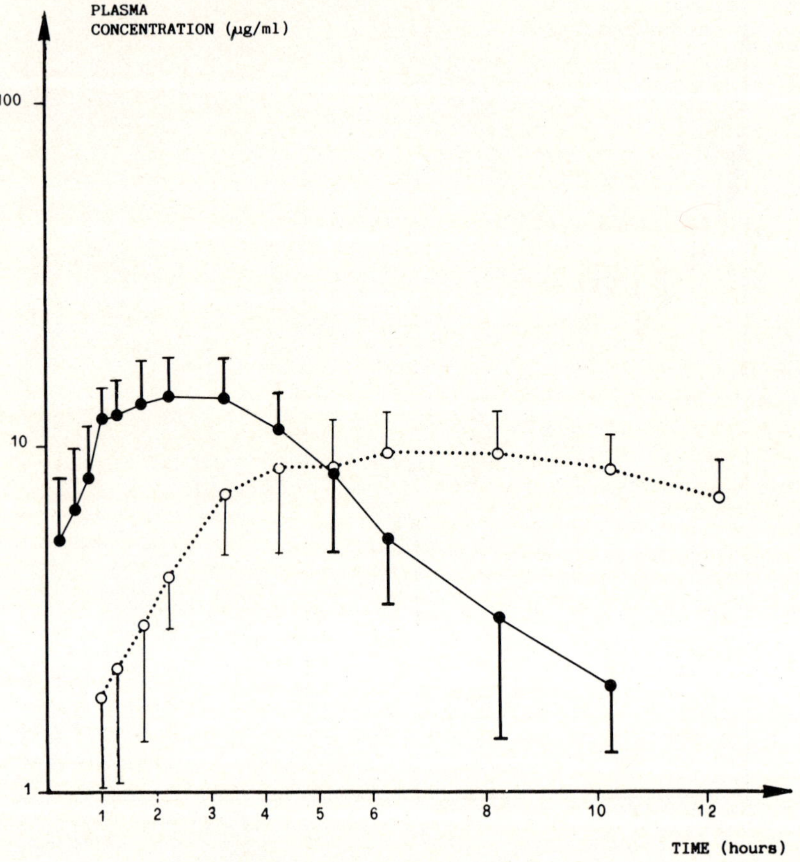

Fig. 2. Mean (± SD) plasma concentrations of cefotaxime and desacetylcefotaxime after intraperitoneal injection of 1 gm (n = 8).

absorbed into systemic circulation, plasma drug concentrations would be determined by the rate absorption and elimination constants k_a and k_e. The apparent calculated k_a was found to be 0.656 ± 0.121 hours^{-1} by regression analysis and in our subjects the absorption $t_{1/2}$ was 1.3 ± 0.2 hours. The total amount of cefotaxime remaining at the end of the first 4-hour dwell time was 371 ± 59 mg (37% ± 6%), and the percent absorption of cefotaxime from the peritoneal space was 58.7% ± 6.4%.

DISCUSSION

Our results demonstrate that when given intraperitoneally, cefotaxime was rapidly and effectively absorbed into the vascular compartment. The absorption of cefotaxime was rapid, with an absorption rate constant (k_a) of 0.656 ± 0.121 hours^{-1}. Plasma cefotaxime concentrations reach therapeutic levels in 0.5 to 1 hours, and these levels are maintained for 5 to 6 hours. Our results suggest that effective peritoneal and plasma drug levels can be achieved by intraperitoneal instillation of 1 gm cefotaxime. This suggested route of dosing for the treatment of peritonitis would be especially important in patients undergoing CAPD, because peritonitis and infections of the catheter are the most frequent complications of CAPD.

Cefotaxime is partially metabolized before excretion. The principal metabolite is a microbiologically active product, desacetylcefotaxime. Cefotaxime is normally rapidly eliminated from the body by glomerular filtration and active renal tubular secretion. About 50% to 60% of an intravenous dose of 1 or 2 gm is excreted as unchanged cefotaxime over a 24-hour period. The mean $t_{1/2}$ of cefotaxime is 0.9 to 1.1 hours after intravenous administration of single 500 to 2000 mg doses to healthy subjects[5,6] and does not change after repeated doses.[10] After cefotaxime dosing, the $t_{1/2}$ of desacetylcefotaxime is reported to be about 1.3 hours in healthy adults. In patients with severe renal dysfunction,[9] CL, renal clearance, and urinary recovery of unchanged cefotaxime are decreased, but the plasma $t_{1/2}$ of cefotaxime appeared to change little as renal function decreased: Mean $t_{1/2}$ values were 2.55 ± 0.73, 1.95 ± 0.31, and 2.04 ± 0.72 hours when creatinine clearance was 45.7 ± 10.5, 16.8 ± 6, and 4.9 ± 2.4 ml/min/1.73 m^2, respectively. The changes in desacetylcefotaxime kinetics were more pronounced, as the $t_{1/2}$ is increased to about 10 to 15 hours. The elimination of cefotaxime is improved by hemodialysis, as the $t_{1/2}$ decreased significantly from 3.4 ± 1.7 to 1.6 ± 0.6 hours. The decrease in the desacetylcefotaxime $t_{1/2}$ is more marked, from 14.4 ± 12.7 to 3.16 ± 1.00 hours. It was calculated that 52.8% ± 4.4% of desacetylcefotaxime and 38.7% ± 25.2% of cefotaxime were extracted by hemodialysis. In our subjects undergoing CAPD, the cefotaxime $t_{1/2}$ was 2.31 ± 0.20 hours and that of desacetylcefotaxime was 11.4 ± 1.9 hours after intravenous administration. These results suggest that peritoneal dialysis can effectively remove cefotaxime, but CAPD does not appear to be as effective as hemodialysis in removing cefotaxime and its main metabolite. The rate of cefotaxime peritoneal elimination suggests that the maximum rate of transfer from plasma to dialysate occurs during the first 4-hour dwell time.

Our data show a bidirectional exchange of cefotaxime between the blood and peritoneal compartments; however, this antibiotic appears to transfer well from the peritoneal to the plasma side of the peritoneal filtration barrier but poorly in the opposite direction. The reasons for these transfer characteristics are not known, but similar results have been found with gentamicin,[11] tobramycin,[2] cefazolin,[1] ceftizoxime,[8] and vancomycin.[3] Many factors such as concentration gradient, protein binding, molecular size, lipid solubility, and drug ionization may influence the rate and the extent of the peritoneal excretion of antibiotics.

In conclusion, peritoneal clearance of cefotaxime is poor. CAPD may require little alteration of the dose conventionally used in renal failure. It is possible that peritonitis alters the transfer characteristics of cefotaxime. Instillation of cefotaxime in CAPD fluid may permit rapid absorption to achieve therapeutic plasma concentrations.

References

1. Bunke CM, Aronoff GR, Brier ME, Sloan RS, Luft FC: Cefazolin and cephalexin kinetics in continuous ambulatory peritoneal dialysis. CLIN PHARMACOL THER **33:**66-72, 1983.
2. Bunke CM, Aronoff GR, Brier ME, Sloan RS, Luft FC: Tobramycin kinetics during continuous ambulatory peritoneal dialysis. CLIN PHARMACOL THER **34:**110-116, 1983.
3. Bunke CM, Aronoff GR, Brier ME, Sloan RS, Luft FC: Vancomycin kinetics during continuous ambulatory peritoneal dialysis. CLIN PHARMACOL THER **34:**631-637, 1983.
4. Demotes-Mainard F, Vincon G, Jarry C, Albin H: A micromethod for determination of cefotaxime and desacetylcefotaxime in plasma and urine by high-performance liquid chromatography. J Chromatogr **336:**438-445, 1984.
5. Esmieu F, Guibert J, Rosenkilde HC, Ho I, Le Go A: Pharmacokinetics of cefotaxime in normal human volunteers. J Antimicrob Chemother **6**(suppl):A83-A92, 1980.
6. Fu KP, Aswapokee P, Ho I, Mattnijssen C, Neu HC: Pharmacokinetics of cefotaxime. J Antimicrob Chemother **16:**592-597, 1979.
6a. Gibson TP, Matusals E, Nelson LD, Briggs WA: Artificial kidneys and clearance calculations. CLIN PHARMACOL THER **20:**720-726, 1976.
7. Gomeni R: IGPHARM—An interactive graphic program for individual and population pharmacokinetic parameter estimation. Comput Biol Med **14:**25-34, 1984.
8. Gross ML, Somani P, Ribner BS, Raeader R, Freimer EH, Higgins JT: Ceftizoxime elimination kinetics in continuous ambulatory peritoneal dialysis. CLIN PHARMACOL THER **34:**673-680, 1983.
9. Ings RMJ, Fillastre JP, Godin M, Leroy A, Humbert G: The pharmacokinetics of cefotaxime and its metabolites in subjects with normal and impaired renal function. Rev Infect Dis **4**(suppl):S379-S391, 1982.
10. Neu HC, Aswapokee P, Fu KP, Ho I, Mattnijssen C: Cefotaxime kinetics after intravenous and intramuscular injection of single and multiple doses. CLIN PHARMACOL THER **27:**677-685, 1980.
11. Somani P, Shapiro R, Stockard H, Higgins J: Unidirectional absorption of gentamicin from the peritoneum during continuous ambulatory peritoneal dialysis. CLIN PHARMACOL THER **32:**113-121, 1982.

A new dosing regimen in renal insufficiency: Application to cephalexin

We describe a new method of drug dosage adjustment. The method simultaneously considers glomerular and tubular functions as parameters, because nonparallel decreases in both functions limit the use of the conventional endogenous creatinine clearance (CL_{CR}) method for dosage adjustment. In the new method, CL_{CR} and the 15-minute phenolsulfonphthalein (PSP15′) test were used and applied to patients with renal insufficiency with cephalexin (CEX) as a model drug for renal tubular secretion. The results clearly demonstrate good control of plasma CEX concentrations by the CL_{CR}-PSP15′ method, whereas there were marked changes in plasma CEX levels with the CL_{CR} method alone. Our method appears to be more useful for patients with renal impairment than the conventional CL_{CR} method for CEX, which is mainly excreted in urine by renal tubular secretion. A nomogram for the CEX dosing interval is proposed for application to clinical practice. (Clin Pharmacol Ther 38:290-295, 1985.)

Ryohei Hori, Ph.D., Katsuhiko Okumura, Ph.D., Hiromi Nihira, M.D., Hiroshi Nakano, M.D., Kazuyoshi Akagi, M.S., and Akira Kamiya, Ph.D.
Kyoto and Hiroshima, Japan

Adjustment of a dosage regimen is necessary in patients with renal impairment, as delayed renal excretion in these patients is related to adverse reactions. Several methods have been proposed on the basis of experiential data, but most of these cannot be applied to a wide variety of drugs. Renal impairment is general divided into stages according to the extent of reduced endogenous CL_{CR}, and the patient's dosage schedule is subsequently corrected for those stages.[1,5,9] Although dosage adjustment methods for many drugs based on CL_{CR} with simple equations have been reported,[2,16] our previous study[6] disclosed that correction of the dosage schedule with the use of the CL_{CR} value alone was inadequate for ampicillin and CEX dosing in some patients with renal insufficiency. Similar findings have been reported with chlorpropamide in patients with glomerulonephritis.[15] Because all of these drugs are excreted in the urine mainly by tubular secretion, it has been speculated that the urinary excretion of these drugs

Abbreviations

a	Nonrenal elimination factor
b	Renal tubular secretion factor
CL_{CR}	Endogenous creatinine clearance
D	Dose
f	Unbound fraction of drug in plasma
GFR	Glomerular filtration rate
K	Mean elimination rate constant in plasma
k_{NR}	Nonrenal elimination rate constant
Km	Michaelis constant for renal tubular secretion
P	Drug concentration in plasma
P′	Drug concentration in plasma when K is given
P_0	Drug concentration in plasma at time 0
P_T	Drug concentration in plasma at time T
PSP	Phenolsulfonphthalein
PSP15′	Phenolsulfonphthalein test 15-minute value
R	Renal reabsorption fraction
T	Dosing interval
t	Time
U	Drug concentration in urine
V	Urine flow rate
V_{max}	Maximum velocity of renal tubular secretion
V_z	Volume of distribution
^	Disease state

From the Department of Pharmacy, Kyoto University Hospital and Faculty of Medicine, Kyoto University, Kyoto, and Department of Urology, Hiroshima University School of Medicine, Hiroshima.
Received for publication Dec. 24, 1984; accepted May 5, 1985.
Reprint requests to: Dr. Ryohei Hori, Department of Pharmacy, Kyoto University Hospital, Sakyo-ku, Kyoto 606, Japan.

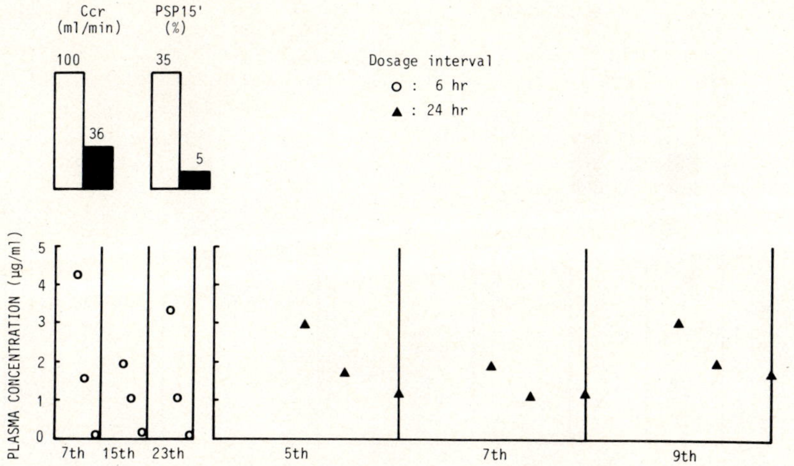

Fig. 1. Plasma cephalexin concentrations in healthy subjects *(open symbols)* and in a patient with renal insufficiency *(closed symbols)* whose dosage interval was determined by the CL_{CR}-PSP15′ method. *Abscissa* refers to number of dosing.

changes in a nonparallel manner with CL_{CR}, which is a good index of the GFR.

We describe a new method for adjustment of the CEX dosage regimen in which glomerular filtration and renal tubular secretion were simultaneously considered. The method was then applied to patients with renal insufficiency.

METHODS

Details of the method. To derive the equation for dosage adjustment, a one-compartment open model is applied to drug pharmacokinetics. Renal excretion of a drug in which tubular secretion is involved is expressed by Eq. 1[7,8,10]:

$$U \cdot V = (GFR \cdot P \cdot f + \frac{V_{max} \cdot P \cdot f}{Km + P \cdot f}) \cdot (1 - R) \quad (1)$$

Nonrenal elimination is assumed to be a first-order process.[2,16] Thus drug elimination from plasma after intravenous injection is expressed as:

$$-\frac{dP}{dt} = k_{NR} \cdot P + \frac{U \cdot V}{V_z} = k_{NR} \cdot P + \frac{1 - R}{V_z} \cdot (GFR \cdot P \cdot f + \frac{V_{max} \cdot P \cdot f}{Km + P \cdot f}) \quad (2)$$

This equation does not permit an explicit solution for P. Therefore, K is assumed to derive the dosage adjustment equation:

$$K = k_{NR} + \frac{1 - R}{V_z} \cdot (GFR \cdot f + \frac{V_{max} \cdot f}{Km + f \cdot P'}) \quad (3)$$

As this P′ is equal to the average concentration of drug in plasma at steady state during multiple dosing,[4] P′ is easily estimated experimentally. Eqs. 2 and 3 yield Eq. 4:

$$-\frac{dP}{dt} = K \cdot P \quad (4)$$

For dosing interval changes, the intervals are calculated under the assumption that the highest and lowest concentrations of the drug in each interval are equal in normal and disease states. That is, $\hat{T}$ is accordingly selected by the following conditions: $\hat{D} = D$, $\hat{T} \neq T$, $\hat{P}_0 = P_0$, and $\hat{P}_{\hat{T}} = P_T$. When V_z does not change in disease states, the highest concentration in plasma ($\hat{P}_0$) equals P_0, because $\hat{D} = D$. Therefore, $\hat{P}_0 = \hat{D}/\hat{V}_z = D/V_z = P_0$. In these conditions, $K \cdot T = \hat{K} \cdot \hat{T}$ is necessary[2] to meet the dosing condition, $P_T = \hat{P}_{\hat{T}}$. Therefore,

$$\frac{\hat{T}}{T} = \frac{K}{\hat{K}} \quad (5)$$

From Eqs. 3 and 5 we can derive Eq. 6:

$$\frac{\hat{T}}{T} = \frac{k_{NR} + \frac{1 - R}{V_z} \cdot (GFR \cdot f + \frac{V_{max} \cdot f}{Km + f \cdot P'})}{\hat{k}_{NR} + \frac{1 - \hat{R}}{\hat{V}_z} \cdot (\hat{GFR} \cdot \hat{f} + \frac{\hat{V}_{max} \cdot \hat{f}}{\hat{Km} + \hat{f} \cdot \hat{P}'})} \quad (6)$$

We have demonstrated in renal insufficiency that little or no change in Km and R occurs, but there are substantial reductions in V_{max} and GFR.[6,11] It is assumed

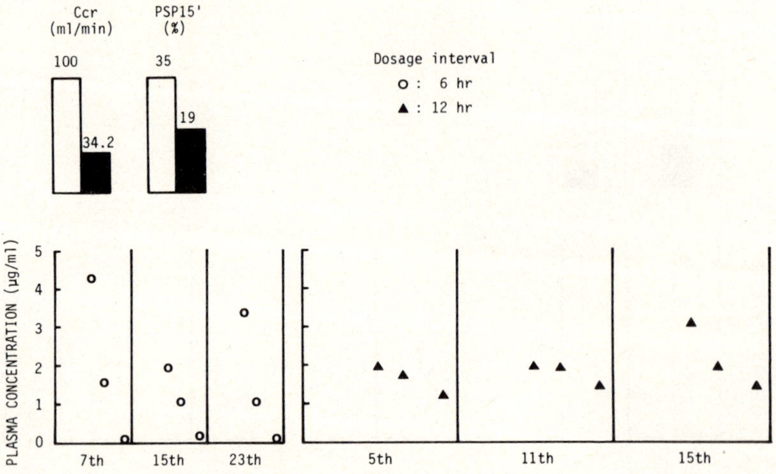

Fig. 2. Plasma cephalexin concentrations in healthy subjects *(open symbols)* and in a patient with renal insufficiency *(closed symbols)* whose dosage interval was determined by the CL_{CR}-PSP15′ method. *Abscissa* refers to number of dosing.

that k_{NR} and f do not change in disease states. It is obvious that $P' = \hat{P}'$, because $P_0 = \hat{P}_0$ and $P_T = \hat{P}_{\hat{T}}$. From these considerations, K and $\hat{K}$ are expressed as $(k_{NR} + A \cdot GFR + B \cdot V_{max})$ and $(k_{NR} + A \cdot \hat{GFR} + B \cdot \hat{V}_{max})$, respectively, where $A = (1 - R) \cdot f/V_z$ and $B = (1 - R) \cdot f/[(Km + f \cdot P') \cdot V_z]$.

When a and b are defined as follows, Eq. 6 is rewritten as Eq. 9:

$$a = \frac{V_z}{(1 - R) \cdot GFR \cdot f} \cdot k_{NR} \quad (7)$$

$$b = \frac{V_z}{(Km + f \cdot P') \cdot GFR} \quad (8)$$

$$\frac{\hat{T}}{T} = \frac{a + 1 + b}{a + \frac{\hat{GFR}}{GFR} + b \cdot \frac{\hat{V}_{max}}{V_{max}}} \quad (9)$$

The parameters a and b for CEX were estimated from the data of an earlier report[6] (V_{max} = 4.9 mg/min; Km = 5.9 µg/ml; R = 0.47; f = 0.8; and GFR = 100 ml/min), from data of Wagner[16] (k_{NR} = 0.0005 minutes^{-1}), and from results of preliminary experiments (P′ = 12.5 µg/ml and V_z = 20 L). This is the general equation for the dosing interval change. Hence, GFR and V_{max} are replaced by the clinical test values for application to clinical practice, i.e., GFR is replaced by CL_{CR}.

The PSP test is taken to reflect renal tubular secretory function, since most of the PSP excretion in the urine depends on tubular secretion. The PSP15′ value is considered to relate to the maximal renal tubular transport[3] and, therefore, Eq. 10 is derived from Eq. 9 with CL_{CR} and PSP15′ instead of GFR and V_{max}, respectively:

$$\frac{\hat{T}}{T} = \frac{a + 1 + b}{a + \frac{\hat{CL}_{CR}}{CL_{CR}} + b \cdot \frac{\hat{PSP15'}}{PSP15'}} \quad (10)$$

This equation is the practical form of the dosing interval adjustment. In clinical practice we use the mean values of CL_{CR} (100 ml/min) and PSP15′ (35%) in healthy subjects and, therefore,

$$\frac{\hat{T}}{T} = \frac{a + 1 + b}{a + \frac{\hat{CL}_{CR}}{100} + b \cdot \frac{\hat{PSP15'}}{35}} \quad (11)$$

is used for the adjustment of dosing interval in patients with renal insufficiency.

Although these equations for dosing intervals are derived on the basis of kinetics after intravenous injection, plasma steady-state concentrations of drugs after oral dosing (assuming complete bioavailability) are the same as those after intravenous injection.[4]

Subjects. To test the method, we applied it to data from five healthy subjects (three men and two women) and eight patients with renal insufficiency (six men and two women). Before CEX dosing the CL_{CR} and PSP15′ were determined for each subject. CEX, 500 mg, was taken by mouth. Dosing intervals were every 6 hours for healthy subjects. Dosing intervals in the patients were calculated by the CL_{CR}-PSP15′ equation (Eq. 11)

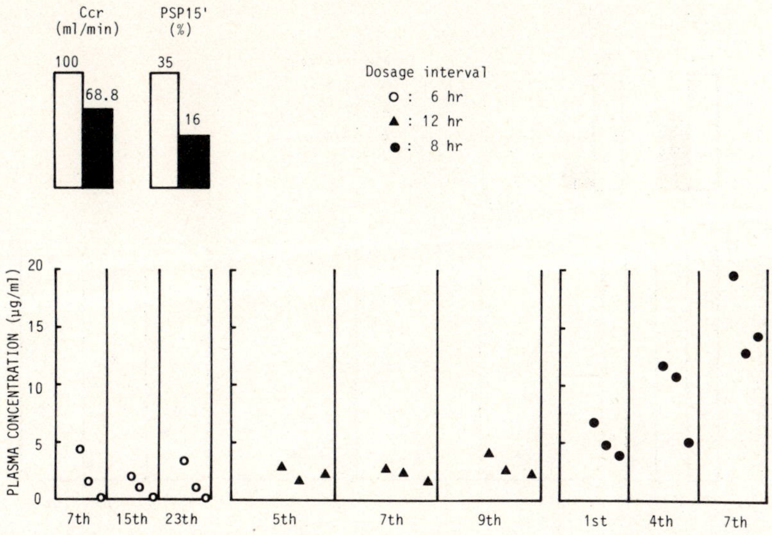

Fig. 3. Plasma cephalexin concentrations in healthy subjects (○) and in a patient with renal insufficiency whose dosage intervals were measured by the CL_{CR}-PSP15′ method (▲) and the CL_{CR} method (●). *Abscissa* refers to number of dosing.

or by the CL_{CR} equation.[16] Blood samples were drawn three times from an antecubital vein during the latter half of each interval.

CEX concentrations in plasma were assayed fluorometrically.[12] Creatinine concentrations in plasma and urine samples were determined by the alkaline picrate method, and PSP in urine was analyzed colorimetrically with the use of 1N sodium hydroxide.

RESULTS

The proposed method was first applied to two patients. The patient depicted in Fig. 1 showed good control of plasma CEX concentrations with a 24-hour dosing interval instead of the 6-hour interval for healthy subjects. If the CL_{CR} method had been applied to this patient, whose PSP15′ was markedly more reduced than the CL_{CR}, the calculated interval would be shorter, about 15 hours, than that calculated by our method, possibly leading to increased plasma CEX concentrations. The other patient with the exact same CL_{CR} and PSP15′ values had similar results (data not shown).

A third patient (Fig. 2) had greater reduction in CL_{CR} than in PSP15′ (CL_{CR} was 34% and PSP15′ was 54% of normal). Thus the relationship between these two renal function parameters was reduced in this patient compared with values in patient 1 (Fig. 1). In this case there was good control of CEX plasma concentrations with the 12-hour dosing interval calculated by the CL_{CR}-PSP15′ method.

Both our method and the CL_{CR} method were used in two patients. One patient (Fig. 3) had a CL_{CR} of 69% and a PSP15′ of 45% compared with control. The dosing intervals were calculated to be 12 hours by the CL_{CR}-PSP15′ method and 8 hours by the CL_{CR} method. These results clearly demonstrated that the plasma CEX concentrations were well controlled by our method, whereas they were much higher as measured by the CL_{CR} method. This increase in plasma CEX concentration was not induced by the declining renal function, because both CL_{CR} and PSP15′ after CEX dosing were checked in all patients and there were no changes between values before and after CEX dosing. The patient in Fig. 4 who had a CL_{CR} of 55% and a PSP15′ of 23% of normal had a marked increase in plasma CEX concentrations derived from the CL_{CR} method, whereas control was good with the 24-hour interval calculated by our CL_{CR}-PSP15′ method.

DISCUSSION

CEX was used as a model drug because it is almost completely absorbed after oral dosing[13,14] and is mainly excreted in the urine by the contributions of all the transport processes of the kidney: glomerular filtration, tubular secretion, and tubular reabsorption.[10,17]

In another study[6] we demonstrated that dosage adjustment of single oral doses of ampicillin and CEX based on the conventional CL_{CR} method was not sufficient for some patients with renal impairment because

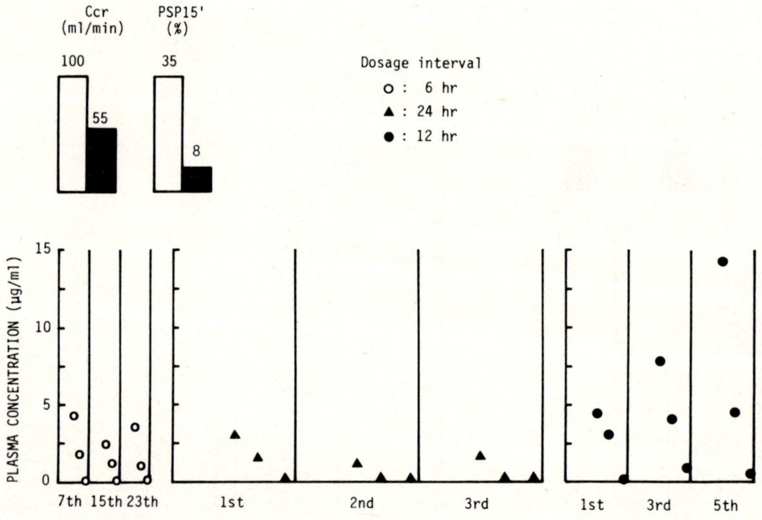

Fig. 4. Plasma cephalexin concentrations in healthy subjects (○) and in a patient with renal insufficiency whose dosage intervals were measured by the CL_{CR}-PSP15′ method (▲) and the CL_{CR} method (●). *Abscissa* refers to number of dosing.

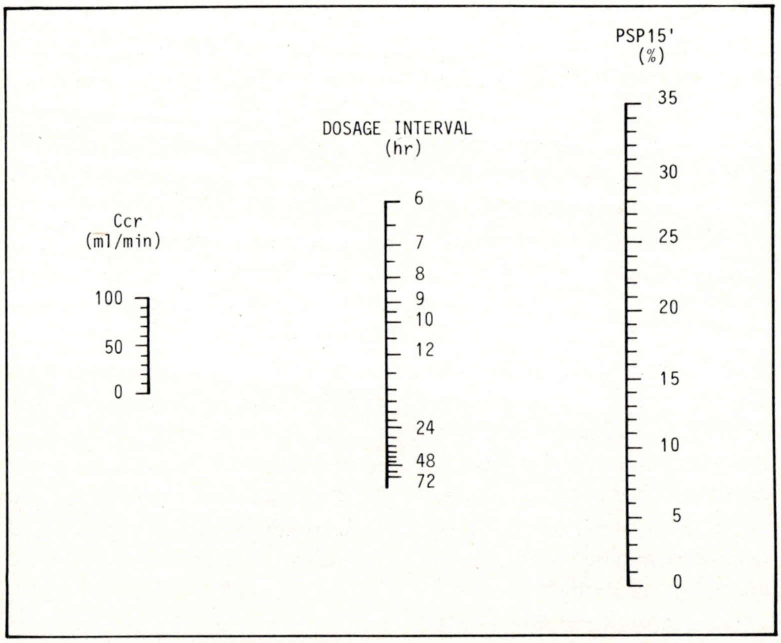

Fig. 5. Nomogram for cephalexin dosing intervals in patients with renal insufficiency (see text for use).

of nonparallel decreases in glomerular and tubular functions. This finding has been confirmed in dogs[11] and rabbits* with acute renal insufficiency after single or multiple intravenous doses of CEX and other drugs. Therefore, we developed a new dosage regimen adjustment equation with CL_{CR} and PSP15′ as parameters of glomerular and tubular functions, respectively. This equation was then applied to such patients. The values of 0.25 for a and 3.1 for b were calculated by Eqs. 7 and 8, and then Eq. 11 was used with these parameters in patients with renal insufficiency.

From our results, our newly proposed method for

*Hori R, Okumura K, Akagi K, Kamiya A: Unpublished data, 1984.

dosage adjustment could be used for better control of the plasma CEX concentrations in patients with renal insufficiency whose CL_{CR} and PSP15′ did not decrease in parallel. The validity of selection of the parameters CL_{CR} and PSP15′ instead of GFR and V_{max} was established. Although data from patients who had nonparallel decreases in glomerular and tubular functions were presented, the dosage regimens were similar to those calculated with the CL_{CR} method when these decreases were essentially parallel in three other patients (data not shown). This method can therefore be applied to patients with any kind of renal insufficiency. It is speculated from another report[6] and our current results that the dosage adjustment regimen of drugs excreted mainly by renal tubular secretion such as ampicillin[6] and chlorpropamide[15] will be made without difficulty with the use of this method.

The nomogram shown in Fig. 5 is for use in clinical practice. It permits determination of individual dosing intervals without calculation from the equation. CL_{CR} and PSP15′ are plotted on the left and right ordinates. These points should be connected by a straight line. The point of intersection is the individual dosing interval.

References

1. Bennet WM, Muther RS, Parker RA, Feig P, Morrison G, Golper TA, Singer I: Drug therapy in renal failure; Dosing guidelines for adults. Parts I and II. Ann Intern Med **93:**62-89, 286-325, 1980.
2. Dettli L: Drug dosage in renal failure. Clin Pharmacokinet **1:**126-134, 1976.
3. Gault MH, Koch B, Dossetor JB: Phenolsulfonphthalein (PSP) in assessment of renal function. JAMA **200:**871-873, 1967.
4. Gibaldi M, Perrier D: Pharmacokinetics. New York, 1975, Marcel Dekker, Inc.
5. Giusti DL: A review of the clinical use of antimicrobial agents in patients with renal and hepatic insufficiency. Drug Intell Clin Pharm **7:**63-74, 252-262, 540-556, 1973.
6. Hori R, Okumura K, Kamiya A, Nihira H, Nakano H: Ampicillin and cephalexin in renal insufficiency. CLIN PHARMACOL THER **34:**792-798, 1983.
7. Hori R, Sunayashiki K, Kamiya A: Pharmacokinetic analysis of renal handling of sulfamethizole. J Pharm Sci **65:**463-465, 1976.
8. Hori R, Sunayashiki K, Kamiya A: Tissue distribution and metabolism of drugs. I. Quantitative investigation on renal handling of phenolsulfonphthalein and sulfonamides in rabbits. Chem Pharm Bull **26:**740-745, 1978.
9. Jacobson EA, McLeod DC: Pharmacokinetics and dosing of antimicrobial agents in renal impairment. Parts 1 and 2. Am J Hosp Pharm **31:**36-52, 137-148, 1974.
10. Kamiya A, Okumura K, Hori R: Quantitative investigation on renal handling of drugs in rabbits, dogs, and humans. J Pharm Sci **72:**440-443, 1983.
11. Kamiya A, Okumura K, Hori R: Quantitative investigation of renal handling of drugs in dogs with renal insufficiency. J Pharm Sci **73:**892-896, 1984.
12. Miyazaki K, Ogino O, Arita T: Fluorometric determination of cephalexin, cephradine, and cephatrizine in biological fluids. Chem Pharm Bull **27:**2273-2280, 1979.
13. Muggleton PW, O'Callaghan CH, Foord RD, Kirby SM, Ryan DM: Laboratory appraisal of cephalexin. Antimicrob Agents Chemother **1968:**353-360, 1969.
14. Nightingale CH, Greene DS, Quintiliani R: Pharmacokinetics and clinical use of cephalosporin antibiotics. J Pharm Sci **64:**1899-1927, 1975.
15. Petitpierre B, Perrin L, Rudhardt M, Herrera A, Fabre J: Behaviour of chlorpropamide in renal insufficiency and under the effect of associated drug therapy. Int J Clin Pharmacol Ther Toxicol **6:**120-124, 1972.
16. Wagner JG: Relevant pharmacokinetics of antimicrobial drugs. Med Clin North Am **58:**479-492, 1974.
17. Welles JS, Froman RO, Gibson WR, Owen NV, Anderson RC: Toxicology and pharmacology of cephalexin in laboratory animals. Antimicrob Agents Chemother **1968:**489-496, 1969.

Cyclosporine kinetics in renal transplantation

The pharmacokinetics of cyclosporine were evaluated in 41 recipients of a cadaveric renal transplant. Cyclosporine was taken by mouth (mean dose 14 mg/kg) on one study day and was intravenously infused over 2 hours (mean dose 4.7 mg/kg) on the next study day. Cyclosporine was extracted from whole blood and analyzed by HPLC. After intravenous infusion, cyclosporine exhibited multicompartmental behavior. The mean (±SD) terminal disposition rate constant was 0.065 ± 0.036 hours^{-1} and the harmonic mean $t_{1/2}$ was 10.7 hours. The harmonic mean total body clearance of cyclosporine was 5.73 ml/min/kg and the mean apparent volume of distribution was 4.5 ± 3.6 L/kg. The absorption of oral cyclosporine was slow and incomplete. Peak blood cyclosporine concentrations ($\overline{X}$ = 1,103 ng/ml) were reached between 1 and 8 hours after oral dosing ($\overline{X}$ = 4 hours). The mean relative bioavailability was 27.6% ± 20%. Oral bioavailability was <10% in 17% of our subjects. The absorption and clearance of cyclosporine were highly variable. We conclude that the variability in the kinetics of cyclosporine makes trough blood level monitoring essential in the management of patients who receive renal transplants. (CLIN PHARMACOL THER 38:296-300, 1985.)

Richard J. Ptachcinski, Pharm.D., Raman Venkataramanan, Ph.D., J. Thomas Rosenthal, M.D., Gilbert J. Burckart, Pharm.D., Rodney J. Taylor, M.D., and Thomas R. Hakala, M.D. *Pittsburgh, Pa.*

Immunosuppression with cyclosporine is now established as a major factor in the recent success in clinical organ transplantation,[5,19] but the optimal dose required to prevent organ rejection while avoiding toxicity has not yet been determined. Cyclosporine kinetics and the determination of factors that influence these kinetics are essential to its optimal use in transplant recipients.[22] Age, disease, or concurrent administration of other drugs may alter the kinetics of cyclosporine.

To our knowledge there have been no properly designed studies of cyclosporine kinetics. Thus our objective was to determine the pharmacokinetics of cyclosporine in recipients of cadaveric renal transplants.

METHODS

Our subjects were 24 men and 17 women between the ages of 12 and 62 years ($\overline{X}$ = 31 years). During the study period, immunosuppression after cadaveric renal transplantation was achieved with cyclosporine and corticosteroids. Subjects received 5 mg/kg iv cyclosporine and 17.5 to 20 mg/kg po cyclosporine before surgery. After transplantation they received intravenous cyclosporine (9 mg/kg/day) in three divided doses and a single oral dose (17.5 to 20 mg/kg/day) for 3 days. On day 4 after surgery, intravenous cyclosporine was discontinued and the subjects were maintained on a single dose of 17.5 to 20 mg/kg/day oral cyclosporine. The oral dose was tapered in accordance with the subject's clinical status. Attempts were made to achieve trough whole blood cyclosporine concentrations >100 ng/ml by HPLC.

Our studies were performed within the first 2 weeks after transplantation. Subjects were studied after at least 3 days of the same oral maintenance dose of cyclosporine. No dietary restrictions were imposed during the study. Subjects received the cyclosporine along with their regular breakfast. On the first day of the study, subjects received oral cyclosporine mixed with 240 ml chocolate milk. Blood samples were drawn into heparinized tubes at 0, 1, 2, 3, 4, 5, 6, 8, 12, 18, and 24 hours after dosing. The next day subjects received approximately 30% of the maintenance oral dose as a 2-hour intravenous infusion. Blood samples were drawn at 0, 1, 2, 2.5, 3, 4, 5, 6, 8, 12, 18, and 24 hours after

From the Departments of Pharmacy Practice, Pharmaceutics, and Surgery, University of Pittsburgh School of Pharmacy and Medicine.

Supported by funds from Sandoz Inc., East Hanover, N. J., and the University of Pittsburgh.

Presented in part at the Annual Meeting of the American College of Clinical Pharmacology, San Diego, Calif., June 28, 1984.

Received for publication Nov. 19, 1984; accepted May 6, 1985.

Reprint requests to: Richard J. Ptachcinski, Pharm.D., Clinical Pharmacokinetics Laboratory, 807 Salk Hall, University of Pittsburgh, Pittsburgh, PA 15261.

Table I. Cyclosporine kinetics after oral and intravenous dosing in recipients of cadaveric renal transplants

	Intravenous			*Oral*		
	*Mean**	*±SD/range†*	*Median*	*Mean**	*±SD/range†*	*Median*
Observed time to peak concentration (hr)				4.03	1.83	3.92
Observed peak (ng/ml)				1103	570	1152
F (%)				27.6	18.1	21.2
V_{ss}						
(L)	266	219	207			
(L/kg)	4.54	3.59	3.92			
(L/m^2)	160	127	207			
CL						
(ml/min)	339	101-1303	364			
(ml/min/kg)	5.73	0.63-23.9	6.51			
($ml/min/m^2$)	207	72-853	236			
Disposition rate constant (hr^{-1})	0.065	0.036	0.059	0.069	0.041	0.057
Disposition $t_{1/2}$ (hr)	10.7	4.3-53.4	12	10	3.8-49.6	12.1

*All values except CL and disposition $t_{1/2}$ are expressed as arithmetic means; CL and disposition $t_{1/2}$ are expressed as harmonic means.
†Standard deviation is reported for all parameters except CL and disposition $t_{1/2}$; range is reported for CL and disposition $t_{1/2}$ because standard deviations cannot be determined for harmonic means.

the start of the infusion. Whole blood samples were stored at 4° C until analysis.

Cyclosporine was extracted from whole blood and analyzed by an HPLC method similar to that of Sawchuck and Cartier.[18] Cyclosporin D (Sandoz, Inc.) was used as the internal standard. The drug was initially extracted into diethyl ether. After drying, the residue was taken up in methanol, combined with hydrochloric acid, and washed twice with hexane. After neutralization the drug and internal standard were reextracted into ether and dried. Samples were reconstituted with mobile phase before injection onto a 15 cm, 5 μ, C-18 column heated to 70° C. The mobile phase was acetonitrile: water (68:32) delivered at a rate of 1.5 ml/min. Column eluents were monitored at 214 nm by an ultraviolet detector. Retention times were 8.3 minutes for cyclosporine and 11.2 minutes for cyclosporin D. In 1 ml blood the lower limit of sensitivity of the assay was 25 ng/ml. The coefficient of variation was 3.25% for spiked samples at 600 ng/ml. All samples and standards were assayed in duplicate.

The terminal disposition rate constant was determined by least-squares linear regression analysis of the terminal phase of the blood concentration-time curves.[10] The principle of reverse superposition was used to generate single-dose curves from the observed blood concentrations.[1] The total blood AUC (AUC_0^∞) and the area under the first moment curve ($AUMC_0^\infty$) values were then calculated from the single-dose curve by standard kinetic procedures.[10] Cyclosporine clearance (CL) was calculated by dividing the intravenous dose by the AUC_0^∞. The volume of distribution at steady state (V_{ss}) was calculated as[17]:

$$V_{ss} = \frac{(k_0T)AUMC_0^\infty}{(AUC_0^\infty)^2} - \frac{T(k_0T)}{2\ AUC_0^\infty}$$

in which k_0 is the infusion rate, T is the infusion time, and k_0T is the administered dose. The bioavailability (F) of oral cyclosporine was calculated in all but two subjects as: $F = (AUC_0^\infty oral/AUC_0^\infty iv) \times (dose_{iv}/dose_{oral}) \times 100\%$. The other two subjects received a combination of intravenous and oral cyclosporine on the first study day and their bioavailability was calculated as: $F = [(AUC_0^\infty(oral + iv) - AUC_0^\infty iv)]/AUC_0^\infty iv \times (dose_{iv}/dose_{oral}) \times 100\%$.

The arithmetic means and standard deviations were calculated for all kinetic parameters except CL and the $t_{1/2}$, for which arithmetic mean calculations were not appropriate and hence harmonic means were determined.[6,7]

RESULTS

The variability in response to cyclosporine resulted in a wide range of doses. The mean oral dose of cyclosporine was 14 mg/kg (range 6 to 22 mg/kg). The mean intravenous dose was 4.7 mg/kg (range 2.0 to 6.7 mg/kg). Cyclosporine kinetics were variable in our subjects (Table I). Whole blood cyclosporine concen-

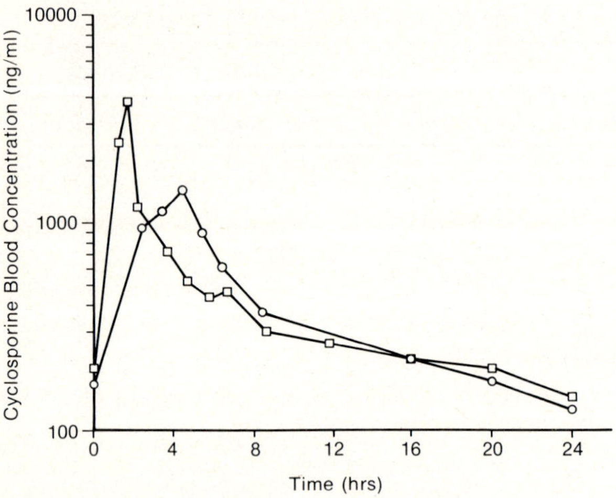

Fig. 1. Cyclosporine blood concentration-time curves for one subject after intravenous (□) and oral (○) cyclosporine. Cyclosporine CL was 5.3 ml/min/kg, V_{ss} was 3.7 L/kg, $t_{1/2}$ was 15.2 hours, and F was 17.9% in this subject.

tration-time curves after oral and intravenous dosing in one subject are shown in Fig. 1. After intravenous infusion, cyclosporine exhibited multicompartmental behavior, with a rapid distribution phase followed by a slower elimination phase. The mean terminal disposition rate constant in our subjects was 0.065 $hours^{-1}$ and the harmonic mean $t_{1/2}$ was 10.7 hours (range 4.3 to 53.4 hours). The harmonic mean CL of cyclosporine was 5.73 ml/min/kg (range 0.6 to 23.9 ml/min/kg). The mean apparent V_{ss} was 4.5 L/kg (range 0.12 to 15.5 L/kg).

The absorption of oral cyclosporine was slow and incomplete. Peak blood cyclosporine concentrations occurred between 1 and 8 hours after dosing ($\overline{X}$ = 4 hours). The peak blood concentration ranged from 165 to 3,431 ng/ml ($\overline{X}$ = 1,103 ng/ml). Mean relative bioavailability was 27.6% ± 20%. Bioavailability after oral dosing was <10% in seven subjects (17%).

DISCUSSION

Cyclosporine has made a major contribution to the recent improvements in the success of organ grafting. Marked variability in blood concentrations achieved with a fixed dose of cyclosporine presents a major problem in the postoperative management of transplant recipients.[22] Differences in response to a fixed dose of cyclosporine and reports of poor bioavailability after oral doses prompted our study.

There are very few reports on the kinetics of cyclosporine in man.[3,9,11,13-15] Previous kinetic studies of cyclosporine were limited by a number of methodologic problems. Several investigators analyzed plasma or serum.[3,11,14,15] The partition of cyclosporine between blood cells and plasma is greatly altered by temperature and time of equilibration. Plasma separated from the red blood cells at a temperature <37° C would lead to underestimation of the drug level in plasma,[21] which would result in an overestimation of cyclosporine CL. RIA has been used in several studies of cyclosporine kinetics,[11,14,15] but the antibody used in the RIA cross-reacts with cyclosporine metabolites,[8] which results in overestimations of cyclosporine concentrations and AUC determinations and reduced CL and V_{ss} estimates.[23] Previous studies were also limited by the small number of blood samples drawn in the terminal elimination phase (leading to inaccurate kinetic parameter estimates).[11,13,14]

We studied cyclosporine kinetics in 41 recipients of renal transplants. Whole blood concentrations were determined by an HPLC assay that measured cyclosporine without interference from the metabolites. Intravenous and oral studies were performed within 2 days, so that time-dependent changes in cyclosporine kinetics[11] would not markedly influence results. The subjects required chronic immunosuppression to prevent graft rejection and had to receive daily doses of cyclosporine. Our methodology was therefore limited to study of the patients for only 24 hours after a dose. This limitation resulted in fewer data points in the terminal disposition phase than desirable. Three or more data points with a linear correlation (r) >0.90 were used to calculate the terminal disposition rate constant and $t_{1/2}$.

There was wide variability in all kinetic parameters. The cyclosporine terminal disposition $t_{1/2}$ after intravenous infusion was 10.7 hours. Follath et al.[9] reported a cyclosporine $t_{1/2}$ of 15.8 hours in four patients with renal failure who were studied for 48 hours; the harmonic mean $t_{1/2}$ in this patient group was 12.2 hours. Beveridge et al.[3] reported an arithmetic mean $t_{1/2}$ of 27 hours in medical patients and bone marrow recipients studied for 48 hours; the harmonic mean $t_{1/2}$ in serum in this patient population was 24 hours. The consistency of our $t_{1/2}$ estimate with that in a 48-hour study demonstrates the validity of our 24-hour design. Other investigators have reported $t_{1/2}$ values of 4.2 to 10.6 hours for cyclosporine.[13,14] Inadequate blood sampling in the terminal disposition phase in the dosing interval studied may have contributed to the short $t_{1/2}$ estimates in those reports. Because cyclosporine has such a long $t_{1/2}$, approximately 2 to 3 days of maintenance dosing are necessary before steady-state levels are achieved. Hence in patients with normal hepatic function, cyclosporine blood concentrations should be measured 2 to 3 days after any change in dosing to determine a new steady-state drug level.

Cyclosporine CL was variable after intravenous infusion, with a harmonic mean of 5.73 ml/min/kg. This value is higher than the values we have noted in recipients of liver transplants (5.5 ml/min/kg) and in patients with liver disease (2.4 ml/min/kg).* In contrast, our subjects had a lower CL than pediatric liver transplant recipients, who have a CL of 8.4 ml/min/kg.[4] Cyclosporine CL was sensitive to microsomal enzyme induction by phenobarbital and phenytoin. This was seen in two subjects who had accelerated cyclosporine CL while receiving an enzyme inducer. This confirms the observation of Keown et al.,[14] who reported a 50% decrease in the AUC and trough concentrations in five patients receiving phenytoin for convulsive disorders. Cyclosporine CL may be impaired by high doses of steroids,[16] but in our subjects there was no difference in CL between patients receiving maintenance doses and those receiving high doses of steroids.

The cyclosporine V_{ss} was 4.5 L/kg. A large V_{ss} is compatible with reports of extensive distribution of cyclosporine throughout the body tissues.[12] The cyclosporine V_{ss} is 3.5 L/kg in patients with renal failure[9] and 2.7 L/kg in bone marrow recipients.[23] These are all significantly lower than the 13 L/kg reported by Beveridge et al.[2] based on serum measurements.

The absorption of cyclosporine after oral dosing was slow and incomplete (relative bioavailability was 27.6%). There was malabsorption (bioavailability <10%) in 17% of our subjects. Poor absorption of cyclosporine has been reported before.[2] The wide variability in bioavailability and CL demonstrates the need to monitor blood concentrations of cyclosporine in recipients of renal transplants. The precise dose or blood level of cyclosporine needed to prevent graft rejection while avoiding toxicity is not known, but adequate levels of immunosuppression with cyclosporine or conventional drugs are essential for graft survival in the early postoperative period. Patients receiving cyclosporine who absorb poorly or who have high metabolic clearance of the drug are at high risk for graft rejection. Twice-weekly monitoring of trough concentrations is usually adequate to avoid complications resulting from unexpected changes in the drug's absorption or elimination. Patients with consistently low trough concentrations may benefit from kinetic analysis after an intravenous dose of cyclosporine. From such an analysis the patient's cyclosporine clearance could be calculated to determine whether accelerated metabolic clearance of the drug is the cause of the low trough concentrations. Whole blood samples should be analyzed by HPLC to indicate cyclosporine CL accurately. Patients with accelerated cyclosporine CL might benefit from a continuous intravenous infusion[20] or divided daily oral doses of cyclosporine. Patients with normal cyclosporine CL but low trough concentrations may have poor absorption of the oral preparation. They might benefit from combined intravenous and oral cyclosporine for several days. The intravenous infusion may be gradually tapered until the patient can receive adequate maintenance therapy with the oral drug alone.

Considerable variability exists in the pharmacokinetics of cyclosporine in recipients of renal transplants. This variability makes trough blood cyclosporine level monitoring an essential tool in the management of transplant recipients.

*Ptachcinski RJ, Burckart GJ, Venkataramanan R: Unpublished observations, 1985.

References

1. Bauer LA, Gibaldi M: Computation of model-independent pharmacokinetic parameters during multiple dosing. J Pharm Sci **72:**978-979, 1983.
2. Beveridge T: Pharmacokinetics and metabolism of cyclosporin A. *In* White DJG, editor: Cyclosporin A. Oxford, 1982, Elsevier Biomed Press, pp 35-44.
3. Beveridge T, Gratwohl A, Michot F, et al: Cyclosporine A: Pharmacokinetics after a single dose in man and serum levels after multiple dosing in recipients of allogenic bone-marrow grafts. Curr Ther Res **30:**5-17, 1981.
4. Burckart G, Starzl T, Williams L, et al: Cyclosporine monitoring and pharmacokinetics in pediatric liver transplant patients. Transplant Proc **17:**1172-1175, 1985.
5. Canadian Multicentre Transplant Study Group: A randomized clinical trial of cyclosporine in cadaveric renal transplantation. N Engl J Med **309:**809-815, 1983.
6. Chiou WL: New calculation method of the mean total body clearance of drugs and its applications to dosage regimens. J Pharm Sci **69:**90-91, 1980.
7. Croxton FE, Cowden DJ, editors: Applied general statistics. New York, 1939, Prentice-Hall, Inc.
8. Donatsch P, Abish E, Homberger M, Trabar R, Trapp M, Voges R: A radioimmunoassay to measure cyclosporin A in plasma and serum. J Immunoassay **2:**19-32, 1981.
9. Follath F, Wenk M, Vozeh S, et al: Intravenous cyclosporin kinetics in renal failure. CLIN PHARMACOL THER **34:**638-643, 1983.
10. Gibaldi M, Perrier D, editors: Pharmacokinetics, ed 2. New York, 1982, Marcel Dekker, Inc.

11. Kahan BD, Ried M, Newburger J: Pharmacokinetics of cyclosporine in human renal transplantation. Transplant Proc **15:**446-453, 1983.
12. Kahan BD, VanBuren CT, Boileau M, et al: Cyclosporin A tissue levels in a cadaveric renal allograft recipient. Transplantation **35:**96-99, 1983.
13. Kennedy MS, Yee GC, Deeg HJ, Storb R, Thomas ED: Pharmacokinetics and toxicity of cyclosporine in marrow transplant patients. Transplant Proc **15:**2416-2418, 1983.
14. Keown PA, Stiller CR, Laupacis AL, et al: The effects and side effects of cyclosporine: Relationship to drug pharmacokinetics. Transplant Proc **14:**659-661, 1982.
15. Keown PA, Stiller CR, Sinclair NR, et al: The clinical relevance of cyclosporine blood levels as measured by radioimmunoassay. Transplant Proc **15:**2438-2441, 1983.
16. Klintmalm G, Sawe J: High dose methylprednisolone increases plasma cyclosporine levels in renal transplant recipients. Lancet **1:**731, 1984.
17. Perrier D, Mayershon M: Noncompartmental determination of the steady state volume of distribution for any mode of administration. J Pharm Sci **72:**372-373, 1982.
18. Sawchuk RJ, Cartier LL: Liquid-chromatographic determination of cyclosporin A in blood and plasma. Clin Chem **27:**1368-1371, 1981.
19. Starzl TE, Iwastsuki S, Van Thiel DH, et al: Evolution of liver transplantation. Hepatology **2:**614-636, 1982.
20. Wall WJ, Keown P, Stiller CR, et al: Efficacy and safety of low dose continuous cyclosporine. Transplant Proc **17:**1256-1257, 1985.
21. Wenk M, Follath F, Abisch E: Temperature dependency of apparent cyclosporin A concentrations in plasma. Clin Chem **26:**1865, 1983.
22. Wood AJ, Maurer G, Niederberger W, Beveridge T: Cyclosporine: Pharmacokinetics, metabolism and drug interactions. Transplant Proc **15:**2409-2412, 1983.
23. Yee GC, Gmur DJ, Kennedy MS: Liquid-chromatographic determination of cyclosporine in serum with use of a rapid extraction procedure. Clin Chem **28:**2269-2271, 1982.

Influence of transdermal scopolamine on motion sickness during 7 days' exposure to heavy seas

We conducted a double-blind, placebo-controlled study to evaluate the efficacy and tolerability of transdermal scopolamine in the prevention of motion sickness (MS) aboard a frigate during 7 days of continuously moderate or heavy seas. Forty-nine healthy sailors with a previous history of MS were randomly assigned to receive a transdermal therapeutic system of scopolamine (TTS-S) or transdermal placebo (TD-P). Patches were placed behind the ears at least 4 hours before departure and were removed 72 hours later. Subjects were observed on days 1 to 4 and 6. In the TTS-S group, both subjective feeling of MS and the incidence of nausea were reduced during the first 2 days. Because of adaptation, differences in signs and symptoms of MS between subjects receiving TTS-S and TD-P disappeared after the second day. During the first 3 days, vomiting occurred less often in the TTS-S group. On day 6, 3 days after removal of the patch, vomiting occurred in 23% of the TTS-S group, probably due to delay in adaptation, but none of the subjects in the TD-P group vomited. Concentration was not adversely influenced, since the ability to work increased in the TTS-S group. During prolonged continuous exposure to heavy and moderate seas, 2.5 cm² TTS-S discs proved to be efficacious in preventing MS, with xerostomia as a tolerable side effect and no significant ocular side effects. (CLIN PHARMACOL THER 38:301-305, 1985.)

W. F. van Marion, M.D., M. C. M. Bongaerts, M.D., J. C. Christiaanse, M.D., H. G. Hofkamp, M.D., and W. van Ouwerkerk, M.D. *Overveen, The Netherlands*

Motion sickness (MS) refers to a complex of symptoms, principally pallor, cold sweating, nausea, and vomiting, that may follow the perceptions of real or putative motion. All forms of travelling may cause MS, and usually continuous exposure to constant conditions will produce adaptation within 2 or 3 days.[7,8] Drowsiness and MS may appear in the same circumstances but are considered to be different expressions of the same vestibular stimulation and, therefore, drowsiness should not be regarded as a symptom of MS.

Effective drugs are available to prevent the development of MS, but they are neither completely effective nor without side effects. Scopolamine (*l*-hyoscine) is the best single drug for protection, especially for brief exposure to severe motion.[8,10] The antinauseant effect of scopolamine does not depend on its peripheral parasympathetic blocking capacity; it is caused by a central effect.[1] This central effect of scopolamine can be clearly associated with blood levels below those required to elicit the peripheral parasympatholytic effects associated with it.

Probably, the sudden entry of scopolamine into systemic circulation by conventional administration induces peak levels responsible for the unwanted peripheral effects. The development of so-called "therapeutic systems," which are drug delivery systems that provide a defined rate of drug release over a defined period of time, is a step forward in overcoming those problems. A transdermal therapeutic system for scopolamine (TTS-S) was developed that provides a constant release of 0.5 mg scopolamine over 72 hours. It is designed for application behind the ear.[9]

Side effects of the TTS-S system include dry mouth, drowsiness, and blurred vision.[3-6] Blurred vision occurs only after prolonged TTS-S use, either after longer periods on a single patch or after successive applications of TTS-S.[3,5] TTS-S does not induce impairments in psychomotor or information processing tasks.[4,5]

We designed a double-blind, placebo-controlled, crossover study to determine the efficacy, tolerability, and aftereffects of TTS-S during 7 days of continuous exposure to moderate or heavy seas aboard a Dutch naval standard frigate.

From the Department of Internal Medicine, Marine Hospitaal.
Received for publication Dec. 5, 1984; accepted May 19, 1985.
Reprint requests to: Dr. W. F. van Marion, Department of Internal Medicine, Marine Hospitaal, Bloemendaalseweg 287, 2050 AE Overveen, The Netherlands.

Table I. Percentage of subjects with the four principal symptoms of MS

	Day				
	1	*2*	*3*	*4*	*6*
Cold sweating					
TTS-S (n = 26)	15	8	4	0	4
TD-P (n = 23)	39	30	9	5	5
Pallor					
TTS-S	31	19	5	0	15
TD-P	48	30	17	9	13
Nausea					
TTS-S	27*	31*	19	12	27
TD-P	70	78	26	17	26
Vomiting					
TTS-S	27	19	8	8	23†
TD-P	30	30	13	0	0

*P < 0.01; †P < 0.05.

METHODS

Our subjects had not been sailing for 4 weeks before the test periods. Fifty-one healthy sailors ranging in age from 17 to 45 years with a history of MS for which they used MS drugs were randomly assigned to a group starting with TTS-S or a group that received a transdermal placebo (TD-P) of identical appearance. Patches of 2.5 cm^2 containing 0.5 mg scopolamine or placebo were used. The subjects applied the patches behind their ear at least 4 hours before leaving the harbor and removed them 72 hours later. No restraints in taking a shower, bath, or washing were imposed on the subjects. On request, subjects received 50 mg cyclizine tablets as supplemental medication; the number of tablets taken by the subjects was recorded. On days 1, 2, 3, 4, and 6 of the study, subjects scored the subjective severity of MS, drowsiness, and the ability to perform tasks on a visual analog scale (VAS). At the same time they were questioned about the relative incidence of cold sweating, nausea, vomiting, and the subjective feeling of MS in comparison with previous experiences.

Side effects reported included salivation, headache, dizziness, concentration problems, diplopia, blurred vision, palpitations, and local tolerability of the patch. The following were determined at each control examination: blood pressure, pulse rate, pupil size and reaction to light, and degree of pallor. On the day before departure and on the first test day, all subjects performed a Bourdon-Wiersma test, representing an information processing task.[2] The time per line and total errors comprised the performance assessments. The VAS (10 cm long) were divided into five classes with a width of 2 cm each. To each class a score was awarded to permit testing according to Yates and Cochran. All other variables were tested by chi-square analysis.

RESULTS

During the first test period sea conditions were moderate to severe. Swells ranged from 1 to 6 m in height, and the wind was from 5 to 9 Beaufort in force. Contrary to expectations, sea conditions were very light during the second test period, and no subject developed MS. Thus only between-subject analysis of efficacy was possible. Side effects were analyzed during both test periods. Of the original 51 subjects, two dropped out, one because of renal colic and the other because of transfer to another ship.

The TTS-S group (n = 26) and the TD-P group (n = 23) did not differ in previous experience of MS, ability to perform work, or drowsiness during sea voyages. The percentages of subjects reporting cold sweating, nausea, vomiting, and those found to be pale are listed in Table I. During the first 2 days nausea occurred less frequently in the TTS-S group, but there was no difference in the frequency of vomiting. On day 6, 3 days after removal of the patch, vomiting occurred in six subjects (23%) of the TTS-S group and in none of the TD-P group ($P < 0.05$). The scores of subjective feeling of MS are listed in Table II. On the first 2 days, 77% and 81%, respectively, of the subjects in the TTS-S group felt less sick than previously, in contrast with 26% and 39% in the TD-P group (Table III). The overall incidence of dizziness and headache with both TTS-S and TD-P is summarized in Table III. As shown in Table IV, in the TTS-S group the ability to perform everyday work was significantly ($P < 0.03$) better on

Table II. Number of subjects with subjective feelings of MS scored on a VAS

	No. of subjects											
	Pretest		*Day 1*		*Day 2*		*Day 3*		*Day 4*		*Day 6*	
*VAS**	*TTS-S*	*TD-P*	*TTS-S*	*TD-P*	*TTS-S*	*TD-P*	*TTS-S*	*TD-P*	*TTS-S*	*TD-P*	*TTS-S*	*TD-P*
0-1.9	1	0	19	7	21	7	22	18	24	19	22	19
2-3.9	2	3	2	4	3	3	2	1	1	2	3	2
4-5.9	8	8	1	5	1	8	2	4	0	2	0	0
6-7.9	11	8	2	2	1	4	0	0	1	0	0	0
8-10	4	4	2	5	0	1	0	0	0	0	1	0
Missing data	0	0	0	0	0	0	0	0	0	0	0	2
	NS		t = 2.29 P < 0.03		t = 3.39 P < 0.001		NS		NS		NS	

NS = Not significant.
*0 = Not sick; 10 = Severely sick.

Table III. Percentages of subjects with dizziness, headache, and less MS compared with previous experiences

	Day				
	1	*2*	*3*	*4*	*6*
Dizziness					
TTS-S	15	27	12	7	15
TD-P	26	22	9	9	13
Headache					
TTS-S	12*	27	12	12	27
TD-P	43*	43	35	13	13
Less MS					
TTS-S	77†	81†	81		
TD-P	26	39	87		

*P < 0.05; †P < 0.01.

the second day. The VAS scores of drowsiness are also presented in Table IV.

On the first day two subjects and on the second day nine subjects (39%) in the TD-P group required cyclizine tablets. Only one subject from the TTS-S group required cyclizine, on the second day (P < 0.02). The Bourdon-Wiersma test, performed before application of the patch and 24 hours thereafter, revealed no differences between the TTS-S and TD-P groups. At the second testing all subjects performed better, probably because of a learning effect. Ocular side effects (blurred vision and diplopia) were reported during days 2 to 3 in seven subjects and during days 4 to 6 in three subjects in the TTS-S group, compared with three and no subjects, respectively, in the TD-P group.

Cycloplegia was not observed. Dry mouth was reported in the TTS-S group more often than in the TD-P group on the third and fourth days (P < 0.01; Table V). There was no significant difference in decreased alertness. There were 14 reports of local irritation, nine in the TTS-S group and five in the TD-P group. Local tolerability was good in 86%, moderate in 12.7%, and poor in 1.2% of all the applications. Five subjects (6%) lost their patch.

No differences in mean blood pressure and resting pulse rate between the two groups were observed.

DISCUSSION

We evaluated the protection against MS produced by TTS-S 2.5 cm^2 discs during prolonged and continuous exposure to moderate or heavy seas. During the first 2 days, the overall feeling of MS in the TTS-S group was reduced, the difference being maximal on the second day. Reliability of the results is confirmed by the parallel course of the diminished frequency of nausea, an objective end point of MS. The increased ability to perform daily work on the second day reflects the decline of MS.

The efficacy of TTS-S is also demonstrated by the decrease in subjective feelings of MS and the reduced

Table IV. Ability to perform daily work and drowsiness scored on a VAS during the first 2 days of the test period

	Ability to perform daily work (no. of subjects)						Drowsiness (no. of subjects)					
	Pretest		Day 1		Day 2		Pretest		Day 1		Day 2	
VAS*	TTS-S	TD-P	TTS-S	TD-P	TTS-S	TD-P	TTS-S	TD-P	TTS-S	TD-P	TTS-S	TD-P
0-1.9	4	3	19	16	23	12	10	5	16	9	18	9
2-3.9	9	5	1	0	1	6	3	2	2	1	3	2
4-5.9	11	7	3	0	2	2	3	7	2	5	5	7
6-7.9	1	5	1	3	0	2	9	2	4	5	0	3
8-10	1	3	2	4	0	1	1	7	2	3	0	2
	NS		NS		$t = 2.17$, $P = 0.03$		NS		NS		$t = 2.49$, $P < 0.02$	

NS = Not significant.
*0 = Normal capability, no drowsiness; 10 = total incapability, severe drowsiness.

Table V. Percentage of subjects reporting dry mouth

	Moderate		Severe		Total	
Day	TTS-S*	TD-P†	TTS-S*	TD-P†	TTS-S*	TD-P†
1	19	18	7	5	26	23
2	29	23	7	2	36	25
3	24	7‡	10	0‡	34‡	7‡
4	29	9	2	0	31§	9§
6	14	2	0	0	14	2

*n = 42.
†n = 44.
‡$P < 0.01$; §$P < 0.05$.

need for additional cyclizine tablets. In our study the lesser protection represented by the overall feeling of MS on the first day compared with that on the second day can be explained by the time of application of TTS-S before departure (4 hours). Because signs of MS, nausea, and subjective feelings of MS did not diminish in the TD-P group, adaptation did not contribute to the greater protection in the TTS-S group during the second day. From 48 to 72 hours after application, the four principal symptoms of MS occurred less frequently in the TTS-S group than in the TD-P group, but the differences were not significant because of a substantial reduction in symptoms due to adaptation in the TD-P group.

On day 6, 3 days after removal of the TTS-S patch, vomiting occurred in six subjects (23%) in the TTS-S group; all these six had an increased subjective feeling of MS, were nauseated, and were pale. The phenomenon is probably due to a delay in adaptation because of the use of TTS-S.

A withdrawal effect of scopolamine is not likely, because vomiting on the sixth day was not reported under light sea conditions. The absence of signs and symptoms of MS on the fourth day, 1 day after removal of the TTS-S patch, can be ascribed to the lasting effect of effective amounts of scopolamine, as can the persistence of dry mouth reported by one third of the subjects in the TTS-S group 1 day after removal of the TTS-S disc. The lasting presence of scopolamine after removal of the TTS-S may have implications for the reiterated use of TTS-S. A new patch applied within 24 hours after removal of the last one may increase unwanted side effects. The most frequently reported unwanted effect is dry mouth. The persistence of dry mouth 1 day after removal of the TTS-S patch can also be ascribed to the lasting effect of scopolamine. Five of the 88 patches used, all from the TTS-S group, became dislodged. Skin irritation was noted in 17% of all applications, a finding comparable with that of Homick et al.[3] However, skin irritation did not become more frequent after 72 hours of continuous patch use.

We conclude that TTS-S applied at least 4 hours, but

preferably longer, before exposure to moderate or heavy seas offers effective protection against MS during at least 48 hours and probably longer, leading to improved ability to perform daily work during exposure. Dry mouth, the only side effect associated with TTS-S, is mild. Visual disturbances were reported infrequently and never negatively influenced the ability to perform daily work aboard a frigate. Because of the lasting presence of scopolamine, a new TTS-S patch should not be applied within 24 hours after removal of an earlier patch.

We thank A. J. P. Flikweert, M.D., for his encouraging support and CIBA-GEIGY for providing the test medications.

References

1. Brand JJ. The time course of action of (−)-hyoscine after intramuscular injection. Br J Pharmacol **35:**202-208, 1969.
2. Nederlands inst. van Psychologen. Documentatie van Tests en Testresearch in Nederland. Amsterdam: Nederlands inst. van Psychologen, 1969:134.
3. Homick JL, Kohl RL, Reschke MF, Degioanni J, Cintron-Trevino NM. Transdermal scopolamine in the prevention of motion sickness: Evaluation of the time course of efficacy. Aviat Space Environ Med **54:**994-1000, 1983.
4. Hordinsky JR, Beier J, Schwarz E, Martin J. Relative efficacy of the proposed space shuttle antimotion sickness medications. Acta Astraunaut 1982;9:375-83.
5. Parrott AC, Jones R. Effects of transdermal scopolamine upon psychological test performance and feeling states in a double blind placebo controlled trial at sea. Alverstoke: Institute of Naval Medicine 1984; publication no. 3/84.
6. Price NM, Schmitt LG, McGuire J, Shaw JE, Trobough G. Transdermal scopolamine in the prevention of motion sickness at sea. CLIN PHARMACOL THER **29:**414-419, 1981.
7. Reason JT. Motion sickness. Some theoretical considerations. Int J Man-Machine Studies **1:**21-38, 1969.
8. Reason JT, Brand JJ. Motion sickness. London, 1975, Academic Press.
9. Urquhart J. Rate controlled drug dosage. Drugs **23:**207-226, 1982.
10. Wood CD. Antimotion sickness and anti-emetic drugs. Drugs **17:**471-479, 1979.

Oral triamterene disposition

Earlier studies of triamterene (T) disposition in man have reported hydroxytriamterene (T-OH) and hydroxytriamterene sulfate (T-O-SO_3H) conjugate to be the major metabolites. We describe T kinetics through use of an HPLC method and confirm that after hydroxylation, T is rapidly converted to T-O-SO_3H. The intermediate T-OH metabolite could not be detected in urine or plasma. Plasma concentrations of T-O-SO_3H exceeded those of T by sevenfold to 26-fold, whereas concentrations of that metabolite in the urine were fourfold to thirteenfold higher than those of the parent. Renal clearance of T was 314.5 ± 121.6 ml/min, exceeding that of the metabolite, which was 206.1 ± 93.6 ml/min. Coadministration of hydrochlorothiazide increased urine flow and urinary pH, but it did not affect renal clearance of the parent drug or the metabolite. T bioavailability from capsules was poorer and more variable than that from a suspension. Hydrochlorothiazide did not influence the bioavailability of T. (Clin Pharmacol Ther 38:306-312, 1985.)

Fritz Sörgel, Ph.D.,* Jiro Hasegawa, Ph.D., Emil T. Lin, Ph.D., and Roger L. Williams, M.D.** *San Francisco, Calif.*

In 1977 Pruitt et al.[12] described the use of radiolabeled and nonlabeled triamterene (T) to study its fate in healthy subjects. Their conclusion that T is converted to hydroxytriamterene (T-OH) and not further conjugated to the sulfate (T-O-SO_3H) was in contrast to the earlier finding of Lehmann.[10] However, reinvestigation by Grebian et al.[3] and by us[13-16] verified Lehmann's results. Despite the work of Grebian et al., a recent analytic method describes assays only for the unchanged drug and the hydroxy metabolite, rather than for the sulfate conjugate.[20] Presumably, the work of Grebian et al., which was published in German, has not been recognized by American investigators. Gundert-Remy et al.[4] reported T kinetics in healthy subjects through use of the assay methodology of Grebian et al. They reported that large variations in plasma levels after a commercial capsule could be partially explained by variations in bioavailability and perhaps by variability in the analytic procedures used.

From the Department of Pharmacy, School of Pharmacy, University of California.

Presented in part at the Eighty-third Annual Meeting of the American Society for Clinical Pharmacology and Therapeutics, Orlando, Fla., March 17-20, 1982.

Supported in part by National Institutes of Health Grant No. AM 20884.

Received for publication Dec. 30, 1982; accepted May 19, 1985.

Reprint requests: F. Sörgel, Ph.D., Department of Pharmacy, University of California, San Francisco, CA 94143.

*Supported by the German Research Foundation (Deutsche Forschungsgemeinschaft).

**Present address: Eisai Co. Ltd., Tokyo, Japan.

The first part of our study was originally designed to investigate the true disposition of T and the variations in its renal clearance after oral dosing. For this part of the study we used the commercial T capsule available in the United States. Because our data suggested that there was great variability in T bioavailability, we performed a second study of its bioavailability in more detail. Since T is usually administered in combination with another drug, we chose to compare a noncommercial capsule preparation (50 mg T and 25 mg hydrochlorothiazide) with a suspension of the same composition as well as with T alone. This allowed us to study the effect of hydrochlorothiazide on T absorption and the influence of increased urine flow and urinary pH caused by hydrochlorothiazide on renal clearance of T and its metabolite.

METHODS

Subjects. A total of 13 healthy male subjects participated in two studies. Each subject was healthy on the basis of medical history, physical examination, and standard laboratory test results. Subjects took no drugs during the 2 weeks before the study.

In study 1, seven subjects fasted overnight for at least 10 hours before drug dosing. In the morning after voiding completely, subjects took a 100 mg T capsule (Dyrenium, lot no. 257H07; Smith Kline & French Laboratories) with 100 ml tap water. Subjects did not eat breakfast, continuing to fast until 4 hours after drug dosing (except for drinking 100 ml water each hour). No dietary or fluid restrictions were imposed after lunch, which was eaten 4 hours after dosing.

During the study subjects maintained normal physical activity.

In study 2, six different subjects took three oral preparations at weekly intervals in a crossover fashion. Subjects fasted overnight and until 4 hours after dosing. Subjects drank 250 ml water before each dosing. At 2, 6, and 8 hours after dosing, the subjects were given 250 ml fruit juice and at 4 hours after dosing they received a clear liquid lunch. After lunch, fluid intake was not controlled, but subjects were not permitted to engage in strenuous exercise. The subjects followed an identical protocol on three different occasions, taking (A) two noncommercial capsules each containing 50 mg T and 25 mg hydrochlorothiazide; (B) a suspension containing 100 mg T and 50 mg hydrochlorothiazide; and (C) a suspension containing 100 mg T.

In both studies, blood samples (10 ml) were drawn through an indwelling heparinized scalp vein needle 15 times between 0.5 and 24 hours. Voided urine was collected from the intervals −1 to 0 hours, hourly thereafter up to 4 hours after dosing, and from 4 to 6, 6 to 8, 8 to 10, 10 to 14, 14 to 24, 24 to 36, 36 to 48, and 48 to 72 hours. Plasma and urine samples were stored at −20° C until analyzed.

Materials. T was obtained from Mylan Pharmaceuticals, Inc. T-O-SO_3H and T-OH were provided by Dr. Bruce Ettinger, Kaiser Permanente Medical Center, San Francisco, Calif., who originally obtained the compounds from Röhm Pharma. Internal standards were from P. Magnusson, Leo Pharmaceuticals (hydroflumethiazide), from Hoechst Pharmaceuticals, Inc. (furosemide), and from Eli Lilly & Co. (cefamandole). Acetonitrile for the HPLC measurements was glass distilled; butanol, chloroform, methanol, ammonia (25%), and all inorganic salts were analytic reagent grade. High-performance TLC plates were from E. Merck AG.

Drug formulations. In study 2, 100 mg of T crystals were suspended in 60 ml water at the time of dosing; the resulting suspension was swallowed, followed by two 60 ml draughts of water. Hydrochlorothiazide was dissolved in a small amount of 0.25% bicarbonate solution before addition to the T suspension.

Analytic methods. Plasma concentrations of T and T-O-SO_3H were analyzed by a rapid and sensitive HPLC assay developed in our laboratory.[15] In brief, after protein precipitation of plasma samples (0.2 ml) with CH_3CN containing internal standards, drug and metabolite were separated from endogenous compounds on a Micropak-MCH 10 μm column (Varian Instruments Division) with a 30% CH_3CN in 0.02% H_3PO_4 (pH 4.0) solvent system for T and a 12% CH_3CN in 0.02% H_3PO_4 (pH 5.5) solvent system for T-O-SO_3H

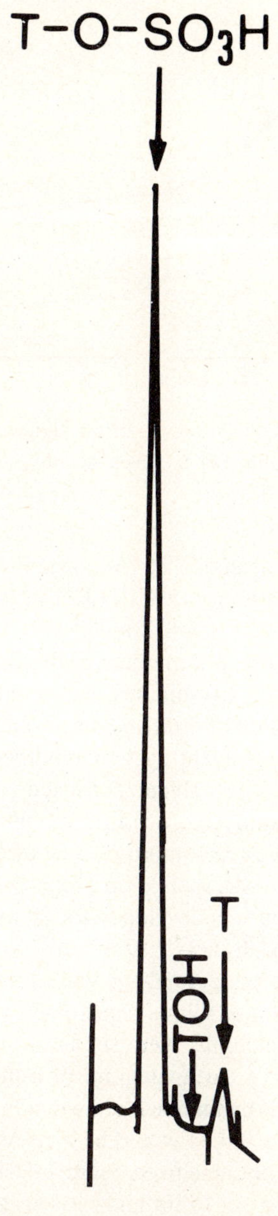

Fig. 1. Representative chromatogram of a urine sample by the TLC technique. *Arrow* for T-OH indicates where T-OH would be located if it were present.

at flow rates of 2.0 ml/min. Measurements were made with a Perkin-Elmer HPLC Series 3 equipped with a flourescence spectrometer and an ultraviolet detector. T, T-O-SO_3H, and furosemide were measured by fluorescence detection at an excitation wavelength of 365 nm and an emission wavelength of 440 nm. In the T plasma assay, rentention times were 4.7 minutes for T and 8.1 minutes for furosemide; in the T-O-SO_3H plasma assay, retention times were 5.1 minutes for T-O-SO_3H and 9.1 minutes for cefamandole (measured

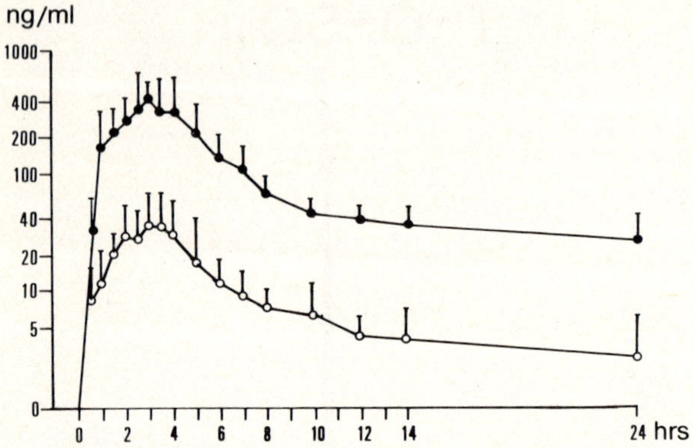

Fig. 2. Plasma concentrations of unchanged T (○) and its T-O-SO_3H metabolite (●) in seven healthy subjects after 100 mg commercial T.

by ultraviolet detection at 254 nm). For urine, a modified solvent system (13% CH_3CN in 0.02% H_3PO_4 at pH 5.3) was used for both T and its metabolite (retention times: T-O-SO_3H, 3.2 minutes; hydroflumethiazide [internal standard], 7.0 minutes; and T, 11.1 minutes).

TLC separation of drug and metabolites in urine samples was by a solvent system modified from that of Pruitt et al.[12] The solvent consisted of a mixture of butanol:methanol:chloroform:ammonia (25%) in a 4:1:1:1 ratio. A maximum of 2 μl of either undiluted or diluted urine was spotted on a high-performance TLC plate. The plate was developed for 30 minutes and then evaporated to dryness. After the compounds were marked on the plate, analysis with fluorescence detection was performed with a densitometer. Excitation and emission wavelengths were set as in the HPLC assay. A representative chromatogram of a urine sample analyzed with this technique is shown in Fig. 1. The arrow indicates where T-OH would be located if it were present. We were not able to measure T-OH even when the instrument was set to its highest sensitivity. From the sensitivity limit of our method we conclude that the excretion of T-OH is <5% of the dose. It is clear from our TLC investigations that T-OH is not the major metabolite excreted in the urine.

For study 1 we used TLC for analysis of T and T-OH in urine. This was done because both Pruitt et al.[12] and Grebian et al.[3] used this methodology and we suspected that the TLC technique used by Pruitt et al. was carried out under inappropriate conditions. In study 2 we used HPLC techniques; again, T-OH was not detectable in plasma and urine.

Data analysis. Plasma AUCs from 0 to 24 hours for T and T-O-SO_3H were calculated by the trapezoidal rule. Renal clearance (CL_R) of T and T-O-SO_3H was estimated as: $CL_R = Ae_{0\text{-}24}/AUC_{0\text{-}24}$, where $Ae_{0\text{-}24}$ is the amount of unchanged drug or metabolite recovered in the urine in 24 hours.

Bioavailability data in study 2 were analyzed by the paired t test. Data from study 2 were compared with data from study 1 by a two-sample t test.

RESULTS

Both in urine and plasma, the only metabolite we detected was T-O-SO_3H. T-OH was not detected in plasma and was found in urine only at concentrations below our quantification limit (1 μg/ml). Mean plasma concentrations of T-O-SO_3H exceeded those of T by sevenfold to 26-fold (mean ratio 13.0 ± 4.8) when the ratios are calculated by dividing the AUCs for T-O-SO_3H by those for T (Fig. 2; Tables I and II). In the urine, the average amount of T-O-SO_3H excreted was approximately four to 13 ($\overline{X}$ = 6.1 ± 2.3) times that of unchanged T (Table III).

In study 1, oral T yielded large coefficients of variation for the AUCs of both T and T-O-SO_3H. The variable bioavailability of T was also manifest in the urinary recovery of T and T-O-SO_3H. Results of study 2 (relative bioavailability) are listed in Tables II and III. The AUCs were higher for the preparations in which T was given as a suspension than when a capsule formulation was taken. Like the T capsule, coefficients of variation were larger for the noncommercial capsule. Urinary excretion data are in accord with a lower bioavailability of T when given as a capsule. Both the AUC and urine data indicate that hydrochlorothiazide did not influence the bioavailability of T.

When average CL_R values (0 to 24 hours) of T and T-O-SO_3H are compared (Table IV), the CL_R of T was found to be higher than that of the metabolite ($P < 0.01$). Coadministration of hydrochlorothiazide did not change the CL_R of T and its metabolite when the two suspension doses (formulations B and C) were compared (Table IV). CL_R of T and T-O-SO_3H were compared over time within subjects (data not shown). No time-dependent variation in CL_R was noted for either compound, even though T induces variation in urine pH (control pH = 5.5 ± 0.4; maximum, at 3 hours = 7.2 ± 0.1) and hydrochlorothiazide causes significant variation in urine flow rate (control = 43.5 ml/hr; maximum, at 1 hour = 342 ± 148 ml/hr).

DISCUSSION

The metabolism and kinetics of T have been the subject of conflicting reports. As early as 1965, Lehmann[10] reported that after hydroxylation T is conjugated to the sulfate, which he had detected in the

Table I. T and T-O-SO_3H kinetics in study 1

Subject No.	Compound	$AUC_{0\text{-}24}$ (ng · hr/ml)	Urinary excretion, 0-72 hr (mg)*	% Dose excreted (T + T-O-SO_3H), 0-72 hr
1	T	298.8	6.54	36.9
	T-O-SO_3-H	2586	30.4	
2	T	187.7	4.56	27.8
	T-O-SO_3-H	1248	23.2	
3	T	225.9	3.65	20.0
	T-O-SO_3-H	2108	16.4	
4	T	98.1	1.80	11.5
	T-O-SO_3-H	1371	9.7	
5	T	346.6	12.13	59.0
	T-O-SO_3-H	3556	46.9	
6	T	213.9	2.22	17.2
	T-O-SO_3-H	3084	15.0	
7	T	99.1	2.97	27.9
	T-O-SO_3-H	2033	24.9	
T				
$\bar{X}$		210.0	4.84	
SD		93.2	3.59	
CV%		44.4	74.1	$\bar{X}$ 28.6
				SD 15.8
T-O-SO_3-H				CV% 55.2
$\bar{X}$		2284	23.8	
SD		852	12.3	
CV%		37.3	51.7	

CV = Coefficient of variation.
*T-O-SO_3-H expressed as T equivalents.

Table II. Plasma AUCs for T and T-O-SO_3H in study 2

Subject No.	$AUC_{0\text{-}24}$ (ng · hr/ml) T A	T B	T C	T-O-SO_3H A	T-O-SO_3H B	T-O-SO_3H C
1	295.7	421.6	435.6	4009	6454	5783
2	510.2	607.0	599.8	6077	7447	8860
3	309.3	640.1	473.9	4135	6317	5005
4	762.7	686.2	595.5	8186	6154	6375
5	61.0	309.5	278.6	1739	6085	7355
6	176.1	437.8	546.8	2504	5433	5195
$\bar{X}$	352.5	517.0	488.4	4442	6315	6429
SD	250.7	148.5	121.9	2368	657	1465
CV%	71.1	28.7	25.0	53.3	10.4	22.8

T: A vs B, $P < 0.05$. T-O-SO_3H: A vs B, $P < 0.05$; A vs C, $P < 0.05$.

A = Noncommercial capsule; B = T/hydrochlorothiazide suspension; C = T suspension; CV = coefficient of variation.

urine. Several years after Lehmann's original finding, Andrasch et al.[1] and Pruitt et al.[12] reported parahydroxylation to be the primary metabolic pathway for T in man, being excreted in the urine. However, Grebian et al.[3] and Gundert-Remy et al.[4] have shown that T is sulfated after hydroxylation. Their findings were substantiated by comparison of the experimental analysis with the synthesized sulfate conjugate. The synthesized

Table III. Urinary excretion of T and T-O-SO_3H in study 2

Subject No.	Urinary excretion, 0-72 hr (mg)*: T A	T B	T C	T-O-SO_3H A	T-O-SO_3H B	T-O-SO_3H C	% Dose excreted, 0-72 hr A	B	C
1	6.48	7.1	7.12	37.4	54.0	48.2	43.9	61.2	55.3
2	6.70	9.34	6.67	38.4	41.3	28.2	45.1	50.6	34.9
3	6.93	7.67	9.18	27.1	34.5	41.6	34.0	42.2	50.8
4	12.48	9.11	10.49	62.2	46.8	47.7	74.7	55.9	58.2
5	1.43	6.19	4.55	20.1	58.3	58.5	21.5	64.5	63.1
6	4.17	5.81	7.38	26.2	44.1	40.8	30.4	49.9	48.2
$\overline{X}$	6.37	7.55	7.57	35.2	46.5	44.2	41.6	54.1	51.8
SD	3.66	1.46	2.06	14.9	8.6	10.1	18.4	8.2	9.8
CV%	57.4	19.4	27.2	42.6	18.4	22.7	44.3	15.2	18.9

A = Noncommercial capsule; B = T/hydrochlorothiazide suspension; C = T suspension; CV = coefficient of variation.
*T-O-SO_3H expressed as T equivalents.

Table IV. CL_R of T and T-O-SO_3H

	CL_R (ml/min): T	T-O-SO_3H
All subjects (n = 13)	314.5 ± 121.6	206.1 ± 93.6
T* (n = 6)	247.0 ± 45.3	156.3 ± 42.3
T with hydrochlorothiazide† (n = 6)	237.2 ± 47.8	159.8 ± 39.3

*Preparation C.
†Preparation B.

conjugate was made available to us and used as a standard in both the TLC and HPLC methods we used. We confirmed the findings of Grebian et al. and Gundert-Remy et al. that T-O-SO_3H is the major metabolite of T.[13-16] The metabolite was found in plasma at concentrations approximately 13 times those of the parent drug. Our mean metabolite-to-parent plasma concentration ratio determined by the HPLC method was slightly higher than the mean ratio of 10 reported by Gundert-Remy et al. with a TLC method. With neither our highly sensitive HPLC procedure nor our TLC technique did we detect T-OH as an intermediate metabolite of T in plasma or urine. We conclude that after hydroxylation of T, the sulfate conjugation step is very rapid. In urine the ratio of sulfate conjugate to unchanged drug averaged 6.1, just slightly higher than the 6.0 ratio reported by Gundert-Remy et al. The difference in ratios in plasma and urine may also be explained by an expected difference in volumes of distribution of T and T-O-SO_3H. Knauf et al.[9] found that the volume of distribution of T was double that of T-O-SO_3H in the rabbit.

CL_R of both T and T-O-SO_3H exceeded the glomerular filtration rate. Hasegawa et al.[5] reported that T is 60% protein bound, while T-O-SO_3H is 90% bound. Thus both are apparently secreted by the renal tubular system. Because CL_R of the metabolite is less than that of the parent, Knauf et al.[7] concluded that the more lipophilic T has a greater affinity for the carrier system in the proximal tubule, but we believe that this may not be the case, since the difference in CL_R may be due to the much higher protein binding of the metabolite than of the parent. If the CL_R of unbound drug and metabolite are calculated (CL_R/fraction free), the unbound clearance of the metabolite would be about 2.5 times that of the parent, indicating a greater affinity of the metabolite for the carrier system.

Kau[6] reported that in perfused kidneys, the percent of the filtered T load that is reabsorbed depends on urine flow and pH. We gave hydrochlorothiazide together with T (study 2) to evaluate the effects of urine flow on the clearance of T and its metabolite. Our data indicate that urine flow and urine pH did not influence the elimination of either T or T-O-SO_3H. With neither a highly sensitive HPLC procedure nor the TLC technique could we detect T-OH as an intermediate metabolite of T in either plasma or urine. We therefore conclude that after hydroxylation, T-OH sulfation is very rapid.

Our data indicate marked variability in T absorption after capsules. The T capsule had poor and variable bioavailability (range 11.5% to 59.0%; $\overline{X}$ = 28.6%). Variable T plasma levels from the T capsule may cause unpredictable effects in the clinical use of the formulation. Hyperkalemia during chronic therapy is probably the most severe side effect and may result from high oral bioavailability (as in subject 5 in study 2). In contrast, refractory diuretic-induced hyperkalemia may result from low T bioavailability (as in subject 4 in study 1). Further studies of absorption and effects of hydrochlorothiazide are needed before conclusions can be made about the clinical use of the new capsule formulation we tested in study 2. The fact that the noncommercial capsule and the commercial T capsule have lower and more variable bioavailability suggests that there is a formulation problem with T capsules. This is supported by recent reports of low and variable bioavailability of Dyazide (Smith Kline & French Laboratories) capsules.[2,17] From our results with a suspension of T, we conclude that hydrochlorothiazide in a 1:2 dose ratio to T does not influence T absorption. Similar results were reported for a 1:1.5 dose ratio.[18]

A most interesting finding reported by Leilich et al.[11] is that in rats, T-O-SO_3H has approximately the same pharmacologic natriuretic activity as T. If this were to be true for man, accurate measurements of T-O-SO_3H would be critical in comparisons of bioavailability and when attempting to correlate dynamics with kinetics. Although others[12,20] have incorrectly identified T-OH[8] as the major metabolite, the data reported as T-OH levels probably reflected hydrolyzed T-O-SO_3H concentrations. Future studies should measure both the parent drug and the potentially active metabolite with an accurate and sensitive method.

In conclusion, T undergoes rapid hydroxylation in the body, followed by immediate conjugation to the sulfate. CL_R of the parent compound is higher than that of its metabolite, indicating that the T metabolite is handled in a unique manner in the kidney, most probably because of the higher degree of binding for T-O-SO_3H than for T. The variable bioavailability of T from commercial preparations should be considered when evaluating the effectiveness of the drug.

We acknowledge the excellent technical assistance of Mrs. Regina Sörgel.

References

1. Andrasch H, Fink T, Schmid E: Uber die Harnausscheidung des Antikaliuretikums Triamteren und seines phenolischen Metaboliten 2,4,7-Triamino-6-p-hydroxy phenylpteridin bei Lebergesunden und kranken mit Leberzirrhose. Z Gastrenterol **9:**240-245, 1971.
2. Blume CD, Williams RL, Upton RA, Lin ET, Benet LZ: Bioequivalence study of a new tablet formulation of triamterene and hydrochlorothiazide. Am J Med **77** (suppl 5A):59-61, 1984.
3. Grebian B, Geissler HE, Mutschler E: Über die Bestimmung von Triamteren, Hydroxytriamteren und Hydroxytriamterenschwefelsäureester in biologischem Material durch direkte Auswertung von Dünnschtchromatogrammen. Arzneimittelforsch (Drug Res) **26:**2125-2127, 1976.
4. Gundert-Remy U, von Kenne D, Weber E, Geissler HE, Grebian B, Mutschler E: Plasma and urinary levels of triamterene and certain metabolites after oral administration to man. Eur J Clin Pharmacol **16:**39-44, 1979.
5. Hasegawa J, Lin ET, Williams RL, Sörgel F, Benet LZ: Pharmacokinetics of triamterene and its metabolites in man. J Pharmacokinet Biopharm **10:**507-523, 1982.
6. Kau ST: Handling of triamterene by the isolated perfused rat kidney. J Pharmacol Exp Ther **206:**701-709, 1978.
7. Knauf H, Kraft H, Leilich G, Mutschler E, Schäfer M, Völger K-D, Vollmer G, Wais U: Untersuchungen zum verbesserten therapeutisschen Einsatz kaliumsparender Diuretika. Therapiewoche **30:**6831-6847, 1980.
8. Knauf H, Mutschler E, Völger K-D, Wais U: Pharmakologische Wirksamkeit von Phase I and Phase II Metaboliten des Triamteren. Arzneimittelforsch (Drug Res) **28:**1417-1420, 1978.
9. Knauf H, Mutschler E, Wais S, Wais U: Verteilungsvolumen und Elimination von Triamteren und seinen wirksmen Metaboliten beim Kaninchen. Arzneimittelforsch (Drug Res) **28:**1414-1416, 1978.
10. Lehmann K: Isolierung und Identifizierung von Stoffwechselprodukten des Triamteren. Arzneimittelforsch (Drug Res) **15:**812-816, 1965.
11. Leilich G, Knauf H, Mutschler E, Völger K-D: Influence of triamterene and hydroxytriamterene sulfuric acid ester on diuresis saluresis in rats after oral and intravenous application. Arzneimittelforsch (Drug Res) **30:**949-953, 1980.
12. Pruitt AW, Winkel JS, Dayton PG: Variations in the fate of triamterene. CLIN PHARMACOL THER **21:**610-619, 1979.
13. Sörgel F, Kiefl H, Hasegawa J, Geldmacher-v Mallinckrodt M, Mutschler E, Benet LZ: Variability of triamterene's fate in the human body. CLIN PHARMACOL THER **31:**D35, 1982.
14. Sörgel F, Lin ET, Benet LZ: Solubility and metabolic fate of triamterene—Not an explanation for triamterene nephrolithiasis. J Pharm Sci. (In press.)
15. Sörgel F, Lin ET, Hasegawa J, Benet LZ: HPLC analysis of triamterene and its major metabolite hydroxytriamterene-sulfate. J Pharm Sci **73:**831-833, 1984.
16. Sörgel F, Lin ET, Mutschler E, Ettinger B, Hropot M, Fabian W, Benet LZ: Triamterene metabolism—A reinvestigation. Presented at the First World Conference on

Clinical Pharmacology and Therapeutics, London, Aug 3-9, 1980. (Abst. No. 542).
17. Tannenbaum PJ, Rosen E, Flanagan T, Crosley AP: The influence of dosage form on the activity of a diuretic agent. CLIN PHARMACOL THER **9:**598-604, 1968.
18. Upton RA, Williams RL, Lin ET, Gee WL, Blume CS, Benet LZ: Absence of a significant pharmacokinetic interaction between hydrochlorothiazide and triameterene when coadministered. J Pharmacokinet Biopharm **12:** 575-586, 1984.
19. Werness PG, Borgert JH, Smith LH: Triamterene urolithiasis: Solubility pK, effect on crystal formation, and matrix binding of triamterene and its metabolites. J Lab Clin Invest **99:**254-262, 1982.
20. Yakatan GJ, Cruz JE: High performance liquid chromatographic analysis of triamterene and *p*-hydroxytriamterene in plasma. J Pharm Sci **70:**949-951, 1981.

Controlled trial of acifran in type II hyperlipoproteinemia

The hypolipidemic effects of acifran were evaluated in a randomized, double-blind, placebo-controlled study of 30 patients with type IIa hyperlipoproteinemia. Plasma lipid and lipoprotein values were determined at baseline (mean of three values), again after a 2-week single-blind period of acifran dosing, and at 2-week intervals during a 10-week period of double-blind drug dosing. At week 8, subjects who received the lower dose of acifran (100 mg t.i.d.) showed significantly lower levels of total and low-density lipoprotein cholesterol and triglycerides compared with their baseline levels ($P < 0.01$) or the placebo group ($P < 0.05$). At week 12, subjects who received the higher dose of acifran (300 mg t.i.d.) had an increase in high-density lipoprotein levels of 16% ($P < 0.01$) and a decrease in the ratio of low- to high-density lipoproteins of 22% compared with their baseline levels ($P < 0.01$). There were no significant differences in lipid responses between the two groups receiving acifran. Transient mild flushing and pruritus were experienced by some subjects, but no subject failed to complete the study because of drug intolerance or side effects. The safety and efficacy demonstrated in this short-term therapeutic trial justify additional long-term studies with acifran. (CLIN PHARMACOL THER 38:313-317, 1985.)

Donald B. Hunninghake, M.D., K. David G. Edwards, M.D., Ph.D., George S. Sopko, M.D., and Robert L. Tosiello, M.S.
Minneapolis, Minn., and New York, N. Y.

A substantial body of evidence supports the positive correlation of elevated plasma total cholesterol (PTC), low-density lipoprotein (LDL) cholesterol, and triglyceride (TG) levels with the risk of coronary heart disease (CHD).[4,12,15] On the other hand, an inverse relationship exists between levels of high-density lipoprotein (HDL) cholesterol and the risk of CHD.[4,7,8] Although diet modification remains a first-line therapy for the patient with hyperlipidemia, there is a continuing need for drugs that will lower cholesterol, TG, and LDL levels and either elevate or have no effect on HDL levels.[9,15,16]

Acifran (4,5-dihydro-5-methyl-4-oxo-5-phenyl-2-furancarboxylic acid) is a novel hypolipidemic agent with potent lipid-lowering properties in both normal and hyperlipidemic rats.[5,6,10,11] In these studies the lipid-lowering activity of acifran closely resembled that of nicotinic acid but not that of clofibrate. Levels of cholesterol, TGs, and LDL were decreased without a lowering of HDL levels or an increase in liver weight or mitochondrial and peroxisomal enzymes; acifran did not affect biliary cholesterol or bile acid concentrations.

The following double-blind study was undertaken to assess the lipid-lowering efficacy and acceptability of two dose levels of acifran compared with placebo in asymptomatic patients with type II hyperlipoproteinemia.

METHODS

Thirty-five outpatients known to have uncomplicated primary type II hyperlipoproteinemia participated. Preliminary testing confirmed that PTC levels were within the required range of 260 to 600 mg/dl or that plasma LDL levels were between 180 and 500 mg/dl. Individuals with diabetes mellitus (fasting plasma glucose level >130 mg/dl), hypothyroidism, renal failure, CHD, or cerebrovascular disease were excluded from study; no subject had received lipid-lowering drugs for at least 8 weeks before the study. Preadmission testing included complete clinical history, physical examination, and laboratory profiles of plasma and urine. The protocol was approved by the Institutional Review Board at the University of Minnesota and written informed consent was obtained from all subjects.

All subjects had previously been instructed and stabilized on phase I of the American Heart Association

From the Lipid Research Clinic, University of Minnesota, Minneapolis, and Ayerst Laboratories, New York.
Received for publication Jan. 18, 1985; accepted May 18, 1985.
Reprint requests to: Donald B. Hunninghake, M.D., Department of Pharmacology, 3-260 Millard Hall, University of Minnesota, Minneapolis, MN 55455.

Table I. Fasting plasma lipid profiles at baseline (average of weeks −2, −1, and 0), week 8 (average of weeks 6 and 8), and week 12 (average of weeks 10 and 12) in subjects with type IIa hyperlipoproteinemia

	PTC (mg/dl)	*LDL cholesterol (mg/dl)*	*HDL cholesterol (mg/dl)*
Placebo (n = 10)			
Baseline	279.0 ± 21.4	198.8 ± 23.2	45.2 ± 10.5
Week 8	283.8 ± 21.8 (1.7%)	198.6 ± 25.6 (−0.1%)	45.1 ± 10.0 (−0.0%)
Week 12	276.0 ± 14.6 (−1.1%)	194.1 ± 20.9 (−2.4%)	45.9 ± 9.5 (1.7%)
Acifran, 100 mg t.i.d. (n = 9)			
Baseline	306.4 ± 49.3	228.1 ± 50.1	44.7 ± 9.7
Week 8	283.7 ± 46.7 (−7.4%)†‡	208.3 ± 50.8 (−8.7%)†‡	48.4 ± 13.0 (8.5%)
Week 12	287.1 ± 49.5 (−6.3%)†	208.2 ± 56.2 (−8.7%)*	52.1 ± 16.2 (16.5%)*‡
Acifran, 300 mg t.i.d. (n = 11)			
Baseline	303.2 ± 39.3	226.0 ± 41.1	42.9 ± 9.8
Week 8	286.4 ± 59.1 (−5.6%)‡	206.1 ± 59.1 (−8.8%)*‡	49.7 ± 9.1 (15.8%)†‡
Week 12	284.1 ± 61.1 (−6.3%)	206.5 ± 59.2 (−8.6%)*	49.9 ± 6.9 (16.1%)†‡

Data are $\overline{X}$ ± SD; numbers in parentheses are the percent change from baseline.
*P < 0.05, †P < 0.01 compared with baseline.
‡P < 0.05 compared with placebo.
§P < 0.001 compared with baseline.

diet or a more stringent diet for at least 3 months before enrolling in our study. Subjects were instructed to maintain their current dietary habits throughout the study. During stage I, which consisted of a 3-week, single-blind pretreatment baseline period (weeks −3 to 0), each subject received one placebo tablet thrice daily. Fasting blood samples were drawn at weekly intervals for analysis of baseline plasma lipid profiles. At the end of stage I, on the basis of fasting plasma TG levels <300 mg/dl, 32 subjects (28 men and four women; age range 31 to 65 years; $\overline{X}$ = 51.5 years) were classified as having type IIa hyperlipoproteinemia, and three subjects (all men; 47, 53, and 64 years old) with fasting plasma TG levels >300 mg/dl were classified as having type IIb hyperlipoproteinemia.[1]

In the following 2-week single-blind period (stage II, weeks 1 to 2), all subjects received acifran, 100 mg t.i.d., during the first week and acifran, 300 mg t.i.d., during the second week. This regimen allowed for evaluation of any minor cutaneous side effects, to which tolerance develops in most cases after the first few doses, thus permitting double-blinding to be maintained during the subsequent stage III.

At stage III, the 10-week double-blind therapy period (weeks 3 to 12), subjects were randomized into one of three treatment groups: group I (n = 11) received placebo thrice daily; group II (n = 11) received acifran, 100 mg t.i.d.; and group III (n = 13) received acifran, 300 mg t.i.d. All tablets used were identical in appearance. During this double-blind therapy period, blood samples were drawn approximately every 2 weeks for analysis of plasma lipid profiles. At all study visits vital signs, body weight, drug adherence determined by tablet count, and laboratory tests including plasma glucose, uric acid, fibrinogen, and liver function tests were performed. All blood samples were collected after a 12-hour overnight fast. Lipid and lipoprotein determinations were carried out by methods of the Lipid Research Clinics.[14]

For each subject, the average of three baseline values (weeks −2, −1, and 0) was subtracted from the week 8 (mean of weeks 6 and 8) or the week 12 (mean of weeks 10 and 12) end points to obtain the variable used to test for within-group and between-group differences. Baseline comparability and differences between groups were tested by ANOVA. Differences within each of the three groups were tested by the two-tailed paired t test.

A separate statistical analysis was performed for subjects who responded to therapy according to the following definitions: PTC responder: a subject with a fall in PTC levels ≥7% (from baseline) at week 8 or ≥10% more at week 12; LDL responder: a subject with a fall in LDL levels ≥10% at week 8 or ≥15% at week 12. A 2 × 2 Fisher's exact test was used to test for differences in numbers of responders in the placebo group and the combined acifran groups.

RESULTS

The random assignment of subjects to acifran or placebo produced comparable groups that did not differ significantly with respect to age, sex, weight, or baseline lipid and lipoprotein concentrations. Thirty-three subjects completed the study; two dropped out for unrelated reasons. The 30 subjects with type IIa hyper-

LDL/HDL ratio	*TG (mg/dl)*
4.63 ± 1.17	175.1 ± 55.9
4.60 ± 1.16 (−0.7%)	200.4 ± 92.4 (14.4%)
4.36 ± 0.99 (−5.8%)*	183.8 ± 73.4 (5.0%)
5.45 ± 2.08	163.4 ± 52.9
4.72 ± 2.06 (−13.4%)†	134.7 ± 44.8 (−17.6%)‡§
4.59 ± 2.50 (−15.8%)*	133.7 ± 53.9 (−18.2%)*‡
5.65 ± 2.21	171.7 ± 69.1
4.33 ± 1.61 (−23.3%)†‡	152.4 ± 56.7 (−11.2%)‡
4.38 ± 1.67 (−22.4%)†‡	138.8 ± 51.6 (−19.2%)*‡

lipoproteinemia who completed the study are described in detail and the three subjects with type IIb hyperlipoproteinemia are briefly summarized.

Administration of acifran to the type IIa group at a dose of 100 mg t.i.d. significantly lowered PTC levels at week 8 and week 12 (P < 0.01 compared with baseline; P < 0.05 compared with placebo for week 8; Table I). The fall in PTC levels was due to a decrease in levels of LDL, which at week 8 were significantly below both baseline levels (P < 0.01) and placebo group levels (P < 0.05). In contrast, acifran, 100 mg t.i.d., caused HDL levels to increase by 8.5% at week 8, and at week 12 a further increase to 16.5% had occurred (P < 0.05 compared with baseline and with placebo). The LDL/HDL ratio declined in both dosage groups and with acifran, 300 mg t.i.d., was 22.4% below baseline levels at week 12 (P < 0.01 compared with baseline; P < 0.05 compared with placebo). TG levels were reduced with both dosages at both week 8 and week 12; this reduction was significant (P < 0.05 compared with placebo group). There were no significant differences between the two acifran groups in any of the lipid and lipoprotein parameters analyzed.

There was no significant change in weight for week 8 or week 12 compared with the baseline values for the Type IIa placebo or acifran groups. The mean change in weight for the various treatments varied from −0.28 to +0.18 kg (−0.62 to +0.40 lb). Adherence to medication based on tablet return was uniformly good for all groups. The mean adherence for week 8 was 90%, 94%, and 97% for the placebo, 100 mg acifran, and 300 mg acifran groups, respectively. Corresponding week 12 values were 94%, 92%, and 93%.

The number of subjects responding to therapy by the defined criteria for PTC and LDL responder status is

Table II. Number (%) of subjects with type IIa hyperlipoproteinemia who responded (PTC and LDL) at week 8 and week 12, and mean percent change from baseline

	No. of subjects responding (%) and mean percent change from baseline	
	PTC responders	*LDL responders*
Week 8	Fell ≥7%	Fell ≥10%
Placebo	1/10 (10%) −7.6%	2/10 (20%) −13.1%
Acifran*	10/20† (50%) −12.9%	10/20 (50%) −17.8%
Week 12	Fell ≥10%	Fell ≥15%
Placebo	0/10 (0%) 0%	0/10 (0%) 0%
Acifran*	8/20† (40%) −13.8%	6/20 (30%) −21.7%

*Data from the two acifran groups (group II, 100 mg t.i.d., and group III, 300 mg t.i.d.) were combined.
†P < 0.05 compared with placebo.

shown in Table II. At both week 8 and week 12, the numbers of PTC responders in the combined acifran groups were significantly (P < 0.05) greater than that in the placebo group. The numbers of LDL responders showed similar trends but did not reach statistical significance. At week 12, PTC responders showed a mean 13.8% decrease in PTC levels from baseline; LDL responders reached a mean 21.7% decrease in LDL levels from baseline.

Lipid profile data from the three subjects with type IIb hyperlipoproteinemia were too limited for statistical analyses; however, acifran did appear to improve lipid profiles in the two subjects who received the drug. The subject who received placebo showed an increase in PTC and LDL levels and LDL/HDL ratios and a decrease in HDL levels during the 10-week double-blind period, while the two receiving acifran showed a decline in PTC, TG, and LDL levels and LDL/HDL ratios and an increase in HDL levels. In the one subject with type IIb hyperlipoproteinemia who received acifran, 300 mg t.i.d., TG levels were reduced from 429 mg/dl at baseline to 175 mg/dl at week 12, and the LDL/HDL ratio decreased from 5.66 at baseline to 4.08 at week 12.

There were no significant changes in the other parameters monitored, including plasma levels of glucose, uric acid, fibrinogen, alkaline phosphatase, SGOT, and SGPT. All subjects were followed for at least 6 months after the end of the study and no adverse effects were noted.

During the stage II single-blind acifran dosing period, 22 of 35 subjects (62.9%) reported flushing and 13 of 35 (37.1%) experienced pruritus. These minor cutaneous effects of acifran were transient and in most cases were associated with the development of tolerance. During the double-blind treatment period, some subjects continued to report flushing on at least one occasion, as follows: group I (placebo): 18%, 0%, and 0% at weeks 4, 8, and 12, respectively; group II (acifran, 100 mg t.i.d.): 9%, 0%, and 40%; and group III (acifran, 300 mg t.i.d.): 23%, 33%, and 42%.

DISCUSSION

In our study acifran was shown to induce modest reductions in levels of PTC and LDL in subjects with type IIa hyperlipoproteinemia. Of primary importance is that, in addition to reducing PTC, TG, and LDL levels, HDL levels were significantly elevated over baseline levels after a 10-week trial with either acifran dosage regimen. A significant improvement in the lipid profile occurred at an acifran dosage of as little as 100 mg t.i.d., which is substantially less than the usual recommended daily dose of nicotinic acid (3 to 6 gm/day).[9] This confirms data from animal studies[6] comparing acifran and nicotinic acid that the minimal lipid-lowering dose of nicotinic acid is five times higher than the effective dose of acifran. Although some subjects receiving acifran experienced transient flushing and pruritus, these side effects were not severe and did not result in any therapy terminations. This is in contrast to the effects of nicotinic acid. Carlson and Oro[2] reported in a trial of the hypolipidemic effects of nicotinic acid that 13% of men and 21% of women failed to complete trials because of intolerance to the side effects. Vessby et al.[16] reported that 32% of patients were unable to take a daily dose of 3 gm nicotinic acid because of subjective side effects. Nicotinic acid therapy has also been associated with a rebound effect when therapy is discontinued.[3] Although we did not analyze lipid levels after the end of the trial, Cayen et al.[5] reported an absence of rebound in plasma levels of free fatty acids and TGs after acifran in rats, in contrast to results after nicotinic acid.

The Lipid Research Clinics Coronary Primary Prevention Trial has shown that reduction in PTC and LDL levels in men receiving cholestyramine results in a significantly lowered incidence of CHD.[15] A 19% reduction in the risk of CHD was associated with each decrement of 8.5% in PTC or of 12.6% in LDL levels. In addition, the small increases in HDL levels (2.8%) that accompanied cholestyramine therapy independently accounted for a 2% reduction in the risk of CHD. The benefits associated with an increase in HDL, combined with a decrease in LDL (or PTC), were more evident in the type II secondary intervention study conducted at the National Institutes of Health.[13] Changes in the HDL/PTC or LDL/HDL ratios were the best predictors of CHD risk.

One cannot directly extrapolate the benefits of reduced risk of CHD from one drug study to another. However, if one postulates that the same degree of reduced risk of CHD observed in the Lipid Research Clinics program can be applied to other studies, then one can calculate a theoretic reduction in risk. At week 12, the 13.8% reduction in PTC levels in responders would result in a 30.8% reduced risk of CHD; similarly, the 21.7% reduction in LDL levels would result in a 32.7% reduced risk of CHD. Also, the mean increase of 16% in HDL levels at week 12 that occurred in all subjects who received acifran would result in an additional 11% reduction in risk of CHD. The projected reduction in CHD risk would be less for all patients who might receive acifran, but would still be substantial.

Acifran was well tolerated without serious adverse effects. The observed changes in plasma lipid and lipoprotein levels suggest that acifran could be associated with a reduction in CHD. Additional studies are needed to define the long-term safety and efficacy of acifran.

References

1. Beaumont JL, Carlson LA, Cooper GR, et al: Classification of hyperlipidaemias and hyperlipoproteinaemias. WHO Bull **43:**891-908, 1970.
2. Carlson LA, Oro L: Effect of treatment with nicotinic acid for one month on serum lipids in patients with different types of hyperlipidemia. Atherosclerosis **18:**1-9, 1973.
3. Carlson LA, Oro L: The effect of nicotinic acid on the plasma free fatty acids—Demonstration of a metabolic type of sympathicolysis. Acta Med Scand **172:**641-645, 1962.
4. Castelli WP, Doyle JT, Gordon T, et al: HDL cholesterol and other lipids in coronary heart disease. The cooperative lipoprotein phenotyping study. Circulation **55:**767-772, 1977.
5. Cayen MN, Kallai-Sanfacon MA, Dubuc J, et al: Effect of AY-25,712 on fatty acid metabolism in rats. Atherosclerosis **45:**281-290, 1982.
6. Cayen MN, Kallai-Sanfacon MA, Dubuc J, et al: Evaluation of the lipid-lowering activity of AY-25,712 in rats. Atherosclerosis **45:**267-279, 1982.
7. Gordon T, Castelli WP, Hjortland MC, et al: High density lipoprotein as a protective factor against coronary heart

disease. The Framingham study. Am J Med **62:**707-714, 1977.

8. Heiss G, Johnson NJ, Reiland S, et al: The epidemiology of plasma high density lipoprotein cholesterol levels. The Lipid Research Clinics Program Prevalence Study Summary. Circulation **62**(suppl 4):116-136, 1980.
9. Hunninghake DB: Pharmacologic therapy for the hyperlipidemic patient. Am J Med **74:**19-22, 1983.
10. Jirkovsky I, Cayen MN: Hypolipidemic 4,5-dihydro-4-oxo-5,5-disubstituted-2-furancarboxylic acids. J Med Chem **25:**1154-1156, 1982.
11. Kallai-Sanfacon MA, Cayen MN, Dubuc J, et al: Effect of AY-25,712 and other lipid-lowering agents on liver catalase and liver carnitine acetyltransferase in rats. Proc Soc Exp Biol Med **173:**367-371, 1983.
12. Kannel WB, Castelli WP, Gordon T, et al: Serum cholesterol, lipoproteins, and the risk of coronary heart disease. The Framingham study. Ann Intern Med **74:**1-12, 1971.
13. Levy RI, Brensike JF, Epstein SE, et al: The influence of changes in lipid values induced by cholestyramine and diet on progression of coronary artery disease: Results of the NHLBI Type II Coronary Intervention Study. Circulation **69:**325-337, 1984.
14. Lipid Research Clinics Program: Manual of Laboratory Operations, vol I, Lipid and Lipoprotein Analysis. Department of HEW publication No. 75-628. Bethesda, Md, 1974, National Heart, Lung, and Blood Institute.
15. Lipid Research Clinics Program: The Lipid Research Clinics Coronary Primary Prevention Trial results. I. Reduction in incidence of coronary heart disease; II. The relationship of reduction in incidence of coronary heart disease to cholesterol lowering. JAMA **251:**351-364, 365-374, 1984.
16. Vessby B, Lithell H, Gustafsson I-B, et al: Pronounced lipoprotein lipid reduction obtained by combined lipid-lowering treatment in patients with atherosclerotic disease. Atherosclerosis **33:**457-477, 1979.

Errata

Please note the following correction in the article by Hicks et al. entitled, "Tolrestat Kinetics" (**36:**493-499, 1984). The t½β values for tolrestat after a single 50 or 200 mg dose were erroneously reported in Table V as 14.5 and 9.0 hours. The correct values are 11.2 and 9.2 hours, respectively.

Also, please note the following correction in the article by White et al. entitled "Alpha-Methyldopa Disposition in Mothers with Hypertension and in Their Breast-Fed Infants" (**37:**387-390, 1985). Lines 3 and 4 of the abstract should list the peak excretion of free α-methyldopa in breast milk as ranging from 0.20 to 1.14 μg/ml.

Kinetics of cocaine distribution, elimination, and chronotropic effects

The pharmacokinetics of cocaine were studied in five subjects with histories of drug abuse who were otherwise healthy. A two-compartment system was used to model the distribution kinetics of the drug. The steady-state volume of distribution averaged 131.8 L or 1.96 L/kg, elimination clearance was 2.10 L/min, and the $t_{1/2}$ was 48 minutes. Cocaine concentrations in a hypothetic biophase were estimated to correlate the chronotropic effects of this drug with its pharmacokinetics. The experimentally determined kinetic parameters indicate that the peak chronotropic effect would occur 7.3 minutes after intravenous bolus injection of cocaine, and that biophase cocaine concentrations would initially accelerate the heart rate by 0.3 bpm for each 1 ng/ml. The kinetic analysis also demonstrated that the chronotropic effects of cocaine decline more rapidly than either plasma levels or biophase concentrations. This progressive attenuation in intensity of the chronotropic effect of a given biophase cocaine concentration could be modeled as a first-order process and is compatible with either the intervention of homeostatic reflex mechanisms or the phenomenon of acute tolerance. (Clin Pharmacol Ther 38:318-324, 1985.)

May J. Chow, M.D., John J. Ambre, M.D., Ph.D., Tsuen Ih Ruo, Ph.D., Arthur J. Atkinson, Jr., M.D., Dennis J. Bowsher, M.D., and Marian W. Fischman, Ph.D. *Chicago, Ill.*

Despite the widespread use of cocaine, there have been few quantitative attempts to relate its disposition kinetics to the responses it elicits. Euphoric and cardiovascular effects decline more rapidly than cocaine plasma levels after a single dose.[9,16] It has been proposed that this phenomenon may represent acute tolerance, because a second dose of cocaine induces a less intense response than the first dose administered 1 hour earlier.[5] Such a phenomenon is of considerable pharmacologic interest and is of critical importance in interpreting cocaine plasma concentrations. These considerations have prompted us to use kinetic modeling techniques to correlate the chronotropic effects of cocaine with its pharmacokinetics, and to extend the application of these techniques to include formal kinetic analysis of the phenomenon of acute tolerance.

From the Clinical Pharmacology Center and Departments of Medicine and Pharmacology, Northwestern University Medical School, and the Department of Psychiatry, Pritzker Medical School, The University of Chicago.

Supported in part by Grants No. RR-00048 and RR-00055 from the Division of Research Resources, No. GM-07842 from the National Institute of General Medical Sciences, National Institutes of Health, and No. DA-01494 from the National Institute on Drug Abuse and by the Louise D. Roland Memorial Fund.

Submitted for publication Feb. 2, 1985; accepted May 18, 1985.

Reprint requests to: John Ambre, M.D., Ph.D., Clinical Pharmacology Center, Northwestern Memorial Hospital, 303 E. Superior St., Chicago, IL 60611.

METHODS

Chemical compounds. Vials containing a sterile, nonpyrogenic, 32 mg/ml solution of cocaine HCl in physiologic saline solution were prepared in the University of Chicago Pharmacy Department. *N*-Propylbenzoylecgonine was synthesized in our laboratory by the method of Jatlow and Bailey[8] and was dissolved in 3:1-methylene chloride:2-propanol to prepare a 40 ng/ml internal standard solution. A 0.7 mol/L carbonate buffer solution was prepared by mixing 26.1 parts K_2CO_3 with 17.5 parts $NaHCO_3$, then dissolving 800 mg of this mixture in 10 ml water. The pH of this buffer solution ranged from 9.5 to 9.7.

Cocaine assay. Concentrations of cocaine in plasma and urine were measured by a modification of the method of Jatlow and Bailey.[8] Into a 10 ml glass-stoppered, conical centrifuge tube were pipetted 1 ml plasma or urine, 0.5 ml buffer, and 6 ml internal standard solution. The tube was shaken and then centrifuged at 700 × g for 5 minutes. The lower layer was then transferred to a second centrifuge tube and 1 ml 50 mmol/L H_2SO_4 was added. Mixing and centrifugation were carried out as before, and the aqueous layer was pipetted into a third centrifuge tube and alkalinized by adding 0.5 ml of the buffer and sufficient carbonate powder mixture to bring the pH to between 9.3 and 9.6. Cocaine was extracted from this aqueous layer by adding 6 ml of 3:1-methylene chloride:2-propanol, then mixing and centrifuging as before. The organic layer was transferred to a 10 ml pear-shaped flask and evaporated at 25 torr in a 20° C water bath. The residue was dissolved in 30 μl 1-propanol and 1.5 to 4.5 μl aliquots were analyzed by gas chromatography.

A Varian model 1400 gas chromatograph (Varian Associates) was fit with a thermionic specific detector and connected to a Linear model 355 recorder (Linear Instrument Corp.). A 2.4 m × 2.2 mm id nickle column packed with 3% SP-2100 DB on 100/120 mesh Supelcoport solid support (Supelco, Inc.) was used for chromatography. The flow of helium carrier gas was 20 ml/min and injector, column, and detector temperatures were 220°, 225°, and 280° C, respectively. The detector was operated with a bead current of 4.5 A and a bias voltage of 4 V.

Cocaine concentrations were determined by comparing the ratio of the height of the cocaine and internal standard peaks measured on each chromatogram with a standard curve that had been prepared by analyzing a series of analytic standards on the same day that the plasma and urine samples were analyzed. These analytic standards were prepared on the day of use by adding 100 μl methanol stock solutions containing cocaine in concentrations of 0.05, 0.1, 0.3, 0.5, 1, 3, and 5 μg/ml to 1 ml drug-free plasma that had been treated with sodium fluoride to inactivate plasma esterase.[11,14] The stock solutions were stable for at least 1 year when stored frozen at − 15° C. Standard curves were linear over a concentration range of 5 to 500 ng/ml. The coefficient of variation was <10% for repeated analysis of standard plasma samples ranging from 10 to 500 ng/ml and between 10% and 20% for samples ranging from 5 to 10 ng/ml.

Study protocol. The study protocol was approved by the Institutional Review Committees of the University of Chicago and of Northwestern University. The subjects were healthy adults whose cocaine use averaged at least once per week for the 2 months before the study. Their medical history was otherwise normal and they had normal physical examination, chest roentgenogram, ECG, and laboratory evaluation (complete blood count, SMA-20, and urinalysis) results. Subjects were clinically well nourished and weighed within 10% of the ideal weight as estimated for their height and sex (Table I).[6] Subjects typically participated in several protocols requiring cocaine administration while hospitalized on the Clinical Research Unit at the University of Chicago Hospital and Clinics. However, they were not allowed other drugs and received no cocaine for 24 hours before the study.

Table I. Subject characteristics

Subject No.	*Age (yr)*	*Sex*	*Height (cm)*	*Weight (kg)*	*% Ideal body weight*
1	36	M	173	76.2	109
2	30	M	175	72.7	100
3	27	F	160	51.6	99
4	34	M	178	74.8	99
5	21	M	165	59.1	96

M = Male; F = female.

On the study day, a heparin lock was placed in a forearm vein for blood sampling and an intravenous line was established in the other arm for drug injection. One milliliter of the cocaine solution, containing 32 mg cocaine HCl, was drawn into a tuberculin syringe for injection. An aliquot of this solution also was reserved for analysis of cocaine concentration and precise determination of the administered dose. The cocaine dose was then infused over 2 minutes. Blood samples were drawn into Vacutainer tubes (Becton-Dickinson) containing sodium fluoride and potassium oxalate at 2, 3, 5, 7, 10, 15, 20, 30, 45, 60, 90, 120, and 180 minutes after the start of the cocaine infusion. All urine voided during the study period was collected, the volume was measured, and aliquots were frozen for later analysis. Blood samples were promptly centrifuged and the plasma was separated and frozen until the day of analysis. Each subject received continuous ECG monitoring during the first 60 to 90 minutes of the study. Heart rate was determined directly from the ECG each time blood was sampled.

Pharmacokinetic analysis. Kinetic analyses were with the SAAM 23 digital computer program developed by Berman and Weiss[3] and implemented on a Control Data Corporation Cyber 170/730 computer. Cocaine distribution and elimination kinetics were modeled with a two-compartment open system with elimination from the central compartment (Fig. 1). The *triangle* in Fig. 1 designates a summer compartment that was used to calculate cocaine renal clearance from the directly proportional relationship between the renal excretion rate and the cocaine plasma concentration.[13] Intercompartmental clearance was calculated by multiplying the volume of the central compartment by the intercompart-

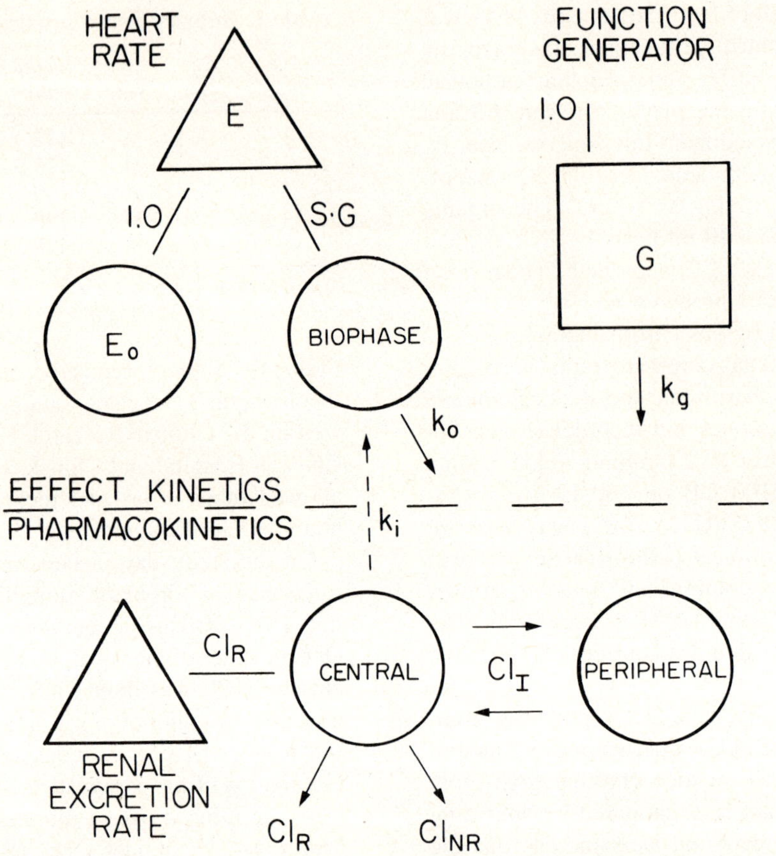

Fig. 1. Multicompartmental system used to model the kinetics of cocaine distribution and elimination and to analyze its effects on heart rate. Cocaine infused into the central compartment distributes to the peripheral compartment at a rate determined by the intercompartmental clearance (Cl_I) and is cleared from the body by both renal (Cl_R) and nonrenal (Cl_{NR}) mechanisms. The renal excretion rate is symbolized by a *triangle* and equals the product of Cl_R and the plasma cocaine concentration. The rise and fall in cocaine concentrations in the biophase compartment is determined by central compartment concentrations and the parameters k_i and k_o. A third parameter (S) relates biophase cocaine concentrations to the initial intensity of chronotropic effect. The intensity of this effect is progressively attenuated by multiplying S by a function (G) that has an initial value of 1.0 and an exponential decay rate (k_g). Observed heart rate (E) is analyzed as the sum of the initial heart rate (E_0) and the chronotropic effect of cocaine.

mental transfer rate directed from that compartment to the peripheral compartment.[12]

The chronotropic effects of cocaine were analyzed with the linear-effect pharmacodynamic model described by Holford and Sheiner,[7] modified so that there was no net cocaine transfer from the central compartment to the hypothetic biophase.[4] The parameters k_i and k_o in Fig. 1 were used to relate the rise and fall of plasma cocaine concentrations to the waxing and waning of cocaine-induced cardioacceleration. The parameter S was used to relate biophase concentrations to the observed intensity of this effect.

Preliminary inspection of the data (Fig. 2) indicated that the intensity of the chronotropic effects of cocaine declined at a greater rate than the decline in plasma concentrations. However, biophase and plasma concentrations of cocaine would be expected to fall in parallel, after distribution equilibrium with the biophase was attained. This indicated a progressive attenuation in the intensity of the observed chronotropic effect of a given biophase concentration of cocaine. We incorporated this in our model as a first-order process using the function generator shown in Fig. 1 as a *square*. The contents of the function generator (G) have an initial

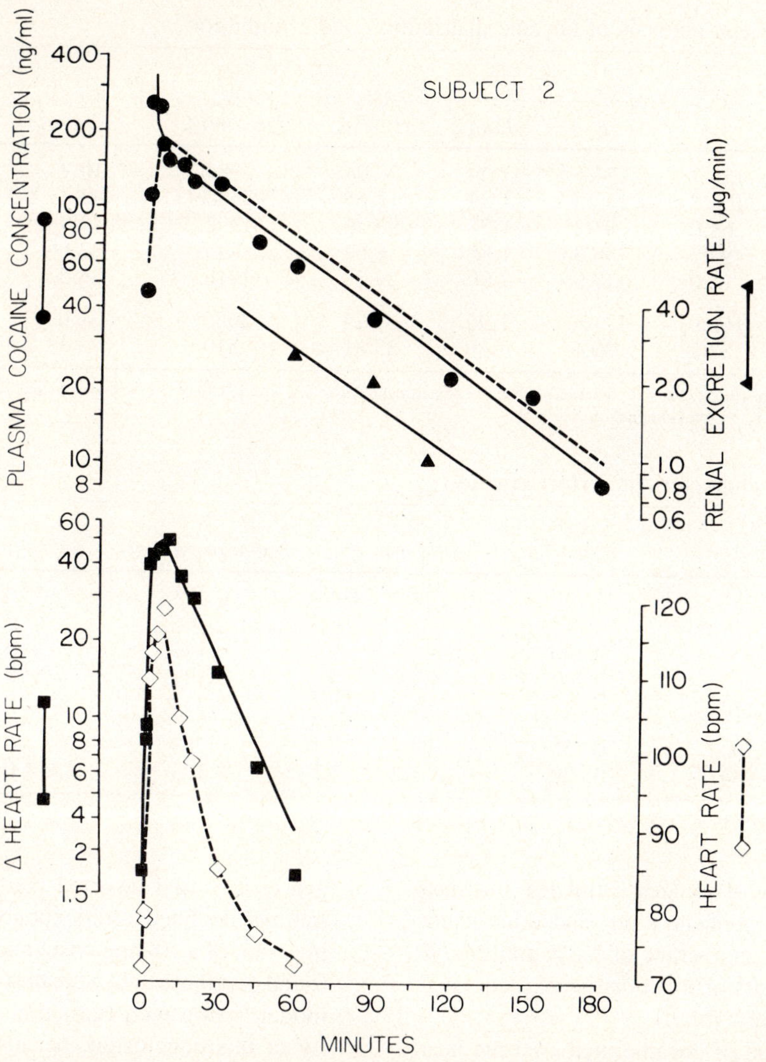

Fig. 2. Kinetic analysis in subject 2 of **(top)** plasma cocaine concentrations *(circles)* and renal excretion rate *(triangles)* and **(bottom)** the observed heart rate *(open diamonds)* and the change in heart rate attributed to the chronotropic effect of cocaine *(solid squares)*. The *lines* are least-squares fits of the measured values. Hypothetic biophase cocaine concentrations are indicated in the top panel by the *dashed line*. Progressive attenuation of the chronotropic effect of cocaine is evident because the acceleration in heart rate declines faster than biophase cocaine concentrations.

value of 1, then fall exponentially at a rate determined by k_g. The chronotropic effects of cocaine (ΔE) are thus described by the equation: $\Delta E = (G)(S)(C_b)$, where C_b is the biophase concentration of cocaine. Accordingly, measured heart rate (E) could be analyzed from the relationship:

$$E = E_0 + [(G)(S)(C_b)] \quad (1)$$

where E_0 is the baseline heart rate before cocaine administration. Kinetic parameters calculated for each subject were also used in a computer simulation to estimate the lag (t_{lag}) that would be observed between instantaneous injection of cocaine and the observation of maximal chronotropic response.

RESULTS

The plasma concentration-time curve from each subject could be resolved into two exponential components and was analyzed with the two-compartment model shown in the lower part of Fig. 1. Parameter values for this model were iteratively adjusted by the computer program to optimize the fit of the theoretic plasma level and urine excretion rate curves to the experimental data, as shown for a representative subject in Fig. 2. For all

Table II. Results of kinetic analysis of cocaine distribution and elimination

Subject No.	V_C (L)	V_P (L)	V_T		CL_I (L/min)	CL_{NR} (ml/min)	CL_R (ml/min)	CL_E (ml/min)	$t_{1/2}$ (min)
			L	L/kg					
1	17.8	156.7	174.5	2.29	20.04	2084	10.7	2095	63
2	28.5	108.8	137.3	1.89	12.65	2585	42.5	2628	42
3	23.2	68.0	91.2	1.77	90.36	1992	42.9	2035	31
4	39.1	99.2	138.3	1.85	6.64	1845	32.6	1878	57
5	20.9	97.0	117.9	2.00	29.26	1818	26.5	1845	45
$\overline{X}$	25.9	105.9	131.8	1.96	31.79	2065	31.0	2096	48
±SD	8.3	32.2	30.6	0.20	33.81	310	13.3	315	13

V_C = Volume of central compartment; V_P = volume of peripheral compartment; V_T = V_C + V_P; CL_I = intercompartmental clearance; CL_{NR} = nonrenal clearance; CL_R = renal clearance; CL_E = total elimination clearance.

Table III. Parameters characterizing effect kinetics

Subject No.	k_i (min^{-1})	k_o (min^{-1})	E_0 (bpm)	S (bpm per ng/ml)	k_g (min^{-1})	t_{lag} (min)
1	2.257	0.127	72.0	0.315	0.0685	3.6
2	1.426	0.112	72.0	0.365	0.0332	8.1
3	1.457	0.190	86.0	0.178	0.0119	8.1
4	0.660	0.200	75.0	0.129	0.0183	3.6
5	3.170	0.147	86.0	0.453	0.0150	13.3
$\overline{X}$	1.794	0.155	78.2	0.288	0.0294	7.3
±SD	0.954	0.039	7.2	0.133	0.0233	4.0

subjects, calculated least-squares estimates and measured cocaine plasma concentrations and urine excretion rates deviated by an average of 5.3% and 23.7%, respectively. The results of this pharmacokinetic analysis are summarized in Table II.

Intravenous injection of cocaine increased the heart rate in all subjects. Heart rate was maximally accelerated within 5 to 15 minutes after the start of the 2-minute injection and returned to baseline within approximately 60 minutes. The kinetics of this effect were analyzed in each subject by Eq. 1 and the model system shown in the upper part of Fig. 1. The mean deviation between computer estimates of heart rate and measured values was 3.3%. Calculated values for the parameters of this system are summarized in Table III, along with estimates of t_{lag}. The constant characterizing the rate of attenuation in intensity of this effect (k_g) had a mean value of 0.0294 $minutes^{-1}$, corresponding to a $t_{1/2}$ of 23.6 minutes.

DISCUSSION

There is continuing controversy as to whether the distribution of intravenous cocaine is best modeled by a one-compartment or a two-compartment system. Kogan et al.[11] first reported that cocaine plasma concentrations declined multiexponentially after intravenous injection of a 100 mg dose, and other investigators have found that these data were best fit by a two-compartment model.[15] However, Barnett et al.[2] questioned the validity of this conclusion, because plasma concentrations defining the terminal exponential component fell below the concentration range for which assay precision and accuracy data were provided. In addition, Javaid et al.[10] found that cocaine plasma concentrations declined monoexponentially after an intravenous injection of 32 mg. Barnett et al. administered 200 mg cocaine doses to two subjects and found that the resulting plasma concentration data were best described by a biexponential function in one subject and by a monoexponential function in the other. Data from three patients who received a 100 mg intravenous dose declined monoexponentially, prompting Barnett et al. and other investigators[10] to speculate that the distribution kinetics of cocaine are dose dependent. However, our results clearly demonstrate that cocaine kinetics are best described by a two-compartment system, even after the administration of a relatively low, 32 mg dose. It is possible that the very rapid distribution phase of this drug was missed in some of the earlier studies because blood samples were not obtained early enough after cocaine administration.

Because of this disparity, the volume of distribution during the terminal phase (V_{area}) was selected for comparison of our estimates of cocaine distribution volume with the results obtained by other investigators after intravenous administration of this drug. Our estimate of 132 L or 1.96 L/kg for the steady-state volume of distribution corresponds to a value of 143 L or 2.11 L/kg for V_{area}. This is greater than the value of 121 L or 1.59 L/kg reported by Barnett et al.[2] but less than the value of 161 L calculated from the results obtained by Javaid et al.[10] Our estimate of 48 ± 13 minutes (±SD) for the mean cocaine $t_{1/2}$ is within the range of 16 to 87 minutes initially reported by Javaid et al.[9] and is similar to the mean values of 58 and 43 minutes subsequently reported by Barnett et al. and by Javaid et al.[10] The value of 2.8 hours reported by Kogan et al.[11] for the cocaine $t_{1/2}$ after intravenous administration is probably not an accurate estimate, given the inability of their assay to reliably measure low cocaine plasma concentrations.[2]

We obtained a mean value of 2.10 L/min for the elimination clearance of cocaine, which lies between the value of 2.45 L/min that can be calculated from the results of Javaid et al.[10] and the value of 1.57 L/min reported by Barnett et al.[2] Our calculated values for renal and nonrenal cocaine clearance indicate that nonrenal mechanisms account for 98.5% of total cocaine elimination. This is consistent with results of a previous study in which between 1% and 15% of an administered cocaine dose was recovered as unchanged drug in the urine of two subjects given cocaine by the intravenous or intranasal route.[1]

Our analysis of the relationship between cocaine plasma levels and observed changes in heart rate is based on a standard pharmacokinetic-pharmacodynamic approach.[7] A linear-effect model was used to estimate two parameters (k_i and k_o) that characterize the waxing and waning of cocaine concentrations in a hypothetic biophase, as well as a parameter (S) that relates these biophase concentrations to the initial intensity of the observed effect. We have not attempted to attach physiologic significance to individual differences in these values, but estimates of S indicate that biophase cocaine concentrations will initially accelerate heart rate by 0.3 bpm, on the average, for each 1 ng/ml.

Further analytic difficulty results from the fact that there is a progressive reduction in the intensity of the observed chronotropic response to a given biophase concentration of cocaine. Javaid et al.[9] first found that the cardiovascular effects of cocaine decline at a faster rate than its plasma concentrations, and other investigators have used a distributed-lags method to analyze the phenomenon.[16] We have taken an alternative approach of using a function generator to attenuate the intensity parameter at an exponentially decreasing rate, and have thus been able to characterize this process while retaining the salient features of conventional effect-kinetic analysis. Our results make no presumption about the mechanistic basis of this phenomenon. However, plausible explanations include triggering of counterregulatory compensatory mechanisms[9] or the development of acute tolerance.[5] In any case, by showing that only a slight modification of standard pharmacokinetic-pharmacodynamic methods is needed to analyze the chronotropic effects of cocaine, we believe that we have demonstrated the feasibility of applying the quantitative rigor of these methods to further mechanistic studies.

References

1. Ambre J, Fischman M, Ruo TI: Urinary excretion of ecgonine methyl ester, a major metabolite of cocaine in humans. J Anal Toxicol **8**:23-25, 1984.
2. Barnett G, Hawks R, Resnick R: Cocaine pharmacokinetics in humans. J Ethnopharmacol **3**:353-366, 1981.
3. Berman M, Weiss MF: SAAM manual. PHS publication No. 1703. Washington, DC, 1967, US Government Printing Office.
4. Eudeikis JR, Henthorn TK, Lertora JJL, Atkinson AJ Jr, Chao GC, Kushner W: Kinetic analysis of the vasodilator and ganglionic blocking actions of *N*-acetylprocainamide. J Cardiovasc Pharmacol **4**:303-309, 1982.
5. Fischman MW, Schuster CR: Acute tolerance to cocaine in humans. Nat Inst Drug Abuse Res Monogr Ser **34**:241-242, 1981. (Abst.)
6. Hamwi GJ: Therapy: Changing dietary concepts. *In* Danowski TS, editor: Diabetes mellitus: Diagnosis and treatment. New York, 1964, American Diabetes Association, Inc, vol 1, pp 73-78.
7. Holford NHG, Sheiner LB: Understanding the dose-effect relationship: Clinical application of pharmacokinetic-pharmacodynamic models. Clin Pharmacokinet **6**: 429-453, 1981.
8. Jatlow PI, Bailey DN: Gas-chromatographic analysis for cocaine in human plasma with use of a nitrogen detector. Clin Chem **21**:1918-1921, 1975.
9. Javaid JI, Fischman MW, Schuster CR, Dekirmenjian H, Davis JM: Cocaine plasma concentration: Relation to physiological and subjective effects in humans. Science **202**:227-228, 1978.

10. Javaid JI, Mahmoud NM, Fischman M, Schuster CR, Davis JM: Kinetics of cocaine in humans after intravenous and intranasal administration. Biopharm Drug Dispos **4:**9-18, 1983.
11. Kogan MJ, Verebey KG, DePace AC, Resnick RB, Mulé SJ: Quantitative determination of benzoylecgonine and cocaine in human biofluids by gas-liquid chromatography. Anal Chem **49:**1965-1969, 1977.
12. Perrier D, Gibaldi M: Clearance and biologic half-life as indices of intrinsic hepatic metabolism. J Pharmacol Exp Ther **191:**17-24, 1974.
13. Stec GP, Ruo TI, Thenot J-P, Atkinson AJ Jr, Morita Y, Lertora JJL: Kinetics of *N*-acetylprocainamide deacetylation. CLIN PHARMACOL THER **28:**659-666, 1980.
14. Stewart DJ, Inaba T, Tang BK, Kalow W: Hydrolysis of cocaine in human plasma by cholinesterase. Life Sci **26:**1557-1564, 1977.
15. Wilkinson P, Van Dyke C, Jatlow P, Barash P, Byck R: Intranasal and oral cocaine kinetics. CLIN PHARMACOL THER **27:**386-394, 1980.
16. Zahler R, Wachtel P, Jatlow P, Byck R: Kinetics of drug effect by distributed lags analysis: An application to cocaine. CLIN PHARMACOL THER **31:**775-782, 1982.

Lack of pharmacokinetic interaction between cimetidine and pirenzepine

The oral administration of pirenzepine (PRZ), an antimuscarinic agent, has a variable effect on gastric acid secretion in patients with duodenal ulcer, and it seems to potentiate cimetidine-induced inhibition of secretion. The possibility of a pharmacokinetic interaction between these drugs was examined in eight patients who received cimetidine and PRZ alone and in combination in a crossover fashion. Cimetidine, 600 mg b.i.d., PRZ, 50 mg b.i.d., or combination therapy were each given for 1 week before the study. Serum samples were serially drawn during each dosing interval for determination of cimetidine and PRZ concentrations by HPLC and RIA, respectively. Cimetidine given alone or with PRZ exhibited diurnal variation, as the peak serum concentration was lower after the nighttime dose than after the morning dose. PRZ showed intersubject variation. However, each drug failed to alter the pharmacokinetic indices of the other. The times to attain the peak serum concentration were not significantly different for cimetidine alone or with PRZ, arguing against an effect of PRZ on gastric motility in the doses we used. The greater and prolonged acid inhibition with the combination of cimetidine and PRZ, therefore, may stem from a synergistic action of both drugs on receptor sites on gastric parietal cells. (Clin Pharmacol Ther 38:325-330, 1985.)

F. Jamali, Ph.D., V. Mahachai, M.D., Paul A. Reilly, Ph.D., and A. B. R. Thomson, M.D. *Edmonton, Alberta, Canada*

Pirenzepine (PRZ) is an antimuscarinic agent shown to inhibit gastric acid secretory volume in animals[15] and in healthy man.[1,21] Its effect is through a peripheral antiacetylcholine property, and hence it is expected to act more selectively than centrally acting drugs on acid secretion.[21] Because of its high hydrophilicity, PRZ has limited gastrointestinal absorption,[14] yet it is highly effective in the treatment of duodenal ulcer.[7,16] Treatment with PRZ, 50 mg b.i.d., has no significant effect on gastric secretion in patients with duodenal ulcer.[22] Other studies have shown reductions of 30% to 60% in total acid output with doses of 50 to 150 mg.[3,8,9,11,18,19,21,24,29] PRZ significantly potentiates the cimetidine-induced reduction in acid secretion.[21,22] For example, other investigators have reported that the combination of 25 mg PRZ with 200 mg cimetidine was more effective under basal conditions and during pentagastrin-stimulated acid secretion than 200 mg cimetidine used alone in patients with duodenal ulcer.[10] At submaximal cimetidine doses, poldine, an anticholinergic agent, has a direct additive effect on the gastric parietal cell.[4] The mechanism of this interaction is not known. Both cimetidine and PRZ are basic drugs and are predominantly eliminated by the kidneys. Cimetidine is known to prolong the residence of other drugs in the body by inhibiting their metabolism[27] or by reducing the renal clearance of basic drugs.[28] PRZ undergoes limited metabolism, and its renal clearance seems to be limited to glomerular filtration.[14] Cimetidine, therefore, may have only a limited effect on PRZ pharmacokinetics. On the other hand, cimetidine absorption has been suggested to be sensitive to changes in gastrointestinal motility.[26] At the doses of PRZ used, it has no effect on gastric motility or emptying.[2,17] We have therefore examined the possibilities of pharmacokinetic drug interaction between cimetidine and PRZ in patients with duodenal ulcer.

From Boehringer Ingelheim (Canada) Ltd. and Faculty of Pharmacy and Division of Gastroenterology, Department of Medicine, University of Alberta and University of Alberta Hospital.

Supported in part by a grant from Boehringer Ingelheim (Canada) Ltd.

Received for publication Feb. 26, 1985; accepted May 18, 1985.

Reprint requests to: Dr. A. B. R. Thomson, 8-104B Clinical Sciences Building, University of Alberta, Edmonton, Alberta T6G 2G3, Canada.

METHODS

Our subjects were eight patients with asymptomatic duodenal ulcer previously documented by endoscopy. There were five men and three women ranging in age from 29 to 63 years. Mean duration of disease was 4.9

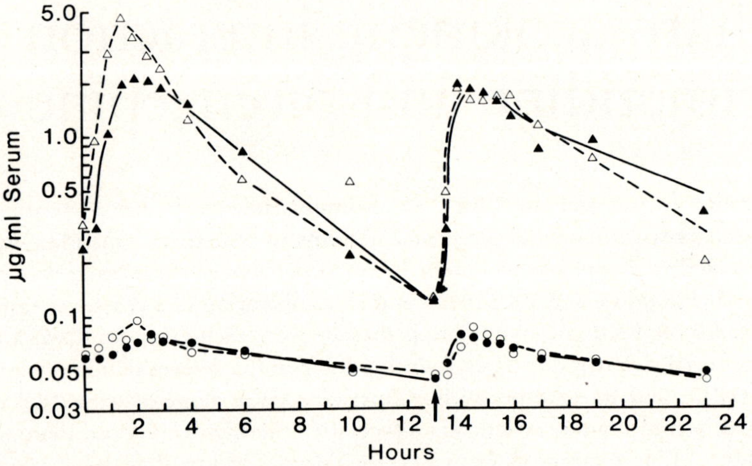

Fig. 1. Serum concentrations of PRZ *(circles)* and cimetidine *(triangles)* given alone *(open symbols)* or in combination *(closed symbols)* in a representative subject (no. 4).

years. Physical examination, routine laboratory tests (complete blood count, serum electrolytes, biochemical profile, and urinalysis), chest x-ray, and ECG results of each subject were normal. The objective and implications of the experiment were explained to each subject and signed informed consent was obtained. The project was approved by the Ethics Committee of the Department of Medicine, University of Alberta. Subjects were not currently taking any other medications or antiulcer medications during the study. Subjects received PRZ, cimetidine, or PRZ plus cimetidine in random sequence. Each regimen was administered for 1 week, after which serum samples were drawn for determinations of cimetidine and PRZ concentrations. Each subject received PRZ tablets (Boehringer-Ingelheim), 50 mg b.i.d. (8 AM and 9 PM), cimetidine tablets (Smith Kline & French Laboratories), 600 mg b.i.d. (8 AM and 9 PM), and the combination of 50 mg PRZ and 600 mg cimetidine twice daily (8 AM and 9 PM). Blood samples were drawn every 30 minutes for 3 hours and then at 4, 5, 10 (after each dosing regimen), and 13 (after morning dosing only). Each sample was immediately centrifuged and the serum was separated and kept frozen until analyzed.

Concentrations of PRZ in serum were measured by a selective RIA.[5] The immunogen was a protein conjugate prepared from human serum albumin and the 5-*N*-propionic acid derivative of PRZ. The antiserum was obtained from one rabbit from a group of four that were identically immunized with the immunogen. All four rabbits had comparable antiserum activities. Four more rabbits were immunized with a conjugate with bovine serum albumin as the carrier protein, which also produced similar antiserum activities. No significant cross-activity was observed from blank plasma or specimens spiked with metabolites of PRZ. The serum cimetidine concentrations were measured by HPLC.[25]

Serum PRZ and cimetidine concentrations were plotted against time and the $t_{1/2}$ of the log-linear portion of the resulting curves was calculated by linear least-square regression. The serum AUC during one dosing interval ($AUC_{0\text{-}t}$) was calculated by the trapezoidal rule. Although our studies have been carried out during steady state, in which $AUC_{0\text{-}t}$ equals the total serum AUC after a single dose ($AUC_{0\rightarrow\infty}$), the latter parameter was calculated as $(AUC_{0\text{-}t}) - (C_0/\beta) + (C_{last}/\beta)$, where β is the rate constant of the log-linear portion of the curve and C_0 and C_{last} are serum drug concentrations taken just before the dose and at the end of the dosing interval. We found this calculation appropriate, as the dosing-time intervals were not equal (13 hours for morning and 11 hours for evening doses).

Statistical significance of the observed differences was tested by the paired Student's t test at $\alpha = 0.05$. Data are expressed as the $\overline{X} \pm SD$.

RESULTS

Fig. 1 shows the PRZ and cimetidine serum concentration curves in a representative of the sample population (subject 4). Tables I to IV contain the calculated pharmacokinetic values in all subjects. There were no diurnal variations in PRZ pharmacokinetics when given alone or in combination with cimetidine, as the values during the two dosing intervals did not differ significantly (Tables I and II). PRZ is absorbed rapidly, as the peak concentration (C_{max}) was attained within 2

Table I. PRZ pharmacokinetics after PRZ alone

Subject No.	t_{max} (hr) AM	t_{max} (hr) PM	C_{max} (ng/ml) AM	C_{max} (ng/ml) PM	$t_{1/2}$ (hr) AM	$t_{1/2}$ (hr) PM	$AUC_{0\rightarrow\infty}$ (ng · hr/ml) AM	$AUC_{0\rightarrow\infty}$ (ng · hr/ml) PM
1	1.0	1.0	64	50	11.80	9.75	369.17*	536.21*
2	1.0	1.0	128	149	21.65	16.13	115.92*	886.04*
3	2.0	1.0	60	67	15.43	20.11	410.11*	614.05*
4	2.0	1.5	93	87	19.21	14.71	109.98†	512.79†
5	1.5	1.5	123	146	12.43	15.48	819.52*	967.82*
6	2.5	1.0	65	58	11.48	18.37	841.74†	412.85†
7	1.0	1.5	57	86	11.65	9.81	443.73*	537.09*
8	2.0	3.0	115	101	11.85	11.70	704.20†	1029.13†
$\overline{X}$	1.61	1.44	88.13	93.00	14.44	14.51	476.80	687.06
SD	0.58	0.68	30.31	37.50	3.96	3.83	288.91	236.42

*Multiexponential plasma concentration-time in postabsorption phase.
†Monoexponential plasma concentration-time in postabsorption phase.

Table II. PRZ pharmacokinetics after PRZ in combination with cimetidine

Subject No.	t_{max} (hr) AM	t_{max} (hr) PM	C_{max} (ng/ml) AM	C_{max} (ng/ml) PM	$t_{1/2}$ (hr) AM	$t_{1/2}$ (hr) PM	$AUC_{0\rightarrow\infty}$ (ng/ml · hr) AM	$AUC_{0\rightarrow\infty}$ (ng/ml · hr) PM
1	2.0	1.0	31	30	*	*	*	*
2	1.0	1.0	101	164	17.70	19.42	196.75†	1067.66†
3	1.0	4.0	45	41	14.29	9.04	438.09†	341.29‡
4	2.5	1.0	80	78	13.64	17.04	471.60‡	715.72†
5	1.0	3.0	82	78	13.53	15.52	897.62‡	899.65‡
6	2.5	1.0	68	49	13.08	20.90	768.00‡	367.98‡
7	1.0	1.5	64	61	10.58	11.54	458.06‡	380.58†
8	2.5	2.0	96	98	9.15	20.61	895.58‡	1211.45†
$\overline{X}$	1.69	1.81	70.87	74.87	13.14	16.30	589.38	712.05
SD	0.75	1.13	24.09	42.29	2.74	4.58	267.34	359.81

*No data because of considerable variation in experimental points.
†Multiexponential plasma concentration-time in postabsorption phase.
‡Monoexponential plasma concentration-time in postabsorption phase.

hours (t_{max}) after dosing (Table I). However, the PRZ serum AUC, which depends on the extent of absorption, showed substantial inter- and intrasubject variations, indicating erratic absorption (Table I).

In five of our eight subjects the plasma PRZ concentration-time curves were multiexponential, as steeper declines preceded the log-linear terminal phases (Table I). PRZ pharmacokinetics also seem to follow characteristics of a multicompartment open model in healthy subjects.[14]

The serum cimetidine concentration-time curve exhibited diurnal variation in pharmacokinetic values, as we have observed.[23] All subjects except nos. 2 and 7 had lower C_{max} values during the night than in the daytime (Table III). The observed mean differences become statistically insignificant if these two subjects are included in the analysis. No significant diurnal variations were found in the observed $AUC_{0\rightarrow\infty}$ values (Table III). However, the serum cimetidine concentration-time curves generally had sharp peaks during the day but not during the night.

After the concomitant administration of PRZ and cimetidine, the pharmacokinetics of both drugs were similar to those observed when either agent was administered alone (Fig. 1; Tables II and IV). Thus there was no indication of an interaction between the two drugs.

DISCUSSION

Hammer and Koss[14] and Bozler and Hammer[6] reported pharmacokinetic indices of PRZ in healthy subjects similar to ours. After a single oral dose of 50 mg PRZ, Bozler and Hammer[6] found a mean t_{max} of 2.0 hours, a C_{max} of 51 ng/ml, and $AUC_{0\text{-}48}$ of 574 ng/hr/ml. Our mean steady-state C_{max} values were 88.1 ±

Table III. Cimetidine pharmacokinetics after cimetidine alone

Subject No.	t_{max} (hr)		C_{max} (μg/ml)		$t_{1/2}$ (hr)		$AUC_{0\to\infty}$ (μg · hr/ml)	
	AM	PM	AM	PM	AM	PM	AM	PM
1	1.5	0.5	4.16	2.56	2.02	4.09	12.85	12.273
2	0.5	1.0	4.68	6.21	2.75	3.33	14.62	14.298
3	2.5	2.0	3.43	0.98	3.36	2.81	15.24	11.042
4	1.5	1.0	4.62	1.85	2.78	2.301	14.25	7.386
5	1.0	2.5	12.26	3.44	2.19	2.01	33.91	14.823
6	1.0	1.0	4.08	2.44	2.29	2.52	11.83	11.572
7	1.0	1.0	5.35	6.08	4.63	4.48	20.47	23.523
8	1.5	1.5	5.61	4.62	3.09	3.03	15.30	17.340
$\bar{X}$	1.31	1.31	5.52	3.52	2.89	3.07	17.31	14.09
SD	0.59	0.65	2.81	1.94	0.85	0.86	7.18	4.82

Table IV. Cimetidine pharmacokinetics after cimetidine in combination with PRZ

Subject No.	t_{max} (hr)		C_{max} (μg/ml)		$t_{1/2}$ (hr)		$AUC_{0\to\infty}$ (μg · hr/ml)	
	AM	PM	AM	PM	AM	PM	AM	PM
1	1.0	1.5	4.61	2.54	3.27	3.68	15.801	21.300
2	1.0	1.0	4.85	7.47	3.28	3.20	12.999	15.647
3	1.0	2.5	4.91	0.43	4.42	2.73	13.503	11.620
4	2.0	1.0	2.08	1.84	2.40	4.44	10.696	10.949
5	1.5	1.5	3.92	3.86	2.16	2.35	17.041	20.055
6	1.0	1.0	3.24	2.27	2.48	3.67	11.853	12.405
7	1.0	1.0	4.71	5.80	3.23	2.76	16.721	24.711
8	1.5	1.5	5.38	3.51	2.64	3.51	19.850	17.614
$\bar{X}$	1.25	1.37	4.21	3.46	2.98	3.29	14.808	16.788
SD	0.38	0.52	1.08	2.26	0.72	0.67	3.063	5.011

30.3 and 93.0 ± 37.5 ng/ml for the morning and evening doses, respectively. The greater C_{max} values observed by us than by Bozler and Hammer[6] indicate accumulation of PRZ after repeated dosing, as is expected with a drug with a log-linear $t_{1/2}$ of approximately 14 hours (Table I). As PRZ was given twice daily, the serum drug concentrations could only be followed for a relatively short period of time, as compared with the $t_{1/2}$ of the postdistribution phase. Nevertheless, our values are similar to those of Bozler and Hammer,[6] who followed PRZ concentrations in serum 48 hours after administration of single doses and reported a mean PRZ $t_{1/2}$ of approximately 11 hours. The similarities observed in PRZ pharmacokinetic indices in healthy subjects[6,14] and in patients with duodenal ulcer may indicate that the disease has no significant influence on the disposition kinetics of this drug.

The underlying mechanism of the observed diurnal variation has not yet been identified. Nevertheless, as the diurnal variation seems to be limited to C_{max} and the pattern of the absorption phase, it is reasonable to suggest that the circadian changes in physiologic factors determining absorption, such as gastrointestinal motility and mesenteric blood flow, may be responsible. Absorption rates of benzodiazepine[12] and sustained-release theophylline[20] also seem to be subject to diurnal variations, as both drugs appear to be absorbed slower during the evening than during the daytime.

Cimetidine is a known inhibitor of the hepatic metabolism of many drugs.[27] Cimetidine-induced inhibition, which seems to take a few days to reach its maximum effect, usually results in a prolongation of the $t_{1/2}$ and thereby increases serum concentration.[30] We concurrently administered cimetidine and PRZ for 1 week to allow time for the onset of the H_2-receptor antagonist action on the metabolic system. Therefore, the lack of a pharmacokinetic interaction cannot be attributed to a limited exposure of subjects to cimetidine. The total body clearance of PRZ is approximately 255 ml/min, which is reported to consist of equal contributions of biliary and renal clearances.[14] Thus, because only 10% of the given dose is metabolized in the body, even if inhibition of the metabolic pathway takes place, the influence on the pharmacokinetic indices of the drug may be insignificant.

It has been shown[28] that cimetidine inhibits tubular secretion of procainamide when the two medications are taken concomitantly. Both of these drugs are predominantly eliminated by the renal route. The renal clearances of approximately 400 ml/min indicate involvement of tubular secretion along with glomerular filtration of these drugs. On the other hand, the renal elimination of PRZ seems to be limited by glomerular filtration.[14] Therefore, inhibition of the renal elimination of PRZ by cimetidine appears unlikely.

As mentioned previously, the diurnal variation in cimetidine pharmacokinetics may be a result of circadian changes in the absorption process. Also, the absorption rate of the drug may depend on gastrointestinal motility.[26] Thus motility-modifying agents such as anticholinergics[13] and metoclopramide[26] may influence the rate of absorption of drugs. PRZ is an antimuscarinic agent with peripheral actions,[21] but at the doses we used, it does not influence normal gastric motility or emptying.[2,19] This is supported by our observation of no significant differences in the pharmacokinetics of cimetidine given alone (Table III) or with PRZ (Table IV). Diurnal variations in cimetidine C_{max} were noted in the same subjects (excluding nos. 2 and 7) in the presence and absence of PRZ. This may indicate that either PRZ elicits no effect on gastrointestinal motility, or that the dose of PRZ we used was not high enough to cause alteration in gastric emptying, thus not influencing cimetidine absorption.

As we noted no pharmacokinetic interactions between cimetidine and PRZ, it seems reasonable to suggest that potentiation of the cimetidine-induced reduction in gastric secretion by coadministration of PRZ[21,22] may be caused by a synergistic action on receptor sites on parietal cells.

We thank Mrs. P. Kirdeikis, Mrs. D. Fisher, Mrs. L. Zuk, Mrs. K. Brunet, and the staff of the Special Investigation Unit of the University of Alberta Hospital.

References

1. Berardi RR, Caplan NB: Agents with tricyclic structures for treating peptic ulcer disease. Clin Pharmacol **2:**425-431, 1983.
2. Bianchi Porro G, Prada A, Parente F, Sangaletti O, Lazzaroni M: The effect of pirenzepine on meal-stimulated gastric acid secretion, gastrin release and gastric emptying. Scand J Gastroenterol **17**(suppl 72):159-161, 1982.
3. Bianchi Porro G, Prada A, Petrillo M, Grossi M: Inhibition of pentagastrin- and insulin-stimulated gastric secretion by pirenzepine in healthy and duodenal ulcer subjects. Scand J Gastroenterol **14**(suppl 57):63-67, 1979.
4. Blackwood WS, Northfield TC: Nocturnal gastric acid secretion: Effect of cimetidine and interaction with anticholinergics. *In:* Burland WL, Simkins MA, editors: Cimetidine. Amsterdam, 1977, Excerpta Medica, chap 11, pp 124-134.
5. Bozler G: The specific radioimmunoassay in pharmacokinetics. Proceedings of the International Symposium on Radioimmunoassay and Related Procedures in Medicine. Vienna, 1978, International Atomic Energy, pp 299-308.
6. Bozler G, Hammer R: An international pharmacokinetic study on pirenzepine following a single oral dose. Scand J Gastroenterol **15**(suppl 66):27-32, 1980.
7. Brunnen H: Pirenzepine and cimetidine in the treatment of peptic ulcer. Scand J Gastroenterol **17**(suppl 71):207-210, 1982.
8. Corinaldesi R, Miglioli M, Daniotti S, Stranghellini V, Borghi E, Barbara L: Inhibition by pirenzepine of nocturnal gastric acid secretion in duodenal ulcer patients. Scand J Gastroenterol **16:**929-931, 1981.
9. Eugenides N, Stockbrugger RW, Hobsley M, Cotton PB: Effect of two doses of pirenzepine on histamine-stimulated gastric acid secretion in man. Scand J Gastroenterol **17**(suppl 72):125-128, 1982.
10. Fritsch WP, Scholten T: Effects of cimetidine, anticholinergic compounds and pirenzepine on gastric secretion. *In* Creutzfeldt W, editor: Cimetidine. Amsterdam-Oxford, 1977, Excerpta Medica, pp 61-69.
11. Fritsch WP, Scholten T, Muller J, Hengels KJ, Hanrath KD: The effect of a 100 mg pirenzepine treatment on acid secretion and serum gastrin. Scand J Gastroenterol **17**(suppl 72):125-128, 1982.
12. Guentert TW: Time-dependence in benzodiazepine pharmacokinetics, mechanism and clinical significance. Clin Pharmacol **9:**203-210, 1984.
13. Hammer R: Muscarinic receptors in the stomach. Scand J Gastroenterol **15:**5-11, 1980.
14. Hammer R, Koss FW: The pharmacokinetic profile of pirenzepine. Scand J Gastroenterol **14**(suppl 57):1-6, 1979.
15. Heathcote BV, Parry M: Pirenzepine selectively inhibits gastric secretion: A comparative pharmacological study between pirenzepine and seven other antiacetylcholine drugs. Scand J Gastroenterol **15**(suppl 66):15-24, 1980.
16. Ishimori A, Yamagata S: Double-blind controlled clinical study of pirenzepine in gastric and duodenal ulcer. *In* Dotevall G, editor: Proceedings of the Symposium on Advances in Gastroenterology with the Selective Antimuscarinic Component Pirenzepine. Amsterdam, 1982, Excerpta Medica, pp 188-204.
17. Jaup BH, Dotevall G: The effect of pirenzepine and *l*-hyoscyamine on gastric emptying and salivary secretion in healthy volunteers. Scand J Gastroenterol **16:**769-773, 1981.
18. Jaup BH, Stockbrugger RW, Dotevall G: Comparison

between the effects of pirenzepine and *l*-hyoscyamine in man. Scand J Gastroenterol **17**(suppl 72):119-122, 1982.

19. Jaup BH, Stockbrugger R, Dotevall G: The effect of pirenzepine on basal, pentagastrin- and insulin-stimulated gastric acid secretion in patients with peptic ulcer disease. Scand J Gastroenterol **14:**621-624, 1979.
20. Jonkman JHG, van der Boon WJV, Balant LP, Schoenmaker R, Holtkamp A: Chronopharmacokinetics of theophylline after sustained release and intravenous administration to adults. Eur J Clin Pharmacol **26:**215-222, 1984.
21. Londong W, Londong V, Prechtl R, Weber T, von Werder K: Interaction of cimetidine and pirenzepine on peptone-simulated gastric acid secretion in man. Scand J Gastroenterol **15**(suppl 66):103-112, 1980.
22. Mahachai V, Reilly P, Thomson ABR: Comparative effects of pirenzepine and cimetidine alone and in combination on 24-hour gastric acidity in duodenal ulcer disease. Clin Ther **7:**98-111, 1984.
23. Mahachai V, Walker K, Jamali F, Navert H, Cook D, Symes A, Thomson ABR: Comparative effects of two cimetidine regimens on 24-hour intragastric acidity in patients with asymptomatic duodenal ulcer. Clin Ther **6:**259-261, 1984.
24. Mignon M, Vatier J, Bauer P, Bonfils S: Effect of pirenzepine on meal-stimulated acid secretion and gastrin release in normal man. Scand J Gastroenterol **17**(suppl 72):145-151, 1982.
25. Soldin SJ, Fingold DR, Fenje PC, Mahon WA: High performance liquid chromatographic analysis of cimetidine in serum. Ther Drug Monitor **1:**371-379, 1979.
26. Somogyi A, Gugler R: Clinical pharmacokinetics of cimetidine. Clin Pharmacokinet **8:**463-495, 1983.
27. Somogyi A, Gugler R: Drug interactions with cimetidine. Clin Pharmacokinet **7:**23-41, 1982.
28. Somogyi A, McLean A, Heinzow B: Cimetidine-procainamide pharmacokinetic interaction in man: Evidence of competition for tubular secretion on basic drugs. Eur J Clin Pharmacol **25:**339-345, 1983.
29. Stockbrugger RW, Jaup BH, Dotevall G: The effect of different doses of pirenzepine on gastric secretion stimulated by modified sham-feeding in man. Scand J Gastroenterol **17**(suppl 72):111-116, 1982.
30. Vestal RE, Thummel KE, Musser B: Cimetidine inhibits theophylline clearance in patients with chronic obstructive pulmonary disease: A study using stable isotope methodology during multiple oral dose administration. Br J Clin Pharmacol **15:**411-418, 1983.

Gastrointestinal absorption as a function of age: Xylose absorption in healthy adults

Xylose oral absorption was examined in 24 healthy male subjects ranging in age from 32 to 85 years. Absorption was evaluated from xylose plasma concentration-time data after administration of a 25 gm po or a 5 gm iv dose. There was no relationship between various estimates of the rate of absorption and age. The absolute oral bioavailability or the extent of xylose absorption showed no relationship to age in our population. In contrast with previous suggestions, xylose absorption does not decline with age. General statements of decreased gastrointestinal absorption efficiency as a function of age may not be correct. (Clin Pharmacol Ther 38:331-335, 1985.)

Stephen L. Johnson, Ph.D., Michael Mayersohn, Ph.D., and Kenneth A. Conrad, M.D. *Tucson, Ariz.*

The elderly, generally but rather arbitrarily considered to be persons >65 years of age, currently represent about 11% of the United States population.[6] The percentage is expected to increase substantially by the end of this century. As a group, geriatric subjects have unique medical needs resulting from a wide variety of chronic age-related illnesses and altered physiologic functions. The provision of optimal drug therapy to the aged individual represents a particular challenge because of age-related changes in drug disposition (i.e., absorption, distribution, and elimination) and the potential for altered inherent response. Therapy is further complicated by the presence of disease and by the concomitant use of several medications. Although about 25% of drug consumption is by the elderly,[6] currently used standard dosing regimens are generally based on data obtained from clinical trials in younger individuals. In recent years attention has been focused on these concerns, but there remains a large void of clinically relevant information.

One process for which there is little quantitative information is that of gastrointestinal (GI) absorption. Changes in the efficiency of that process with age may have considerable impact on both nutritional status and oral drug therapy. Based on a variety of age-related alterations in the GI tract, such as reduced blood flow,[1] reduced gastric emptying rate,[5] and decreased mucosal surface area,[24] one may postulate a priori impaired absorption with age. Indeed, the literature contains numerous suggestions to that effect. At present, however, there is little, if any, rigorous information to support that general conclusion. Many studies that have attempted to examine GI absorption as a function of age suffer from flaws in experimental design or in the methods of data analysis. The two most common errors are incomplete sample collection and the failure to contrast the results from oral dosing with those after intravenous administration. Consideration of the disposition characteristics of the compound and basic principles of pharmacokinetics would, for the most part, avoid those criticisms.

The purpose of our study was to evaluate the GI absorption of D-xylose as a function of age in healthy male subjects. D-Xylose was chosen as a model compound because it has been used for many years in assessing GI absorptive function and because several investigators have previously attempted to use the compound to study absorption in the elderly. Although the mechanism of absorption may be in doubt, D-xylose is thought to be passively absorbed, and it might therefore serve as a useful model for certain nutrients and drugs.

METHODS

Twenty-four healthy male subjects ranging in age from 32 to 85 years participated after giving written

From the Colleges of Pharmacy and Medicine, The University of Arizona.

Supported by Grant No. AG03460 from The National Institute on Aging.

Received for publication March 15, 1985; accepted May 18, 1985.

Reprint requests to: Dr. Michael Mayersohn, College of Pharmacy, The University of Arizona, Tucson, AZ 85721.

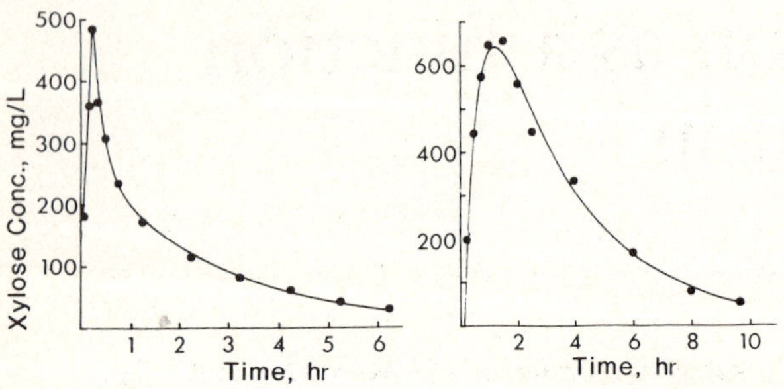

Fig. 1. Representative plot in one subject of xylose plasma concentration as a function of time after a 15-minute 5 gm iv infusion *(left)* and a 25 gm oral solution dose *(right)*. The *solid line* is the nonlinear regression fit of the data.

informed consent. Health status was established by medical history, physical examination, and clinical laboratory findings. Subjects were nonsmokers and were not taking any medication before and during the study.

Subjects fasted overnight before the experiment and for 5 hours after dosing. There were no dietary restrictions after that time, except that foods high in xylose content, such as citrus fruit, were not ingested. Each subject received an intravenous and an oral solution dose of xylose on two separate occasions. Xylose was infused intravenously into an arm vein over 15 minutes, such that exactly 5 gm was delivered in a total fluid volume of 50 ml. An indwelling venous catheter was placed in the arm opposite to the infusion apparatus. Blood samples were drawn through this catheter and collected into Vacutainer tubes (Becton-Dickinson) containing sodium oxalate and sodium fluoride. Heparin was used to prevent clotting. One milliliter of fluid was removed and discarded before the blood sample was drawn and then heparin was reinstilled. Blood was sampled at frequent intervals during and after infusion for a total of 6 hours. Plasma was obtained and immediately frozen until assayed. Complete urine samples were obtained at frequent intervals for a total of 24 hours. Sodium fluoride was added to the urine containers to produce a concentration of about 1% (w/v). Urine volumes were measured and aliquots were frozen until assayed. Subjects drank water during the day to maintain adequate urine output.

Oral doses of xylose were ingested as 25 gm in 200 ml water. The cup was rinsed with an additional portion of water and the contents were swallowed. Blood and urine samples were obtained as described above, except that blood sampling continued for 8 hours. Frozen samples were shown to be stable for at least 2 months based on repeated assays of samples of known concentrations.

Plasma samples were analyzed for D-xylose by a specific capillary column gas chromatographic procedure developed in our laboratory.[10] This assay is sensitive to plasma concentration <10 mg/L. Urine samples were analyzed by a modification of the colorimetric method by Eberts et al.[4] after we demonstrated the reliability of this procedure by a comparison with our gas chromatographic method. Details of that comparison are given elsewhere.[9]

Xylose plasma concentration-time data were analyzed by compartmental and by model-independent area methods. In the former method the data were fit to the appropriate model equation in the form of a sum of linear exponential terms with a nonlinear regression algorithm.[17] All disposition processes were assumed to be first order and the appropriate model was determined by a statistical test.[2] The computer-generated parameter values were used to calculate the total AUC. The equation describing the oral data included a term for a lag time (t_{lag}), which was allowed to vary as a parameter and which represents the time between dose ingestion and the time when xylose first appears in blood. The apparent first-order absorption rate constant was determined by two methods. One value was generated as a parameter in fitting the oral data (Ka_{fit}) and the other value was calculated according to Wagner's modification[23] of a method[14] that attempts to eliminate the influence of distribution on the calculation of the rate constant ($Ka_{L\text{-}R}$).

Model-independent area methods were also applied in data analysis. The value for AUC was determined by a combination of the linear and logarithmic trapezoidal rules and the terminal elimination rate constant was obtained by linear regression of the concentration-time data in the postabsorptive and postdistributive phases.

The absolute systemic oral bioavailability, which reflects the extent of absorption, was calculated as the ratio of the oral to the intravenous AUCs and corrected for differences in dose. That ratio was also corrected for any differences in xylose renal clearance between the oral and intravenous experiments.[13] Xylose renal clearance was calculated as the ratio of the amount of unchanged xylose excreted in urine during 24 hours to the AUC during the same time period.

RESULTS

Xylose plasma concentration-time data after intravenous infusion were best described by a two-compartment model, while the oral data were consistent with a one-compartment model, as no distributive phase

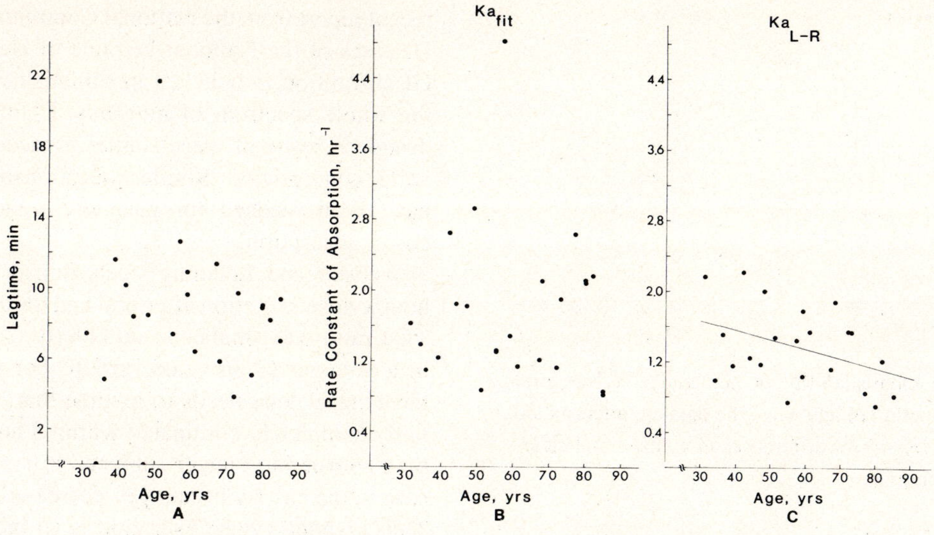

Fig. 2. A, t_{lag} for xylose absorption after a 25 gm oral dose as a function of age. **B,** Xylose absorption rate constant as a function of age after a 25 gm oral dose determined by a nonlinear regression fit of the xylose plasma concentration-time data. **C,** Xylose absorption rate constant as a function of age after a 25 gm oral dose determined by a modification[23] of the method of Loo and Riegelman[14] (r^2 = 0.15).

was apparent. A representative plot from one subject is shown in Fig. 1. Because the longest $t_{1/2}$ was 2.7 hours, the blood sampling and urine collection times were sufficient to describe nearly total xylose elimination.

There was no age-related dependence in the t_{lag} for oral absorption, with values ranging from 0.06 to 0.36 hours (Fig. 2, *A*). Of the two methods used for calculating the apparent absorption rate constant of xylose, Ka_{fit} showed no dependence on age, while Ka_{L-R} demonstrated only a modest relationship (r^2 = 0.15), as illustrated in Fig. 2, *B* and *C*.

The extent of absorption or bioavailability shows no relationship with age in our subject population whether the data are uncorrected or corrected for differences in renal clearance between experiments (Fig. 3).

DISCUSSION

The xylose plasma concentration-time data after oral dosing permit an evaluation of the absorption process as a function of age. The t_{lag} for absorption indicates no relationship with age (Fig. 2). That parameter, which is an indication of the time needed for the onset of absorption, reflects the processes of dissolution, gastric emptying, and transport across the GI membrane into blood. Because xylose is water soluble and was ingested as a solution, any differences in t_{lag} would reflect the two latter processes. With the exception of one subject, the t_{lag} values calculated occurred earlier than the time of the first blood sampling (15 minutes), indicating a rapid onset for absorption. The absence of a relationship between t_{lag} and age does not preclude an age-related difference in gastric emptying, as emptying rate must be evaluated with sequential measurements over time after oral dosing. Several investigators report longer gastric emptying times in the elderly than in younger subjects.[5,19]

A frequently used means of assessing GI absorption rate is with reference to the apparent absorption rate constant. This is a relatively complex parameter for which there are a variety of methods of calculation, each based on some simplifying assumptions. The values obtained from nonlinear regression analysis of the concentration-time data (Ka_{fit}) showed no dependence on age, while the constant determined by another approach (Ka_{L-R}) showed a modest but statistically not significant relationship (r^2 = 0.15; Fig. 2). Therefore, our data suggest no age-related change in the absorption rate of xylose in normal healthy men.

The literature is somewhat confusing with regards to how the absorption rate changes with age. To some extent this reflects the different subject characteristics within and among studies, especially with regard to health status, and the methods used to assess absorption rate. For example, the time required to achieve the maximum plasma concentration after an oral dose is

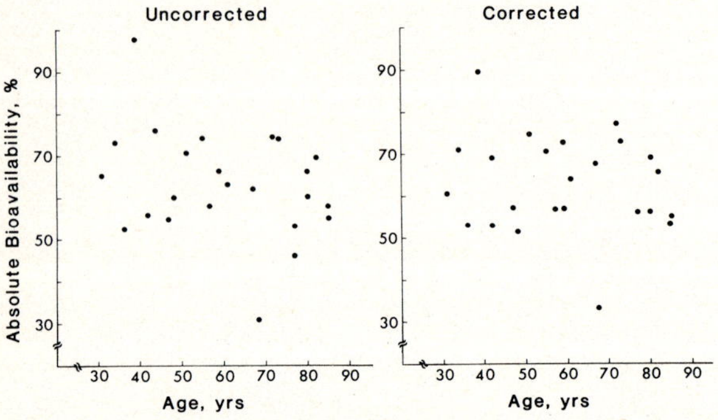

Fig. 3. Absolute bioavailability or percentage xylose oral absorption as a function of age when the data are uncorrected *(left)* or corrected *(right)* for differences in xylose renal clearance between experiments.

often used as an index of absorption rate; however, that value depends on both absorption and elimination constants. If the latter changes with age, as it is known to do for a variety of compounds, then the time to peak concentration will change whether or not there is an alteration in the absorption rate constant. Several studies indicate no change in absorption rate as a function of age for a variety of drugs such as acetaminophen,[22] phenylbutazone,[22] propoxyphene,[16] aspirin,[16] and lorazepam.[7] Our findings with xylose are consistent with those observations. An age-related decrease in the absorption rates of digoxin[3] and propylthiouracil[11] have been reported.

We determined the absolute percentage of the oral dose absorbed (or percent bioavailability) by reference to an intravenous dose. The results (Fig. 3) indicate no age relationship in absorption whether the values for bioavailability are uncorrected or corrected for differences in xylose renal clearances between experiments. Although xylose renal clearance changed little between experiments, it is appropriate to correct for clearance because the method for calculating bioavailability (the ratio of oral to intravenous AUCs) depends in part on the clearance value.

Xylose, which is used clinically to assess malabsorption syndromes, has been used as a model compound to examine absorption in the elderly. Many investigators have suggested an age-related decrease in xylose absorption[8,20,25] based on several observations, including a smaller maximum serum concentration, a longer time to achieve that concentration, and reduced xylose excretion during a urine collection 5 hours after dosing. Those studies, among others, are frequently cited in the literature to support a general statement of diminished GI absorptive capacity with age. Indeed, a recent report from the National Committee on Digestive Diseases of the National Institute of Health stated that GI absorption is believed to diminish with age across the whole spectrum of nutrients.[21] Unfortunately, the design of many of these studies is inadequate to allow valid conclusions. Similar questionable conclusions have been reached for galactose[18] and 3-methylglucose[20] absorption.

Webster and Leeming[25] determined the ratio of 5-hour xylose excretion after oral and intravenous dosing. That ratio was smaller in an elderly (>62 years) than in a younger (<36 years) group. For that ratio to be meaningful, one needs to assume that xylose is essentially completely eliminated within 5 hours. While that may be true in younger subjects, it is probably not the case in the elderly because of decreased renal function. Thus, 5-hour xylose excretion is an incorrect measure of the completeness of absorption, especially in older subjects. This is best illustrated from the work of Kendall,[12] who showed an age-related decrease in the 5-hour xylose excretion after intravenous dosing, which can only be explained by reduced renal function. Several investigators have recognized the importance of renal function in evaluating xylose absorption as a function of age.[15]

Our data on xylose in healthy men indicate no age dependence in absorption over the age range of 32 to 85 years. This finding is in contrast with the generally held belief that GI absorptive function decreases with age. The extent to which our findings reflect the absorption of drugs that are less water soluble than xylose or of nutrients that are chemically more similar to xylose is not known at present. Such studies need to be conducted, but they must be designed with appropriate consideration to a pharmacokinetic analysis.

We gratefully acknowledge the assistance of Mr. James Morse and Mr. J. C. Poe for the preparation of the xylose parenteral solution; Robyn Kessler, R.N., for her assistance during the clinical phase of our study; and Ms. Marla Bliss for assistance with analytic aspects.

References

1. Bender AD: The effect of increasing age on the distribution of peripheral blood flow in man. J Am Geriatr Soc **13:**192-198, 1965.
2. Boxenbaum HG, Riegelman S, Elashoff RM: Statistical estimations in pharmacokinetics. J Pharmacokinet Biopharm **2:**123-148, 1974.
3. Cusack B, Kelly J, O'Malley K, Noel J, Lavan J, Horgan J: Digoxin in the elderly: Pharmacokinetic consequences of old age. CLIN PHARMACOL THER **25:**772-776, 1979.
4. Eberts TJ, Sample RHB, Glick MR, Ellis GH: A sim-

plified, colorimetric micromethod for xylose in serum or urine, with phloroglucinol. Clin Chem **25:**1440-1443, 1979.

5. Evans MA, Triggs EJ, Cheung M, Broe GA, Creasey H: Gastric emptying rate in the elderly: Implications for drug therapy. J Am Geriatr Soc **29:**201-205, 1981.
6. Gibson RM, Mueller MS, Fisher CR: Age differences in health care spending, fiscal year 1976. Soc Secur Bull **40:**3-19, 1977.
7. Greenblatt DJ, Allen MD, Locniskar A, Harmatz JS, Shader RI: Lorazepam kinetics in the elderly. CLIN PHARMACOL THER **26:**103-113, 1979.
8. Guth PH: Physiologic alterations in small bowel function with age—The absorption of D-xylose. Am J Dig Dis **13:**565-571, 1968.
9. Johnson SL, Bliss M, Mayersohn M, Conrad KA: Phloroglucinol-based colorimetry of xylose in plasma and urine compared with a specific gas-chromatographic procedure. Clin Chem **30:**1571-1574, 1984.
10. Johnson SL, Mayersohn M: Quantitation of xylose from plasma and urine by capillary column gas chromatography. Clin Chim Acta **137:**13-20, 1984.
11. Kampmann JP, Mortensen HB, Bach B, Waldorff S, Kristensen MB, Hansen JM: Kinetics of propylthiouracil in the elderly. Acta Med Scand [Suppl] **624:**93-98, 1979.
12. Kendall MJ: The influence of age on the xylose absorption test. Gut **11:**498-501, 1970.
13. Kwan KC, Till AE: Novel method for bioavailability assessment. J Pharm Sci **62:**1494-1497, 1973.
14. Loo JCK, Riegelman S: New method for calculating the intrinsic absorption rate of drugs. J Pharm Sci **57:**918-928, 1968.
15. Mayersohn M: The "Xylose Test" to assess gastrointestinal absorption in the elderly: A pharmacokinetic evaluation of the literature. J Gerontol **37:**300-305, 1982.
16. Melander A, Bodin N-O, Danielson K, Gustafsson B, Haglund G, Westerlund D: Absorption and elimination of D-propoxyphene, acetylsalicylic acid, and phenazone in a combination tablet (Doleron): Comparison between young and elderly subjects. Acta Med Scand **203:**121-124, 1978.
17. Metzler CM: A users manual for NONLIN. Kalamazoo, Mich, 1969, The Upjohn Company.
18. Meyer J, Sorter H, Oliver J, Necheles H: Studies in old age. VII. Intestinal absorption in old age. Gastroenterology **1:**876-881, 1943.
19. Moore JG, Tweedy C, Christian PE, Datz FL: Effect of age on gastric emptying of liquid-solid meals in man. Dig Dis Sci **28:**340-344, 1983.
20. Sapp OL, Sessions JT, Rose JW: Effect of aging on intestinal absorption of sugars. Clin Res **12:**31, 1964.
21. Schnaper HW: Nutrition and aging: Gastrointestinal function changes, their relationship to anatomic and physiological changes and to nutrition in older individuals—Epidemiology and impact. DHEW publication No. (NIH) 79-1887. Washington, DC, 1978, National Commission on Digestive Disease, National Institutes of Health, pp 121-124.
22. Triggs EJ, Nation RL, Long A, Ashley JJ: Pharmacokinetics in the elderly. Eur J Clin Pharmacol **8:**55-62, 1975.
23. Wagner JG: Pharmacokinetic absorption plots from oral data alone or oral/intravenous data and an exact Loo-Riegelman equation. J Pharm Sci **72:**838-842, 1983.
24. Warren PM, Pepperman MA, Montgomery RD: Age changes in small intestinal mucosa. Lancet **2:**849-850, 1978.
25. Webster SGP, Leeming JT: Assessment of small bowel function in the elderly using a modified xylose tolerance test. Gut **16:**109-113, 1975.

Efficacy of clonidine and of methadone in the rapid detoxification of patients dependent on heroin

The efficacy of a rapid detoxification schedule (8 to 10 days) with clonidine or methadone was evaluated in 30 patients addicted to heroin. The dose of study drug was preestablished according to the subject's weight and the amount of opioid consumption, and the total daily dose was reduced by approximately 15% during the study. All subjects completed the detoxification program and stayed in the hospital for at least 12 days. Clonidine and methadone therapies proved to be highly effective. There was a marked reduction in anxiety during opioid detoxification, although subjects' experiences differed according to the drug used. On the day of discharge, subjects who had received methadone still had attenuated withdrawal symptoms, whereas there were no such symptoms in the clonidine group. Muscular aching, flatulence, and daily drowsiness were more common among subjects in the methadone group, while subjects in the clonidine group had more sleep disturbances and weeping. Syncopal episodes and bradycardia occurred more frequently in the clonidine group. (CLIN PHARMACOL THER 38:336-341, 1985.)

Jordi Camí, M.D., Santiago de Torres, M.D., Lluís San, M.D., Àngels Solé, D.Psychol., Diana Guerra, D.Psychol., and Balbina Ugena, R.N.
Barcelona, Spain

Recent studies have established the effectiveness of clonidine, an α-adrenergic blocker, in suppressing the signs and symptoms of opioid withdrawal in methadone, heroin, and synthetic opioid addictions.[4,5,7,8,10,11] Clonidine induces rapid opioid detoxification in subjects receiving methadone maintenance and allows subjects addicted to methadone to begin a maintenance program with naltrexone directly.[2] Ginzburg[3] published a detailed review of the use of clonidine or lofexidine to detoxify from opioids. We used short therapy schedules of clonidine or methadone in a double-blind fashion to detoxify patients addicted to heroin.

METHODS

Our subjects were heroin addicts who had been hospitalized in the Detoxification Unit of our hospital before their admission to a Drug-Free Therapeutic Community. The study was carried out in a voluntary admission unit that accepts individuals under controlled inpatient conditions provided that at discharge, the individual will arrange his or her admission to a Therapeutic Community. In our six-bed unit, patients were treated for physical dependence and associated organic complications, and during the 2-week hospitalization period they received neither telephone calls nor visitors. A series of inpatient regulations including random supervision of urine specimens was established.

Our subjects were heroin addicts of either sex whose age ranged between 18 and 35 years and who fit the DSM-III criteria for opioid dependence. None of the 45 patients originally admitted to the study has psychopathologic antecedents before drug addiction; all were in good health with no signs of cardiovascular disease. Two groups of 15 patients who completed the detoxification program and who remained hospitalized for a minimum of 12 days were studied.

The study was conducted in a double-blind fashion. Subjects were informed that they would be receiving methadone with clonidine placebo or clonidine with methadone placebo, and that they would be opioid free by the end of the study. Six different therapy schedules

From the Division of Clinical Pharmacology, Hospital Nuestra Señora del Mar, Autonomous University of Barcelona.

Supported by a grant from Comisión Asesora de Investigación Científica y Técnica (1391/82) and by Boehringer Ingelheim, S.A., Spain.

Received for publication Dec. 23, 1984; accepted May 21, 1985.

Reprint requests to: Dr. Jordi Camí, Division of Clinical Pharmacology, Hospital Nuestra Señora del Mar, Paseo Maritimo s/n 08003 Barcelona, Spain.

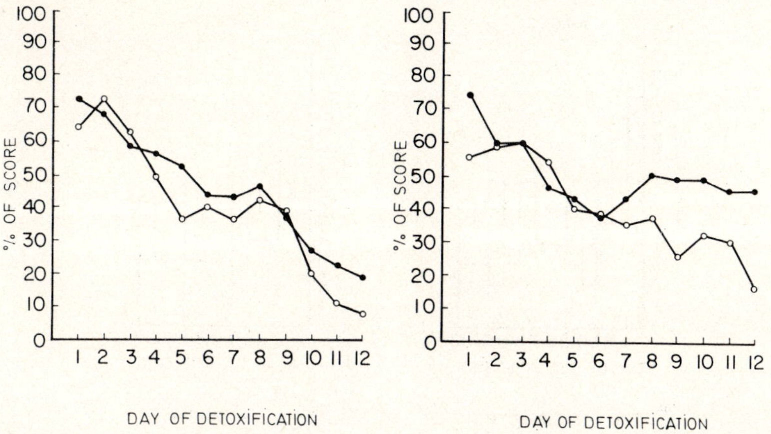

Fig. 1. Percentage of mean positive symptoms of withdrawal *(right)* and adverse effects *(left)* in the methadone (●) and clonidine (○) groups.

Table I. Dosing schedule

Subject weight (kg)	*Daily street heroin use during the last month (gm)*	*Initial daily dose (mg) at 8-hr intervals*	
		Clonidine	*Methadone*
≤55	≤0.25	0.90	30
≤55	>0.25 to <1	1.05	35
≤55	≥1	1.20	40
>55	≤0.25	1.05	35
>55	>0.25 to <1	1.20	40
>55	≥1	1.35	45

were preestablished according to the subject's weight and the amount of heroin consumed during the last month before study (Table I).

On treatment days 1 and 2, subjects received the same total dose (in fragments) at 8 AM and 4 and 12 PM. On day 3 and until discharge, the doses of clonidine and methadone were reduced (by 0.15 mg/day and 5 mg/day, respectively), with a tendency to decrease the afternoon dose first and then the morning dose, and finally the midnight dose. Placebo was given during the days of dose reduction and for 2 days after discontinuance of the drugs. Flunitrazepam, up to 4 mg, and acetylsalicylic acid, up to 2 gm, were prescribed for some subjects for nighttime sedation and analgesia. On the day of discharge (day 13 or 14), 0.4 mg naloxone was injected subcutaneously to evaluate residual withdrawal symptoms. The same team of three counsellors were responsible for the psychotherapeutic support of the subjects during the study.

A team of research nurses measured blood pressure, heart rate, and axillary temperature every day at 9 AM and 5 PM while the subjects lay in bed. The nurses completed daily abstinence rating scales recording the presence or absence of 19 signs associated with opioid withdrawal (craving, muscular aching, spontaneous ejaculation, insomnia, nightmares, hot/cold flashes, anxiety, restlessness, yawning, sweating, weeping, rhinorrhea, mydriasis, gooseflesh, tremors, anorexia, nausea, vomiting, and diarrhea) and 17 items related to adverse effects of the drugs (headache, mental clouding, asthenia, dizziness on standing, dry mouth, vertigo, buzzing, fatigue during walking, discomfort after ingestion, pyrosis, flatulence, salivation, hot flashes, generalized pruritus, visual abnormalities, daily drowsiness, and unstable walk). Subjects completed the State

Table II. Schedule for daily doses of clonidine and methadone

Detoxification day	*Clonidine (mg)*	*No. of subjects*	*Methadone (mg)*	*No. of subjects*
1*	0.780 ± 0.101	15	24.0 ± 3.4	15
2	1.083 ± 0.125	15	35.3 ± 6.4	15
3	0.960 ± 0.095	15	32.3 ± 6.5	15
4	0.810 ± 0.095	15	26.6 ± 4.0	15
5	0.664 ± 0.097	15	21.5 ± 3.5	15
6	0.510 ± 0.095	15	16.3 ± 2.9	15
7	0.360 ± 0.095	15	11.3 ± 2.9	15
8	0.210 ± 0.095	15	6.3 ± 2.9	15
9	0.180 ± 0.067	5	6.6 ± 2.8	3
10	0.150 ± 0.000	1	5.0 ± 0.0	1

Data are the $\overline{X}$ ± SD.
*Dosing began at 4 PM.

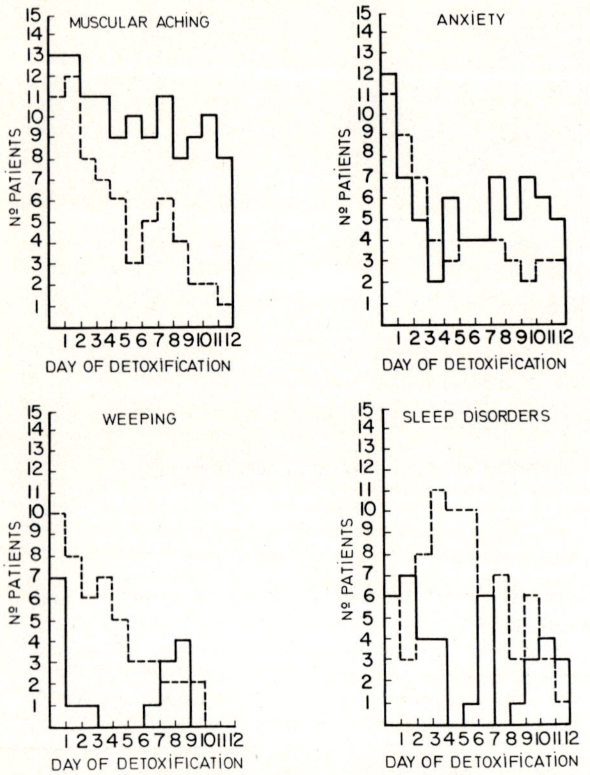

Fig. 2. Number of subjects with signs and symptoms of withdrawal during methadone *(solid line)* and clonidine *(dashed line)* therapy.

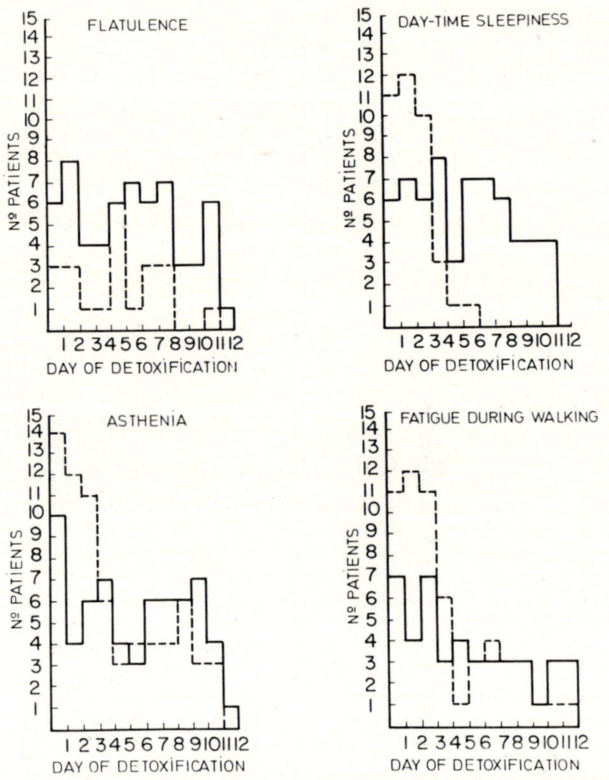

Fig. 3. Number of subjects with adverse effects attributed to methadone *(solid line)* and clonidine *(dashed line)* therapy.

Trait Anxiety Inventory questionnaire to measure state of anxiety[9] on treatment days 1, 2, 3, 4, 7, and 10 at 10 AM. Supervised urine specimens were collected daily for evidence of illicit drug use.

Results were assessed by ANOVA after logarithmic transformation of the original data. The Scheffé test was applied for mean comparisons. The Wilcoxon test and the median test with later application of the chi-square test and Yates correction were used in cases of nonparametric magnitudes. The maximum acceptable error was 5%.

RESULTS

Thirty of the 45 patients who began the study completed the therapy and were discharged drug free. Of the 30, 24 were men and six were women ranging in age from 18 to 30 years ($\overline{X}$ = 23.5 years). Subjects had a mean 4.2-year history of heroin consumption (range 1 to 10 years) and the mean number of previous supervised attempts to discontinue heroin was 1.8. Twelve patients decided that they did not want to continue with the research study and left before treatment day 10; three patients completed therapy after being shifted from the clonidine to the methadone group. Patients who failed to complete the study did not differ from the subjects with respect to previous attempts at detoxification and length of opioid dependence. Our final analysis applies to the 30 subjects (15 in the clonidine group and 15 in the methadone group) who completed the protocol. They were discharged from 12 to 17 days after admission ($\overline{X}$ = 13 days).

On treatment day 1, the initial clonidine dose of 0.78 mg and methadone dose of 24 mg were well tolerated. As shown in Table II, larger doses of drug were required on treatment days 2 and 3; after the first 3 days, however, clonidine and methadone dosage could be reduced (by 15%) and tapered without the recurrence of withdrawal symptoms on treatment day 9 in most subjects. Flunitrazepam was used preferentially by subjects in the clonidine group on the first and last days of detoxification, but the difference as compared with the methadone group was not significant. Acetylsalicylic acid was prescribed to relieve headache and toothache in nine subjects who received methadone and in seven who

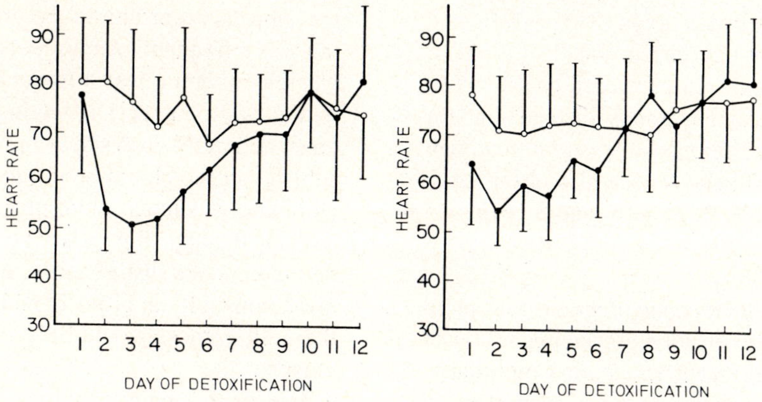

Fig. 4. Mean (± SD) changes in pulse rate at 9 AM *(left)* and 5 PM *(right)* in the clonidine (●) and methadone (○) groups.

received clonidine. On the morning of the day of discharge, 0.4 mg sc naloxone was given to all subjects to assess the extent of withdrawal signs.

The clonidine and methadone regimen we used was effective in rapid opioid detoxification. Fig. 1 shows the percentage of the mean number of abstinence and adverse effects rating scores reported daily. ANOVA showed a significant progressive decrease in the score along the days of detoxification ($F = 13.67$; $P < 0.001$). Although there were no significant differences between the groups, there were significant group-by-treatment day ($F = 3.82$; $P < 0.001$) and group-by-subjects ($F = 8.05$; $P < 0.001$) interactions. In the first half of the study there was a reduction in the score in the methadone group; in the second half, there was a greater reduction in the clonidine group. By the end of the study, withdrawal symptoms had practically disappeared in the clonidine group. An individualized analysis of the items on the withdrawal questionnaire (item/subject/day) revealed differences in some signs (Fig. 2). The subjects who received methadone had higher scores for muscular aching ($\chi^2 = 8.17$; $P < 0.01$) and anxiety ($\chi^2 = 4.17$; $P < 0.05$), whereas in the clonidine group the scores for weeping were higher ($\chi^2 = 6.04$; $P < 0.025$). There were no significant differences between the groups with respect to the remaining items.

In relation to the state of anxiety, ANOVA indicated a progressive decrease in the score along the days of treatment ($F = 11.12$; $P < 0.001$) and a group-by-treatment day interaction ($F = 2.36$; $P < 0.05$). There was a marked reduction in anxiety symptoms during the first days of therapy in the methadone group, whereas the reduction was more progressively constant throughout the treatment period in the clonidine group. In the methadone group, the only differences in daily scores corresponded to treatment days 7 and 12 as compared with treatment day 1; for the clonidine group there were differences between the scores on treatment day 12 and those on treatment days 1, 2, 3, and 4. The naloxone test did not reveal signs of interest in either of the groups.

There was a progressive decrease in the adverse effects rating score during the days of detoxification (Fig. 1), but there were no significant differences between both drugs with respect to days of treatment or to subjects in the groups. Analysis of each item on the adverse effects questionnaire (item/subject/day) revealed differences in some signs (Fig. 3). In the methadone group the scores were higher for flatulence ($\chi^2 = 4.69$; $P < 0.05$) and daily drowsiness ($\chi^2 = 6.04$; $P < 0.025$).

ANOVA of the effect of clonidine and methadone on supine systolic and diastolic blood pressures and heart rate indicated no differences in blood pressure between days, except for systolic blood pressure at 9 AM on treatment day 3 in the clonidine group ($F = 6.17$). During the study four subjects had orthostatic hypotension that was reversed with recumbency. One episode occurred on treatment day 7 in a subject receiving methadone, but there was doubt whether the fall in blood pressure was directly related to the drug. The three other episodes occurred on days 1 and 2 in subjects receiving clonidine. Systolic blood pressure was 50 mm Hg. There was a transient loss of consciousness in one subject receiving clonidine.

ANOVA of mean heart rates showed that at 9 AM and 5 PM there were significant differences between days ($P < 0.001$; in the clonidine group, between the first

5 and the last 5 days), between drugs ($P < 0.001$), and in the drug-by-treatment day interaction ($P < 0.001$). Comparison of mean heart rates for each day between the clonidine and methadone groups showed that for both drugs there was a difference at 9 AM on treatment days 2, 3, 4, and 5. Differences were also observed at 5 PM on treatment days 1, 2, 3, 4, 6, and 8 (Fig. 4).

DISCUSSION

In Spain, most of the therapeutic programs for opioid addicts are based on detoxification procedures followed by admittance to a Drug-Free Therapeutic Community. Methadone maintenance programs have been recently started because of legal regulations and their use is not established.[1] Our study was designed to compare the advantages and disadvantages of methadone and clonidine as agents of detoxification.

Clonidine or methadone therapy enabled 30 of 45 patients to be completely withdrawn from heroin addiction within 12 days after abrupt discontinuation of heroin. Eight of the 12 patients who requested to leave the Unit before treatment day 10 had started the protocol of detoxification with clonidine. Patients who failed to complete the study did not differ from the subjects with respect to previous attempts at detoxification and length of opioid dependence. One might speculate that clonidine precipitated some type of psychopathologic reaction[6] that resulted in a request for voluntary discontinuance of therapy.

The preestablished dosing schedules according to the subject's weight and heroin consumption allowed for maximum individualization of dosages while preserving the double-blind research design. We used these criteria because of the difficulty in ascertaining the seriousness of physical dependence.

Our results show that clonidine and methadone therapies made rapid opioid withdrawal possible, although the personal experiences of each subject differed for each drug. As indicated by the withdrawal rating scores, subjects receiving methadone had mild withdrawal symptoms at the end of the study, while subjects receiving clonidine appeared to be free of withdrawal signs and symptoms. The slowness in the decrease of the abstinence rating scale for the methadone group could be explained by eventual cumulation of the drug.

The adverse effects rating scores were similar in both groups and followed a curve related to the dose of drug. One of the aspects we most carefully considered was the differentiation between signs and symptoms attributable to adverse effects. Our results permit the documentation of the different sensations experienced by the subjects according to the drug used. Muscular aching was a frequent symptom of methadone withdrawal, whereas weeping was a frequent sign during clonidine withdrawal. Subjects receiving methadone had flatulence and daily drowsiness in a higher proportion than subjects in the clonidine group. The sedative effect of clonidine was much more prominent during the first 3 days of therapy. Subjects who received clonidine also had more sleep disturbances, usually manifest as early awakenings. If our protocol had included more subjects, these differences would have probably been more conclusive.

One of the main symptoms of opioid withdrawal is anxiety, a phenomenon difficult to evaluate objectively. Behavioral rating of anxiety recorded by the research nurses suggested the presence of this symptom more frequently in the methadone group. However, the self-rated STAI scale for anxiety completed by the subjects indicates an equal reduction in anxiety for both drugs as therapy progressed.

Clonidine had clinically important effects on blood pressure in three subjects on treatment days 1 and 2, despite the absence of significant differences in supine blood pressures at 9 AM and 5 PM. There were significant differences in the mean heart rates between the clonidine and the methadone groups. This was probably the main difficulty in the use of clonidine under the preestablished conditions of our study. Clonidine should be used in rapid opioid detoxification programs only by experienced personnel who can guarantee close surveillance, especially with respect to cardiovascular complications.

Our results indicate that the use of clonidine or methadone is effective in the treatment of heroin withdrawal syndrome, although symptoms presented by the subjects differed according to the drug used, whether we refer to the alleviation of the signs or symptoms of withdrawal or to the adverse effects related to each type of therapy. Further studies are needed to evaluate the distinct action of opioid substitutes and adrenergic agonists.

We thank the nurses of the Detoxification Unit; J. Aznar, M.D., for skillful statistical advice; J. Cembrano, M.D., of Boehringer Ingelheim, S.A., who supplied the clonidine placebo; and L. Rodriguez, Ph.D., of Laboratorios Dr. Esteve, SA, who supplied the methadone placebo.

References

1. Camí J: A propósito de la orden ministerial por la que se regulan los tratamientos con metadona. Med Clin (Barc) **81:**911-913, 1983.

2. Charney DS, Riordan CE, Kleber HD, Murburg M, Braverman P, Sternberg DE, Heninger GR, Redmond DE: Clonidine and naltrexone. A safe, effective, and rapid treatment of abrupt withdrawal from methadone therapy. Arch Gen Psychiatry **39:**1327-1332, 1982.
3. Ginzburg HM: Use of clonidine or lofexidine to detoxify from methadone maintenance or other opioid dependencies. *In* Cooper JR, editor: Research on treatment of narcotic addiction. National Institute on Drug Abuse, Department of Health and Human Services. Washington, DC, 1983, US Government Printing Office, pp 174-211.
4. Gold MS, Kleber, HD: A rationale for opiate withdrawal symptomatology. Drug Alcohol Depend **4:**419-424, 1979.
5. Gold MS, Pottash ALC, Extein I, Stroul A: Clinical utility of clonidine in opiate withdrawal. *In* Harris LS, editor: Problems of drug dependence. National Institute on Drug Abuse, Department of Health and Human Services. Washington, DC, 1979, US Government Printing Office, pp 95-100.
6. Gold MS, Pottash ALC, Sweeney DR, Kleber HD, Redmond DE: Rapid opiate detoxification: Clinical evidence of antidepressant and antipanic effects of opiates. Am J Psychiatry **136:**982-983, 1979.
7. Gold MS, Redmond DE, Kleber HD: Clonidine in opiate withdrawal. Lancet **1:**929-930, 1978.
8. Kleber HD, Gold MS, Riordan CE: The use of clonidine in detoxification from opiates. Bull Narc **32:**1-10, 1980.
9. Spielberger CD, Gorsuch RL, Lushene RE: Manual for the state-trait anxiety inventory. Palo Alto, Calif, 1970, Consulting Psychologists Press.
10. Washton AM, Resnick RB: Clonidine in opiate withdrawal: Review and appraisal of clinical findings. Pharmacotherapy **1:**140-146, 1981.
11. Washton AM, Resnick RB, LaPlaca RW: Clonidine hydrochloride: a nonopiate treatment for opiate withdrawal. Psychopharmacol Bull **16:**50-52, 1980.

Lack of interaction between verapamil and cimetidine

Nine healthy normal subjects received verapamil, 10 mg iv, before (control) and during cimetidine dosing (300 mg every 6 hours), and verapamil, 120 mg po, twice in the same manner. After intravenous doses, the $t_{1/2}$ ($\bar{X}$ ± SE: control, 3.60 ± 0.40 hours; cimetidine trial, 4.30 ± 0.60 hours), volume of distribution (5.8 ± 0.6 vs. 6.6 ± 0.9 L/kg), and total clearance (19.2 ± 1.5 vs. 18.4 ± 1.6 ml/min/kg) did not change during cimetidine dosing. After oral doses, the $t_{1/2}$ (4.25 ± 0.57 vs. 4.60 ± 0.70 hours), plasma AUC (585 ± 113 vs. 506 ± 82 ng/ml · hr) and absolute bioavailability (35% ± 7% vs. 30% ± 5%) did not differ between control and cimetidine trials, respectively. Five of the subjects also received lidocaine, 25 mg iv, once in the control state and once during the cimetidine regimen described above. Lidocaine clearance fell (665 ± 216 vs. 527 ± 134 ml/min; $P < 0.05$) during cimetidine therapy, resulting in a trend toward a longer $t_{1/2}$ (1.81 ± 0.41 vs. 2.44 ± 0.42 hours; $0.1 > P > 0.05$) with no change in volume of distribution (1.77 ± 0.66 vs. 1.99 ± 0.81 L/kg). Verapamil pharmacodynamics (ECG PR interval, blood pressure, and heart rate) were evaluated after intravenous doses. A decrease in mean arterial pressure (8 ± 1 vs. 9 ± 2 mm Hg) and a reflex increase in heart rate (14 ± 3 vs. 17 ± 2 bpm) were no different in the control and cimetidine trials. After intravenous doses under a sigmoid E_{max} pharmacodynamic model, verapamil concentration at 50% maximal prolongation of PR interval from baseline did not differ between trials (27.5 ± 2.8 [control] vs. 24.3 ± 2.1 ng/ml), nor did the maximal PR prolongation differ (94 ± 36 [control] vs. 85 ± 20 msec). After oral verapamil doses under a linear pharmacodynamic model, the slope of the line describing the verapamil concentration vs. PR interval relationship (1.10 ± 0.61 [control] vs. 1.15 ± 0.56 msec/ng · mg^{-1}) and the defined y-intercept (−37 ± 21 [control] vs. −28 ± 15 msec) were no different between trials. Our data indicate that neither a pharmacokinetic nor a pharmacodynamic interaction between verapamil and cimetidine occur in vivo in man when therapeutic doses are administered, and that verapamil hepatic extraction after oral dosing is not affected by cimetidine, unlike extraction processes described for other high-clearance drugs. (CLIN PHARMACOL THER 38:342-349, 1985.)

Darrell R. Abernethy, M.D., Ph.D., Janice B. Schwartz, M.D., and Elizabeth L. Todd, Ph.D. *Houston, Tex.*

Verapamil, a widely prescribed antiarrhythmic and antianginal drug,[11,17,19] undergoes extensive first-pass hepatic extraction after oral dosing[22,31] and is biotransformed to a number of metabolites.[7,10,20] A major route of metabolic clearance is by oxidative *N*-demethylation to norverapamil. It has therefore been predicted that cimetidine, which inhibits hepatic drug oxidation in vivo by competitive inhibition of the cytochrome P-450 hepatic drug metabolizing enzyme system[21,26,27] and additionally impairs hepatic extraction of drugs with high first-pass hepatic extraction,[3,5,8,9] would have a demonstrable pharmacokinetic drug-drug interaction with verapamil.[23,24] Such an interaction has recently been reported,[26] but no significant changes in verapamil pharmacodynamics could be demonstrated during concurrent cimetidine dosing. Verapamil-induced inhibition of arteriovenous (AV) nodal conduction has been described as a concentration-dependent process, with a good correlation between verapamil plasma concentration and AV nodal conduction delay after single verapamil doses.[6] This AV conduction delay has been measured by a surface ECG and therefore can be repetitively measured and related to simultaneous drug plasma concentrations.[6,17,22]

From the Section on Hypertension-Clinical Pharmacology, Department of Medicine, Baylor College of Medicine.

Supported in part by Grant No. AM-34479 from the United States Public Health Service.

Received for publication Feb. 7, 1985; accepted May 26, 1985.

Reprint requests to: Darrell R. Abernethy, M.D., Ph.D., Section on Hypertension/Clinical Pharmacology, Department of Medicine, Baylor College of Medicine, Suite 826E, Houston, TX 77030.

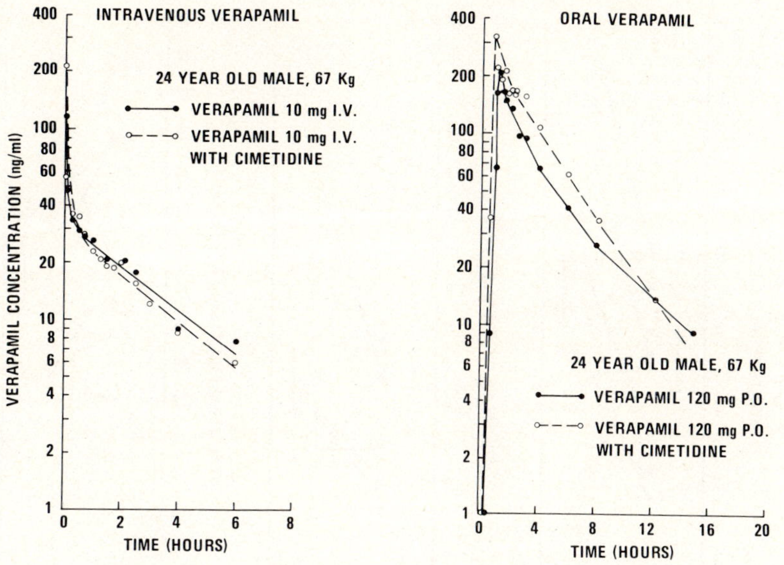

Fig. 1. Plasma concentrations of verapamil after intravenous *(left)* and oral *(right)* dosing in a healthy man in the control state and during cimetidine dosing.

We report the absence of a pharmacokinetic or pharmacodynamic drug-drug interaction between cimetidine and verapamil. The experimental design is verified by documenting the previously described cimetidine-lidocaine interaction in the same subjects under conditions identical to those used in our present study.

METHODS

Subjects. Nine healthy subjects aged 23 to 40 years who were taking no other medications participated after giving written informed consent. All were within 20% of their ideal body weight (46 to 90 kg) and had no evidence of medical illness as determined by physical examination, ECG, and laboratory determinations of complete blood count, urinalysis, serum electrolyte levels, liver function tests, and serum creatinine levels.

Study design

Study 1. Each subject participated in four separate verapamil trials in random sequence, separated by at least 1 week.

In trial I, verapamil HCl (10 mg) was given by intravenous infusion over 10 minutes.

In trial II, after an overnight fast, 120 mg verapamil HCl was taken by mouth with 100 ml water. Fasting was maintained for 3 hours after dosing.

In trial III, cimetidine, 300 mg po every 6 hours, was administered starting 12 hours before and for 24 hours after the verapamil doses. Verapamil was then administered intravenously as described in trial I.

In trial IV, cimetidine, 300 mg po every 6 hours, was administered starting 12 hours before the verapamil dose and for 24 hours after the dose. After an overnight fast, verapamil was taken by mouth as described in trial II.

Before each verapamil dose, at the end of drug dosing (time 0), and at 5, 15, 30, and 45 minutes and 1, 1.25, 1.5, 1.75, 2, 2.25, 2.5, 3, 4, 6, 8, 10 and 24 hours after dosing, venous blood samples were drawn into Venoject heparinized tubes (Terumo Medical Corp.). Simultaneous with each blood sample, blood pressure, heart rate, and ECG lead II strips at 25 and 50 mm/sec paper speed were obtained. An indwelling 20-guage venous catheter, kept patent by 1 ml irrigation with a dilute heparin solution (10 U/ml) after each sample, was used to draw blood samples during the first 10 hours after the verapamil dose. The 24-hour sample was obtained by venipuncture. Blood specimens were centrifuged and the plasma was separated and stored at −20° C until analyzed.

Concentrations of verapamil and norverapamil were analyzed by GLC with nitrogen-phosphorous detection.[4] The extent of verapamil binding to plasma protein was determined from single samples obtained in the nonfasting state at least 8 hours after the verapamil dose. Binding was determined with and without addition of a therapeutic concentration of cimetidine (3.3 μg/ml) by equilibrium dialysis with duplicate 1 ml plasma samples. Plasma was spiked with 167 ng/ml verapamil. Dialysis was performed at 37° C for 5 hours. Recovery of verapamil from the dialysis system was

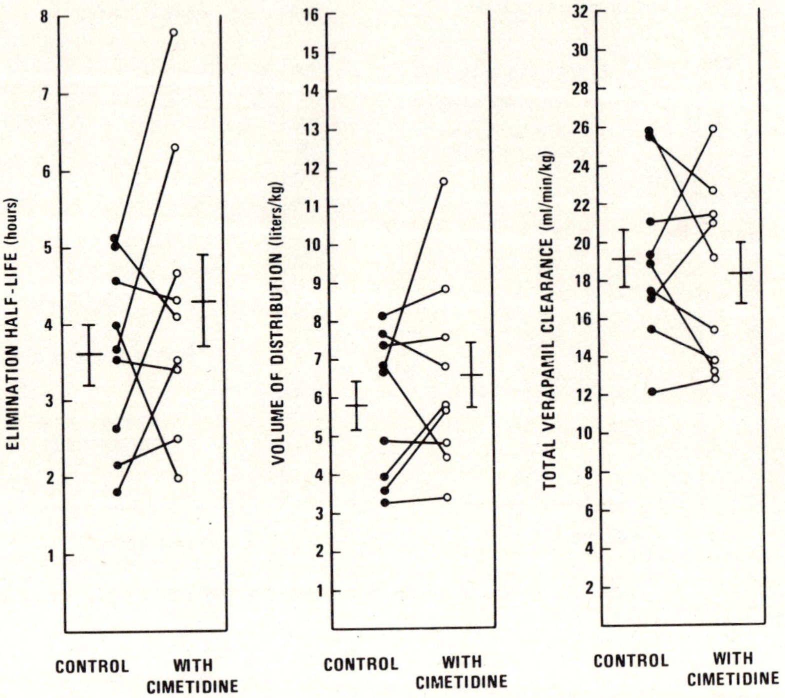

Fig. 2. Effect of cimetidine on verapamil $t_{1/2}$ *(left)*, volume of distribution *(center)*, and total clearance *(right)* after intravenous verapamil. Individual and mean ($\pm$SE) values are shown.

complete. Variation between replicate samples was always <8%. Equilibrium between bound and unbound verapamil was complete at 5 hours and verapamil binding was concentration independent to 500 ng/ml.[18]

Study 2. Five of the nine subjects who participated in the verapamil study also participated in a two-trial lidocaine study. These trials were also randomly sequenced and separated by 1 week.

In trial I, lidocaine HCl (25 mg) was given by intravenous bolus infusion.

In trial II, cimetidine, 300 mg po every 6 hours, was administered 12 hours before lidocaine dosing and for 8 hours after lidocaine dosing. Lidocaine was then administered intravenously as described in trial I.

Before each lidocaine dose, immediately after bolus administration of lidocaine, and at 5, 15, and 30 minutes and 1, 2, 3, 4, 5, 6, 7 and 8 hours after the dose, venous blood samples were drawn into Venoject heparinized tubes. Samples were obtained and stored in the same manner as described for the verapamil study.

Lidocaine concentrations were analyzed by GLC with nitrogen-phosphorous detection.[2]

Pharmacokinetic data analysis. After intravenous verapamil and lidocaine doses, postinfusion plasma drug concentrations were fit to equations formed by a linear sum of exponential terms through the use of iterative weighted nonlinear least-squares regression analysis.[12,16] For verapamil, after correction of the coefficients for the infusion time,[15] and for lidocaine, with the coefficients derived after bolus drug dosing, the functions were used to calculate the $t_{1/2}$, total apparent volume of distribution by the area method, and total clearance. The AUC from time zero was determined by the trapezoidal method. To this was added the residual area extrapolated to infinity, calculated as the final concentration divided by the slope of the terminal phase of the plasma concentration-time curve, to give total AUC. The AUC was used to calculate model-independent parameters for volume of distribution and total clearance, and was also used for estimation of verapamil absolute bioavailability.[29]

After oral verapamil, the AUC was determined as described above and the $t_{1/2}$ was determined by linear regression analysis of the terminal log-linear phase of the plasma concentration-time curve. Absolute bioavailability of verapamil was determined as the dose-normalized ratio of oral AUC and intravenous AUC in the same subject during the various trials. Trial I AUC (verapamil without cimetidine) was used for all comparisons of absolute bioavailability.[29] Differences in pharmacokinetics between control and cimetidine trials for both verapamil and lidocaine were analyzed by the

Table I. Effect of cimetidine on verapamil pharmacokinetics and pharmacodynamics

	Control	*During cimetidine dosing*
Subjects		
Number	9	
Age (yr)	27 ± 2	
Weight (kg)	60 ± 5	
Sex (M/F)	2/7	
Intravenous kinetic parameters		
$t_{1/2}$ (hr)	3.60 ± 0.40	4.30 ± 0.60
Volume of distribution (L/kg)	5.81 ± 0.63	6.56 ± 0.85
Total clearance (ml/min/kg)	19.2 ± 1.5	18.4 ± 1.6
Free fraction (% not bound to plasma protein)	6.4 ± 0.6	6.3 ± 0.6
Oral kinetic parameters		
$t_{1/2}$ (hr)	4.25 ± 0.57	4.60 ± 0.70
Time to peak plasma concentration (hr)	1.6 ± 0.2	1.4 ± 0.3
Peak concentration (ng/ml)	142 ± 26	146 ± 32
AUC (ng/ml · hr)	585 ± 113	506 ± 82
Absolute bioavailability (%)	35.0 ± 7.3	30.1 ± 5.0
Intravenous pharmacodynamic parameters (Sigmoid E_{max} model)		
EC_{50} (ng/ml)	27.5 ± 2.8	24.3 ± 2.1
E_{max} (msec)	94.1 ± 36.0	85.0 ± 19.8
Decrease in mean arterial pressure (mm Hg)	8 ± 1	9 ± 2
Increase in heart rate (bpm)	14 ± 3	17 ± 2
Oral pharmacodynamic parameters (linear model)		
Slope of line (msec/ng · ml^{-1})	1.10 ± 0.61	1.15 ± 0.56
Intercept with ordinate (PR, in msec)	−37 ± 21	−28 ± 15
Correlation coefficient (r)	0.95 ± 0.01	0.87 ± 0.04

Data are $\bar{X}$ ± SE.
M = Male; F = female.

paired Student's t test. A level of $P < 0.05$ was used as the criterion for establishing a significant difference.

Pharmacodynamic data analysis. After each verapamil dose, three pharmacodynamic parameters (ECG PR interval, blood pressure, and heart rate) were determined at the time of each blood sampling for analysis of verapamil concentration. The ECG PR interval was measured for 10 successive cardiac cycles, and the mean was used for the individual data point. Blood pressure was determined with the subject in the sitting position and was expressed as: Mean arterial pressure = [(Systolic − diastolic pressure)/3] + diastolic pressure. Heart rate was determined as the mean of five cardiac cycles by measurement of the R-R interval.

The PR interval was related to verapamil plasma concentration after intravenous doses by a sigmoid E_{max} pharmacodynamic model of the form: $E = (E_{max} \cdot C^n)/EC_{50}{}^n + C^n$, where E is the prolongation of PR interval from baseline (predrug), E_{max} is the maximal prolongation in PR interval, C is the drug concentration at the measured effect (E), EC_{50} is the verapamil plasma concentration associated with 50% maximal prolongation in PR interval, and n is a "sigmoidicity" factor that introduces curvature into the concentration-response curve and permits fitting with less residual error at concentrations approaching no effect and maximal effect.[13,25] Data fitting was performed by unweighted iterative nonlinear least-squares regression analysis and iterating the variables E_{max}, EC_{50}, and n. Data were graphically examined before fitting, and no significant hysteresis could be ascertained after intravenous verapamil doses. In some subjects, however, there was definite hysteresis after oral doses. Therefore, after oral verapamil we used a linear pharmacodynamic model of the form: $E - E_0 = S \cdot C$, where E is the measured PR interval, E_0 is the baseline PR interval, S is the slope, and C is the verapamil concentration at the measured effect ($E - E_0$). Only effect-concentration data after the appearance of peak effect until disappearance of effect were used to minimize the influence of the apparent initial delay in equilibration between the plasma compartment and the effector site.[6]

After intravenous verapamil, changes in mean arterial pressure were transient and maximal in all subjects by the end of drug infusion or 5 minutes thereafter. Therefore, only the maximal decrease from preinfusion baseline was used from each trial. The change in heart rate was also transient, and after intravenous doses

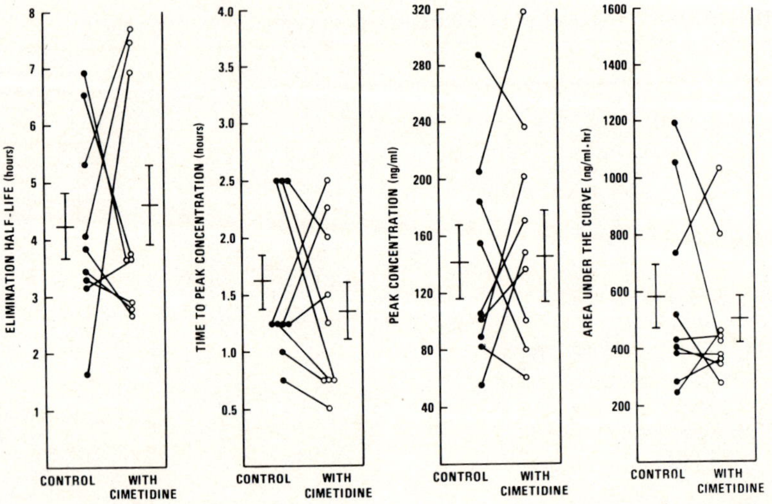

Fig. 3. Effect of cimetidine on verapamil $t_{1/2}$ *(left)*, time to peak concentration *(center-left)*, peak concentration *(center-right)*, and total verapamil plasma AUC *(right)* after oral verapamil. Individual and mean (±SE) values are shown.

again only maximal changes were used. After single oral doses, changes in both mean arterial pressure and heart rate were highly variable and inconsistent, and therefore were not formally evaluated.

RESULTS

Fig. 1 shows verapamil plasma concentrations during each of the four trials for one subject. After intravenous doses, the $t_{1/2}$, volume of distribution, and total clearance were similar between control and cimetidine trials (Fig. 2; Table I). Similarly, after oral doses, the $t_{1/2}$, time to peak verapamil concentrations, peak verapamil concentrations, and total AUC were no different between control and cimetidine treatment trials (Fig. 3; Table I). Furthermore, cimetidine did not alter verapamil binding to plasma proteins (Table I).

Five of the same subjects with identical cimetidine dose and pretreatment schedules received intravenous lidocaine. Fig. 4 shows lidocaine plasma concentrations during control and cimetidine trials for one subject. The $t_{1/2}$ tended to be longer during cimetidine dosing because of significantly decreased total lidocaine clearance with no change in volume of distribution (Fig. 5; Table II).

Verapamil-induced prolongations in the PR interval after intravenous and oral doses were related to plasma concentrations (Fig. 6). The concentration-effect relationship was not changed by cimetidine after intravenous or oral verapamil (Fig. 6; Table I). Similarly, the relative decrease in verapamil effect after oral doses (Fig. 7) was uniform in all subjects and was not changed by cimetidine.

After intravenous verapamil the decrease in mean blood pressure and the reflex increase in heart rate were maximal at the end of infusion or at 5 minutes thereafter for all subjects, and were not changed by concurrent cimetidine dosing (Table I).

DISCUSSION

Verapamil undergoes oxidative *N*-demethylation as a major route of biotransformation[7] and has significant first-pass hepatic extraction.[22,32] Cimetidine, extensively reported both to inhibit hepatic cytochrome P-450–mediated oxidative drug biotransformation[1] and to impair first-pass hepatic extraction of high-clearance drugs,[3,5,8,9] might be expected to have an in vivo kinetic interaction with cimetidine.[23] Such an interaction after oral verapamil was recently reported,[23] but was interpreted not to have pharmacodynamic consequences.

A close relationship between a verapamil-induced delay in AV nodal conduction and verapamil plasma concentrations within a subject has been reported.[6,10] Multiple measurements of effect and concentration may then be formally evaluated by pharmacodynamic modeling techniques such as a sigmoid E_{max} pharmacodynamic model, if the following requirements are fulfilled: (1) There is a maximal effect (in this case represented by a maximum prolongation of surface ECG PR interval before progression to higher degrees of AV blockade); (2) the concentration-effect relationship is independent of duration of exposure to drug; (3) the rate constant describing the transfer of drug between plasma and effector compartments is larger than the distribution or elimination rate constants, such that no lag time is interposed between measured plasma concentrations and

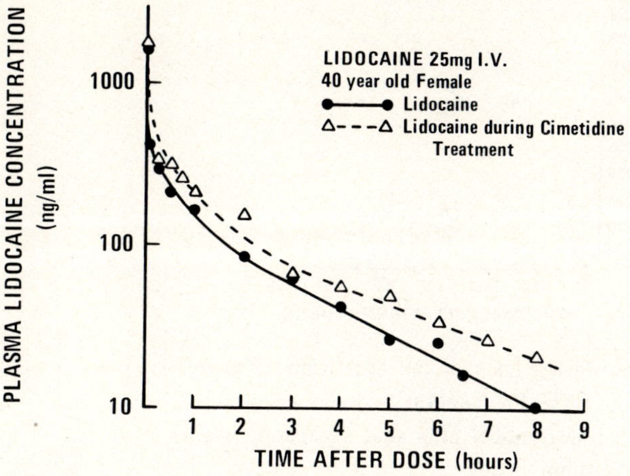

Fig. 4. Plasma concentrations of lidocaine after intravenous dosing in a healthy woman in the control state and during cimetidine dosing.

the quantitatively appropriate effect response; and (4) the pharmacodynamic effect is exclusively due to the pharmacologically active substance being measured, since metabolite effects invalidate the model.

These criteria are fulfilled for the relationship between plasma verapamil concentration after intravenous dosing and the prolongation of AV nodal conduction as measured by surface ECG PR interval. Existence of a maximal PR prolongation (high-grade first-degree AV blockade) over a range of verapamil concentrations before achieving second-degree blockade is verified by the presence of several points approaching 100% effect at different verapamil concentrations measured at different points in time. Constancy of the concentration-effect relationship over time (lack of adaptation or sensitization) has been documented by chronic dosing studies during which PR prolongation at a steady-state verapamil concentration was constant.[6] Equilibration of drug between the central (plasma) compartment and the effect compartment is rapid, as shown by the lack of hyteresis in the concentration-effect relationship after intravenous dosing. Finally, norverapamil, the demethylated metabolite of verapamil, may cause peripheral vasodilation with about 20% of the potency of the parent drug,[20] but at least in animal models it has not been demonstrated to impair cardiac electrophysiologic properties. Other metabolites have no pharmacologic activity.[20]

After oral verapamil, reverse hysteresis in the concentration-effect relationship was consistently observed. Therefore, a linear pharmacodynamic model that uses only concentration-effect points after the time of maximal effect was used as described by Eichelbaum et al.[6]

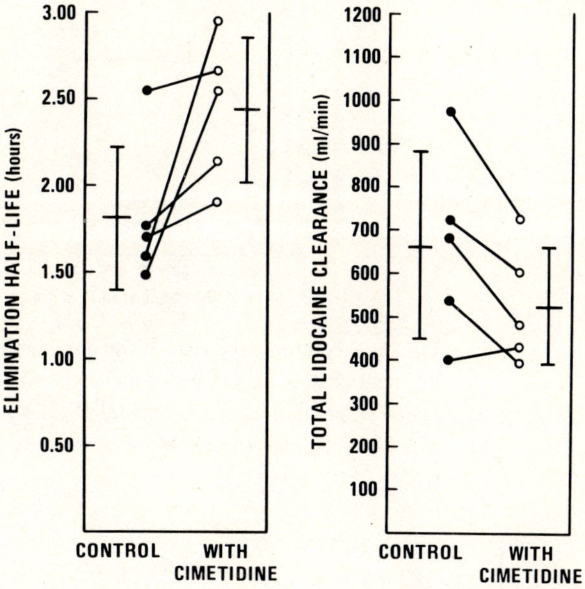

Fig. 5. Effect of cimetidine on lidocaine $t_{1/2}$ *(left)* and total clearance *(right)* after intravenous lidocaine. Individual and mean (±SE) values are shown.

Table II. Effect of cimetidine on lidocaine pharmacokinetics

	Control	*During cimetidine dosing*
Subjects		
Number	5	
Age (yr)	28 ± 3	
Weight (kg)	58 ± 3	
Sex (M/F)	1/4	
Kinetics		
$t_{1/2}$ (hr)	1.81 ± 0.41	2.44 ± 0.42*
Volume of distribution (L/kg)	1.77 ± 0.66	1.99 ± 0.81
Total clearance (ml/min)	665 ± 216	527 ± 134†

Data are $\bar{X}$ ± SE.
M = Male; F = female.
*0.1 > P > 0.05 (paired Student's t test).
†P < 0.05.

These models empirically fit the data well and the theoretic justification for their use has been extensively described.[13,30] The decreased effect of verapamil on PR interval prolongation after oral dosing has been previously reported and ascribed to stereoselective first-pass hepatic extraction, such that the pharmacologically more active (−)-verapamil isomer undergoes more extensive hepatic extraction than does the much less active (+)-verapamil isomer after oral dosing.[6] This has recently been confirmed by determination of oral clear-

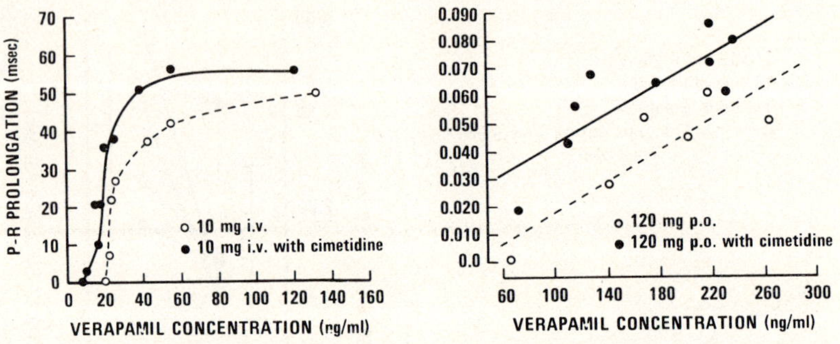

Fig. 6. Representative data from one subject studied during each of the four trials. Shown is the relationship of verapamil-induced prolongation in ECG PR interval under a sigmoid E_{max} model after intravenous verapamil *(left)* and under a linear model after oral verapamil *(right)*. o- - - -o = Control trials; •——• = trials during cimetidine dosing.

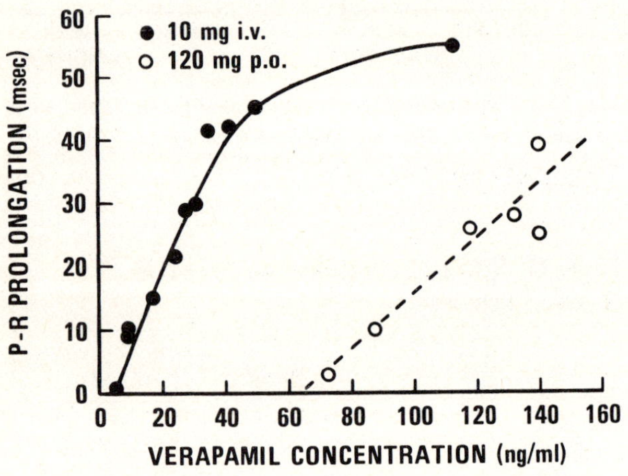

Fig. 7. Comparison of verapamil-induced prolongation in ECG-PR interval related to verapamil concentration after an intravenous and an oral dose to the same subject on different occasions. Verapamil effect at a given plasma concentration was much less after oral dosing in all subjects.

ance of each stereoisomer individually after oral dosing of a pseudoracemic mixture of (−)-verapamil and deuterated (+)-verapamil.[28]

The total absence of a kinetic interaction between verapamil and cimetidine in our study, in contrast to the previous report of increased verapamil bioavailability during concurrent cimetidine dosing,[26] cannot be explained by the present data. In the previous report, 300 mg cimetidine was taken every 6 hours for 8 days before the verapamil trial,[26] whereas we gave pretreatment for 12 hours. However, in our present study, to document that the cimetidine pretreatment and dosing regimen was sufficient, five of the same subjects underwent a lidocaine-cimetidine interaction study. Decreased lidocaine clearance with prolonged $t_{1/2}$ during cimetidine dosing indicates the cimetidine dose regimen is adequate to demonstrate an interaction if it exists. Furthermore, this difference was established by study of only five subjects. Because no difference, or even a trend toward a difference, could be identified during the verapamil-cimetidine trials by the study of nine subjects (Table I), a clinically meaningful interaction between verapamil and cimetidine is extremely unlikely.

Our data suggest that verapamil and lidocaine, both high-clearance drugs with extensive first-pass hepatic extraction,[32] have hepatic extraction mechanisms that are differentially sensitive to cimetidine impairment. One (lidocaine) is impaired during cimetidine dosing, while the other (verapamil) is resistant to the effect of cimetidine, at least at the doses used in this study. To date, other high-clearance drugs evaluated, including imipramine,[3] propranolol,[9] and indocyanine green,[9] have had impaired hepatic extraction in the presence of cimetidine.

Clinically, if our results from young healthy subjects can be extrapolated to a patient population that requires verapamil therapy, the absence of either a pharmacokinetic or pharmacodynamic interaction between verapamil and cimetidine indicates concurrent administration should result in no change in verapamil therapeutic or toxic effects.

We are grateful for the technical assistance of Maya Sadhukhan and the support of Dr. Jerry R. Mitchell.

References

1. Abernethy DR, Greenblatt DJ, Divoll M, Ameer B, Shader RI: Differential effect of cimetidine on drug oxidation (antipyrine, diazepam) versus conjugation (ac-

etaminophen, lorazepam): Prevention of acetaminophen toxicity by cimetidine. J Pharmacol Exp Ther **224:**508-513, 1983.

2. Abernethy DR, Greenblatt DJ, Ochs HR: Lidocaine determination in human plasma with application to single low-dose pharmacokinetic studies. J Chromatogr **232:** 180-185, 1982.
3. Abernethy DR, Greenblatt DJ, Shader RI: Imipramine-cimetidine interaction: Impairment of clearance and enhanced absolute bioavailability. J Pharmacol Exp Ther **229:**702-705, 1984.
4. Abernethy DR, Todd EA, Mitchell JR: Verapamil and norverapamil determination in human plasma by gas-liquid chromatography using nitrogen-phosphorous detection: Application to single-dose pharmacokinetic studies. Pharmacology **29:**264-268, 1984.
5. Bauer LA, Edwards WAD, Randolph FP, Blouin RA: Cimetidine-induced decrease in lidocaine metabolism. Am Heart J **108:**413-415, 1984.
6. Eichelbaum M, Birkel P, Grube E, Gutegemann U, Somogyi A: Effects of verapamil on P-R intervals in relation to verapamil plasma levels following single i.v. and oral administration and during chronic treatment. Klin Wochenschr **58:**919-925, 1980.
7. Eichelbaum M, Ende M, Remberg G, Schomerus M, Dengler HJ: The metabolism of DL-^{14}C-verapamil in man. Drug Metab Dispos **7:**145-148, 1979.
8. Feely J, Wilkinson GR, McAllister CB, Wood AJJ: Increased toxicity and reduced clearance of lidocaine by cimetidine. Ann Intern Med **96:**592-594, 1982.
9. Feely J, Wilkinson GR, Wood AJJ: Reduction of liver blood flow and propranolol metabolism by cimetidine. N Engl J Med **304:**692-695, 1981.
10. Hamann SR, Blouin RA, McAllister RG: Clinical pharmacokinetics of verapamil. Clin Pharmacokinet **9:**26-41, 1984.
11. Henry PD: Comparative pharmacology of calcium antagonists: Nifedipine, verapamil, and diltiazem. Am J Cardiol **46:**1047-1058, 1980.
12. Holford NHG: Drug model. *In* Perry HM, editor: Public proceedings notebook. Cambridge, Mass, 1982, Bolt, Beranek, Newman.
13. Holford NHG, Sheiner LB: Pharmacokinetic and pharmacodynamic modeling in vivo. CRC Crit Rev Bioeng **5:**273-322, 1981.
14. Keefe DL, Yee YG, Kates RE: Verapamil protein binding in patients and in normal subjects. CLIN PHARMACOL THER **29:**21-26, 1981.
15. Loo JCK, Riegelman S: Assessment of pharmacokinetic constants from postinfusion blood curves obtained after i.v. infusion. J Pharm Sci **59:**53-55, 1970.
16. Marquardt DW: An algorithm for least-squares estimation of non-linear parameters. J Soc Ind Appl Math **11:**431-441, 1963.
17. McAllister RG: Clinical pharmacology of slow channel blocking agents. Prog Cardiovasc Dis **25:**83-102, 1982.
18. McGowan FX, Reiter MJ, Pritchett ELC, Shand DG: Verapamil plasma binding: Relationship to alpha-1-acid glycoprotein and drug efficacy. CLIN PHARMACOL THER **33:**485-490, 1983.
19. Mitchell LB, Shroeder JS, Mason JW: Comparative clinical electrophysiologic effects of diltiazem, verapamil and nifedipine: A review. Am J Cardiol **49:**629-635, 1982.
20. Neugebauer G: Comparative cardiovascular actions of verapamil and its major metabolites in the anesthetized dog. Cardiovasc Res **12:**247-254, 1978.
21. Pelkonen O, Puurunen J: The effect of cimetidine on *in vitro* and *in vivo* microsomal drug metabolism in the rat. Biochem Pharmacol **29:**3075-3080, 1980.
22. Schomerus M, Speigelholder B, Stieren B, Eichelbaum M: Physiological disposition of verapamil in man. Cardiovasc Res **10:**605-612, 1976.
23. Schwartz JB: Verapamil in atrial fibrillation: The expected, the unexpected and the unknown. Am Heart J **106:**173-176, 1983.
24. Schwartz JB, Keefe DL, Kirsten E, Kates RE, Harrison DC: Prolongation of verapamil elimination kinetics during chronic oral administration. Am Heart J **104:**198-203, 1982.
25. Sheiner LB, Stanski DR, Vosch S, Miller RD, Ham J: Simultaneous modeling of pharmacokinetics and pharmacodynamics: Application to d-tubocurarine. CLIN PHARMACOL THER **25:**358-371, 1979.
26. Smith MS, Benyunes MC, Bjornsson TD, Shand DG, Pritchett ELC: Influence of cimetidine on verapamil kinetics and dynamics. CLIN PHARMACOL THER **36:**551-554, 1984.
27. Speeg KV, Patwardhan RV, Avant GR, Mitchell MC, Schenker S: Inhibition of microsomal drug metabolism by histamine H2-receptor antagonist studied in vivo and in vitro in rodents. Gastroenterology **82:**89-96, 1982.
28. Vogelgesang B, Echizen H, Schmidt E, Eichelbaum M: Stereoselective first-pass metabolism of highly cleared drugs: Studies of the bioavailability of L- and D-verapamil examined with a stable isotope technique. Br J Clin Pharmacol **18:**733-740, 1984.
29. Wagner JG: Fundamentals of clinical pharmacokinetics. Hamilton, Ill, 1975, Drug Intelligence Publications.
30. Wagner JG: Kinetics of pharmacologic response. I. Proposed relationships between response and drug concentration in the intact animal and man. J Theor Biol **20:**173-201, 1968.
31. Wagner JG: Predictability of verapamil steady-state plasma levels from single-dose data explained. CLIN PHARMACOL THER **36:**1-4, 1984.
32. Wilkinson GR, Shand DG: A physiological approach to hepatic drug clearance. CLIN PHARMACOL THER **18:**377-390, 1975.

Lack of effect of oral activated charcoal on imipramine clearance

The effect of oral activated charcoal on the pharmacokinetics of intravenous imipramine was studied in a randomized, crossover trial. Four normal men received intravenous imipramine (12.5 mg/70 kg) on two separate occasions, followed by either water or water plus high-surface-area activated charcoal (180 gm) in divided doses over 24 hours. Serum imipramine concentrations were measured from 0 to 24 hours after the imipramine infusion. There was no difference in the mean (±SE) $t_{1/2}$ (9.0 ± 0.8 vs. 10.9 ± 1.6 hours), apparent volume of distribution (11.2 ± 2.1 vs. 12.4 ± 2.1 L/kg), or systemic clearance (992.2 ± 138.3 vs. 930.3 ± 101.9 ml/min/70 kg) of imipramine after dosing without and with oral activated charcoal, respectively ($P > 0.05$; paired t test). These results suggest that multiple oral doses of activated charcoal do not increase the clearance of imipramine in man. (CLIN PHARMACOL THER 38:350-353, 1985.)

Mark J. Goldberg, M.D.,* Glen D. Park, Pharm.D., Reynold Spector, M.D., Lawrence J. Fischer, Ph.D., and Ross D. Feldman, M.D.** *Iowa City, Iowa*

The treatment of tricyclic antidepressant overdose, the most common serious drug overdose seen in many hospitals, consists mainly of supportive care. At present there is no known practical method to increase substantially the clearance of tricyclic antidepressants from the body. Several authors have suggested that multiple oral doses of activated charcoal may enhance the elimination of tricyclic antidepressants from the body by interrupting enterogastric or enterohepatic cycling of these drugs.[4,7] One group administered activated charcoal (repeated doses) in several patients with amitriptyline overdose and claimed that the $t_{1/2}$ of the drug was shortened.[19] In previous studies, we and others have shown that the oral administration of multiple doses of activated charcoal will greatly increase the clearance of intravenously administered phenobarbital and theophylline in normal subjects.[1,2,11] Furthermore, we and others have shown that therapy with activated charcoal (multiple doses) will increase the clearance of phenobarbital and theophylline in patients intoxicated with these drugs.[9,15,16]

Based on the hypothesis that multiple oral doses of activated charcoal would increase the clearance of imipramine, we studied the effect of this therapy on the pharmacokinetics of intravenous imipramine in normal subjects. We used an activated charcoal with a higher surface area (which is two to four times more "potent" in decreasing the absorption and increasing the clearance of certain drugs) than standard activated charcoal to maximize the likelihood of obtaining a positive result.[13]

METHODS

Four nonsmoking men between 20 and 30 years of age and proved healthy by a history and physical examination participated after giving informed consent in accord with standards of the Human Subjects Review Committee at the University of Iowa. All subjects took no drugs including over-the-counter drugs, alcohol, or marijuana for at least 3 days before and throughout the study. After an overnight fast, each subject received imipramine HCl (Tofranil; Geigy Pharmaceuticals), 12.5 mg per 70 kg body weight, intravenously over 60 minutes on two separate occasions separated by at least 7 days. ECG monitoring and frequent measurement of vital signs were performed during and for 1 hour after

From the Departments of Internal Medicine and Pharmacology, College of Medicine and the Division of Clinical/Hospital Pharmacy, College of Pharmacy, The University of Iowa and the Veterans Administration Medical Center.

Supported in part by National Institutes of Health General Clinical Research Center Support Grant No. RR0059, United States Public Health Service Junior Faculty Research Grant No. RR 07035-16, and the Veterans Administration.

Received for publication March 3, 1985; accepted June 3, 1985.

Reprint requests to: Dr. Mark Goldberg, Department of Internal Medicine, University of Iowa Hospitals, Iowa City, IA 52242.

*Teaching and Research Scholar of the American College of Physicians.

**George Morris Piersol Research and Teaching Scholar of the American College of Physicians.

Table I. Pharmacokinetics of imipramine with and without activated charcoal therapy

	$t_{1/2}$ (hr)		V_{area} (L/kg)		CL (ml/min/70 kg)	
Subject No.	*Without charcoal*	*With charcoal*	*Without charcoal*	*With charcoal*	*Without charcoal*	*With charcoal*
1	10.1	14.4	16.5	17.4	1324.4	973.5
2	7.2	6.7	9.5	8.6	1067.8	1036.5
3	10.5	10.6	11.9	14.2	911.3	1079.4
4	8.2	11.8	6.7	9.2	665.4	631.7
$\overline{X}$	9.0	10.9	11.2	12.4	992.2	930.3
SE	0.8	1.6	2.1	2.1	138.3	101.9

the imipramine infusion. Also, on each occasion each subject ingested, in a randomized block design, either 20 gm of a high-surface-area activated charcoal (Super-Char; Gulf Bio-Systems) in 300 ml water at 0, 2, 4, 6, 9, 12, 16, 20, and 24 hours after the end of the imipramine infusion or 300 ml water (without charcoal) at the same time schedule. Two of the four subjects (chosen at random) received charcoal after the first imipramine infusion and two received charcoal after the second imipramine infusion. Each subject drank water ad libitum and took sodium sulfate, 10 gm po, at 2 and 14 hours after the imipramine infusion to prevent constipation. At 3, 7.5, and 14 hours after the imipramine infusion, each subject received 0.25 L fruit juice. At 10.5 hours after the imipramine infusion, each subject received 0.5 L fruit juice and unbuttered toast. At 22 hours after the imipramine infusion, each subject received a light, low-fat breakfast.

For the determination of the concentration of imipramine in serum, blood samples were drawn through heparinized catheters from each subject before and 0, 0.75, 1.5, 2.5, 4, 8, 12, 18, 24, 30, 36, and 48 hours after the end of the imipramine infusion. Imipramine concentrations in 1.0 ml serum were determined by a previously reported drug extraction procedure and gas chromatography-mass spectrometry.[18,20] For each analysis, a deuterated internal standard (D_4-imipramine) was added to serum samples from subjects and to blank human plasma to which known amounts of imipramine (1, 2, 5, 10, and 20 ng/ml) had been added. Linear standard curves were obtained with the following instrumental conditions: fused silica capillary GC column, 5% phenylmethyl silicone, 0.2 mm × 25 m operated at 260° C; Ross-type injector at 270° C, mass spectrometer; Riber R10-10C with Nermag Model 40 data system operated in the chemical ionization mode (NH_3) with single-ion monitoring at m/z 282 (imipramine) and 286 (D_4-imipramine). Retention time for imipramine under these conditions was 4.5 minutes. Concentrations of the imipramine metabolite desipramine (retention time 6.7 minutes) were not determined because they were <6 ng/ml and could not be reliably measured in the underivitized form. Samples were analyzed in duplicate.

Because a plot of the logarithms of the imipramine serum concentration-time data from 4 to 24 hours after the end of the imipramine infusion appeared linear, we concluded that the distribution phase was complete and analyzed this data assuming linear pharmacokinetics.[8,12] For each subject the serum elimination rate constant (k, in $hours^{-1}$) and $t_{1/2}$ (in hours) of imipramine for each treatment (with and without charcoal) were calculated by linear regression analysis.[8] For each subject the serum AUC (in microgram-hours per liter) of imipramine for each treatment was calculated by summing the AUC from 0 to 24 hours after the end of the infusion (calculated by the trapezoidal rule) and the AUC from 24 hours to infinity (assuming log-linear decline and calculated by dividing the serum concentration at 24 hours by k).[8] For each subject the apparent volume of distribution (V_{area}; in liters per kilogram) of imipramine for each treatment was calculated by dividing the dose of imipramine administered by $k \cdot AUC$.[8] For each subject the systemic clearance (CL; in milliliters per minute per 70 kg body weight) of imipramine for each treatment was calculated by dividing the dose of imipramine administered by the AUC.[8]

The difference between two related sample means was analyzed by a paired t test.[3]

RESULTS

The values of $t_{1/2}$, V_{area}, and CL for the four subjects with and without activated charcoal therapy are listed in Table I. There was no significant difference in $t_{1/2}$, V_{area}, or CL between treatments ($P > 0.05$; paired t test).

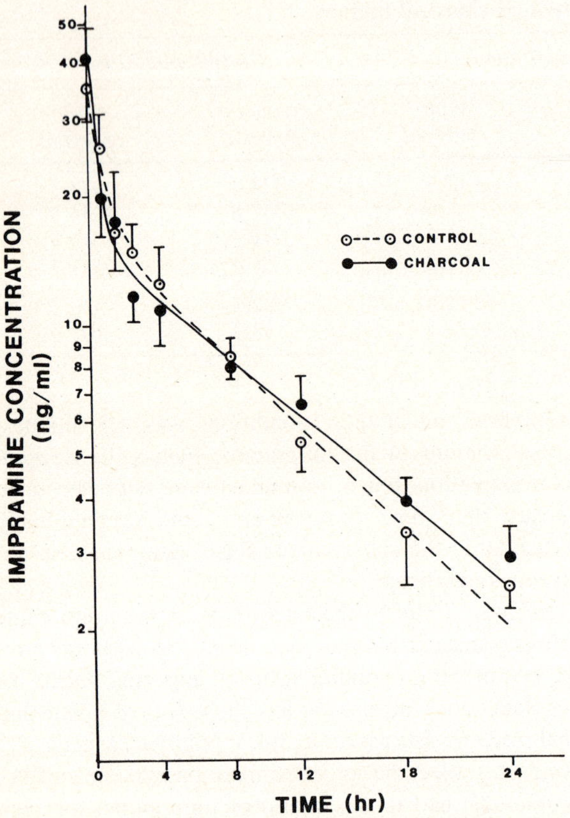

Fig. 1. Mean (± SE) serum imipramine concentrations plotted against time after the end of the intravenous imipramine infusion with and without the oral administration of activated charcoal. Lines of best fit were generated from the mean serum data by a nonlinear least-squares regression program for a two-compartment open pharmacokinetic model.

In Fig. 1, the logarithms of the mean serum concentrations of imipramine for the four subjects with and without activated charcoal therapy are plotted against time after the end of the imipramine infusion.

Other than mild sedation and dry mouth experienced transiently by all subjects, there were no adverse effects of imipramine or charcoal administration.

DISCUSSION

Our principal finding is that the oral administration of multiple doses of high-surface-area activated charcoal had no effect on the serum $t_{1/2}$ or systemic clearance of imipramine. Although an effect may have been missed due to the few subjects studied, it is not likely that oral activated charcoal therapy significantly increases imipramine clearance in man. Implicit in this statement is the assumption that high serum concentrations of imipramine (as in the setting of an imipramine overdose) are not eliminated differently from the body than low serum concentrations (as in this study).

We speculate that there are several possible reasons for the lack of effect of activated charcoal on imipramine clearance. First, the inability of activated charcoal to bind imipramine in the gastrointestinal tract is not likely, since activated charcoal has been shown to bind imipramine in vitro.[17] Second and most probable, the lack of effect is due to the very large volume of distribution of imipramine. Other investigators have reported similarly high values.[12] Due to the extensive tissue distribution of imipramine, there is relatively little imipramine present in blood available for "gastrointestinal dialysis" across the gut wall and subsequent binding by activated charcoal in the gut lumen.[10] Furthermore, our results suggest that enterogastric or enterohepatic cycling does not contribute substantially to imipramine elimination kinetics in man. It is worth noting that hemoperfusion (or hemodialysis) does not appreciably increase the clearances of imipramine or amitriptyline from the body, presumably because of the large volumes of distribution of these drugs.[6,14]

Despite the lack of effect of oral activated charcoal on imipramine clearance, activated charcoal is still important in the treatment of tricyclic antidepressant overdose. Single oral doses of activated charcoal have been shown to decrease significantly the absorption of nortriptyline after therapeutic doses in normal subjects, and multiple charcoal doses have an even greater effect.[5] Therefore, we still recommend the oral administration of one or more doses of activated charcoal for patients who overdose with tricyclic antidepressants to decrease drug absorption. However, unlike the case of certain drugs with smaller volumes of distribution (e.g., phenobarbital and theophylline), it is not likely that multiple doses of activated charcoal will increase the systemic clearance of imipramine or other tricyclic antidepressants in patients who overdose with these drugs.

References

1. Berg MJ, Berlinger WG, Goldberg MJ, Spector R, Johnson GF: Phenobarbital clearance: Acceleration by oral activated charcoal. N Engl J Med **307:**642-644, 1982.
2. Berlinger WG, Spector R, Goldberg MJ, Johnson GF, Quee CK, Berg MJ: Enhancement of theophylline clearance by oral activated charcoal. CLIN PHARMACOL THER **33:**351-354, 1983.
3. Colquhoun D: Lectures on biostatistics. Oxford, 1971, Clarendon Press.
4. Cramer J, Davies B: Activated charcoal in tricyclic drug overdoses. Br Med J **3:**527, 1972.

5. Crome P, Dawling S, Braithwaite RA: Effect of activated charcoal on absorption of nortriptyline. Lancet **2:**1203-1205, 1977.
6. Crome P, Hampel G, Vale JA, Volans GN, Widdop B, Goulding R: Haemoperfusion in treatment of drug intoxication. Br Med J **1:**174, 1978.
7. Gard H, Knapp D, Walle T, Gaffney T: Qualitative and quantitative studies on the disposition of amitriptyline and other tricyclic antidepressant drugs in man as it relates to the management of the overdosed patient. Clin Toxicol **6:**571-584, 1973.
8. Gibaldi M, Perrier D: Pharmacokinetics, ed 2. New York, 1982, Marcell Dekker, Inc.
9. Goldberg MJ, Berlinger WG: Treatment of phenobarbital overdose with activated charcoal. JAMA **247:**2400-2401, 1982.
10. Levy G: Gastrointestinal clearance of drugs with activated charcoal. N Engl J Med **307:**677-678, 1982.
11. Mahutte CK, True RJ, Michiels TM, Berman JM, Light RW: Increased serum theophylline clearance with orally administered activated charcoal. Am Rev Respir Dis **128:**820-822, 1983.
12. Nagy A, Johansson R: Plasma levels of imipramine and desipramine in man after different routes of administration. Naunyn Schmiedebergs Arch Pharmacol **290:**145-160, 1975.
13. Park GD, Spector R, Goldberg MJ, Johnson GF, Feldman R, Quee CK: Effect of the surface area of activated charcoal on theophylline clearance. J Clin Pharmacol **24:**289-292, 1984.
14. Pentel PR, Bullock ML, DeVane CL: Hemoperfusion for imipramine overdose: Elimination of active metabolites. J Toxicol Clin Toxicol **19:**239-248, 1982.
15. Pond SM, Olson KR, Osterlok JD, Tong TG: Randomized study of the treatment of phenobarbital overdose with repeated doses of activated charcoal. JAMA **251:** 3104-3108, 1984.
16. Radomski L, Park G, Goldberg M, Spector R, Johnson G, Quee C: A model for treatment of theophylline overdose with oral activated charcoal. CLIN PHARMACOL THER **35:**402-408, 1984.
17. Rauws AG, Olling M: Treatment of experimental imipramine and desipramine poisoning in the rat. Arch Toxicol **35:**97-106, 1976.
18. Scoggins BA, Maguire KP, Narman TR, Burrows GD: Measurement of tricyclic antidepressants. I. A review of methodology. Clin Chem **26:**5-17, 1980.
19. Swartz CM, Sherman A: The treatment of tricyclic antidepressant overdose with repeated charcoal. J Clin Psychopharmacol **4:**336-340, 1984.
20. Wold JS, Fischer LJ: The tissue distribution of cyproheptadine and its metabolites in rats and mice. J Pharmacol Exp Ther **183:**188-196, 1972.

Notes of the American Society for Clinical Pharmacology and Therapeutics

Nominations for awards

The Scientific Awards Committee wishes to solicit nominations from the membership of the American Society for Clinical Pharmacology and Therapeutics for the following awards. Send nominations to: John L. McNay, M.D., Chairman, Scientific Awards Committee, Clinical Pharmacologist, Lilly Laboratory for Clinical Research, Eli Lilly and Company, Wishard Memorial Hospital, Indianapolis, IN 46202.

1987 OSCAR B. HUNTER AWARD

This award honors individual scientists for outstanding contributions to clinical pharmacology and therapeutics. It is the premier award of the American Society for Clinical Pharmacology and Therapeutics and recognizes a meritorious career in drug research, excellence in patient care, and a distinguished teaching career. The awardee, who may or may not be a member of the Society, presents an oration at the annual meeting of the Society summarizing the work forming the basis for the award. Appended is a list of previous recipients of the award.

The award consists of a bronze medal mounted on a plaque struck in the likeness of Dr. Hunter and engraved with the name of the recipient and the date. An honorarium is provided and travel expenses to the meeting of the Society are reimbursed.

Members interested in making nominations may do so by sending to the Scientific Awards Committee a letter of nomination for each candidate stating the reasons supporting the nomination and accompanied by a curriculum vitae and bibliography. Members wishing to reactivate a nomination submitted in a previous year should submit an updated curriculum vitae and bibliography for the candidate. Deadline for receipt of nominations is December 1, 1985.

Previous recipients of the Oscar B. Hunter Memorial Award in Therapeutics of the American Society for Clinical Pharmacology and Therapeutics

1955	Jonas E. Salk, M.D.
1956	E. M. K. Geiling, M.D.
1957	Robert W. Wilkins, M.D.
1958	C. Walton Lillehei, M.D.
1959	Tom D. Spies, M.D.
1960	John H. Moyer, III, M.D.
1961	Hattie E. Alexander, M.D.
1962	Charles B. Huggins, M.D.
1963	Albert B. Sabin, M.D.
1964	Henry K. Beecher, M.D.
1965	William B. Castle, M.D.
1966	Irvin H. Page, M.D.
1967	George W. Thorn, M.D.
1968	Sidney Farber, M.D.
1969	Arthur Grollman, M.D.
1970	Bernard B. Brodie, M.D.
1971	Maxwell Finland, M.D.
1972	Edward D. Freis, M.D.
1973	George C. Cotzias, M.D.
1974	Raymond P. Ahlquist, Ph.D.
1975	Louis Lasagna, M.D.
1976	Louis Goodman, M.D. and Alfred Gilman, Ph.D.
1977	Harris Isbell, M.D.
1978	Walter Modell, M.D.
1979	Ray W. Gifford, Jr., M.D.
1980	John A. Oates, M.D.
1981	Albert Sjoerdsma, M.D., Ph.D.
1982	Gerhard Levy, Pharm.D.
1983	C. Gordon Zubrod, M.D.
1984	George H. Hitchings, Ph.D., Sc.D.
1985	Raymond W. Houde, M.D.
1986	To be announced

1987 RAWLS-PALMER AWARD

Each year this award recognizes a clinical pharmacologist for significant contributions to drug investigation that bring the efforts of modern drug research to the care of patients. The awardee delivers a lecture at the annual meeting of the Society on "Progress in Medicine."

The award was founded because of the generosity of Dr. W. B. Rawls, an Honorary Director, and Mrs. Rawls, and honors the memory of their parents, who dedicated themselves to providing a full education for their children.

The major selection criterion is that the candidate be an investigator actively engaged in high-quality clinical pharmacologic research. It is preferable, but not a requirement, that the candidate be a member of the Society. In addition, he or she should be capable of delivering an engaging, lucid lecture with wide audience appeal on recent developments in drug sciences. Appended is a list of previous recipients of the award.

The award consists of a plaque expressly struck for the occasion engraved with the name of the recipient and an honorarium. In addition, travel expenses to the annual meeting of the Society are reimbursed.

Members interested in making nominations may do so by sending to the Scientific Awards Committee a letter of nomination for each candidate stating the reasons supporting the nomination and accompanied by a curriculum vitae and bibliography. Members wishing to reactivate a nomination submitted in a previous year should submit an updated curriculum vitae and bibliography for the candidate. Deadline for receipt of nominations is December 1, 1985.

Previous Recipients of the Rawls-Palmer Award and Lectureship

1979	Richard M. Weinshilboum, M.D.
1980	David J. Greenblatt, M.D.
1981	Marcus M. Reidenberg, M.D.
1982	William A. Pettinger, M.D.
1983	Arthur J. Atkinson, Jr., M.D.
1984	Henry R. Bourne, M.D.
1985	Alan S. Nies, M.D.
1986	To be announced

1987 YOUNG INVESTIGATOR AWARD

The purpose of this award is to encourage and recognize young scientists active in the field of clinical pharmacology. There are no restrictions concerning the scientific field in which nominees have earned their doctoral degrees. Nominees must not be more than 36 years of age by March 1 of the year of presentation of the award. It is not required that candidates be members of the Society.

The award consists of a plaque engraved with the name of the recipient and an honorarium. In addition, travel expenses to the annual meeting of the Society are reimbursed.

Members interested in making nominations may do so by sending to the Scientific Awards Committee a letter supporting the nomination accompanied by a curriculum vitae and bibliography. In addition, please submit copies of up to five reprints or manuscripts in press that are representative of the candidate's work. Deadline for receipt of nominations is December 1, 1985.

USAN Council

List No. 264

New Names

The following nonproprietary names for the compounds described have been adopted by the United States Adopted Names (USAN) Council, which is sponsored by the American Medical Association, the American Pharmaceutical Association, and the US Pharmacopeial Convention, Inc., in cooperation with the respective pharmaceutical manufacturers. The designation USAN (United States Adopted Name) distinguishes these formally adopted nonproprietary names from other names. The information given under the category Therapeutic Claim is based on the manufacturer's claims at the time of publication. Adoption of USAN does not imply endorsement of the claims or products by the AMA, the US Pharmacopeia, or the APhA.

In some instances, the drugs listed are available only from the manufacturer to properly qualified investigators for clinical study.

USAN QUADAZOCINE MESYLATE

Pronunciation kwăd ā′ zō sēn″

Therapeutic claim opioid antagonist

Chemical names

(1) [2*R*-(2α,6α,11*S**)]-1-cyclopentyl-5-(1,2,3,4,5,6-hexahydro-8-hydroxy-3,6,11-trimethyl-2,6-methano-3-benzazocin-11-yl)-3-pentanone methanesulfonate (salt)

(2) (−)-(2*R*,6*S*,11*S*)-1-cyclopentyl-5-(1,2,3,4,5,6-hexahydro-8-hydroxy-3,6,11-trimethyl-2,6-methano-3-benzazocin-11-yl)-3-pentanone methanesulfonate (salt)

Structural formula

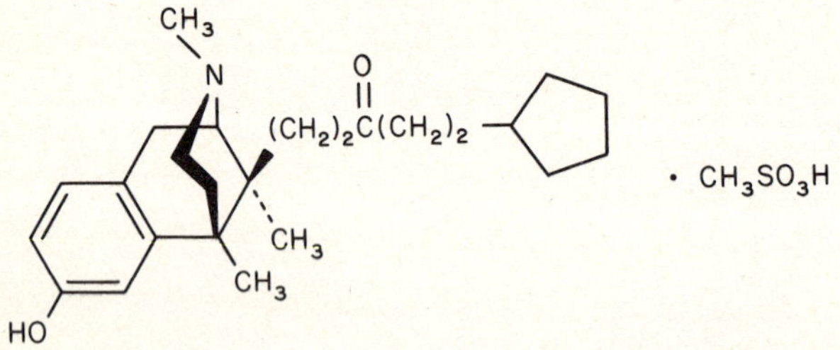

Molecular formula $C_{25}H_{37}NO_2 \cdot CH_4O_3S$ or $C_{26}H_{41}NO_5S$

Molecular weight 479.68

Manufacturer Sterling Drug Inc.

Code designation Win 44,441-3

CAS registry No. 71276-44-3

USAN FUREGRELATE SODIUM

Pronunciation fūr ĕ grĕl′ āt

Therapeutic claim thromboxane synthetase inhibitor

Chemical names

(1) sodium 5-(3-pyridinylmethyl)-2-benzofurancarboxylate monohydrate

(2) sodium 5-(3-pyridylmethyl)-2-benzofurancarboxylate monohydrate

Structural formula

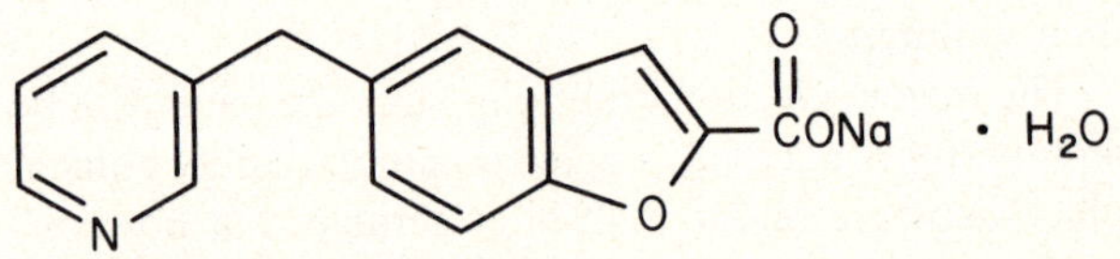

Molecular formula $C_{15}H_{10}NNaO_3 \cdot H_2O$

Molecular weight 293.25

Manufacturer The Upjohn Company

Code designation U-63,557A

CAS registry No. 87463-91-0

USAN LAMOTRIGINE

Pronunciation lȧ mō′ trĭ gēn

Therapeutic claim anticonvulsant

Chemical names

(1) 6-(2,3-dichlorophenyl)-1,2,4-triazine-3,5-diamine

(2) 3,5-diamino-6-(2,3-dichlorophenyl)-*as*-triazine

Structural formula

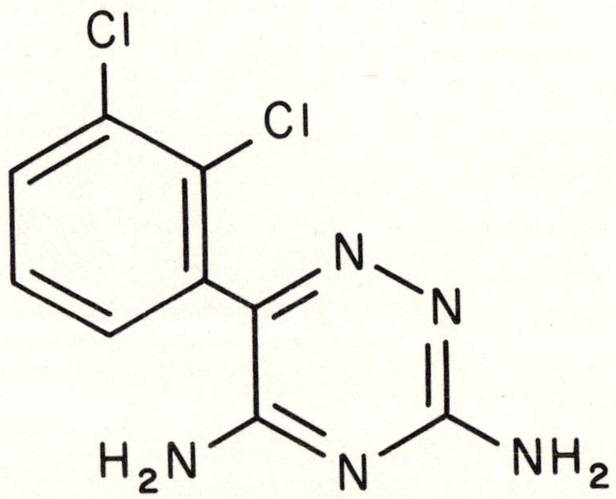

Molecular formula $C_9H_7Cl_2N_5$

Molecular weight 256.09

Manufacturer Burroughs Wellcome Co.

Code designation BW 430C

CAS registry No. 84057-84-1

USAN	NAPAMEZOLE HYDROCHLORIDE
Pronunciation	nă pă mĕ′ zōl
Therapeutic claim	antidepressant

Chemical names

(1) 2-[(3,4-dihydro-2-naphthalenyl)methyl]-4,5-dihydro-1*H*-imidazole monohydrochloride

(2) 2-[(3,4-dihydro-2-naphthyl)methyl]-2-imidazoline monohydrochloride

Structural formula

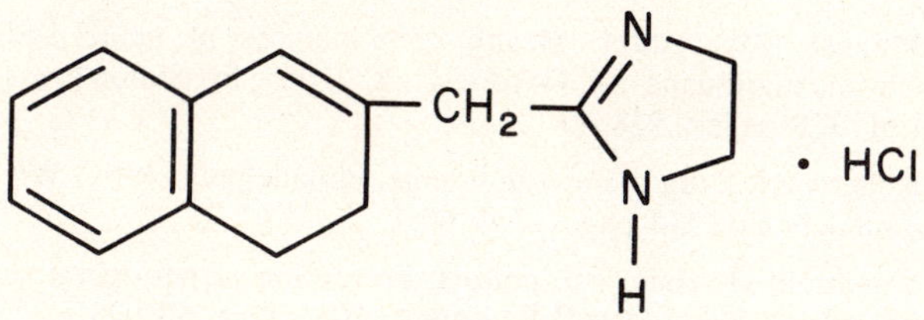

Molecular formula	$C_{14}H_{16}N_2 \cdot HCl$
Molecular weight	248.75
Manufacturer	Sterling Drug Inc.
Code designation	Win 51,181-2
CAS registry No.	87495-33-8

USAN	RECAINAM HYDROCHLORIDE
Pronunciation	rĕ kān′ ăm
Therapeutic claim	antiarrhythmic

Chemical names

(1) *N*-(2,6-dimethylphenyl-*N′*-[3-[(1-methylethyl)amino]propyl]urea monohydrochloride

(2) 1-[3-(isopropylamino)propyl]-3-(2,6-xylyl)urea monohydrochloride

Structural formula

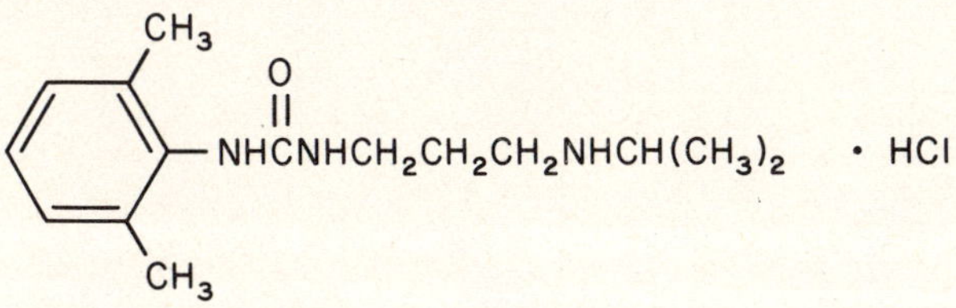

Molecular formula	$C_{15}H_{25}N_3O \cdot HCl$
Molecular weight	299.84
Manufacturer	Wyeth Laboratories Inc.
Code designation	WY-42,362 HCl
CAS registry No.	74752-07-1

USAN	FOSARILATE
Pronunciation	fŏs′ ă rīl″ āt
Therapeutic claim	antiviral

Chemical name

diethyl [6-(2-chloro-4-methoxyphenoxy)hexyl]phosphonate

Structural formula

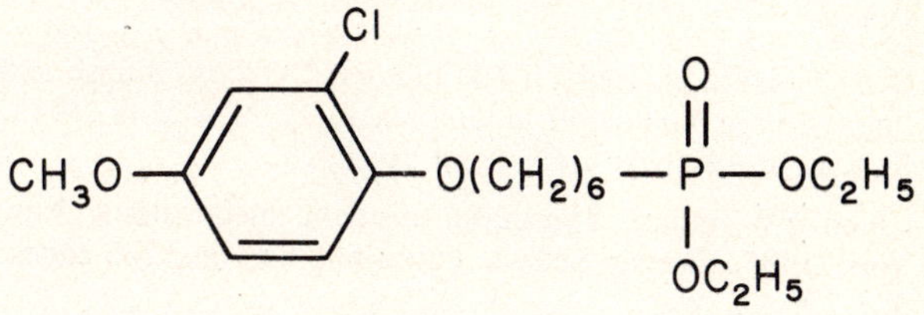

Molecular formula	$C_{17}H_{28}ClO_5P$
Molecular weight	378.83
Manufacturer	Sterling Drug Inc.
Code designation	Win 42,202
CAS registry No.	73514-87-1

USAN	VIPROSTOL
Pronunciation	vī prŏst′ ōl
Therapeutic claim	hypotensive (vasodilator)

Chemical names

(1) (±)-methyl (5*Z*,11α,13*E*)-16-ethenyl-11,16-dihydroxy-9-oxoprosta-5,13-dien-1-oate

(2) (±)-methyl *(Z)*-7-[(1*R*,2*R*,3*R*)-2-[*(E)*-(4*RS*)-4-butyl-4-hydroxy-1,5-hexadienyl]-3-hydroxy-5-oxocyclopentyl]-5-heptenoate

Structural formula

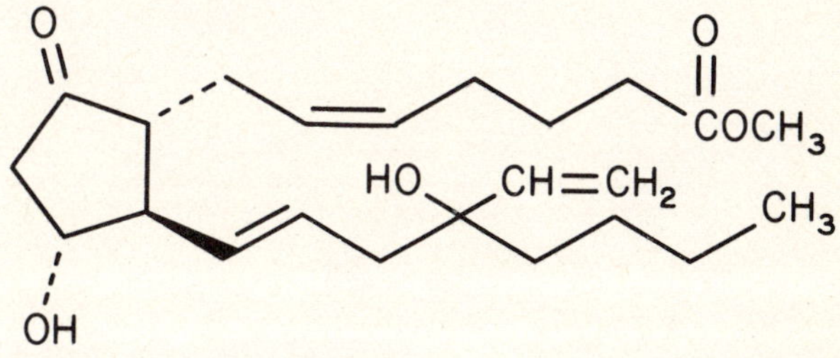

Molecular formula	$C_{23}H_{36}O_5$
Molecular weight	392.54
Manufacturer	Lederle Laboratories
Code designation	CL 115,347
CAS registry No.	73647-73-1

BOOKS RECEIVED

Aronoff GM, editor: Evaluation and treatment of chronic pain. Baltimore, 1985, Urban & Schwarzenberg. 684 pages. $65.00.

Balfour DJK, editor: Nicotine and the tobacco smoking habit. Elmsford, NY, 1984, Pergamon Press Inc. 221 pages. $65.00.

Barbagallo-Sangiorgi G, Exton-Smith AN, editors: Aging and drug therapy. New York, 1984, Plenum Press. 521 pages. $85.00.

Berti F, Hurd S, Hegyeli RJ, editors: Cyclooxygenase and lipoxygenase modulators in lung reactivity. New York, 1985, S. Karger. 146 pages. Price not given.

Chien YW, editor: Transnasal systemic medications. New York, 1985, Elsevier Science Publishing Co. Inc. 226 pages. $53.75.

Cogan MG, Garovoy MR, editors: Introduction to dialysis. New York, 1984, Churchill Livingstone Inc. 303 pages. $38.50.

Csaky TZ, editor: Pharmacology of intestinal permeation. New York, 1984, Springer-Verlag. 708 pages. Price not given.

Engquist A, editor: Fluids, electrolytes, nutrition. Copenhagen, 1985, Munksgaard International Publishers Ltd. 230 pages. Price not given.

Fuchs F, Stubblefield PG, editors: Preterm birth. New York, 1984, MacMillan Publishing Co. 392 pages. $48.00.

Grahame-Smith DG, Aronson JK, editors: The Oxford textbook of clinical pharmacology and drug therapy. New York, 1984, Oxford University Press. 843 pages. Price not given.

Griffin JP, D'Arcy PF, editors: Adverse drug interactions. Bristol, U. K., 1984, John Wright & Sons Ltd. 419 pages. $56.00.

Hansten PD: Drug interactions. Philadelphia, 1985, Lea & Febiger. 460 pages. $30.00.

Lindgren B, editor: Pharmaceutical economics. Sweden, 1984, Institute for Health Economics. 286 pages. Price not given.

Matsumura F, editor: Differential toxicities of insecticides and halogenated aromatics. Elmsford, NY, 1984, Pergamon Press Inc. 5,888 pages. $140.00.

Maykut MO, editor: Health consequences of acute and chronic marihuana use. Oxford, U. K., 1984, Pergamon Press Ltd. 328 pages. $28.00.

Roberts RJ: Drug therapy in infants. Philadelphia, 1984, WB Saunders Co. 414 pages. $49.00.

Schonfeld H, Hahn FE, editors: Prevention of perioperative infections, Basel, 1985, S. Karger. 208 pages. $89.25.

Shugar E, editor: Viral chemotherapy, vol 1. Elmsford, NY, 1984, Pergamon Press Inc. 573 pages. Price not given.

Spilker B: Guide to clinical studies and developing protocols. New York, 1984, Raven Press. 302 pages. $45.00.

Trimble MR, Zarifian E, editors: Psychopharmacology of the limbic system. New York, 1984, Oxford University Press. 266 pages. $35.00.

Tucker D, editor: The world health market. London, 1984, Euromonitor Publications Ltd. 220 pages. $60.00.

Urquhart J, Heilmann K, editors: Risk watch. New York, 1984, Kindler-Verlag. 214 pages. $16.95.

CLINICAL PHARMACOLOGY & THERAPEUTICS
VOLUME 38 NUMBER 4 OCTOBER 1985

COMMENTARY

The computerized on-line Medicaid pharmaceutical analysis and surveillance system: A new resource for postmarketing drug surveillance

Brian L. Strom, M.D., M.P.H., Jeffrey L. Carson, M.D., M. Lee Morse, Pharm.B., and Aida A. LeRoy, Pharm.D. *Philadelphia, Pa., Camden, N. J., and Arlington, Va.*

Postmarketing drug surveillance (PMS) assesses the use of drugs and monitors their beneficial and harmful effects after marketing.[1,2] Traditionally, PMS has been performed by: (1) physicians voluntarily reporting suspected adverse drug reactions either to the Food and Drug Administration (FDA), to pharmaceutical companies, or in the medical literature; (2) intensive hospital-based research systems; and (3) a few large-scale cohort studies conducted by pharmaceutics companies. Clearly, no single data resource will meet all needs for PMS studies. However, there remains a need for a large, relatively inexpensive, yet comprehensive system of collecting data on drug effects. To that end, the FDA has funded the development and testing of the Computerized On-Line Medicaid Pharmaceutical Analysis and Surveillance System (COMPASS) over the past 6 years. We will describe COMPASS and outline its advantages and disadvantages, providing a perspective on its potential in the investigation of effects of marketed drugs.

From The Clinical Epidemiology Unit, Section of General Medicine, Departments of Medicine and Pharmacology, University of Pennsylvania School of Medicine, Philadelphia; Department of Medicine, University of Medicine and Dentistry of New Jersey/Rutgers Medical School, Camden; and Health Information Designs, Inc., Arlington.

Supported in part by funds from the United States Food and Drug Administration, The Andrew W. Mellon Foundation, and The Rockefeller Foundation.

Received for publication Jan. 26, 1985; accepted June 19, 1985.

Reprint requests to: Brian L. Strom, M.D., M.P.H., Clinical Epidemiology Unit, 225L NEB/S2, University of Pennsylvania School of Medicine, Philadelphia, PA 19104.

DESCRIPTION OF THE COMPASS SYSTEM

COMPASS is a very large computerized data base of Medicaid billing data. It is designed to permit a researcher to enroll and analyze cohorts of patients ex-

Table I. Selected frequently used drugs—1984 COMPASS system*

Generic drug name	*Estimated No. of patients*†
Codeine phosphate	1,487,646
Amoxicillin	1,247,862
Penicillin	1,213,320
Sulfamethoxazole	682,492
Hydrocortisone	656,157
Cephalexin	653,928
Trimethoprim	645,247
Ergocalciferol	630,033
Promethazine HCl	579,209
Hydrochlorothiazide	480,886
Ibuprofen	432,617
Ethinyl estradiol	416,246
Norethindrone	366,093
Miconazole nitrate	350,586
Furosemide	318,992
Clotrimazole	306,130
Mestranol	259,439
Cefaclor	256,613
Metronidazole	249,725
Cimetidine	247,755
Digoxin	243,893
Propoxyphene HCL	239,798
Doxycycline hyclate	239,379
Hydroxyzine HCl	234,274
Chlordiazepoxide HCl	230,875
Potassium chloride	225,435
Betamethasone valerate	216,225
Norgestrel	199,666
Flurazepam HCl	199,055
Thiamine mononitrate	196,909
Diazepam	190,724
Amitriptyline HCl	190,016
Propoxyphene napsylate	173,599
Hydrocortisone acetate	158,670
Gentamicin sulfate	158,215
Naproxen	157,334
Propranolol HCl	155,543
Nitroglycerin	155,515
Methyldopa	149,759
Prednisone	149,407
Sulindac	136,523
Diphenoxylate HCl	134,559

*System population 5.3 million.
†Estimates based on COMPASS generic drug ranking reports.

posed to a drug or patients with specific diseases, and to compare them with matched or unmatched control groups. COMPASS derives its data as a by-product of the Medicaid Management Information System (MMIS), a computerized claims processing and management information system created in 1972 by the U.S. Department of Health, Education, and Welfare for fiscal and administrative control of Medicaid. This system collects data on all aspects of a Medicaid patient's interaction with the health care system.

MMIS data have been found to be useful to researchers in a variety of health care research areas. Buck and White[3] used California Medi-Cal data to study the impact of professional standards review organizations on practice patterns of physicians. Federspiel et al.[4] used the Tennessee Medicaid data base to analyze physician practice and drug prescribing habits and to review the effects of physician education programs. Eisenberg and Nicklin[5] used Pennsylvania Medicaid data to evaluate the use of diagnostic services by physicians in the community. Morse et al.[6] continue to use multistate Medicaid data to assess the impact of inappropriate drug therapy on hospitalizations. More recently, Avorn and Sumerai[7] have used Medicaid data to assess the impact of various physician drug information interventions on physician prescribing patterns.

COMPASS was originally conceived by Health Information Designs, Inc. (HID) and has been under development by HID since 1979. Initially, HID undertook on-site evaluation of the MMIS system of six states, and chose the data from Michigan and Minnesota (with an initial Medicaid population of 1.2 million, now increased to 2.0 million). More recently, Medicaid data from Florida, Missouri, Nebraska, Arkansas, Mississippi, Ohio, and Virginia have been added. HID provides these states an MMIS-based drug utilization review program and, as part of this program, obtains the right to use the MMIS data it receives for PMS. With these additions, the total COMPASS population is now approximately 5.3 million patients. Negotiations are under way to add other states and to add non-Medicaid sources of data, such as health maintenance organizations.

HID has created software to abstract that part of the MMIS data useful for a PMS system, store the data, retrieve it, and process it. COMPASS software is currently installed on a mini-computer manufactured by Wang Laboratories. Drug and diagnosis data processed by each state's MMIS are extracted and forwarded to the HID offices. Patient and provider identities are kept strictly confidential. The extract tape is sorted by patient identification number, service type/code, and date of service and then edited for incomplete or erroneous data elements. During the edit stage, specifically developed binary codes are assigned to each National Drug Code (NDC) and International Classification of Diseases (ICD-9-CM) code. This maximizes the on-line storage capacity of the patient history files. Data are organized by patient history files and can be accessed interactively or by batch processing. Currently available billing data for each patient include: state, age (as of any year specified by the investigator), sex, race, county, inpatient and outpatient diagnoses, outpatient drugs, and death. Data on procedures (laboratory, radiologic, etc.) are also available. Tables I and II list some of the most frequently used drugs and the most frequent diagnoses, respectively, in the 1984 COMPASS system.

Information on drugs and diagnoses can be accessed by a variety of coding methods. For drug information, data can be accessed with NDC codes, generic codes, specific therapeutic class codes, or user-defined code groupings. Similarly, it is possible to access diagnosis information with ICD-9-CM codes, disease category class codes, or user-defined code groupings.

Interaction with the system is menu driven. The user may choose between a number of epidemiologic routines displayed on the terminal screen. A selected list of these epidemiologic routines is presented in Table III. For example, the relative risk signal generator takes a user-defined cohort of patients exposed to a drug and a user-defined control group and automatically calculates relative risks and 95% confidence intervals for all ICD-9-CM diagnosis codes, all NDC generic codes, and all procedure codes or any defined subset of these. Analogously, the odds ratio signal generator takes a user-defined case group of patients with a particular disease and a user-defined control group and calculates odds ratios and 95% confidence intervals.

Primary medical records can be obtained from physicians, hospitals, and other sources as long as the number of requests is relatively limited. These requests are submitted to the states through use of the confidential patient and provider identification numbers. The states translate the numbers into personal identifications and submit the requests to the providers. The providers, in turn, are asked to delete identifying information when they provide the primary records.

ADVANTAGES OF COMPASS

The principal advantage of COMPASS is its very large population, currently over 5 million. This allows the study of relatively uncommonly used drugs and relatively uncommon illnesses. Second, COMPASS is population based, allowing the calculation of incidence rates. Third, unlike most alternative data systems, it includes both inpatient and outpatient diagnoses. Fourth, COMPASS data are not subject to recall or interviewer bias. Finally, because the data are collected in an ongoing way as a by-product of an administrative process, it is relatively inexpensive and can be used to

Table II. Selected frequent diagnoses—1984 COMPASS system*

ICD9-CM diagnoses	*Estimated No. of patients*†
Acute upper respiratory infection	1,432,799
Acute pharyngitis	1,096,469
Otitis media NOS	824,223
Bronchitis NOS	772,676
Abdominal pain	766,796
Urinary tract infection NOS	710,501
Chest pain NOS	578,024
Noninfectious gastroenteritis NEC	565,555
Pneumonia, organism NOS	548,076
Anemia NOS	511,299
Vaginitis NOS	510,457
Acute tonsillitis	502,471
Dermatitis NOS	467,326
Acute bronchitis	431,911
Headache	376,211
Hypertension NOS	368,403
Chronic sinusitis NOS	344,235
Flu with respiratory manifestations NEC	305,074
Normal delivery	286,697
Pregnancy, incidental	280,989
Cystitis NOS	270,942
Diabetes, uncomplicated adult	269,379
Absence of menstruation	267,901
Respiratory abnormality NEC	262,098
Strep sore throat	246,416
Myalgia and myositis NOS	230,799
Supervised other normal pregnancy	224,168
Gastritis/duodenitis NOS	215,594
Single liveborn in hospital	199,630
Coronary atherosclerosis	199,072
Nonspecific skin eruption NEC	194,371
Cervicitis	191,483
Allergic rhinitis NOS	189,502
Hypothyroidism NOS	183,381
Viral infection NOS	183,283
Anxiety state NOS	179,160
Female pelvic inflammatory disease NOS	179,151
Pregnancy examination—pregnancy unconfirmed	178,446
Diabetes mellitus, uncomplicated	177,522
Backache NOS	176,186
Asthma NOS	171,141
Benign hypertension	141,436
Cardiac dysrhythmia NOS	139,430
Asthma without status asthmaticus	138,055
Congestive heart failure	136,746
Death	118,804
Acne NEC	118,162

NOS = Not otherwise specified; NEC = not elsewhere classifiable.
*System population 5.3 million.
†Estimates based on COMPASS diagnosis ranking reports.

Table III. Selected epidemiologic procedures available on-line in COMPASS

Procedure	*Description*
Admissibility screenings	A requirement that patients must have had a medical service of some type before and after a specified time period, to assure they were probably eligible for Medicaid benefits in the interim
Cohort enrollment	Enrollment of all patients exposed to a certain drug or with a certain disease
Challenge/rechallenge analysis	After finding an apparent drug-disease association, this routine searches for those patients who have a second appearance of the disease subsequent to a second drug exposure
Diagnosis rankings	A count of the number of people suffering from each diagnosis in any specified group of patients, ranked by disease incidence, code number, etc.
Drug exposure rankings	A count of the number of people exposed to each drug in any specified group of patients, ranked by use, code number, etc.
Odds ratio signal generation	See text
Period of exposure analysis	Analysis of exposures in a specified time interval relative to an illness or another exposure, e.g., in the first trimester of pregnancy
Random age/sex/morbidity matched-control patient selection	Development of control groups for any specified cohort, matched for age, sex, diagnosis, or drug
Relative risk signal generation	See text
Temporal analysis	Examination of the temporal relationship between a drug and a subsequent diagnosis

address questions of clinical or regulatory importance quickly.

COMPASS has an advantage specific to conducting cohort studies, i.e., studies comparing patients receiving therapy with a drug with patients not receiving that drug or with patients taking a different drug, looking for differences in clinical outcomes. The major disadvantage of the cohort design is that it generally requires a large number of subjects to be followed over a long period of time. This is not a problem when an existing data base like COMPASS is used to perform cohort studies.

COMPASS also has advantages specific to conducting case-control studies, i.e., studies comparing patients with disease to those without, looking for differences in antecedent drug exposures. First, there is no opportunity for recall bias; drug exposure is determined from billing data rather than from patient recall. Second, the risk of selecting a biased control group can be reduced. In COMPASS, controls may be randomly selected from the entire population of individuals without the disease of interest, with or without matching for age, sex, race, drug(s), or other disease(s). These can be hospital-based controls (i.e., patients admitted to the hospital for a different reason), community-based controls, or both.

DISADVANTAGES OF COMPASS

It is also important to keep in mind the system's limitations. First, COMPASS does not include any data on inpatient drug use and only limited data on over-the-counter drug use (only those over-the-counter drugs that were prescribed).

Second, there is a 2-month lag period between the time a drug is dispensed and the time that it appears on the system. The analogous time delay for diagnoses can be as long as 6 months. This could be important in prospective cohort studies of newly marketed drugs, delaying for additional months the detection of drug effects.

Third, despite its size, COMPASS cannot be used to study very rarely prescribed drugs or extremely rare adverse reactions. When using COMPASS, as in any study, one must perform sample size calculations to determine whether the available sample sizes will be sufficient for the intended purposes.[8] On the other hand, when interpreting COMPASS-based studies, as with any study with very large sample sizes, one must be careful to distinguish between clinically significant differences and statistically significant but clinically trivial differences.

Fourth, to date COMPASS contains only Medicaid patients and thus its results may not be generalizable to other populations. This may be a significant problem for descriptive studies. It is less likely to be a problem for analytic (controlled) studies, inasmuch as both the study group and the control group will be drawn from the same population. The imminent addition of the first of a number of health maintenance organizations, with about 100,000 patients, should help alleviate this problem.

Fifth, COMPASS is limited to data collected since its initiation in January 1980. There are no data on drug exposures or illnesses that occurred before its initiation. Even if an exposure or illness persisted into the 1980s and thus appears in COMPASS, one cannot determine from COMPASS when the illness began. The only method of filling these gaps is getting past records from physicians currently administering to the patients under study.

Sixth, when using billing data, especially Medicaid data, one must always keep in mind the potential for gaps in the data due to eligibility changes. This will be a particular problem when one of the study groups is chosen by the absence of a disease or the absence of an exposure, rather than by its presence. One approach to this problem of eligibility changes is to choose both study and control groups by the presence of an exposure or disease, when possible, rather than by its absence. Then the investigator knows that the patient was eligible as of the date of that defined medical service. Alternatively, one can use software created to apply an admissability screen, requiring that patients must have a medical service of some type both before and after a specified time period to establish that they were probably eligible for medical service in the interim period.

Seventh, and importantly, COMPASS is limited to billing data. Thus it may be impossible to control for some potentially important confounding variables such as smoking, diet, parity, and occupation. In anticipating the use of COMPASS data, it is extremely important to consider all possible confounding variables and whether or not the data base includes data regarding each of them. If not, and if one cannot design any alternative approach, one must seriously question the utility of COMPASS in investigating the drug-disease association of interest.

Finally, the most important limitation in a system that uses billing data concerns the validity of its data. An FDA-funded validation study of COMPASS was recently completed, comparing COMPASS data with those from its primary sources, i.e., data from hospitals, physicians, pharmacies, and the like.[9] Within preestablished limits, year of birth agreed in 94% of sampled patients and could not be determined from the medical records in another 2.5%; sex agreed in 95% of patients and could not be determined from the medical records in another 4%; and the date of pharmacy dispensation of each drug agreed in 97% of sampled prescriptions. However, data regarding medical services were more questionable. Of the records that could be evaluated, looking within 1 week of the COMPASS date, 93% of the services in COMPASS could be found in the provider records. In 17% of those the provider record also included a previous or subsequent visit that was not in COMPASS. Diagnostic agreement to at least three digits of the ICD9-CM code occurred in 41% of these, and agreement within a broad diagnostic category (i.e., same body system or type of illness) in only another 16%.

Clearly, this study raises important doubts about the validity of the diagnostic data in COMPASS. However, this validation study has serious methodologic problems itself. First, physicians were sampled from only two urban areas, which may not reflect the accuracy of the diagnostic information in the entire system. Second, only 55% of physicians participated. Of the other 45%, 9% could not be located, 5% had no records available, and the remainder refused to participate. Third, the study checked records only from the physicians' primary practice site and never attempted to get information from sites such as other offices or an emergency room. In Michigan and Minnesota, 50% of physicians have such other practice sites. Fourth, the FDA study sampled claims rather than patients. If a patient with diabetes and hypertension had diabetes listed in his medical record on June 15 and hypertension on June 30, but COMPASS had a claim for hypertension listed on June 15 and one for diabetes listed on June 30, the validation study would have considered either the June 15 claim or the June 30 claim, or both, "disagreements" if it had included them in its sample. Fifth, this was not a study of validity, but a study of disagreement. This is especially important in view of a previous study of billing data suggesting that when there was disagreement, the claims diagnoses were more useful than the chart diagnoses.[10] As examples from the COMPASS validation study, included within the 43% disagreements were 12% (28% of the disagreements) in which the provider record had no diagnosis and 3% (7% of the disagreements) in which the provider record was probably missing diagnoses. Finally, even the remaining 28% disagreements await additional analyses regarding the seriousness of the discrepancy, since included as a disagreement would be situations such as a diagnosis of myocardial infarction in one of the data sources and a diagnosis of chest pain in the other.

Thus this study is inadequate to answer definitively the question about the validity of the COMPASS diagnostic data. Contradicting its apparent findings are the facts that the data appear to have face validity, i.e., the right drugs appear with the right diagnoses and in the right sequence. Also, the findings of the FDA-funded validation study must be interpreted in the context of the drug utilization review program that enables HID to obtain the COMPASS data. Each month thousands of patient-specific alerts are sent to the physicians and pharmacists providing the patients' medical care. These alerts request that the practitioner verify the accuracy of the billing data and, if they agree with the basis of the alert, modify their patients' drug therapy regimen to minimize the risks for a possible drug-induced illness. Over 70% of the alerts are responded to by the practitioners involved, and less than 1% of their responses indicate that the medical event data, upon which the risk was generated, was erroneous. Finally, there have been two formal studies[11,12] and a number of informal unpublished studies performed with COMPASS by both the FDA and the Clinical Epidemiology Unit of the University of Pennsylvania School of Medicine. In all cases, COMPASS confirmed known associations including, in some of them, a dose response.

If there is significant error in the diagnostic data, it may be random and overpowered by the available sample size. However, this remains an open question. Therefore, in using COMPASS, one must always remain aware of the potential for invalidity, building into each study tests for validation. Some examples of such tests would be: (1) preliminary case-control studies to document the system's ability to reproduce known drug causes of the disease(s) in question; (2) use of drugs and procedures that are more reliable in combination with diagnoses to define illnesses; (3) stratification of cases by the certainty of their diagnosis (e.g., the presence or absence of hospitalization, drug treatment, multiple appearances of the same or related diagnoses, etc.); and (4) procurement of copies of the primary records of patients of particular interest and importance.

ROLE OF COMPASS IN PMS

COMPASS provides a large and growing source of data on the relationships between drug exposures and illnesses. Its most important advantages are its size, its ability to provide population-based information, and the fact that the data already exist as a by-product of the Medicaid billing process. Its most important limitations are the question that has been raised about the validity of its diagnostic data, the potential for gaps in information due to changes in eligibility, and the absence of data on some potentially important confounding variables. However, used carefully, COMPASS may represent a useful new resource for PMS.

References

1. Strom BL, Melmon KL. Can postmarketing surveillance help to effect optimal drug therapy? JAMA 1979; 242:2420-3.
2. Strom BL: Postmarketing Drug Surveillance: an idea whose time has come. In: Melmon KL, ed. Drug therapeutics: concepts for physicians. New York: Elsevier-North Holland, 1982.
3. Buck CR, White KC. Peer review: impact of a system based on billing claims. N Engl J Med 1974;291: 877-83.
4. Federspiel CF, Wayne RA, Schaffner W. Medicaid records as a valid data source: the Tennessee experience. Med Care 1976;14:166-72.
5. Eisenberg JM, Nicklin D. Use of diagnostic services by physicians in community practice. Med Care 1981; 19:297-309.
6. Morse ML, LeRoy AA, Gaylord TA, Kellenberger T. Reducing drug therapy-induced hospitalizations: impact of drug utilization review. Drug Info J 1982;16:199-202.
7. Avorn J, Sumerai S. Improving drug-therapy decisions through educational outreach. N Engl J Med 1983; 308:1457-63.
8. Cohen J. Statistical power analysis for the behavioral sciences. Revised ed. New York: Academic Press, 1977.
9. Lessler JT, Harris BSH. Medicaid data as a source for post marketing surveillance information. Final report. Research Triangle Park, NC: Research Triangle Institute, 1984.
10. Studney DR, Hakstian AR. A comparison of medical record with billing diagnostic information associated with ambulatory medical care. Am J Public Health 1981; 71:145-9.
11. Van de Carr SW, Kennedy DL, Rosa FW, Anello C, Jones JK. Relationship of oral contraceptive estrogen dose to age. Am J Epidemiol 1983;117:153-9.
12. Strom BL, Tamragouri RN, Morse ML, Lazar EL, West SL, Stolley PD, Jones JK. Oral contraceptives and other risk factors for gallbladder disease. CLIN PHARMACOL THER. (Submitted for publication)

ORIGINAL ARTICLES

Morphine-induced skin wheals: A possible model for the study of histamine release

We evaluated the ability of morphine to release histamine when injected intradermally in man. Mathematic analysis of the dose-response (wheal) relationship suggested that two different effects were involved. The effect of low doses of morphine (0.05 to 1 μg) was clearly antagonized by naloxone (0.4 or 1.2 mg im 30 minutes before), whereas the effect of higher doses (5 to 50 μg) was not modified. The median effective doses of morphine (ED_{50}) for the low dose range effect were 0.07 ± 0.01 and 0.08 ± 0.01 μg before naloxone and 0.14 ± 0.02 and 0.15 ± 0.03 μg after 0.4 and 1.2 mg doses, respectively. Astemizole (45 mg po 30 minutes before) and oxatomide (60 mg po 120 minutes before) produced similar inhibition of histamine-induced wheals, but there were clear differences in their effects on wheals elicited by morphine. Morphine ED_{50} values for the low dose range effect rose from 0.09 ± 0.01 to 0.20 ± 0.01 μg after astemizole and from 0.08 ± 0.01 to 0.46 ± 0.04 μg after oxatomide. Opiate receptors may be involved in some of the effects produced by morphine injection in the human skin, but morphine-induced wheals seem to offer a suitable model for the evaluation of agents capable of inhibiting histamine release in man. (CLIN PHARMACOL THER 1985;38:365-70.)

Roberto Saucedo, M.D., and Sergio Erill, M.D.* *Granada, Spain*

Although the ability to release histamine is assumed to be a common feature of many drugs, few quantitative studies in man have been performed. In vitro studies with human basophils have been conducted to evaluate histamine release by radiocontrast materials,[1,2] and measurement of plasma histamine levels has been used in the evaluation of histamine release after intravenous injection of narcotic analgesics.[3,4] Morphine,[5] as well as meperidine,[6] produces "triple response" effects in human skin, which could provide a model for the study of agents capable of inhibiting histamine release in man.

Our study was undertaken to investigate the dose-dependence of morphine-induced wheals in human skin and the possible participation of opiate receptors in this effect. The usefulness of this model in the differentiation of antihistamines that act solely as histamine receptor blockers, such as astemizole,[7] from those that are also capable of inhibiting histamine release, such as oxatomide,[8,9] was also explored.

METHODS

Our subjects were 30 healthy men of normal weight ranging in age from 22 to 28 years. The study was approved by the Clinical Trials Board of the University Hospital and participants gave written informed consent. In each experiment subjects rested for 1 hour in a temperature-controlled room (20° ± 1° C) before morphine dosing and for 15 minutes thereafter. Morphine HCl was dissolved in 0.1 ml saline solution and was injected intradermally in the volar surface of the forearm. Each subject received six injections (0.05, 0.1, 1, 5, 10, and 50 μg), 3 cm apart, plus a control injection of 0.1 ml saline solution and two or three injections of histamine phosphate in an equal volume. Doses of histamine were 1 and 4 μg in the study of the effects of naloxone and 0.5, 1, and 2 μg in the studies with antihistamines (see below). Solutions were freshly prepared for each experiment. Fifteen minutes after the

From the Department of Pharmacology, University of Granada Medical School.

Received for publication April 8, 1985; accepted July 10, 1985.

Reprint requests to: Roberto Saucedo, M.D., Department of Pharmacology, University of Granada Medical School, Avda. de Madrid s/n, 18012 Granada, Spain.

*Present address: Esteve Foundation, Barcelona, Spain.

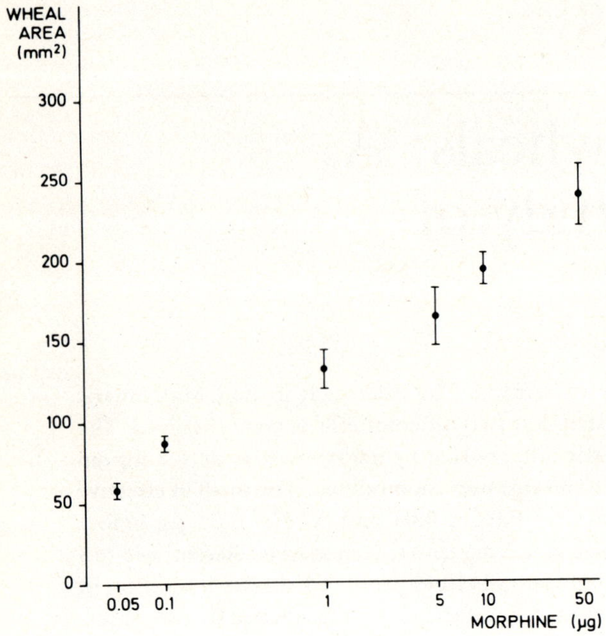

Fig. 1. Areas of wheals elicited by intradermal injection of morphine in 0.1 ml saline solution. Data are $\overline{X} \pm$ SE (n = 6).

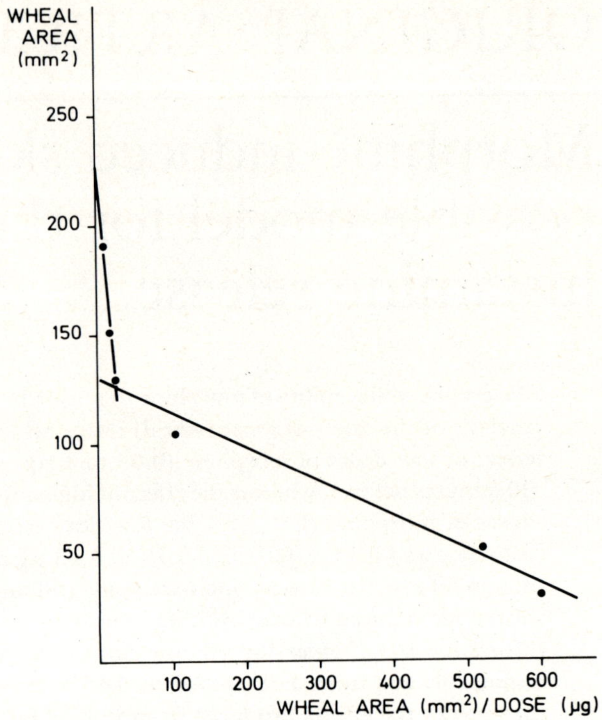

Fig. 2. Plot of effect vs. effect/dose for the analysis of morphine effects in human skin. A graph with two straight lines is quite apparent (same data as in Fig. 1).

injections, wheals were mapped out with ink and their patterns were transcribed onto cellophane paper. Two photocopies of the transcripts were made; one was kept as a permanent record and the other was carefully cut and weighed. The same batch of paper was used throughout the study, and surface area was calculated as a direct function of weight. Surface areas of the corresponding saline solution control subjects were subtracted from morphine and histamine areas in all cases. The sequence of injections along the forearm was random in each subject, and the mapping out of the areas was done by an investigator unaware of the sequence.

Systemic medications were given in a double-blind manner. In the experiments with naloxone, the drug or placebo was given by intramuscular injection at a dose of 0.4 or 1.2 mg 30 minutes before morphine injection. Astemizole (45 mg) or placebo was taken by mouth 30 minutes before morphine, and oxatomide (60 mg) was also taken by mouth 120 minutes before morphine. A series of preliminary experiments in healthy subjects had shown that at these doses and times, the antihistaminic potency of astemizole and oxatomide was roughly equal.

Each dose of naloxone, astemizole, and oxatomide were evaluated in a different group of six subjects. Thus five experimental groups of six subjects each were studied: morphine alone, low-dose naloxone, high-dose naloxone, astemizole, and oxatomide. The study was performed twice in the last four groups, with morphine injection in alternate forearms. Student's t tests for paired and group data were used in the statistical analysis of results. Analysis of the dose-response relationship was by the double-reciprocal plot and by plotting effect vs. effect/dose (see Appendix).

RESULTS

Morphine effects in normal subjects. Intradermal injection of morphine in the forearm of normal subjects produced triple response effects in a dose-related manner, with apparent good linearity for the relationship of wheal surface area vs. dose (Fig. 1). However, a double-reciprocal plot of data failed to give a straight line. A plot of effect vs. effect/dose was then used, but again no straight line was obtained in any of the subjects, and indeed a graph with two straight lines was quite apparent (Fig. 2). The theoretic maximum effect (E_{max}) for the lower doses of morphine (0.05 to 1 µg) was 129.3 ± 7.4 mm^2 and the dose producing half-maximal effect (ED_{50}) was 0.12 ± 0.02 µg. The theoretic E_{max} for the higher doses (5 to 50 µg) was 227.2 ± 17.6 mm^2, with an ED_{50} of 3.13 ± 0.65 µg.

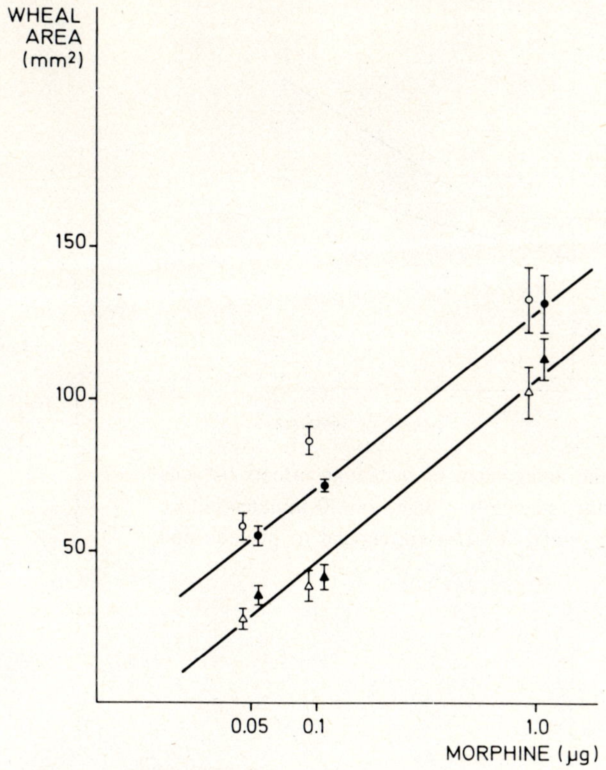

Fig. 3. Areas of wheals elicited by intradermal injection of low doses of morphine after pretreatment with placebo *(circles)* or naloxone *(triangles)*. *Open* and *solid* symbols show data from two different studies with either 0.4 or 1.2 mg naloxone, respectively. Only regression lines for the second study are shown. Data are $\overline{X} \pm$ SE (n = 6).

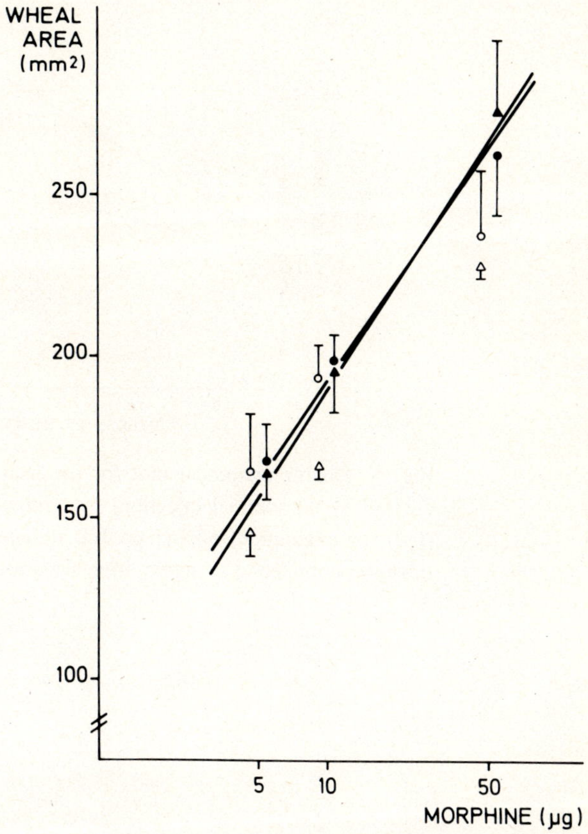

Fig. 4. Areas of wheals elicited by intradermal injection of high doses of morphine after pretreatment with placebo *(circles)* or naloxone *(triangles)*. *Open* and *solid* symbols show data from two different studies (same as in Fig. 3) with 0.4 or 1.2 mg naloxone, respectively. Only regression lines for the second study are shown. Data are $\overline{X} \pm$ SE (n = 6).

Effect of naloxone on morphine-induced histamine release. Pretreatment with naloxone (0.4 or 1.2 mg) had different effects on the production of wheals by low or high doses of morphine. In the group of six subjects receiving 0.4 mg naloxone, the log dose-response curve for low doses of morphine was clearly displaced to the right (Fig. 3) and the ED_{50} shifted from 0.07 ± 0.01 to 0.14 ± 0.02 µg ($P < 0.01$). Similar results were obtained in the group who received 1.2 mg naloxone (ED_{50} increased from 0.08 ± 0.01 to 0.15 ± 0.03 µg; $P < 0.05$). The theoretic E_{max} did not change (142.4 ± 12.8 and 141.0 ± 11.6 mm^2 after placebo and 115 ± 11.3 and 130.2 ± 10.4 mm^2 after 0.4 and 1.2 mg naloxone, respectively).

The effect of higher doses of morphine was not altered by naloxone (Fig. 4). ED_{50} values were 3.58 ± 1.23 and 3.59 ± 0.65 µg after placebo and 3.78 ± 0.40 and 4.02 ± 0.56 µg after naloxone, 0.4 and 1.2 mg, respectively. The theoretic E_{max} for this range of morphine doses was 256.2 ± 25.3 and 278.2 ± 21.4 mm^2 after placebo and 239.8 ± 4.7 and 290.5 ± 26.5 mm^2 after 0.4 and 1.2 mg naloxone, respectively. Neither dose of naloxone modified the size of control wheals produced by saline solution or of wheals elicited by 1 or 4 µg histamine in the same subjects.

Effect of astemizole and oxatomide on wheals elicited by histamine or morphine. The surface area of wheals produced by the intradermal injection of 0.5, 1, and 2 µg histamine was similarly reduced by pretreatment with oral astemizole or oxatomide (Fig. 5). Histamine ED_{50} values calculated from a plot of wheal surface area vs. wheal surface area/dose increased from 0.27 ± 0.02 to 0.56 ± 0.05 µg ($P < 0.001$) after astemizole and from 0.32 ± 0.04 to 0.78 ± 0.10 µg ($P < 0.001$) after oxatomide.

There were clear differences between astemizole and oxatomide in the effect on wheal surface area after intradermal morphine injection (Figs. 6 and 7). Esti-

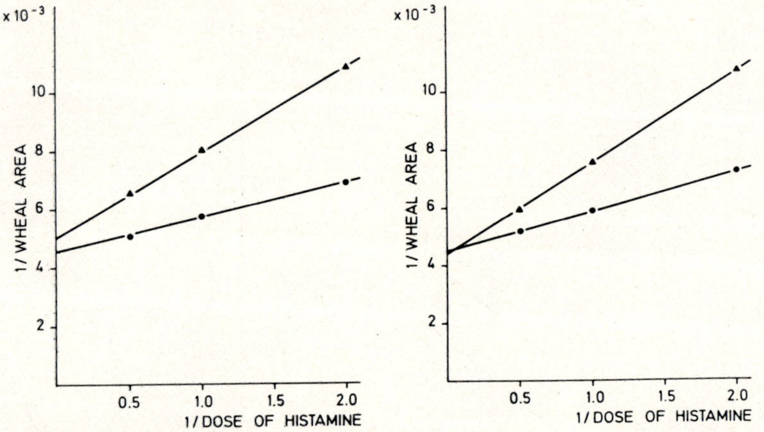

Fig. 5. Double-reciprocal plot for the analysis of the antagonism of histamine effects (wheals elicited by intradermal injection) by pretreatment with astemizole, 45 mg po 30 minutes before *(left)*, or oxatomide, 60 mg po 120 minutes before *(right)*. *Circles* correspond to placebo and *triangles* correspond to active drug. Data are $\overline{X}$ (n = 6).

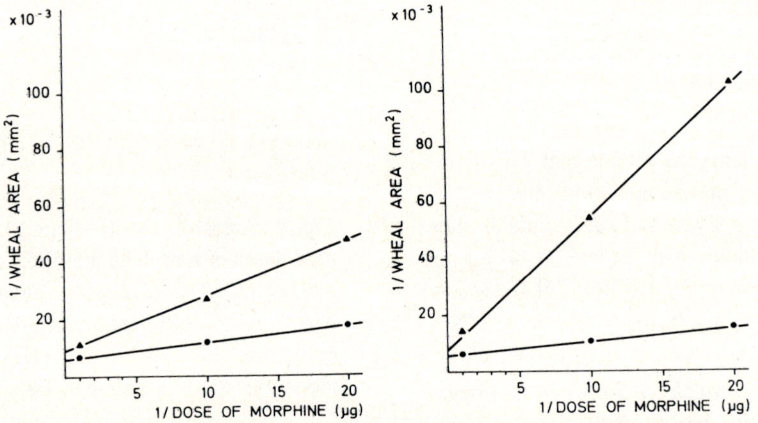

Fig. 6. Double-reciprocal plot for the analysis of the antagonism of morphine effects (wheals elicited by intradermal injection of low doses, 0.05 to 1 µg) by astemizole, 45 mg po 30 minutes before *(left)*, or oxatomide, 60 mg po 120 minutes before *(right)*. *Circles* correspond to placebo and *triangles* correspond to active drug. Data are $\overline{X}$ (n = 6).

mated ED_{50} values in the low-dose range of morphine were 0.09 ± 0.01 µg after pretreatment with placebo and 0.20 ± 0.01 µg after astemizole ($P < 0.001$), whereas ED_{50} values in the placebo-oxatomide group were 0.08 ± 0.01 and 0.46 ± 0.04 µg ($P < 0.001$), respectively ($P < 0.01$ for the difference between astemizole and oxatomide). ED_{50} values for the higher doses of morphine were 2.16 ± 0.49 and 4.91 ± 0.99 µg ($P < 0.01$) in the placebo-astemizole study and 2.49 ± 0.60 and 8.29 ± 0.40 µg ($P < 0.001$) in the placebo-oxatomide series ($P < 0.05$ for the difference between astemizole and oxatomide).

DISCUSSION

The ability of narcotics to release histamine is well known,[4,10,11] although the potency of the different agents in therapeutic use probably differs.[3] Histamine release by morphine is well documented[4,5,12,13] and it is generally assumed to be related directly to its basic nature.[14,15] Many basic compounds, including a number of widely used drugs such as codeine,[13] guanethidine,[14] stilbamidine,[12] and tubocurarine,[13] cause histamine release from mast cells.[16] Our results confirm the ability of morphine to release histamine in human skin and its dose dependence. However, our data suggest that two

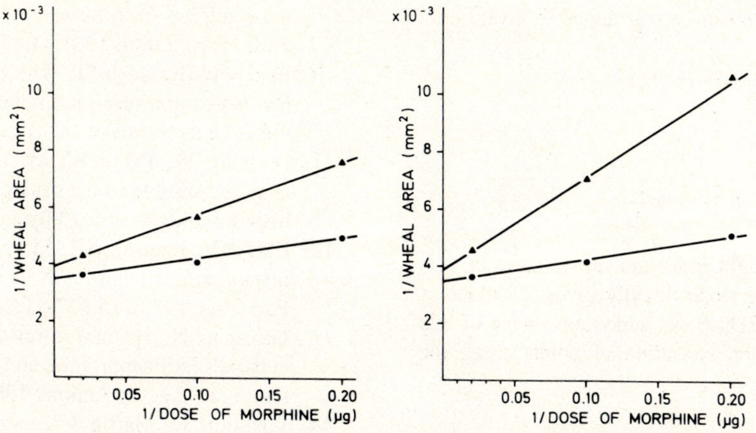

Fig. 7. Double-reciprocal plot for the analysis of the antagonism of morphine effects (wheals elicited by intradermal injection of high doses, 5 to 10 μg) by astemizole, 45 mg po 30 minutes before *(left)*, or oxatomide, 60 mg po 120 minutes before *(right)*. *Circles* correspond to placebo and *triangles* correspond to active drug. Data are $\overline{X}$ (n = 6).

different effects are involved. This is evidenced by the lack of linearity of the plot of effect (wheal area) vs. effect/dose, which consistently produces a graph with two straight lines, and by the differential influence of naloxone on these apparent effects. It seems likely that the basic nature of morphine plays a major role in the release of histamine by this drug, but the antagonist effect of naloxone on low doses of morphine suggests possible participation of opiate receptors. Naloxone did not modify the size of wheals induced by saline solution or histamine, and this makes highly unlikely any explanation of the observed antagonism through antihistaminic activity or through a direct effect on capillary permeability. On the other hand, it has been reported[16] that naloxone, 10 to 20 μg/kg, does not prevent the changes in resistance and capacitance vessels induced by intra-arterial morphine. These changes are presumably due to histamine release, but the morphine doses that elicit them (0.5 to 1 mg/kg intra-arterially) are probably more in accord with the high-dose range than with the low-dose range in our study. Therefore, it is tempting to postulate involvement of opiate receptors, as well as the basic nature of morphine, in the release of histamine by this drug. Although any attempt to interpret the role of these opiate receptors in mast cells would be too speculative, it is appropriate to mention that opiate receptors have been found in human phagocytic leukocytes,[17] lymphocytes,[18,19] and platelets.[19]

Our data also suggest that morphine effects on the intact skin may offer a suitable model for the evaluation of agents capable of inhibiting histamine release. Oxatomide is an H_1-receptor blocker[20] shown to inhibit anaphylactic histamine release from human lung tissue and basophilic leukocytes,[8,9] whereas astemizole is an H_1-competitive antihistamine devoid of this additional activity.[7] The pharmacokinetics as well as the antihistaminic potencies of these two drugs differ, but when used at times and dosages that allow for an equal antagonist activity on the effects of intradermally injected histamine, the activity of oxatomide is superior to that of morphine. This discrimination between oxatomide and astemizole is elicited with either low or high concentrations of morphine and, unless further studies prove the contrary, either of the two ranges we used seems equally suitable for the evaluation of agents capable of inhibiting histamine release in man.

APPENDIX

Analysis of the dose-response relationships was carried out under the assumption that there is a relationship between drug concentration (or dose) and effect elicited:

$$E = \frac{E_{max} A}{A + K}$$

where E stands for effect, A is the concentration or dose given, and K is the apparent dissociation constant of the drug receptor complex. This equation graphs as an hyperbola in rectangular coordinates, but a plot of 1/E vs. 1/A produces a straight line, because when both sides of the equation are inverted:

$$\frac{1}{E} = \frac{K}{E_{max}} \cdot \frac{1}{A} + \frac{1}{E_{max}}$$

Similarly, the first equation can be rearranged to give:

$$\frac{E\,(A + K)}{A} = E_{max}$$

and this leads to:

$$E = E_{max} - K\frac{E}{A}$$

This also produces a straight line, and the y-intercept corresponds to E_{max} while the slope directly gives K, which is numerically equal to the ED_{50}.[21] An added advantage of this plot is that it gives a good spreading of points along the graph.[22]

References

1. Rockoff SD, Brasch R, Kuhn C, Chraplyvy M. Contrast media as histamine liberators. I. Mast cell histamine release in vitro by sodium salts of contrast media. Invest Radiol 1970;6:503-9.
2. Ring J, Simon RA, Arroyave CM. Increased in vitro histamine release by radiographic contrast media in patients with history of incompatibility. Clin Exp Immunol 1978;34:302-9.
3. Flacke JW, Van Etten A, Flacke WE. Greatest histamine release from meperidine among four narcotics: double blind study in man. Anesthesiology 1983;39:A-51.
4. Fahmy NR, Sunder BS, Soter NA. Role of histamine in the hemodynamic and plasma catecholamine responses to morphine. CLIN PHARMACOL THER 1983;33:615-20.
5. Sollman T, Pilcher JD. Morphine evokes the triple response in human skin. J Pharmacol 1917;9:309-14.
6. Finer BL, Partington MW. Pethidine and the triple response. Br Med J 1953;1:431-3.
7. Richards DM, Brogden RN, Heel RC, et al. Astemizole. A review of its pharmacodynamic properties and therapeutic efficacy. Drugs 1984;28:38-61.
8. Church MK, Gradidge CF. Inhibition and stimulation of histamine release from human lung and leucocytes in vitro. Agents Actions 1980;10:4-7.
9. Rademecker M. Inhibition of allergen-mediated histamine release from human cells by ketotifen and oxatomide. Respiration 1981;41:45-55.
10. Eckenoff JE, Oech SR. The effects of narcotics and antagonists upon respiration and circulation in man. A review. CLIN PHARMACOL THER 1960;1:483-524.
11. Feldberg W, Paton WDM. Release of histamine from skin and muscle in the cat by opium alkaloids and other histamine liberators. J Physiol 1951;114:490-509.
12. Ellis HV, Johnson AR, Moran NC. Selective release of histamine from mast cells by several drugs. J Pharmacol Exp Ther 1970;175:627-31.
13. Grosman N. Histamine release from isolated rat mast cells: effect of morphine and related drugs and their interaction. Agents Actions 1981;11:196-203.
14. Lagunoff D, Martin TW. Agents that release histamine from mast cells. Ann Rev Pharmacol Ther 1983;23:331-51.
15. Paton WDM. Histamine release by compounds of simple chemical structure. Pharmacol Rev 1959;9:269-328.
16. Hsu-Ho, Hickey RF, Forbes AR. Morphine decreases peripheral vascular resistance and increases capacitance in man. Anesthesiology 1979;50:98-102.
17. Lopker A, Abood LG, Hoss W, Lionetti FJ. Stereoselective muscarinic acetylcholine and opiate receptors in human phagocytic leukocytes. Biochem Pharmacol 1980; 29:1361-5.
18. McDonough RJ, Madden JJ, Falek A, et al. Alteration of T and null lymphocyte frequencies in the peripheral blood of human opiate addicts: in vivo evidence for opiate receptor sites on T lymphocytes. J Immunol 1980;125: 2539-43.
19. Mehrishi JN, Mills IH. Opiate receptors on lymphocytes and platelets in man. Clin Immunol Immunopathol 1983;27:240-9.
20. Richards DM, Brogden NN, Heel RC, et al. Oxatomide. A review of its pharmacodynamic properties and therapeutic efficacy. Drugs 1984;27:210-31.
21. Tallarida RJ, Jacob LS. The dose-response relation in pharmacology. New York: Springer-Verlag, 1979:49-84.
22. Dixon M, Webb EC. Enzymes. London: Longman, 1979:47-206.

Interactions between ethanol and oral contraceptive steroids

We investigated the effect of oral contraceptive steroids (OCSs) on plasma ethanol disposition and tolerance to ethanol. Fifty-four healthy women between 18 and 40 years old were classified as light (31) or moderate (23) drinkers. Each group was further subdivided into controls (no OCS; 10 light, seven moderate drinkers), 30 or 35 μg estrogen OCS (14 light, 11 moderate drinkers), and 50 μg estrogen OCS (seven light, five moderate drinkers). Four of the subjects were studied on a second occasion, thus acting as their own controls with and without OCS use. All women were studied between days 14 and 21 of their pill/menstrual cycle. Plasma ethanol concentrations and two simple tests of motor function were measured for 6 hours after ethanol, 0.9 gm/kg in orange juice drank over a 30-minute period. The groups were well matched for age and weight. There were no significant differences between any of the six subgroups in mean peak plasma ethanol concentration, mean time to peak, mean AUC, or mean rate of ethanol disappearance. This was also the case for the four women who acted as their own controls. Analyses between those receiving high and low progestogen OCSs and between smokers and nonsmokers showed no significant differences. There was acute deterioration in functional performance as measured by two motor function tests in all subjects, regardless of OCS use. Moderate drinkers were significantly less functionally impaired than light drinkers whether with or without OCS use, indicating acquired tolerance. The mean degree of impairment and mean recovery time for both tests were significantly less in the OCS groups than in the control groups. The same trend was seen in the four women who were their own controls. Our results suggest that OCS use may induce some form of "tolerance" to ethanol. However, because there is no evidence of any change in ethanol disposition even at high plasma ethanol concentrations (>100 mg/dl), women taking OCSs should not attempt to drink more than usual. (Clin Pharmacol Ther 38:371-380, 1985.)

Joy Hobbes, M.Sc., John Boutagy, Ph.D., and Gillian M. Shenfield, D.M.
St. Leonards, Australia

Many drugs are metabolized by liver enzymes and there may be competition between drugs that use the same pathways; either induction or inhibition may result. The oral contraceptive steroids (OCSs) stimulate or do not change the metabolism of drugs metabolized principally by hepatic conjugation, such as paracetamol, oxazepam, and lorazepam.[1,4,21] In contrast, OCSs inhibit the metabolism of a variety of drugs that undergo oxidative biotransformation in the liver, such as antipyrine,[2] diazepam,[3] theophylline,[27] caffeine,[23] metoprolol,[14] and imipramine.[5] It is believed, but not established, that these inhibitory interactions are due to the estrogen component of the OCS.[7,16]

Ethanol is metabolized in the liver by cytoplasmic alcohol dehydrogenase to form acetaldehyde, which is further converted to acetate by aldehyde dehydrogenase. Conversion of ethanol to acetaldehyde is the rate limiting step because of a limited rate of oxidation of NADH to NAD.[24] It is thought that at high ethanol doses, alcohol dehydrogenase becomes saturated and that catalases and microsomal oxidizing enzymes become additional pathways for the metabolism of ethanol.[17,25] It is reported that cimetidine, a potent inhibitor of microsomal enzyme activity, increases plasma ethanol concentrations.[10] At high ethanol concentrations it is therefore possible that OCSs could have a similar effect. This has been supported by anecdotal evidence of some women who observe decreased subjective ethanol tolerance while taking OCS and by a report that women taking OCSs had a decreased rate of ethanol metabolism, although the peak plasma ethanol concentrations were lower in the OCS group than in controls.[12] Others have also found that women taking OCSs had

From the Department of Clinical Pharmacology, The Royal North Shore Hospital.
Submitted for publication Dec. 3, 1984; accepted March 8, 1985.
Reprint requests to: Professor G. M. Shenfield, Department of Clinical Pharmacology, Royal North Shore Hospital, St. Leonards NSW 2065, Australia.

Table I. Subject characteristics

	Light drinkers' estrogen intake			*Moderate drinkers' estrogen intake*		
	Control	*30 or 35 μg*	*50 μg*	*Control*	*30 or 35 μg*	*50 μg*
No. of subjects	10	14	7	7	11	5
Age (yr)	27.7(21-35)	26.9(21-35)	30.3(23-39)	29.0(19-38)	26.5(19-40)	25.0(22-33)
Weight (kg)	56.5(50-77)	56.9(48-74)	57.4(46-64)	54.9(51-58)	55.1(48-65)	55.2(55-76)
No. of smokers	2	6	1	3	6	4
No. taking low progestogen OCS (50 to 250 μg)	—	13	2	—	10	2
No. taking high progestogen OCS (500 to 1000 μg)	—	1	5	—	1	3
Baseline reaction time (msec)	660 ± 20	680 ± 30	700 ± 40	670 ± 20	680 ± 20	—
Baseline bead count (no.)	27.1 ± 0.84	27.2 ± 0.61	23.6 ± 1.60	24.8 ± 1.30	25.8 ± 1.38	26.5 ± 1.19

Data are $\overline{X}$ ± SE (range).

lower peak plasma ethanol concentrations than a control group, but no data on ethanol elimination were reported.[32] Both groups used breath alcohol measurements.

In view of the widespread use of OCSs and ethanol and the potential medicolegal implications of any interaction between them, we performed a controlled study with blood ethanol measurements. We also investigated the effect of OCSs on tolerance to ethanol.

METHODS

Our subjects were women 18 to 40 years old who regularly drank ethanol and had normal hepatic and renal function. Their existing method of contraception had been in use for at least 3 months, with good compliance. They were not taking any medication known to modify the central nervous system action of ethanol or its hepatic metabolism. Pregnant women were excluded. Details of the 54 healthy subjects recruited are listed in Table I. Subjects were allocated to two major drinking categories determined from a grid described in the first report of a Risk Factor Prevalence Study[22] that takes into account frequency of drinking, the number of drinks consumed, and sex. For example, one or two ethanol drinks 4 or 5 days a week classify a woman as a light drinker, while three to four drinks every day indicate a moderate drinker. The subjects were further divided into subgroups based on the estrogen content of their OCS (30 or 35 μg and 50 μg). Control subjects were not taking OCSs. There were no statistically significant differences in age, weight, and progestogen content of the OCS between the groups, but fewer controls were smokers.

Subjects were studied during days 14 to 21 of the menstrual/pill cycle. They drank no alcohol for 24 hours and fasted for 12 hours before the study. Subjects were weighed and given 0.9 gm/kg ethanol (rectified spirit B.P.) diluted in orange juice to give a 10% (w/v) drink and flavored with peppermint to reduce nausea. The ethanol was drunk at as uniform a rate as possible over a 30-minute period. Blood samples were collected from an indwelling cannula (with a heparin lock) inserted in a forearm vein. Sampling times were zero (before ethanol), every 15 minutes for the first hour after ceasing to drink ethanol, then every 30 minutes for 2 hours, and hourly for the last 3 hours of the study. Coffee and a biscuit were eaten at 90 minutes and a light lunch was eaten at 3 hours after ceasing to drink ethanol. Each time blood was drawn, tests of functional performance were carried out with a simple reaction time apparatus and a bead threading test. Before the study subjects were given a short period in which to familiarize themselves with the equipment. Baseline performance was taken as the reaction time (in milliseconds) or bead count (number) just before starting to drink ethanol. Table I lists baseline results for all groups. There were no significant differences. For the purpose of analyzing any changes, these values were

Table II. Plasma ethanol results for the six major groups

	Light drinkers' estrogen intake			Moderate drinkers' estrogen intake		
	Control	*30 or 35 μg*	*50 μg*	*Control*	*30 or 35 μg*	*50 μg*
Peak concentration (mg/dl)	130(5)	126(4)	125(9)	126(4)	128(6)	113(4)
Time to peak (min)	27(6)	33(5)	32(5)	30(7)	28(8)	45(7)
AUC (mg · hr/dl)	727(177)	715(136)	642(129)	679(96)	725(150)	640(56)
β_{60} (gm/L/hr)	0.22(0.03)	0.22(0.04)	0.23(0.04)	0.23(0.04)	0.22(0.05)	0.23(0.04)

Data are $\bar{X}$ ($\pm$SE).

standardized to zero. During the studies in the moderate drinking 50 μg OCS group, the reaction time apparatus was not functioning and only bead counts were performed.

Four of the women taking 30 or 35 μg OCSs underwent study a second time while not taking OCSs, thus acting as their own controls. These studies were at least 3 months apart and the protocol was identical to that detailed above.

To determine the effects of learning on functional performance, 20 women matched for age who were not given ethanol performed the reaction time test at intervals for 6 hours.

All blood collected was immediately centrifuged and the plasma transferred to sterile Vacutainers (Becton-Dickinson) with 1% sodium fluoride and 1% potassium oxalate added as preservatives. Plasma samples were stored at −20° C until analysis. The assay for plasma ethanol was essentially that described by Cooper,[9] in that 0.2 ml plasma was deproteinized by treatment with 0.2 ml 10% (w/v) sodium tungstate and 0.2 ml 0.3 mol/L sulphuric acid. The internal standard (isopropanol) was added as 1.5 ml (15 mg/dl) solution and the samples were mixed and centrifuged. The supernatant (5 μl) was analyzed by gas chromatography on a Hewlett-Packard Model No. 5839A fitted with a flame ionization detector and a prepacked Porapak Q column (4′ × 1/8″; Australian Analytical Laboratories). Samples were injected by an automatic sampler and chromatograms were recorded on a recording integrator. Quantitation was by peak area determination of the ratio of ethanol to that of isopropanol. Average percentage recovery for a plasma ethanol concentration of 45 mg/dl was 97.8% and for 120 mg/dl it was 99.4% ($n = 6$). The average coefficients of variation for plasma ethanol concentrations of 45, 120, and 150 mg/dl were 3.8%, 2.0%, and 3.8%, respectively ($n = 8$ for each concentration). Sensitivity of the method for quantitation was 10 mg/dl. Loss of ethanol at −20° C from storage containers over a period of 3 months was <5%.

The mean peak plasma ethanol concentrations and time to reach peak concentrations were calculated for the six groups. The plasma ethanol AUCs were calculated by the trapezoidal method and extrapolated to infinity. The rate of ethanol disappearance was estimated by the slope of the regression line fit by the method of least squares to the pseudolinear portion of the elimination curve (1 to 5 hours after completion of ethanol absorption). This is referred to as the β_{60}.[31] All measurements were analyzed for the six groups, for smokers and nonsmokers, and for those taking an OCS with a low (50 to 250 μg) or high (500 to 1000 μg) progestogen content.

Results for functional performance measured with the reaction time apparatus were recorded as the number of milliseconds to achieve a correct response, and for the bead threading test results are expressed as the number of beads threaded in a given sequence in 1 minute. Thus an increase in milliseconds represented a deterioration in reaction time, while a decrease in the count per minute indicated deterioration in the bead test. There were wide variations in baseline performance, so to compare results the predrinking starting point for each test was taken as zero and changes were recorded as incremental increases or decreases from baseline. These results were plotted against time and analyzed by least-squares regression of the portion of the curve before return to baseline, so that the y-intercept gave a measure of degree of impairment, the x-intercept a measure of recovery time, and the slope a measure of rate of recovery.

Statistical analyses between groups were by ANOVA and Student's unpaired two-tailed t test.

RESULTS

Table II lists mean peak plasma ethanol concentrations, time to reach peak concentration, AUC, and rate of ethanol elimination (β_{60}) for the six major groups. There were no significant differences between light and moderate drinkers overall or in any subcategory. There

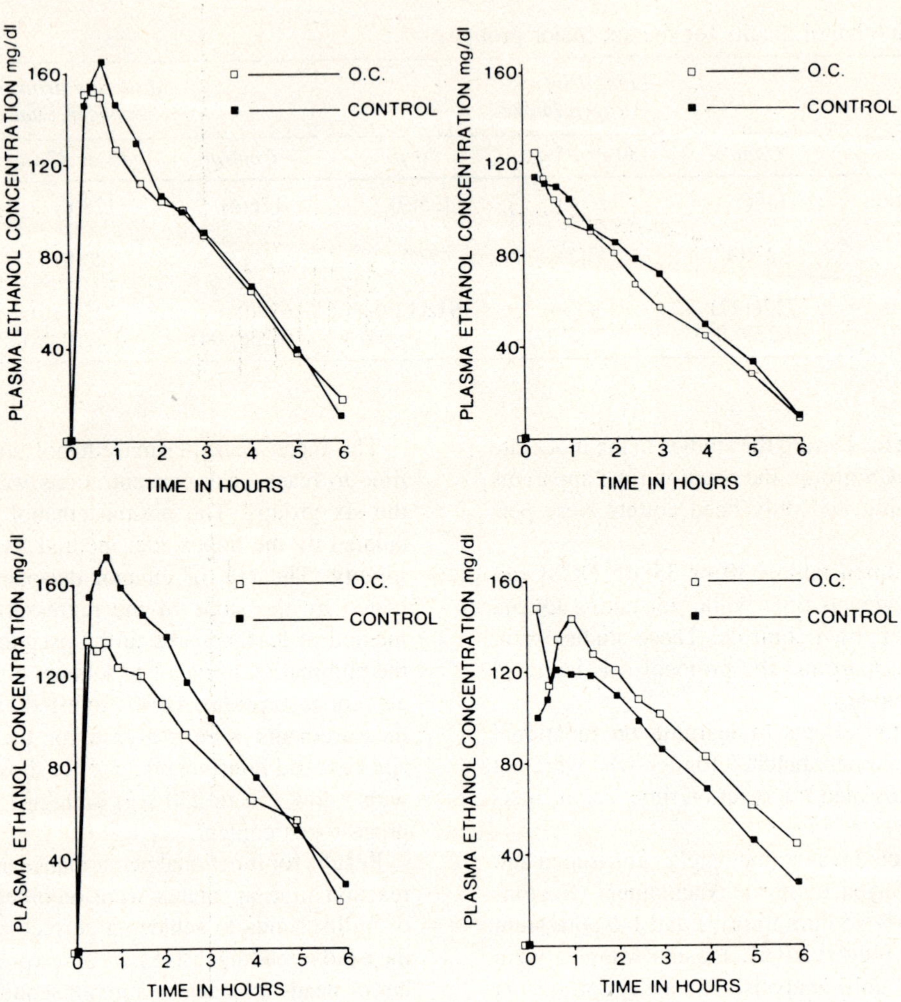

Fig. 1. Plasma ethanol concentrations in four women acting as their own controls while receiving and not receiving OCSs.

were also no significant differences between those taking OCSs and controls in either drinking category. Analysis for differences related to smoking or progestogen intake showed no significant differences. The power of the study to detect a difference in plasma ethanol of 20 mg/dl between any of the six major groups was 60%.

Fig. 1 shows individual plasma ethanol concentrations of the four subjects who acted as their own controls. Two of them showed no change with OCS use, and one had higher and one had lower plasma ethanol concentrations while taking an OCS. Mean peak ethanol concentrations and AUCs for the four subjects were slightly higher than those listed in Table II (144 ± 15 mg/dl without and 142 ± 6 mg/dl with and 718 ± 114 mg · hr/dl without and 717 ± 179 mg · hr/dl with). There were no significant differences between these mean results. Mean β_{60} was 0.25 ± 0.03 gm/L/hr without and 0.23 ± 0.04 gm/L/hr with OCSs.

The "sober" control group of 20 subjects all showed a learning effect lasting for 2 to 3 hours for the reaction time test, during which reaction times improved (decreased) by 30 msec, after which time the response leveled out. All subjects given alcohol had a marked initial deterioration, indicating a genuine effect of alcohol. In all cases the reaction time increased and the bead count decreased in parallel. After return to baseline, all groups showed an "overshoot" in performance that may have represented a delayed learning effect.

Figs. 2 to 4 show representative results for the light and moderate drinking control groups and the 30 or 35 μg OCS moderate drinking group. The mean plasma ethanol concentrations are plotted together with mean reaction times, for which an increase indicates deteri-

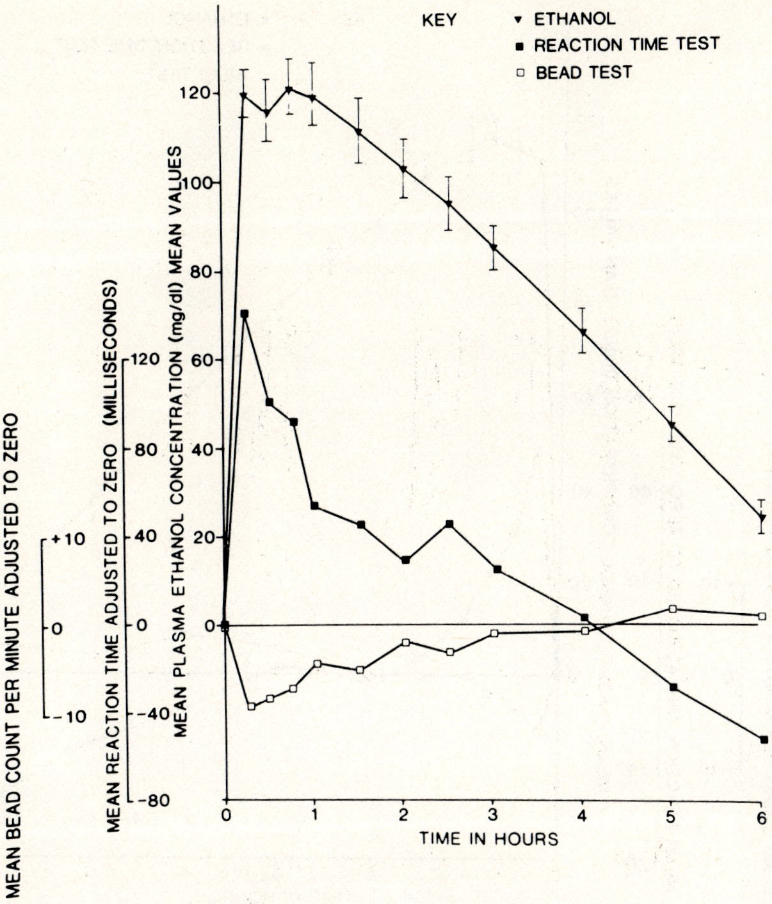

Fig. 2. Mean (±SE) plasma ethanol concentrations, changes in reaction times, and changes in bead count for the control light drinking group.

oration, and mean bead counts, for which a decrease indicates deterioration. All groups show acute tolerance, i.e., recovery of motor function at plasma ethanol concentrations at which there was impairment on the upslope of the ethanol curve. Table III lists the mean computed values for the y-axis (peak deterioration), x-axis (recovery time), and slope (rate of recovery) for reaction times and bead counts for the six groups. There were statistically significant differences between these parameters.

In all cases in the two control groups when there was a significant difference, moderate drinkers were less impaired than light drinkers. There was also a trend in both the 30 or 35 μg and 50 μg OCS groups for the moderate drinkers to be less impaired than the light drinkers, but this achieved statistical significance only for the three parameters for bead count between the light and moderate drinking 30 or 35 μg OCS groups. In both drinking categories when there were significant differences, the 30 or 35 μg OCS groups were significantly less impaired than their matched controls. For bead counts, subjects in both of the 50 μg OCS groups were significantly less impaired than their respective controls. Reaction times were not available for the moderate drinking 50 μg OCS group, but the light drinking 50 μg OCS group had significantly less impairment than their controls. The trend for the 50 μg OCS groups to be less impaired than their respective 30 or 35 μg OCS groups achieved significance only for rate of recovery of bead count.

The four subjects who acted as their own controls showed exactly the same trends, i.e., significantly faster recovery times for both tests while taking OCSs (3 hours) than while not taking OCSs (5 hours; $P < 0.01$).

DISCUSSION

We found no effect of OCSs on ethanol absorption or elimination, but did find a significant OCS-related improvement in tolerance to ethanol. Our results for the effect of OCSs on plasma ethanol concentrations

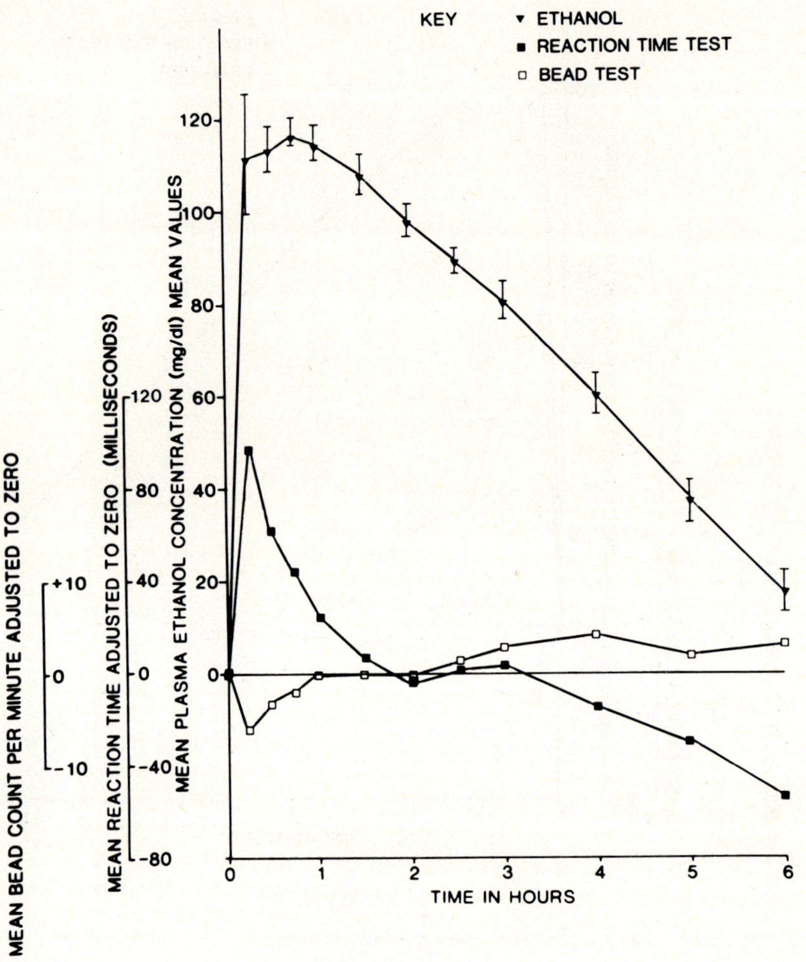

Fig. 3. Mean (±SE) plasma ethanol concentrations, changes in reaction times, and changes in bead count for the control moderate drinking group.

are at variance with those of Jones and Jones,[12] who not only found a reduced ethanol elimination rate in their OCS group but also lower peak plasma ethanol concentrations, even after correction for weight. These investigators used only breath analysis for ethanol and did not classify their subjects by hormonal content of OCS or by drinking status. All our subjects were studied at the same stage of the menstrual or pill cycle, took no additional medications, and were grouped according to the estrogen content of their OCSs. Plasma ethanol concentrations were the same for light and moderate drinkers and for both estrogen OCS groups. We also found no differences between those women taking high- and low-progestogen OCSs or between the smokers and nonsmokers. The similar findings for the four women acting as their own controls with and without OCSs supported the group results.

The dose of ethanol we used was higher than that of Jones and Jones,[12] but this should have ensured saturation of alcohol dehydrogenase and allowed metabolism by microsomal enzymes.[19] Our dose was the same as that used by Feely and Wood[10] in their cimetidine study. However, the increase in blood alcohol in the latter study could well have been due to altered ethanol absorption rather than inhibition of ethanol metabolism. This interpretation has been offered by another group who did not find any effect of cimetidine on the ethanol disposition rate.[26] This suggests that microsomal oxidizing enzymes play only a minor role in ethanol metabolism, a view held by others.[24] It has been stated that ethanol kinetics can be completely explained by the alcohol dehydrogenase pathway and that there is no need to postulate alternative oxidation pathways.[11] Our results certainly indicate that OCSs, and by implication

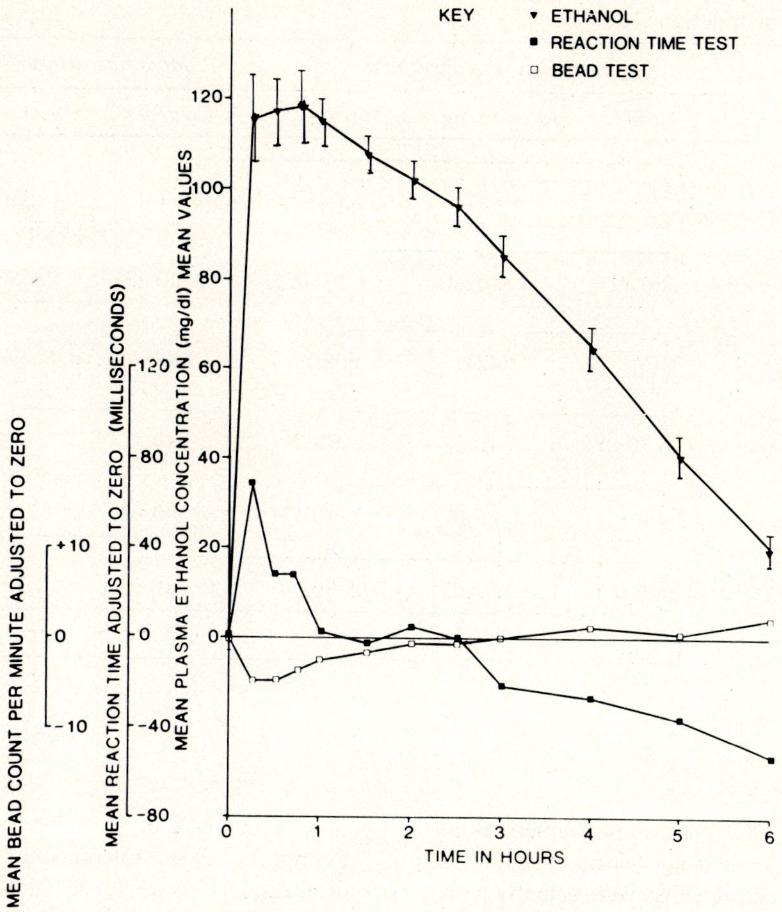

Fig. 4. Mean (±SE) plasma ethanol concentrations, changes in reaction times, and changes in bead count for the 30 or 35 μg OCS moderate drinking group.

microsomal oxidases, have no major effect on ethanol clearance.

Although we are confident that our classification was as accurate as possible, we also did not find any evidence of induction of metabolism in our moderate drinkers. However, even our moderate drinkers drank only three to four drinks a day, which is probably insufficient to induce significant enzyme metabolism. Induction of ethanol metabolism has usually been demonstrated only in chronic alcoholics who drink >250 gm ethanol daily for ≥2 weeks.[20] In confirmation of this, there is another report that ethanol in a daily dose of 0.95 gm/kg for 21 days significantly increased antipyrine metabolism but failed to induce a consistent change in ethanol metabolism.[28] Our results are quite consistent with these findings.

Because of its complex kinetics,[6,29,30] methods for analyzing ethanol elimination are controversial. A recent detailed analysis suggests that β_{60} is the best available measurement and that the many correction factors that have been described are likely to compound rather than reduce errors.[31] Our β_{60} values averaged 0.2 gm/L/hr, which lies in the middle of the accepted range of 0.1 to 0.3 gm/L/hr.[18,31] In this context it is relevant to note that Jones and Jones[12] used the breathalyzer to estimate a "zero" blood ethanol level from which they calculated time to reach zero and the slope of the line from peak to zero concentration.[12] Conversion of their data to our units produces β_{60} values of 0.8 to 1.0 gm/L/hr, which suggests an error either in analysis or calculation.

We are satisfied that OCSs have no significant effect on plasma ethanol concentration or elimination rate. Women taking OCSs are therefore not at extra risk of failing to comply with legal requirements for driving. Although many women claim to have reduced ethanol

Table III. Tests of motor function

	Light drinkers' estrogen intake			Moderate drinkers' estrogen intake		
	Control	*30 or 35 μg*	*50 μg*	*Control*	*30 or 35 μg*	*50 μg*
Reaction times						
Peak deterioration (msec)	112(13)	59(27)	53(4)	73(14)	55(13)	NR
Recovery time (hr)	3.2(0.12)	1.4(0.21)	1.2(0.02)	2.2(0.13)	1.5(0.15)	NR
Rate of recovery (msec/hr^{-1})	31(6)	26(22)	50(5)	29(8)	29(12)	NR
Bead count						
Peak deterioration (no.)	8 (0.8)	7(0.6)	5(0.7)	8(0.7)	5(0.3)	5(0.6)
Recovery time (hr)	3.4(0.12)	2.3(0.07)	2.0(0.13)	2.9(0.03)	2.8(0.06)	2.0(0.20)
Rate of recovery (no/hr^{-1})	0.38(0.02)	0.29(0.02)	0.37(0.04)	0.13(0.03)	0.37(0.06)	0.49(0.02)

Data are $\bar{X}$ ± SE.
NR = Not recorded.
$*P < 0.05$; $**P < 0.01$; $\dagger P < 0.001$.

tolerance while taking OCSs and some women taking OCSs drink less than women not taking OCSs,[12] our data show that women taking OCSs were actually more tolerant to ethanol than women not taking OCSs. We found a highly statistically significant effect of OCSs on tolerance to ethanol as measured by tests of motor function. This was confirmed in the four women acting as their own controls. Furthermore, these changes in tolerance occurred without any significant change in plasma ethanol concentrations and must therefore be due to a "central" effect. We recognize that tests of motor function are subject to a number of variables, but our nondrinking control subjects consistently improved for the first 2 hours of reaction time testing, indicating a learning effect. All our ethanol subjects showed marked deterioration for at least the first 2 hours. The moderate drinkers, whether or not they were taking OCSs, showed less deterioration, quicker recovery times, and more tolerance than the light drinkers in both reaction time and bead tests. This correlated well with how "intoxicated" they appeared. We consider that this provides validation both of our drinking categories and of the tests of motor function that we used. Our methods were also sensitive and specific enough to detect the well-known phenomenon of "acute" tolerance.[13]

It is therefore of great interest that OCSs appeared to improve ethanol tolerance in both light and moderate drinkers. For example, a light drinker taking a 30 or 35 μg OCS was impaired only to the same extent as a moderate drinking control, and was considerably less impaired than a light drinking control; in particular, recovery time, measured as a return to baseline performance, was significantly shorter. These changes bore no relation to any subjective assessment by the subjects of the effect of the OCS on their tolerance to ethanol. This discrepancy between subjective and objective assessment of tolerance was also present in the four subjects who acted as their own controls.

In all groups there was "overshoot" after returning to baseline performance values (Figs. 2 to 4). It is probable that this represents the learning phase that in the sober controls occurred at an earlier stage. We cannot rule out the possibility that some additional factor was operating and that a true improvement in performance was occurring. We cannot explain our observations, and there appears to be no consensus about the mechanisms of central nervous system tolerance to ethanol.[13,15] Possibilities include alterations in formation and release of neurotransmitters such as catecholamines, serotonin, γ-aminobutyric acid, and the opioids. It is therefore of interest that a recent report indicates prolonged elevation of hypothalamic opioid peptide activity in women taking OCSs.[8] Another possibility is that OCSs alter the transfer of ethanol across the blood-brain barrier. There is no available data on whether OCSs themselves will alter and improve performance in tests of motor function, although the baseline values in our subjects suggest not. A prospective study of women with and without OCS use needs to be done. Further studies are also needed to establish the relative roles of estrogens and progestogens in this effect.

Although we have demonstrated that OCSs improved tolerance to ethanol, we do not recommend that women taking OCS increase their ethanol intake. Their plasma ethanol concentrations and ethanol elimination rates remain unchanged, and they are therefore at the same risk as women not taking OCS of exceeding the limits legally determined for driving.

We thank Dr. Edith Weisberg and the Family Planning Association of New South Wales for assistance with recruitment of subjects.

References

1. Abernethy DR, Divoll M, Ochs HR, Ameer B, Greenblatt DJ: Increased metabolic clearance of acetaminophen with oral contraceptive use. Obstet Gynecol **60:**338-341, 1982.
2. Abernethy DR, Greenblatt DJ: Impairment of antipyrine metabolism by low-dose oral contraceptive steroid use. CLIN PHARMACOL THER **26:**106-110, 1981.
3. Abernethy DR, Greenblatt DJ, Divoll M, Arendt R, Ochs HR, Shader RI: Impairment of diazepam metabolism by low-dose estrogen oral contraceptive steroids. N Engl J Med **306:**791-792, 1982.
4. Abernethy DR, Greenblatt DJ, Ochs HR, Weyers D, Divoll M, Hormatz JS, Shader RI: Lorazepam and oxazepam kinetics in women on low-dose oral contraceptives. CLIN PHARMACOL THER **33:**628-632, 1983.
5. Abernethy DR, Greenblatt DJ, Shader RI: Imipramine disposition in users of oral contraceptive steroids. CLIN PHARMACOL THER **35:**792-797, 1984.
6. Auty RM, Branch RA: Pharmacokinetics and pharmacodynamics of ethanol, whiskey and ethanol with *n*-propyl, *n*-butyl and iso-amyl alcohols. CLIN PHARMACOL THER **22:**242-249, 1977.
7. Breckenridge AM, Back DJ, Orme M: Interactions between oral contraceptives and other drugs. Pharmacol Ther **7:**617-626, 1979.
8. Casper RF, Bhanot R, Wilkinson M: Prolonged elevation of hypothalamic opioid peptide activity in women taking oral contraceptives. J Clin Endocrinol Metab **58:**582-584, 1984.
9. Cooper JDH: Determination of blood ethanol by gas chromatography. Clin Chim Acta **33:**483-485, 1971.
10. Feely J, Wood AJJ: Effects of cimetidine on the elimination and actions of ethanol. JAMA **247:**2819-2821, 1982.
11. Havre P, Abrams MA, Corrall RJM, Yu LC, Szczepanik PA, Feldman HB, Klein P, Kong MS, Mongolis JM, Landau BR: Quantitation of pathways of ethanol metabolism. Arch Bichem Biophys **182:**14-23, 1977.
12. Jones MK, Jones BM: Ethanol metabolism in women taking oral contraceptives. Alcoholism **8:**24-28, 1984.
13. Kalant H, LeBlanc AE, Gibbins RJ: Tolerance to and dependence on some non-opiate psychotropic drugs. Pharmacol Rev **23:**135-191, 1971.
14. Kendall MJ, Quarterman CP, Jack DB, Beeley L: Metoprolol pharmacokinetics and the oral contraceptive pill. Br J Clin Pharmacol **14:**120-122, 1982.
15. Khanna JM, Kalant H, Le AD, LeBlanc AE: The role of serotonin in drug tolerance and general adaptation. Acta Psychiatr Scand [Suppl] **286:**161-170, 1980.
16. Knodell RG, Richard G, Allen C, Kyner WT: Effects of ethinyloestradiol on pharmacokinetics of meperidine and pentobarbital in the rat. J Pharmacol Exp Ther **221:**1-6, 1982.
17. Lieber CS, DeCarli LM: The role of the hepatic microsomal ethanol oxidising system for ethanol metabolism in vivo. J Pharmacol Exp Ther **181:**279-287, 1972.
18. Martin E, Moll W, Schmid P, Dettli L: The pharmacokinetics of alcohol in human breath, venous and arterial blood after oral ingestion. Eur J Clin Pharmacol **26:**619-626, 1984.
19. Mezey E: Ethanol metabolism and ethanol drug interactions. Biochem Pharmacol **25:**869-875, 1976.
20. Mezey E, Tobon F: Rates of ethanol clearance and activities of the ethanol-oxidizing enzymes in chronic alcoholic patients. Gastroenterology **61:**707-715, 1971.
21. Mitchell MC, Hanew T, Meredith CG, Schenker S: Effects of oral contraceptive steroids on acetaminophen metabolism and elimination. CLIN PHARMACOL THER **34:**48-53, 1983.
22. National Heart Foundation of Australia: Risk Factor Prevalence Study Report No. 1, Melbourne, 1980.
23. Patwardhan RV, Mitchell MC, Johnson RF, Schenker S: Differential effects of oral contraceptive steroids on the metabolism of benzodiazepines. Hepatology **3:**248-253, 1983.
24. Peters TJ: Ethanol metabolism. Br Med Bull **38:**17-20, 1982.
25. Rangno RE, Kreeft JH, Sitar DS: Ethanol dose-dependent elimination: Michaelis-Menten v classical kinetic analysis. Br J Clin Pharmacol **12:**667-673, 1981.
26. Seitz HK, Bosche J, Czygan P, Veith S, Simon B, Kommerell B: Increased blood ethanol levels following cimetidine but not ranitidine. Lancet **1:**760, 1983.
27. Tornatore KM, Kanarkowski R, McCarthy TL, Gardner MJ, Yurchak AM, Jusko WJ: Effect of oral contraceptive

steroids on theophylline disposition. Eur J Clin Pharmacol **23:**129-134, 1982.

28. Vessell ES, Page JG, Passanan GT: Genetic and environmental factors affecting ethanol metabolism in man. CLIN PHARMACOL THER **12:**192-201, 1971.
29. Wagner JG, Wilkinson PK, Sedman AJ, Kay DR, Weidler DJ: Elimination of alcohol from human blood. J Pharm Sci **65:**152-154, 1976.
30. Wilkinson PK: Pharmacokinetics of ethanol: A review. Alcoholism **4:**6-21, 1980.
31. Wilson JR, Erwin VG: Rate of alcohol metabolism; Do not "correct" the β_{60} estimate for comparisons among ethnic groups. J Stud Alcohol **44:**1093-1096, 1983.
32. Zeiner AR, Kegg PS: Effects of sex steroids on ethanol pharmacokinetics and autonomic reactivity. Prog Biochem Pharmacol **18:**130-142, 1981.

The acute effects of acrivastine (BW825C), a new antihistamine, compared with triprolidine on measures of central nervous system performance and subjective effects

The new H_1-antagonist acrivastine (BW825C) in doses of 4, 8, and 16 mg was compared with triprolidine HCl (2.5 and 5 mg) in a double-blind crossover study in 12 subjects. Adaptive tracking performance 1.5 hours after dosing was impaired by triprolidine, 2.5 and 5 mg; the impairment was still detectable 3.5 hours after 5 mg. Acrivastine did not impair adaptive tracking after any of the doses. Triprolidine increased reaction times after 1.5 hours (2.5 and 5 mg) and 3 hours (5 mg), but acrivastine did not have any effect on reaction time at any dose. Both doses of triprolidine caused subjective central nervous system effects after 1.5 hours, and triprolidine, 5 mg, still had some detectable effects on subjective rating scales after 3 hours. No subjective effects were noted after acrivastine. We conclude that acrivastine at doses causing more peripheral H_1-antagonism than tripolidine has considerably reduced central nervous system activity. (Clin Pharmacol Ther 38:381-386, 1985.)

A. F. Cohen, M.D., M. Hamilton, Ph.D., R. Philipson, and A. W. Peck, Ph.D.
Kent, United Kingdom

The most common side effect of H_1-antagonists is drowsiness.[5] Although there are differences between the various antihistamines in their ability to cause sedation, there are only two H_1-antagonists, terfenadine and astemizole, currently available that are claimed to be virtually free of sedative side effects.[2,7,9]

Acrivastine (see structure) is a new antihistamine with peripheral H_1-antagonist potency equal to that of triprolidine, but in doses up to 4 mg acrivastine does not impair performance on a vigilance task or increase reaction time.[3] Even at a 2.5 mg dose, triprolidine showed significant differences from placebo on the measures of performance examined.

Our study was designed to detect possible effects of acrivastine doses up to 16 mg on subjective rating scales, visual motor coordination as measured by adaptive tracking, and reaction time. Triprolidine was included as a positive control because it has significant effects on adaptive tracking,[9] reaction time,[1,3,6] and subjective rating scales.[3]

From The Wellcome Research Laboratories.
Received for publication Feb. 23, 1985; accepted June 19, 1985.
Reprint requests to: A. F. Cohen, M.D., The Wellcome Research Laboratories, Langley Court, Beckenham, Kent, United Kingdom.

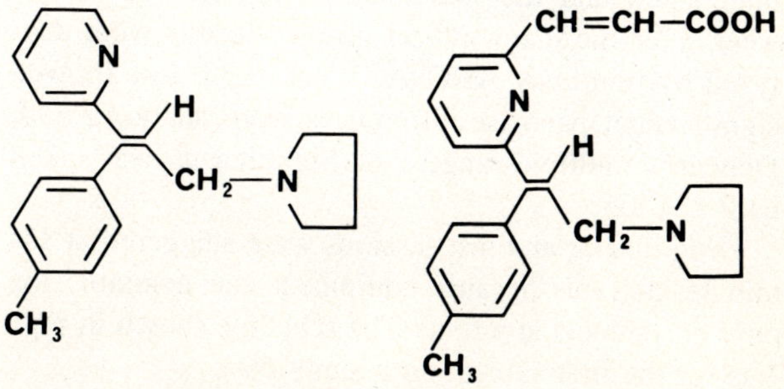

Triprolidine *(left)* and acrivastine *(right)*

METHODS

Twelve subjects (six men and six women) were recruited for the study. Ages ranged between 20 and 55 years. The women weighed 60.5 ± 5.6 kg ($\overline{X}$ ± SD) and the men weighed 68.5 ± 8.5 kg. Subjects received a medical interview and physical examination, ECG, hematology, and plasma biochemistry tests. They gave informed consent and were paid, and were transported to and from the laboratory on study days. A light breakfast was allowed but no smoking, caffeine-containing beverages, or alcohol were allowed on the experimental day.

7:45 AM	Arrival at laboratory
8:00 AM	Predosing test battery:
	Adaptive tracking (10 minutes)
	Reaction time test (5 minutes)
	Visual analog lines
8:30 AM	Drug dosing
10:00 AM	Test battery 1 (1.5 hours after dosing)
11:30 AM	Test battery 2 (3 hours after drug dosing)
1:00 PM	Lunch
1:30 PM	Test battery 3 (5 hours after drug dosing)
	Recording of side effects
2:00 PM	End of study

Fig. 1. Sample dosing schedule.

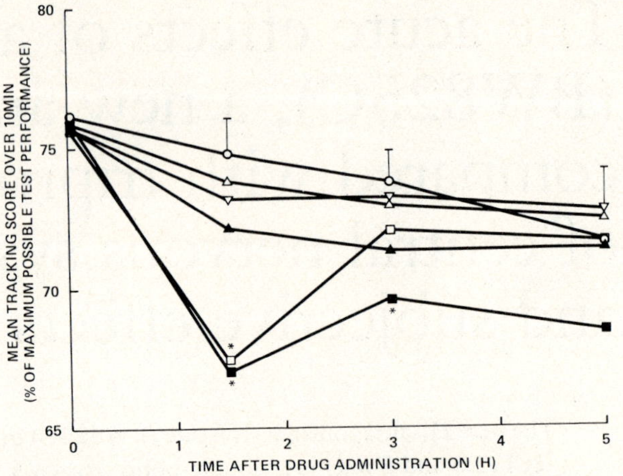

Fig. 2. Mean (±SE) tracking score (expressed as percentage of maximum possible performance). ○ = Placebo; △ = acrivastine, 4 mg; ▽ = acrivastine, 8 mg; ▲ = acrivastine, 16 mg; □ = triprolidine, 2.5 mg; ■ = triprolidine, 5 mg. *Significantly different from placebo ($P < 0.05$).

The study was conducted as a double-blind, placebo-controlled, crossover trial. All subjects received each of the following treatments at intervals of at least 5 days according to two 6 × 6 Latin squares balanced for the treatment and preceding treatment: (1) acrivastine, 4 mg; (2) acrivastine, 8 mg; (3) acrivastine, 16 mg; (4) triprolidine HCl, 2.5 mg; (5) triprolidine HCl, 5 mg; and (6) lactose dummy.

All treatments were administered in identical gelatin capsules with 150 ml water. Subjects were studied on 2 separate days in two groups of six subjects each. If a subject missed a treatment, the treatment order was maintained and the individual completed the trial 1 week after the main subject group. Results were analyzed by multiway ANOVA. When the F test showed significance, pairwise differences were analyzed with Duncan's multiple range test. Significance was taken as $P < 0.05$.

Drug dosing and test sessions were staggered at 15-minute intervals because equipment was available for only one subject at a time. The schedule shown in Fig. 1 is for the first subject on a study day.

A modified adaptive tracking test as described by Borland and Nicholson[1] was used. In this test the subject attempts to position a dot inside a moving circle by means of a joystick. The movement of the circle in two dimensions was determined by two sequences of numbers read independently. In this way a pseudorandom movement was generated. When the dot was positioned in the circle, a factor determining the magnitude of its excursions (called the difficulty factor) increased until a maximum excursion situation was reached or the dot moved outside the circle. In such case the difficulty factor was decreased. The position of the dot was assessed every 15 msec and the difficulty factor was adjusted accordingly. The score was calculated for the 10-minute test, as were the summed difficulty factors over that time divided by the maximum score possible (presented as a percentage). A graph was also presented by the instrument in which the difficulty factor was plotted against time elapsed from the start of the run. This allows the study of variability in performance during the test. Variability was also expressed by the standard deviation of the scores. The duration of the test was 10 minutes excluding the first 30 seconds, which allowed the subject to reach stable performance. Subjects were not aware of their results until the end of the study. To eliminate possible practice effects, subjects were trained on the instrument until stable performance was reached.

A microprocessor-controlled portable reaction timer adapted from Wilkinson and Houghton[11] was used. The digital clock on the instrument was turned on at random intervals from 1 to 20 seconds, after which the subject pressed a button as rapidly as possible. The display then showed the subjects' reaction time, which was stored in the instrument's memory. The test lasted for 5 minutes, during which approximately 30 reaction times were measured and stored in the memory together with an identifying code. Data were processed by a microcomputer. Mean reaction times and standard deviations were calculated after discarding reaction times <100 msec that occasionally occurred when the subject pressed the reaction button prematurely and reaction times that were >1.5 times the crude mean reaction time. Unduly long reaction times occurred only infrequently, when the subject did not pay attention to the

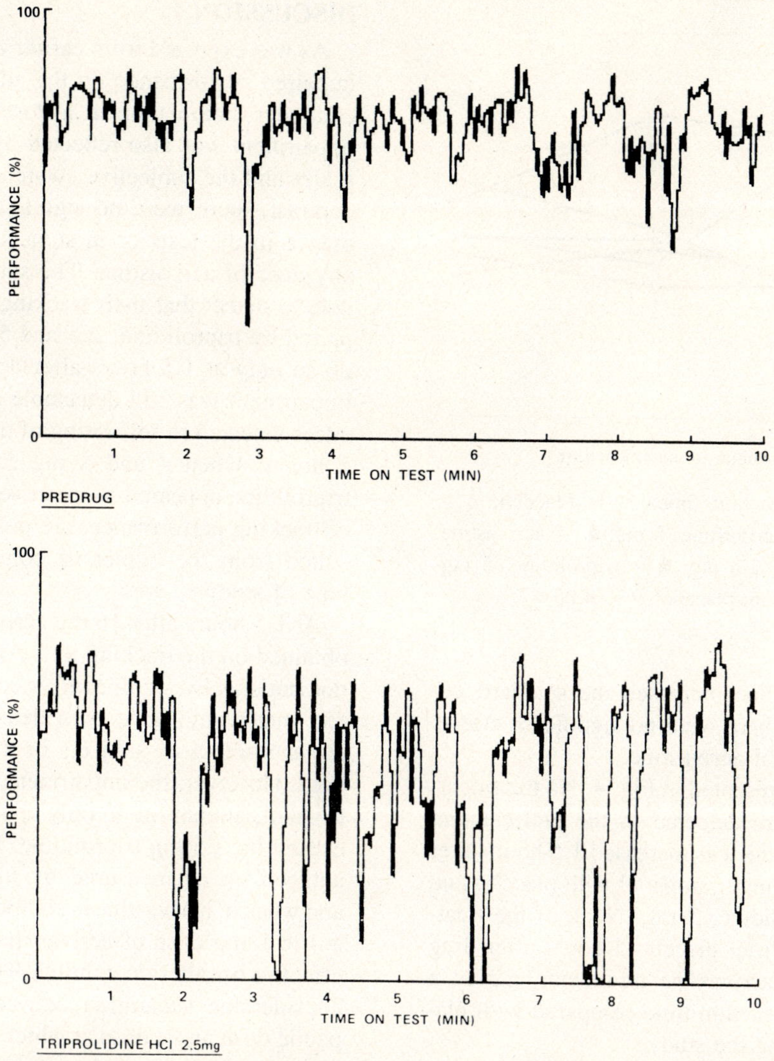

Fig. 3. Performance plotted against time on test for subject 6 before and 1.5 hours after 2.5 mg triprolidine. Note the increased variability.

display or improperly pressed the buttons, but such mistakes have a great influence on the average. Subjects were familiarized with the instrument on three occasions before the study.

Subjective effects were recorded on 19 horizontal visual analog lines (100 mm). On the same form the subjects were asked to indicate if they thought they received an active drug. Side effects were recorded on a standard form at the end of each study day.

RESULTS

The mean scores over the 10-minute tracking test for different treatments are shown in Fig. 2. No occasion differences were noted, showing that training effects were effectively eliminated by the prestudy training sessions, and there were no treatment differences detected in the pretreatment tests.

Triprolidine at both dose levels decreased the tracking score at 1.5 hours after drug dosing compared with placebo and all the acrivastine treatments. The mean tracking score was still impaired 3 hours after triprolidine, 5 mg. None of the acrivastine treatments caused any significant impairment compared with placebo. Visual inspection of the performance-time curve on test traces showed a marked increase in variability after triprolidine (Fig. 3). This effect is reflected in the standard deviation of the mean 10-minute score, a measure of variability in performance during the test (Table I).

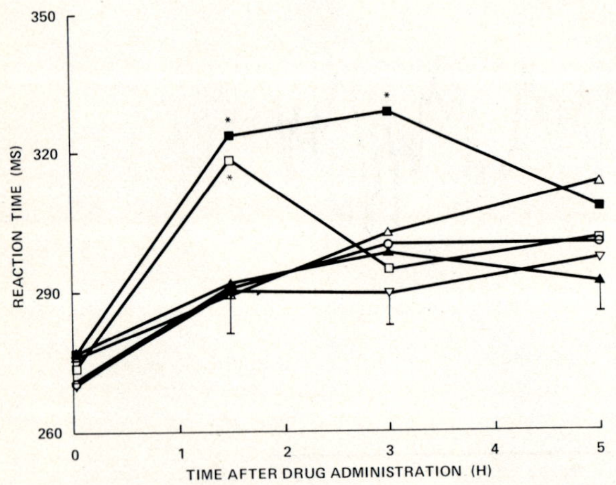

Fig. 4. Mean (±SE) reaction times. ○ = Placebo; △ = acrivastine, 4 mg; ▽ = acrivastine, 8 mg; ▲ = acrivastine, 16 mg; □ = triprolidine, 2.5 mg; ■ = triprolidine, 5 mg. *Significantly different from placebo ($P < 0.05$).

Both doses of triprolidine increased the standard deviation at 1.5 hours. There were no significant effects after any of the doses of acrivastine.

Reaction times are presented in Fig. 4. No treatment-related differences were detected in the pretreatment test results. Reaction time was increased 1.5 hours after triprolidine, 2.5 and 5 mg, compared with placebo and at 3 hours after triprolidine, 5 mg. None of the treatments were different from placebo 5 hours after drug dosing. None of the acrivastine treatments caused a significant change in reaction time compared with placebo at any time during the study.

Table II shows only the visual analog scales on which significant drug effects were noted. At 1.5 hours after drug dosing both doses of triprolidine made the subjects feel more drowsy, clumsy, lethargic, mentally slow, dreamy, and bored than placebo. Triprolidine, 5 mg, also made them feel muzzier and more incompetent. They rated their performance on the tracker as impaired after both doses of triprolidine. No effects were noted after any of the acrivastine doses. Effects were still seen 3 hours after triprolidine, 5 mg, as the subjects felt clumsy, lethargic, and mentally slow.

Answers to the questions, ''Did you receive an active drug?'' were analyzed by the sign test for comparing placebo with each other treatment. Only after 5 mg triprolidine were the subjects able to indicate correctly that they had received an active treatment ($P < 0.03$).

Side effects experienced by the subjects at any time during the study day were always minor, and the main side effect was drowsiness after triprolidine dosing.

DISCUSSION

As was expected from earlier work,[3,6,9,10] triprolidine impaired performance on the adaptive tracker and increased reaction time in a dose-related manner. This impairment was also reflected by the subjective rating scales and the subjective awareness of active drug. By contrast, there were no significant changes in performance in the tests or in subjective rating scales after any dose of acrivastine. The subjects as a group were able to detect that their tracking performance was impaired by triprolidine, 2.5 and 5.0 mg, but they could do so only at 1.5 hours after dosing, while the actual impairment was still detectable at 3 hours. The differences detected in self-rating of tracking performance at 5 hours, when 4 and 8 mg acrivastine and 2.5 mg triprolidine appeared to improve subjective impression of tracking performance, are probably spurious and resulted from the numerous comparisons made in this type of study.

At 1.5 hours after 16 mg acrivastine a low score was obtained on the tracking test. Although this decrease is not statistically significant, it could indicate a drug effect that would have been detected as significant if a larger number of subjects or a higher dose had been used. However, the impairment after 16 mg acrivastine is small, amounting to only approximately 30% of that caused by 2.5 mg triprolidine. In peripheral histamine antagonism as measured by histamine-induced flares and wheals, acrivastine is equipotent to triprolidine[3] and a 4 to 8 mg dose of acrivastine has been shown to be effective in allergic rhinitis. This means that there is considerable separation between the expected therapeutic dose and a dose at which central nervous system impairment might occur.

Many tests for psychomotor performance are notoriously insensitive to drug effects, as has been shown in a recent study[8] in which effects on only a few tests were seen even after 10 mg diazepam or 0.75 gm/kg of ethanol. Both reaction time tests and the adaptive tracker we used were slight modifications of existing tests with proved relevance for detecting drug effects.[6,9] Both tests were shown to be reliable measures for detecting sedative effects induced by triprolidine. It is noteworthy that both tests are relatively short and that the adaptive tracker might be expected to prove interesting to the subjects, raising their motivation and possibly decreasing their sensitivity to drugs. In a recent study[3] the Wilkinson vigilance test showed comparable results. Differences in sensitivity of the tests caused by increased interest appear not to be very great, although in another study the vigilance test has detected effects of doses as low as 1.25 mg triprolidine.[10]

Table I. Standard deviation of adaptive tracking performance score (%)

Time after dosing	*Treatments (in rank order)*						*Overall SE*
1.5 hr	LAC	B8	B4	B16	T5	T2.5	
	6.84	7.25	7.39	7.59	9.08*	9.42*	0.54
3 hr	B8	LAC	B4	B16	T2.5	T5	
	7.17	7.29	7.53	7.65	8.29	8.43	0.59
5 hr	B4	B16	B8	LAC	T2.5	T5	
	7.57	7.79	7.85	8.35	8.40	9.01	0.62

B = Acrivastine; T = triprolidine; LAC = placebo.
*P < 0.05 compared with other scores for that measure.

Table II. Subjective effects assessed from visual analog scale

Time after dosing	*Scores (ranked in ascending order)*					
1.5 hr						
Alert/drowsy	B16	B8	LAC	B4	T5	T2.5
Clear headed/muzzy	B8	B4	B16	LAC	T2.5	T5
Well coordinated/clumsy	B8	LAC	B16	B4	T2.5	T5
Energetic/lethargic	LAC	B4	B16	B8	T2.5	T5
Quick witted/mentally slow	LAC	B8	B4	B16	T2.5	T5
Attentive/dreamy	LAC	B8	B16	B4	T5	T2.5
Proficient/incompetent	B8	B4	LAC	B16	T2.5	T5
Interested/bored	LAC	B16	B8	B4	T2.5	T5
Tracking good/poor	B8	B4	B16	LAC	T2.5	T5
3 hr						
Well coordinated/clumsy	B4	B8	LAC	B16	T2.5	T5
Energetic/lethargic	B4	LAC	T2.5	B8	B16	T5
Quick witted/mentally slow	B8	B4	LAC	T2.5	B16	T5
5 hr						
Tracking good/poor	B4	B8	T2.5	B16	LAC	T5

B = Acrivastine; T = triprolidine; LAC = placebo.
Treatments not underlined by the same score differ from each other (P < 0.05).

Although it is held that the adaptive tracker measures only visual motor coordination,[1] our results suggest that additional factors are involved. The decrease in mean score (the only measure examined on the original instrument) caused by drugs is associated with an increase in variability of performance during the time of testing, and was only detectable with this more sophisticated instrument. This suggests that at least part of the impairment is caused by intermittent lapses of attention. This problem should be studied more extensively by testing drugs with a predominant action on coordination without being sedative (e.g., phenytoin), and possibly by monitoring electroencephalographic patterns during the test. The relationship between our test battery and real-life situations like driving a car is not clear, but it has recently been shown that the test battery used was more sensitive to the effects of diphenhydramine than are "off-road" tests of car driving.[4]

In conclusion, we have shown that acrivastine in doses of at least 16 mg has no effects on reaction time and adaptive tracking and causes no subjective sedative side effects.

We gratefully acknowledge the technical support of Mr. A. G. R. Strutt, Mr. R. Tubridy, Mr. K. Hobbs, and Mr. B. Littlechild.

References

1. Borland RG, Nicholson AN: Human performance after a barbiturate (heptabarbitone). Br J Clin Pharmacol **1:**209-215, 1974.
2. Clarke CH, Nicholson AN: Performance studies with antihistamines. Br J Clin Pharmacol **6:**31-35, 1978.
3. Cohen AF, Hamilton MS, Liao SMT, Findlay JWA, Peck AW: Pharmacodynamics and pharmacokinetics of BW825C: A new antihistamine. Eur J Clin Pharmacol **28:**197-204, 1985.
4. Cohen AF, Posner J, Ashby L, Smith R, Peck AW: A comparison of methods for assessing the sedative effects of diphenhydramine on skills related to car driving. Eur J Clin Pharmacol **27:**477-482, 1984.
5. Faingold CL: Antihistaminics as central nervous depressants. *In* Rocha e Silva M, editor: Handbook of experimental pharmacology: Histamine, vol 2. Berlin, 1978, Springer Verlag. p 561.
6. Hamilton MJ, Burke C, Strutt A, Peck AW: A brief portable reaction time test and automated visual analogue scales: Sensitivity to antihistamines in man. Br J Clin Pharmacol **15:**613P, 1983.
7. Kulshrestna VK, Gupta PP, Turner P, Wadsworth J: Some clinical pharmacological studies with terfenadine, a new antihistamine drug. Br J Clin Pharmacol **6:**25-29, 1978.
8. Moser L, Huther KJ, Koch-Weser J, Lundt PV: Effects of terfenadine and diphenhydramine alone or in combination with diazepam or alcohol on psychomotor performance and subjective feelings. Eur J Clin Pharmacol **14:**417-423, 1978.
9. Nicholson AN, Stone BM: Performance studies with the H_1-histamine receptor antagonists astemizole and terfenadine. Br J Clin Pharmacol **13:**199-202, 1982.
10. Peck AW, Fowle ASE, Bye C: A comparison of triprolidine and clemastine on histamine antagonism and performance tests in man: Implications for the mechanism of drug induced drowsiness. Eur J Clin Pharmacol **8:**455-463, 1975.
11. Wilkinson RT, Houghton D: Portable four choice reaction time test with magnetic tape memory. Behav Res Methods Instrument **7:**444-446, 1975.

Sulindac metabolism: The importance of an intact colon

The pharmacokinetics of sulindac have been studied after a single 200 mg oral dose in six normal subjects and five patients with surgical ileostomies. The plasma concentration-time curves for sulindac were similar in both groups up to 12 hours after dosing, indicating similar absorption of the drug. Higher plasma concentrations of sulindac were found in normal subjects after 12 hours, but this late phase accounted for only 12% of the total AUC in the subjects. The sulfone metabolite showed a similar pattern, with no statistically significant difference in the total AUC, but in patients with ileostomy there was a halving of the AUC after 12 hours. Plasma concentrations of the active sulfide metabolite were similar in both groups up to 12 hours, but negligible concentrations were detected in the plasma of patients with ileostomy after 12 hours. Thus the AUC after 12 hours, which represented 55% of the total AUC in normal subjects, was reduced to only 7% in patients with ileostomy. The rate of reduction of sulindac in vitro by ileostomy effluent was only one hundredth that by normal feces. Our results suggest that the gut microflora are an important site of reduction of sulindac in man. Comparison of AUC values suggests that about half the total sulfide is formed by the gut bacteria, probably from sulindac excreted in the bile. (Clin Pharmacol Ther 38:387-393, 1985.)

H. A. Strong, B.Sc.,* N. J. Warner, A. G. Renwick, Ph.D., and C. F. George, M.D.
Southampton, United Kingdom

Sulindac (see structure) is a substituted indeneacetic acid chemically related to indomethacin. It is a relatively new nonsteroidal anti-inflammatory antipyretic and analgesic agent used in the treatment of rheumatoid arthritis, osteoarthritis, gout, and periarticular diseases.[1] Its biotransformation has been studied extensively in man and animals[5-7] and consists of irreversible oxidation to the sulfone metabolite, reversible reduction to the sulfide metabolite, and acylglucuronide conjugation of the three redox forms (see structure). In man the drug is eliminated extensively in the urine as unchanged sulindac, its sulfone metabolite, and their respective glucuronides.[5]

The sulfide metabolite is an active moiety and is about five times more potent than sulindac, while the sulfone elicits no pharmacologic response.[8] Thus sulindac may be regarded as a prodrug, with the sulfide as the active species or pharmacophore.[4] The long $t_{1/2}$ of the sulfide results in its cumulation during chronic dosing.[5,12] After a single oral dose of sulindac to man, the peak plasma concentrations of both the sulfide and the sulfone occur about 2 hours after that of the parent compound.[5,12,17] This suggests that the tissues rather than the gut flora are the site of both the reduction and oxidation of sulindac. Studies with liver preparations from rats,[13] guinea pigs,[11,18] and rabbits[16,18] have demonstrated both reductive and oxidative metabolism of sulindac in vitro.

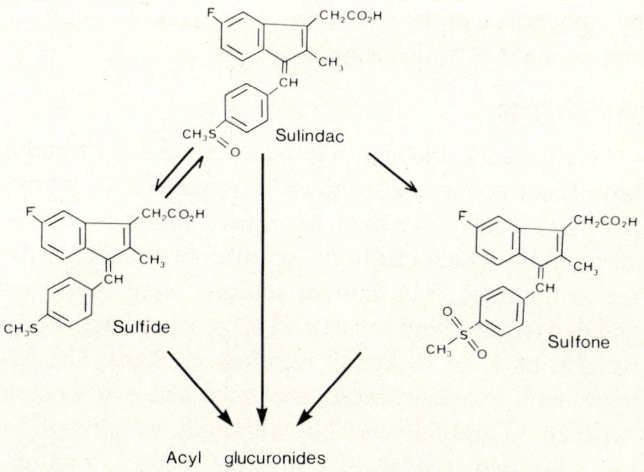

Sulindac and its sulfide and sulfone metabolites

From the Clinical Pharmacology Group, Faculty of Medicine, University of Southampton.
Received for publication March 20, 1985; accepted June 19, 1985.
Reprint requests to: Dr. A. G. Renwick, Clinical Pharmacology, Medical and Biological Sciences Building, Bassett Crescent East, Southampton S09 3TU, United Kingdom.
*Supported by a grant from Ciba-Geigy through the Wessex Medical School Trust.

These data contrast with those of sulfinpyrazone. Although sulfinpyrazone undergoes both oxidation and reduction of the sulfoxide group in vivo, negligible reduction occurred in vitro with rat[14] or rabbit[16] liver preparations. The principal site of reduction of sulfinpyrazone was shown to be the gut flora in man[15] and animals.[14,16] Because sulindac undergoes extensive elimination in the bile of man[2,9] and animals[7] and the sulfide was formed on incubation of sulindac with rat colon contents or human feces,[5] it is possible that the gut microflora may contribute to the formation of the active metabolite.

The role of the gut flora in the reduction of sulfinpyrazone in man was demonstrated[15] by comparison of its metabolism in normal subjects and in patients who had undergone surgical removal of the large bowel with formation of an ileostomy. Negligible sulfide was formed in vivo in patients with ileostomy despite normal absorption of sulfinpyrazone.[15] In contrast to the extensive reduction of sulfinpyrazone in vitro by fecal homogenates, only trace amounts of the sulfide were formed by ileostomy effluent, indicating that the difference in vivo was due to the absence of microbial metabolism. In this study we investigated the contribution of the gut microflora to the reduction of sulindac by comparison of the fate of this drug in normal subjects and patients with ileostomy.

METHODS

Five patients who had undergone removal of the large bowel and six normal subjects took part in the study. All participants gave their informed consent to the investigation, which had been approved by the local Ethical Committee. The normal subjects were four men and two women between 21 and 42 years old with body weights of 47 to 80 kg; all were nonsmokers. The patients with ileostomy were three men and two women between 33 and 53 years old with body weights of 54 to 76 kg; two were regular smokers. Patients had undergone colectomy and ileostomy at least 2 years before the study. Only one subject and one patient had taken any other medication (paracetamol and codeine, respectively) within 1 week of the study.

Participants were given a single oral dose of sulindac (200 mg in tablet form) after an overnight fast. Samples of blood, urine, and feces or ileostomy effluent were collected before drug dosing. Blood samples (10 ml) were taken into lithium heparin tubes hourly up to 8 hours and at 12, 14, 24, 28, 32, 48, and 55 hours after drug dosing. Plasma was separated by centrifugation. Urine was collected for 48 hours after dosing. Plasma and urine samples were stored at −20° C until analyzed. Reanalysis of plasma and urine samples about 9 months after initial measurement indicated negligible decomposition under these conditions.

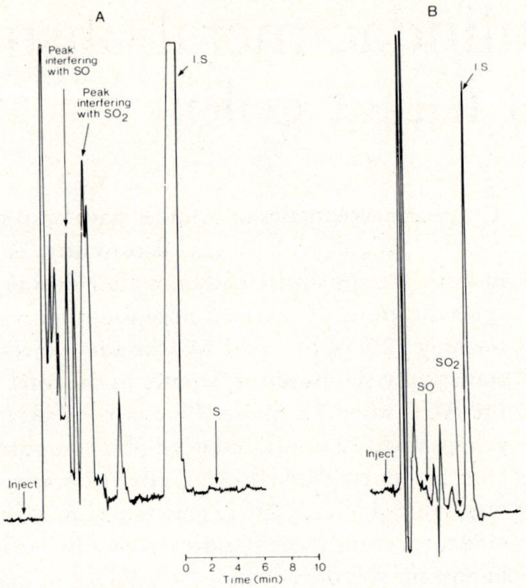

Fig. 1. HPLC traces of predose plasma by the two methods used. **A,** Analyzed by method A showing peaks interfering with sulindac *(SO)* and sulfone *(SO_2)* but not sulfide *(S)*. The internal standard *(IS)* was sulfinpyrazone sulfide. **B,** Analyzed by method B showing position of sulindac, its sulfone, and internal standard (fenbufen).

Samples (3 to 5 gm) of feces from normal subjects and ileostomy effluent from patients were collected either immediately before the study or between 7 and 14 days after sulindac dosing. The samples were homogenized with 2 to 11 volumes of phosphate buffer (0.1 mol/L at pH 7.4) and an aliquot (1 ml) was incubated with substrate (50 μg sulindac in 1 ml phosphate buffer) for 1 hour at 37° C under an atmosphere of oxygen-free nitrogen. The reaction was stopped by the addition of 2 mol/L HCl (1 ml) and internal standard (10 μg in 50 μl methanol). The incubates and appropriate controls, i.e. substrate, homogenate, and substrate with boiled homogenate, were extracted and analyzed by HPLC for sulindac and its sulfide. The sulfide was not detected in any of the control incubations.

The samples of plasma (1 ml), urine (0.5 ml), urine (0.5 ml) treated with alkali (3 mol/L NaOH; 200 μl) to hydrolyze the acyl conjugates,[5] and ileostomy and fecal incubates were analyzed in duplicate by reversed-phase HPLC (method A). The samples were mixed with the internal standard (the sulfide metabolite of sulfinpyrazone; 5 μg in 50 μl methanol; 10 μg for incubates) acidified by the addition of 2 mol/L HCl (200 μl; 1 ml

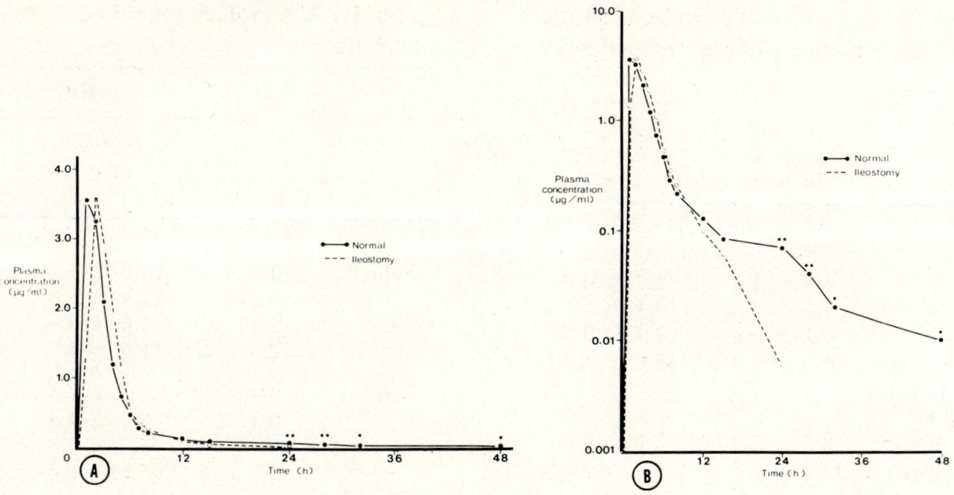

Fig. 2. Mean plasma concentration-time curve for sulindac in normal subjects and patients with ileostomy. **A,** Linear plot. **B,** Semilogarithmic plot. *$P < 0.05$, **$P < 0.01$ (Student's t test). Sulindac was not detectable in the plasma of patients with ileostomy after 24 hours.

for incubates) and extracted with chlorobutane:1,2-dichloroethane (4:1, v/v; 5 ml) by shaking for 10 minutes. The upper organic layer was separated by centrifugation and the acidic drug and metabolites were back extracted into 0.1 mol/L NaOH (400 μl). An aliquot (50 to 100 μl) of the alkali solution was injected into an HPLC system consisting of a Waters Associates Inc. Model U6K or WISP injector, a model M6000A pump, a μ-Bondapak C-18 column (30 cm; 3.9 mm id), and a model 450 ultraviolet detector set at 254 mm. The mobile phase was 0.2 mol/L ammonium phosphate buffer at pH 3.5 and acetonitrile (50:50, v/v) at a flow of 2 ml/min. Peak areas were measured by an integrator and the ratio of sulindac or metabolite to internal standard was calculated. The concentrations of sulindac and its metabolites were calculated by comparison with standards added to control samples and analyzed with each batch of samples (one standard for each four to five samples). Within the range of concentrations we report there was a linear relationship ($r > 0.998$) between the area ratios and the concentration of sulindac and its metabolites added. However, control plasma samples contained small ultraviolet absorbing peaks that interfered with the measurement of sulindac and its sulfone but not that of the sulfide at low concentrations (i.e., <0.3 μg/ml; Fig. 1). Thus samples containing <0.5 μg/ml of sulindac and its sulfone were also analyzed by a modified method (method B) that separated these compounds from the interference (Fig. 1). However, this modified assay did not allow simultaneous measurement of the sulfide, which was retained on the column. In this method the extraction procedure was similar except that the internal standard was fenbufen (5 μg in 50 μl methanol) and up to 200 μl of the alkaline solution was injected. HPLC separation was achieved with a Hypersil 3μ ODS column (17 cm; 4.6 mm id; HPLC Technology) and an increased proportion of buffer to acetonitrile (57:43, v/v) as the mobile phase. The peaks were detected by ultraviolet absorption at 332 nm and quantitated by measurement of peak height ratio to that of the internal standard. There was a linear relationship ($r > 0.998$) between peak height ratio and concentration of sulindac or sulfone. The increased sensitivity and specificity allowed measurement of concentrations as low as 5 ng/ml. Accumulated sulfide was removed by washing the column with 100% acetonitrile after every six assays.

The plasma AUCs were calculated by the trapezoidal rule with extrapolation to infinity. The peak plasma concentrations and times to peak are reported as the observed values. The $t_{1/2}$ values were derived by least-squares regression analysis on the terminal phase of the plasma concentration-time curve. Statistical analysis was by Student's t test for unpaired data.

RESULTS

Sulindac was absorbed rapidly after oral administration to normal subjects, and in three individuals the first sample (1 hour) contained the peak concentration. The plasma concentration-time curve (Fig. 2) showed a rapid exponential initial decrease during the first 12 hours. This was followed by a slower and less linear

Table I. The pharmacokinetics of sulindac (200 mg) and its metabolites in normal subjects and patients with ileostomy

	Normal subjects (n = 6)	*Patients (n = 5)*
Sulindac		
Plasma		
C_{max} (μg/ml)	4.7 ± 2.6	3.7 ± 0.9
t_{max} (hr)	1.6 ± 0.8	2.1 ± 0.6
$t_{1/2}$ (hr)	9.7 ± 6.8	2.7 ± 0.7*
AUC(0 − ∞) (μg/ml · hr)	14.0 ± 6.0	13.0 ± 6.3
Urine (0-48 hr)		
Free (% dose)	8.2 ± 2.9	3.6 ± 4.6
Total (% dose)	13.3 ± 2.3	6.2 ± 3.1†‡
Sulfone		
Plasma		
C_{max} (μg/ml)	1.5 ± 1.1	1.6 ± 0.5
T_{max} (hr)	2.9 ± 0.9	4.0 ± 0.8
$t_{1/2}$ (hr)	20.1 ± 4.8	5.4 ± 2.4§
AUC(0 − ∞) (μg/ml · hr)	23.2 ± 8.8	18.3 ± 12.2
Urine (0-48 hr)		
Free (% dose)	3.0 ± 0.8	1.6 ± 1.3
Total (% dose)	16.1 ± 2.5	10.0 ± 6.8†
Sulfide		
Plasma		
C_{max} (μg/ml)	2.7 ± 1.2	2.6 ± 1.1
t_{max} (hr)	3.1 ± 0.8	3.1 ± 0.5
$t_{1/2}$ (hr)	14.0 ± 7.7	2.5 ± 1.2‡
AUC(0 − ∞) (μg/ml · hr)	33.9 ± 14.9	14.8 ± 9.4
Urine (0-48 hr)		
Free (% dose)	0.4 ± 0.4	0.1 ± 0.1

Data are $\overline{X}$ ± SD.
C_{max} = Maximum observed plasma concentration; t_{max} = time to reach C_{max}.
*$P < 0.05$ (Student's t test).
†Only four samples available for analysis.
‡$P < 0.01$, §$P < 0.001$ (Student's t test).

Table II. AUC values for sulindac and its metabolites

		AUC (μg/ml · hr)	
	Interval	*Normal subjects (n = 6)*	*Patients (n = 5)*
Sulindac	0-∞	14.0 ± 6.0	13.0 ± 6.3
	0-12	12.4 ± 5.5	12.4 ± 5.6
	12-∞	1.6 ± 0.8	0.6 ± 0.7
	12-∞ (%)	11.5 ± 4.5	3.5 ± 3.1
Sulfone	0-∞	23.2 ± 8.8	18.3 ± 12.2
	0-12	8.3 ± 4.4	10.2 ± 4.3
	12-∞	15.0 ± 4.8	8.1 ± 8.2
	12-∞ (%)	65.6 ± 6.4	34.8 ± 22.2*
Sulfide	0-∞	33.9 ± 14.9	14.8 ± 9.4†
	0-12	15.7 ± 8.9	13.2 ± 7.6
	12-∞	18.2 ± 7.2	1.6 ± 1.9‡
	12-∞ (%)	55.3 ± 10.5	7.0 ± 7.1‡

Data are $\overline{X}$ ± SD.
12-∞ (%) = AUC (12-∞)/AUC (0-∞) × 100.
*$P < 0.01$, †$P < 0.05$, ‡$P < 0.001$ (Student's t test).

decrease until 48 hours, by which time plasma concentrations approached the limit of detection. The $t_{1/2}$ values (Table I) were estimated from the data between 12 and 48 hours. However, in most subjects one or two distinct secondary peaks of sulindac and its metabolites were detected between these times (Fig. 3). Thus the $t_{1/2}$ values calculated by least-squares regression analysis should be regarded as estimates only, and they showed wide interindividual variations (mean 9.7 hours; range 3.5 to 21.9 hours). The AUC showed less variability (mean 14.0 μg/ml · hr; range 8.2 to 24.9 μg/ml · hr) and most of the area (88%) was derived from the first 12 hours (Table II). The plasma concentration-time curve for sulindac in patients with ileostomy (Fig. 2) was similar to normal subjects during the first 12 hours. There were no significant differences in either the peak concentration, time to peak, or AUC (Table I). However, the irregular late phase detected in normal subjects was not found in patients with ileostomy (Fig. 2, *B*). This resulted in a shorter $t_{1/2}$ (Table I), and a reduced proportion of the total AUC was found between 12 hours and infinity (Table II). About 13% of the dose was recovered in the urine of normal subjects as sulindac; over half was recovered as the free drug (Table I) and most (12.0% ± 2.2% of the dose) was recovered within the first 24 hours. In patients, significantly less sulindac was recovered in the urine (Table I). Almost all sulindac was excreted within the first 24 hours, which is consistent with the plasma data.

The sulfone metabolite reached a peak plasma concentration at 3 to 4 hours after dosing in both normal subjects and patients with ileostomy (Table I). The subsequent decrease (Fig. 4) showed a complex pattern, with secondary peaks characteristic of enterohepatic circulation detected in both groups. Although the $t_{1/2}$ (averaged over two or three secondary peaks) was shorter in the patients, (Table I), only the plasma concentrations at 48 and 55 hours showed a statistically significant difference between the two groups. The AUC values (Tables I and II) were similar in each group, but the proportion of the AUC that occurred after 12 hours in

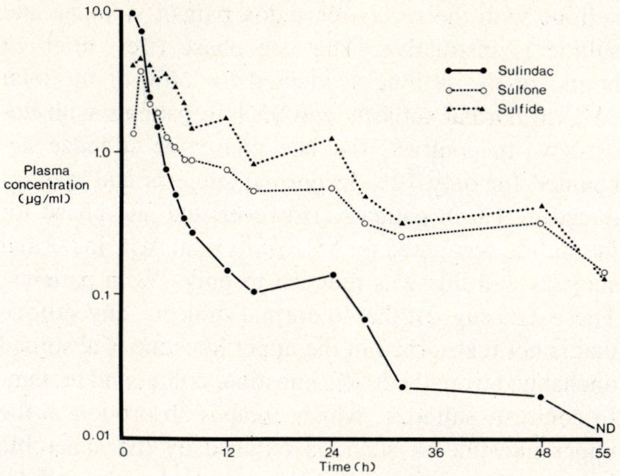

Fig. 3. Plasma concentration-time curves for sulindac and its sulfone and sulfide metabolites in a normal subject. *ND* = Not detectable.

patients (35% of total) was only about half that in subjects (66% of total). The excretion of sulfone was greater than that of the parent drug in both normal subjects (16.1% ± 2.5% of dose) and patients (10.0% ± 6.8% of dose; Table I); most of this was excreted as the conjugate. In contrast to sulindac, a higher proportion of the total (31% in normal subjects and 19% in patients) was excreted between 24 and 48 hours, which is consistent with the plasma data.

The plasma concentration-time curves for the sulfide (Fig. 5) showed a marked difference between the two groups. Between 0 and 10 hours the plasma concentration-time curves were almost superimposable, and thus there were no significant differences in peak concentration, time to peak (Table I), or AUC (0-12) (Table II). In patients with ileostomy there was a rapid decrease in plasma levels ($t_{1/2}$ of 2.5 ± 1.2 hours), so that negligible concentrations were present after 12 hours. In contrast, normal subjects showed a much slower and more complex decrease ($t_{1/2}$ of 14.0 ± 7.7 hours) consistent with an enterohepatic cycling process. This resulted in a significantly higher ($P < 0.001$) AUC after 12 hours in normal subjects, which represented about 55% of the total AUC (Table II). In patients the period from 12 hours was associated with a greatly reduced AUC that corresponded to only 7% of the total AUC in these patients.

Incubation of sulindac with the feces of the normal subjects resulted in extensive reduction to the sulfide (576 ± 177 µg/hr/gm feces). In contrast, ileostomy effluent showed a very limited capacity for sulfide for-

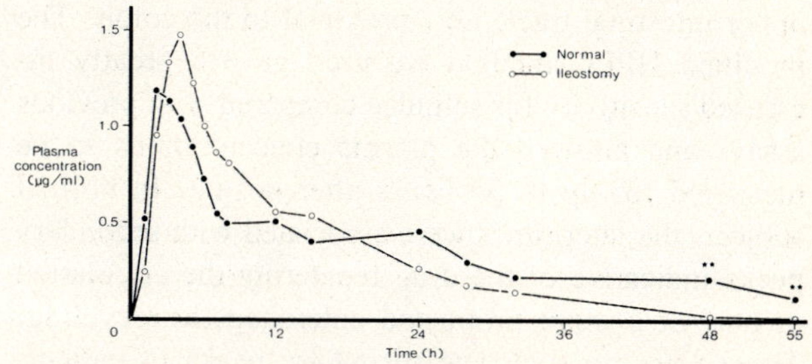

Fig. 4. Mean plasma concentration-time curve for sulindac sulfone in normal subjects and patients with ileostomy. **$P < 0.01$ (Student's t test). Sulfone was measurable in only two of the five patients at 48 hours.

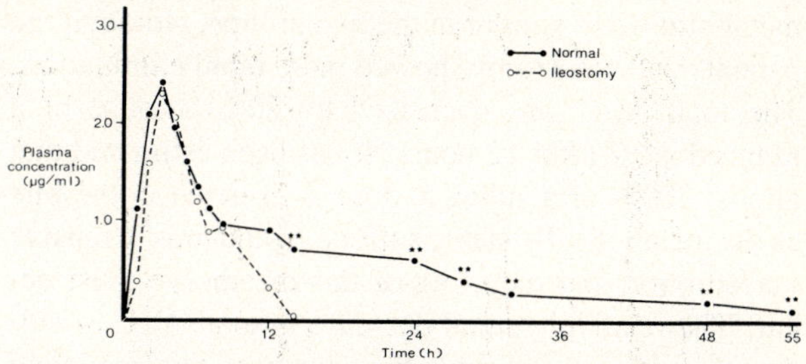

Fig. 5. Mean plasma concentration-time curves for sulindac sulfide in normal subjects and patients with ileostomy. **$P < 0.01$ (Student's t test). Sulfide was not detectable in the plasma of patients at 24 hours or thereafter.

mation (7 ± 6 µg/hr/gm effluent), with no detectable sulfide formation in one individual.

DISCUSSION

The peak plasma concentration, time to peak, and AUC of sulindac after a single 200 mg dose in normal subjects were similar to previously published data.[5,10,12,17] Based on these parameters, the absorption of sulindac in patients with ileostomy was similar to that in normal subjects.

A total of over 300% of a dose of sulindac is excreted in the bile of man[2,9] as sulindac and its sulfone. Because about 140% of the dose is eliminated as sulindac per se,[2,9] there must be extensive reabsorption and enterohepatic recycling of the excreted drug. The similarity in AUC values for sulindac in normal subjects (14.0 µg/ml · hr) and patients with ileostomy (13.0 µg/ml · hr) indicates that most of the normal enterohepatic recycling must occur in these patients. Thus sulindac reabsorption, which is part of its enterohepatic circulation and contributes to its AUC, must occur in the upper intestinal tract, i.e., proximal to the colon. The modified HPLC method we used gave a greatly increased sensitivity for sulindac compared with previous assays and allowed the plasma concentrations to be measured for up to 55 hours after dosing. In normal subjects the later times were associated with secondary peaks indicative of the drug reentering the circulation as part of a more protracted enterohepatic recycling. There were no such late secondary peaks in patients with ileostomy. It is possible that the secondary peaks of sulindac arose in normal subjects from the reoxidation of sulfide formed by the gut flora. This late phase (12 hours to infinity) contributed only 12% to the total AUC for sulindac in normal subjects.

The plasma concentration-time curves for the sulfone metabolite were similar in the two groups, although the patients with ileostomy showed more rapid elimination. The total AUC was decreased by 20% because of a reduced AUC after 12 hours. It has been estimated that almost 200% of a sulindac dose is excreted in the bile as the metabolically stable sulfone,[2,9] and thus extensive reabsorption and recycling of this metabolite must occur. The relatively small decrease in total AUC of sulfone in patients indicates that much of this recycling occurs in the upper intestine. However, the more marked decrease in AUC between 12 hours and infinity suggests that reabsorption from the colon and rectum contributes to the recycling of the sulfone metabolite. The late phase (12 hours to infinity) contributed 66% to the total AUC for the sulfone metabolite in normal subjects.

The initial peak of the sulfide metabolite in plasma was detected in both the normal subjects and the patients, which is consistent with its formation by tissues such as the liver rather than the gut flora. However, there was negligible sulfide in the plasma of patients after 12 hours, while clearly measurable plasma concentrations were maintained in the normal subjects throughout the study. This very marked difference in vivo was also found in vitro; unlike feces, ileostomy effluent showed a very limited capacity for the reduction of sulindac. Ileostomy effluents are not sterile but contain greatly reduced numbers of strict anaerobes.[3] Because the sulfide undergoes little biliary excretion per se[2,9] and the sulfone is metabolically stable,[7] it is probable that the late phase of sulfide present in plasma is formed from sulindac, which is excreted in bile but incompletely reabsorbed in the upper intestine. The importance of the gut microflora as an essential part of this process is indicated by the marked contrast in the AUC data for the sulfide between normal subjects and patients with ileostomy.

Comparison of the data for the metabolically stable sulfone with the reversible redox pair of sulindac and sulfide is instructive. The late phase (i.e., after 12 hours) of the sulfone accounted for 66% of the total AUC in normal subjects and 35% in patients with ileostomy. In contrast, the late phase for sulindac accounted for only 12% in normal subjects and was reduced to 4% in patients. However, the late phase for the sulfide accounted for 55% of its total AUC in normal subjects and this was reduced to only 7% in patients. These data suggest that in normal subjects, any sulfone that is not reabsorbed in the upper intestine is absorbed unchanged from the lower intestine, colon, and rectum. In contrast, sulindac, which escapes absorption in the upper intestine as such, is reduced by the anaerobic bacteria of the lower gut and reabsorbed as the sulfide. It is also possible that the higher plasma levels of sulindac and sulfone detected in the normal subjects after 12 hours may have arisen in part from the sulfide, which is readily oxidized.[4,7,16]

Our results suggest that about 50% of the active sulfide metabolite found in normal subjects given sulindac is formed by the bacteria of the gastrointestinal tract. The substrate is probably sulindac excreted in the bile and not absorbed from the upper intestine. The differences in $t_{1/2}$ of the sulfide in normal subjects and patients with ileostomy suggest that the extent of accumulation after chronic dosing will be determined by the extent of microbial reduction. In view of the wide inter- and intraindividual differences in the nature of the gut flora, it is likely that wide variations in therapeutic responses will result, especially in patients receiving chronic sulindac therapy.

We are grateful to Merck, Sharpe and Dohme Ltd., Hoddesdon, U.K., for gifts of sulindac and its metabolites; to Geigy Pharmaceuticals, Horsham, U.K., for sulfinpyrazone sulfide; and to Lederle Laboratories, Gosport, U.K., for fenbufen. We thank Drs. S. Karran, F. McGinn, and H. Steer for allowing us to study patients under their care.

References

1. Brogden RN, Heel RC, Speight TM, Avery GS: Sulindac: A review of its pharmacological properties and therapeutic efficiency in rheumatic diseases. Drugs **16**:97-114, 1978.
2. Dobrinska MR, Furst DE, Spiegel T, Vincek WC, Tompkins R, Duggan DE, Davies RO, Paulus HE: Biliary secretion of sulindac and metabolites in man. Biopharm Drug Dispos **4**:347-358, 1983.
3. Drasar BS, Hill MJ: Human intestinal flora. New York, 1974, Academic Press.
4. Duggan DE: Sulindac: Therapeutic implications of the prodrug/pharmacophore equilibrium. Drug Metab Rev **12**:325-337, 1981.
5. Duggan DE, Hare LE, Ditzler CA, Lei BW, Kwan KC:

The disposition of sulindac in man. CLIN PHARMACOL THER **21**:326-335, 1977.

6. Duggan DE, Hooke KF, Hwang S: Kinetics of the tissue distribution of sulindac and metabolites. Drug Metab Dispos **8**:241-246, 1980.
7. Duggan DE, Hooke KF, Noll RM, Hucker HB, Van Arman CG: Comparative disposition of sulindac and metabolites in five species. Biochem Pharmacol **27**:2311-2320, 1978.
8. Duggan DE, Hooke KF, Risley EA, Shen TY, Van Arman CG: Identification of the biologically active form of sulindac. J Pharmacol Exp Ther **201**:8-12, 1977.
9. Dujovne CA, Pitterman A, Vincek WC, Dobrinska MR, Davies RO, Duggan DE: Enterohepatic circulation of sulindac and metabolites. CLIN PHARMACOL THER **33**:172-177, 1983.
10. Juhl RP, Van Thiel DH, Dittert LW, Albert KS, Smith RB: Ibuprofen and sulindac kinetics in alcoholic liver disease. CLIN PHARMACOL THER **34**:104-109, 1983.
11. Kitamura J, Tatsumi K, Yoshimura H: Metabolism *in vitro* of sulindac. Sulfoxide-reducing enzyme systems in guinea pig liver. J Pharm Dyn **3**:290-298, 1980.
12. Mattila J, Mantyla R, Vuoreln A, Lamminsivu U, Mannisto P: Pharmacokinetics of graded oral doses of sulindac in man. Arzneimittelforsch/Drug Res **34**:226-229, 1984.
13. Ratnayake JH, Hanna PE, Anders MW, Duggan DE: *In vitro* reduction of sulindac by rat hepatic cytosolic enzymes. Drug Metab Dispos **9**:85-87, 1981.
14. Renwick AG, Evans SP, Sweatman TW, Cumberland J, George CF: The role of the gut flora in the reduction of sulphinpyrazone in the rat. Biochem Pharmacol **31**:2649-2656, 1982.
15. Strong HA, Oates J, Sembi J, Renwick AG, George CF: Role of the gut flora in the reduction of sulfinpyrazone in humans. J Pharmacol Exp Ther **230**:726-732, 1984.
16. Strong HA, Renwick AG, George CF: The site of reduction of sulphinpyrazone in the rabbit. Xenobiotica **14**:815-826, 1984.
17. Swanson BN, Boppana V: Measurement of sulindac and its metabolites in human plasma and urine by high-performance liquid chromatography. J Chromatogr Biomed Appl **225**:123-130, 1981.
18. Tatsumi K, Kitamura S, Yamada S: Sulfoxide reductase activity of liver aldehyde oxidase. Biochim Biophys Acta **747**:86-92, 1983.

A family study of genetic and environmental factors determining polymorphic hydroxylation of debrisoquin

Debrisoquin hydroxylation capacity determined as the ratio of debrisoquin to 4-OH-debrisoquin (DMR) in urine after a single oral dose (10 mg) was studied in 52 nuclear families comprising 226 subjects. The relative importance of genetic and environmental factors for DMR was studied by path analysis. There was a significant negative correlation between DMR and coffee intake but no significant correlations between DMR and sex, age, alcohol intake, or smoking habits. Path analysis showed that genetic heritability was 0.79 while cultural heritability was only 0.06. Complex segregation analysis gave evidence for a major locus with incomplete dominance (d = 0.28) between a recessive and an additive gene. The frequency of the major gene was 0.31, allowing an estimate of the frequency of slow hydroxylators in the Swedish population of 9.4%. There was also evidence for a multifactorial component accounting for 14% of the total variation. It was not possible to distinguish between the different genotypes within the rapid hydroxylator phenotype. Our data agree with previous studies in British and German populations showing that two alleles at a major autosomal locus can explain most of the observed variation in DMR. The frequency of slow hydroxylators in Sweden is very similar to that reported in other European studies. The debrisoquin metabolic phenotype seems to be extensively controlled by a monogenic system and not significantly influenced by environmental factors or age. (Clin Pharmacol Ther 38:394-401, 1985.)

E. Steiner, M.D., L. Iselius, M.D., G. Alván, M.D., J. Lindsten, M.D., and F. Sjöqvist, M.D. *Stockholm, Sweden*

Interindividual differences in the rate of drug metabolism will lead to differences between patients in steady-state plasma concentrations and drug responses during long-term therapy. If distinct phenotypes, e.g., slow and rapid metabolizers, can be distinguished, the distribution of steady-state concentrations will be affected and it might be possible to relate clinical effects and side effects to specific genetic factors.

Traditionally, twin studies have been used to search for a genetic influence on the disposition of drugs.[32] In a second step, family studies have been used to define the mode of genetic transmission.[2,8] Such studies necessitate the selection of subjects at basal or near basal conditions and do not usually take environmental influences into account.[33]

The oxidative metabolism of some drugs seems to be polymorphic, i.e., the metabolic capacity can be divided into more or less discrete groups. Among these are the benzylic hydroxylation of debrisoquin,[17,30] *N*-oxidation of sparteine,[6] and *p*-hydroxylation of mephenytoin.[13] The polymorphic hydroxylation of debrisoquin is one of the most extensively studied conditions. Defining the drug metabolic ratio (DMR) as: Percent dose excreted as debrisoquin/percent dose excreted as 4-hydroxy-debrisoquin in the 0 to 8–hour urine collection after a single oral dose of 10 mg, it was possible to differentiate two phenotypes in the British white population.[17,30] This polymorphism gives rise to wide interindividual variations in the kinetics of oral debriso-

From the Department of Clinical Pharmacology, Huddinge University Hospital and the Department of Clinical Genetics, Karolinska Hospital, Karolinska Institute.

Supported by Grants No. 3681 and 3902 from the Swedish Medical Research Council and by the Karolinska Institute.

Received for publication March 23, 1985; accepted June 19, 1985.

Reprint requests to: Eugen Steiner, M.D., Department of Clinical Pharmacology, Huddinge University Hospital, S-141 86 Huddinge, Sweden.

quin[26,28] and in the response to a given dose.[27] In a family study the frequency of slow debrisoquin hydroxylators was estimated to 8.9% in British white subjects, and a deficient capacity to hydroxylate debrisoquin appeared to be an autosomal recessive trait.[10] Studies in small groups from different ethnic populations have suggested geographic variations in the frequency of the two phenotypes.[18]

We investigated the importance of genetic and environmental factors to the hydroxylation of debrisoquin in man. Path analysis[25] was used to resolve the relative contribution of genetic and cultural heritability, while segregation analysis[14] was used to search for evidence of a major locus.

METHODS

Subjects. The study was approved by the local Ethics Committee. Medical students and staff members together with their families were asked to participate in the investigation. All subjects were informed in writing about the purpose and experimental design of the study. Altogether 52 white families comprising 226 subjects (119 men and 107 women) were studied. Men ranged in age between 14 and 76 years ($\bar{X} \pm SD = 38.7 \pm 17.5$ years), in weight between 52 and 97 kg ($\bar{X} \pm SD = 74.3 \pm 9.9$ kg), and in height between 162 and 192 cm ($\bar{X} \pm SD = 179 \pm 5.67$ cm). Women ranged in age between 14 and 72 years ($\bar{X} \pm SD = 38.9 \pm 15.7$ years), in weight between 43 and 91 kg ($\bar{X} \pm SD = 60.5 \pm 8.5$ kg), and in height between 155 and 182 cm ($\bar{X} \pm SD = 166 \pm 5.6$ cm). There were 175 nonsmokers and 30 subjects who smoked ≥ 10 cigarettes a day. There were 20 total alcohol abstainers (9%). Forty subjects were taking daily medication, six of whom were taking drugs that are known inducers of drug metabolism. Nineteen women used contraceptive steroids or were receiving postmenopausal estrogen therapy. Five subjects were vegetarians. There was one monozygotic and one dizygotic twin pair among the children. One of the monozygotic twins was excluded from the genetic analysis.

Debrisoquin phenotyping test. The subjects received 10 mg debrisoquin (Declinax; Roche Laboratories) by mouth after an overnight fast. Urine was collected during 6 hours and was analyzed by gas chromatographic procedures.[15] The capacity to hydroxylate debrisoquin was expressed as the MDR.[17] A report on the reproducibility of the measurement of the MDR will be published separately.

Cultural and environmental variables. Because family environment is not easily measurable, an estimate of the environment was created for the different variables by stepwise multiple regression on obesity (defined as Quetelet's index: weight/height^2), smoking habits (number of cigarettes per day; 1 gm pipe tobacco was taken as equal to one cigarette), use of alcohol (measured in grams of alcohol per kilogram body weight), type of work (on a scale from 1 to 4, 1 corresponding to light and 4 to hard work), physical exercise (hours per week), amount of stress in work (on a scale from 1 to 3), number of cups of coffee per day, current medication, prior and current state of health, and known hypersensitivity to drugs. The information on these variables was obtained by a standardized questionnaire previously used in a family study of propranolol protein binding.[1] The part of the environment estimated in this way is called the indexed environment, while the remaining part is called the residual environment.

Table I. Correlation coefficients (r) and sample sizes

	r	*No. of subjects*
P_F, P_M	0.081	52
I_F, I_M	0.437	52
P_FI_M, P_MI_F	0.002	104
P_FI_F, P_MI_M	0.103	104
P_{C_1}, P_{C_2}	0.510	68
I_{C_1}, I_{C_2}	0.262	74
P_C, I_C	0.268	102
P_{C_1}, I_{C_2}	0.172	112
P_F, P_C	0.380	76
I_F, P_C	0.099	68
P_F, I_C	0.009	95
I_F, I_C	0.324	89
P_M, P_C	0.421	71
I_M, P_C	0.076	73
P_M, I_C	0.338	89
I_M, I_C	0.361	99

P = Phenotype; F = father; M = mother; I = index; C = child.

Path analysis. A path analytic model was applied to resolve genetic and cultural inheritance. The model used is a special case of the general model presented by Rao et al.[24] It is assumed that environment acts additively without interactions to produce the phenotype. Support for this view is given by Morton and Rao.[22]

Nuclear families yield 16 correlations (Table I) when an environmental index is created for father, mother, and child. We assume no dominance deviation, no direct effect of parental phenotype on child's phenotype, and no genetic correlation between mates. The parameters to be estimated are as follows:

Table II. Descriptive statistics of the families

		Age (yr)		*DMR*			*ln (DMR)*		
	n	$\bar{X} \pm SD$	*Range*	$\bar{X} \pm SD$	*Range*	*Skewness*	$\bar{X} \pm SD$	*Range*	*Skewness*
Parents	104	54.8 ± 8.6	37-76	3.46 ± 9.55	0.12-62.32	4.21	−0.119 ± 1.30	−2.12 to 4.13	1.56
Children	121	25.1 ± 6.6	14-43	5.95 ± 18.91	0.11-124.8	4.34	−0.064 ± 1.45	−2.21 to 4.83	1.83
Total	225	38.8 ± 16.7	14-76	4.80 ± 15.3	0.11-124.8	4.93	−0.090 ± 1.38	−2.21 to 4.83	1.73

c Effect of child's indexed environment on child's phenotype
cy Effect of adult's indexed environment on adult's phenotype
h Effect of genotype on child's phenotype
hz Effect of genotype on adult's phenotype
u Correlation between indexed environments of spouses
f_F Effect of father's indexed environment on child's indexed environment
f_M Effect of mother's indexed environment on child's indexed environment
i Effect of child's indexed environment on the index
i_F Effect of father's indexed environment on his index
i_M Effect of mother's indexed environment on her index
B Nontransmitted common environment for siblings

The genetic and cultural heritabilities are h^2 and c^2 in children and $(hz)^2$ and $(cy)^2$ in adults. Cases of special interest include:

$f_F = f_M = f$ (No maternal effect)
$y = z = 1$ (No intergenerational differences)
$u = 0$ (No marital correlation)
$h = z = 0$ (No genetic heritability)
$c = y = 0$ (No cultural heritability)
$B = 0$ (No nontransmitted common environment for siblings)

The 16 correlations (r_i) in nuclear families and the appropriate samples sizes (N_i) in terms of independent pairs were estimated by maximum likelihood with the computer program PATHMIX.[19] The correlations are treated as independent, giving

$$\chi^2 = \sum_{i=1}^{16} N_i(z_i - \bar{z}_i)^2$$

where z_i is the z score transformation of the expected correlation ρ_i and N_i is the sample size. Ignoring correlations of correlations does not lead to unreliable results.[25]

Estimation of parameters and tests of hypotheses were carried out in terms of the log-likelihood function: $\ln L = -\chi^2/2 + \text{constant}$. The residual χ^2 after estimating k parameters follows a chi-square distribution with 16 − k degrees of freedom. By specifying ρ_i as a function of parameters, χ^2 is made a function of the parameters. Therefore, by minimizing χ^2 we can estimate all or some parameters and use the residual χ^2 for tests of hypotheses.

Segregation analysis. The DMR exhibited positive skewness (Table II). Not allowing for this skewness can give spurious evidence for a major locus. Skewness was therefore removed by use of the power transformation

$$y = \frac{6}{p}\left[\left(\frac{X}{6} + 1\right)^p - 1\right]$$

where X is the standardized ln(DMR), y is the transformed DMR, and p is a parameter chosen to abolish skewness obtained from the data by the computer program SKUMIX.[19]

To test for a major locus we used the mixed model for complex segregation analysis.[14] This model postulates an underlying scale of liability to which a major locus (a gene of large effect), polygenes (genes of small effect), and environment contribute independently. The major locus is assumed to be biallelic, producing three genotypes. The distribution within each major locus genotype is assumed to be normal and homoscedastic. The model is specified by the following seven parameters: V, variance of the quantitative trait; U, mean of the quantitative trait; H, polygenic heritability for children; HZ, polygenic heritability for adults; q, gene frequency of the major locus; d, degree of dominance at the major locus (position of the heterozygous mean relative to the means of the two homozygous classes); and t, displacement due to major locus (measured in standard deviation units). The general model is specified by these seven parameters, while specific subhypotheses concerning certain parameters can be tested by likelihood ratios.

The present case selection was through the parents and should therefore be regarded as complete. Both joint and conditional likelihoods were used for the analysis and the results were compared. Joint likelihood is suitable for this data set because sampling is unconditional and disjoint families are used. Conditional likelihood can, however, serve as an internal check.

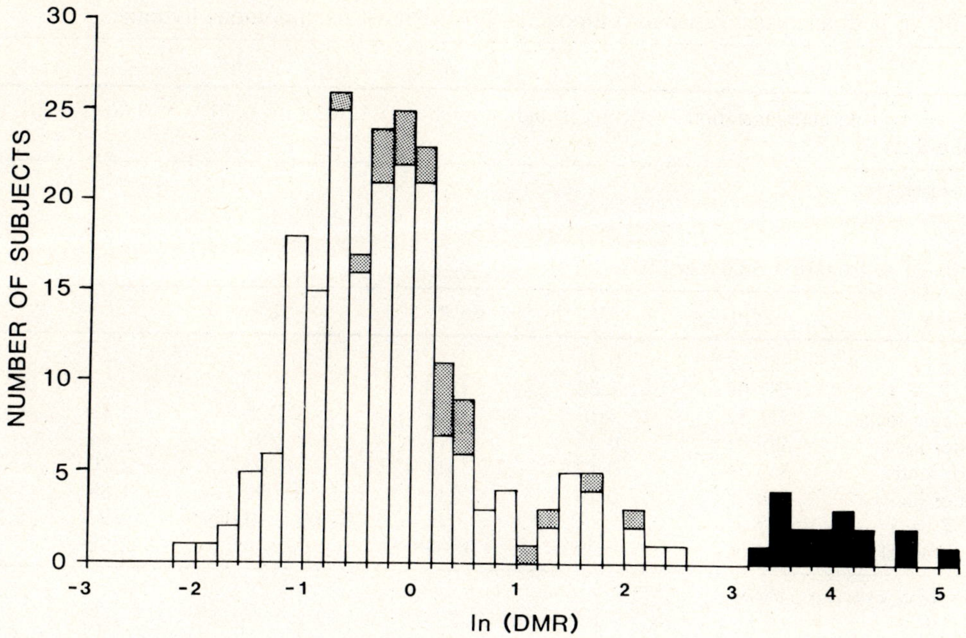

Fig. 1. Frequency distribution of ln (DMR) in all subjects in the study. □ = Dominant phenotype, unknown genotype; ▨ = dominant phenotype, obligate heterozygous genotype (see Fig. 2); ■ = recessive phenotype, homozygous genotype.

RESULTS

Descriptive statistics of the DMR are listed in Table II. Because of the pronounced skewness, the natural logarithm of DMR was taken as variable for the rest of the analysis. A frequency distribution histogram of ln(DMR) indicates a bimodal distribution with an antimode appearing at around 12 (ln(DMR) $\simeq$ 2.5; Fig. 1). Stepwise multiple regression on a cubic polynomial of sex (men coded as 1, women as 2) and age gave no evidence for age and sex effects. No correction was therefore made.

Only coffee intake was found to correlate with ln(DMR) ($r = -0.19$; $P < 0.01$), and path analysis with coffee intake as an index was therefore made. The maximum likelihood estimates of the 16 correlations in nuclear families are listed in Table I. Table III presents the testing of different hypotheses. The general model gave a good fit. There was no evidence for intergenerational differences or maternal effects. As can be seen from the most parsimonious hypothesis, genetic heritability was high (0.79) while cultural heritability was much lower (0.06; Table IV). Segregation analysis was therefore carried out to elucidate the mode of inheritance.

Before segregation analysis, ln(DMR) was standardized to mean zero and variance one and skewness was eliminated. There was significant evidence for two distributions ($\chi^2_6 = 25.46$; $P < 0.001$). Three distributions did not give a better fit. The two distributions could be due to a major locus but this can only be tested by segregation analysis.

A preliminary segregation analysis (data not shown) with joint likelihood and a P value corresponding to one distribution ($P = -2.98$) gave significant evidence for a major gene ($\chi^2_3 = 8.88$; $P < 0.05$). Since this conservative analysis gave evidence for a major locus, we turned to a segregation analysis with the

Table III. Results of path analysis: Tests of hypotheses

Hypothesis	*df*	χ^2
$h = z = 0$ (no genetic heritability)	9	30.24
$c = y = 0$ (no cultural heritability)	9	24.77
$u = 0$ (no assortative mating)	8	19.60
$f_F = f_M$ (no maternal effects)	8	9.42
$y = z = 1$ (no intergenerational differences)	9	10.73
$y = 1$ (no intergenerational difference for cultural heritability)	8	9.74
$z = 1$ (no intergenerational difference for genetic heritability)	8	9.53
$B = 0$ (no sibling environment)	8	8.92
General	7	8.91

df = Degrees of freedom.

Table IV. Results of path analysis: Variance components for the most parsimonious hypothesis

Model	*df*	χ^2	h^2	c^2	*u*	*f*
$y = z = 1$, $f_F = f_M$ (no intergenerational differences and no maternal effect)	11	11.63	0.79	0.06	0.71	0.40

df = Degrees of freedom.

Table V. Results of segregation analysis

Hypothesis	*−21nL*	*H*	*Z*	*q*	*t*	*d*
Multifactorial Z = 1	582.37	0.76	(1)	—	—	—
Multifactorial Z ≠ 1	580.09	1.00	0.61	—	—	—
Generalized single locus	515.32	(0)	(1)	0.325	2.88	0.29
Recessive major locus	529.91	0.37	(1)	0.291	2.44	(0)
Additive major locus	552.74	0.12	(1)	0.203	2.70	(0.5)
Dominant major locus	556.25	0.18	(1)	0.099	1.88	(1)
Mixed model Z = 1	509.53	0.14 ± 0.12*	(1)	0.306 ± 0.059*	2.94	0.28 ± 0.03*
General mixed model	504.64	0.29	0.088	0.316	2.90	0.28

Noniterated parameters are given in parentheses.
*X ± SD.

P value for two distributions (P = −0.56; Table V). There was strong evidence for a major locus (χ^2_3 = 580.09 − 504.64 = 75.45; P < 0.001) with incomplete dominance (d = 0.28), i.e., between a recessive and an additive gene. There was also evidence for a multifactorial component (χ^2_1 = 515.32 − 509.53 = 5.79; P < 0.05).

The evidence for the multifactorial component was evenly distributed over the families. The data also gave evidence of an intergenerational difference for this component (χ^2_1 = 509.53 − 504.64 = 4.89; P < 0.05). However, this evidence came almost entirely from one family. The mother in this family had a DMR of 1.06, which in itself is not remarkably high but was high in relation to that of the other family members (father 0.24; offspring 0.27, 0.17, and 0.11). This woman was receiving thyroid hormones and had a previous history of excessive alcohol intake and psychotropic drug use. When she was excluded, no significant evidence for an intergenerational difference remained (χ^2_1 = 3.07).

The mixed model with Z = 1 was therefore used as the most parsimonious model, with a major gene with frequency q = 0.306 and incomplete dominance d = 0.28 explaining 70.8% of the variation in the population. In addition, there was a small multifactorial component with heritability 0.14, which is smaller than the value for childhood heritability obtained under the general model with Z ≠ 1 (H = 0.29). However, the parameters for the major gene were not influenced by differences in Z. The use of conditional likelihood instead of joint likelihood did not alter results to any major extent. The best model with conditional likelihood was H = 0.12, Z = 1, q = 0.335, t = 2.90, and d = 0.27.

As an additional test to the major locus, the τ parameter of Elston and Stewart[7] was used. In short, τ_{AAA}, τ_{AaA}, and τ_{aaA} are the probabilities that a parent with genotype AA, Aa, and aa, respectively, will transmit A to an offspring. For Mendelian inheritance these probabilities are 1, 0.5, and 0, respectively. We fixed τ_{AAA} and τ_{aaA} to 1 and 0, respectively, and τ_{AaA} = 0.5 was tested. No significant evidence was found against this hypothesis (χ^2_1 = 0.08), strengthening our hypothesis of a major locus.

DISCUSSION

We have shown that the greatest part of the interindividual variation in DMR can be explained by genetic heritability (79%). This is a high figure compared with the 21% genetic heritability of plasma protein binding of propranolol estimated with the same technique.[1] Cultural heritability accounted for only 6% of the variation, leaving 15% to technical and random factors. Surprisingly, coffee intake was the only specific environmental factor correlating with DMR. The mechanism for this possible interaction is highly intriguing. If tea consumption was also taken into account the correlation increased, although no significant correlation was found between cups of tea and DMR. Caffeine might possibly influence the tubular secretion of debrisoquin or act as an inducer of a cytochrome P-450 isozyme.

Complex segregation analysis gave evidence for a major locus with incomplete dominance (d = 0.28)

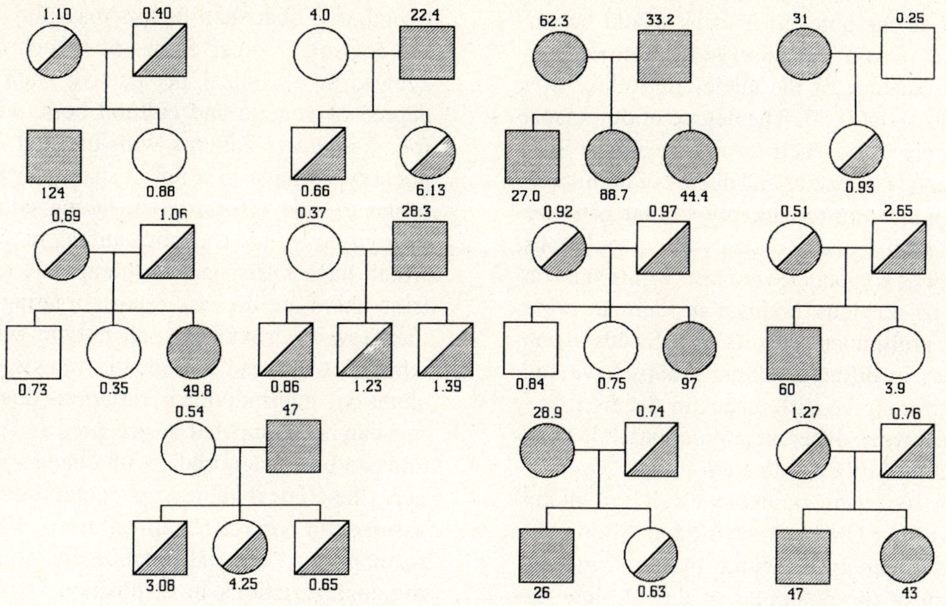

Fig. 2. Pedigrees of the families of propositi with the slow metabolizer phenotype. DMR is given for each subject. ◐, ◪ = Obligate heterozygous genotype.

Table VI. Results of segregation analysis with an oligogenic model

Hypothesis	$-2 l nL$	*q*	*d*	*t*	q_m	d_m	t_m
No modifier	515.32	0.325	0.29	2.88	—	—	—
Recessive modifier	506.04	0.317	0.24	2.86	0.363	(0)	1.09
Additive modifier	501.05	0.308	0.25	3.00	0.086	(0.5)	1.98
Dominant modifier	502.61	0.321	0.25	2.97	0.070	(1)	1.01
General model	500.78	0.300	0.25	3.03	0.098	0.45	2.12

Noniterated parameters are given in parentheses.

between a recessive and an additive gene. The calculated frequency of the major gene was 0.306, allowing us to estimate the frequency of the homozygous recessive and dominant genotypes (aa and AA) as 0.09 and 0.48, respectively, and the heterozygous genotype as 0.42.

The genetic model applied explains 71% of the interindividual variation in DMR. The remaining genetic heritability is explained by a small multifactorial component evenly spread out over all the families. The evidence obtained for a multifactorial component indicates that there is a residual family resemblance in addition to the family resemblance caused by the major gene. This residual family resemblance might be due to an additional major gene, a modifier, polygenes, common environment, or a mixture of these factors. At present there is no method to distinguish between these alternatives. However, it is possible to model this residual resemblance in terms of a single modifier locus. In this oligogenic model a major locus with parameters q, t, and d is interacting with a modifier locus with parameters q_m, t_m, and d_m. No polygenic component is allowed for. This model has been implemented in the computer program COMBIN. Results of the COMBIN analysis, again with joint likelihood, are listed in Table VI. There is significant evidence for a modifier ($\chi^2_3 = 515.32 - 500.78 = 14.54$; $P < 0.01$). However, it was not possible to elucidate the degree of dominance, although a recessive modifier seems less likely. The parameters for the major locus were stable regardless of the parameters of the modifier locus. For the general model the variances due to the major locus and modifying locus were 0.72 and 0.17, respectively. It should be stressed that this analysis has not shown the existence of a modifier; it has only suggested likely values of the parameters in an assumed modifying locus.

In previous investigations the mode of inheritance of DMR was studied without taking environmental factors into account. Evans et al.[10] suggested that two alleles of major effect at one autosomal locus would be sufficient to explain most of the observed variation. They estimated the frequency of the allele controlling slow hydroxylation to about 0.30. The degree of dominance was approximately 30%. Their results are almost identical with the gene frequencies and degree of dominance we estimated, indicating remarkably similar gene frequencies in the British and Swedish white populations. The estimated gene frequencies are also within the confidence limits of previous findings in German populations[6] and in preliminary reports of a Swedish population.[4] Studies in different ethnic groups have suggested that there may be differences in the frequency of these genes between different populations,[10,18] a suggestion warranting further evaluation.

From a pharmacogenetic point of view, it is of interest to determine whether DMR can be used to differentiate between different genotypes within the rapid metabolizers. By study of the pedigrees of the 17 slow metabolizers (Fig. 2) it was possible to identify 21 subjects who are obligate heterozygotes. In this group DMR varied between 0.4 and 6.13, indicating that it is not possible to differentiate between the two genotypes through the use of the DMR. This is in contrast to the suggestion of Mahgoub et al.[18] which was based on data from one family.

It has been proposed that the metabolism of several other drugs, notably sparteine,[5,11] nortriptyline,[4,21] desmethylimipramine,[3,29] metoprolol,[16] and propranolol,[23] may be controlled by genetic factors similar to those of debrisoquin. Further family and in vitro studies with several of these substrates are needed to clarify the relationships between the metabolism of these drugs, since crossover studies comparing the capacity to metabolize debrisoquin and sparteine have given conflicting results. Thus there are reports of individuals with dissimilar phenotypes of debrisoquin and sparteine metabolic ratios. Evans et al.[9,10] performed debrisoquin and sparteine tests in 15 families. Four of the subjects did not agree with respect to the debrisoquin and sparteine phenotypes. Woolhouse et al.[31] did not find any slow sparteine metabolizers in a Ghanian population sample, while slow debrisoquin metabolizers were not uncommon. Possible explanations for these anomalies could be errors in the phenotyping method, influences of modifier alleles acting to magnify what may be minor pathways of metabolism, or two closely linked loci for alleles of major effect.

Path analysis gave evidence that only a minor part of family resemblance is actually due to common environment. Because other drug oxidative processes are readily influenced by environmental factors, we can hypothesize that such factors may play a larger role in the control of other forms of cytochrome P-450 enzymes. In a clinical perspective such differences in degree of genetic and cultural heritability are of profound interest. Patients with unusual drug metabolic phenotypes have in a few instances been shown to be prone to side effects when taking common doses of phenytoin[12] and tricyclic antidepressants,[4] both of which have fairly narrow therapeutic ranges. By contrast, there are no case reports relating side effects to the slow hydroxylation phenotype with β-blockers, which have broad therapeutic ranges. In the clinical situation, interindividual variations due to genetic factors can be anticipated by prepared and aware clinicians and can be "diagnosed" with phenotyping tests. However, the clinical value of phenotyping patients must be assessed in controlled clinical trials. Far more difficult to manage in clinical practice are drugs with intraindividual variations in disposition caused by environmental factors. Such variations are the rationale for repeated therapeutic drug monitoring, while phenotyping in these cases is of questionable value.

We used path analysis and complex segregation analysis to assess the relative importance of genetic and environmental factors to interindividual differences in debrisoquin hydroxylation. Family studies with other drug substrates thought to be metabolized by enzymes under genetic control similar to that of debrisoquin hydroxylase may, together with in vitro studies, clarify interrelationships between cytochrome P-450–mediated drug metabolic processes.

The genetic analyses were performed at the Population Genetics Laboratory, University of Hawaii.

Authors' note

Tabulated data from all subjects participating in the study can be obtained from the authors on request.

References

1. Alván G, Bergström K, Borgå O, Iselius L, Pedersen N: Family study of genetic and environmental factors determining the protein binding of propranolol. Eur J Clin Pharmacol **25**:437-441, 1983.
2. Åsberg M, Price Evans DA, Sjöqvist F: Genetic control of nortriptyline kinetics in man—A study of relatives of proposity with high plasma concentrations. J Med Genet **8**:129-135, 1971.
3. Bertilsson L, Åberg-Wistedt A: Debrisoquine hydroxylation test predicts steady state plasma levels of desipramine. Br J Clin Pharmacol **15**:388-390, 1983.
4. Bertilsson L, Mellström B, Sjöqvist F, Mårtenson B, Åsberg M: Slow hydroxylation of nortriptyline and con-

comitant poor debrisoquine hydroxylation: Clinical implications. Lancet **1**:560-561, 1981.

5. Eichelbaum M, Bertilsson L, Säwe J, Zekorn C: Polymorphic oxidation of sparteine and debrisoquine: Related pharmacogenetic entities. CLIN PHARMACOL THER **31**:184-186, 1982.
6. Eichelbaum M, Spannbrucher N, Steinecke B, Dengler HJ: Defective N-oxidation of sparteine in man. A new pharmacogenetic defect. Eur J Clin Pharmacol **16**:183-187, 1979.
7. Elston RC, Stewart J: A general method for the genetic analysis of pedigree data. Hum Hered **21**:523-542, 1971.
8. Evans DAP: Individual variations of drug metabolism as a factor in drug toxicity. Ann NY Acad Sci **123**:178-187, 1965.
9. Evans DAP, Hammer D, Daunham DY, Whibley EJ, Idle JR, Ritschie J, Smith RL: The genetic control of sparteine and debrisoquine metabolism in man with new methods of analyzing bimodal distributions. J Med Genet **20**:321-329, 1983.
10. Evans DAP, Mahgoub A, Sloan TP, Idle JR, Smith RL: A family and population study of the genetic polymorphism of debrisoquine in white British population. J Med Genet **17**:102-105, 1980.
11. Inaba T, Vinks A, Otton SV, Kalow W: Comparative pharmacogenetics of sparteine and debrisoquine. CLIN PHARMACOL THER **33**:394-399, 1983.
12. Kutt H, Wolk M, Scherman R, McDowell F: Insufficient parahydroxylation as a cause of diphenylhydantoin toxicity. Neurology (Minneap) **14**:542-548, 1964.
13. Küpfer A, Desmond P, Patwardhan R, Schenker S, Branch RA: Mephenytoin hydroxylation deficiency: Kinetics after repeated doses. CLIN PHARMACOL THER **35**:33-39, 1984.
14. Lalouel JM, Morton NE: Complex segregation analysis with pointers. Hum Hered **31**:312-321, 1981.
15. Lennard MS, Silas JH, Smith AJ, Tucker GT: Determination of debrisoquine and its 4-hydroxy metabolite in biological fluids by gas chromatography with flame-ionization and nitrogen-selective detection. J Chromatogr **133**:161-166, 1977.
16. Lennard MS, Tucker GT, Silas JH, Freestone S, Ramsay LE, Woods HF: Differential stereoselective metabolism of metoprolol in extensive and poor debrisoquine metabolizers. CLIN PHARMACOL THER **34**:732-737, 1983.
17. Mahgoub A, Idle JR, Dring LG, Lancaster R, Smith RL: Polymorphic hydroxylation of debrisoquine in man. Lancet **2**:584-586, 1977.
18. Mahgoub A, Idle JR, Smith RL: A population and familial study of defective alicyclic hydroxylation of debrisoquin among Egyptians. Xenobiotica **9**:51-56, 1979.
19. MacLean CJ, Morton NE, Elston RC: Skewness in comingled distributions. Biometrics **32**:695-699, 1976.
20. MacLean CJ, Morton NE, Yee S: Combined analysis of segregation linkage and association under an oligogenic model. Comput Biomed Res **17**:471-480, 1984.
21. Mellström B, Bertilsson L, Säwe, J, Schulz H-U, Sjöqvist F: E-and Z-hydroxylation of nortriptyline—relationship to polymorphic debrisoquine hydroxylation. CLIN PHARMACOL THER **30**:189-193, 1981.
22. Morton NE, Rao DC: Quantitative inheritance in man. Yearbook Physical Anthropol **21**:12-41, 1978.
23. Raghuram TC, Koshakji RP, Wilkinson GR, Wood AJJ: Polymorphic ability to metabolize propranolol alters 4-hydroxy-propranolol levels but not beta-blockade. CLIN PHARMACOL THER **36**:51-56, 1984.
24. Rao DC, Morton NE, Cloninger CR: Path analysis under generalized assortative mating. I. Theory. Genet Res **33**:175-188, 1979.
25. Rao DC, Morton NE, Yee S: Resolution of cultural and biological inheritance by path analysis. Am J Hum Genet **28**:228-242, 1976.
26. Silas JH, Lennard MS, Tucker GT, Smith AJ: The disposition of debrisoquine in hypertensive patients. Br J Clin Pharmacol **5**:27-34, 1978.
27. Silas JH, Lennard MS, Tucker GT, Smith AJ, Malcolm SL, Marten TR: Why hypertensive patients vary in the response to oral debrisoquine. Br Med J **1**:422-425, 1977.
28. Sloan TP, Lancaster R, Shah RR, Idle JR, Smith RL: Genetically determined oxidation capacity and disposition of debrisoquine. Br J Clin Pharmacol **15**:443-450, 1983.
29. Spina E, Birgerson C, von Bahr C, Eriksson Ö, Mellström B, Steiner E, Sjöqvist F: Phenotypic consistency in hydroxylation of desmethylimipramine and debrisoquine in healthy subjects and in human liver microsomes. CLIN PHARMACOL THER **36**:677-682, 1984.
30. Tucker GT, Silas JH, Iyun AO, Lennard MS, Smith AJ: Polymorphic hydroxylation of debrisoquine. Lancet **2**:718, 1977.
31. Woolhouse NM, Eichelbaum M, Oates NS, Idle JR, Smith RL: Dissociation of co-regulatory control of debrisoquin/phenformin and sparteine oxidation in Ghanaians. CLIN PHARMACOL THER **37**:512-521, 1985.
32. Vesell ES: Selection of subjects for investigation of host factors affecting drug response: A method to identify new pharmacogenetic conditions. CLIN PHARMACOL THER **35**:1-11, 1984.
33. Vesell ES, Penno MB: Assessment of methods to identify sources of interindividual pharmacokinetic variations. Clin Pharmacokinet **8**:378-409, 1983.

Interethnic differences in genetic polymorphism of debrisoquin and mephenytoin hydroxylation between Japanese and Caucasian populations

Interethnic differences in debrisoquin and mephenytoin hydroxylation have been compared between normal white (n = 183) and Japanese (n = 100) subjects with the 8-hour urinary metabolic ratio of debrisoquin and the urinary *S/R* enantiomeric ratio of mephenytoin to identify extensive (EM) and poor (PM) metabolizers. In white subjects the frequency of PMs was 8.7% and 2.7% for debrisoquin and mephenytoin, respectively. In contrast, in Japanese subjects no PMs of debrisoquin were identified, while the incidence of PMs of mephenytoin was 18%. These substantial differences ($P < 0.001$) in polymorphic distributions of oxidative drug metabolizing ability have implications for interethnic efficacy and toxicity of drugs and other xenobiotics that are metabolized by the involved cytochrome P-450 isozymes. (CLIN PHARMACOL THER 38:402-408, 1985.)

K. Nakamura, M.D., F. Goto, M.D., W. A. Ray, Ph.D., C. B. McAllister, M.S., E. Jacqz, M.D., G. R. Wilkinson, Ph.D., and R. A. Branch, M.D.

Nashville, Tenn., and Tsukuba, Japan

The activities of a number of enzymes involved in the metabolism of xenobiotics is known to be monogenetically regulated and to exhibit polymorphism. These include pseudocholinesterase,[14] alcohol and aldehyde dehydrogenases,[25,31] paraoxonase,[20] *N*-acetyltransferase,[28] and certain mixed-function oxidases.[5] In many instances the gene frequencies for the involved loci vary among racial and ethnic groups, resulting in differences in the polymorphic distribution.[11,16] For example, with debrisoquin 4-hydroxylase activity the incidence of a poor metabolizer (PM) phenotype ranges from about 1% to 10% and appears to decline in moving from Western to middle-Eastern/African population groups.[9] Recently, a new oxidative polymorphism involving the 4-hydroxylation of *S*-mephenytoin has been described in white populations, in which the frequency of the PM phenotype is about 3% to 5%.[10,19,30] The present study compares the distributions of these two polymorphisms in a white population to that in a Japanese population.

From the Departments of Pharmacology and Preventive Medicine, Vanderbilt University, Nashville, and Department of Anesthesiology, University of Tsukuba, Tsukuba.

Supported in part by United States Public Health Service Grants No. GM 31304 and RR 00095.

Received for publication April 29, 1985; accepted June 19, 1985.

Reprint requests to: Dr. R. A. Branch, Department of Pharmacology, Vanderbilt University, Nashville, TN 37232.

METHODS

Studies were performed in 183 (14 women) unrelated and randomly selected normal white subjects 18 to 50 years old who resided in middle Tennessee, and in a similar group of 100 (14 women) Japanese 18 to 40 years old from Tsukuba, Japan. Most of the white group had been studied before.[30] Subjects had had no recent illness, were receiving no drugs, and had no abnormalities on physical examination or biochemical evidence of renal or hepatic dysfunction. On the day of the study, urine was voided immediately before oral dosing with either 10 mg (57 μmol) debrisoquin (Declinax tablet; Roche Laboratories) or 100 mg (460 μmol) racemic mephenytoin (Mesantoin tablet; Sandoz Pharmaceuticals). Urine was collected over the subsequent 8 hours, its volume was measured, and aliquots were stored frozen until analysis (samples from Japan were transferred over dry ice and were still frozen on receipt in Nashville). The order of dosing was random and at least 3 days elapsed between each study.

Oxidative phenotypes for the two drugs were determined by previously described methods.[30] For debrisoquin the urinary metabolic ratio of unchanged drug to its 4-hydroxy metabolite was used, whereas the urinary *S/R* enantiomeric ratio was taken as an index of *S*-mephenytoin 4-hydroxylation.

Interethnic differences in distribution of the phenotypes was based on three approaches. The first was the ordinary frequency histogram. The second was the cumulative frequency distribution, rescaled by applying the inverse normal transformation, i.e., probit values less the value 5.0. If the variable under consideration is normally distributed, then such a "normit plot" produces a linear relationship, the slope of which is a function of the standard deviation.[23,26] This type of analysis, therefore, provides a visual means of detecting departures from normality by comparing distributions in different populations and detecting subgroups with different distributions. For example, discontinuous populations will produce separate lines that are horizontally displaced from each other. In contrast, overlapping populations will lead to a curvilinear relationship with a clear breakpoint, whereas a skewed distribution yields a smooth continuous curve. Heterogeneity of distribution was also assessed by Fisher's exact test on the difference in the proportion of PMs in the two populations.[27]

RESULTS

With mephenytoin, the urinary *S/R* enantiomeric ratio values indicated two discrete populations separated by a large antimodal gap in both whites and Japanese (Fig. 1). Five subjects (2.7%) of the white population could be classified as PMs, with *S/R* ratios ≥0.95, whereas 18 of the Japanese subjects (18%) exhibited impairment in the 4-hydroxylation of mephenytoin. This interethnic difference in PM frequency was highly significant ($P < 0.001$). If a phenotypic trait is inherited by a single allele pair with dominant and recessive genes, then it should be possible to identify homozygous dominant from heterozygous genotypes within the extensive metabolizer (EM) group. The distribution of the EM phenotype, characterized by *S/R* ratios <0.6, appeared to be skewed to the right and further analysis indicated a log-normal distribution. There was, however, no evidence even in the Japanese population that subgroups possibly corresponding to genotypic distributions could be discriminated within the EM phenotype. One of the white subjects had an *S/R* ratio of 0.72, which was about in the middle of the antimodal gap (Fig. 1). This individual has been tentatively classified as an "intermediate metabolizer."

Pronounced interethnic differences were also noted in the distribution of debrisoquin's metabolic ratio (Fig. 2). The Japanese population exhibited a unimodal fre-

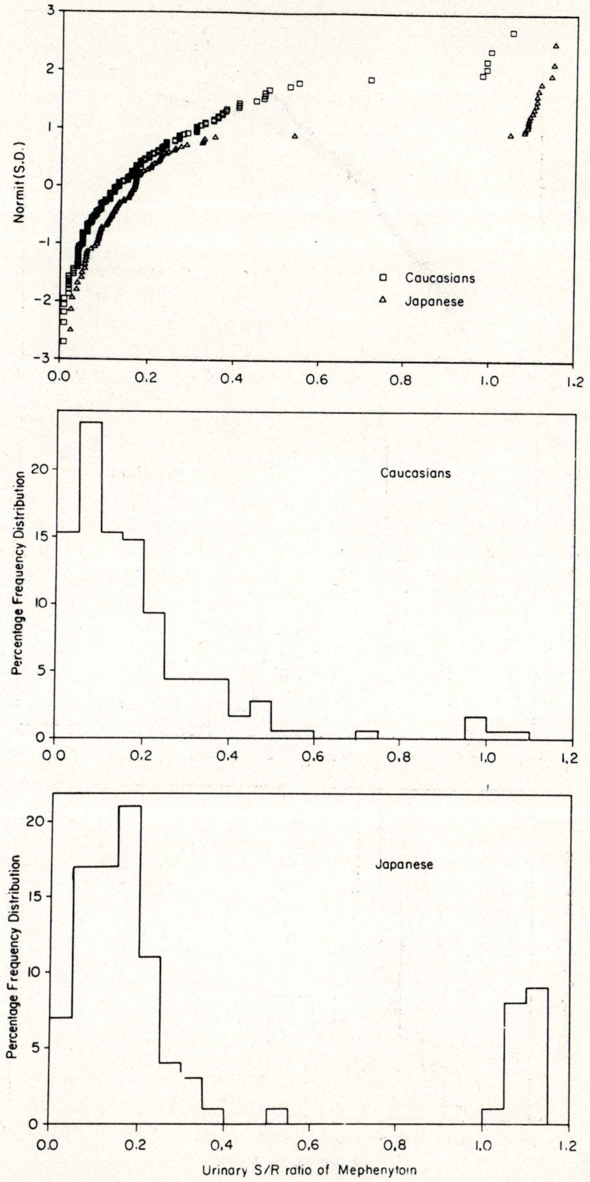

Fig. 1. Distributions of the urinary *S/R* ratio of mephenytoin in white and Japanese populations.

quency distribution that was log-normally distributed. No metabolic ratio value >10 was observed, indicating the absence of any subject of the PM phenotype. In distinct contrast, distribution in the white population was bimodal, with 16 of the subjects (8.7%) demonstrating a PM phenotype with metabolic ratios above an antimode of 13. The interethnic difference in the frequency of the PM phenotype was highly significant ($P < 0.001$). When the separate PM population was excluded from analysis, the distribution of the debrisoquin metabolic ratio for the white EMs was identical

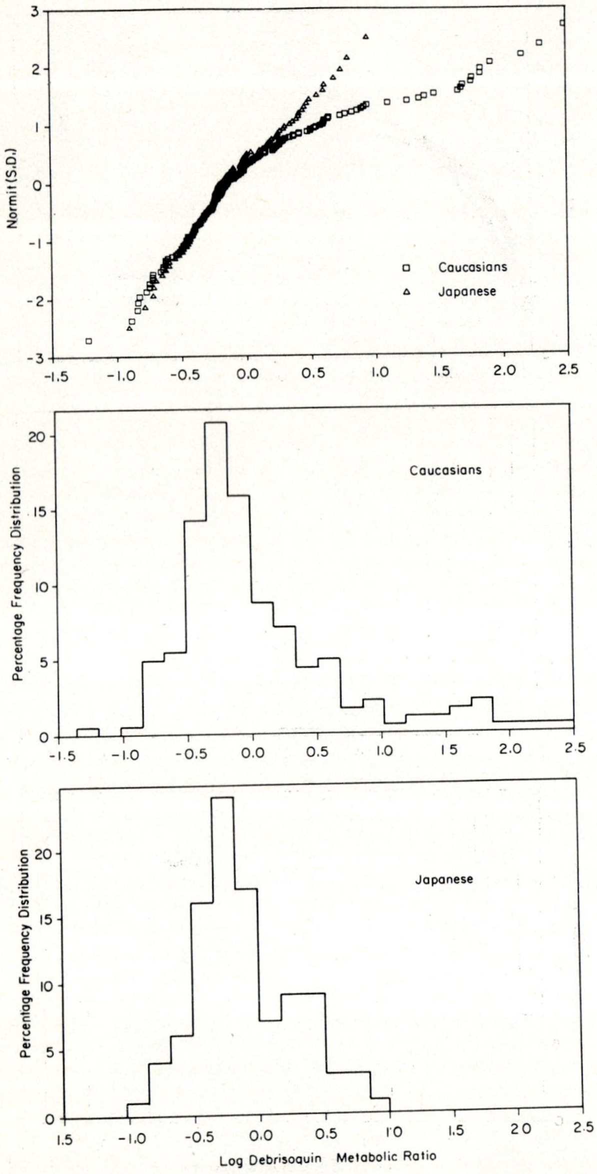

Fig. 2. Distributions of debrisoquin urinary metabolic ratio in white and Japanese populations.

to that for the entire Japanese population (Fig. 3). The same findings were obtained when the ratio of recovered debrisoquin to that of the sum of debrisoquin and 4-hydroxydebrisoquin was examined.

Separate comparisons of the urinary recoveries of debrisoquin and its 4-hydroxy metabolite showed that the distributions were log-normal in both populations, with the Japanese excreting a slightly higher but not significantly different mean amount of both compounds with a smaller standard deviation (Table I; Fig. 4).

DISCUSSION

Many examples exist of interethnic differences in gene frequency for a variety of proteins; this study as it relates to drugs and their action has been termed pharmacoanthropology.[12] Well-established differences between Caucasians and Orientals include the responsiveness to ethanol involving differences in both alcohol and aldehyde dehydrogenases,[25,31] and also the different distribution of slow and fast acetylators of *N*-arylamines determined by *N*-acetyltransferase.[28] More recently, cytochrome P-450–mediated oxidative metabolism of a number of drugs such as amobarbital[15] has also been shown to differ between the two ethnic groups. Our present observations extend these findings to two further pathways. Debrisoquin 4-hydroxylation was bimodally distributed in whites, with 8.7% of the population having the PM phenotype, a frequency consistent with previous studies in this ethnic group.[7,9] In contrast, this pathway was unimodally distributed in the Japanese, with no PMs being identified in 100 subjects. Furthermore, the incidence of the PM phenotype for mephenytoin 4-hydroxylation was sixfold higher in the Japanese population than in the white population. These disparate findings confirm the independence of the two oxidative metabolizing traits[10,19,30] and also demonstrate the wide variability in polymorphism that can occur between populations of different ethnic origin.

Concern has been expressed over the use of the debrisoquin urinary metabolic ratio in pharmacoanthropologic studies because it may not necessarily reflect drug metabolizing ability.[13] For example, the mean amount of drug that is excreted unchanged shows wide population differences suggestive of possible genetic differences in the renal tubular secretion of debrisoquin.[13] Other interethnic discrepancies also exist. In our study the urinary recoveries of unchanged drug, its 4-hydroxy metabolite, and their sum were very similar in the two populations. This would suggest that the same drug metabolizing ability and disposition are being measured in both groups.

A number of mechanisms could account for the reduced 4-hydroxylation of debrisoquin in the PM phenotype.[6] The isolation, purification, and characterization of the cytochrome P-450_H isozyme responsible for the formation of virtually all of this metabolite in rat liver suggested that impaired metabolism was associated with the absence of this quantitatively minor isozyme.[21] On the other hand, similar studies with a human liver isozyme, cytochrome P-450_{DB}, are more consistent with the impairment being due to a qualitative differ-

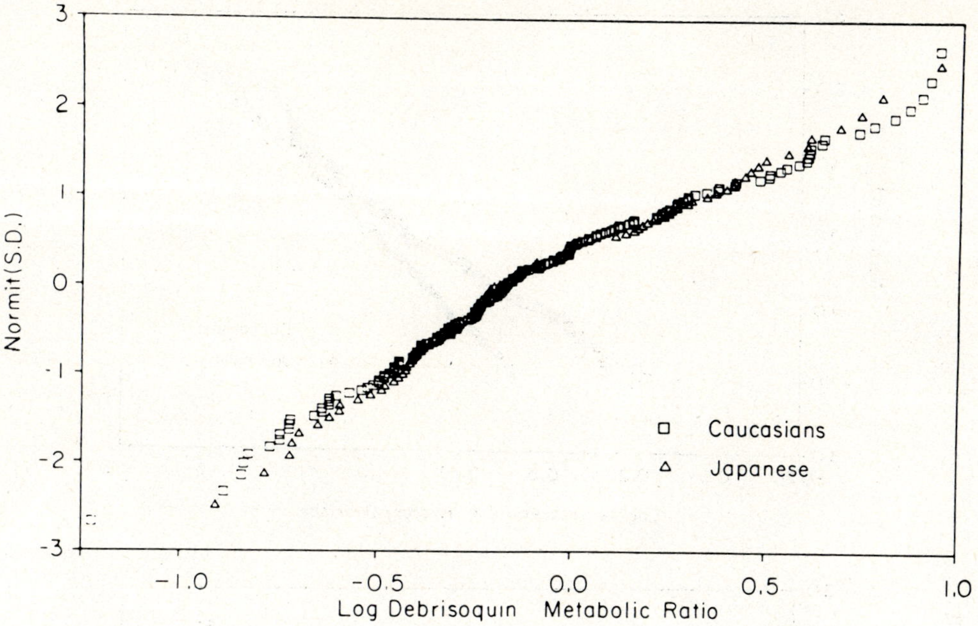

Fig. 3. Comparison of the cumulative frequency distributions of the debrisoquin metabolic ratio in white and Japanese EMs.

Table I. Percentage of dose excreted in 8 hours as debrisoquin and 4-hydroxydebrisoquin in white and Japanese subjects

	Debrisoquin	*4-Hydroxydebrisoquin*	*Total*
White EM phenotype (n = 167)	8.00 ± 6.36	9.67 ± 6.87	17.68 ± 10.66
White PM phenotype (n = 16)	12.78 ± 8.66	0.26 ± 0.17	13.04 ± 8.64
Japanese (n = 100)	9.34 ± 5.74	10.93 ± 4.63	20.26 ± 6.04

Data are $\overline{X}$ ± SD.

ence(s) in the isozyme.[3] Additional studies with liver preparations from subjects of known in vivo phenotype will be required to resolve the mechanism further.

Family studies in white subjects indicate that the deficient trait for debrisoquin hydroxylation is inherited in an autosomal-recessive Mendelian fashion that is determined by at least two alleles at a single gene locus.[24] Accordingly, the PM phenotype represents the homozygous recessive genotype and the EM population is a mixed distribution of heterozygous and homozygous dominant individuals. Attempts have been made to identify these genotypic distributions within the dominant phenotype in white populations assuming diallelic regulation and a log-normal distribution of the metabolic ratio in each population.[1,18] Our present findings, however, indicate that the distribution of the EM phenotype in white subjects is superimposable on that of the Japanese population, who are presumably genetically homogenous. Accordingly, it appears that discrimination of genotypes within the EM phenotype on the basis of the metabolic ratio is not possible. A similar conclusion also applies when the ratio of debrisoquin to the sum of debrisoquin and its 4-hydroxy metabolite is considered.

The biochemical basis for the polymorphic 4-hydroxylation of mephenytoin has not yet been elucidated. Presumably, impaired metabolism reflects a quantitative or qualitative difference in catalytic activity of one or more cytochrome P-450 isozymes. The genetic regulation of this isozyme is also less well characterized than that for the debrisoquin trait, although data from limited family studies are consistent with an autosomal recessive trait.[18,19] On this basis, the PM phenotype represents the homozygous recessive genotype, whereas the homozygous dominant and heterozygous genotypes are distributed within the EM phenotype.

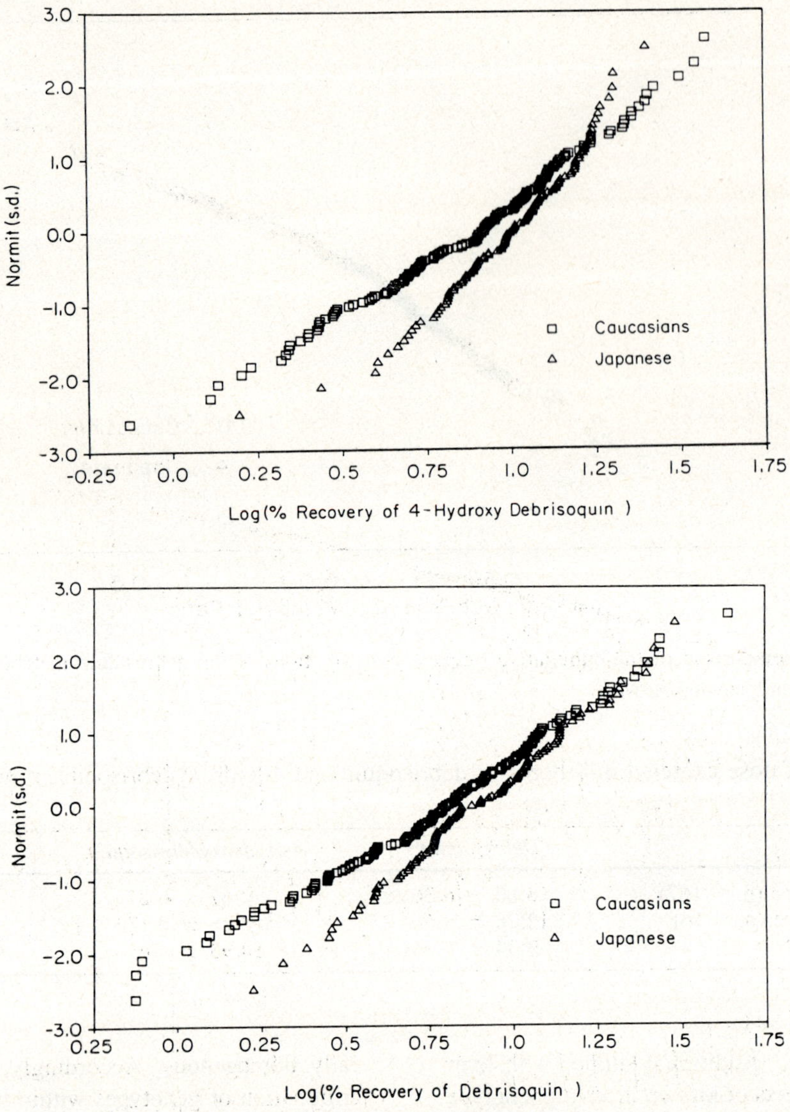

Fig. 4. Cumulative frequency distributions of the urinary recoveries of debrisoquin and its 4-hydroxy metabolite in white and Japanese populations.

Interestingly, even in the Japanese population in which there is a high incidence of PMs, there was no indication that the *S/R* ratio of any subgroups within the EM population might correspond to these genotypes. Furthermore, no individuals were identified in the antimodal region (*S/R* ratio 0.6 to 0.95) who might represent the heterozygote genotype. One white subject, however, had an *S/R* ratio of 0.72, and detailed pharmacokinetic studies have clearly demonstrated that his ability to eliminate *S*-mephenytoin is between that of EMs and PMs.[29] Whether this has a genetic basis or involves some other mechanism such as subclinical liver dysfunction remains to be elucidated.

The in vivo metabolism of an increasing and substantial number of drugs cosegregates with the debrisoquin trait,[9] and a similar situation is emerging with mephenytoin.[8] It would be expected that the described interethnic differences in the distribution of the polymorphisms between white subjects and the Japanese would extend to these cosegregating drugs. In this regard it is important to consider the pharmacokinetic consequences of polymorphic drug metabolizing ability. Dependent on the particular drug and the relative importance of the involved pathway to overall elimination, interphenotypic differences in disposition may range from minor to highly pronounced. If pharmacologically active metabolites are involved, then this may further affect differences in drug responsiveness. In the case of mephenytoin, for example, there is an almost 100-fold interphenotypic difference in the oral clearance of *S*-mephenytoin to its 4-hydroxy metabolite, leading to doubled plasma hydantoin concentrations. As a result, PMs have exaggerated central effects compared with EMs when given the same dose of racemic drug.[17] Interestingly, mephobarbital, a drug whose metabolism cosegregates with the mephenytoin trait,[17] has an incidence of adverse effects of about 3.5% in white subjects living in Australia[4] but approximately 20% in Japanese patients.* Studies in male Hawaiians of different ethnic origins have also noted that the frequency of bladder cancer in whites is over twice that in Japanese.[32] Because bladder cancer is thought to arise by metabolic activation of environmental procarcinogens[22] and is associated with a shift to the left in the frequency distribution of the debrisoquin metabolic ratio (i.e., carcinogenesis is more prevalent in the most extensive metabolizers of the EM phenotype[2]), it is tempting to speculate that this difference in incidence reflects, in part, a genetic predisposition linked to the interethnic difference in xenobiotic metabolism characterized by the debrisoquin trait.

Both anecdotal and experimental reports indicate that drug responsiveness may differ substantially between such ethnic groups as Caucasians and Orientals, so that there are significant differences in dosage requirements. Our findings indicate that one factor that may be involved is the population frequency of genetically determined polymorphisms of certain oxidative biotransformation pathways. The magnitude of such differences between populations of other ethnic origins is largely unknown and cannot be estimated except by empiric determination. Given the international nature of drug development and use and the multiracial nature of the populations of many countries, it appears that the potential for genetically determined interethnic differences in drug responsiveness caused by drug dispositional factors should be given increased recognition.

*Bayer Yakuhin, Ltd., data on file for Comital.

References

1. Ayesha R, Idle JR, Ritchie JC, Crothers MJ, Hetezel MR: Metabolic oxidation phenotypes as markers for susceptibility for lung cancer. Nature **312:**169-170, 1984.
2. Branch RA, Wilkinson GR, McAllister CB, Ray WA, Kaisary A, Smith P: Association of polymorphic oxidative drug metabolism, cigarette smoking and alcohol consumption with bladder cancer. Clin Res **33:**527A, 1985.
3. Distlerath LM, Reilly PEB, Martin MV, Davis GD, Guengerich FP: Purification and characterization of the human liver cytochromes P-450 involved in debrisoquine 4-hydroxylation and phenacetin O-deethylation, two prototypes for genetic polymorphism in oxidative drug metabolism. J Biol Chem **260:**9057-9067, 1985.
4. Eadie MJ, Bochner F, Hooper WD, Tyrer JH: Preliminary observations on the pharmacokinetics of methylphenobarbitone. Clin Exp Neurol **15:**131-144, 1978.
5. Eichelbaum M: Defective oxidation of drugs; Pharmacokinetic and therapeutic implications. Clin Pharmacokinet **7:**1-22, 1982.
6. Eichelbaum M: Polymorphic drug oxidation in humans. Fed Proc **43:**2298-2302, 1984.
7. Evans DAP, Harmer D, Downham DY, Whibley EJ, Idle JR, Ritchie J, Smith RL: The genetic control of sparteine and debrisoquine metabolism in man with new methods of analyzing biomodal distributions. J Med Genet **20:**321-329, 1983.
8. Hall SD, Branch RA, Guengerich FP, Wilkinson GR: Inhibition of S-mephenytoin hydroxylation in human liver microsomes by anticonvulsants and other drugs. Fed Proc **44:**1257, 1985.
9. Idle JR, Smith RL: The debrisoquine hydroxylation gene: A gene of multiple consequence. Presented at the Second World Conference on Clinical Pharmacology and Therapeutics, Washington, D.C., July 31-Aug 5, 1983, pp 148-164.
10. Inaba T, Jurima M, Nakano M, Kalow W: Mephenytoin and sparteine pharmacogenetics in Canadian Caucasians. CLIN PHARMACOL THER **36:**670-676, 1984.
11. Kalow W: Ethnic differences in drug metabolism. Clin Pharmacokinet **7:**373-400, 1982.
12. Kalow W: Pharmacoanthropology: Outline, problems and the nature of case histories. Fed Proc **43:**2314-2318, 1984.
13. Kalow W: Pharmacoanthropology: Drug metabolism. Fed Proc **43:**2326-2331, 1984.
14. Kalow W, Genest K: A method for the detection of atypical forms of human serum cholinesterase. Determination of dibucaine numbers. Can J Biochem Physiol **35:**339-340, 1957.
15. Kalow W, Tang BK, Kadar D, Inaba T: Distinctive patterns of amobarbital metabolites. CLIN PHARMACOL THER **24:**576-582, 1978.
16. Karim AKMB, Elfellah MS, Evans DAP: Human acetylator polymorphism: Estimate of allele frequency in Libya and details of global distribution. J Med Genet **18:**325-330, 1981.
17. Küpfer A, Branch RA: Stereoselective mephobarbital hydroxylation cosegregates with mephenytoin hydroxylation. CLIN PHARMACOL THER **38:**414-418, 1985.
18. Küpfer A, Desmond P, Patwardhan R, Schenker S, Branch RA: Mephenytoin hydroxylation deficiency: Kinetics after repeated doses. CLIN PHARMACOL THER **35:** 33-39, 1984.
19. Küpfer A, Preisig R: Pharmacogenetics of mephenytoin:

A new drug hydroxylation polymorphism in man. Eur J Clin Pharmacol **26:**753-759, 1984.

20. LaDu BN, Eckerson HW: The polymorphic paraxonase/arylesterase isozyme in human serum. Fed Proc **43:**2338-2341, 1984.
21. Larrey D, Distelrath LM, Dannan GA, Wilkinson GR, Guengerich FP: Purification and characterization of the rat liver microsomal cytochrome P-450 involved in the 4-hydroxylation of debrisoquine, a prototype of genetic variation in oxidative drug metabolism. Biochemistry **23:**2787-2794, 1984.
22. Lower GM: Arylamines and bladder cancer causality: Application of conceptual and operational criteria. CLIN PHARMACOL THER **34:**129-135, 1983.
23. Pearson ES, Hartley HO: Biometrika tables for statisticians, vol 2. Cambridge, 1972, Cambridge University Press, pp 27-32.
24. Price-Evans DA, Mahgoub A, Sloan TP, Idle JR, Smith RL: A family and population study of the genetic polymorphism of debrisoquine hydroxylation in a white British population. J Med Genet **127:**102-105, 1980.
25. Rowat AK: Genetic aspects of ethanol disposition and dependence. Neurobehav Toxicol Teratol **5:**198-199, 1983.
26. Snedecor GW, Cochrane WG: Normal distribution. *In* Statistical methods, ed 7. Ames, Iowa, 1980, Iowa State University Press, pp 59-63.
27. Steel RDG, Torrie JH: Principles and procedures in statistics, ed 2. New York, 1980, McGraw Hill, pp 504-506.
28. Weber WW: Acetylation of drugs. *In* Fishman WH, editor: Metabolic conjugation and metabolic hydrolysis, vol 3. New York, 1973, Academic Press, pp 249-296.
29. Wedlund PJ, Aslanian WA, Jacqz E, McAllister CB, Branch RA, Wilkinson GR: Phenotypic differences in mephenytoin pharmacokinetics in normal subjects. J Pharmacol Exp Ther **234:**662-669, 1985.
30. Wedlund PJ, Aslanian WS, McAllister CB, Wilkinson GR, Branch RA: Mephenytoin hydroxylation deficiency in Caucasians: Frequency of a new oxidative drug metabolism polymorphism. CLIN PHARMACOL THER **36:**773-780, 1984.
31. Yoshida A: Molecular basis of difference in alcohol metabolism between Orientals and Caucasians. Jpn J Hum Genet **27:**55-70, 1982.
32. Young JL, Percy CL, Asire AJ: Surveillance, epidemiology and end-results: Incidence and mortality data. Natl Cancer Inst Monogr **57:**1-1081, 1981.

Pharmacokinetics and beta-blocking effects of timolol in poor and extensive metabolizers of debrisoquin

We studied the pharmacokinetics and β-blocking effects of a single, oral 20 mg dose of timolol in six poor metabolizers (PMs) and six extensive metabolizers (EMs) of debrisoquin. The plasma timolol concentration was significantly higher in PMs than in EMs. There was a fourfold difference in mean AUC (1590 ± 1133 vs. 394 ± 239 ng · hr/ml; P < 0.01) and a twofold difference in mean $t_{1/2}$ (7.5 ± 3 vs. 3.7 ± 1.7 hours; P < 0.01), reflecting differences in oral clearance (13.1 ± 7.8 vs. 48.5 ± 23.2 L/hr; P < 0.01). The degree of β-blockade was greater in PMs than in EMs at 12 hours (30.9% vs. 18.2%; P < 0.05) and at 24 hours (28.3% vs. 13.1%; P < 0.05). In the group as a whole the metabolic ratio correlated positively with both kinetic data and β-blockade, but some overlap was observed. Hence timolol metabolism appears to be subject to debrisoquin-type polymorphism, which results in interphenotypic variation in plasma concentration and β-blocking effect. (CLIN PHARMACOL THER 38:409-413, 1985.)

John C. McGourty, M.B., Joseph H. Silas, M.D., Jude J. Fleming, Ph.D., Alan McBurney, M.Phil., and John W. Ward, M.B.
Merseyside and Leicester, United Kingdom

Polymorphic drug oxidation was first described for the antihypertensive drug debrisoquin, which has since been used as a probe to determine oxidation phenotype.[11] After a 10 mg oral dose of debrisoquin the ratio of debrisoquin to 4-hydroxydebrisoquin (metabolic ratio) recovered in an 8-hour urine collection is <12.5 for extensive metabolizers (EMs, median 0.5) and >12.5 in poor metabolizers (PMs, median 65). About 9% of the white British and North American populations are PMs and the defect is transmitted as an autosomal recessive trait.[5,12] In addition to defective alicyclic hydroxylation, other oxidative pathways are impaired in PMs, including aromatic hydroxylation, *N*-oxidation, and *O*-dealkylation.

Many β-adrenoceptor antagonists are eliminated principally by oxidative metabolism. Interphenotypic differences in the metabolism of metoprolol, propranolol, and bufuralol have already been documented.[4,7,8] Clinical implications have included enhanced β-blockade in metoprolol PMs with a diminished antihypertensive effect in metoprolol EMs receiving once-daily therapy.[7,13] Bufuralol PMs experience more toxicity, presumably because of higher plasma concentrations.[4]

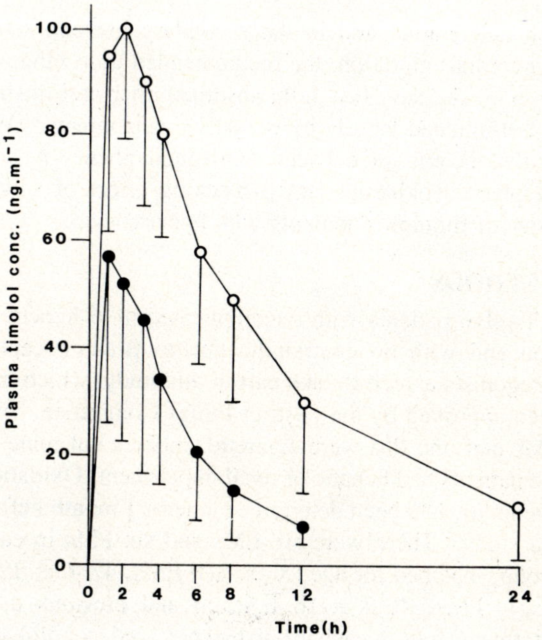

Fig. 1. Mean (±SD) plasma timolol concentration plotted against time in PMs (○) and EMs (●) of debrisoquin.

Timolol is widely used in the treatment of hyperten-

From the Hypertension Unit, Clatterbridge Hospital, Merseyside, and Department of Clinical Pharmacology, Glenfield General Hospital, Leicester.

Supported in part by Leo Laboratories Ltd., Sandoz Pharmaceuticals, and ICI Pharmaceuticals.

Received for publication Feb. 10, 1985; accepted May 26, 1985.

Reprint requests to: John C. McGourty, M.B., Hypertension Unit, Clatterbridge Hospital, Bebbington, Wirral, Merseyside L63 4JY, United Kingdom.

Table I. Pharmacokinetic parameters after 20 mg oral timolol maleate in debrisoquin EMs and PMs

	Dose (mg/kg)	t_{max} (hr)	C_{max} (ng/ml)	C_{24} (ng/ml)	AUC(0-∞) (ng · hr/ml)	$t_{1/2}$ (hr)	CL_o (L/hr)	CL_R (ml/min)	T_{ur} (%)
PMs	0.26	1.83	113.8*	11.3	1590†	7.5†	13.1†	39.9	14.7
	±0.04	±0.75	±20.6	±9.6	±1133	±3.0	±7.8	±26.9	±8.4
EM	0.30	1.17	60.7	Below assay	394	3.7	48.5	62.8	7.9
	±0.09	±0.41	±38.6	sensitivity	±239	±1.7	±23.2	±32.4	±3.7

Data are $\bar{X}$ ± SD.
t_{max} = Time to maximum timolol plasma concentration; C_{max} = maximum plasma concentration; C_{24} = plasma concentration at 24 hours; T_{ur} = 24-hour urinary timolol recovery (% dose).
*$P < 0.05$; †$P < 0.01$.

Table II. Exercise heart rate and degree of β-blockade before and 4, 12, and 24 hours after timolol

	PMs		EMs		
Time after dosing (hr)	Heart rate (bpm)	β-blockade (%)	Heart rate (bpm)	β-blockade (%)	P
0	141.5 ± 9.5	—	143 ± 7.8	—	NS
4	90.2 ± 8.8	36.2	94.7 ± 10.9	33.5	NS
12	97.8 ± 9.2	30.9	116.6 ± 10.7	18.2	<0.05
24	101 ± 13.6	28.3	124.3 ± 13.8	13.1	<0.05

Data are $\bar{X}$ ± SD.
NS = Not significant.

sion and angina and in the secondary prevention of myocardial infarction; the recommended dose range is 10 to 40 mg/day. It is fully absorbed after oral dosing and eliminated largely by oxidative metabolism.[17] We studied the relation between debrisoquin phenotype and the pharmacokinetics and β-blocking effect of single doses of timolol in patients with hypertension.

METHODS

Twelve patients with uncomplicated mild hypertension and with no contraindication to β-adrenoceptor antagonists agreed to take part in this study, which had been approved by the District Ethics Committee. Two EMs and one PM were cigarette smokers but none of the patients had hepatic or renal impairment. Oxidation phenotype had been determined at least 1 month before the study.[9] There were six EMs and six PMs in each group, matched for age ($\bar{X}$ ± SD: EMs, 47.4 ± 12.4 years; PMs, 46.0 ± 16.4 years) and previous drug treatment (four in each group had received atenolol and a diuretic). There were two male EMs and three male PMs. The PMs were slightly heavier (79.1 ± 13.8 vs. 71.7 ± 17.9 kg), but this difference was not statistically significant. The metabolic ratio was 0.22 to 1.22 (median 0.55) in EMs and 29.1 to 181 (median 57.5) in PMs.

Subjects receiving atenolol stopped therapy 72 hours before the study. Oral timolol maleate, 20 mg, was taken with 50 ml water about 2 hours after a light breakfast. No food or drink was permitted for another 2 hours. Blood (10 ml) for timolol level estimation was drawn from an indwelling cannula immediately before dosing and 1, 2, 3, 4, 6, 8, 12, and 24 hours thereafter. Urine was collected for 24 hours. Exercise was performed on a motorized treadmill immediately before and 4, 12, and 24 hours after drug dosing.

Subjects had previously been familiarized with the treadmill exercise (4 minutes) and the work load required to achieve an exercise heart rate of approximately 140 bpm without β-blocker therapy was individually determined. Each subject repeated his or her predetermined exercise on the study day and the heart rate was measured after 4 minutes from a continuous ECG recording. The β-blocking effect of timolol at 4, 12, and 24 hours was calculated as the percentage change in heart rate in comparison with the exercise heart rate before drug dosing.

Blood samples were spun immediately, and plasma and urine were stored at −20° C until assayed. Urinary and plasma timolol maleate concentrations were measured by HPLC with an ESA Coulochem model 5100A electrochemical detector (LDC/Milton Roy) in the oxidation mode with guard cell, detector 1, and detector 2 potentials of 1.1, 0.5, and 1.1 V, respectively, and a gain setting of 10 × 40. The column was a 25 cm × 4.6 mm Spherisorb 5 phenyl column (Severn

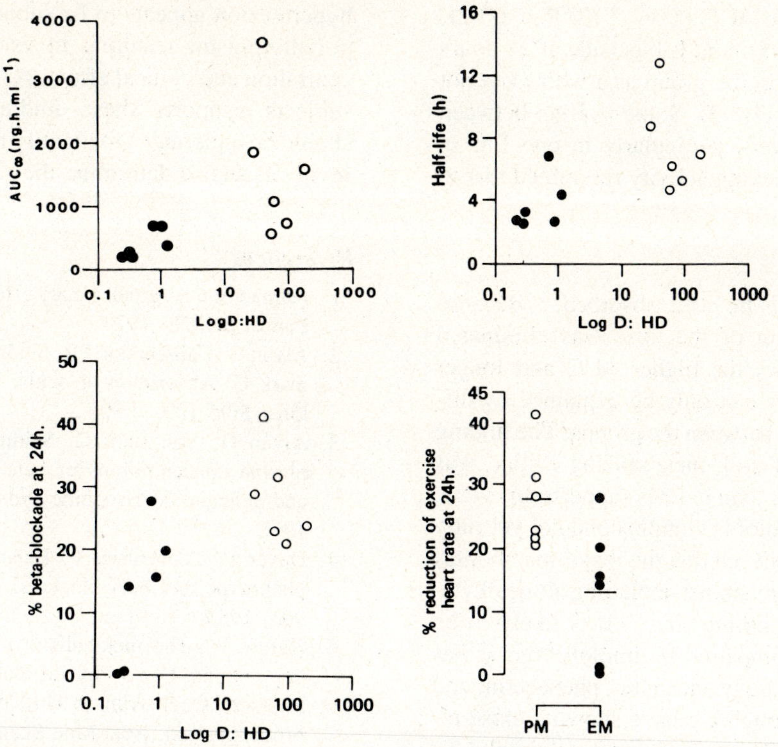

Fig. 2. Correlations between the log debrisoquin:4-hydroxydebrisoquin *(D:HD)* ratio and timolol AUC, $t_{1/2}$, and β-blockade at 24 hours, and a scattergram of β-blockade at 24 hours. ○ = PM; ● = EM.

Analytical) with orthophosphoric acid (0.1 mol/L): methanol (70:30) as eluent. Flow rate was 1.5 ml/min. The internal standard was 1(tert-butylamino)3[(4-piperidino-1,2,5-thiadiazol-3-yl)oxy]2 propranolol maleate (Leo Laboratories Ltd.). Timolol was extracted from plasma or urine (1.0 ml) plus 20 μl internal standard (2 μg/ml) and 50 μl sodium hydroxide (1.0 mol/L) by 10 1-second interruptions of the vortexing procedure with methyl tertbutyl ether (1.0 ml). The organic layer was evaporated to dryness at 55° C, reconstituted in methanol (100 μl), and 20 to 80 μl was injected into the column. Where necessary, urine samples were diluted with water before extraction. Retention times of the drug and internal standard were 9 and 11 minutes, respectively. The assay was linear to a concentration of 600 ng/ml, with 79% recovery of timolol from serum and 72% from urine. The lower limit of sensitivity of the assay was 1.0 ng/ml and the coefficient of variation between assays was 9.4% for plasma and 7.0% for urine. Results are expressed as the concentration of timolol (timolol maleate × 0.732). The plasma AUC was calculated by the trapezoidal rule with extrapolation to time infinity. The $t_{1/2}$ was calculated by linear regression analysis from the slope of the terminal phase. Oral clearance (CL_o) was calculated as: CL_o = Dose · F/AUC(0-∞), where F is the fraction of the dose absorbed. For purposes of comparison between EMs and PMs, F was assumed to be one (i.e., complete absorption). Renal clearance (CL_R) was calculated as: CL_R = Urinary recovery of timolol from 0 to 24 hours/AUC(0-24).

Differences between PMs and EMs were analyzed by the Mann-Whitney U test. Correlations were performed with the Spearman rank correlation test (r_s).

RESULTS

At all time points measured, plasma timolol concentrations were higher in PMs than in EMs (Fig. 1). Twenty-four hours after dosing the mean plasma timolol concentration was 11.3 ± 9.6 ng/ml in PMs but below the sensitivity of the assay in four EMs. There was a fourfold difference in mean AUC and a twofold difference in mean $t_{1/2}$. CL_o was significantly reduced in PMs when compared with EMs. There was no significant difference in CL_R and as expected only a small proportion of the dose was eliminated unchanged in the urine (Table I). The reduction in exercise tachycardia was similar in both groups at 4 hours, but was significantly greater in PMs than EMs at 12 and 24 hours after dosing (Table II; Fig. 2).

The debrisoquin:4-hydroxydebrisoquin ratio correlated positively with the AUC ($r_s = 0.73$; $P < 0.02$), $t_{1/2}$ ($r_s = 0.63$; $P < 0.05$), and β-blockade at 24 hours ($r_s = 0.72$; $P < 0.02$) in the group as a whole but not within each subgroup (Fig. 2). Some overlap between phenotypes was observed, particularly in one EM in whom the $t_{1/2}$ and β-blocking activity resembled that in PMs.

DISCUSSION

Timolol is known to be well absorbed.[17] Because only a small proportion of the dose was eliminated unchanged in the urine, the higher AUC and longer $t_{1/2}$ in PMs than in EMs can only be explained by differences in metabolism between the groups. The finding that CL_o, a measure of drug metabolizing ability, was four times lower in PMs than in EMs supports this view. The metabolism of timolol is complex and not yet fully understood, but it is believed that the major metabolites result from oxidative reactions including *O*-dealkylation cleaving the morpholino ring.[18] It is likely to be *O*-dealkylation that is impaired in timolol PMs, as has been described for the drugs encainide, phenacetin, and metoprolol.[14,15,19] Although we have shown a close relationship between oxidation phenotype and timolol kinetics, this is less marked than that seen with metoprolol, in which the metabolic ratio correlates with kinetic parameters and β-blockade both in the group as a whole and also in each subgroup.[8] Presumably this reflects the influence of monomorphic metabolism through other pathways.

The observed inhibition of exercise tachycardia suggests that in angina, hypertension, and secondary prevention of myocardial infarction, once-daily timolol would provide an adequate degree of β-blockade in PMs, and in fact a small dose (10 mg) should suffice. In contrast, EMs usually require twice-daily dosing, as currently suggested. Timolol, 10 mg b.i.d., was used in the Norwegian multicenter postinfarction study and the implications of unexpectedly high plasma timolol concentrations in PMs receiving this dose are uncertain, particularly as that study was performed in a population in which the frequency of PM phenotype is only 3%.[3,16] Hence it is important to determine whether PMs are more likely to develop dose-related side effects after oral therapy. Timolol is also used topically in the treatment of glaucoma. Significant systemic absorption may occur, leading to asthma and heart failure in predisposed individuals.[1,2,6] However, peak plasma concentrations are likely to be similar in all patients, and it is therefore not likely that PMs would be at a greater risk than EMs from these complications.

In conclusion, timolol metabolism in patients with hypertension appears to be subject to debrisoquin-type polymorphism, resulting in variation in plasma concentration and clinical effect. A recent report in healthy subjects supports these findings.[10] Further studies should be undertaken to identify the metabolic pathways involved and to determine the clinical significance.

References

1. Ahmad S: Cardiopulmonary effects of timolol eye drops. Lancet **2:**1028, 1979.
2. Alván G, Calissendorff B, Seidman P, Widmark K, Widmark G: Absorption of ocular timolol. Clin Pharmacokinet **5:**95-100, 1980.
3. Alván G, Von Bahr C, Seidman P, Sjoqvist F: High plasma concentrations of beta receptor blocking drugs and deficient debrisoquine hydroxylation. Lancet **1:**333, 1982.
4. Dayer P, Courvoisier F, Balant L, Fabre J: Oxidation phenotype and beta blockers. N Engl J Med **308:**964-965, 1983.
5. Kalow W: The metabolism of xenobiotics in different populations. Can J Physiol Pharmacol **60:**1-12, 1982.
6. Laursen SO, Bjerrum P: Timolol eye drop induced severe bronchospasm. Acta Med Scand **211:**505-506, 1982.
7. Lennard MS, Jackson PR, Freestone S, Ramsay LE, Tucker GT, Woods HF: The oral clearance and beta adrenoceptor antagonist activity of propranolol after single dose are not related to debrisoquine oxidation phenotype. Br J Clin Pharmacol **17:**106-107S, 1984.
8. Lennard MS, Silas JH, Freestone S, Ramsay LE, Tucker GT, Woods HF: Oxidation phenotype—A major determinant of metoprolol metabolism and response. N Engl J Med **307:**1558-1560, 1982.
9. Lennard MS, Silas JH, Smith AJ, Tucker GT: Determination of debrisoquine and its 4-hydroxy metabolite in biological fluids by gas chromatography with flame-ionization and nitrogen sensitive detection. J Chromatogr **133:**161-166, 1977.
10. Lewis RV, Lennard MS, Jackson PR, Tucker GT, Ramsay LE, Woods HF: Timolol, atenolol and oxidation phenotype. Br J Clin Pharmacol **18:**2, 287P, 1984.
11. Maghoub A, Idle JR, Dring LG, Lancaster R, Smith RL: Polymorphic hydroxylation of debrisoquine in man. Lancet **2:**584-586, 1977.
12. Price Evans DA, Maghoub A, Sloan TP, Idle JR, Smith RL: A family and population study of the genetic polymorphism of debrisoquine oxidation in a white British population. J Med Genet **17:**102-105, 1980.
13. Silas JH, Freestone S, Lennard MS, Ramsay LE: Chronic dosing comparison of three formulations of metoprolol and atenolol in hypertensive patients. Br J Clin Pharmacol **18:**2, 270P, 1984.
14. Silas JH, McGourty JC, Lennard MS, Tucker GT, Woods HF: Genetic polymorphism of beta blocker metabolism. Eur J Clin Pharmacol. (In press.)

15. Sloan TO, Maghoub A, Lancaster R, Idle JR, Smith RL: Polymorphism of carbon oxidation of drugs and clinical implications. Br Med J **2:**655-657, 1978.
16. The Norwegian Multicentre Study Group. Timolol induced reduction in mortality and reinfarction in patients surviving acute myocardial infarction. N Engl J Med **304:**801-807, 1981.
17. Tocco DJ, Duncan AEW, de Luna FA, Hucker HB, Gruber VF, Vanden Heuval WJA: Physiological disposition of timolol in man and laboratory animals. Drug Metab Dispos **3:**361-370, 1975.
18. Wasson BK, Scheiyetz J, Rooney CS, Hall RA, Share NN, Vanden Heuval WJA, Avison BH, Hensens OD, Ellsworth RL, Tocco DJ: Urinary metabolites of timolol from humans and laboratory animals syntheses and beta adrenergic blocking activities. J Med Chem **23:**1178-1184, 1980.
19. Woosley RL, Roden DM, Duff HJ, Carey EL, Wood AJ, Wilkinson JR: Coinheritance of deficient oxidative metabolism of encainide and debrisoquine. Clin Res **29:**501A, 1981.

Stereoselective mephobarbital hydroxylation cosegregates with mephenytoin hydroxylation

The 8-hour urinary recovery of 4-hydroxy-mephobarbital has been measured after oral administration of racemic mephobarbital (90 mg) in 17 extensive (EM) and six poor (PM) metabolizer phenotypes of mephenytoin. The recovery of this metabolite was measurable in every EM and ranged from 2.5% to 48% (10.9% ± 1.9% of dose), but was not detected in any PM (<1% of dose). In EMs, the 8-hour urine recovery of 4-OH-mephobarbital after mephobarbital was approximately half that of 4-OH-mephenytoin over the same time after mephenytoin administration. One EM received similar doses of *R*- and *S*-mephobarbital on separate occasions. Urinary recovery of 4-OH-mephobarbital was 33% and <1%, respectively. These results suggest that mephobarbital is stereoselectively hydroxylated by the same drug metabolizing enzyme that is responsible for the stereoselective aromatic hydroxylation of mephenytoin.
(CLIN PHARMACOL THER 38:414-418, 1985.)

A. Küpfer, Ph.D., and R. A. Branch, M.D. *Nashville, Tenn., and Bern, Switzerland*

Mephenytoin is a chiral hydantoin, as indicated by the spatial arrangement of its substituents (see structure). In man, mephenytoin undergoes two main routes of metabolism. One route is aromatic hydroxylation to 4-hydroxy-mephenytoin, which is highly stereoselective[12,17] and occurs almost exclusively with *S*-mephenytoin with a high intrinsic metabolic clearance.[16] The alternative route of metabolism is *N*-demethylation to the anticonvulsant phenyl-ethylhydantoin (PEH), which has low intrinsic clearances for both *S*- and *R*-enantiomers without evidence of stereoselective metabolism.[16] Recently, individuals have been identified who have defective hydroxylation of *S*-mephenytoin. This defect occurs in approximately 3% to 5% of Caucasians[7,14,17] but with a higher frequency in Japanese populations.[7] The defect also occurs with a higher frequency within family members of an identified poor metabolizer (PM),[11,14] suggesting a genetic basis for this defect. It is, however, independent of the polymorphic distribution of debrisoquin oxidation,[14,17] indicating that different drug metabolizing enzymes are responsible for metabolizing mephenytoin and debrisoquin.

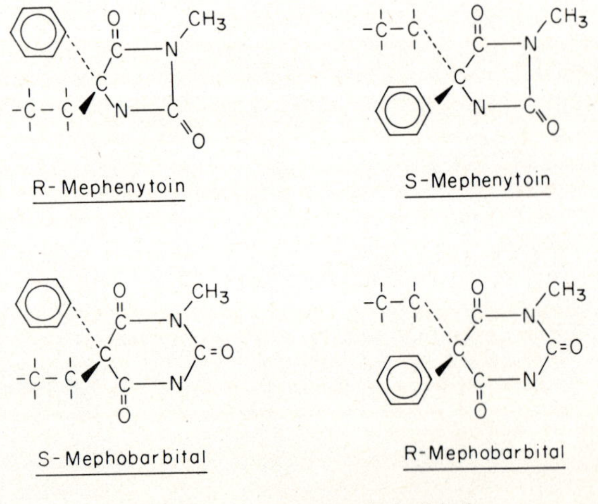

Mephenytoin and mephobarbital

If a single species of isoenzyme is responsible for mephenytoin hydroxylation, then this enzyme should also metabolize other substrates. We have previously shown that PEH, the demethylated analog of mephenytoin, also undergoes stereoselective hydroxylation of *S*-PEH; furthermore, this route of metabolism is deficient in PMs of *S*-mephenytoin.[13] Thus PEH is likely to be metabolized by this isozyme. Mephobarbital is an optically active barbituric analog with phenyl, ethyl,

From the Division of Clinical Pharmacology, Vanderbilt University, Nashville, and Department of Clinical Pharmacology, University of Bern, Bern.

Supported by Schweizerisch Stiftung für Medizinische-Biologische Stipendien and United States Public Health Service Grants No. GM-31304 and RR00099.

Received for publication March 22, 1985; accepted June 3, 1985.

Reprint requests to: R. A. Branch, M.D., Division of Clinical Pharmacology, Vanderbilt University, Nashville, TN 37232.

and methyl constituents similar to those of mephenytoin, even though the Cahn, Ingold, Prelog nomenclature of enantiomers reverses the *S*- and *R*-assignment for equivalent molecules (see structure). Mephobarbital is known to be metabolized by both aromatic hydroxylation and demethylation[9] and might be a suitable substrate for the drug metabolizing enzyme responsible for mephenytoin hydroxylation.

We report an investigation of whether mephobarbital hydroxylation occurs in PMs of mephenytoin. We have obtained preliminary information about the stereoselectivity of mephobarbital hydroxylation.

METHODS

Subjects had participated in a previous study that had identified their ability to hydroxylate mephenytoin. Each subject had taken 100 mg racemic mephenytoin by mouth and had a urine sample collected over the subsequent 8 hours. The urinary recovery of 4-OH-mephenytoin was measured by HPLC[15] and from this the hydroxylation index was calculated[14] as: Hydroxylation index = (0.5 × Dose)/recovery of 4-OH-mephenytoin.

Extensive metabolizers (EMs) of mephenytoin were defined as having a hydroxylation index between 0.6 to 9.6 and mephenytoin PMs were defined as having a ratio between 16 and 1000.

Seventeen EMs and six PMs received a single, oral, 90 mg dose of racemic mephobarbital. Urine was collected for the subsequent 8 hours. 4-OH-mephobarbital concentrations in urine were measured after acid hydrolysis by the HPLC method of Kunze et al.[9,10] and recovery was estimated from the product of urine volume and concentration.

In further observations in one EM, 90 mg *R*-mephobarbital and 90 mg *S*-mephobarbital were administered on separate occasions. Similar urinary recoveries of 4-OH-mephobarbital were measured after each dosing.

RESULTS

In mephenytoin EMs, the 8-hour urinary recovery of 4-OH-mephobarbital ranged from 2.5% to 48% ($\overline{X}$ = 10.9%; Table I) of the total racemic dose administered. In contrast, in all six mephenytoin PMs the concentrations of 4-OH-mephobarbital were below the level of detection (<2 μg/ml), so that <1% of the dose administered was eliminated as this metabolite. Thus there was a clear dissociation in urinary recovery of 4-OH-mephobarbital between EMs and PMs (Fig. 1). In EMs the percentage of racemic dose of mephobarbital recovered as 4-OH-mephobarbital in 8 hours was approximately half that recovered as 4-OH-mephenytoin after mephenytoin administration in each subject (Table I).

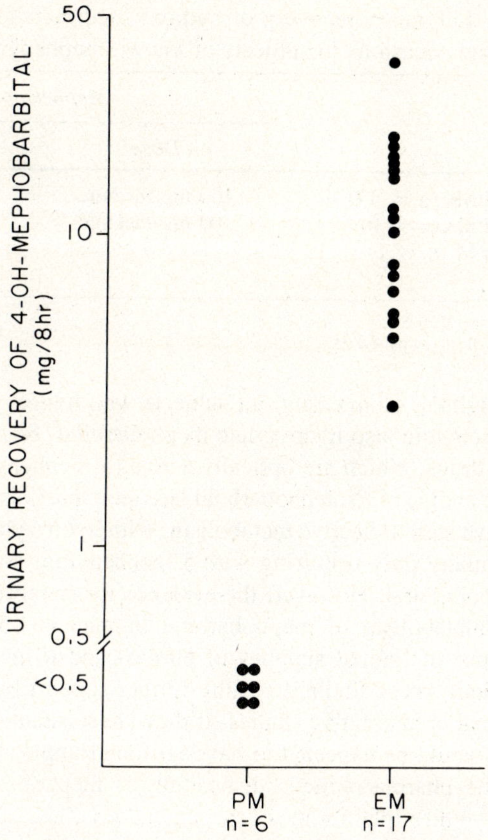

Fig. 1. Recovery of 4-OH-mephobarbital in urine in the 8 hours after oral racemic mephobarbital to mephenytoin EMs and PMs.

Only a small amount of pure *R*- and *S*-mephobarbital was available for study, but we were able to undertake one study. When this subject, who was a mephenytoin EM, received 90 mg *R*-mephobarbital, the 8-hour urinary recovery of 4-OH-mephobarbital was 33% of the dose, which was approximately twice that when the same dose of racemic mephobarbital was administered to the same subject (17.4%). In contrast, the urinary recovery of 4-OH-mephobarbital after the same dose of *S*-mephobarbital to this subject was undetectable (Table I).

DISCUSSION

Our data provide evidence that the same drug metabolizing enzymes are involved in the aromatic hydroxylation of mephobarbital and mephenytoin. This conclusion can be inferred from two observations. First, subjects who have a defect in hydroxylation of mephenytoin also have a defect in hydroxylation of me-

Table I. Urinary recovery of hydroxylated metabolite after administration of mephenytoin and mephobarbital on separate occasions to subjects of known mephenytoin hydroxylation phenotype

	Mephenytoin		*Mephobarbital*	
	Dose	*% Recovery*	*Dose*	*% Recovery*
EMs (n = 17)	100 mg racemic	25.8 ± 2.6	90 mg racemic	10.8 ± 1.9*
PMs (n = 6)	100 mg racemic	<1	90 mg racemic	<1
EM (n = 1)			90 mg *R*-epimer	33.1
			90 mg *S*-epimer	<1

Data are $\bar{X}$ ± SE.
*$P < 0.01$ (paired t test).

phobarbital. Conversely, all subjects who hydroxylate mephenytoin also hydroxylate mephobarbital. Second, both drugs, which are optically active (*S*-mephenytoin is the anolog of *R*-mephobarbital [see structure]) appear to have stereoselective metabolism, with hydroxylation essentially only occurring with *S*-mephenytoin and *R*-mephobarbital. However, the evidence for stereoselective metabolism of mephobarbital in man is limited because of limited supplies of pure *S*- and *R*-mephobarbital. These findings require further support by additional or alternative studies. If they are substantiated, they would be expected to have profound implications on the pharmacokinetic disposition of mephobarbital and would explain some of the anomalous observations and toxicologic implications observed in subjects who are mephenytoin PMs.[3]

Mephobarbital, the *N*-methyl derivative of phenobarbital, has been used as an anticonvulsant since its introduction in the 1930s.[1] Initially, mephobarbital was considered to be a rather poorly absorbed prodrug for phenobarbital, as approximately twice the mephobarbital dose was required to produce equivalent plasma concentrations of phenobarbital,[3,4] and the major circulating barbiturate during chronic therapy was phenobarbital. More recently, 4-OH-mephobarbital has been identified as a major urinary metabolite, accounting for up to 30% of urinary recovery of a single dose administered over a 10-day urine collection.[5] Interestingly, the shape of the cumulative urinary excretion curve of 4-OH-mephobarbital shows a large proportion of metabolite excreted within the first 2 days, with little subsequent excretion despite continued appreciable levels of mephobarbital in plasma. This suggests rapid absorption and metabolism that is sustained only for a short time. This situation is similar to that of mephenytoin, where *S*-mephenytoin is largely excreted within 24 hours of administration as *S*-4-OH-mephenytoin. This metabolite accounts for almost half of the racemic dose administered.[15,16] In contrast, *R*-mephenytoin is not appreciably metabolized by this route of metabolism. Instead, *R*-mephenytoin is demethylated to PEH, which is not further metabolized, has very low clearance, and has the potential to cumulate during chronic therapy. The doubling of urinary recovery of 4-OH-mephobarbital after *R*-mephobarbital dosing in comparison with racemic administration and the complete absence of 4-OH-mephobarbital after *S*-mephobarbital dosing in one subject indicates almost complete stereoselective hydroxylation of mephobarbital in this individual. This would suggest that *R*-mephobarbital is largely hydroxylated and eliminated such that it does not contribute to circulating barbiturate levels, while *S*-mephobarbital is only demethylated to phenobarbital and this product is largely responsible for the anticonvulsant efficacy of the drug. It has previously been shown that, although the production of phenobarbital is not large after a single dose, phenobarbital does accumulate to three to 10 times the mephobarbital levels during chronic therapy.[3,6] Our results suggest that the circulating phenobarbital has almost exclusively been formed from *R*-mephobarbital.

In Caucasian populations the ability to hydroxylate *S*-mephenytoin is absent in approximately 5% of unrelated individuals and in a higher proportion in families with a family member with defective hydroxylation.[14,17] This defect would be expected to influence markedly the pharmacokinetic disposition of mephobarbital. The defect in *R*-mephobarbital hydroxylation would be expected to make more *R*-mephobarbital available for the alternative route of metabolism by demethylation. With both *R*- and *S*-mephobarbital contributing to phenobarbital formation, plasma concentrations of phenobarbital should be twice as high in PMs than in EMs. It is interesting that in a comparison of mephobarbital dose to phenobarbital steady-state plasma concentrations in 77 Australian patients with epilepsy, four patients (5%) had phenobarbitone levels that were approximately twice the levels expected from the linear regression obtained from the entire population.[4] Another observation that supports the clinical relevance of differences between EMs and PMs is the detailed report by Butler and Waddell[3] in 1958. These investigators administered mephobarbital to three subjects and observed that after 5 days of dosing, phenobarbital levels were approximately 12 mg/L. They also found that they could only account for approximately 50% of the dose administered as mephobarbital and phenobarbital in blood and urine. They studied a different subject twice with the same results despite a year's interval. This subject had a steep rise in phenobarbital concentration, with levels of 25 mg/L after 5 days and the onset of sedation requiring withdrawal of therapy on each occasion. In this subject essentially all of the dose was accounted for as mephobarbital and phenobarbital. It is probable that this individual was not able to hydroxylate *R*-mephobarbital and that this defect effectively doubled the dose of drug available for conversion to phenobarbital. This would suggest that the dosage requirement for PMs of mephobarbital or mephenytoin is half that of EMs. Although the frequency of the PM phenotype is low in Caucasian populations, it would be relevant in affected individuals. The recent report of a higher frequency in Japanese subjects[7] suggests that it might also provide a basis for an interethnic difference in adverse effects due to this drug.

There is now evidence that the close structural analogs mephobarbital, mephenytoin, and PEH are metabolized by the same drug metabolizing enzyme. It is not yet known which other compounds also use this enzyme, and the enzyme has not yet been purified to homogeneity. It is of interest that there appear to be substantial differences in the efficiency with which this enzyme metabolizes different substrates, with mephenytoin being more rapidly metabolized than PEH.[13] In our study the percentage of dose recovered in urine over 8 hours as hydroxylated metabolite was approximately twice as great for mephenytoin than for mephobarbital in every mephenytoin EM, suggesting that mephenytoin has a higher affinity for this enzyme than mephobarbital. The demethylated metabolite of mephobarbital, phenobarbital, has lost its chirality and is only metabolized to a minor extent by aromatic hydroxylation.[2] A similar structure-activity relationship whereby modification of an *N*-group alters the hydroxylation potential at a distant site in the molecule has been observed with a homologous series of phenacetin analogs in rat microsomes.[8] The molecular basis for these interactions is not clearly understood, but appears to be relevant in determining the metabolic fate of barbiturates and hydantoins in man.

In conclusion, measurements of urinary recovery of 4-OH-mephobarbital after administration of racemic mephobarbital to mephenytoin EMs and PMs and after *R*- and *S*-mephobarbital administration to a mephenytoin EM, suggest that mephobarbital has stereoselective hydroxylation of the *R*-enantiomer by the same enzyme responsible for the stereoselective metabolism of *S*-mephenytoin. This stereoselective metabolism means that in most subjects only *S*-mephobarbital is a prodrug for phenobarbital formation, while in a few PMs both enantiomers are prodrugs for phenobarbital and there is an effective doubling of barbiturate available to achieve a therapeutic or toxic response.

We thank Professor J. Knabe, University of Saarland, Saarbrücken, West Germany, for the *R*- and *S*-mephobarbital.

References

1. Blum E: Die bekempfung epileptischer Anfelle und ihrer Folger-Erscheinungen mit prominal. Deutch Med Wochenschr **58:**230-236, 1932.
2. Butler TC: The metabolic hydroxylation of phenobarbital. J Pharmacol Exp Ther **116:**326-336, 1956.
3. Butler TC, Waddell WJ: *N*-Methylated derivatives of barbituric acids, hydantoin and oxazolidine used in the treatment of epilepsy. Neurology **8**(suppl 1):106-112, 1958.
4. Eadie MJ, Bochner F, Hooper WD, Tyrer JH: Preliminary observations on the pharmacokinetics of methylphenobarbitone. Clin Exp Neurol **15:**131-144, 1978.
5. Hooper WD, Kunze HE, Eadie MJ: Pharmacokinetics and bioavailability of methylphenobarbital in man. Ther Drug Monitor **3:**39-44, 1981.
6. Hooper WD, Kunze HE, Eadie MJ: Qualitative and quantitative studies of methylphenobarbital metabolism in man. Drug Metab Dispos **9:**381-385, 1981.
7. Jacqz E, Goto F, Nakamura K, Wilkinson GR, Branch RA: Interethnic differences in polymorphism of S-mephenytoin hydroxylation between Japanese and Caucasions. CLIN PHARMACOL THER. (In press.)
8. Kapetanovic IM, Strong JM, Mieyal JJ: Metabolic structure activity relationship for homologous series of phenacetin anologues. J Pharmacol Exp Ther **209:**20-24, 1979.
9. Kunze HE, Hooper WD, Eadie MJ: The metabolism of methylphenobarbitone in man. Asian J Clin Sci **1:**115-119, 1980.
10. Kunze HE, Hooper WD, Eadie MJ: High performance liquid chromatographic assay of methylphenobarbital metabolites in urine. Ther Drug Monitor **3:**45-49, 1981.
11. Küpfer A, Desmond PV, Patwardhan R, Schenker S, Branch RA: Mephenytoin hydroxylation deficiency: Kinetics after repeated doses. CLIN PHARMACOL THER **35:** 33-39, 1984.

12. Küpfer A, Desmond PV, Schenker S, Branch RA: Stereoselective metabolism and disposition of the enantiomers of mephenytoin during chronic oral administration of the racemic drug in man. J Pharmacol Exp Ther **221**:590-597, 1982.
13. Küpfer A, Patwardhan R, Ward S, Schenker S, Preisig R, Branch RA: Stereoselective metabolism and pharmacogenetic control of 5-phenyl-5-ethylhydantoin (nirvanol) in humans. J Pharmacol Exp Ther **230**:28-33, 1984.
14. Küpfer A, Preisig R: Pharmacogenetics of mephenytoin: A new drug hydroxylation polymorphism in man. Eur J Clin Pharmacol **26**:753-759, 1984.
15. Küpfer A, Roberts RK, Schenker S, Branch RA: Stereoselective metabolism of mephenytoin in man. J Pharmacol Exp Ther **218**:329-335, 1981.
16. Wedlund PJ, Aslanian WA, Jacqz E, McAllister B, Branch RA, Wilkinson GR: Phenotypic differences in mephenytoin pharmacokinetics in normal subjects. J Pharmacol Exp Ther. (In press.)
17. Wedlund PJ, Aslanian WS, McAllister CB, Wilkinson GR, Branch RA: Mephenytoin hydroxylation deficiency in Caucasians: Frequency of a new oxidative drug metabolizing polymorphism. CLIN PHARMACOL THER **36**:773-776, 1984.

Effects of long-term therapy with naltrexone on body weight in obesity

The endogenous opiate system is thought to be associated with the regulation of food intake and body weight. Opiate antagonists decrease food intake in animals, but there are no controlled studies in obese man to evaluate body weight response to naltrexone. Sixty obese people were randomized into three groups and given 0, 50, or 100 mg of the opiate antagonist naltrexone for 8 weeks in an outpatient, double-blind study. Weight loss was not significant in either the 50 or 100 mg groups as compared with placebo. However, when broken down by sex, women had a significant ($P < 0.05$) weight loss of 1.7 kg, while men did not lose weight. Side effects were modest, but six subjects had one or more abnormal liver function test results; in one subject these abnormalities appeared to be clinically significant. The effects of naltrexone on weight loss were less than expected in light of prior animal studies, but further studies with a wider dose range of naltrexone may be indicated. (CLIN PHARMACOL THER 38:419-422, 1985.)

Richard L. Atkinson, M.D., Lisa K. Berke, M.S.N., F.N.P., Charles R. Drake, M.D., Mary Lynn Bibbs, M.S.N., F.N.P., Frederick L. Williams, M.D., and Donald L. Kaiser, Ph.D. *Charlottesville, Va.*

A large body of literature suggests that the endogenous opiate system is involved in the regulation of food intake. In animals, administration of both exogenous and endogenous opiates increases food intake,[4,8,14,19-22] and this increased intake may be blocked by opiate antagonists.[4-6,9,12,18,21-23] Holtzman[12] first demonstrated that naloxone, a "pure" opiate antagonist, decreased food intake in rats. Margules et al.[18] found that genetically obese mice (ob/ob) and rats (fa/fa) were 10 times as sensitive to the anorectic effects of naloxone than were their lean littermates.

There are only a few studies of the effects of opiates and opiate antagonists on feeding behavior in man.[3,7,11,15,26,27] In a controlled study of obese and lean people we demonstrated that naloxone in large doses (15 mg) decreased single-meal food intake in obese but not lean subjects.[3] Smaller doses (2 mg) had no effect in obese people. Trenchard and Silverstone[27] demonstrated a dose-related suppression of food intake, maximal 2.5 hours after drug dosing.

From the Department of Internal Medicine, University of Virginia Medical Center.

Supported by a grant from the E. I. DuPont de Nemours Company and by National Institutes of Health Grant No. 5 P60 AM 22125 to the Diabetes Research and Training Center at the University of Virginia.

Received for publication April 8, 1985; accepted June 19, 1985.

Reprint requests to: Richard L. Atkinson, M.D., Division of Clinical Nutrition, School of Medicine, TB-156, University of California, Davis, CA 95616.

There are no published controlled studies of the effects of naltrexone on food intake in man. Hollister et al.[11] reported reduced food intake in six of 10 normal subjects given naltrexone, but food intake was not actually measured, the study was not blinded, and no placebo was given. Sternbach et al.[26] reported decreased food intake and weight loss in two former narcotics addicts who received naltrexone therapy, but food intake was not measured and there was no control group. All the above studies focused predominately on food intake. There have been no long-term controlled studies of the effects of naltrexone on body weight in man. In this study we administered placebo and two doses of naltrexone to 60 obese subjects over an 8-week period and noted a small but significant weight loss in the women taking naltrexone but no significant effect in men. Side effects were mild in most subjects and the drug was generally well tolerated.

METHODS

Sixty obese subjects were recruited from the patient population of the weight reduction program of the Clinical Nutrition Center at the University of Virginia Medical Center. All subjects were fully informed of the nature and risks of the study and signed a consent form approved by the Human Investigation Committee of the University of Virginia. Inclusion criteria were age between 21 and 60 years, weight ≥30% over ideal, and weight loss <10 pounds in the 3 months before the

Table I. Weight change at visit 9 among male and female subjects taking naltrexone or placebo

	Women		Men	
	n	*Weight change (kg)*	*n*	*Weight change (kg)*
Placebo	14	+0.1 ± 0.4	5	−0.9 ± 2.1
50 mg naltrexone	8	−1.7 ± 0.7*	9	−1.5 ± 0.9
100 mg naltrexone	14	−1.7 ± 1.0	4	+3.4 ± 1.8
Combined (50 + 100 mg)	22	−1.7 ± 0.6*	13	0.0 ± 1.0

Data are X ± SE.
*P < 0.05.

study. Furthermore, subjects had to be men or women incapable of becoming pregnant (postmenopausal, hysterectomy, or bilateral tubal ligation). Exclusion criteria included known or suspected history of drug or alcohol abuse; current therapy with narcotic analgesics; known sensitivity to naltrexone, naloxone, or acetaminophen (used as a placebo); use of any drug known to alter body weight; presence of significant systemic disease; and necessity for therapy with any endocrine replacement drug. Twenty men and 40 women entered the study. Mean (±SE) body weight for the men was 135.2 ± 8.5 kg and for the women it was 101.4 ± 2.8 kg. There were 54 white and six black subjects. All subjects underwent an initial history and physical examination with laboratory tests, ECG, and chest x-ray photography. Subjects were randomized by computer into three groups of 20 each and assigned in a double-blind fashion to placebo, 50 mg naltrexone daily, or 100 mg naltrexone daily. The identification code was not broken until all subjects had completed the study. The subjects were given a test dose of 25 mg naltrexone at their first visit after the history and physical examination and were observed for 1 hour to uncover any immediate reactions.

The study medication was supplied each week in two bottles each containing 10 identical, scored tablets. Subjects took one pill from each bottle each day. Subjects receiving placebo had two tablets containing 50 mg acetaminophen to mimic the bitter taste of naltrexone. Subjects receiving 50 mg naltrexone had one bottle with 50 mg naltrexone tablets and the other bottle with placebo tablets. The 100 mg naltrexone group had 50 mg naltrexone in both bottles, except during the first week when these subjects received only 50 mg/day in an attempt to increase the dose gradually. They began the full 100 mg dose at the start of the second week of the study. Subjects were asked to take their pills once each day at approximately the same time of day, usually in the morning. At the weekly visits the pills remaining in each bottle were counted and recorded to assess compliance. If significant side effects occurred, subjects were given the option of discontinuing the drug or changing to a lower dose of the drug.

At visit one, subjects were asked to choose a target weight between ideal (as determined by 1959 Metropolitan Life Insurance Tables) and 30% above ideal weight. A target daily calorie intake was then calculated by the formula: 12 kcal/lb × target weight = Daily intake. An adjustment of −100 kcal/day per decade of age over 35 years was made. Subjects were asked to try to maintain this calorie intake, but no attempts were made to ensure their dietary compliance during the study and no further nutritional counseling was given.

Subjects returned to the Clinical Nutrition Center weekly for 9 weeks, thus receiving medication for 8 full weeks. At each visit they were weighed, had blood pressure and pulse recorded, and were asked if they noted any side effects, illnesses, or had taken any other medications during the week. Repeat physical examination and laboratory tests were performed at visit nine. Groups were compared by ANOVA, and correlation coefficients were calculated where appropriate.

RESULTS

Fifty-four of the initial 60 subjects completed the study, for a completion rate of 90%. Three subjects were removed from the study because of side effects. Three subjects (one from each of the three groups) left the study voluntarily because of boredom or perceived lack of sufficiently rapid weight loss. Of the 54 subjects who completed the study, one missed a single visit that was not made up, but the other 53 completed all nine visits as scheduled. Compliance with the medication schedule as assessed by counts of the remaining pills and by questioning each week was excellent.

Comparison of the body weights of the combined population of men and women reveals no significant weight loss during the 8 weeks of medication. The changes in weight were −0.02, −1.65, and −0.5 kg for the placebo, 50 mg naltrexone, and 100 mg naltrexone groups, respectively. However, when the data are evaluated by sex a different picture emerges (Table I). Women taking 50 or 100 mg naltrexone lost a mean of 1.7 kg, compared with a gain of 0.1 kg in the placebo group (P < 0.05). Men were more variable and had no significant weight changes (Table I). Although dosages were fixed and there were great differences in weight, there was no correlation of weight loss with initial body weight in any of the groups for either sex.

The three subjects who were dropped from the study

complained of nausea and vomiting within the first 24 hours of medication. These symptoms did not respond to a halving of the dose. Two of the three were women taking 50 mg naltrexone and one was a man taking 100 mg naltrexone per day. All three also complained of changes in mentation such as decreased mental acuity, depression, and anxiety. Their symptoms resolved after discontinuing medication. In the 54 subjects completing the protocol there were no significant differences in adverse reactions in the drug groups as compared with the placebo group. The most common side effects were headache, nausea, or vomiting, nervousness or anxiety, and weakness or lethargy.

At baseline 28 of our subjects had mild abnormalities of liver function. Such abnormalities are common in very obese subjects and are probably due to the fatty liver seen in obesity.[1,2] Six subjects had elevations in one or more liver function parameters while taking naltrexone; three of the six were taking 50 mg naltrexone a day and three were taking 100 mg/day. Five of the six had at least one minimally abnormal test result at baseline. All five of these subjects had a rise in SGPT, with a mean increase of 35 ± 12 U/L (range 21 to 48 U/L). Two of the five subjects had slight rises in SGOT (18 and 19 U/L, respectively), and one had a rise in lactate dehydrogenase levels from 199 to 372 U/L. The sixth subject, who was taking 50 mg naltrexone, had significant abnormalities, with increases in SGOT from 32 to 155 U/L, in SGPT from 51 to 370 U/L, and in lactate dehydrogenase from 177 to 258 U/L. Five subjects in the placebo group had increases in one or more liver function test results from normal baseline to abnormal values during the 8 weeks of the study. The subjects with abnormal values during naltrexone dosing were followed and the abnormal values returned to baseline levels or below over a period of a few weeks to months after naltrexone was discontinued.

DISCUSSION

The weight loss observed in women in this study suggests that naltrexone or similar drugs may have a role in the clinical treatment of obesity, although the lack of a dose-response curve in women and the paradoxic increase in body weight in men taking 100 mg naltrexone are disturbing. The observed weight loss (1.7 kg over 8 weeks) is similar to that induced by currently marketed weight reduction drugs that are derivatives of the amphetamine molecule.[24] If our study defines the limits of the drug response, naltrexone provides no great advantage over these drugs. Further studies with larger doses of naltrexone and other opiate antagonists may be carried out in the future, but our results are important to temper the high expectations of the usefulness of naltrexone that were raised by previously published studies in animals. The occurrence of significantly elevated liver function parameters in at least one subject in our study mandates that future studies very carefully assess a variety of liver function tests at frequent intervals. It is not clear why man does not appear to respond as well to naltrexone as do animals. It is possible that naltrexone is less effective than other opiate antagonists in man. In our previous study with naloxone[3] we observed that a 2 mg dose had no effect on food intake, but doses of 15 mg reduced single-meal intake by 29%. Since 0.4 mg is the standard initial dose to overcome morphine or heroin overdose, it is apparent that doses far in excess of those required to reverse the analgesic effect of opiates are necessary to see an effect on food intake. The naltrexone dosages of 50 and 100 mg we used were sufficient to block the narcotic effects in addicts,[10] but may not be adequate to induce a full response on food intake and body weight. Dosages of 2.5 to 10 mg/kg were necessary to see effects on food intake or body weights in rats, and lower doses were ineffective.[23] The explanation of the difference in dose response is not clear, but Morley et al.[23] have suggested that opiate antagonists may have different selectivities for different opiate receptors, and that κ-receptors may be the most important in feeding. Naloxone and naltrexone bind mainly to μ-receptors and only slightly to κ-receptors.[13,16] but other drugs that bind more avidly to these receptors may be more effective in decreasing food intake or body weight.

Naltrexone was generally well tolerated and side effects were usually short lived. The changes noted in liver function are bothersome and any future studies with naltrexone should evaluate liver function more carefully. Other studies with higher doses of naltrexone appear to have resulted in an increased incidence of liver abnormalities.*

Our observations of sex differences in response to naltrexone were unexpected, as there has been little evidence to suggest that the endogenous opiate system functions differently in men and women. The small number of men in each group may explain the lack of a statistically significant effect on weight change, as there was wide individual variation among the men. An alternate explanation for the sex difference is that the dose-response curve may differ between the sexes. Finally, the sex differences might be explained by observations that energy expenditure and defense of body

*Pfohl D: Personal communication, 1985.

weight may differ between the sexes in animals, possibly because of an opiate-dependent mechanism. In response to exercise, female rats are more resistant to change and usually maintain their body weight: Male rats may decrease food intake with exercise, but female rats do not change or may increase food intake.[25] Mandenoff et al.[17] observed that naloxone reduced body weight in male rats by an amount greater than could be explained by decreased food intake and postulated that naloxone increases energy expenditure. Further studies will be necessary to determine if there are changes in energy expenditure in response to opiate antagonists, and if such changes differ between the sexes.

We thank Carolyn Russ and Paula Ciavarella for assistance with patient care and Faye Raybon, Carol Blake-Scott, and David Dworaczyk for administrative assistance.

References

1. Andersen T, Christoffersen P, Gluud C: The liver in consecutive patients with morbid obesity: A clinical, morphological, and biochemical study. Int J Obesity **8:**107-115, 1984.
2. Andersen T, Gluud C: Liver morphology in morbid obesity: A literature study. Int J Obesity **8:**97-106, 1984.
3. Atkinson RL: Naloxone decreases food intake in obese humans. J Clin Endocrinol Metab **55:**196-198, 1982.
4. Baile CA, Keim DA, Della-Fera MA, McLaughlin CL: Opiate antagonists and agonists and feeding in sheep. Physiol Behav **26:**1019-1023, 1981.
5. Brands B, Thornhill JA, Hirst M, Gowdey CW: Suppression of food intake and body weight gain by naloxone in rats. Life Sci **24:**1773-1778, 1979.
6. Brown DR, Holtzman SG: Suppression of deprivation-induced food and water intake in rats and mice by naloxone. Pharmacol Biochem Behav **11:**567-573, 1979.
7. Dunger DG, Leonard JV, Wolff OH, Preece MA: Effect of naloxone in a previously undescribed hypothalamic syndrome. Lancet **1:**1277-1281, 1980.
8. Grandison L, Guidotti A: Stimulation of food intake by muscimol and beta endorphin. Neuropharmacology **16:**533-536, 1977.
9. Herman BH, Holtzman SG: Repeated administration of naltrexone and diprenorphine decreases food intake and body weight in squirrel monkeys. Life Sci **34:**1-12, 1983.
10. Hollister LE, Bearman JE, Duster TS, et al: Clinical evaluation of naltrexone treatment of opiate-dependent individuals. Arch Gen Psychiatry **35:**335-340, 1978.
11. Hollister LE, Johnson K, Boukhabza D, Gillespie HK: Aversive effects of naltrexone in subjects not dependent on opiates. Drug Alcohol Depend **8:**37-41, 1981.
12. Holtzman S: Behavioral effects of separate and combined administration of naloxone and d-amphetamine. J Pharmacol Exp Ther **189:**51-60, 1974.
13. Kosterlitz HW: Opioid peptides and their receptors. Progr Biochem Pharmacol **16:**3-10, 1980.
14. Kumar R, Mitchell E, Stolerman IP: Disturbed patterns of behavior in morphine tolerant and abstinent rats. Br J Pharmacol **42:**473-484, 1971.
15. Kyriakides M, Silverstone T, Jeffcoate W, Laurance B: Effect of naloxone on hyperphagia in Prader-Willi syndrome. Lancet **1:**876-877, 1980.
16. Magnan J, Paterson SJ, Tavani A, Kosterlitz HW: The binding spectrum of narcotic analgesic drugs with different agonist and antagonist properties. Naunyn Schmiedebergs Arch Pharmacol **319:**197-205, 1982.
17. Mandenoff A, Fumeron F, Apfelbaum M, Margules DL: Endogenous opiates and energy balance. Science **215:** 1536-1538, 1982.
18. Margules DL, Lewis MJ, Shibuya H, Pert CG: β-Endorphin is associated with overeating in genetically obese mice (ob/ob) and rats (fa/fa). Science **202:**988-991, 1978.
19. Martin WR, Wikler A, Eades CG, Pescor FT: Tolerance to and physical dependence on morphine in rats. Psychopharmacologia (Berlin) **4:**247-260, 1963.
20. McKay D, Kenney NJ, Edens NK, Williams RH, Woods SC: Intracerebroventricular beta-endorphin increases food intake of rats. Life Sci **29:**1429-1434, 1981.
21. Morley JE, Levine AS: Dynorphin-(1-13) induces spontaneous feeding in rats. Life Sci **29:**1901-1903, 1981.
22. Morley JE, Levine AS, Grace M, Kneip J: Dynorphin-(1-13), dopamine and feeding in rats. Pharmacol Biochem Behav **16:**701-705, 1982.
23. Morley JE, Levine AS, Yim GK, Lowy MT: Opioid modulation of appetite. Neurosci Biobehav Rev **7:**281-305, 1983.
24. Scoville BA: Review of amphetamine-like drugs by the Food and Drug Administration. *In:* Obesity in perspective. DHEW Publ No (NIH) 75-708. Washington, DC 1974, pp 441-443.
25. Stern JS: Is obesity a disease of inactivity? *In* Stunkard AJ, Stellar E, editors: Eating and its disorders. New York, 1984, Raven Press, pp 131-139.
26. Sternbach HA, Annitto W, Pottash AL, Gold MS: Anorexic effects of naltrexone in man. Lancet **1:**388-389, 1982.
27. Trenchard E, Silverstone T: Naloxone reduces the food intake of normal human volunteers. Appetite: J Intake Res **4:**43-50, 1983.

Terazosin kinetics after oral and intravenous doses

Terazosin kinetics were followed in normal subjects after intravenous doses of 0.5, 1.0, and 2.0 mg and oral doses of 1.0 mg. Plasma and urine samples were collected for the first 48 and 24 hours. The samples were analyzed by a sensitive HPLC assay developed in our laboratory. Mean calculated peak plasma levels from the 0.5, 1.0, and 2.0 mg intravenous doses were 25.0, 44.1, and 83.3 ng/ml. After a 1 mg oral dose the mean peak level was 19.6 ng/ml. Data were fit to a two-compartment open model with mean elimination phase $t_{1/2}$ values of 7.9, 8.9, and 10.1 hours for the ascending intravenous doses and 11.6 hours for the oral dose. Mean 0 to 24–hour urinary recovery after the intravenous doses was 14%, 13%, and 11%. It is concluded that terazosin kinetics are linear after oral and intravenous doses. (CLIN PHARMACOL THER 38:423-427, 1985.)

Sean E. Patterson, Ph.D. *Abbott Park, Ill.*

Terazosin (see structure) has been shown to have antihypertensive effects.[2,3] It is thought to exert these effects by means of peripheral vasodilation through α-sympathetic blockade. Terazosin is orally effective in the spontaneously hypertensive rat, which is a predictive animal model for the therapy of essential hypertension in man,[5] and has been administered to more than 90 normotensive adult men in phase I studies.

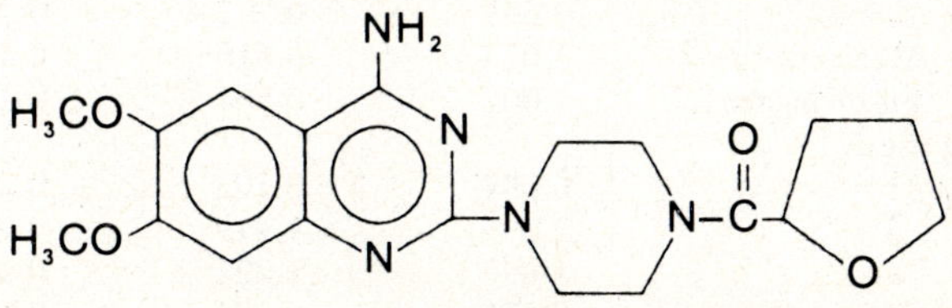

Terazosin

This report details the results of two pharmacokinetic studies in normotensive adult men. In the first study, terazosin hydrochloride dihydrate (THD) was administered as an intravenous bolus in three single, progressively increasing doses (0.5, 1, and 2 mg terazosin free base). In the second study, THD was taken by mouth as a tablet (1 mg terazosin free base).

METHODS

Eight subjects participated in the intravenous study and 18 subjects participated in the oral study. All subjects were healthy adult men between the ages of 18 and 40 years. They were subjected to extensive clinical examinations including ECGs and a range of laboratory screening tests before the study and after its conclusion. Subjects fasted for 8 hours before dosing but were allowed water ad libitum until 1 hour before dosing.

The eight subjects in the intravenous study received three single, progressively increasing doses of THD (equivalent to 0.5, 1, and 2 mg terazosin free base) as an intravenous bolus on days 1, 4, and 7 of the study. Blood samples (7 ml) were drawn before dosing and 0.25, 0.5, 0.75, 1, 2, 3, 4, 8, 12, 24, 36, and 48 hours thereafter. Total urine output was collected over 0 to 2, 2 to 4, 4 to 6, 6 to 8, 8 to 10, 10 to 12, 12 to 14, and 14 to 24 hours after dosing. Meals were served after the 2-hour blood collection and at approximately 6 and 10 hours after dosing. Subjects were required to drink about 500 ml water after each urine collection and to remain supine for 4 hours after dosing.

The 18 subjects in the oral study received a single oral dose of THD (1 mg terazosin free base) as a tablet. Blood samples (7 ml) were drawn before dosing and at 0.5, 1, 1.5, 2, 3, 4, 6, 9, 12, 24, 36, and 48 hours thereafter. Meals were served after the 2-hour blood collection and at approximately 5 and 10.5 hours after dosing.

All blood samples were drawn into heparinized Vacutainer tubes (Becton Dickinson). The specimens were centrifuged within 1 hour of collection and the plasma was decanted and immediately frozen. Urine volumes were measured and 20 ml aliquots were immediately frozen.

From the Department of Drug Metabolism, Abbott Laboratories.
Received for publication Dec. 27, 1984; accepted July 1, 1985.
Reprint requests to: Sean E. Patterson, Ph.D., Department of International Clinical Research, Abbott Laboratories D-6RH/AP6A, Abbott Park, IL 60064.

Table I. NONLIN-estimated pharmacokinetics from 0 to 48–hour curves after intravenous dosing

Subject No.	k_{12} (hr^{-1})	k_{21} (hr^{-1})	k_e (hr^{-1})	V_C (L)	$t_{1/2\alpha}$ (hr)	$t_{1/2\beta}$ (hr)	CL (ml/min)
0.5 mg iv							
1	0.482	0.395	0.169	29.7	0.7	10.2	83.7
3	2.108	1.069	0.253	18.2	0.2	8.6	76.7
4	0.100	0.157	0.152	40.0	2.1	9.8	101.3
6	0.054	0.170	0.156	36.6	2.4	7.6	95.2
7	7.092	1.827	0.689	7.0	0.1	5.2	80.4
9	0.357	0.440	0.175	44.0	0.8	8.0	128.3
11	1.282	1.114	0.185	23.6	0.3	8.4	72.8
12	1.214	1.185	0.178	19.3	0.3	8.2	57.3
Means of fits	1.586	0.795	0.245	27.3	0.9	7.9*	87.0
Fit of means	0.685	0.799	0.169	28.9	0.4	8.1	81.4
1 mg iv							
1	1.363	0.732	0.237	20.6	0.3	9.0	81.4
3	0.858	0.794	0.170	19.9	0.4	9.0	56.4
4	0.531	0.935	0.122	39.9	0.5	9.2	81.1
6	0.994	0.874	0.177	25.8	0.4	8.8	76.1
7	2.867	0.864	0.359	10.2	0.2	9.0	61.0
9	0.960	0.941	0.158	39.6	0.3	9.2	104.3
11	0.349	0.647	0.131	37.8	0.7	8.6	82.5
12	0.663	0.742	0.169	24.6	0.5	8.2	69.3
Means of fits	1.073	0.816	0.190	27.3	0.4	8.9*	76.5
Fit of means	1.007	0.861	0.174	25.1	0.4	9.1	72.8
2 mg iv							
1	0.084	0.103	0.220	29.6	2.0	10.4	108.5
3	2.096	1.419	0.214	17.2	0.2	8.3	61.3
4	1.897	1.222	0.199	18.1	0.2	9.2	60.0
6	0.071	0.095	0.142	32.1	2.8	13.1	76.0
7	0.106	0.106	0.170	26.1	2.1	12.6	74.0
9	0.063	0.090	0.126	42.8	3.0	14.0	89.9
11	0.489	0.449	0.185	24.4	0.7	8.7	75.2
12	0.890	0.678	0.221	19.1	0.4	7.9	70.4
Means of fits	0.712	0.520	0.185	26.2	1.4	10.1*	76.9
Fit of means	0.204	0.238	0.155	28.7	1.3	9.9	74.1

k_{12}, k_{21}, k_e = Rate constants; V_C = volume of the central compartment; $t_{1/2\alpha}$ = distribution phase $t_{1/2}$; $t_{1/2\beta}$ = elimination phase $t_{1/2}$; CL = total body clearance.
*Calculated from corresponding mean value of β.

Plasma and urine concentrations were determined by the method of Patterson.[6] This HPLC procedure involved basic extraction of samples with benzene/ethyl acetate, which contained an internal standard. A portion of the organic phase was evaporated and the residue was redissolved in 0.1 mol/L phosphoric acid. An aliquot of the phosphoric acid solution was then injected onto a 150 × 3.9 mm IBM C-1 column with a solvent system of 22% (v/v) acetonitrile and 6% (v/v) tetrahydrofuran in 0.02 mol/L sodium phosphate buffer at pH 5.0. The plasma calibration curves consisted of six terazosin standards ranging in concentration from 1 to 60 ng/ml; the lower quantifiable concentration under these conditions was about 0.25 ng/ml. Urine calibration curves consisted of five terazosin standards ranging from 5 to 600 ng/ml; the lower quantifiable concentration under these conditions was about 3 ng/ml. The assay has been demonstrated to have mean intra-assay coefficients of variation of about 7% and 3% for plasma and urine, respectively. With prazosin as internal standard, the peak area ratios (terazosin/prazosin) of these standards yielded linear regression correlation coefficients that averaged >0.99.

For the intravenous doses, individual and mean plasma concentration-time data were subjected to sequential polyexponential regression analyses by the program STRIP, a slightly modified version of the computer program CSTRIP.[7] Selection of the model that provided the best description of the data was based on criteria outlined by Sedman and Wagner.[8] Output from the STRIP program was also used for generation of initial estimates of the microscopic rate constants of the appropriate pharmacokinetic model to be used by the program NONLIN,[4] which performed iterative nonlinear regressions to fit the experimental data for each subject to the model. During the NONLIN fitting process, data from individual subjects were weighted by the reciprocals of the squared observed concentrations

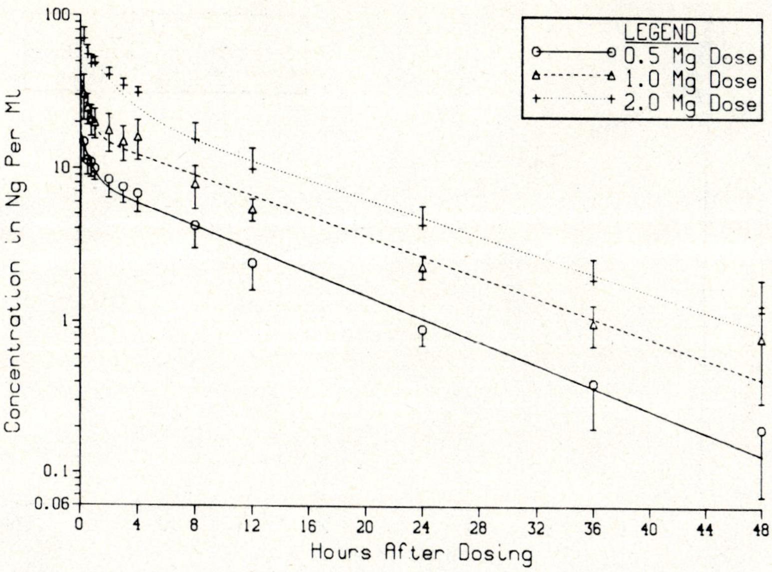

Fig. 1. Mean (±SD) plasma terazosin levels after intravenous doses with best-fit curves generated by NONLIN.

Table II. Mean urinary excretion of terazosin after intravenous dosing

	Interval after dosing (hr)								
	0-2	*2-4*	*4-6*	*6-8*	*8-10*	*10-12*	*12-14*	*14-24*	*Total*
0.5 mg iv									
Volume (ml)	239	493	403	773	780	773	500	1052	4973
Concentration (ng/ml)	45.2	23.7	18.5	9.1	2.9	16.2	17.2	19.2	
Amount excreted (μg)	10.8	11.7	7.5	7.0	2.3	11.9	8.6	20.2	80.0
1.0 mg iv									
Volume (ml)	273	422	338	639	563	460	559	838	4092
Concentration (ng/ml)	111.3	66.0	66.6	20.4	23.0	23.8	20.0	23.6	
Amount excreted (μg)	30.4	27.9	22.5	13.0	12.9	10.9	11.2	19.8	148.6
2.0 mg iv									
Volume (ml)	266	369	229	410	334	393	291	757	3049
Concentration (ng/ml)	230.0	140.6	121.2	89.9	44.3	40.0	36.6	49.9	
Amount excreted (μg)	61.2	51.9	27.8	36.9	14.8	15.7	10.7	37.8	256.8

($1/C^2$). The $1/C^2$ weighting factor was determined to approximate most closely the analytic reciprocal variances. Mean data, weighted by the reciprocal intersubject concentration variances, were also fit.

For the oral doses, individual and mean plasma concentration-time data were fit in a fashion similar to that for the intravenous doses. The model that best described the data after intravenous dosing was also used for the data obtained from oral dosing.

RESULTS AND DISCUSSION

Intravenous doses. The decline in the plasma levels of terazosin after intravenous injection was found by STRIP to be biphasic. The estimated preexponential and exponential terms were then expressed as microscopic rate constants for a two-compartment open model under the assumptions and equations described by Gibaldi and Perrier.[1]

Results of the NONLIN-generated kinetic analyses are summarized in Table I. A comparison of the results obtained from the fits of mean data and the mean values of individual fits shows no appreciable differences, suggesting a Gaussian distribution of observed terazosin levels at each sampling point. The best-fit curve of the mean plasma level data is plotted for each dose in Fig. 1. The plots of mean data show a biphasic first-order decline for plasma terazosin, with $t_{1/2}$ values of 0.9 hours for the initial (distributive) phase and 9.2 hours for the terminal phase.

The estimated zero-hour plasma levels ($\overline{X}$ = 25.0,

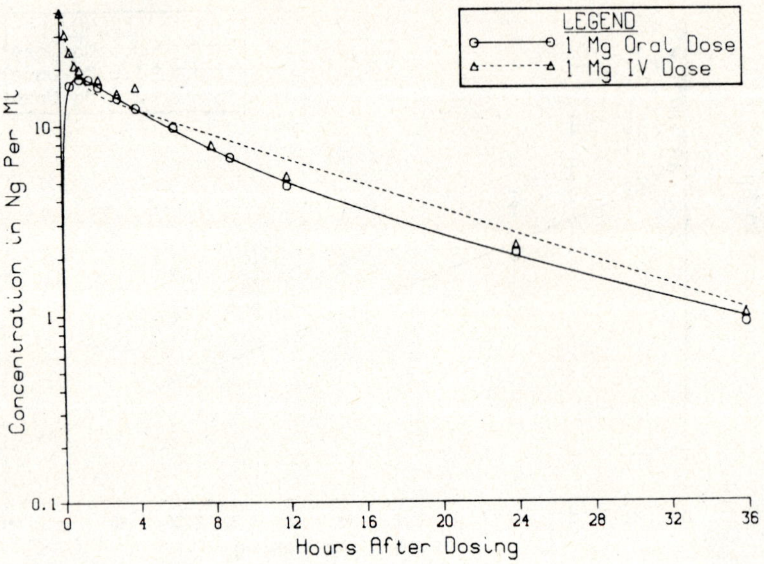

Fig. 2. Mean plasma terazosin levels after 1 mg oral and intravenous doses with best-fit curves generated by NONLIN.

Table III. NONLIN-estimated pharmacokinetics from 0 to 48–hour curves after oral dosing

No. Subject	k_a *(hr⁻¹)*	k_{21} *(hr⁻¹)*	k_{12} *(hr⁻¹)*	k_e *(hr⁻¹)*	V_C/F *(L)*	$t_{1/2\alpha}$ *(hr)*	$t_{1/2\beta}$ *(hr)*	*CL (ml/min)*	C_{max} *(ng/ml)*	t_{max} *(hr)*
1	2.5	0.077	0.042	0.101	40.4	3.9	15.7	68.0	20.8	1.2
2	5.2	1.171	0.098	0.200	54.9	0.5	3.8	183.0	15.5	1.1
3	5.0	0.173	0.066	0.109	49.1	2.5	10.3	89.2	18.1	0.7
4	4.3	0.204	0.129	0.162	31.9	1.7	8.7	86.1	25.8	0.7
5	8.8	0.075	0.020	0.091	53.7	5.1	13.7	81.4	17.6	0.5
6	1.8	0.180	0.085	0.125	40.6	2.2	9.9	84.6	18.7	1.4
7	1.7	0.170	0.112	0.120	48.0	2.0	11.6	96.0	15.3	1.4
8	2.5	0.175	0.119	0.131	42.3	1.9	10.9	92.4	18.3	1.1
9	5.0	0.216	0.121	0.128	38.8	1.8	9.9	82.8	22.1	0.7
10	22.3	0.352	0.111	0.099	48.5	1.4	9.8	80.0	19.7	0.2
11	4.1	0.194	0.136	0.159	23.7	1.7	9.3	62.8	34.6	0.7
12	1.1	0.085	0.022	0.096	48.2	4.7	12.5	77.1	15.8	2.4
13	3.3	0.056	0.025	0.080	60.5	5.5	19.3	80.7	14.8	2.0
14	65.7	0.127	0.088	0.142	50.9	2.3	11.4	120.5	19.2	0.1
15	8.2	0.125	0.045	0.087	42.8	3.4	13.0	62.1	21.9	0.5
16	21.0	0.229	0.115	0.117	36.3	1.8	10.2	70.8	26.2	0.2
17	1.1	0.147	0.056	0.080	71.4	3.0	13.7	95.2	10.6	2.2
18	90.0	0.103	0.102	0.122	55.3	2.4	15.6	112.4	17.8	0.1
Means of fits	14.1	0.214	0.083	0.119	46.5	2.0	11.6*	90.3	19.6	1.0
Fit of means	3.4	0.111	0.045	0.107	47.9	3.4	12.0	85.4	18.1	1.0

k_a, k_{21}, k_{12}, k_e = Rate constants; V_C = volume of the central compartment; F = bioavailability; $t_{1/2\alpha}$ = distribution phase $t_{1/2}$; $t_{1/2\beta}$ = terminal phase $t_{1/2}$; CL = apparent total body clearance; C_{max} = maximum plasma concentration; t_{max} = time to reach C_{max}.
*Calculated from corresponding mean value of β.

44.1, and 83.3 ng/ml) correlated linearly (r = 0.852) with the respective doses of 0.5, 1, and 2 mg. Linearity of the kinetics was also suggested by the correlation (r = 0.965) of the 0 to infinity AUCs ($\overline{X}$ = 101, 225, and 448 hr · ng/ml). The mean 0 to infinity plasma clearances of terazosin were 87, 77, and 77 ml/min for the 0.5, 1, and 2 mg doses, respectively. There were no significant systematic trends in the kinetic parameters with increasing doses.

Mean 0 to 24–hour urinary excretions of terazosin, in order of increasing doses, were 16%, 15%, and 13% of the respective doses. Mean renal terazosin clearance, calculated from 0 to 24–hour urinary excretion and 0 to 24–hour trapezoidal AUC values, was 12.5, 10.6, and 9.0 ml/min for the doses. Related to these changes were decreases in mean 0 to 24–hour urine volume, from 4.97 L in the 0.5 mg dose group to 3.05 L in the 2 mg dose group (Table II). The decreases in mean 0 to 24–hour urine volume, fractional terazosin excretion, and renal clearance of terazosin between the low- and high-dose groups were significant ($P < 0.05$). These changes may reflect altered renal hemodynamics, which have been reported after the administration of antihypertensive drugs.[9]

Oral doses. Results of NONLIN analyses of the data after oral dosing are listed in Table III. A semilogarithmic plot of the best-fit curve for the mean plasma level data is presented in Fig. 2.

Terazosin levels tended to peak at approximately 20 ng/ml about 1 hour after a 1 mg tablet (means of fits = 19.6 ng/ml and 1.0 hour, respectively). A lag time before absorption was not required for fitting the data from most of the subjects. Fig. 2 shows a biphasic log-linear decline in mean terazosin plasma levels after the peak, with mean distribution and terminal phase $t_{1/2}$ values of 3.4 and 12.0 hours, respectively. The mean apparent body clearance for terazosin of 90.3 ml/min was similar to that after intravenous dosing.

Comparison of intravenous and oral kinetics. Superimposed semilogarithmic plots of the best-fit curves of mean plasma terazosin levels after 1 mg oral and intravenous doses are shown in Fig. 2. The curves are quite similar from 2 to 36 hours after dosing, indicating rapid and complete absorption of the 1 mg tablet. The mean AUC after oral dosing was 82% that after intravenous dosing.

The distribution and terminal phase $t_{1/2}$ values were longer after oral (3.4 and 12 hours) than after intravenous (0.4 and 9.1 hours) dosing. These differences cannot be readily explained and it would be inappropriate to compare statistically the means of two sample populations in different studies. After oral dosing, however, it is often difficult to discern the distributive phase of drugs that display two-compartment kinetics after intravenous dosing.

I thank Lajos L. Varga and Gail E. Baldwin for technical assistance.

References

1. Gibaldi M, Perrier D: Pharmacokinetics. New York, 1975, Marcel Dekker Inc.
2. Kyncl JJ, Bush EN, Buckner SA: Alpha adrenergic blocking properties of terazosin. Fed Proc **41:**1648, 1982.
3. Kyncl JJ, Hollinger RE, Oheim KW, Winn M: (ABBOTT-45975), 2-[4-[(tetrahydro-2-furanyl)carbonyl]-1-piperazinyl]-6,7-dimethoxy-4-quinazolinamine HC1, a new antihypertensive agent of the quinazoline type. Pharmacologist **3:**272, 1980.
4. Metzler CM, Elfring GL, McEwen AJ: A package of computer programs for pharmacokinetic modeling. Biometrics **30:**562-563, 1974.
5. Mizogami S, Hanazuka M: Antihypertensive effect of 2-[4-[(tetrahydro-2-furanyl)carbonyl]-1-piperazinyl]-6,7-dimethoxy-4-quinazolinamine hydrochloride dihydrate (terazosin). Jpn J Pharm **32**(suppl):174P, 1982.
6. Patterson SE: Rapid and sensitive analysis of terazosin in plasma, peritoneal dialysis solution, and urine using HPLC with fluorescence detection. J Chromatogr **311:**206-212, 1984.
7. Sedman AJ, Wagner JG: CSTRIP, a FORTRAN IV computer program for obtaining initial polyexponential parameter estimates. J Pharm Sci **65:**1006-1010, 1976.
8. Sedman AJ, Wagner JG: AUTOAN, A decision making pharmacokinetic computer program. Ann Arbor, 1976, Publication Distribution Service.
9. Warren SE, O'Connor DT, Cohen IM, Mitas JA: Renal hemodynamic changes during long-term antihypertensive therapy. CLIN PHARMACOL THER **29:**310-317, 1980.

Ventilatory effects of atenolol and bevantolol in asthma

The cardioequipotency of 400 mg bevantolol and 100 mg atenolol was determined by measuring the exercise heart rate in healthy subjects. The β-blockers were then used in these doses to investigate their ventilatory effects in patients with asthma. The effects of both drugs on forced expiratory flow parameters for large and small airways were assessed at rest and during and after exercise. A dose-response curve was then plotted after inhalation of the β_2-adrenoceptor agonist terbutaline. Bevantolol significantly decreased the forced expiratory volume in 1 second (FEV_1) and the peak expiratory flow rate (PEFR) at rest, while there was no such change with placebo or atenolol. Both β-blockers decreased the maximal expiratory flow rates at 50% of forced vital capacity (MEF_{50}) and after expiration of 75% of the forced vital capacity (MEF_{25}) at rest; the decrease was larger after bevantolol than after atenolol. During atenolol there was a decrease in FEV_1 and in PEFR ($P < 0.01$) 15 minutes after exercise in comparison with preexercise values. There was no significant difference between pre- and postexercise values of MEF_{50} and MEF_{25} during atenolol dosing. After bevantolol there was only a small change in PEFR after exercise, probably because of the low preexercise values of the ventilatory indices with this drug. Inhalation of terbutaline up to a dose of 2 mg significantly improved all ventilatory indices measured, but with bevantolol the values after 2 mg inhaled terbutaline were lower than the initial values. We conclude that atenolol and bevantolol have different effects on large and small airways function in patients with asthma and that the effect of exercise on bronchoconstriction can be enhanced by β-blockade. Furthermore, 100 mg atenolol appears to be more β_1-adrenoceptor–selective than 400 mg bevantolol. (CLIN PHARMACOL THER 38:428-433, 1985.)

Jan-Willem J. Lammers, M.D., Hans T. M. Folgering, M.D., and Cees L. A. van Herwaarden, M.D. *H. Landstichting, The Netherlands*

Studies of the ventilatory effects of β-adrenoceptor antagonists in patients with asthma and reversible bronchial obstruction have proved to be good models for assessment of the β_1-adrenoceptor selectivity of these drugs.[9,11] Atenolol has been shown to be a β_1-adrenoceptor–selective blocker, inducing a limited decrease in airway conductance that can easily be reversed by a β_2-adrenoceptor agonist.[6,14] Bevantolol is a new β-adrenoceptor antagonist with β_1-adrenoceptor–selective effects in animals.[8] Our aim was to investigate the β_1-adrenoceptor selectivity of bevantolol in comparison with atenolol in patients with asthma. In many studies of the effects of β-blockade on lung function, only parameters of large airways function are measured. We were interested whether the influence of these drugs on large airways function on the one hand and conductance in the more peripheral airways on the other hand would differ.

Abbreviations

FEV_1	Forced expiratory volume in 1 second
FVC	Forced vital capacity
MEF_{25}	Maximal expiratory flow rate after expiration of 75% of FVC
MEF_{50}	Maximal expiratory flow rate at 50% of FVC
PEFR	Peak expiratory flow rate

The effects of β-blockers on lung function in patients with asthma can be enhanced by exercise.[15,22,23] This phenomenon is probably caused by more effective β-blockade during a state of increased sympathetic tone. We therefore measured lung function at rest and during exercise. To compare cardioequipotent doses of both drugs, we first determined in healthy subjects which dose of bevantolol induced the same reduction in exercise-induced tachycardia as 100 mg atenolol.

From the Department of Pulmonary Diseases and Pulmonary Function Laboratory, University of Nymegen, Medical Centre Dekkerswald.
Received for publication Dec. 19, 1984; accepted May 30, 1985.
Reprint requests to: Jan-Willem J. Lammers, M.D., Department of Pulmonary Diseases, University of Nymegen, Medical Centre Dekkerswald, 6564CA H. Landstichting, The Netherlands.

Table I. Patient characteristics

Patient No.	Age (yr)	Asthma type	Height (cm)	Weight (kg)	FEV_1 L	FEV_1 % Increase with terbutaline	Therapy
1	36	I	176	85	3.1(74)	16	C
2	21	E	178	61	2.6(55)	29	—
3	20	E	177	62	2.7(57)	56	C
4	20	E	185	73	3.7(71)	24	—
5	35	E	177	73	1.9(45)	21	CBS
6	23	E	171	62	2.3(53)	35	—
7	46	E	164	62	2.7(83)	22	B
8	20	E	180	60	2.4(50)	42	CS
$\bar{X}$ ± SE	27.6 ± 3.5		176 ± 2.2	67.3 ± 3.1	2.68 ± 0.19	30.6 ± 4.7	

Values in parentheses are the percentage of predicted values.[21]
I = Intrinsic; C = cromoglycate; E = extrinsic; B = beclomethasone; S = salbutamol.

METHODS

The study to determine cardioequipotency was carried out in six healthy men 21 to 25 years old. Each subject was studied on 4 days at intervals of at least 1 week; a training effect could thus be discounted. After arrival at the hospital at 9 AM, the subjects rested 30 minutes before the first exercise test began. Each exercise test consisted of 5 minutes of bicycling on an electrically braked ergometer at an individually determined load that induced a heart rate of approximately 150 bpm before drug dosing. After the first test the study drugs were taken by mouth. On the first day the subjects took (single-blind) a placebo; on the 3 other days they received (double-blind in random order) 200 mg bevantolol, 400 mg bevantolol, and 100 mg atenolol. Subsequent exercise tests were performed 1, 2, 3, 5 and 7 hours after dosing. At each test the heart rate was recorded by a continuous ECG tracing and blood samples were drawn for determination of the plasma levels of the β-blockers. Samples were stored at −20° C until analyzed by HPLC.

To compare the ventilatory effects of bevantolol and atenolol, we studied eight men with bronchial asthma.[1] Clinical data of these patients are listed in Table I. Seven patients had atopic extrinsic asthma with one or more positive skin tests. Two patients (nos. 1 and 5) were cigarette smokers and the others were nonsmokers. All patients were in a stable respiratory state (no respiratory infection or increase in bronchoconstriction within the past month). Salbutamol was stopped in the two patients who used this drug regularly at least 2 days before the study; four patients continued cromoglycate therapy and two continued beclomethasone therapy without a change in dose during the study. In all patients the FEV_1 increased by >15% after stimulation with the β_2-adrenoceptor agonist terbutaline. Patients with cardiovascular diseases other than arterial hypertension were excluded. The study was approved by the local Ethical Committee and informed consent was obtained from each patient.

The study was designed as a placebo-controlled, double-blind, crossover comparison of single doses of 400 mg bevantolol and 100 mg atenolol. Every patient was studied on 3 different days, separated by intervals of at least 2 days as washout periods. All experiments started at noon to minimize variation in baseline lung function and to avoid the "morning dip" that frequently occurs in patients with asthma.[3]

The following measurements were determined each day: After a resting period of 30 minutes the patients exercised for 5 minutes on a bicycle ergometer at an individually fixed load that induced a heart rate of approximately 150 bpm after placebo. Heart rate and blood pressure were measured before, during the last minute of exercise, and 15 minutes after exercise. At the same time lung function was assessed with flow-volume equipment. Several components of air flow rate were recorded: FEV_1 and PEFR as parameters of large airways function, and MEF_{50} and MEF_{25} mainly as parameters of smaller airways conductance.[20] These indices were obtained from the curve yielding the largest sum of FVC and FEV_1.[5,19] Immediately after this first exercise test the medication was taken by mouth 30 minutes before a standard meal to avoid differences in bioavailability within each individual.[16] Two hours after dosing a second exercise test was performed, which consisted of 5 minutes of bicycling at the same load as during the first exercise test. The same measurements were assessed before, during the last minute of exercise, and 15 minutes after exercise. Twenty-five minutes after

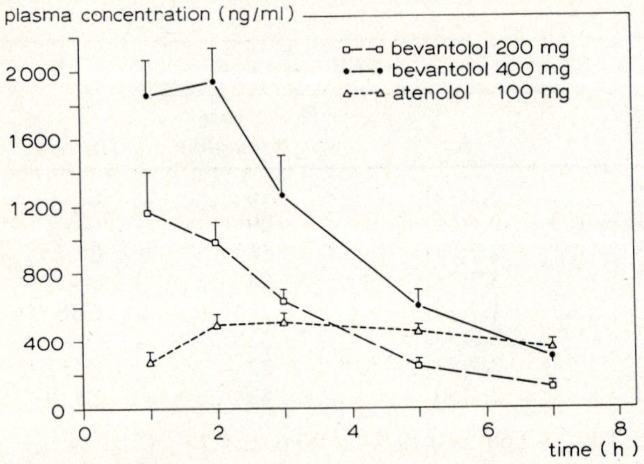

Fig. 1. Mean (±SE; n = 6) plasma concentrations after oral dosing with 200 mg bevantolol, 400 mg bevantolol, and 100 mg atenolol.

this second exercise period (i.e., 2.5 hours after drug dosing) a dose-response curve was constructed by measuring the forced expiration indices, heart rate, and blood pressure 15 minutes after terbutaline inhalation. Terbutaline was inhaled three times from a metered-dose aerosol, each puff containing 0.5 mg terbutaline sulphate in cumulative doses of 0.5, 1, and 2 mg.

Statistical analysis was by the Wilcoxon test for paired observations and correlations were calculated by the Pearson method.[2] Statistical significance was defined as $P < 0.05$.

RESULTS

Study in healthy subjects. Both β-blockers induced significant decreases in exercise-induced tachycardia in comparison with placebo ($P < 0.01$). The largest reduction in exercise-induced tachycardia was measured 2 hours after drug dosing, at which time the effects of 400 mg bevantolol and 100 mg atenolol were identical (−37 bpm) and greater than that of 200 mg bevantolol (−34 bpm). The curves of the plasma concentrations of the β-blockers are shown in Fig. 1. The mean time of peak plasma concentrations was 1 hour 8 minutes for 200 mg bevantolol, 1 hour 40 minutes for 400 mg bevantolol, and 2 hours 40 minutes for 100 mg atenolol. The $t_{1/2}$ for both doses of bevantolol was approximately 2 hours, but the study period was too short to calculate a precise $t_{1/2}$ for atenolol. There was good correlation between plasma levels of the β-blockers and the reduction in exercise-induced tachycardia (r = 0.87 for bevantolol and r = 0.84 for atenolol). Because 400 mg bevantolol could be regarded as cardioequipotent to 100 mg atenolol, the drugs were used in these doses to compare their ventilatory effects in patients with asthma.

Study in patients with asthma. There were no significant differences between the initial values of the indices measured on the different days of the study. At rest 2 hours after drug dosing, mean (±SE) heart rate decreased by 10 ± 2.4 bpm after 400 mg bevantolol ($P < 0.01$) and by 12.8 ± 2.5 bpm after 100 mg atenolol ($P < 0.01$). Systolic blood pressure at rest decreased 9.5 ± 3.2 mm Hg after bevantolol ($P < 0.05$) and 12.3 ± 2.3 mm Hg after atenolol ($P < 0.01$). There was no significant change in diastolic blood pressure during β-blockade at rest.

Results of the forced expiratory flow measurements are presented in Table II and Figs. 2 to 4. Bevantolol, 400 mg, induced a decrease in FEV_1 of 1.07 ± 0.26 L and in PEFR of 2.35 ± 0.69 L/sec ($P < 0.01$), whereas atenolol and placebo did not decrease these parameters (Table II). MEF_{50} and MEF_{25} fell significantly after both β-blockers, but the decline after bevantolol was significantly larger than that after atenolol. During exercise there was a significant increase ($P < 0.01$) in the forced expiratory flow indices measured during placebo, bevantolol, and atenolol dosing (Fig. 2, *upper panel*). Fifteen minutes after the second exercise test during atenolol dosing, FEV_1 significantly fell from 2.61 ± 0.24 L before exercise to 1.99 ± 0.21 L after exercise, and PEFR declined from 6.45 ± 0.56 to 5.33 ± 0.62 L/sec (Table II; Fig. 2, *lower panel*). Bevantolol significantly decreased PEFR after exercise (from 4.63 ± 0.58 to 4.28 ± 0.60 L/sec), whereas FEV_1 did not change. During placebo there were no significant changes in either FEV_1 or PEFR 15 minutes after exercise (Table II; Fig. 2, *lower panel*). There were no significant decreases in MEF_{50} and MEF_{25} after exercise as compared with preexercise values during placebo, bevantolol, and atenolol dosing. However, the decrease in MEF_{50} and MEF_{25} after exercise during atenolol dosing was significant as compared with the effect of bevantolol on these indices (Fig. 2, *lower panel*). The absolute values for FEV_1, PEFR, MEF_{50}, and MEF_{25} before and after the second exercise test, 2 hours and 2 hours 20 minutes, respectively after bevantolol dosing, were significantly lower than the corresponding values during placebo and atenolol dosing ($P < 0.05$; Table II).

Inhalation of terbutaline up to a cumulative dose of 2 mg significantly increased the ventilatory indices measured (Table II; Figs. 3 and 4). The bronchodilatory effect of terbutaline was smaller during bevantolol dosing than during placebo and atenolol dosing (Figs. 3 and 4). During bevantolol dosing the absolute values of FEV_1, PEFR, MEF_{50}, and MEF_{25} after terbutaline inhalations were almost at the same level as the initial values before drug dosing, whereas during placebo and

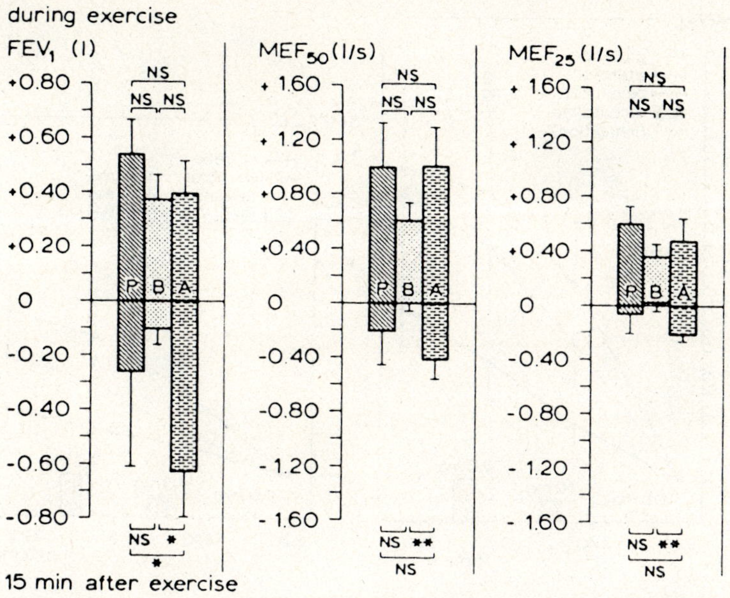

Fig. 2. Mean (±SE; n = 8) rise and fall in FEV_1, MEF_{50}, and MEF_{25} during and after the second exercise test 2 hours after drug dosing. Measurements were performed during the last minute of exercise *(upper panel)* and 15 minutes after exercise *(lower panel)* and differences were calculated from preexercise values 2 hours after drug dosing during placebo *(P)*, 400 mg bevantolol *(B)*, and 100 mg atenolol *(A)*. *NS* = Not significant; $^*P < 0.05$; $^{**}P < 0.01$.

atenolol dosing the values after terbutaline were significantly higher than the inital values (Table II).

After the second exercise test all patients had at least one minor asthmatic attack. This happened seven times during bevantolol dosing and only once after atenolol. All complaints disappeared immediately after the first inhalation of terbutaline, and all patients left the clinic without complaints.

DISCUSSION

From our study in healthy subjects we conclude that 2 hours after drug dosing, 400 mg bevantolol was cardioequipotent to 100 mg atenolol, because at that time both β-blockers induced equal decreases in exercise-induced tachycardia. We therefore used both β-blockers at these two doses to compare their effects on forced expiration parameters. The study was carried out in patients with asthma with >15% reversibility of the FEV_1, because β-blockers usually induce bronchospasm in such patients while this effect is much smaller or absent in normal subjects and in patients with low reversible or fixed bronchoconstriction.[17,18,24] In the patients with asthma both β-blockers induced the same reduction in heart rate at rest and during exercise, indicating the same degree of cardiac β-blockade. However, the two β-blockers had significantly different effects on lung function.

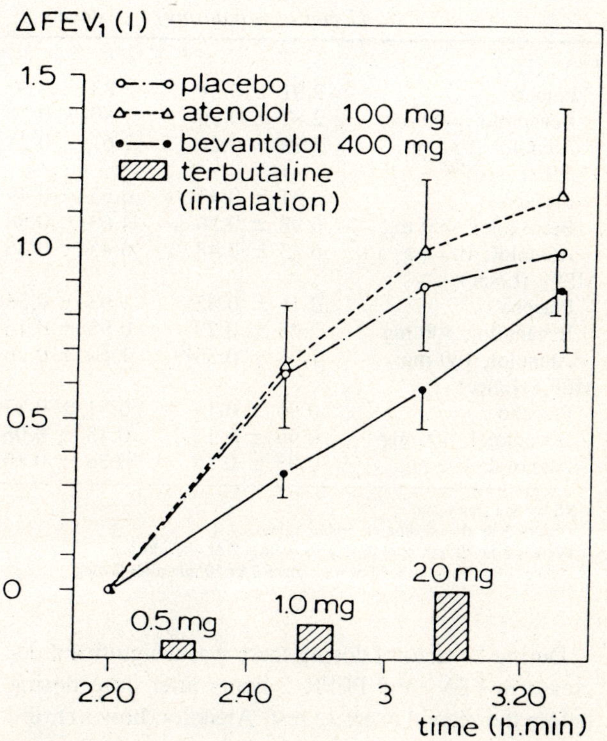

Fig. 3. Mean (±SE; n = 8) changes in FEV_1 induced by inhalation of terbutaline in cumulative doses after placebo, 400 mg bevantolol, and 100 mg atenolol.

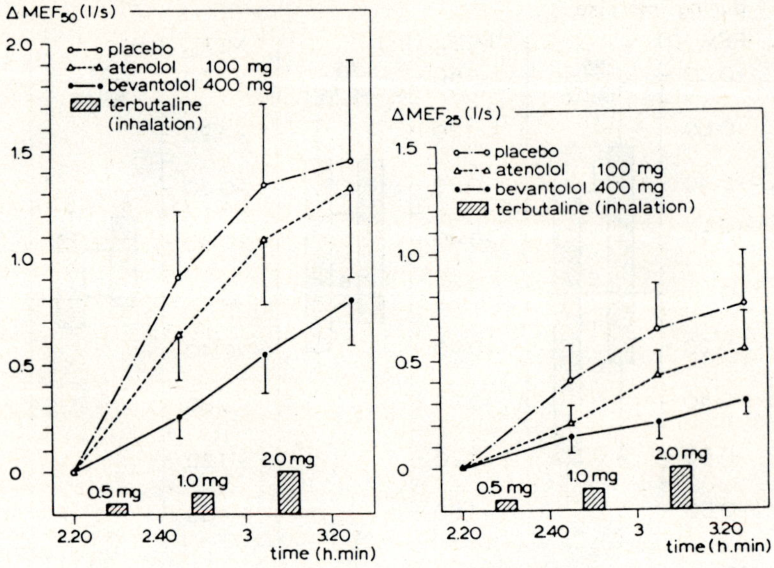

Fig. 4. Mean (±SE; n = 8) changes in MEF_{50} and MEF_{25} induced by inhalation of terbutaline in cumulative doses after placebo, 400 mg bevantolol, and 100 mg atenolol.

Table II. Ventilatory indices before and after placebo, 400 mg bevantolol, and 100 mg atenolol after exercise and after inhalation of terbutaline

	Initial values (5 min before dosing)	*2 hr after dosing*	*P value**	*2 hr 20 min after dosing (15 min after second exercise test)*	*P value†*	*After inhalation of 2 mg terbutaline*	*P value‡*
FEV_1 (L)							
Placebo	2.91 ± 0.31	2.83 ± 0.30	NS	2.60 ± 0.22	NS	3.58 ± 0.29	<0.01
Bevantolol, 400 mg	2.87 ± 0.26	1.80 ± 0.21	<0.01	1.70 ± 0.22	NS	2.58 ± 0.31	<0.01
Atenolol, 100 mg	2.79 ± 0.26	2.61 ± 0.24	NS	1.99 ± 0.21	<0.01	3.14 ± 0.33	<0.02
PEFR (L/sec)							
Placebo	6.81 ± 0.43	6.53 ± 0.49	NS	6.33 ± 0.45	NS	8.31 ± 0.51	<0.01
Bevantolol, 400 mg	6.98 ± 0.56	4.63 ± 0.58	<0.01	4.28 ± 0.60	<0.05	6.49 ± 0.73	<0.01
Atenolol, 100 mg	6.33 ± 0.48	6.45 ± 0.56	NS	5.33 ± 0.62	<0.01	8.00 ± 0.80	<0.01
MEF_{50} (L/sec)							
Placebo	2.16 ± 0.42	1.93 ± 0.38	NS	1.79 ± 0.23	NS	3.24 ± 0.55	<0.01
Bevantolol, 400 mg	2.05 ± 0.29	0.98 ± 0.16	<0.01	0.99 ± 0.16	NS	1.79 ± 0.28	<0.01
Atenolol, 100 mg	1.98 ± 0.35	1.60 ± 0.26	<0.05	1.24 ± 0.17	NS	2.56 ± 0.49	<0.01
MEF_{25} (L/sec)							
Placebo	0.96 ± 0.19	0.81 ± 0.17	NS	0.80 ± 0.08	NS	1.56 ± 0.28	<0.01
Bevantolol, 400 mg	0.96 ± 0.15	0.45 ± 0.06	<0.01	0.46 ± 0.05	NS	0.78 ± 0.10	<0.01
Atenolol, 100 mg	0.93 ± 0.15	0.76 ± 0.10	<0.05	0.60 ± 0.07	NS	1.15 ± 0.21	<0.01

NS = Not significant.
*Values 2 hr after dosing vs. initial values.
†Values 2 hr 20 min after dosing vs. values 2 hr after dosing.
‡Values after 2 mg terbutaline vs. values 2 hr 20 min after dosing.

During bevantolol dosing there was a significant decrease in FEV_1 and PEFR 2 hours after drug dosing before the second exercise test. Atenolol, however, did not induce such a decrease in these large airways parameters at rest. Although both bevantolol and atenolol significantly decreased MEF_{50} and MEF_{25}, the reduction after bevantolol was larger than that after atenolol. Small airways function at rest, therefore, seems to be more sensitive to β-adrenoceptor blockade than large airways function in these patients with asthma.

The normal rise in airway conductance during exercise, probably due to increased sympathetic tone,[12] was not influenced by either bevantolol or atenolol; this is in accord with results of other studies.[6,10] During atenolol dosing there was a significant decrease in FEV_1 and PEFR after exercise in comparison with the preexercise values 2 hours after drug dosing, while the differences in MEF_{50} and MEF_{25} between pre- and postexercise values were not significant. This increase in bronchoconstriction, especially in the larger airways, by exercise was not demonstrated during placebo dosing. During bevantolol dosing there was only a small decrease in PEFR after exercise, while FEV_1 remained unchanged. The different effects of atenolol and bevantolol on bronchomotor tone after exercise are probably explained by the fact that bevantolol had already induced considerable bronchoconstriction before the second exercise test. Therefore, exercise-induced bronchoconstriction can be enhanced by β-adrenoceptor blockade, an effect that seems to depend on the preexercise bronchomotor tone.

During therapy with 400 mg bevantolol the dose-response curves with terbutaline for FEV_1, PEFR, MEF_{50}, and MEF_{25} shifted downward in comparison with placebo and atenolol, indicating less β_1-adrenoceptor selectivity for bevantolol at this dose than for atenolol.[7,9] β_1-Adrenoceptor selectivity is, however, a dose-dependent phenomenon,[4,13] and a smaller dose of bevantolol might show more β_1-adrenoceptor selectivity.

Test drugs were kindly provided by Warner Lambert International Drug Development, Ann Arbor, Mich., where the plasma level determinations were also performed.

References

1. American Thoracic Society: Chronic bronchitis, asthma, and pulmonary emphysema. A statement by the committee on diagnostic standards for nontuberculous respiratory diseases. Am Rev Respir Dis **85:**762-768, 1962.
2. Colton T. Statistics in medicine. Boston, 1974, Little, Brown and Co.
3. Conolly DK: Diurnal rhythms in airway obstruction. Br J Dis Chest **73:**357-366, 1979.
4. Fleming GM, Chester EH, Schwartz HJ, Jones PK: Beta-adrenergic blockade of the lung. Dose-dependent cardioselectivity of tolamolol in asthma. Chest **73:**807-812, 1978.
5. Gardner RM (Chairman): ATS statement-Snowbird Workshop on Standardization of Spirometry. Am Rev Respir Dis **119:**831-838, 1979.
6. Greefhorst APM, Van Herwaarden CLA: Comparative study of the ventilatory effects of three β_1-selective blocking agents in asthmatic patients. Eur J Clin Pharmacol **20:**417-421, 1981.
7. Greefhorst APM, Van Herwaarden CLA: Ventilatory and haemodynamic effects of terbutaline infusion during $beta_1$-selective blockade with metoprolol and acebutolol in asthmatic patients. Eur J Clin Pharmacol **23:**203-208, 1982.
8. Hoefle ML, Hastings SG, Meyer RF, Corey RM, Holmes A, Stratton CD: Cardioselective β-adrenergic blocking agents. I. 1-[(3,4-dimethoxyphenetyl)amino]-3-aryloxy-2-propanols. J Med Chem **18:**148-152, 1975.
9. Johnsson G, Svedmyr N, Thiringer G: Effects of intravenous propranolol and metoprolol and their interaction with isoprenaline on pulmonary function, heart rate and blood pressure in asthmatics. Eur J Clin Pharmacol **8:**175-180, 1975.
10. Kumana CR, Marlin GE, Kaye CM, Smith DM: New approach to assessment of cardioselectivity of beta-blocking drugs. Br Med J **4:**444-447, 1974.
11. Lammers JWJ, Folgering HTM, Van Herwaarden CLA: Ventilatory effects of $beta_1$-receptor–selective blockade with bisoprolol and metoprolol in asthmatic patients. Eur J Clin Pharmacol **27:**141-145, 1984.
12. Lefcoe NM: The time course of maximum ventilatory performance during and after moderately heavy exercise. Clin Sci **36:**47-52, 1969.
13. Lertora JJL, Mark AL, Johannsen UJ, Wilson WR, Abboud FM: Selective beta-1 receptor blockade with oral practolol in man. J Clin Invest **56:**719-724, 1975.
14. Löfdahl C-G, Svedmyr N: Cardioselectivity of atenolol and metoprolol. Eur J Respir Dis **62:**396-404, 1981.
15. McDevitt DG: The assessment of β-adrenoceptor blocking drugs in man. Br J Clin Pharmacol **4:**413-425, 1977.
16. Melander A, Danielson K, Schersten B, Wählin E: Enhancement of the bioavailability of propranolol and metoprolol by food. CLIN PHARMACOL THER **22:**108-112, 1977.
17. Nordstrom LA, MacDonald F, Gobel FL: Effect of propranolol on respiratory function and exercise tolerance in patients with chronic obstructive lung disease. Chest **67:**287-292, 1975.
18. Perks WH, Chatterjee SS, Croxson RS, Cruickshank JM: Comparison of atenolol and oxprenolol in patients with angina or hypertension and co-existent chronic airways obstruction. Br J Clin Pharmacol **5:**101-106, 1978.
19. Peslin R, Bohadana A, Hannhart B, Jardin P: Comparison of various methods for reading maximal expiratory flow-volume curves. Am Rev Respir Dis **119:**271-277, 1979.
20. Pride NB: Assessment of changes in airway calibre. I. Tests of forced expiration. Br J Clin Pharmacol **8:**193-203, 1979.
21. Quanjer PH, editor: Standardized lung function testing. Clin Respir Physiol **19**(suppl 5):1-95, 1983.
22. Ruffin RE, McIntyre ELM, Latimer KM, Ward HE, Crockett AJ, Alpers JH: Assessment of β-adrenoceptor antagonists in asthmatic patients. Br J Clin Pharmacol **13:**325S-335S, 1982.
23. Sue DY, Hansen JE, Wasserman K: The value of exercise in testing beta blockade and airway reactivity in asthmatic patients. Am Heart J **104:**442-445, 1982.
24. Woods KL, Linton SP, Kendall MJ, Faragher EB, Grieve RJ: Exercise responses of healthy subjects in the evaluation of cardioselectivity of β-blockers. Eur J Clin Pharmacol **15:**229-233, 1979.

Antihypertensive and cardiovascular effects of nitrendipine: A controlled study vs. placebo

The antihypertensive and cardiovascular effects of nitrendipine, a calcium entry blocker similar to nifedipine, have been evaluated in a double-blind, placebo-controlled study in 20 patients with hypertension. At baseline and at the end of the 8-week period (nitrendipine, 20 mg once a day, or placebo, 1 tablet once a day) the following parameters were measured: systolic and diastolic blood pressure (BP) and heart rate (HR) at rest by an automatic recorder; BP, HR, and cardiac workload (systolic BP × HR) during exercise testing on a bicycle; left ventricular mass (LVMe according to the method of Devereux) and cross-sectional area (CSA), and main parameters of systolic function (end diastolic volume, end systolic volume [ESV], and ejection fraction [EF]) by M mode echocardiography. There was a significant decrease in BP at rest (163/108 vs. 144/92 mm Hg; $P < 0.001$) and during exercise in subjects receiving nitrendipine, while placebo did not modify these parameters. LVMe (from 195 to 188 gm; $P < 0.01$) and CSA (from 20.2 to 19.8 cm^2; $P < 0.05$) were reduced by nitrendipine, which also improved cardiac performance (ESV fell from 44 to 38 ml [$P < 0.001$] and EF fell from 62% to 66% [$P < 0.01$]). No effect was observed in the placebo group. Our results indicate that nitrendipine is a powerful antihypertensive agent that also improves cardiac performance and slightly but significantly reduces left ventricular mass. (CLIN PHARMACOL THER 38:434-438, 1985.)

Liberato Aldo Ferrara, M.D., Maria Luisa Fasano, M.D., Giovanni de Simone, M.D., Stefano Soro, M.D., and Renato Gagliardi, B.Sc.
Naples, Italy

Arterial hypertension is treated with several drugs. In particular, calcium entry blockers (alone or in combined therapy) are useful in the treatment of mild or moderate arterial hypertension.[4,13] Nitrendipine (Bay e 5009) is a calcium entry blocker similar in structure to nifedipine. It is a dihydropyridine derivative (1,4-dihydro-2,6-dimethyl-4-(3-nitrophenyl)-3,5-pyridinedicarboxylic acid, ethyl methyl ester) shown in preliminary studies in animals and man to have a powerful antihypertensive activity more pronounced than that of other calcium antagonists.[1,2,8,17] Its kinetics allow an adequate antihypertensive effect after single, oral daily doses.[10]

Our aims were to investigate: (1) the antihypertensive activity of long-term therapy with a single oral dose of nitrendipine (20 mg) in comparison with placebo; (2) the effects on cardiac workload during ergometric exercise on a bicycle; and (3) the effects on left ventricular mass and on the main parameters of systolic function of the left ventricle, noninvasively determined by M mode echocardiography.

From the Institute of Internal Medicine and Metabolic Disease, Clinica Medica, Second Medical School, University of Naples, and Medical Department, Bayer Italia S.p.A.
Received for publication March 25, 1985; accepted June 17, 1985.
Reprint requests to: L. A. Ferrara, M.D., Clinica Medica, 2 Facoltà di Medicina, Università di Napoli, Via S. Pansini 5, 80131 Naples, Italy.

METHODS

Thirty patients (20 men and 10 women) between 24 and 62 years old were studied. Subjects had high blood pressure (BP) determined in at least four separate examinations evaluated at weekly intervals. Criteria for inclusion were: (1) systolic BP <200 mm Hg and diastolic BP <120 mm Hg; (2) absence of target organ damage by the hypertensive disease; and (3) absence of other concomitant chronic diseases (diabetes mellitus, liver disease). Pregnant women or those taking oral contraceptives were excluded.

Patients who gave informed consent to participate were asked to discontinue any previous antihypertensive drugs and to observe a well-balanced normocaloric diet

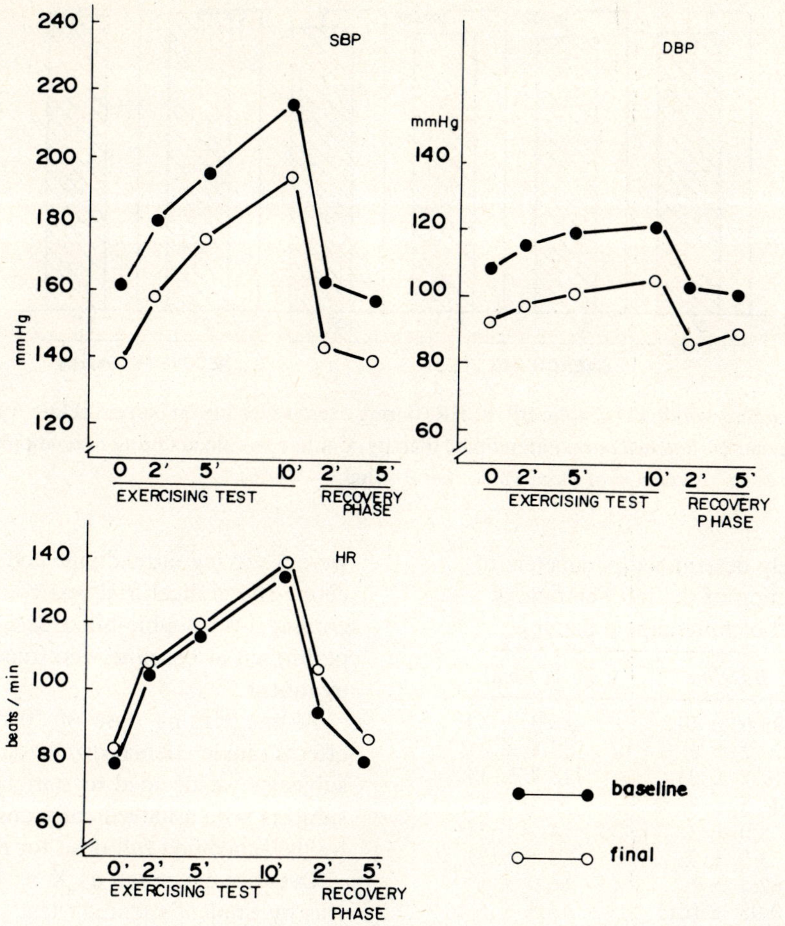

Fig. 1. Systolic *(SBP)* and diastolic *(DBP)* BPs and HR during exercise testing on a bicycle before and at the end of nitrendipine therapy.

Table I. BPs and HR at baseline and at the end of nitrendipine therapy

	Supine			*Standing*		
	Systolic BP (mm Hg)	*Diastolic BP (mm Hg)*	*HR (bpm)*	*Systolic BP (mm Hg)*	*Diastolic BP (mm Hg)*	*HR (bpm)*
Baseline	163 ± 10	108 ± 9	69 ± 8	159 ± 16	113 ± 19	74 ± 8
Final	114 ± 11*	92 ± 4*	77 ± 10†	137 ± 14*	91 ± 6*	84 ± 8‡

*P < 0.001; †P < 0.005; ‡P < 0.01.

(without salt restriction) for 2 weeks. Thereafter they were prescribed placebo, once a day in the morning, for 2 weeks. At the end of the washout the BP and heart rate (HR) were measured twice by an automatic recorder after at least 10 minutes of supine rest and after 5 minutes of standing. BP and HR were also measured during exercise testing on a bicycle. After a 2-minute warm-up at 40 W, the load was increased at 2-minute intervals to 100 W and then continued for 5 minutes. Recovery phase was followed up to 5 minutes afterwards. Cardiac workload (systolic BP × HR) during exercise at the end of treatments was expressed as a percentage of the basal value (basal value = 100%).

Left ventricular mass was noninvasively determined by M mode echocardiography and was expressed as echocardiographic left ventricular mass (LVMe)[5] and

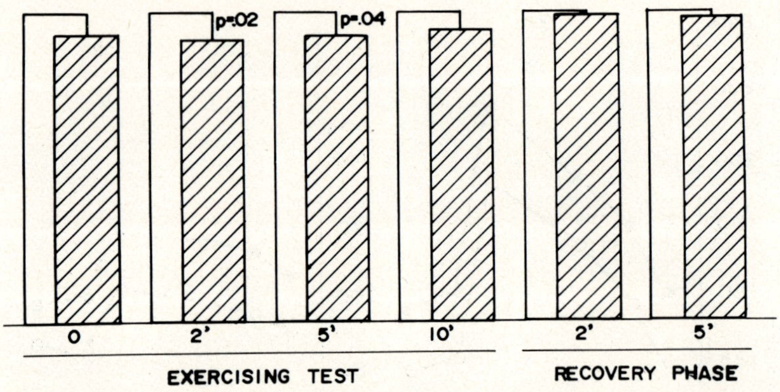

Fig. 2. Cardiac workload (systolic BP × HR) during exercise testing on bicycle before *(open bars)* and at the end of *(hatched bars)* nitrendipine therapy. Cardiac workload during nitrendipine therapy is expressed as percentage of basal value (basal value = 100%).

Table II. Noninvasively determined parameters of mass and systolic function of the left ventricle at baseline and at the end of nitrendipine therapy

	Baseline	*Final*
LVMe (gm)	195.0 ± 49	188.3 ± 49*
CSA (cm^2)	20.2 ± 3	19.8 ± 3*
EDV (ml)	119.7 ± 23	113.7 ± 14
ESV (ml)	44.5 ± 9	38.5 ± 8†
EDD (cm)	5.0 ± 3	4.9 ± 3‡
ESD (cm)	3.3 ± 3	3.1 ± 3†
EF (%)	62.4 ± 6	66.0 ± 6*
vcf (cycles/sec)	0.98 ± 0.15	1.08 ± 0.14*

ESD = End systolic diameter; vcf = velocity of circumferential fiber shortening.
*$P < 0.01$; †$P < 0.001$; ‡$P < 0.05$

cross-sectional area (CSA).[15] Left ventricular dimensions were measured at the level of the chordae tendineae of the mitral valve. Interventricular septal thickness, posterior wall thickness, and end diastolic diameter (EDD) were determined with the Penn convention for the evaluation of LVMe and the standard convention for the evaluation of CSA. Main noninvasively determined parameters of systolic function (end diastolic volume [EDV], end systolic volume [ESV], and ejection fraction [EF]) and mean velocity of circumferential fiber shortening were also measured.[14,18] As frequently observed with calcium entry blockers, possible increases in the volume of the ankle were assessed by the measurement of the volume of water displaced by the subject's foot placed in a basin.

After baseline measurements, subjects were randomly prescribed either 20 mg nitrendipine or a placebo tablet, once a day for a period of 8 weeks. The study design was such that at the end of the study, 20 patients were receiving nitrendipine and 10 were receiving placebo. The clinical trial was completely carried out according to a double-blind design. The measurements performed at baseline were repeated at the end of the treatment.

As the starting dose of 20 mg induced some side effects (ankle edema, dizziness, and headache) in four subjects, we decided to start both treatments in later subjects with a halved daily dose for 1 week followed by the scheduled full dose for 8 weeks.

Data are expressed as $\overline{X}$ ± SD. Statistical analysis was by Student's paired t test.

RESULTS

Placebo and nitrendipine groups at baseline were comparable with respect to age (48 ± 7 and 47 ± 9 years, respectively), body mass index (weight/height^2; 27.2 ± 4 and 27.9 ± 4, respectively), and BP (mean arterial pressure 122 ± 7 and 126 ± 8 mm Hg, respectively).

Body weight was constant throughout the study (77.5 and 77.5 kg in the nitrendipine group and 72.5 and 72.1 kg in the placebo group). There was a highly significant reduction in both supine and standing systolic and diastolic BPs at rest at the end of nitrendipine dosing. A reflex increase in HR was induced by nitrendipine (from 69 ± 8 to 77 ± 10 bpm; $P < 0.005$; Table I). Placebo induced no significant changes in the same parameters (supine BP, from 151 ± 13/104 ± 7 to 152 ± 12/105 ± 7 mm Hg; standing BP, from 149 ± 12/107 ± 8 to 151 ± 16/110 ± 7 mm Hg). There was also no change in HR (78 ± 14 and 73 ± 9 bpm supine; 80 ± 16 and 77 ± 18 bpm standing).

During bicycle exercise testing there was a significant reduction in systolic and diastolic BPs; HR increased only slightly as compared with pretreatment values (Fig. 1). Cardiac workload (systolic BP × HR) was therefore reduced during the bicycle test, in particular in the early steps when differences from baseline were statistically significant (Fig. 2). On the other hand, placebo was absolutely unable to modify the same parameters.

With regard to myocardial mass, nitrendipine induced partial regression of left ventricular hypertrophy, with reductions in LVMe (from 195 ± 49 to 188 ± 49 gm; P < 0.01) and CSA (from 20.2 ± 3.4 to 19.8 ± 3.5 cm^2; P < 0.01) in all subjects. A remarkable reduction in ESV with significant improvement in EF during nitrendipine therapy was also observed (Table II). No effect on the same parameters was shown by placebo (LVMe, from 205 ± 62 to 213 ± 54 gm; CSA, from 22 ± 4 to 22 ± 3 cm^2; ESV, from 54 ± 24 to 48 ± 19 ml; and EF, from 60% ± 7% to 63% ± 5%).

There was a slight increase in the volume of the ankle during nitrendipine therapy. The volume of water displaced by the foot increased from 895 ± 150 ml at baseline to 1034 ± 316 ml at the end of the study (P < 0.03).

DISCUSSION

Nitrendipine, a calcium antagonist with antihypertensive and vasodilating properties, was able to reduce significantly systolic BP and diastolic BPs at rest with a concomitant slight increase in HR in the supine and standing positions. Because of the drug's kinetics, single daily doses will maintain good BP control for 24 hours. It is particularly interesting that the BP during exercise testing on the bicycle was significantly reduced. A reflex increase in HR, which is particularly marked with other vasodilators, was confined to the end of the exercise during nitrendipine therapy; cardiac workload was therefore significantly reduced. Nitrendipine also significantly decreased peripheral resistance as indicated by the reduction in ESV and the increase in EF, therefore improving left ventricular performance.

Unlike other vasodilators, nitrendipine reduced LVMe along with arterial pressure. This is a peculiar characteristic of nitrendipine, since hydralazine or minoxidil did not induce any change in left ventricular size in both man and animal studies.[16] Nifedipine was also recently shown unable to modify left ventricular mass.[3] Our data confirm in man the findings of Kazda et al.[11] and Kobayashi and Tarazi[12] in animals. Because vasodilating drugs, which consequently enhance reflex sympathetic outflow, do not influence myocardial mass, the effects of nitrendipine on left ventricular size might possibly depend on the marked action on intrarenal hemodynamics after increased renal sodium excretion,[9] which might counter the increase in adrenergic activity. This is in keeping with other findings showing that salt depletion induced by severe salt intake restriction or thiazide therapy significantly reduces ventricular mass in patients with hypertension with left ventricular hypertrophy.[6,7]

Side effects never were such to cause subject withdrawal from the study. A starting dose of 10 mg twice a day further avoided the incidence of side effects, although ankle edema and skin flushing were sometimes observed. In conclusion, our data seem to indicate that nitrendipine is a long-acting, powerful antihypertensive agent at rest and during exercise that can induce partial regression of the increased myocardial mass of the left ventricle.

References

1. Andren L, Hansson L, Orö L, Ryman T: Experience with nitrendipine, a new calcium antagonist in hypertension. J Cardiovasc Pharmacol **4**:(suppl 3):387-391, 1982.
2. Burris JF, Notargiacomo AV, Papademetriou V, Freis ED: Acute and short term effects of a new calcium antagonist in hypertension. Hypertension **4**(suppl 2):32-35, 1982.
3. de Simone G, Ferrara LA, Di Lorenzo L, Lauria R, Fasano ML: Effects of slow-release nifedipine on left ventricular mass and systolic function in mild or moderate hypertension. Curr Ther Res **36**:537-543, 1984.
4. de Simone G, Ferrara LA, Fasano ML, Di Lorenzo L, Lauria R: Slow-release nifedipine versus placebo in the treatment of arterial hypertension: A double-blind ergometric evaluation of cardiac workload. Jpn Heart J **26**:219-225, 1985.
5. Devereux RB, Reichek M: Echocardiographic determination of left ventricular mass: Anatomic validation of the method. Circulation **55**:613-618, 1977.
6. Ferrara LA, de Simone G, Mancini M, Fasano ML, Pasanisi F, Vallone G: Changes in left ventricular mass during a double-blind study with chlorthalidone and slow-release nifedipine. Eur J Clin Pharmacol **27**:525-528, 1984.
7. Ferrara LA, de Simone G, Pasanisi F, Mancini M, Mancini M: Left ventricular mass during salt depletion in arterial hypertension. Hypertension **6**:755-759, 1984.
8. Fouad F, Abour-Khair M, Tarazi RC: Heterogeneity of systemic haemodynamic response to a new calcium entry blocker, nitrendipine. J Cardiovasc Pharmacol **4**(suppl 3):383-386, 1982.
9. Garthoff B, Knorr A, Thomas G, Kazda S: Nitrendipine increases sodium excretion in acutely saline-loaded rats. Biochem Pharmacol **31**:3015-3016, 1982.
10. Hansson L, Andren L, Oro L, Ryman T: Pharmacokynetic and pharmacodynamic parameters in patients

treated with nitrendipine. Hypertension **5**(part II):125-128, 1983.

11. Kazda S, Garthoff S, Knorr A: Nitrendipine and other calcium entry blockers (calcium antagonists) in hypertension. Fed Proc **42:**196-200, 1983.
12. Kobayashi K, Tarazi RC: Effect of nitrendipine on coronary flow and ventricular hypertrophy in hypertension. Hypertension **5**(part II):45-51, 1983.
13. Leonetti G, Sala C, Bianchini C, Terzoli L, Zanchetti A: Antihypertensive and renal effects of orally administered verapamil. Eur J Clin Pharmacol **18:**375-380, 1980.
14. Paraskos J, Grossman W, Saltz S, Dalen S, Dexter L: A noninvasive technique for the determination of velocity of circumferential fiber shortening in man. Circ Res **29:**610-616, 1971.
15. Schuler G, Peterson KL, Johnson AD, Francis G, Ashburn W, Dennish G, Daily FC, Ross I: Serial noninvasive assessment of left ventricular hypertrophy and function after surgical correction of aortic regurgitation. Am J Cardiol **44:**585-594, 1979.
16. Sen S, Tarazi RC, Bumpus FM: Cardiac hypertrophy and antihypertensive therapy. Cardiovasc Res **11:**427-433, 1977.
17. Stoepel K, Heise A, Kazda S: Pharmacological studies of the antihypertensive effect of nitrendipine. Arzneimittelforsch/Drug Res **31:**2056-2061, 1981.
18. Teicholtz LE, Kreulen T, Herman MV, et al: Problems in echocardiographic volume determinations: Echocardiographic angiographic correlations in the presence or absence of asynergy. Am J Cardiol **37:**7-11, 1976.

Pefloxacin kinetics in cirrhosis

Pefloxacin pharmacokinetics were evaluated in 16 patients with histologically proved cirrhosis of the liver and compared with those in 12 healthy subjects. In the patients with cirrhosis, the mean (±SD) $t_{1/2}$, although highly variable, was significantly longer (35.10 ± 19.00 hours) than in the normal subjects (11.00 ± 2.64 hours; $P < 0.001$). In the patients, the volume of distribution was decreased by 18% ($P < 0.02$) and total plasma clearance was markedly decreased (2.66 ± 1.85 vs. 8.19 ± 2.80 L/hr · 1.73 m^2; $P < 0.001$). The $t_{1/2}$ was longer in patients with ascites or jaundice than in patients without these complications. The urinary excretion of unchanged pefloxacin was higher in the patients than in the subjects, while the excretion of *N*-desmethyl pefloxacin (a major metabolite of the drug) was lower. It is proposed that the decreased plasma clearance of pefloxacin in patients with cirrhosis is a result of decreased hepatic metabolism of the drug, and that the dosage should probably be modified in these patients. (CLIN PHARMACOL THER 38:439-442, 1985.)

Gaby Danan, M.D., Guy Montay, Rober Cunci, M.D., and Serge Erlinger, M.D.
Clichy and Alfortville, France

Pefloxacin, a new broad-spectrum antibacterial agent of the quinolone group (see structure), was shown effective in a preliminary trial of severe systemic infections.[8,9] Its use in patients with cirrhosis seems justified, since they frequently have gram-negative infections.[1] Pefloxacin is, however, demethylated and oxidized in the liver[7]; in addition, 20% to 30% of a single oral dose is excreted in bile as unchanged drug or metabolites.* Because the liver is the main site of the transformation of pefloxacin, the elimination of this drug could be modified in patients with liver disease. This could lead to accumulation of the drug and its active metabolite, which could be potentially toxic for the central nervous system, as are other quinolones. This study was undertaken to estimate the elimination kinetics of pefloxacin in patients with cirrhosis.

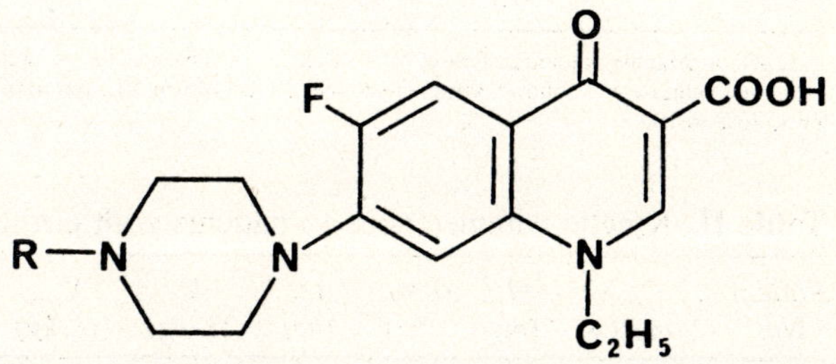

Pefloxacin (R = CH_3) and its main active *N*-desmethylated metabolite (R = H)

METHODS

Sixteen alcoholic patients (nine men and seven women) with histologically proved cirrhosis were included in the study. Informed consent was obtained from all patients. Their clinical and biochemical characteristics are listed in Table I. Nine patients had ascites (nos. 2, 4, 6, and 11 to 16). Except for thiamine and pyridoxine, no drugs were taken for at least 1 week before the study. All male patients were smokers.

After an overnight fast, patients received pefloxacin, 8 mg/kg total body weight. The drug was given as the mesylate salt diluted in 250 ml 5% dextrose solution in water infused intravenously over 1 hour. In all calculations the amount of pefloxacin itself was taken into account. Food was allowed 3 hours after dosing. Venous blood samples were drawn in tubes containing oxalate before and at 1, 1.5, 2, 3, 6, 9, 12, 24, 36, 48, 72, and 96 hours after the start of dosing. Plasma was separated from red blood cells by refrigerated centrifugation immediately after being drawn. Urine was collected for 96 hours from only six patients. Plasma and urine samples were frozen at −20° C until assayed.

Plasma levels of pefloxacin and urinary levels of pefloxacin and its active *N*-desmethylated metabolite were assayed by an HPLC method based on separation by reverse-phase ion-pair chromatography.[6] Two synthe-

From the Service d'Hépatologie and Unité de Recherches de Physiopathologie Hépatique (INSERM U-24), Hôpital Beaujon, Clichy, and Centre de Recherches du Laboratoire Roger Bellon, Alfortville.

Received for publication Jan. 18, 1985; accepted June 19, 1985.

Reprint requests to: S. Erlinger, M.D., Unité de Recherches de Physiopathologie Hépatique (INSERM U-24), Hôpital Beaujon, 92118 Clichy CEDEX, France.

*Gaillot J: Personal communication, 1985.

Table I. Clinical and biochemical characteristics of 16 patients with histologically proved cirrhosis

Patient No.	Sex	Age (yr)	Weight (kg)	Ascites	Serum creatinine (μmol/L)	Serum bilirubin (μmol/L)	ALAT (IU/L)	Serum albumin (gm/L)	Prothrombin level (% normal)
1	M	62	68	−	80	82	22	36	42
2	M	47	60	+	85	221	23	21	34
3	M	56	80	−	70	68	26	34	30
4	M	61	62	+	80	145	29	34	36
5	M	53	60	−	65	34	16	31	57
6	F	65	54	+	100	49	90	23	40
7	F	74	65	−	80	48	11	33	80
8	F	60	57	−	70	19	31	32	80
9	M	57	67	−	80	37	12	37	78
10	F	47	41	−	55	60	56	35	40
11	F	70	50	+	110	26	14	30	65
12	F	32	65	+	60	62	53	29	39
13	M	53	99	+	75	21	33	25	66
14	F	48	68	+	65	11	76	30	60
15	M	70	83	+	80	10	25	37	72
16	M	50	73	+	50	82	60	31	35
$\overline{X}$		56.6	65.8		75.3	59.7	36.1	31.1	53.4
SD		10.7	13.7		15.4	55.3	23.9	4.8	18.2

ALAT = Alanine aminotransferase; M = Male; − = absence; + = presence; F = female.
Normal values are as follows: serum creatinine, 50 to 110 μmol/L; serum bilirubin, <17 μmol/L; ALAT, 5 to 45 IU/L; serum albumin, 40 to 50 gm/L; prothrombin level, 80% to 100%.

Table II. Kinetic parameters in 16 patients with cirrhosis receiving a single dose of pefloxacin, 8 mg/kg iv

Patient No.	C_{max} (mg/L)	AUC (0-∞) (mg/L · hr)	$t_{1/2}$ (hr)	V_C (L/kg)	V_{area} (L/kg)	V_{ss} (L/kg)	CL (L/hr · 1.73 m²)	CL_R (L/hr · 1.73 m²)	CL_{NR} (L/hr · 1.73 m²)
1	11.9	233	31.8	0.31	1.62	1.57	2.40		
2	11.7	454	43.6	0.32	1.11	1.10	1.09		
3	8.2	264	37.3	0.57	1.63	1.61	2.14	0.80	1.34
4	7.5	339	44.7	0.87	1.54	1.52	1.57		
5	6.4	146	23.9	0.93	1.88	1.84	3.38	0.92	2.46
6	13.7	678	90.7	0.28	1.52	1.41	0.72	0.27	0.45
7	9.5	245	34.2	0.32	1.61	1.37	2.09		
8	8.4	110	12.1	0.35	1.27	1.24	4.49		
9	4.3	64	11.2	1.44	2.02	2.00	8.09	0.98	7.11
10	14.0	236	29.7	0.18	1.46	1.40	1.82	0.74	1.08
11	6.2	347	49.7	1.16	1.83	1.74	1.49		
12	8.8	270	26.0	0.84	1.11	1.10	1.96	0.69	1.27
13	7.5	402	47.1	0.96	1.35	1.34	1.62		
14	6.4	197	30.3	1.16	1.78	1.77	2.70		
15	6.9	119	14.5	0.95	1.41	1.39	5.10		
16	6.7	282	35.5	1.03	1.45	1.45	1.90		
mean	8.63	274	35.1	0.73	1.54	1.49	2.66	0.73	2.29
SD	2.82	151	19.0	0.39	0.26	0.25	1.85	0.25	2.45

C_{max} = Plasma concentration at the end of infusion; V_C = volume of central compartment; V_{ss} = steady-state volume of distribution; CL_R = renal clearance; CL_{NR} = nonrenal clearance.

sized analogs were used as internal standards. Sensitivity was 0.05 μg/ml for pefloxacin in plasma and 1 and 3 μg/ml for pefloxacin and its metabolite in urine, respectively. Coefficients of variation ranged from 4.5% to 6.4%.

The plasma concentration-time curves were analyzed according to an open two-compartment model by the ADAPT computer program.[2] For two patients (nos. 6 and 7) a three-compartment model was necessary to fit the data. The $t_{1/2}$ was calculated from the relationship:

Table III. Kinetic parameters of pefloxacin in 12 healthy subjects receiving a single dose of 400 mg iv and in 16 patients with cirrhosis receiving a single dose of 8 mg/kg iv

	Subjects	*Patients*
t½ (hr)	11.00 ± 2.64	35.10 ± 19.00*
V_{area} (L/kg)	1.88 ± 0.37	1.54 ± 0.26†
CL (L/hr · 1.73 m²)	8.19 ± 2.80	2.66 ± 1.85*

*P < 0.001, †P < 0.02.

$t_{1/2} = \ln 2/\beta$, where β is the slope of the last exponential phase. AUC values were calculated by the formula: $AUC = C_i/\lambda_i$, where C_i is the concentration and λ_i is an exponent of time. Total plasma clearance (CL) was calculated as: Dose/AUC. The volume of the central compartment, the area volume of distribution (V_{area}), and the volume of distribution at steady state were calculated according to Gibaldi and Perrier's formulas.[5]

Renal clearance of pefloxacin was calculated as the slope of a plot of the amount of pefloxacin excreted in urine during a time interval t_1 to t_2 $[(Xu)_{t1}^{t2}]$ vs. the AUC during the same time ($\int_{t1}^{t2} Cdt$).

Results are expressed as the $\overline{X}$ ± SD. Comparisons of kinetic parameters in 12 healthy men (mean age 26 years; range, 21 to 33 years) who received a single 400 mg iv dose of pefloxacin as a 1-hour infusion[4] was by the Mann-Whitney U test.

RESULTS

Pefloxacin tolerance was excellent. The plasma concentration-time curves for pefloxacin are shown in Fig. 1. Kinetic values for each patient are listed in Table II. Great variability was noted for AUC and $t_{1/2}$, with an eight- to 10-fold difference between the lowest and the highest values (patients 9 and 6, respectively).

The renal clearance of pefloxacin calculated in six patients (nos. 3, 5, 6, 9, 10, and 12) was 0.73 ± 0.25 L/hr, corresponding to a mean of about 28% of CL. Over the period 0 to 96 hours the urinary excretion of the unchanged pefloxacin was 25.80% ± 9.10% of the dose (Table III) and that of the principal active metabolite *N*-desmethyl pefloxacin was 13.78% ± 5.15%. Another metabolite in man, 4-oxo-*N*-desmethyl pefloxacin, was not detectable.

Because excretion data of pefloxacin and the metabolites were not available for all patients, urinary measurements must be considered only as rough estimates.

There was no significant correlation between CL and any of the liver function tests performed. However, the $t_{1/2}$ tended to increase according to the presence of ascites or jaundice: $t_{1/2}$ was 28 hours when jaundice alone was present (serum bilirubin level >30 μmol/L), 35.4 hours when ascites alone were present, and 48.1 hours when both ascites and jaundice were present.

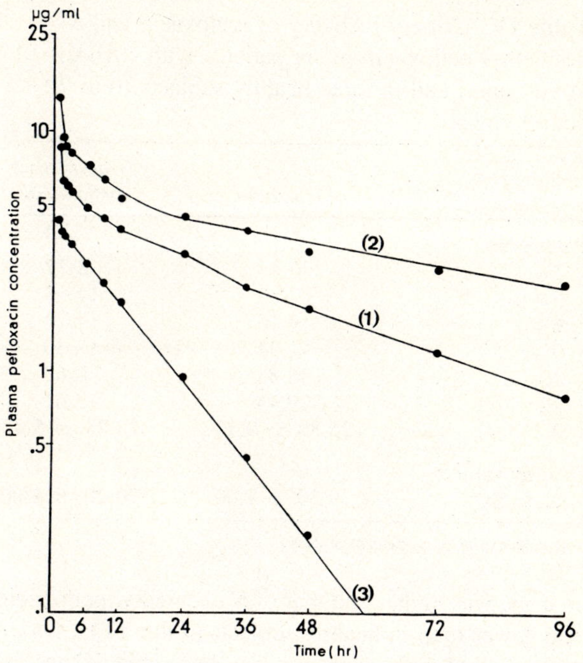

Fig. 1. Mean plasma concentration-time profile *(1)* in 16 patients with cirrhosis after a single intravenous dose of pefloxacin (8 mg/kg). Note the discrepancy between the highest *(2)* (patient 6) and the lowest *(3)* (patient 9) fitted curves.

There was no relationship between the nonrenal clearance of pefloxacin and serum levels of albumin or bilirubin or serum activity of alanine aminotransferase. However, there was a significant correlation between the nonrenal clearance (y) and prothrombin time (x) expressed as a percentage of the normal value; the equation was: $y = 0.13x - 3.88$ ($r = 0.923$; $P < 0.01$).

There was no relationship between V_{area} and serum albumin level.

DISCUSSION

Despite great variability, pefloxacin CL was markedly decreased in patients with cirrhosis (Table III). This clearance was about 30% of normal values. The $t_{1/2}$ increased by 219%. The V_{area} was slightly decreased, by 18% (Table III). Ascites did not significantly modify V_{area}. The renal clearance of pefloxacin was not different in patients and control subjects (0.61 ± 0.09 L/hr). Consequently, the extrarenal clearance of pefloxacin, which is equivalent to hepatic clearance, decreased.

In addition, the amount of the unchanged pefloxacin

Table IV. Urinary recovery of pefloxacin and *N*-desmethyl pefloxacin in six patients with cirrhosis (0 to 96 hours) and in three healthy subjects (0 to 72 hours)

	Pefloxacin	*N-desmethyl pefloxacin*
Patient No.		
3	30.44	8.77
5	27.60	14.65
6	19.16	14.73
9	11.34	18.30
10	36.88	6.60
12	29.44	19.62
$\overline{X} \pm$ SD	25.80 ± 9.10	13.78 ± 5.15
Healthy subjects		
$\overline{X} \pm$ SD	9.30 ± 1.00	20.20 ± 1.00

Results expressed as percent of dose.

in urine was higher and that of *N*-desmethyl pefloxacin was lower than in healthy subjects (Table IV)[7]; 4-oxo-*N*-desmethyl pefloxacin was not detectable. These results suggest that the main factor of the low CL could be the low rate of the hepatic metabolism of pefloxacin in patients with cirrhosis. The low CL explains, in part, the high plasma pefloxacin concentrations at the end of the infusion. However, this concentration did not reach a toxic level and the drug was well tolerated by all the patients.

There was no significant relationship between pefloxacin CL and any of the liver tests performed. However, the prolongation of the $t_{1/2}$ seemed to be related to the presence of jaundice or ascites. In addition, a close relationship was found between nonrenal clearance and prothrombin time; if all these data were confirmed by other studies, in particular with repeated doses, it could be possible to determine the dose of the drug according to biochemical or clinical characteristics of the patient.

CL has been found not to be changed in patients with chronic renal failure.* In our patients, 24-hour creatinine clearance was >60 ml/min. This condition has probably permitted the renal excretion of pefloxacin. There was no relationship between 24-hour creatinine clearance and renal clearance of pefloxacin. However, a correlation was found between these two clearances in patients with chronic renal failure.* Therefore, it can reasonably be assumed that in patients with cirrhosis, low creatinine clearance could exaggerate the decrease in pefloxacin plasma CL.

The minimal inhibitory concentration of pefloxacin ranges between 0.125 and 1 μg/ml for gram-negative bacteria generally encountered in patients with cirrhosis.[3] Since the mean plasma pefloxacin concentration was about 1 μg/ml 24 hours after dosing, it seems sufficient to give these patients a single daily intravenous dose of 8 mg/kg. Nevertheless, studies are warranted to measure the changes in kinetic parameters (in particular the accumulation rate) after repeated doses.

*Montay G: Unpublished observations, 1984.

We thank Mr. J. Gaillot and Mr. A. Frydman for communication of results in control subjects and Ms. M. Lebesgue and Mr. J. P. Tassel for their excellent technical assistance.

References

1. Conn HO: Cirrhosis. *In* Schiff L, Schiff ER, editors: Diseases of the liver. Philadelphia, 1982, JB Lippincott Company.
2. D'Argenio DZ, Schumitzky A: A program package for simulation and parameter estimation in pharmacokinetic systems. Comput Programs Biomed **9:**115-134, 1979.
3. Duval J, Acar JF, Bergogne-Berezin E, Christol D, Courtieu AL, Fleurette J, Lareng MB, Morel C, Thabaut A: In vitro activity of pefloxacin against 3,422 strains. A multicenter study. *In* Spitzy KH, Karrer K, editors: Pefloxacin. Presented at the Thirteenth International Congress of Chemotherapy, Vienna, Aug 28-Sept 3, 1983, part 110, pp 7-9.
4. Gaillot J, Frydman A, Le Roux Y, Fourtillan JB, Lefebvre MA, Duchier J, Djebbar F: Pharmacokinetics of pefloxacin in man during repeated treatment (400 mg b.i.d.) with i.v. infusion. *In* Spitzy KH, Karrer K, editors: Pefloxacin. Presented at the Thirteenth International Congress of Chemotherapy, Vienna, Aug 28-Sept 3, 1983, part 110, pp 18-22.
5. Gibaldi M, Perrier D: Pharmacokinetics. *In* Swarbrick J, editor: Drugs and the pharmaceutical sciences, vol 1. New York, 1975, Marcel Dekker, Inc.
6. Montay G, Blain Y, Roquet F, Le Hir A: High-performance liquid chromatography of pefloxacin and its main active metabolites in biological fluids. J Chromatogr **272:**359-365, 1983.
7. Montay G, Goueffon Y, Roquet F: Absorption, distribution, metabolic fate, and elimination of pefloxacin mesylate in mice, rats, dogs, monkeys, and humans. Antimicrob Agents Chemother **25:**463-472, 1984.
8. Thibault M, Koumare B, Soussy CJ, Duval J: Relations structure-activité dans le groupe des quinolones: Etude de l'activité bactérienne de deux nouveaux composés. Ann Microbiol (Inst Pasteur) **132A:**267-281, 1981.
9. Wolff M, Vittecoq D, Regnier B, Modai J, Vachon F, Sarrazin C, Bure A: Preliminary trial of pefloxacin in the treatment of urinary tract infections and in seriously ill patients treated in hospital. *In* Spitzy KH, Karrer K, editors: Pefloxacin. Presented at the Thirteenth International Congress of Chemotherapy, Vienna, Aug 28-Sept 3, 1983, part 110, pp 60-64.

Inhibition of prostaglandin synthesis by indomethacin interacts with the antihypertensive effect of atenolol

The interaction of inhibition of prostaglandin (PG) synthesis by indomethacin (75 mg/day) with the antihypertensive effect of atenolol (50 mg b.i.d.) was studied in 11 untreated otherwise healthy men 35 to 45 years old with essential hypertension. Atenolol for 3 weeks decreased supine blood pressure (BP) from 157/109 mm Hg during placebo to 148/97 mm Hg. Indomethacin alone for 1 week slightly increased BP and antagonized the antihypertensive action of atenolol. Atenolol reduced plasma renin activity (PRA) to 40% but did not modify either the urinary excretion of vasodilatory PGs (PGE_2 and prostacyclin measured as 6-keto-$PGF_{1\alpha}$) or plasma kininogen and urine kallikrein. Indomethacin suppressed PRA to 27% and PG excretion to approximately 70% but did not markedly change plasma kininogen and urine kallikrein excretion. The decreased excretion of 6-keto-$PGF_{1\alpha}$, the metabolite of the main vasodilatory prostanoid prostacyclin, correlated with the increased BP measured in standing subjects. The effects of indomethacin were practically the same when given with atenolol as when given alone. We conclude that the slight increase in BP by indomethacin in essential hypertension is associated with the reduced production of vasodilatory PGs but not with alterations in activities of the renin-angiotensin or kallikrein-kinin systems. (Clin Pharmacol Ther 38:443-449, 1985.)

Pauli Ylitalo, M.D., Timo Pitkäjärvi, M.D., Maija-Liisa Pyykönen, M.D., Anna-Kaisa Nurmi, M.Sc., Erkki Seppälä, M.D., M.Sc., and Heikki Vapaatalo, M.D.
Tampere, Finland

Indomethacin, an inhibitor of prostaglandin (PG) synthesis, increases blood pressure in hypertensive animals and to some degree also in patients with essential hypertension.[18,27] It also inhibits the antihypertensive effect of β-adrenergic blockers both in animals[7] and in man.[6,21] This effect has been considered to be due to the inhibition of PG synthesis. Watkins et al.[25] have shown that indomethacin decreases the urinary excretion of $PGF_{2\alpha}$ in patients with hypertension receiving propranolol. In our study, β_1-blockade by atenolol did not affect the urinary excretion of $PGF_{2\alpha}$ but it did decrease plasma renin activity (PRA),[19] while indomethacin decreased both of these.[27] Thus under certain conditions PRA seems to depend on the production of PGs, but the decrease in adrenergic β-receptor activity depresses the renin-angiotensin system with no marked effects on PGs. Both the renin-angiotensin system and PGs are closely connected to the kallikrein-kinin system, which has also been assumed to participate in the regulation of blood pressure and possibly even in the pathogenesis of hypertension.[14,16]

Our aim was to investigate the antagonism by indomethacin of the antihypertensive effect of atenolol in patients with essential hypertension, with special reference to inhibition of PG synthesis and the renin-angiotensin and kallikrein-kinin systems.

METHODS

Patients. Twelve male patients gave informed consent. Except for essential hypertension they were healthy and were between 35 and 45 years old ($\bar{X}$ = 40 years). They had been found to have diastolic blood pressure of ≥110 mm Hg in a health screening examination and thereafter on at least two successive visits to the Outpatient Hypertension Clinic. Seven patients had had high blood pressure for from 4 months to 9 years but none of them had received any previous antihypertensive therapy. On clinical examination the patients had no signs of secondary hypertension. Two patients had proteinuria but both of them had normal

From the Department of Biomedical Sciences, University of Tampere and the Community Health Centre.
Supported in part by a grant from Oy Star Ab, Tampere, Finland.
Received for publication March 3, 1985; accepted June 19, 1985.
Reprint requests to: Pauli Ylitalo, M.D., Department of Pharmacology and Toxicology, University of Kuopio, P.O.B. 6, SF-70211 Kuopio, Finland.

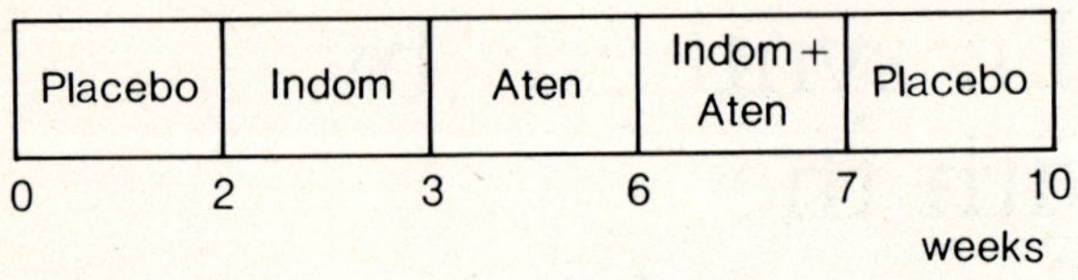

Fig. 1. Study design in 11 men with essential hypertension who received placebo, indomethacin (*Indom;* 75 mg/day), atenolol (*Aten;* 100 mg/day), and indomethacin with atenolol each for 1 to 3 weeks.

nephrography results, serum creatinine concentrations, and urine sediment and stain.

The patients were asked to continue their ordinary life-style throughout the study period, with no dietary restriction except for abstaining from alcoholic beverages and fasting in the mornings of the visits to the clinic. No coffee or tea was allowed on the day before the sampling, and drugs other than study drugs were not allowed. One of the 12 patients stopped the treatment 3 weeks after beginning the study because of misuse of alcohol.

Measurement of blood pressure. The diagnosis of hypertension was confirmed before the beginning of the trial at two or more visits after the screening examination. Blood pressure was measured in the morning both at rest after lying down for 30 minutes and while erect after 2 minutes' standing. Two measurements were made in each position, and heart rate was also determined in both positions. Blood pressure was measured at an accuracy of 2 mm Hg. Diastolic blood pressure was recorded at the fifth Korotkoff sound. Blood pressure was measured by the same physician in the same weekday at the same time in the right arm with the same brachial cuff and mercury manometer. The mean values recorded in both positions were used for analysis. The patients took their morning drug dose 2 hours before blood pressure was measured and laboratory samples were drawn.

Examinations. The following examinations were performed to uncover possible complications of the disease and to exclude secondary hypertension: careful physical examination, inspection of the ocular fundi, ECG, and chest x-ray with the estimation of heart size. Hypertensive changes in the ocular fundi were of 0 or 1 degree. Left ventricular hypertrophy was found in four patients (36%). These four men were considered to have hypertension of WHO stage 2.

Laboratory examinations before the start of the study included the following: hematocrit, hemoglobin, erythrocytes, mean corpuscular hemoglobin, mean corpuscular hemoglobin concentration, mean corpuscular volume, blood glucose, serum cholesterol, serum creatinine, serum sodium, serum potassium, serum calcium, serum urate, urine protein, urine glucose, urine sediment, and urine bacterial stain. None of the above parameters showed any signs of secondary hypertension or any other disease that could be considered to affect blood pressure or other parameters measured in this study.

Design of the trial. The design of the trial is presented in Fig. 1. After the placebo period for 2 weeks, the patients received indomethacin for 1 week with a conventional dose of 75 mg/day. Thereafter they received 50 mg atenolol alone twice a day for 3 weeks, and then atenolol in combination with indomethacin for 1 further week. Finally there was another placebo period of 3 weeks.

For the measurement of various laboratory parameters, venous blood samples were drawn after 30 minutes of supine rest by means of a polyethylene canula. Urine was collected over the preceding night for 12 hours, corresponding to the dose interval of placebo, atenolol, and indomethacin. All serum, plasma, and urine samples were taken at the end of each treatment period and stored at $-20°$ C until analyzed.

After each treatment period, side effects were recorded by asking if the patients had experienced any symptoms during the preceding drug period.

Measurement of laboratory parameters. Urine PGE_2, 6-keto-$PGF_{1\alpha}$ (a metabolite of prostacyclin), and thromboxane (Tx) B_2 were measured by RIA with a modification of the double-antibody procedure[23] and commercial antisera. Before the RIA 6-keto-$PGF_{1\alpha}$ was separated by TLC.[20] Plasma samples for renin determination were drawn into cooled test tubes containing 0.1N Na_2EDTA and were incubated for 1 hour at 37° C in the presence of renin substrate. The generated angiotensin I was measured by RIA according to the method of Fyhrquist et al.[10] Blood samples for kininogen measurement were drawn into ice-cold plastic tubes containing acid-citrate-dextrose anticoagulant solution. Plasma kininogen content was determined indirectly by measuring trypsin-released bradykinin from denatured kininase-free substrates.[11] The generated bradykinin was measured radioimmunologically.[12] Urine kallikrein activity was measured with a method based on *p*-nitroaniline release from the substrate S-2266 (kits of Kabi Diagnostica). The absorbance of *p*-nitroaniline was measured with a spectrophotometer at a wavelength of 405 nm.

The glomerular filtration rate was estimated as endogenous creatinine clearance. Creatinine in serum and urine were measured by a method based on the Jaffe

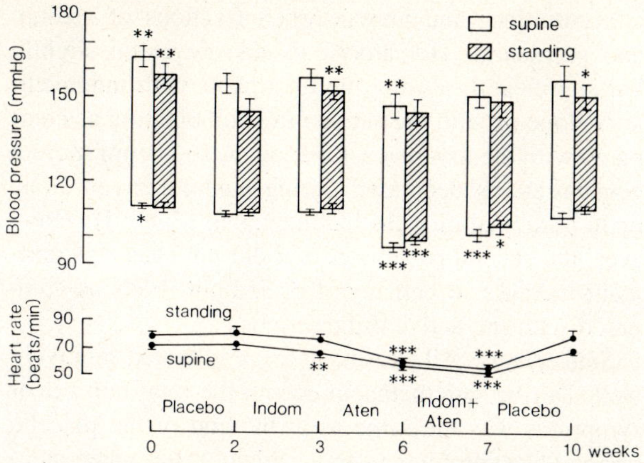

Fig. 2. Mean (± SE) systolic and diastolic blood pressures and heart rate values in supine and standing positions in 11 men with essential hypertension who received placebo, indomethacin (*Indom;* 75 mg/day), atenolol (*Aten;* 100 mg/day), and indomethacin with atenolol each for 1 to 3 weeks. $^{*}P < 0.05$, $^{**}P < 0.01$, $^{***}P < 0.001$ compared with values at the end of the first placebo period.

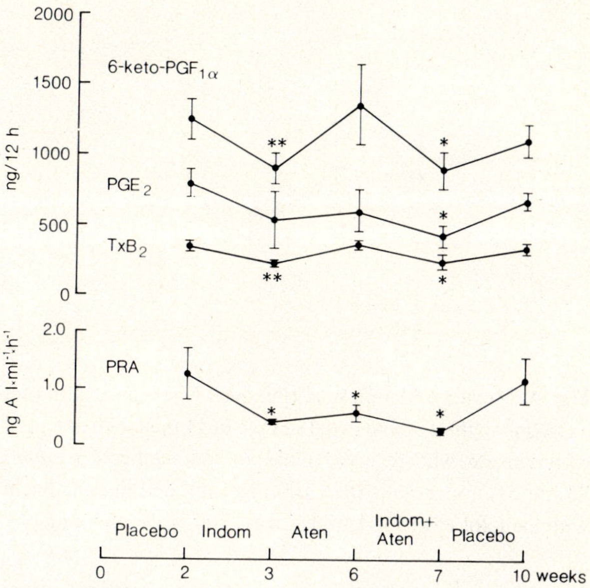

Fig. 3. Mean (± SE) 6-keto-$PGF_{1\alpha}$, PGE_2, and TxB_2 excretions in the 12-hour urine sample and PRA in 11 men with essential hypertension who received placebo, indomethacin (*Indom;* 75 mg/day), atenolol (*Aten;* 100 mg/day), and indomethacin with atenolol each for 1 to 3 weeks. $^{*}P < 0.05$, $^{**}P < 0.01$ compared with values at the end of the first placebo period. *A I* = Angiotensin I.

reaction.[5] The possible effect of drugs on renal handling of sodium and potassium was estimated by the proportion (percentage) of sodium and potassium not reabsorbed according to the following formula: (Na^+ or K^+ in urine × urine volume)/(creatinine clearance × Na^+ or K^+ in serum). Serum and urine sodium and potassium levels were measured by a flame photometer and serum osmolality was determined by the melting point of serum samples. The hematocrit was measured in heparinized centrifuge capillaries.

Statistics. Statistical analysis was by the paired t test. Two-tailed significance results are presented. Regression equations were calculated by the method of least squares.

RESULTS

Blood pressure and heart rate. Blood pressure values during the five different treatment periods are presented in Fig. 2. During the first placebo period there was a significant decrease ($P < 0.01$) in systolic blood pressure in both positions and in diastolic pressure in the supine position ($P < 0.05$). When indomethacin was thereafter given alone for 1 week, the blood pressure tended to increase, but the increase was significant ($P < 0.01$) only in systolic blood pressure in the standing position. During the 3-week atenolol period, except for systolic blood pressure in the standing position, blood pressures decreased significantly compared with values during placebo ($P < 0.01$ or $P < 0.001$). Mean supine blood pressure fell from 157/109 to 148/97 mm Hg and standing values fell from 153/110 to 145/99 mm Hg. When indomethacin was added the diastolic blood pressures rose from the preceding supine ($P < 0.05$) and standing ($P < 0.01$) values but remained below the values during the placebo period ($P < 0.001$ or $P < 0.05$, respectively). After discontinuation of active drug treatment (during the second placebo period), blood pressures rose again and systolic blood pressure in the standing position exceeded even the values after the first placebo period ($P < 0.05$).

There was a decrease ($P < 0.01$) in heart rate in the supine position during indomethacin dosing (Fig. 2). When atenolol was given alone for 3 weeks the heart rate decreased ($P < 0.001$) in both positions compared with values during the placebo period. The addition of indomethacin to atenolol further decreased heart rates in both the supine and standing positions ($P < 0.001$). At the end of the second placebo period heart rate returned to the levels during first placebo treatment.

PG excretion and PRA. Indomethacin reduced urinary excretion of 6-keto-$PGF_{1\alpha}$, PGE_2, and TxB_2 on average to 72%, 68%, and 65%, respectively, of the initial placebo values (Fig. 3). Atenolol alone did not modify the excretion of prostanoids and it did not alter

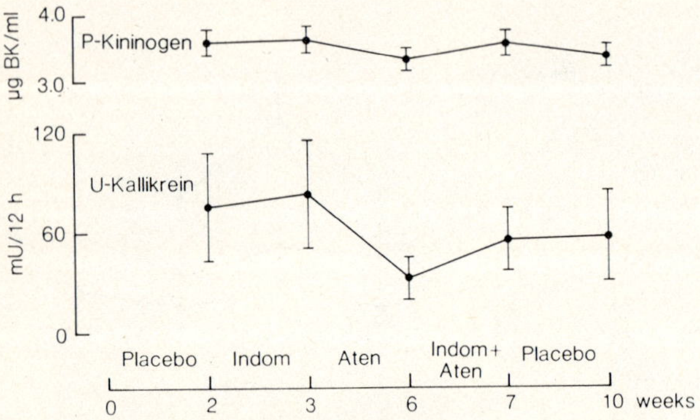

Fig. 4. Mean (±SE) plasma kininogen levels and kallikrein excretion in the 12-hour urine sample in 11 men with essential hypertension who received placebo, indomethacin (*Indom;* 75 mg/day), atenolol (*Aten;* 100 mg/day), and indomethacin with atenolol each for 1 to 3 weeks. *BK* = Bradykinin.

the reduction in prostanoid excretion caused by indomethacin alone. Withdrawal of active drugs reversed prostanoid excretion to about the level measured during the first placebo period. Indomethacin suppressed 6-keto-$PGF_{1\alpha}$ excretion in close correlation with the increase in systolic ($r = -0.714$; $n = 10$; $P < 0.05$) and diastolic ($r = -0.666$; $n = 10$; $P < 0.05$) blood pressures in the standing position. No other significant correlation could be drawn between the suppression of prostanoid excretion and the increased standing and supine blood pressures caused by indomethacin alone or in combination with atenolol.

Both indomethacin and atenolol given alone decreased the PRA to an average of 27% and 40% of the initial placebo values, respectively. The combination of the two drugs reduced PRA slightly but significantly more than either drug alone ($P < 0.05$). Discontinuation of the active drugs reversed PRA to about the initial level during placebo dosing. The alterations in PRA did not correlate with the changes in blood pressure caused by various treatments but did correlate significantly with overall changes in 6-keto-$PGF_{1\alpha}$ ($r = 0.394$; $n = 36$; $P < 0.05$) and TxB_2 ($r = 0.456$; $n = 33$; $P < 0.01$) excretion.

Plasma kininogen and urine kallikrein. There were no statistically significant changes in plasma kininogen and kallikrein excretion in urine in any phase of the trial (Fig. 4), although kallikrein excretion during atenolol dosing tended to be slightly suppressed.

Kidney function and other parameters. There were no changes in urine volume, glomerular filtration rate (evaluated on the basis of endogenous creatinine clearance), body weight, serum osmolality, serum potassium concentration, and unreabsorbed fractions of sodium and potassium. Hematocrit values decreased slightly but significantly during the treatments with indomethacin alone or with the active drug combination as compared with the first placebo period. Also, serum sodium concentrations decreased during atenolol given alone or in combination with indomethacin (Table I). However, the second placebo period did not cause a significant increase in hematocrit or sodium levels as compared with the active drug periods.

Side effects. All treatments were tolerated relatively well. During indomethacin dosing the total number of symptoms was the same as at the end of the placebo period (11 symptoms in four patients), but when atenolol was given alone the number of symptoms increased slightly (15 symptoms in eight patients). During combination therapy with atenolol and indomethacin there were as many symptoms as during the first placebo period (11 symptoms in six patients). All symptoms were quite conventional, such as tiredness, sleep disturbances, dry mouth, headache, dizziness, palpitation, numbness of legs, chest pain, sweating, and gastrointestinal symptoms. All side effects were slight and none were considered sufficient to stop the trial in any of the patients.

DISCUSSION

Our patient population was very homogeneous, which reduced variation. To achieve a situation better corresponding the normal life conditions, the patients had no restrictions in diet during the study. The dosage of indomethacin was not high, but it is the one commonly used in general practice and it effectively decreased prostanoid excretions. The daily dose of atenolol was 100 mg, which is generally recommended for the treatment of hypertension. This dose effectively decreased diastolic blood pressure, while in our experience smaller doses (50 mg/day) are clearly less effective in relatively young otherwise healthy men. With respect to systolic blood pressure, even atenolol, 100 mg/day, induced a decrease only in the supine position. This relatively weak effect on systolic blood pressure was probably because the patients had true diastolic hypertension while their systolic blood pressures were only slightly above normal.

Indomethacin induced a small increase in blood pressure as compared with placebo, but the increase was significant only in systolic blood pressure in the erect position. These results are comparable with those of our earlier study when we used the same daily dose (75 mg) of indomethacin.[27] The antihypertensive effect of

Table I. Kidney function and other parameters during different drug regimens in 11 men with essential hypertension

	Placebo for 2 wk	*Indomethacin for 1 wk*	*Atenolol for 3 wk*	*Indomethacin with atenolol for 1 wk*	*Placebo for 3 wk*
Body weight (kg)	79.8 ± 4.0	79.9 ± 4.0	80.7 ± 4.0	80.9 ± 4.0	81.3 ± 4.2
Urine volume (ml/12 hr)	756 ± 92	693 ± 98	701 ± 128	636 ± 61	595 ± 74
Glomerular filtration rate (ml/sec)	2.4 ± 0.1	2.3 ± 0.1	2.3 ± 0.1	2.3 ± 0.1	2.4 ± 0.1
Hematocrit	0.438 ± 0.008	0.422 ± 0.006*	0.427 ± 0.008	0.422 ± 0.007*	0.427 ± 0.006
Serum osmolality (mosm/kg H_2O)	288.0 ± 1.3	291.0 ± 1.2	288.4 ± 1.3	285.4 ± 1.9	286.1 ± 0.9
Serum sodium (mmol/L)	143.7 ± 0.8	143.2 ± 0.8	140.8 ± 0.7†	141.6 ± 0.9*	142.4 ± 0.8
Serum potassium (mmol/L)	4.4 ± 0.1	4.2 ± 0.1	4.1 ± 0.1	4.3 ± 0.1	4.1 ± 0.1
Unreabsorbed fraction of sodium in urine (%)	0.66 ± 0.05	0.76 ± 0.12	0.71 ± 0.07	0.79 ± 0.08	0.69 ± 0.05
Unreabsorbed fraction of potassium in urine (%)	7.5 ± 0.4	8.4 ± 1.0	7.9 ± 0.7	8.4 ± 0.9	7.9 ± 0.8

Data are $\bar{X}$ ± SE.
*P < 0.05, †P < 0.01 compared with values during the first placebo period.

atenolol also decreased when atenolol was given in combination with indomethacin. Observations like these have previously been made with other β-adrenergic blocking agents. Indomethacin increased blood pressure both in rabbits[7] and in patients receiving pindolol or propranolol.[6] In a study by Watkins et al.,[25] indomethacin, 100 mg/day, significantly ($P < 0.05$) increased blood pressure in patients with hypertension receiving both propranolol and a thiazide diuretic. All these changes in blood pressure have been proposed to be associated with the inhibition of synthesis of vasodilatory PGs. It is possible that the antagonism of an antihypertensive agent by indomethacin may be greater in subjects with more severe hypertension than in our patients, who had WHO stage 1 or 2 essential hypertension. Interactions may also be more marked when larger doses of indomethacin are used. In addition, little is known about the effect of other anti-inflammatory agents in patients receiving antihypertensive medication.[4,15,21] Thus our results cannot be generalized to other anti-inflammatory drugs. Blood pressure must be carefully observed in patients who receive the combination of these drugs. On the other hand, our results show that short-term indomethacin therapy interferes only slightly or moderately with the antihypertensive effect of atenolol in patients with moderate essential hypertension.

Indomethacin decreased heart rate significantly both before and during atenolol dosing. This negative chronotropic effect can be explained by compensatory reflex inhibition due to an increase in blood pressure, while direct cardiac effects of PG synthesis inhibition by indomethacin are of only minor importance.[26]

Both after the first placebo period and during atenolol dosing the increase in blood pressure by indomethacin coincided with the decreased excretion of prostanoids. The blood pressure elevations of individual subjects in the standing position were related to the decreases in the excretion of 6-keto-$PGF_{1\alpha}$, which is an important metabolite of vasodilating prostacyclin, considered to be the most important prostanoid regulating circulation.[24] Indomethacin also decreased the excretion of TxB_2, the stable metabolite of unstable platelet aggregating and vasoconstricting TxA_2, but the suppression in TxA_2 production was not able to abolish the tendency of blood pressure to increase after indomethacin, even if it should have reduced it.

As shown in earlier studies, PRA is significantly decreased both by indomethacin[9,13,27] and by atenolol.[1,3,19,22] In our study indomethacin also markedly suppressed the hypertensive renin-angiotensin system, but it simultaneously inhibited the production of vasodilatory prostanoids and increased blood pressure both after the placebo period and during atenolol dosing. These observations suggest that the increase in blood pressure by indomethacin is associated with reduced prostanoid production. Even the pronounced decrease in PRA could not eliminate the hypertensive effect of indomethacin. Also, atenolol decreased PRA but did not modify the excretion pattern of prostanoids. Thus the decrease in blood pressure by β-blockade was not associated with the PG system but may depend in part on the decrease in PRA. On the other hand, we and others found no significant correlation between the decreases in PRA and blood pressure by atenolol.[2,8,19] The positive correlation between PRA and prostanoid excretion calculated here and in our previous study[27] agrees well with the suggestion that renin release is at least partly mediated by PGs.[9] However, the dissociation between PRA and prostanoid excretion by atenolol and the PRA-decreasing interaction of indomethacin and atenolol support the hypothesis of Oates et al.[17] that renin excretion from the kidneys is regulated by PGs and β-adrenergic mechanisms, independently of each other.

None of the treatments significantly changed kallikrein excretion in urine or the level of plasma kininogen, the substrate for producing vasodilatory kinins. This suggests that the kallikrein-kinin system has no essential role in the antagonism of the antihypertensive effect of atenolol or in the increase in blood pressure caused by indomethacin in patients with mild or moderate essential hypertension.

Both indomethacin and atenolol were well tolerated. The number of symptoms the patient experienced as adverse effects increased only slightly during atenolol therapy but not during therapy with the combination or with indomethacin alone as compared with placebo. Indomethacin and atenolol had no significant effects on kidney function, since glomerular filtration rate, sodium and potassium reabsorption, urine volume, and body weight were not affected by any of the treatments. Thus the present indomethacin dosage caused no marked water retention to explain the increased blood pressure during the indomethacin treatment, but the slight decreases in hematocrit might reflect some minor gastrointestinal bleeding. However, the small decreases caused by active drugs in hematocrit and serum sodium concentration as compared with the first placebo period were probably of no marked biologic significance, since the second placebo period did not result in significant increases in these parameters.

As we and other authors have shown, indomethacin may increase blood pressure and it antagonizes the antihypertensive effect of atenolol. This unfavorable effect of indomethacin is associated with decreased production of vasodilatory PGs but is not related to changes in the activities of the renin-angiotensin and kallikrein-kinin systems.

Indomethacin, atenolol, and identical placebo capsules were supplied by Oy Star Ab, Tampere, Finland. PGE_2 and 6-keto-$PGF_{1\alpha}$ were supplied by Pasteur Institute, Paris, France, and TxB_2 was a gift from Dr. Christel Taube, Martin Luther University, Halle, GDR.

References

1. Åberg H: Plasma renin activity after the use of a new beta-adrenergic blocking agent (I.C.I. 66,082). Int J Clin Pharmacol **9**:98-100, 1974.
2. Amery A, Billiet L, Boel A, Fagard R, Reybrouck T, Willems J: Mechanism of hypotensive effect during beta-adrenergic blockade in hypertensive patients. Hemodynamic and renin response to a new cardioselective agent, Tenormin or ICI 66,082. Am Heart J **91**:634-642, 1976.
3. Balansard P, Chabrillat Y, Paulin R, Libes M, Gérard R: Effect of atenolol, a new cardioselective beta-blocker, on plasma renin activity in the treatment of hypertension. Acta Cardiol **32**:229-243, 1977.
4. Chalmers JP, West MJ, Wing LM, Bune AJ, Graham JR: Effects of indomethacin, sulindac, naproxen, aspirin, and paracetamol in treated hypertensive patients. Clin Exp Hypertens [A] **6**:1077-1093, 1984.
5. Clark LC Jr, Thompson HL: Determination of creatine and creatinine in urine. Anal Chem **21**:1218, 1949.
6. Durao V, Prata MM, Concalves LMP: Modification of antihypertensive effect of β-adrenoceptor–blocking agents by inhibition of endogenous prostaglandin synthesis. Lancet **2**:1005-1007, 1977.
7. Durao V, Rico JMGT: Modification by indomethacin of the blood pressure lowering effect of pindolol and propranolol in conscious rabbits. Eur J Pharmacol **43**:377-381, 1977.
8. Epstein SE, Lubbe WF: Effects of propranolol and atenolol on blood pressure and plasma renin activity in patients with moderate hypertension. S Afr Med J **52**:875-879, 1977.
9. Frölich JC, Hollifield JW, Dormois JC, Frölich BL, Seyberth H, Michelakis AM, Oates JA: Suppression of plasma renin activity by indomethacin in man. Circ Res **39**:447-452, 1976.
10. Fyhrquist F, Soveri P, Puutula L, Stenman U-H: Radioimmunoassay of plasma renin activity. Clin Chem **22**:250-256, 1976.
11. Hamberg U: Kininogen in human plasma after fibrinolytic activation. Scand J Clin Lab Invest **24**(suppl 107):37-47, 1969.
12. Hulthén UL, Borge T: Determination of bradykinin in blood by a sensitive radioimmunoassay. Scand J Clin Lab Invest **36**:833-839, 1976.
13. Lee JB, Patak RV, Mokerjee BK: Renal prostaglandins and the regulation of blood pressure and sodium and water homeostasis. Am J Med **60**:798-816, 1976.
14. Levinsky NG: The renal kallikrein-kinin system. Circ Res **44**:441-451, 1979.
15. Mills EH, Whithworth JA, Andrews J, Kincaid-Smith P: Non-steroidal anti-inflammatory drugs and blood pressure. Aust NZ J Med **12**:478-482, 1982.
16. Nasjletti A, Malik KU: Relationship between the kallikrein-kinin and prostaglandin systems. Life Sci **25**:99-110, 1979.
17. Oates JA, Whorton AR, Gerkens JF, Branch RA, Hol-

lifield JW, Frölich JC: The participation of prostaglandins in the control of renin release. Fed Proc **38:**72-74, 1979.
18. Patak RV, Mookerjee BK, Benzell CJ, Hysert PE, Babej M, Lee JB: Antagonism of effects of furosemide by indomethacin in normal and hypertensive man. Prostaglandins **10:**649-659, 1975.
19. Pitkäjärvi T, Ylitalo P, Metsä-Ketelä T, Vapaatalo H: The effects of a beta$_1$-blocking agent, atenolol, on blood pressure, plasma renin activity and prostaglandin $F_{2\alpha}$ excretion in patients with essential hypertension. Acta Med Scand **206:**107-113, 1979.
20. Riutta A, Seppälä E, Vapaatalo H: A rapid, sensitive method for detecting different arachidonic acid metabolites by thin-layer chromatography: The use of autoradiography. J Chromatogr **307:**185-189, 1984.
21. Salvetti A, Pedrinelli R, Alberici P, Magagna A, Abdel-Haq B: The influence of indomethacin and sulindac on some pharmacological actions of atenolol in hypertensive patients. Br J Clin Pharmacol **17**(suppl 1):108S-111S, 1984.
22. Sassard J, Pozet N, Vincent M, Zech PY: Atenolol and renin release. N Engl J Med **294:**787, 1976.
23. Seppälä E, Pora O, Metsä-Ketelä T: A modified method for extraction and purification of prostaglandins with resin XAD-2. Prostaglandins Leukotrienes Med **14:**235-241, 1984.
24. Vane JR: Prostaglandins and the cardiovascular system. Br Heart J **49:**405-409, 1983.
25. Watkins J, Abbot EC, Hensby CN, Webster J, Dollery CT: Attenuation of hypotensive effect of propranolol and thiazide diuretics by indomethacin. Br Med J **281:**702-705, 1980.
26. Wennmalm Å: Prostaglandin-mediated inhibition of noradrenaline release. VII. Effect of indomethacin on some cardiovascular reflexes in man. Acta Physiol Scand **117:**527-531, 1983.
27. Ylitalo P, Pitkäjärvi T, Metsä-Ketelä T, Vapaatalo H: The effect of inhibition of prostaglandin synthesis on plasma renin activity and blood pressure in essential hypertension. Prostaglandins Med **1:**479-488, 1978.

Transdermal nicotine reduces cigarette craving and nicotine preference

The effects of transdermal nicotine in 10 cigarette smokers were studied in a within-subjects, double-blind design. Either 8 mg nicotine base in a 30% aqueous solution or an inactive placebo solution was applied to intact skin under a polyethylene patch. Subjective reports of cigarette craving were collected every 30 minutes during a 90-minute smoking abstinence period. Immediately before and after this abstinence period subjects smoked through a smoke mixing device that allowed them to select their desired nicotine intake with each puff. Transdermal nicotine significantly increased saliva nicotine levels within 30 minutes after application. Cigarette craving was significantly lower in the nicotine condition than in the placebo condition. Nicotine preference during the initial puffs of the smoke mixer test at the end of 90 minutes of deprivation was also decreased by transdermal nicotine. In contrast, measures of cumulative smoke intake were not affected by the nicotine dose used. Our results suggest that transdermal nicotine may enhance success in smoking cessation by preventing the rise in cigarette craving usually observed after cessation. Transdermal nicotine may be preferable to other routes of nicotine administration because of the relative absence of adverse side effects. (CLIN PHARMACOL THER 38:450-456, 1985.)

Jed E. Rose, Ph.D., Joseph E. Herskovic, Ph.D., Yvonne Trilling, and Murray E. Jarvik, M.D., Ph.D. *Los Angeles, Calif.*

Smokers attempting to give up cigarettes frequently experience the tobacco withdrawal syndrome, which includes craving for cigarettes, irritability, anxiety, and inability to concentrate.[17] Nicotine substitution is a smoking cessation strategy based on the finding that nicotine partially alleviates this syndrome. For example, nicotine chewing gum has been shown to reduce smoking withdrawal symptoms and improve cessation success rates.[7,10,16] However, while nicotine gum may be a promising smoking cessation aid, it presents unpleasant side effects for some individuals, including bad taste, nausea, heartburn, and hiccups.[15] Transdermal nicotine is an alternative nicotine substitution method that would potentially avoid these side effects while delivering adequate doses of nicotine. In a previous study we found that significant systemic levels of nicotine resulted from topical application of 9 mg nicotine to the skin.[12] Nicotine levels peaked 90 minutes after the nicotine was applied and significant levels were maintained for over 3 hours. These findings suggest that transdermal nicotine merits investigation as a smoking cessation tool.

We examined the effects of transdermal nicotine on the early signs of smoking withdrawal during a 90-minute cigarette deprivation period. We also measured nicotine preference before and after this period by having subjects smoke through a smoke mixing device that enabled them to control the nicotine delivery of each puff.[13] Previous studies in our laboratory have shown that nicotine preference increases with cigarette deprivation and decreases with satiation,[11] and we wanted to determine whether transdermal nicotine would decrease nicotine preference and other indices of smoke intake.

From the Psychopharmacology Unit, Veterans Administration Medical Center and Department of Psychiatry and Biobehavioral Sciences, The Neuropsychiatric Institute, University of California School of Medicine.

Supported by the Medical Research Service of the Veterans Administration and by National Institute on Drug Abuse Grant No. DA 02665 from the United States Department of Health and Human Services.

Received for publication March 20, 1985; accepted June 19, 1985.

Reprint requests to: Jed E. Rose, Ph.D., Veterans Administration Medical Center, West Los Angeles Brentwood Division (691/B151D), Los Angeles, CA 90073.

METHODS

Subjects. Ten smokers (three men and seven women) participated in the study. Subjects smoked an average ($\pm$SD) of 29 $\pm$ 10.8 cigarettes per day with a mean nicotine delivery (Federal Trade Commission method) of 0.9 $\pm$ 0.20 mg. Subjects were chosen from a group that showed evidence of nicotine dependence in a preliminary screening session comparing nicotine preference after 12 hours of smoking abstinence with that immediately after smoking 10 puffs from a Marlboro Lights 100s cigarette (Phillip Morris Inc.) delivering 0.7 mg nicotine. We reasoned that transdermal nicotine would be likely to substitute for smoking only in those smokers who were dependent on nicotine. Nicotine preference was determined with a smoke mixing device (described below) with which subjects controlled the nicotine concentration of each puff.

For our purposes subjects were classified as nicotine dependent if nicotine preference was higher after overnight abstinence than after smoking. Fourteen of 23 subjects screened (61%) were classified as nicotine dependent, and 10 of these were chosen at random to complete the study.

Cigarettes. We used high- and low-nicotine cigarettes in a smoke mixing device to measures subjects' nicotine preference. To ensure that cigarettes differed only in nicotine delivery, we used commercial Marlboro Lights 100s cigarettes and added either distilled water or a small amount of nicotine base to the filter. Twenty microliters of water or 30% aqueous nicotine (6 mg) were injected approximately 1 cm axially into the cigarette filters. When smoked, the nicotine delivery of the nicotine-injected cigarettes was enhanced. To quantify nicotine delivery we used artificial smoking procedures that approximated Federal Trade Commission criteria (35 ml puffs, one every minute, to a butt length of 3 mm in excess of filter and overwrap) and analyzed the residue trapped in Cambridge filter pads (Phipps & Bird). Nicotine delivery of the low-nicotine control cigarettes agreed well with published values for that brand (0.73 ± 0.03 vs. 0.75 ± 0.02 mg), whereas nicotine-injected cigarettes delivered 1.5 ± 0.1 mg nicotine. Tar delivery was not affected by the nicotine injection technique.

Smoke mixing device. To control the nicotine delivery of each puff, subjects used an experimental smoke mixing device that blended smoke in graded amounts from the high- and low-nicotine cigarettes. By turning a knob, subjects could select any intermediate nicotine delivery desired. A dial reading ranging from 3.0 to 7.0 in 0.1-unit steps indicated the position of the knob on any given puff. We used a smoke mixer design similar to that described previously,[11,13] but modified the device so that a portion of smoke (15%) delivered through the high- and low-nicotine sides was diverted and trapped in Cambridge filter pads. By weighing the residue we could estimate the total particulate matter drawn into the smoker's mouth as well as the proportion of smoke selected from the high- and low-nicotine cigarettes.

Transdermal nicotine patches. Nicotine or placebo was topically applied under a 5 cm × 5 cm polyethylene patch. Nicotine base was administered in a 30% aqueous solution and the placebo consisted of a solution of food coloring in water that was visually identical to the nicotine solution. The volume of solution (26 μl) was equal to that of the 8 mg nicotine dose. An opaque polyethylene patch covered the area to prevent subjects from observing any changes in skin color (e.g., redness).

Saliva pH and expired air CO measurements. Because the ratio of nicotine concentration in saliva to that in blood depends on the pH,[14] we measured saliva pH to the nearest 0.1 unit. Expired air CO levels were measured with an electrochemical analyzer before and after each nicotine preference test to estimate smoke inhalation.[6] Samples were collected after 20 seconds of breath holding and discarding the first 500 ml of expirate to eliminate dead-space air from the sample.

Procedure. Subjects entered the laboratory on three consecutive afternoons without having abstained from tobacco. Subjects were informed that either nicotine or placebo would be administered transdermally and informed consent was obtained. On all days the session began with a nicotine preference test in which subjects were instructed to first take a puff from the middle, low, and high nicotine settings of the smoke mixer. Then they were allowed to smoke freely for 10 minutes, adjusting the nicotine delivery of each puff to the level desired. The sides of the mixer in which the high- and low-nicotine cigarettes were placed were counterbalanced across subjects. Subjects recorded the mixer dial reading to the nearest 0.1 unit and rated the strength, harshness, and desirability of each puff using 10-point scales ranging from "not at all" (0) to "extremely" (9).

After the preference test subjects received in a double-blind fashion either 0, 4, or 8 mg nicotine in a transdermal patch taped to the volar surface of the nondominant forearm. Our previous study[12] had suggested that due to the relatively slow absorption of nicotine through the skin, a much higher dose than is delivered by a cigarette would be necessary to produce reliable effects. However, because transdermal administration of nicotine is still a relatively new experimental procedure, the 4 mg dose was always administered on the first day as a safety precaution. Data from this day were not included in any analyses because the order of presentation of this screening day was not counterbalanced. No adverse reactions were noted in any subject for either the 4 or 8 mg dose, and hence no subjects were eliminated from the study. The placebo and 8 mg nicotine doses were presented on days 2 and 3 in counterbalanced order. No carryover effects were anticipated, because (1) any residual influence of the transdermal nicotine received the previous day would have been masked by the several cigarettes smoked between sessions, and (2) the nicotine metabolic $t_{1/2}$ is relatively short (2 hours).[3]

The skin was cleansed with 70% isopropyl alcohol before application of the transdermal patch, and after its application subjects were not allowed to smoke for 90 minutes. Every 30 minutes they completed the Shiffman-Jarvik questionnaire to assess smoking withdrawal symptoms.[18] Heart rate, an index of nicotine effects, was also measured at these times by counting the radial pulse for 30 seconds.

To monitor the absorption of transdermal nicotine, saliva samples were collected every 30 minutes for subsequent nicotine analysis. Saliva flow was stimulated by having subjects hold a sugar cube in the mouth and expectorate into a vial. Saliva pH was measured to estimate blood nicotine levels from the expected ratio of nicotine in the free base form (which passes readily between saliva and blood) to that in the positively charged form (which does not readily pass between saliva and blood). Before stimulating saliva flow, subjects rinsed their mouths three times with water to minimize any contamination of saliva by nicotine previously ingested in cigarette smoke.

Ninety minutes after the patch was applied, a second nicotine preference test was administered. Transdermal patches were removed at the end of the session and subjects were asked to indicate whether they believed they had received nicotine or placebo.

Saliva nicotine levels. Saliva samples collected 30 minutes after application of the patch were sent to the Clinical Psychopharmacology Laboratory at the Veterans Administration Medical Center in Sepulveda for nicotine assay. The accuracy of the HPLC technique used was ±10%. Two samples were not analyzed because of apparatus difficulties. The remaining saliva nicotine concentrations were transformed to yield estimated blood levels through use of a correction factor based on the relative pH of saliva and blood. Assuming negligible plasma protein binding,[3] the ratio of nicotine in saliva to that in blood is theoretically estimated[19] by the fraction: $(1 + 10^{(pKa - pH\ saliva)})/(1 + 10^{(pKa - pH\ plasma)})$. The pH of plasma was assumed to be 7.4 and the pKa of nicotine at 37° C was taken to be 7.75.[5]

Withdrawal measures. Withdrawal questionnaire data were scored according to a previous factor analysis validation study,[18] resulting in the following scales: craving, arousal, appetite, psychologic symptoms, and physical symptoms.

Smoking measures. Three indices of nicotine preference during the smoking periods were calculated: (1) the mean proportion of particulate matter obtained from the high-nicotine side of the mixer, determined by weighing residue trapped in the Cambridge filter pad in each barrel of the mixer; (2) the mean preference for the high-nicotine cigarette as calculated from the dial settings recorded for each puff, determined by transforming the dial readings into flow ratios with calibration curves relating dial reading to the proportion of air flowing through each side of the mixer. During calibration tests air flow was measured with spherical float flowmeters. Because the nicotine concentration selected at the end of each smoking period may have been influenced by satiation produced by the early puffs, the mean nicotine preferences for the first two voluntary puffs (after the three mandatory puffs) and the last two puffs were calculated separately; and (3) the change in puff desirability ratings with increasing nicotine content, calculated by plotting for each subject the desirability ratings of each puff against the proportion of smoke taken from the high-nicotine cigarette during that puff. The slope of the regression line reflected the change in puff desirability induced by a change in nicotine content. A more positive slope indicated a greater desire for nicotine.

In addition to these specific measures of nicotine preference, overall smoke intake was estimated by the number of puffs taken during the preference test, the total particulate intake (sum of the high- and low-nicotine sides), and the increase in expired air CO after smoking. These measures were, of course, not specific indices of nicotine preference and could have reflected the reinforcing characteristics of other aspects of the habit (puffing, "tar," handling, etc.).

RESULTS

Smoking withdrawal. Each measure of smoking withdrawal from the Shiffman-Jarvik questionnaire was analyzed by repeated-measures 2 (nicotine dose) × 4 (time) ANOVA. Craving increased significantly over time ($P < 0.001$) and there was a significant nicotine × time interaction ($P < 0.001$). Craving increased differentially on the placebo day (Fig. 1).

Appetite showed a significant increase over time ($P < 0.0001$), and arousal decreased over time ($P < 0.01$), with no effects of nicotine. No effects of either 90 minutes of deprivation or nicotine were noted for physical or psychologic symptoms.

Nicotine preference and smoke intake. In view of the high peak plasma nicotine levels produced by smoking,[14] it seemed logical to assess the effect of transdermal nicotine on nicotine preference during the first

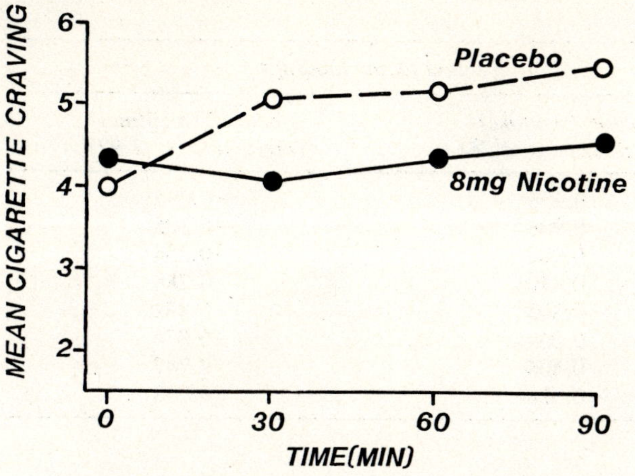

Fig. 1. Mean reported cigarette craving during a 90-minute deprivation period after application of a transdermal patch containing either 8 mg nicotine or placebo.

two puffs of the smoke mixer test, before subsequent puffs overshadowed the effect of transdermal nicotine. A 2 (nicotine dose) × 2 (mixer) repeated-measures ANOVA revealed that nicotine preference was lower in the 8 mg nicotine condition for the second mixer test 90 minutes after the transdermal patch was applied ($P < 0.03$; Fig. 2). A similar analysis was conducted for nicotine preference on the last two puffs in each mixer test, but no effect of deprivation or nicotine dose was found.

Surprisingly, nicotine preference did not increase after the 90-minute deprivation interval for either the first or last puffs. Therefore, we conducted an additional analysis to determine whether a decrease in nicotine preference with satiation occurred across puffs within a mixer test. Visual inspection of the data revealed striking individual differences across subjects, so a separate paired t test was conducted for each subject comparing nicotine preference on the last two puffs with that on the first two puffs for the four smoke mixer tests (mixer tests 1 and 2, nicotine and placebo days). Although the statistical power of these tests was low, there was evidence for a satiation effect across puffs that resulted in a decline in nicotine preference from initial to final puffs for eight of 10 subjects. For three subjects this decline was significant ($P < 0.05$), but one subject showed a consistent increase in nicotine preference across puffs ($P < 0.01$). Thus there were individual differences that confounded an analysis of trends with pooled data, but results strongly suggested that at least some subjects showed the expected decline in nicotine seeking after satiation.

A 2 (nicotine dose) × 2 (mixer) ANOVA was also conducted for the best a priori measure of cumulative

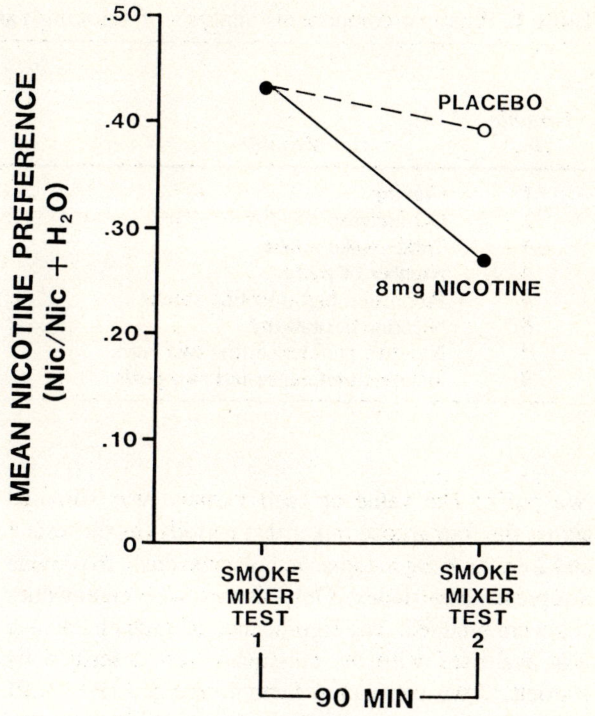

Fig. 2. Effects of transdermal nicotine on nicotine-seeking behavior. Shown are subjects' mean nicotine preference scores (proportion of smoke selected from a nicotine-injected vs. a water-injected cigarette) during the first two puffs of smoke mixer test periods before and 90 minutes after application of either a transdermal nicotine or placebo patch.

smoke intake. This measure was obtained by adding the total estimated smoke particulate intake for both high- and low-nicotine cigarettes as calculated from the weight of the smoke residue trapped in the Cambridge filter pads attached in parallel to each barrel of the mixer. This analysis failed to show any effect of either transdermal nicotine or 90 minutes of deprivation on total particulate intake.

Factor analysis of smoking measures. To examine the interrelationship between the measures of smoking just discussed and the remaining dependent measures collected during the experiment, we conducted a principal components analysis on the following eight dependent variables: (1) cigarette craving reported immediately before the smoke mixer test; (2) increase in expired air CO after smoking; (3) total smoke particulate matter taken from both cigarettes in the mixer; (4) number of puffs taken from the smoke mixer; (5) proportion of smoke obtained from the high-nicotine cigarette (measured by trapped particulate matter); (6) slope of the regression line relating puff desirability to nicotine content; (7) nicotine preference during the first two puffs; and (8) nicotine preference during the last

Table I. Principal components analysis of smoking variables

Variable No.	Variable	Rotated factor loadings: Factor 1 (smoke) (eigenvalue = 3.76)	Factor 2 (nicotine) (eigenvalue = 2.97)
1	Craving	0.938	−0.096
2	CO increase	0.906	−0.305
3	Total smoke intake	0.900	−0.254
4	Number of puffs	0.840	−0.288
5	Proportion high-nicotine smoke	−0.303	0.892
6	Nicotine desirability	0.069	0.874
7	Nicotine preference first two puffs	0.404	0.782
8	Nicotine preference last two puffs	−0.528	0.738

two puffs. The value of each variable was summed across the four smoke mixer test periods (mixer tests 1 and 2 on the 8 mg nicotine and placebo days) to provide a representative index. Only factors with eigenvalues >1 were retained. The significance of each eigenvalue was evaluated with the chi-square test described by Bartlett.[2] Two substantial factors emerged ($P < 0.01$ for factor 1 and $P < 0.02$ for factor 2) that together accounted for 84% of the total variance. Varimax rotation yielded a simplified factor structure (Table I). The first factor (smoke) encompassed variables 1 to 4, which comprised all the cumulative measures of smoke intake and, interestingly, included craving. The second factor (nicotine) consisted of all the variables postulated to be specific measures of nicotine preference (variables 5 to 8). The residual correlation matrix after extraction of these two factors was not significant.

Estimated blood nicotine levels. Blood nicotine levels were estimated from saliva levels as described above. A paired t test comparison between placebo and 8 mg transdermal nicotine confirmed that nicotine levels on the active treatment day (16 ± 12.3 ng/ml) were significantly higher than those during placebo (10 ± 8.5 ng/ml; $P < 0.01$). Thus at least some nicotine was absorbed from the transdermal patch.

Heart rate. A 2 (nicotine dose) × 4 (time) ANOVA showed that heart rate declined steadily over the 90-minute deprivation period, from 81 ± 10.6 to 74 ± 11.1 bpm ($P < 0.00001$) but was not affected by transdermal nicotine. A 2 (nicotine dose) × 2 (mixer) ANOVA on the change in heart rate after each smoking period showed that heart rate increased after the second mixer test after 90 minutes deprivation more than after the first smoking period in each session ($P < 0.05$ for the main effect of mixer). A t test for the mean heart rate change after the first mixer period indicated that the first smoking period did not increase heart rate (mean change −0.8 ± 3.4 bpm). In contrast, the mean heart rate increase after the second mixer test was +2 ± 2.3 bpm ($P < 0.05$).

Efficacy of the double-blind design. Subjects' responses to the questionnaire asking whether they believed they had received nicotine on each day were scored. Responses were counted as correct if subjects stated nicotine was received on the 8 mg day and not on the placebo day. Only four of the 10 subjects guessed correctly on both days, and assuming the probability of success was 0.25 for random guessing, the probability of the observed level of performance or better was 0.22. Thus subjects' ability to discriminate accurately between the placebo and 8 mg nicotine conditions was not significantly better than chance.

DISCUSSION

Transdermal nicotine prevented the increase in craving for cigarettes during a short deprivation period of 90 minutes. It also diminished the preference for nicotine during the initial puffs of the subsequent smoking period. Despite the influence of transdermal nicotine in this experiment, subjects generally were not able to discriminate nicotine from placebo. These findings suggest that like nicotine chewing gum, transdermal nicotine may be a useful smoking cessation aid. However, transdermal nicotine may offer several advantages over nicotine gum that could increase the efficacy of a smoking cessation program. First, transdermal nicotine does not produce the bad taste and gastrointestinal problems sometimes associated with nicotine gum. Further, the dental problems and sore jaw sometimes caused by nicotine gum would be avoided. A transdermal patch containing a large quantity of nicotine (e.g., 50 mg) that has a membrane-limited delivery rate should be capable of sustaining nicotine levels over extended periods of time (e.g., 24 hours). The reduction of adverse side effects and the possibility for sustained release should improve compliance with smoking cessation programs.

With the exception of craving, no effects of 90 minutes of deprivation were observed on most indices of smoking withdrawal, e.g., physical and psychologic symptoms. Thus a longer abstinence period may be required to test the effectiveness of transdermal nicotine in alleviating these tobacco withdrawal complaints. Also, further studies measuring plasma nicotine levels will be necessary to assess the reliability and efficiency of nicotine absorption through the skin.

Results of the principal components analysis supported the view that there are two independent components of smoking behavior—preference for a certain nicotine concentration in smoke (nicotine) and a second factor (smoke) reflecting overall cumulative smoke ingestion. Transdermal nicotine reduced cigarette craving without affecting cumulative smoke intake. One explanation for this may be that the small increase in plasma nicotine levels produced by transdermal nicotine was sufficient to alleviate craving to some extent, but was still far below the amount required to induce complete satiation. Hence when allowed to smoke subjects took roughly the same amount of nicotine as in the placebo condition. An alternative possibility is that cumulative intake may have reflected a nonpharmacologic component of smoking satisfaction. Craving for the pharmacologic effects of nicotine may have been reduced by transdermal nicotine, but craving for the other stimuli associated with smoking (e.g., chemosensory stimulation of the respiratory tract[4]) would not have been satisfied. The latter possibility is consistent with the poor regulation of nicotine levels usually observed in smoking titration studies[1] and the finding that intravenous nicotine induces little if any suppression of smoking behavior relative to cigarette smoke itself.[9] Further research should clarify the relationship between plasma nicotine levels and nicotine preference.

Additionally, nicotine preference and smoke intake might be affected not only by plasma nicotine levels but also by the degree of acute tolerance to nicotine, which varies with cigarette deprivation.[8] In our present study the significantly greater heart rate increase after the second smoke mixer period relative to the first suggests that some tolerance to nicotine was lost after 90 minutes of deprivation. Possibly, an increased sensitivity to nicotine's reinforcing effects could have led to the increased craving for a cigarette after 90 minutes. The loss of tolerance to nicotine also may have prevented an increase in nicotine intake during the second smoke mixer test (Fig. 2). The hypothesis that nicotine tolerance affects preferred nicotine levels and cigarette craving should be evaluated in future studies to further our understanding of tobacco withdrawal and to illuminate its components.

References

1. Ashton H, Stepney R: Smoking: Psychology and pharmacology. London, 1982, Tavistock.
2. Bartlett MS: Tests of significance in factor analysis. I. Description and illustration of a test of significance for analysis into principal components. Br J Psychol **3**(part II):77-85, 1950.
3. Benowitz NL, Jacob P III, Jones RT, Rosenberg J: Interindividual variability in the metabolism and cardiovascular effects of nicotine in man. J Pharmacol Exp Ther **221**:368-372, 1982.
4. Cain WS: Sensory attributes of cigarette smoking. *In* Gori GB, Bock FG, editors: Banbury Report 3: A Safe Cigarette? New York, 1980, Cold Spring Harbor Laboratory, pp 239-249.
5. Domino EF: Behavioral, electrophysiological, endocrine, and skeletal muscle actions of nicotine and tobacco smoking. *In* Remond A, Izard C, editors: Electrophysiological effects of nicotine. Amsterdam, 1979, Elsevier/North Holland Biomedical Press, pp 133-146.
6. Hopkins R, Wood LE, Sinclair NM: Evaluation of methods to estimate cigarette smoke uptake. CLIN PHARMACOL THER **36**:788-795, 1984.
7. Hughes JR, Hatsukami DK, Pickens RW, Krahn D, Malin S, Luknic A: Effect of nicotine on the tobacco withdrawal syndrome. Psychopharmacology **83**:82-87, 1984.
8. Jones RT, Farrell TR III, Herning RI: Tobacco smoking and nicotine tolerance. *In* Krasnegor NA, editor: Self-administration of abused substances: Methods for study. DHEW Publ No (ADM)78-727. Rockville, Md, 1978, National Institute on Drug Abuse.
9. Kumar R, Cooke EC, Lader MH, Russell MAH: Is nicotine important in tobacco smoking? CLIN PHARMACOL THER **21**(5):520-528, 1976.
10. Raw M, Jarvis MJ, Feyerabend C, Russell MAH: Comparison of nicotine chewing-gum and psychological treatments for dependent smokers. Br Med J **281**:481-482, 1980.
11. Rose JE, Jarvik ME, Ananda S: Nicotine preference increases after cigarette deprivation. Pharmacol Biochem Behav **20**:55-58, 1984.
12. Rose JE, Jarvik ME, Rose KD: Transdermal administration of nicotine. Drug Alcohol Depend **13**:209-213, 1984.
13. Rose JE, Lafer RL, Jarvik ME: A smoke-mixing device for measuring nicotine preference. Behav Res Methods Instrument **14**:501-503, 1982.
14. Russell MAH, Feyerabend C: Cigarette smoking: A dependence on high-nicotine boli. Drug Metab Rev **8** (12):29-57, 1978.

15. Russell MAH, Raw M, Jarvis MJ. Clinical use of nicotine chewing-gum. Br Med J **280:**1599-1602, 1980.
16. Schneider NG, Jarvik ME, Forsythe AB: Nicotine vs. placebo gum in the alleviation of withdrawal during smoking cessation. Addict Behav **9:**149-156, 1984.
17. Shiffman SM: The tobacco withdrawal syndrome. *In* Krasnegor NA, editor: Cigarette smoking as a dependence process. DHEW Publ No. (ADM)79-800. Rockville, Md, 1979, National Institute on Drug Abuse.
18. Shiffman SM, Jarvik ME: Smoking withdrawal symptoms in two weeks of abstinence. Psychopharmacology **50:**35-39, 1976.
19. Zylber-Katz E, Granit L, Levy M: Relationship between caffeine concentrations in plasma and saliva. CLIN PHARMACOL THER **36:**133-137, 1984.

Pharmacokinetics of high-dose pentobarbital in severe head trauma

High-dose pentobarbital infusion has been advocated as an effective adjunct in controlling persistent intracranial hypertension after severe head trauma in patients refractory to conventional therapy. Pentobarbital disposition was assessed in 10 adults with severe nonpenetrating head injury after an intravenous loading dose of sodium pentobarbital, 10 mg/kg, infused over 1 hour, followed by a continuous infusion at 0.5 to 3.0 mg/kg/hr provided the cerebral perfusion pressure remained >50 torr. Pharmacokinetic parameters of volume of distribution at steady state (V_{ss}), total body clearance (CL), and $t_{1/2}$ for the patients with trauma were statistically compared with similar estimates reported for seven adult subjects without head injury. On discontinuation of the pentobarbital infusion, serum concentrations in the patients followed a monoexponential decline with a mean (±SD) $t_{1/2}$ and V_{ss} that were significantly less than values reported for the control subjects (15.6 ± 3.9 vs. 22.3 ± 4.0 hours and 44.0 ± 11.7 vs. 63.4 ± 15.2 L, respectively). However, there was no significant difference between the mean pentobarbital CL of the patients (2.0 ± 0.7 L/hr) and the subjects (2.0 ± 0.4 L/hr). To our knowledge this is the first report on the disposition, elimination, and intrasubject variability of high-dose pentobarbital infusion in adult patients with head trauma. (CLIN PHARMACOL THER 38:457-461, 1985.)

Charles D. Bayliff, Pharm.D., Michael L. Schwartz, M.D., and Brian G. Hardy, Pharm.D. *Toronto, Ontario, Canada*

The use of barbiturates to control intracranial pressure in neurosurgical patients is well documented.[7-9,11,13] While the effect of these agents on patient outcome is as yet unresolved, a number of case reports[7,14] and clinical studies[8,9] have demonstrated that barbiturates can reduce elevated intracranial pressure that is refractory to conventional therapy such as fluid restriction, controlled hyperventilation, intravenous mannitol, or high-dose dexamethasone. Marshall et al.[9] effectively used pentobarbital to reduce or normalize intracranial pressure in 76% and 52% of patients, respectively, who had elevated intracranial pressure unresponsive to other treatments. These investigators administered pentobarbital to achieve a steady-state serum concentration of 25 to 35 mg/L (110 to 155 μmol/L), a range extrapolated from observations of comatose patients after drug overdose[2] and values comparable with those reported in subsequent studies.[5,7,13,14] While acknowledging that a wide variation in dose is required to produce a therapeutic concentration, Marshall et al. did not attempt to account for these differences based on intrasubject variabilities in the disposition and elimination of pentobarbital. Schaible et al.[12] compared the pharmacokinetics of pentobarbital in 11 pediatric patients with hypothermia with those reported by Ehrnebo[3] in normal adults. However, to our knowledge there is no study to date that characterizes pentobarbital pharmacokinetics in adult patients with head trauma who are receiving high-dose pentobarbital infusions.

In our present study we examined the steady-state disposition and overall elimination of pentobarbital in adult patients with head injury who were receiving the drug for control of elevated intracranial pressure.

METHODS

Ten adult patients (nine men and one woman) aged 18 to 75 years who were enrolled in a multicenter trial[13] comparing the use of mannitol vs. pentobarbital in severe nonpenetrating head injury were selected. Demographic characteristics and outcome data for these patients are listed in Table I. Patients admitted to the surgical intensive care unit at Sunnybrook Medical Centre with severe head trauma received pentobarbital only if their intracranial pressure was >25 torr for 15 minutes. Each patient received an initial intravenous loading dose of sodium pentobarbital (Nembutal; Abbott Laboratories) of 10 mg/kg infused over 1 hour,

From the Departments of Pharmacy and Surgery, Division of Neurosurgery, Sunnybrook Medical Centre, University of Toronto.
Received for publication Feb. 26, 1985; accepted June 21, 1985.
Reprint requests to: Brian G. Hardy, Pharm.D., Research and Clinical Coordinator, Department of Pharmacy, Sunnybrook Medical Centre, University of Toronto, 2075 Bayview Ave., Toronto, Ontario M4N 3M5, Canada.

Table I. Demographics of the 10 patients with head trauma

Patient No.	Sex	Age (yr)	Incident	Outcome	Infusion duration (hr)
1	M	20	MVA	Alive/well	156
2	M	32	MVA	Died	68
3	M	50	MVA	Died	96
4	M	27	MVA	Died	43
5	M	27	MVA	Alive/well	117
6	M	29	Fall	Alive/well	86
7	F	75	Fall	Died	126
8	M	20	MVA	Died	55
9	M	26	Fall	Alive/decerebrate	33
10	M	18	MVA	Died	81

M = Male; MVA = motor vehicle accident; F = female.

Table II. Pentobarbital pharmacokinetics in the 10 patients with head trauma

Patient No.	V_{ss} (L)	$t_{1/2}$ (hr)	CL (L/hr)
1	23.0	20.1	1.3
2	46.7	19.3	1.6
3	63.4	15.8	2.8
4	45.7	15.6	1.1
5	37.1	11.8	2.1
6	40.4	11.2	2.8
7	54.4	13.5	1.8
8	42.4	22.5	1.2
9	33.0	15.0	2.3
10	54.4	11.5	3.1
$\bar{X}$	44.0	15.6	2.0
SD	11.7	3.9	0.7

followed by a continuous infusion at 0.5 to 3.0 mg/kg/hr provided the cerebral perfusion pressure remained >50 torr. The cerebral perfusion pressure was estimated as the difference between mean arterial pressure and intracranial pressure. Additional increments in the pentobarbital infusion rate were allowed when the intracranial pressure was >20 torr, as long as the serum pentobarbital concentration did not exceed 45 mg/L (200 μmol/L).

Timed blood samples were drawn through an indwelling arterial catheter 1 hour after the loading dose and at a mean (±SD) of 8.2 ± 4.2–hour intervals during pentobarbital infusion. Pentobarbital therapy was continued for at least 24 hours after an episode of intracranial pressure >20 torr. Upon discontinuation of therapy, serum pentobarbital concentrations were measured every 8.6 ± 4.8 hours until the values were below the detectable limits of the assay. A minimum of 10 serum concentration-time data pairs were used to characterize each profile. All blood samples were collected in Vacutainer tubes (Becton-Dickinson) and centrifuged and the serum was analyzed for pentobarbital by a modified gas chromatographic technique.[3] The method had a coefficient of variation <6% and allowed accurate determination of serum pentobarbital concentrations to as low as 0.25 mg/L.

The AUC after intravenous infusion of sodium pentobarbital was determined by the Lagrange technique[15] alone or in conjunction with the linear or log-trapezoidal methods. Total body clearance (CL) and volume of distribution at steady state (V_{ss}) were computed with model-independent calculations.[4] CL was estimated by dividing the total administered dose of pentobarbital acid by the AUC extrapolated from zero to infinity. The V_{ss} was calculated as: (MRT − 0.5T) × CL, where MRT is the mean residence time and T is the duration of pentobarbital infusion. The MRT was computed as: AUMC/AUC, where AUMC is the first moment of the serum concentration-time curve. Whereas AUC, CL, and V_{ss} were estimated by model-independent means, the $t_{1/2}$ was determined by regression of the terminal phase of the serum concentration-time profile after discontinuation of the pentobarbital infusion.

The CL, V_{ss}, and $t_{1/2}$ obtained from the adult patients with head trauma were statistically compared with values reported by Ehrnebo[3] after a single 100 mg intravenous pentobarbital bolus administered to seven healthy adults (four men and three women). These control parameters were calculated by fitting the pentobarbital serum concentration-time data to a two-compartment open model and are comparable with those values derived by model-independent methods.[4] Statistical comparisons were by the unpaired Student's t test with a minimal level of significance defined as $P < 0.05$.

RESULTS

Seven of the 10 patients had received severe closed-head injuries as a result of motor vehicle accidents; the remaining three patients were admitted to the trauma unit after accidental falls (Table I). Of the 10 patients studied, only four are alive, one of whom continues to have severe neurologic impairment. In all but two cases the duration of pentobarbital infusion exceeded 48 hours (range 33 to 156 hours) as a result of at least one episode of intracranial pressure elevation (>20 torr) during this period.

A representative pentobarbital serum concentration-

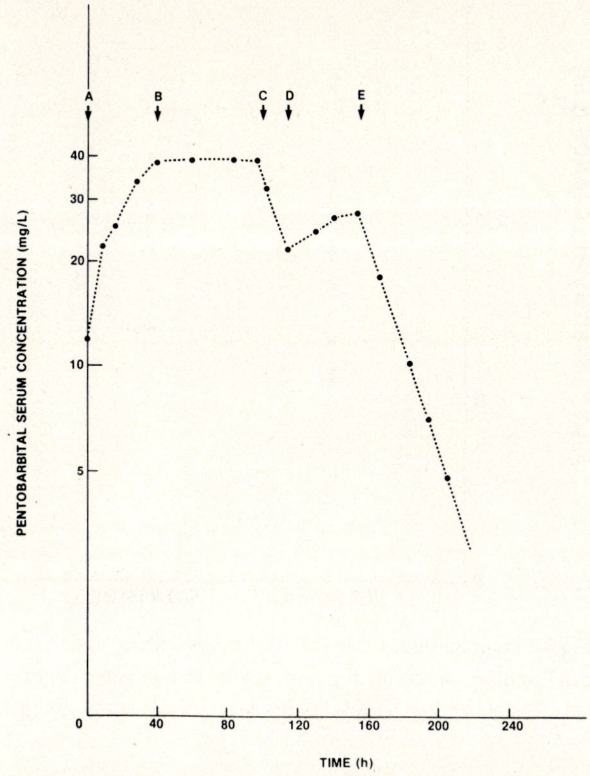

Fig. 1. Representative serum pentobarbital concentration-time profile for patient 1. *A* = Pentobarbital bolus (700 mg over a 1-hour period); *B* = steady-state maintenance infusion (120 mg/hr); *C* = infusion held to reduce levels; *D* = adjusted pentobarbital maintenance infusion (100 mg/hr); *E* = infusion discontinued.

time profile after a 700 mg pentobarbital slow bolus (over a 1-hour period) and a 120 mg/hr maintenance infusion is shown in Fig. 1. In this subject (no. 1), pentobarbital serum concentrations >20 mg/L were achieved within 8 hours of initiating therapy. After 156 hours of therapy the infusion was discontinued and pentobarbital concentrations followed a monoexponential decline, with an apparent $t_{1/2}$ of 20 hours. The individual pharmacokinetic data for the 10 patients are listed in Table II.

The mean (±SD) $t_{1/2}$ for the 10 patients of 15.6 ± 3.9 hours was significantly less than that reported by Ehrnebo[3] (22.3 ± 4.0 hours) in seven healthy adults (Fig. 2). Similarly, the V_{ss} calculated in the patients with trauma was significantly less than that observed in the control subjects (44.0 ± 11.7 vs. 63.4 ± 15.2 L; $P < 0.05$; Fig. 3). However, there was no significant difference between the mean pentobarbital CL of the

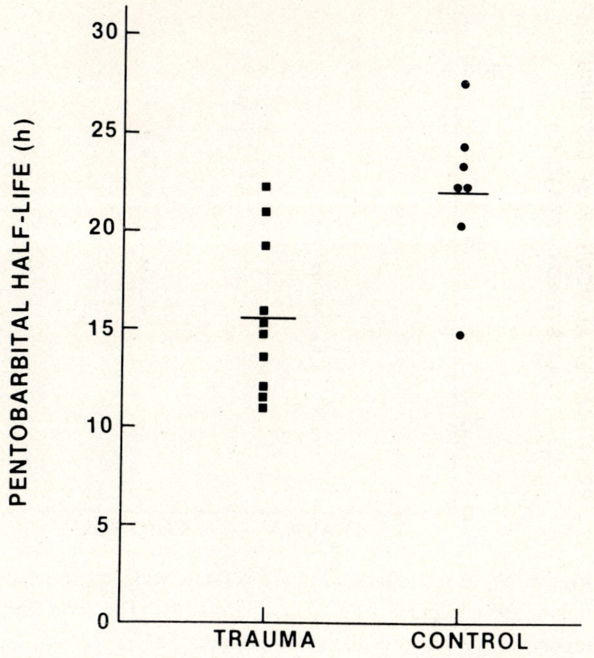

Fig. 2. Pentobarbital $t_{1/2}$ in 10 patients with severe nonpenetrating head injury (■) compared with seven normal adult subjects (●).[3] The *solid line* represents the mean of the study groups.

patients (2.0 ± 0.7 L/hr) and the subjects (2.0 ± 0.4 L/hr; Fig. 4).

DISCUSSION

The therapeutic use of high-dose pentobarbital infusions in patients with severe head trauma refractory to conventional therapy has been advocated as an effective adjunct in controlling persistent intracranial hypertension.[7,9,11,14] Pentobarbital administration and initial dosage are titrated according to changes in intracranial pressure and arterial pressure, with a reduction of intracranial pressure to <15 torr and an estimated cerebral perfusion pressure ranging from 60 to 70 torr. Maintenance doses of pentobarbital required to achieve this effect vary. Generally, an infusion rate is selected that maintains steady-state serum pentobarbital concentrations of 25 to 35 mg/L (110 to 155 μmol/L), with precaution taken to avoid levels >45 mg/L (200 μmol/L).

In view of the widespread clinical use of barbiturate-induced coma, it is surprising that the pharmacokinetics of high-dose pentobarbital in patients with severe closed head injury have not been well documented. As such, a number of questions remain unanswered. For exam-

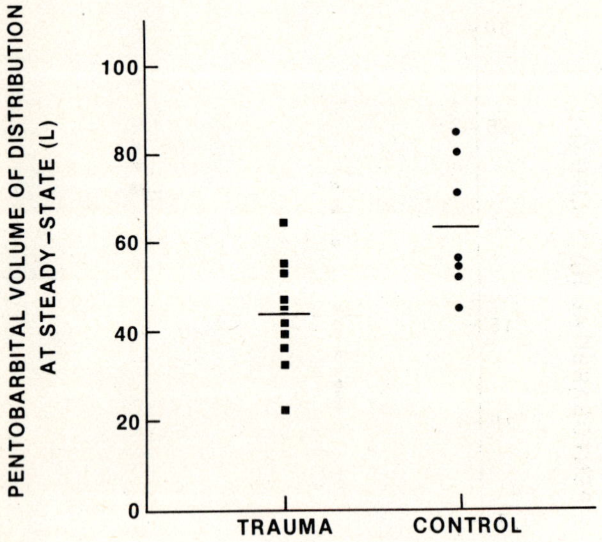

Fig. 3. V_{ss} of pentobarbital in the patients with severe head trauma (■) compared with adult controls (●).[3] The *solid line* represents the mean of the study groups.

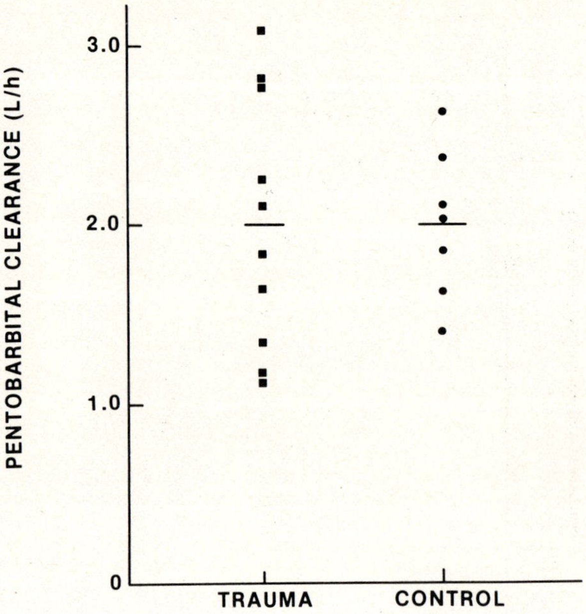

Fig. 4. Pentobarbital CL in the 10 patients with severe closed-head injuries (■) compared with seven normal adult controls (●).[3] The *solid line* represents the mean of the study groups.

ple, Marshall et al.[9] observed considerable variation in the dosage required to achieve therapeutic serum pentobarbital concentrations. The total dose of pentobarbital required to maintain serum levels between 25 to 35 mg/L and reduce intracranial pressure to <15 torr varied from 100 to 200 mg every 30 to 60 minutes. Whether these differences in dosage reflect intersubject variability in disposition or elimination parameters is as yet unknown. Do adult patients with trauma demonstrate different pharmacokinetic traits in pentobarbital clearance when compared with healthy adults? Finally, can pentobarbital be described by a monoexponential decline from high serum concentrations, which would allow predictions on timing of subsequent blood samples or anticipated time to negligible drug levels? This latter question is of profound ethical concern to relatives, physicians, and human transplant personnel awaiting discrimination between brain death and pentobarbital coma.

In our present study we attempted to address the pharmacokinetic issues, in part by examining the steady-state disposition of pentobarbital during constant intravenous infusion and the elimination rate during discontinuation of therapy.

The apparent V_{ss} of the adult patients with head injury was determined under the assumption that the pentobarbital infusion rate remained constant over the administration time. In most patients the infusion rates were increased with time to achieve therapeutic effect. Such rate changes would result in overestimation of the true V_{ss}, suggesting that the actual differences in V_{ss} from control values may be greater than observed. The lower V_{ss} observed in the patients with trauma may have been due to possible pathophysiologic changes from acute injury or drug-induced alterations in factors affecting drug distribution to peripheral binding sites, such as decreased cardiac output and altered regional blood flow.

In our present study there was no significant difference in pentobarbital CL between control subjects and patients with trauma. Unlike V_{ss}, which may be sensitive to changes in perfusion to peripheral sites, pentobarbital CL is thought to be independent of blood flow and limited by low intrinsic clearance.[10] The observation of no change in CL despite the persistent hypotensive action of pentobarbital infusion is consistent with blood flow–independent elimination of the drug. In contrast, Kozlowski et al.[6] observed a positive correlation between the degree of hypotension produced by pentobarbital and the degree of impairment of drug biotransformation in rabbits. They suggested that, depending on the dose and extent of blood pressure depression, impairment of fluid exchange between blood and tissues may initiate metabolic disturbances and subsequent reductions in pentobarbital biotransformation. However, it appears that for such alterations in fluid exchange to occur, blood pressure depressions lower than the osmotic pressure of blood proteins (23 to 30 torr) are required.

The mean $t_{1/2}$ in the patients with trauma was significantly less than that reported in the adult control subjects. As the $t_{1/2}$ depends on drug distribution and clearance ($t_{1/2} = 0.693 \cdot V_{ss}/CL$), any observed decreases in $t_{1/2}$ can be partially or totally accounted for by the decreases in V_{ss}, even though CL remains constant. This is supported by the 30% reduction in both V_{ss} and $t_{1/2}$ observed in the patients with trauma when compared with the subjects. Another possible, although less plausible, explanation for the differences in $t_{1/2}$ may be related to comparing a single 100 mg intravenous dose given to the seven volunteers[3] to a constant pentobarbital infusion received by our patients with head trauma. Baldeo et al.[1] observed a significantly shorter (25%) mean urinary $t_{1/2}$ in men given multiple doses of pentobarbital. It was surmised that pentobarbital is capable of inducing its own metabolism after as few as three therapeutic doses. Differences in the $t_{1/2}$ between groups in our study may then reflect the significantly longer exposure time to pentobarbital (AUC) experienced by the patients, although one would expect that these changes in drug metabolism would have been mirrored by similar changes in CL.

In summary, the 10 adult patients with trauma showed considerable intrasubject variability in the disposition and elimination of pentobarbital, with coefficients of variation for CL, V_{ss}, and $t_{1/2}$ of 35.3%, 26.5%, and 25.0%, respectively. The patients eliminated a given dose of pentobarbital at a more rapid rate but from a smaller V_{ss} than that reported for normal adults. Whatever the mechanisms for these changes, the net effect is not remarkable. Because there is no significant difference in the CL of the two groups, it is anticipated that similar steady-state serum concentrations of pentobarbital would be achieved after a given constant infusion rate. In addition, on discontinuation of pentobarbital therapy serum concentrations fell monoexponentially from therapeutic levels, allowing predictions of the time to negligible drug concentrations. Based on the apparent mean $t_{1/2}$ in our patients, we suggest that, on the average, blood samples for analysis of pentobarbital should not be drawn more frequently than every 24 hours after discontinuation of therapy.

References

1. Baldeo WC, Gilbert JNT, Powell JW: Multidose studies in the human metabolism of pentobarbitone. Eur J Drug Metab Pharmacokinet **5**:75-80, 1980.
2. Bird TD, Plum F: Recovery from barbiturate overdose coma with prolonged isoelectric electroencephalogram. Neurology **18**:456-460, 1968.
3. Ehrnebo M: Pharmacokinetics and distribution properties of pentobarbital in humans following oral and intravenous administration. J Pharm Sci **63**:1114-1118, 1974.
4. Jusko WJ: Guidelines for collection and pharmacokinetic analysis of drug disposition data. *In* Evans WE, Schentag JJ, Jusko WJ, editors: Applied pharmacokinetics. Principles of therapeutic drug monitoring. San Francisco, 1980, Applied Therapeutics, pp 639-680.
5. Kassell NF, Peerless SJ, Drake CG, Boarini DJ, Adams HP: Treatment of ischemic deficits from cerebral vasospasm with high dose barbiturate therapy. Neurosurgery **7**:593-597, 1980.
6. Kozlowski KH, Szaykowski A, Danysz A: Dependence of pentobarbital kinetics upon the dose of the drug and its pharmacodynamic effects. Pol J Pharmacol Pharm **29**:497-508, 1977.
7. Marshall LF, Bruce DA, Bruno L, Schut L: Role of intracranial pressure monitoring and barbiturate therapy in malignant intracranial pressure. Case report. J Neurosurg **47**:481-484, 1977.
8. Marshall LF, Shapiro HM, Rauscher A, Kaufman NM: Pentobarbital therapy for intracranial hypertension in metabolic coma: Reye's syndrome. Crit Care Med **6**:1-5, 1978.
9. Marshall LF, Smith RW, Shapiro HM: The outcome with aggressive treatment in severe head injuries. II. Acute and chronic barbiturate administration in the management of head injury. J Neurosurg **50**:26-30, 1979.
10. Nies AS, Shand DG, Wilkinson GR: Altered hepatic blood flow and drug disposition. Clin Pharmacokinet **1**:135-155, 1976.
11. Piatt JH Jr, Schiff SJ: High dose barbiturate therapy in neurosurgery and intensive care. Neurosurgery **15**:427-444, 1984.
12. Schaible DH, Cupit GC, Swedlow DB, Rocci ML Jr: High dose pentobarbital pharmacokinetics in hypothermic brain-injured children. J Pediatr **100**:655-660, 1982.
13. Schwartz ML, Tator CH, Rowed DW, Reid SR, Meguro K, Andrews DF: The University of Toronto Head Injury Treatment Study: A prospective randomized comparison of pentobarbital and mannitol. Can J Neurol Sci **11**:434-440, 1984.
14. Shapiro HM, Wyte SR, Loeser J: Barbiturate augmented hypothermia for reduction of persistent intracranial hypertension. J Neurosurg **40**:90-100, 1974.
15. Yeh KC, Kwan KC: A comparison of numerical integrating algorithms by trapezoidal, Lagrange, and spline approximation. J Pharmacokinet Biopharm **6**:79-98, 1978.

Pharmacokinetics of a new angiotensin I converting enzyme inhibitor (alacepril) after oral dosing in fasting or fed states

The plasma concentration and urinary excretion of a newly developed angiotensin I converting enzyme inhibitor, alacepril (which is converted to captopril after absorption), were investigated in seven normal healthy subjects. Fifty milligrams of the drug was administered orally either in the fasting or in the fed state. In the fasting state, the time of maximal plasma concentration (t_{max}) was 1 hour for free captopril, 1.7 hours for protein-conjugated captopril, and 1.6 hours for total captopril. The biologic $t_{1/2}$ of free, protein-conjugated, and total captopril was 1.9, 4.2, and 5 hours, respectively. In the fed state, neither t_{max} nor $t_{1/2}$ changed, except that the t_{max} of free captopril was prolonged to 1.9 hours ($P < 0.01$). Cumulative urinary excretion of free captopril at 8 hours was 35% of the drug administered in the fasting state and that of total captopril at 24 hours was 59%. These data did not differ significantly from those obtained after food intake. The biologic $t_{1/2}$ of free captopril after alacepril dosing was longer than in previous studies of captopril per se. Because biologic or clinical effects have not been studied, it should be left conjectural whether alacepril is a longer-acting angiotensin I converting enzyme inhibitor. A prolonged effect of the drug can be expected by its administration after a meal. (CLIN PHARMACOL THER 38:462-468, 1985.)

Kaoru Onoyama, M.D., Hideki Hirakata, M.D., Hiroshi Tsuruda, M.D., Nobuaki Ohchi, M.D., Suguru Tomooka, M.D., Kenichi Motomura, M.D., Teruo Omae, M.D., Kouji Hayashi, Ph.D., and Masatoshi Fujishima, M.D.
Fukuoka, Japan

A new angiotensin I converting enzyme inhibitor, alacepril (1-(D-3-acetylthio-2-methylpropanoyl)-L-prolyl-L-phenylalanine; see structure), was developed recently as an orally active antihypertensive agent.[7] According to studies with ^{14}C-alacepril in rats, alacepril was determined to undergo considerable conversion to its active metabolite, captopril, as captopril and its mixed disulfide were detected in blood and urine.[11] Although a clinical use of the drug is currently under investigation, examination of its pharmacokinetics seems important. Because captopril is a main metabolite of this agent, its pharmacodynamics can be suggested to be similar to previous reports.[1,3,6,9,10,12,13]

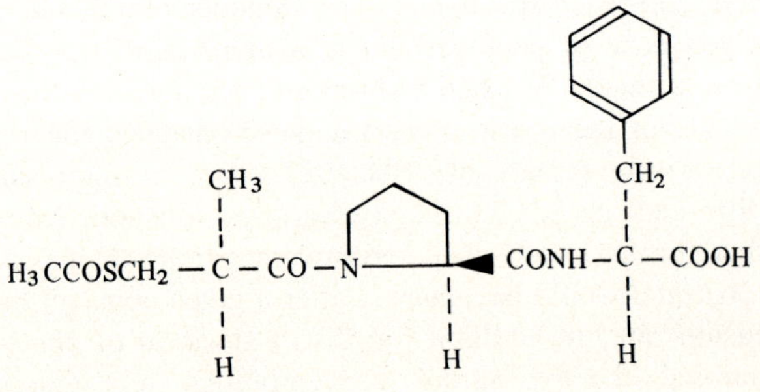

Alacepril

Our study was undertaken to determine blood elimination and urinary excretion of this drug in normal subjects in the fasting or the fed state.

METHODS

Our subjects were seven healthy normal men 33 to 50 years old ($\overline{X}$ = 41 years). Kidney and liver functions were normal (Table I). Subjects in the fasting state

From the Second Department of Internal Medicine, Faculty of Medicine, Kyushu University, National Cardiovascular Center, and Research Laboratories of Dainippon Pharmaceutical Co., Ltd.
Supported by research grants from Glomerular Injury Research Committee and from Renal Body Fluid Volume Regulation Research Committee (59Kou-8), Division of Public Health and Welfare, Japan.
Received for publication April 2, 1985; accepted July 10, 1985.
Reprint requests to: Kaoru Onoyama, M.D., Second Department of Internal Medicine, Faculty of Medicine, Kyushu University, Maidashi 3, Higashi-Ku, Fukuoka City, 812 Japan.

Table I. Profiles of seven normal subjects

	Age (yr)	*Weight (kg)*	*SGOT (U/dl)*	*SGPT (U/dl)*	*Creatinine (mg/dl)*
Mean ± SE	41 ± 2	65.5 ± 2.2	15 ± 1.1	14.8 ± 1.6	0.9 ± 0.03
Range	50-33	76-60	20-13	22-8	1.1-0.8

Table II. Plasma concentrations (ng/ml) of free captopril after 50 mg alacepril

	Time after dosing (hr)							
Subject	*0.5*	*1*	*2*	*3*	*4*	*6*	*8*	*24*
Fasting								
T. S.	156.2	191.3	106.2	82.0	60.6	27.8	12.7	8.5
T. T.	175.3	377.6	139.5	65.3	34.6	19.0	16.9	10.6
I. U.	493.7	285.5	86.5	50.4	22.3	20.2	16.2	9.0
H. S.	63.2	108.1	124.6	100.2	85.3	32.0	21.0	7.1
H. N.	20.6	249.5	210.9	86.7	47.4	30.4	23.0	15.1
S. N.	103.7	111.6	104.8	56.9	32.5	19.9	17.4	15.1
H. M.	313.7	281.6	56.9	47.4	25.8	14.1	13.2	8.3
Mean	189.5	229.3	118.5	69.8	44.1	23.3	17.2	10.5
± SE	61.9	37.3	18.4	7.6	8.5	2.5	1.4	1.2
Fed								
T. S.	23.2	70.4	207.6	69.9	21.1	12.5	0.4	0.0
T. T.	136.7	384.9	140.2	45.3	26.5	10.2	7.4	0.0
I. U.	15.8	105.5	399.5	97.6	28.5	19.7	9.5	1.6
H. S.	30.4	120.2	131.8	75.1	56.9	14.8	13.9	8.1
H. N.	62.3	160.0	175.3	142.0	65.8	34.4	17.6	12.5
S. N.	63.0	148.8	156.2	81.0	54.6	34.4	23.2	15.3
H. M.	42.0	148.6	270.4	104.6	35.3	29.7	27.4	17.8
Mean	53.3	162.6	211.6	87.9	41.2	22.2	14.2	7.9
± SE	15.5	38.8	36.1	11.6	6.6	3.9	3.5	2.8

study were not given any food or drink except water overnight. The study started at 9 AM with the oral intake of 50 mg alacepril and 150 ml water. A 5 ml venous blood sample was drawn just before drug dosing and at 0.5, 1, 2, 3, 4, 6, 8, and 24 hours thereafter. Blood was drawn into a heparinized tube containing a solution of 0.1 mol/L EDTA and 0.1 mol/L ascorbic acid[8] and was immediately centrifuged for 2 minutes.

Urine was collected 2 hours before and at 2, 4, 6, and 8 hours after drug dosing. After the 8-hour sampling, all urine was pooled up to 24 hours. On the first day subjects remained in supine position from 1 hour before the study to the 8-hour sampling. On day 2 they remained supine from 1 hour before the 24-hour sampling until the sampling. Lunch was served after the 4-hour sampling and dinner was taken after the 8-hour sampling. Blood pressure and pulse rate were examined at the same intervals as blood sampling.

The fed state study was performed 1 week after the fasting state study in the same subjects with the same protocol, except that breakfast was served before drug dosing.

Captopril and its disulfides in blood and urine and protein-conjugated captopril in blood were measured according to the newly developed method of Hayashi et al.[5]

To measure free captopril in plasma, 1 ml fresh plasma was mixed with 0.5 ml 0.5% BPM [*N*-(4-benzoylphenyl)-maleimide] solution and 2 ml 0.1 mol/L phosphate buffer and left for 10 minutes at room temperature. After the addition of SA-446 [(4*R*)-2-2-hydroxyphenyl) - 3 - (3-mercaptopropionyl) - 4 - thiazolidinecarboxylic acid] as internal standard, the mixture was acidified, extracted with chloroform, and evaporated. For the cleanup the residue was again dissolved with 0.1 mol/L phosphate buffer, washed with ether twice, acidified, extracted with chloroform, and evaporated. The res-

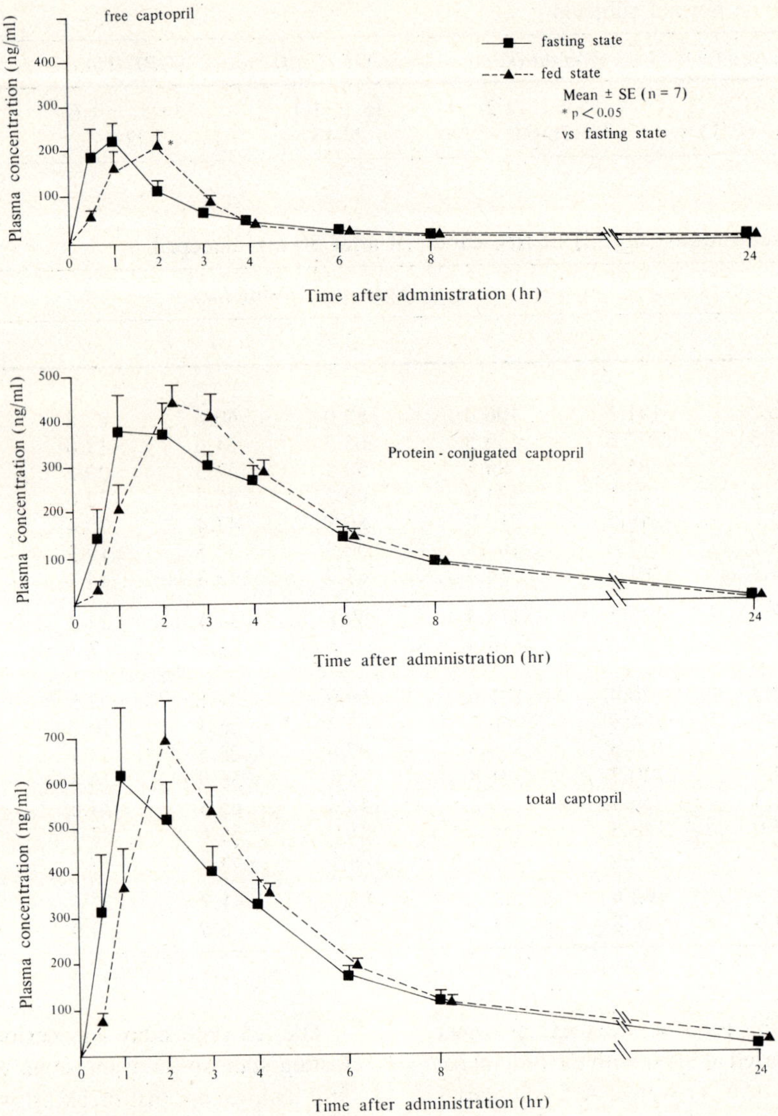

Fig. 1. Plasma concentration of free captopril *(top)*, protein-conjugated captopril *(middle)*, and total captopril *(bottom)* after 50 mg alacepril in the fasting or in the fed state.

idue was dissolved in methanol and examined by HPLC.

To measure total captopril in plasma, 2 ml phosphate buffer, 0.2 ml 0.1 mol/L EDTA, and 0.2 ml 0.8% tributylphosphine methanol were added to 1 ml fresh plasma and incubated at 50° C for 60 minutes. The reaction was stopped in the ice box and the internal standard solution was added. After extraction by ether, 0.5 ml BPM solution was added and kept at room temperature for 30 minutes. The mixture was acidified and extracted with chloroform. The same procedure described above was followed.

To measure protein-conjugated captopril in plasma, 1 ml plasma was mixed with 0.2 ml 3 mol/L perchloric acid and centrifuged. The precipitated pellet was resuspended, neutralized, and mixed with EDTA and tributylphosphine solution. After incubation at 50° C for 30 minutes, captopril was determined with the same method mentioned above.

To measure free captopril in urine, 0.2 ml BPM solution and phosphate buffer was added to 0.2 ml urine and kept at room temperature for 15 minutes. After washing with ether, the internal standard solution was added. The mixture was acidified, extracted with chloroform, and evaporated. The residue was dissolved in

Table III. Plasma concentrations (ng/ml) of protein-conjugated captopril after 50 mg alacepril

	Time after dosing (hr)							
Subject	*0.5*	*1*	*2*	*3*	*4*	*6*	*8*	*24*
Fasting								
T. S.	114.3	393.2	381.9	331.0	313.6	168.2	94.6	16.4
T. T.	31.4	518.3	371.7	370.1	275.2	205.0	149.5	17.4
I. U.	455.9	557.9	324.9	256.3	171.2	108.7	70.9	15.7
H. S.	62.5	72.8	121.4	248.1	366.5	159.5	115.7	8.3
H. N.	0.0	319.0	679.5	454.8	363.1	204.6	103.6	9.3
S. N.	29.1	224.0	466.8	234.1	180.2	76.2	43.4	4.6
H. M.	314.3	608.6	315.4	244.8	236.1	117.0	74.2	5.3
Mean	143.9	384.8	380.2	305.6	272.3	148.5	93.1	11.0
±SE	65.5	73.3	63.9	31.5	30.4	18.7	13.0	2.0
Fed								
T. S.	9.3	107.0	609.9	488.2	306.3	117.7	68.5	8.7
T. T.	126.4	425.3	369.8	260.1	174.5	105.3	90.3	8.0
I. U.	0.0	105.6	368.5	476.2	298.3	135.7	91.3	25.7
H. S.	6.7	98.0	325.7	303.6	222.0	145.4	64.8	0.0
H. N.	33.1	155.5	447.4	524.0	362.5	209.7	114.0	31.4
S. N.	47.1	123.0	358.2	253.8	251.8	141.8	69.5	0.0
H. M.	8.3	423.4	602.6	585.6	383.2	172.5	119.7	20.4
Mean	33.0	205.4	440.3	413.1	285.5	146.9	88.3	13.5
±SE	16.8	57.0	45.0	51.7	28.3	13.2	8.4	4.7

acetonitrile and examined by HPLC. To measure total captopril in urine, 0.1 ml 2% tributylphosphine, 0.1 ml EDTA, and phosphate buffer were added to 0.2 ml urine and the mixture was incubated at 50° C for 60 minutes. After the reaction was stopped by ice cooling, 0.5 ml BPM solution was added. After being kept at room temperature for 30 minutes, the mixture was washed with ether and 0.2 ml of internal standard solution was added. The procedure was the same as that mentioned above.

Data are expressed as the $\overline{X} \pm SE$. Pharmacokinetic analysis was performed with a one-compartment open model. Statistical significance of differences was assessed by Student's t test.

RESULTS

Plasma concentrations of free captopril in the fasting and in the fed states are shown in Table II and Fig. 1, *top*. The highest plasma concentration of free captopril was observed at 1 hour in the fasting state and at 2 hours in the fed state. In both conditions free captopril was not detected at 24 hours.

Plasma concentrations of protein-conjugated captopril in the fasting and in the fed states are shown in Table III and Fig. 1, *middle*. The highest plasma concentration of protein-conjugated captopril was at 1 hour in the fasting state and at 2 hours in the fed state, but this difference is not significant. There was a delay in the time to reach maximal plasma concentrations (t_{max}) in the fed state, but the difference was not significant.

Plasma concentrations of total captopril are shown in Table IV and Fig. 1, *bottom*. The highest plasma concentration of total captopril was at 1 hour in the fasting state and at 2 hours in the fed state.

Pharmacokinetic parameters after 50 mg alacepril in either the fasting or the fed state are listed in Table V. The t_{max} values of free captopril, protein-conjugated captopril, and total captopril were longer in the fed than in the fasting state, and the difference for free captopril reached statistical significance ($P < 0.01$). The maximum concentration, biologic $t_{1/2}$, and AUC of free, protein-conjugated, and total captopril did not differ significantly between the two studies.

Cumulative urinary excretions of free and total captopril in either the fasting or the fed states are shown in Fig. 2. Thirty-three percent of the drug administered in the fasting state and 28% in the fed state was excreted as free captopril at 8 hours. Likewise, 59% of the drug administered in the fasting state and 54% in the fed state was excreted as total captopril at 24 hours. Cumulative urinary excretions were always greater in the

Table IV. Plasma concentrations (ng/ml) of total captopril after 50 mg alacepril

	Time after dosing (hr)							
Subject	*0.5*	*1*	*2*	*3*	*4*	*6*	*8*	*24*
Fasting								
T. S.	286.9	652.9	521.2	457.8	430.6	196.0	119.8	22.9
T. T.	175.8	895.7	525.4	466.8	307.5	223.5	183.0	29.8
I. U.	937.7	856.1	403.9	349.3	193.4	118.0	97.4	24.6
H. S.	91.8	179.6	215.3	327.3	447.0	172.7	115.9	21.6
H. N.	20.7	567.6	919.8	685.5	508.1	274.8	190.8	39.2
S. N.	104.3	318.8	603.0	261.8	207.2	101.2	56.5	20.3
H. M.	599.5	888.8	493.1	285.1	270.9	127.9	81.4	21.6
Mean	316.7	622.8	526.0	404.8	337.8	173.4	120.7	25.7
±SE	126.3	108.3	80.7	55.5	47.0	23.7	18.9	2.5
Fed								
T. S.	35.8	145.2	1144.6	602.9	381.1	199.8	139.6	24.2
T. T.	197.3	8656	527.9	519.8	259.7	154.6	107.7	45.3
I. U.	23.7	298.9	752.8	600.3	318.2	159.4	99.1	24.6
H. S.	40.5	188.2	422.4	391.0	317.8	199.0	110.3	28.0
H. N.	78.0	285.9	640.6	710.4	452.6	259.7	138.3	39.2
S. N.	83.6	228.7	505.5	328.2	297.2	161.1	100.4	19.4
H. M.	49.6	516.8	868.1	626.5	440.5	233.0	137.0	37.1
Mean	72.6	361.3	694.6	539.9	352.4	195.2	118.9	31.1
±SE	22.4	95.4	94.7	51.5	27.9	15.2	7.0	3.6

Table V. Pharmacokinetics of captopril after 50 mg alacepril in normal subjects

	C_{max} (ng/ml)	t_{max} (hr)	$t_{1/2}$ (hr)	AUC(0-24) (ng · hr/ml)
Fasting				
Free	266 ± 53	1.0 ± 0.2	1.9 ± 0.1	807 ± 41
Protein-conjugated	513 ± 43	1.7 ± 0.4	4.2 ± 0.2	2678 ± 224
Total	764 ± 73	1.6 ± 0.4	5.0 ± 0.1	3702 ± 384
Fed				
Free	247 ± 41	1.9 ± 0.1*	1.6 ± 0.2	746 ± 77
Protein-conjugated	475 ± 42	2.1 ± 0.3	4.1 ± 0.5	2648 ± 247
Total	753 ± 92	2.0 ± 0.2	5.3 ± 0.2	3780 ± 251

Data are $\overline{X}$ ± SE.
C_{max} = Maximum concentration.
*$P < 0.01$ compared with free captopril in fasting state.

fasting than in the fed state at all observation periods, but the differences were not statistically significant.

Average values for mean blood pressure and pulse rate are listed in Table VI. Compared with pretreatment values, mean blood pressure slightly decreased after alacepril for approximately 4 hours in the fasting state and for 6 hours in the fed state. Also, the pulse rate slightly decreased for 4 hours and increased afterward in the fasting state, and it slightly increased in the fed state.

DISCUSSION

In our previous study with 50 mg captopril in normal subjects under the fasting state, the t_{max} and $t_{1/2}$ values of free captopril were 0.74 and 0.35 hours,[12] respectively. Using ^{35}S-captopril, Kripalani et al.[10] reported that t_{max} was 0.93 hours. In patients with hypertension who have normal kidney function, t_{max} and $t_{1/2}$ of free unchanged captopril were reported to be 0.98 and 0.45 hours[13] and 0.98 and 0.56 hours.[3]

After oral dosing, alacepril is known to be converted to captopril and its mixed disulfides with thiol compounds such as cysteine, glutathione, and plasma proteins. In the present study of 50 mg alacepril administered under the fasting state, t_{max} and $t_{1/2}$ of free captopril were 1 and 1.9 hours, respectively. The t_{max} was slightly but not significantly longer than that after administration of captopril per se, indicating that the absorption and conversion of alacepril to captopril are considerably rapid.

Table VI. Changes in mean blood pressure (MBP) and heart rate (HR) after 50 mg alacepril in the fasting and in the fed state

	Hr after dosing								
	0	*0.5*	*1*	*2*	*3*	*4*	*6*	*8*	*24*
MBP (mm Hg)									
Fasting	85.6	80.6*	78.7*	79.1*	77.9*	78.7*	82.9	83.9	83.9
	±2.8	±3.7	±3.4	±3.7	±4.0	±3.2	±1.9	±2.1	±2.3
Fed	83.9	80.3	78.3	78.4	74.3*	79.1	78.3	82.0	80.1
	±2.1	±2.7	±3.3	±3.2	±2.2	±1.2	±2.1	±2.6	±2.1
HR (bpm)									
Fasting	63.3	61.9*	62.1	62.1	60.6*	60.7*	65.4	68.6*	73.1*
	±2.1	±1.5	±1.9	±1.7	±1.5	±1.8	±1.1	±3.2	±3.6
Fed	59.4	64.7*	64.4*	62.7	62.0	62.4	66.1*	68.7*	73.9*
	±1.7	±1.9	±1.9	±2.0	±1.9	±2.1	±2.7	±2.5	±4.4

Data are $\overline{X} \pm$ SE.
*$P < 0.05$ compared with pretreatment value.

According to the previously reported studies of captopril, the $t_{1/2}$ of free captopril varied as 0.35,[12] 0.45,[13] and 0.56 hours,[3] while it was 1.9 hours after alacepril in our study. These findings indicate that free captopril converted from alacepril can be retained about four times longer in the plasma. But it is not ascertained by the present study whether biologic or clinical effects of alacepril can last longer. The mechanism of the longer $t_{1/2}$ of this drug cannot be clarified but protein-conjugated captopril, which was demonstrated in a manner similar to that of free captopril, may play a role. Alacepril is expected to have a longer action as a converting enzyme inhibitor than captopril per se. On the other hand, it has been reported that the action of enalapril maleate (MK-421) appears more slowly but its depressor effect continues longer than does captopril, and its $t_{1/2}$ in healthy subjects with normotension is 6 to 7 hours.[4]

Because protein-conjugated captopril has not been measured in any other studies of converting enzyme inhibitors, its biologic significance or mechanism is not clear. Recently, captopril linked with thiol groups of protein as well as captopril disulfide was suggested to act as a reservoir from which captopril could be released slowly.[1] Similar mechanisms for protein-conjugated captopril may be highly valuable.

As is that for captopril, alacepril excretion is mainly by the kidney.[11] In our study of cumulative urinary excretion, 33% of alacepril administered was detected as free captopril and 59% appeared as total captopril at 6 hours. This is quite similar to our previous study of captopril,[12] in which the cumulative urinary excretion was 35% for free captopril and 60% for total captopril.

The time of drug dosing, whether it is in the fasting or in the fed state, is important for the drug to obtain its proper and more effective action. In our study administration during the fed state significantly delayed the t_{max} of free captopril without a difference in maximum concentrations. Other pharmacokinetic parameters as well as cumulative urinary excretion did not differ significantly between the two conditions. The effect of food was only to shift the plasma concentration profile to the right, leaving the AUC unchanged. In our previous study of captopril in patients undergoing

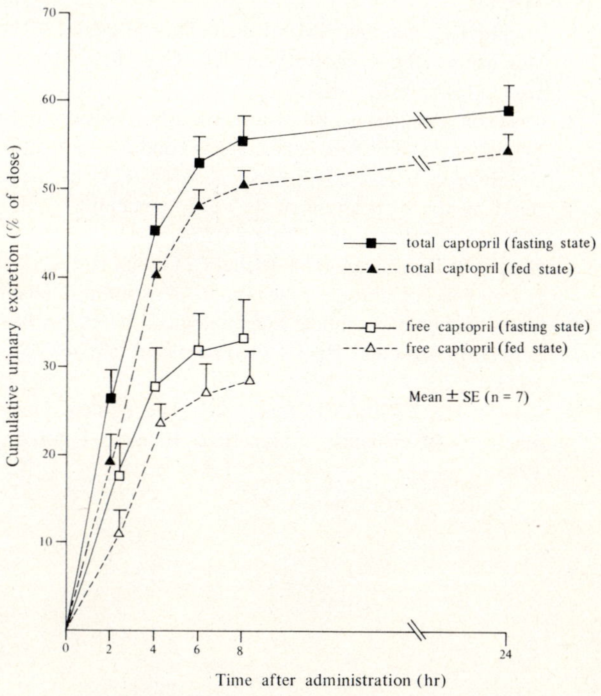

Fig. 2. Cumulative urinary excretion of free and total captopril after 50 mg alacepril in the fasting or in the fed state.

chronic hemodialysis, the maximal blood concentration of free captopril was apparently lower when captopril was administered in the fed state.[6] In contrast, MK-421 administered with food did not affect its bioavailability.[2,4] These discrepancies may be due to the difference in drug specificity, mainly that alacepril is converted to captopril after absorption.

Because we investigated pharmacokinetic aspects of alacepril in normal healthy subjects, we found no remarkable changes in blood pressure or in heart rate. In other words, alacepril has no further lowering action of blood pressure in subjects with normotension, but the depressor effect of the drug should be evaluated in patients with hypertension.

Alacepril was kindly supplied by Dainippon Pharmaceutical Co., Ltd., Japan.

References

1. Duchin KL, Singhvi SM, Willard DA, Migdalof BH, McKinstry DN: Captopril kinetics. CLIN PHARMACOL THER **31:**452-458, 1982.
2. Ferguson RK, Irvin JD, Swanson BN, Vlasses PH, Bergquist PA, Till AE, Feinberg JA: Food does not alter the absorption of enalapril maleate (MK-421) as measured by the disposition of its active metabolite (MK-422). CLIN PHARMACOL THER **33:**254, 1983.
3. Giudicelli JF, Chaignon M, Richer C, Giroux B, Guedon J: Influence of chronic renal failure on captopril pharmacokinetics and clinical and biological effects in hypertensive patients. Br J Clin Pharmacol **18:**749-758, 1984.
4. Gomez HJ, Cirillo VJ, Jones KH: The clinical pharmacology of enalapril. J Hypertens **1**(supple 1):65-70, 1983.
5. Hayashi K, Miyamoto M, Sekine Y: Determination of captopril and its mixed disulfides in plasma and urine by high-performance liquid chromatography. J Chromatogr Biomed App **338:**161-169, 1985.
6. Hirakata H, Onoyama K, Iseki K, Omae T, Fujimi S, Kawahara Y: Captopril (SQ 14225) clearance during hemodialysis treatment. Clin Nephrol **16:**321-323, 1981.
7. Hosoki K, Takeyama K, Okamoto H, Minato H, Kadokawa T: Pharmacological studies on alacepril: Antihypertensive activity and inhibitory effect on angiotensin converting enzyme. Jpn J Pharmacol **31:**116, 1981.
8. Jarrott B, Anderson A, Hooper R, Louis WJ: High-performance liquid chromatographic analysis of captopril in plasma. J Pharm Sci **70:**665-667, 1981.
9. Jarrott B, Drummer O, Hooper R, Anderson AIE, Miach PJ, Louis WJ: Pharmacokinetic properties of captopril after acute and chronic administration to hypertensive subjects. Am J Cardiol **49:**1547-1549, 1982.
10. Kripalani KJ, McKinstry DN, Singhvi SM, Willard DA, Vukovich RA, Migdalof BH: Disposition of captopril in normal subjects. CLIN PHARMACOL THER **27:**636-641, 1980.
11. Matsumoto T, Miyazaki H, Hosoki K, Hashimoto M: Biological distribution of a new antihypertensive compound, alacepril in rats. Abstracts of the One Hundred Third Annual Meeting of the Pharmaceutical Society of Japan, Tokyo, April 3, 1983.
12. Onoyama K, Hirakata H, Iseki K, Fujimi S, Omae T, Kobayashi M, Kawahara Y: Blood concentration and urinary excretion of captopril (SQ 14225) in patients with chronic renal failure. Hypertension **3:**456-459, 1981.
13. Richer C, Giroux B, Plouin PF, Maarek B, Giudicelli JF: Captopril: Pharmacokinetics, antihypertensive and biological effects in hypertensive patients. Br J Clin Pharmacol **17:**243-250, 1984.

New insights into the pharmacokinetics of spironolactone

Four healthy men took a single oral dose of 200 mg spironolactone after a standardized breakfast. Blood samples were drawn until 24 hours after dosing. A specific HPLC method was used to determine the serum concentrations of spironolactone and its metabolites 7α-thiomethylspirolactone, 6β-hydroxy-7α-thiomethylspirolactone, and canrenone. Pharmacokinetic parameters were derived from the serum concentration-time course of each compound. Spironolactone, 7α-thiomethylspirolactone, and canrenone are known to have antimineralocorticoid activity in man. Our study demonstrated that: (1) 7α-Thiomethylspirolactone is the main metabolite of spironolactone after a single oral dose as judged by the AUC(0-24) and the maximum concentration; and (2) unchanged spironolactone was detected in serum, with a maximum concentration at 1 hour and detectable levels up to 8 hours after dosing. Our findings are contrary to the widely accepted belief that spironolactone is metabolized too rapidly to be detected in serum after oral dosing and that canrenone is the principal metabolite of spironolactone. (Clin Pharmacol Ther 1985;38:469-74.)

Hans W. P. M. Overdiek, Pharm.D., Walter A. J. J. Hermens, B.S., and Frans W. H. M. Merkus, Ph.D. *Sittard and Amsterdam, The Netherlands*

The aldosterone antagonist spironolactone is extensively metabolized into many metabolites in man.[1-5] The most likely route of metabolism is shown in Fig. 1.[5,6] Until now, canrenone was quantitatively found through the use of unspecific assays to be the major unconjugated metabolite in serum or plasma after administration of spironolactone.[1-3,7-9] Because canrenone also has aldosterone-blocking properties, the activity of spironolactone was mainly attributed to canrenone.[10,11] For this reason pharmacokinetic studies of spironolactone focus on its kinetic behavior.[12-21]

The fluorimetric method[22-24] most frequently used for measuring canrenone concentrations in plasma and urine was recently proved to be relatively unspecific,[16,21,25-28] as other metabolites were measured concomitantly. Consequently, true canrenone concentrations were much lower than had been previously assumed.[16,21,25-28] Furthermore, it was shown from studies of its pharmacologic activity that canrenone could only explain a minor part of the activity of spironolactone.[26,29,30] Combining these analytic and pharmacologic results led to the unavoidable conclusion that metabolites other than canrenone must be mainly responsible for the antimineralocorticoid activity of spironolactone.[3,21,25,26,29,30] Also, spironolactone itself is mentioned as the possible pharmacologically active principle after its administration.[3,31,32] Among the metabolites, the sulfur-containing metabolites are proposed as the principal pharmacologically active moieties after spironolactone administration.[3,29,31,32] However, very little is known about the pharmacokinetic behavior of these metabolites and the unaltered parent drug. Our objective was to determine the single-dose pharmacokinetics of spironolactone in healthy subjects, with special regard to spironolactone itself and its sulfur-containing metabolites.

From the Clinical Pharmacokinetics and Toxicology Laboratory, Hospital of Sittard, Sittard, and Department of Biopharmaceutics, University of Amsterdam, Amsterdam.

Received for publication May 17, 1985; accepted July 10, 1985.

Reprint requests to: J. W. P. M. Overdiek, Pharm.D., Clinical Pharmacokinetics and Toxicology Laboratory, Hospital of Sittard, Walramstraat 23, 6131 BK Sittard, The Netherlands.

METHODS

Preliminary study. Two healthy men took an oral dose of 200 mg spironolactone as two 100 mg tablets of Aldactone (G. D. Searle & Co.). Pooled serum samples drawn up to 24 hours after dosing were qualitatively analyzed by HPLC for the presence of spironolactone, canrenone, and 6β-hydroxy-7α-thiomethylspirolactone. These are the compounds found by other investigators in the plasma or serum of subjects who took an oral dose of spironolactone,[1,5] although there are conflicting reports about the presence of spironolactone.[5,29] The HPLC method we used has been described previously.[25] However, for the purpose of our study we changed the wavelength of detection from 280

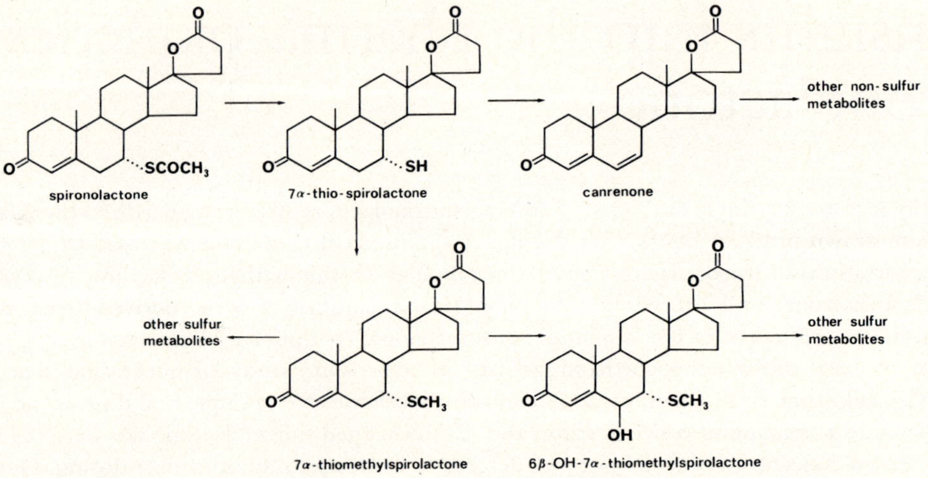

Fig. 1. Metabolic pathway of spironolactone.

Table I. Serum concentrations of spironolactone and its metabolites in four subjects after spironolactone, 200 mg po

	Serum concentration (ng/ml)			
Time after dosing (hr)	*Spironolactone*	*7α-Thiomethylspirolactone*	*6β-Hydroxy-7α-thiomethylspirolactone*	*Canrenone*
0.5	79 ± 33	132 ± 31	8 ± 9	21 ± 7
1	185 ± 51	486 ± 54	71 ± 24	101 ± 14
2	114 ± 32	555 ± 90	158 ± 18	203 ± 14
3	60 ± 21	461 ± 132	194 ± 53	225 ± 57
4	33 ± 14	353 ± 133	190 ± 65	213 ± 62
6	11 ± 6	193 ± 55	174 ± 59	190 ± 44
8	6 ± 4	137 ± 40	155 ± 55	159 ± 36
24	0	37 ± 11	47 ± 9	58 ± 7

Data are $\overline{X}$ ± SD.

to 240 nm. At this latter wavelength, spironolactone and its sulfur metabolites exert their maximum of absorption while canrenone still shows sufficient absorption to be measured. Spironolactone, canrenone, and 6β-hydroxy-7α-thiomethylspirolactone were detected in the serum of the subjects. There was also a large unidentified peak in our HPLC chromatograms, the retention time of which coincided with the retention time of synthetic 7α-thiomethylspirolactone. Isolation of this compound from the column and mass spectrometric analysis confirmed its identity as 7α-thiomethylspirolactone. Mass spectrometric analysis was performed on a Kratos Inc. MS 80 mass spectrometer. The sample was run at 70 eV by direct probe analysis in the electron impact mode.

Although 7α-thiospirolactone has the same retention time as 7α-thiomethylspirolactone in the HPLC system, no 7α-thiospirolactone could be detected in the serum of the two subjects when a reversed-phase HPLC system was applied to separate these compounds. Characteristics of this system are: column, 30 cm μ-Bondapak C-18 (Waters Associates, Inc.); mobile phase, methanol:water (60:40) flow rate, 1.5 ml/min; and detection, ultraviolet absorption at 240 nm. Retention times of the thiol and the thiomethyl compound in this system are 10.9 and 12.7 minutes, respectively.

Main study. Four healthy men ($\overline{X}$ ± SD age = 34 ± 12 years, weight = 76 ± 11 kg) took a single oral dose of 200 mg spironolactone as two 100 mg Aldactone tablets with 250 ml water. Because food has been shown to enhance the absorption of spironolactone,[33] the tablets were taken immediately after a standardized meal and the subjects were not allowed to eat for 2 hours afterwards. Subjects used no other drugs and abstained from alcohol the day before and during the experiment. Blood samples (10 ml) were drawn by venipuncture into nonheparinized Vacutainer tubes (Becton Dickinson) just before and at 0.5, 1, 2, 3, 4,

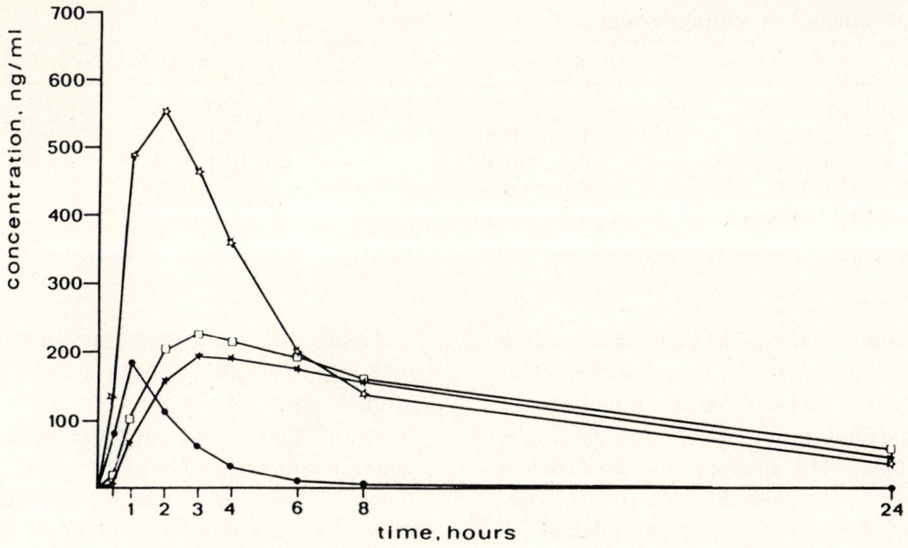

Fig. 2. Mean serum concentrations of spironolactone (●), 7α-thiomethylspirolactone (☆), 6β-hydroxy-7α-thiomethylspirolactone (★), and canrenone (□) after 200 mg po spironolactone in four subjects.

6, 8, and 24 hours after spironolactone dosing. After clotting the serum was separated by centrifugation and stored at −20° C until analyzed.

Serum concentrations of spironolactone, 7α-thiomethylspirolactone, 6β-hydroxy-7α-thiomethylspirolactone, and canrenone were determined by a specific normal phase HPLC method, which is a modification of our previously used method[25] and is described elsewhere.[34] Although 7α-thiospirolactone was not present in the serum in our preliminary study, the absence of this compound should be controlled for in other subjects by the reversed-phase HPLC system used in the preliminary study.

The following pharmacokinetic parameters were derived from the serum concentrations of spironolactone and its metabolites: time of observed maximum serum concentration (t_{max}), observed maximum serum concentration (C_{max}), serum AUC up to 24 hours after dosing calculated by the trapezoidal method, and the elimination $t_{1/2}$ determined by linear regression analysis of the linear terminal phase of the serum concentration-time curve.

Data are expressed as the $\overline{X} \pm$ SD.

RESULTS

7α-Thiospirolactone could not be detected in any serum sample. Serum concentrations of spironolactone, 7α-thiomethylspirolactone, 6β-hydroxy-7α-thiomethylspirolactone, and canrenone are listed in Table I and shown in Fig. 2. The most important findings were the high serum concentrations of 7α-thiomethylspirolactone relative to spironolactone, canrenone, and 6β-hydroxy-7α-thiomethylspirolactone. The mean C_{max} of 7α-thiomethylspirolactone reached a high value of 571 ± 74 ng/ml, far exceeding that of spironolactone (185 ± 51 ng/ml), canrenone (231 ± 49 ng/ml), and 6β-hydroxy-7α-thiomethylspirolactone (202 ± 54 ng/ml) (these C_{max} values are the means of individual C_{max} values).

Despite its relatively short $t_{1/2}$ of 2.8 ± 0.4 hours, the dominant presence of 7α-thiomethylspirolactone is also reflected by its AUC(0-24) value of 3880 ± 869 ng/ml · hr, which is the highest value of all four compounds measured in serum. Before this study 7α-thiomethylspirolactone had never been identified in biologic fluids. Another important finding was that the spironolactone C_{max} (185 ± 51 ng/ml) was the same order of magnitude as the C_{max} of canrenone (231 ± 49 ng/ml) and 6β-hydroxy-7α-thiomethylspirolactone (202 ± 54 ng/ml). Because of its short $t_{1/2}$ of 1.3 ± 0.2 hours, the AUC(0-24) of spironolactone (473 ± 149 ng/ml · hr) is only a fraction of the AUC(0-24) value of its metabolites. The t_{max} values for each compound are in accord with the metabolic pathway of spironolactone (Fig. 1). The pharmacokinetics of spironolactone and its metabolites are summarized in Table II.

DISCUSSION

Published data on the pharmacokinetic behavior of the sulfur-containing metabolites of spironolactone are

Table II. Pharmacokinetics of spironolactone and its metabolites

	Spironolactone	*7α-Thiomethylspirolactone*	*6β-Hydroxy-7α-thiomethylspirolactone*	*Canrenone*
C_{max} (ng/ml)	185 ± 51	571 ± 74	202 ± 54	231 ± 49
t_{max} (hr)	1.0 ± 0	1.8 ± 0.5	3.1 ± 0.9	2.9 ± 0.6
$t_{1/2}$ (hr)	1.3 ± 0.3	2.8 ± 0.4	10.1 ± 2.3*	11.2 ± 2.3*
$AUC_{(0-24)}$ (ng/ml · hr)	473 ± 149	3880 ± 869	2812 ± 785	3107 ± 551

Data are $\overline{X}$ ± SD.
*These data should be interpreted with some reserve, as not enough blood samples may have been drawn during the elimination phase to determine these values accurately.

scarce and are mainly restricted to their identification in biologic fluids.[5,7,9] The generally accepted theory that spironolactone itself is metabolized too rapidly to be detected in biologic fluids is not supported by the results of all investigations.[5] The findings discussed below were only possible in our study because of the availability of the sensitive and specific assay method for simultaneously measuring spironolactone, canrenone, 7α-thiomethylspirolactone, and 6β-hydroxy-7α-thiomethylspirolactone.

The most important result of our study is that in a quantitative sense, 7α-thiomethylspirolactone is the major metabolite of spironolactone in serum after a single oral dose of 200 mg spironolactone to healthy men. Although this metabolite was postulated to be an intermediary product in the metabolism of spironolactone (Fig. 1), its presence even in trace amounts has not been reported before.[6,29,32] The logical question arises as to why high serum concentrations of this metabolite were found by us but not by others. In our opinion the most probable reason is the use of relatively nonspecific analytic methods in previous studies elucidating spironolactone metabolism.

After the conclusion of Gochman and Gantt[22] that the major portion of circulating spironolactone was in the form of canrenone, they developed a fluorimetric assay to measure its concentrations. Since then, this assay (or slight modifications thereof[23]) has been exhaustively used in the study of spironolactone pharmacokinetics and bioavailability. In the past few years it has been clearly shown that the fluorimetric assay is not specific for canrenone and that other metabolites are also measured concomitantly[21,25] by this technique. The fact that other investigators who identified not only canrenone but also other metabolites did not find 7α-thiomethylspirolactone, may be due to: (1) The use of TLC systems that do not separate 7α-thiomethylspirolactone from canrenone[21,35] or 7α-thiomethylspirolactone from spironolactone and 7α-thiospirolactone,[21] and (2) the in vitro conversion of sulfur-containing metabolites to canrenone, especially under gas chromatography.[9,35-37]

Among the sulfur-containing metabolites, 7α-thiomethylspirolactone has been shown to possess a higher affinity than canrenone for aldosterone receptors in vitro.[37] Furthermore, it possesses a remarkably high antimineralocorticoid activity in rats and dogs.[38] In a bioassay model developed to determine the renal antimineralocorticoid activity of orally administered spirolactones in man, 7α-thiospirolactone and 7α-thiomethylspirolactone were found to have an activity of only 0.26 and 0.33, respectively, relative to spironolactone.[32] However, serum concentrations of these substances were not determined, and the authors suggested that the 7α-thio and 7α-thiomethyl side chains might be removed completely either before or immediately after absorption.[32] It is possible that 7α-thiospirolactone and 7α-thiomethylspirolactone have high activity but do not reach the target organ in sufficient quantities. It can be hypothesized that spironolactone is the prodrug for these metabolites.

Another important finding is the presence of high concentration of unchanged spironolactone in serum. There are conflicting results concerning the presence of unchanged spironolactone in biologic fluids. Most investigators report that spironolactone is metabolized too rapidly to be detected in urine or in plasma.[4,29,32] Only two studies have been published in which the parent drug was found in plasma after administration of spironolactone to man, but absolute serum concentrations have never been determined.[5,22]

Our study indicates that spironolactone reaches a C_{max} of the same order of magnitude as those of 6β-hydroxy-7α-thiomethylspirolactone and canrenone. Even 8 hours after spironolactone dosing it could still be detected in the serum of all subjects. The hypothesis that spironolactone itself might be responsible for its activity is supported by the finding that spironolactone has a relatively high affinity for renal aldosterone receptors in vitro[37] and shows antimineralocorticoid action in an isolated toad bladder system.[39] Furthermore, until now no metabolite of spironolactone has been found that is more active than the unaltered parent drug in man.

The logical consequence of rejecting the untenable theory that canrenone is the major active metabolite of spironolactone was to propose sulfur-containing metabolites and/or spironolactone itself as the substance(s) responsible for the action of spironolactone. However, this new theory has never been firmly supported by pharmacokinetic data of these substances. Our study is the first to offer tangible support by identifying 7α-thiomethylspirolactone as the major metabolite after a single oral dose of spironolactone and by showing considerable amounts of the parent drug in serum.

Finally, since our study demonstrates that the $t_{1/2}$ values of spironolactone and 7α-thiomethylspirolactone are much shorter than that of canrenone, one could speculate that after multiple dosing the relative proportion of canrenone at steady state would be higher than that of spironolactone or 7α-thiomethylspirolactone. For this reason, further studies will be carried out after multiple doses of spironolactone.

We thank Dr. Aziz Karim of G. D. Searle & Co. for comments and for the supply of spironolactone and its metabolites, and Dr. Gerard J. Q. van der Peyl and Mr. Leo J. Cremers for the mass spectrometric analysis.

References

1. Karim A. Spironolactone: disposition, metabolism, pharmacodynamics, and bioavailability. Drug Metab Rev 1978;8:151-88.
2. Karim A. Pharmacokinetics and metabolism of aldosterone antagonists: a review. In: Addison GM, Wirenfeldt Asmussen N, Corvol P, et al, eds. Aldosterone antagonists in clinical medicine. Amsterdam-Oxford: Excerpta Medica, 1978:115-29.
3. Ramsay LE. Clinical pharmacology and therapeutic use of aldosterone antagonists. In: Agarwal MK, ed. Hormone antagonists. Berlin-New York: Walter de Gruyter and Co, 1982:335-63.
4. Karim A, Hribar J, Doherty M, et al. Spironolactone: diversity in metabolic pathways. Xenobiotica 1977;7: 585-600.
5. Abshagen U, Rennekamp H, Luszpinski G. Pharmacokinetics of spironolactone in man. Naunyn Schmiedebergs Arch Pharmacol 1976;296:37-45.
6. Ho PC, Bourne DWA, Triggs EJ, Heazlewood V. Pharmacokinetics of canrenone and metabolites after base hydrolysis following single and multiple dose oral administration of spironolactone. Eur J Clin Pharmacol 1984;27:441-6.
7. Karim A, Zagarella J, Hribar J, Dooley M. Spironolactone. I. Disposition and metabolism. CLIN PHARMACOL THER 1976;19:158-69.
8. Sadée W, Dagcioglu M, Schröder R. Pharmacokinetics of spironolactone, canrenone and canrenoate-K in humans. J Pharmacol Exp Ther 1973;185:686-95.
9. Karim A, Hribar J, Aksamit W, Doherty M, Chinn LJ. Spironolactone metabolism in man studied by gas chromatography-mass spectrometry. Drug Metab Dispos 1975;3:467-78.
10. Sadée W, Dagcioglu M, Schröder R. Pharmacokinetics of Aldactone[R] in humans. In: Brendel W, Coraboeuf E, Ebling FJG, et al, eds. Extrarenal activity of aldosterone and its antagonists. Amsterdam: Excerpta Medica, 1972:40-2.
11. Hettiarachchi J, Ramsay LE. Spironolactone response related to plasma canrenone concentration. Br J Clin Pharmacol 1979;7:426P-7P.
12. Portal A, Gaillot J, Bieder A, Rodary C, Bertharion JJ. Des aspects de la biodisponibilité physiologique de la spironolactone et de la canrénone. Semin Hop 1976; 5:465-70.
13. Radó JP, Szende L, Takó J, Nagy O, Kozma C. Application of a simple fluorometric method on absorption of canrenone. Int J Clin Pharmacol Res 1976;13:123-6.
14. Jackson L, Branch R, Levine D, Ramsay L. Elimination of canrenone in congestive heart failure and chronic liver disease. Eur J Clin Pharmacol 1977;11:177-9.
15. Clarke JM, Ramsay LE, Shelton JR, Tidd MJ, Murray S, Palmer RF. Factors influencing comparative bioavailability of spironolactone tablets. J Pharm Sci 1977; 66:1429-32.
16. Besenfelder E, Endele R. High performance liquid chromatographic method for determination of canrenone in serum. J High Resolut Chromatogr Chromatogr Commun 1981;4:419-21.
17. Abshagen U, Platt D, Horn HJ. Zur Pharmakokinetik von Spironolacton im Alter. Klin Wochenschr 1981;59: 909-10.
18. McInnes GT, Asbury MJ, Ramsay LE, Shelton JR, Harrison IR. Effect of micronization on the bioavailability and pharmacologic activity of spironolactone. J Clin Pharmacol 1982;22:410-7.
19. Sponer G, Kaufmann B, Kuhr M. Pharmakokinetik von Aldosteron-Antagonisten. Krankenhausarzt 1976;49: 569-75.
20. Krause W, Karras J, Seifert W. Pharmacokinetics of canrenone after oral administration of spironolactone and intravenous injection of canrenoate-K in healthy man. Eur J Clin Pharmacol 1983;25:449-53.
21. Abshagen U, Besenfelder E, Endele R, Koch K, Neubert B. Kinetics of canrenone after single and multiple doses of spironolactone. Eur J Clin Pharmacol 1979;16:255-62.
22. Gochman N, Gantt CL. A fluorimetric method for the determination of a major spironolactone (Aldactone) metabolite in human plasma. J Pharmacol Exp Ther 1962;135:312-6.
23. Sadée W, Dagcioglu M, Riegelman S. Fluorometric microassay for spironolactone and its metabolites in biological fluids. J Pharm Sci 1972;61:1126-8.
24. Neubert P, Koch K. Simultaneous automated determination of spironolactone metabolites in serum. J Pharm Sci 1977;66:1131-4.

25. Merkus FWHM, Overdiek JWPM, Cilissen J, Zuidema J. Pharmacokinetics of spironolactone after a single dose: evaluation of the true canrenone serum concentrations during 24 hours. Clin Exp Hypertens 1983;5:239-48.
26. Dahlöf CG, Lundborg P, Persson BA, Regårdh CG. Reevaluation of the antimineralocorticoid effect of the spironolactone metabolite, canrenone, from plasma concentrations determined by a new high-pressure liquid-chromatographic method. Drug Metab Dispos 1979; 7:103-7.
27. Neurath GB, Ambrosius D. High-performance liquid chromatographic determination of canrenone, a major metabolite of spironolactone, in body fluids. J Chromatogr 1979;163:230-5.
28. Overdiek JWPM, Cilissen J, Hermens WAJJ, Merkus FWHM. The importance of canrenone in the metabolism of spironolactone. Pharm Weekbl [Sci] 1984;6:270.
29. Ramsay L, Shelton J, Harrison I, Tidd M, Asbury M. Spironolactone and potassium canrenoate in normal man. CLIN PHARMACOL THER 1976;20:167-77.
30. Huston GJ, Turner P. Antagonism of fludrocortisone by spironolactone and canrenone. Br J Clin Pharmacol 1976;3:201-4.
31. Merkus FWHM. Is canrenone the major metabolite of spironolactone? Clin Pharm 1983;2:209-10.
32. McInnes GT, Asbury MJ, Shelton JR, et al. Activity of sulfur-containing intermediate metabolites of spironolactone. CLIN PHARMACOL THER 1980;27:363-9.
33. Melander A, Danielson K, Schersten B, Thulin T, Wåhlin E. Enhancement by food of canrenone bioavailability from spironolactone. CLIN PHARMACOL THER 1977; 22:100-3.
34. Overdiek JWPM, Hermens WAJJ, Merkus FWHM. Determination of the serum concentrations of spironolactone and its metabolites by high-performance liquid chromatography. J Chromatogr 1985;341:279-85.
35. Karim A, Brown EA. Isolation and identification of novel sulfur-containing metabolites of spironolactone (Aldactone[R]). Steroids 1972;20:41-62.
36. Stüber W, Mutschler E, Steinbach D. Zur Spezifität der Bestimmung von Canrenon in biologischen Flüssigkeiten. Arch Pharm 1981;314:148-56.
37. Funder JW, Feldman D, Highland E, Edelman IS. Molecular modifications of anti-aldosterone compounds: effects on affinity of spirolactones for renal aldosterone receptors. Biochem Pharmacol 1974;23:1493-501.
38. Hofmann LM. Aldosterone antagonists in laboratory animals. In: Wesson LG, Fanelli GM, eds. Recent advances in renal physiology and pharmacology. Baltimore: University Park Press, 1974:305-16.
39. Sakauye C, Feldman D. Agonist and antimineralocorticoid activities of spirolactones. Am J Physiol 1976; 231:93-7.

LETTER TO THE EDITOR

Concomitant food intake does enhance the bioavailability and effect of hydralazine

To the Editor:

There is evidence that concomitant food intake can influence the bioavailability of several drugs.[1,2] Such an influence can be exerted not only on their gastrointestinal absorption,[1] but also (and most pronouncedly) on their presystemic metabolic clearance.[2] Indeed, concomitant food intake can enhance the bioavailability of lipophilic, weakly basic drugs such as propranolol, metoprolol, dixyrazine, and hydralazine by 40% to 100% through reduction of their presystemic clearance.[2-6] The most dramatic example is hydralazine, whose food-induced increase in bioavailability may exceed 100%.[5]

In a recent issue of this JOURNAL, Shepherd et al.[6] reported that food intake decreased rather than increased the bioavailability of hydralazine and that this food effect was associated with a diminished increase in heart rate.[6] The authors argued that this discrepancy occurred because the analytic method used in one of our previous studies[5] is nonspecific. We are fully aware of this nonspecificity and accept the data of Shepherd et al. without hesitation. However, their interpretation is inaccurate insofar as concomitant food intake is concerned.

For reasons not stated, Shepherd et al.[6] chose to administer hydralazine 45 minutes after a test meal identical to ours, whereas we have always tested the influence of food by giving the drug together with the meal. This is more important than it may seem, as the food effect is very transient[2] and may wane within 45 minutes. In support of this, a study with a more selective analytic approach[7] confirmed that concomitant food intake does enhance hydralazine bioavailability, but only when given in the conventional rapid-release formulation; when administered in a slow-release formulation there was no such influence.[7] A similar difference has been observed when rapid-release and slow-release formulations of propranolol have been given together with food.[8] Moreover, five subjects in the first food-hydralazine study[5] had higher heart rates 30 minutes after drug intake when hydralazine was administered together with food ($\bar{X} \pm SD = 94 \pm 8$ bpm) than when administered in the fasting state (80 ± 6 bpm; data not given in the report).

Accordingly, the findings of Shepherd et al.[6] do not challenge the contention that concomitant food intake enhances the bioavailability of hydralazine or of some active hydralazine metabolite. Rather, they emphasize the very transient nature of the food effect.

A. Melander, M.D.
H. Liedholm, M.D.
A. McLean, M.D.
Lund University Health Sciences Center and Monash University Department of Medicine
Dalby, Sweden, and Melbourne, Australia

References

1. Melander A. Influence of food on the bioavailability of drugs. Clin Pharmacokinet 1978;3:337-51.
2. Melander A, McLean AJ. Influence of food intake on presystemic clearance of drugs. Clin Pharmacokinet 1983;8:286-97.
3. Melander A, Danielson K, Scherstén B, Wåhlin E. Enhancement of the bioavailability of propranolol and metoprolol by food. CLIN PHARMACOL THER 1977;22:108-12.
4. Liedholm H, Lidén A, Kroon L, Melander A, Wåhlin-Boll E. Pharmacokinetics of dixyrazine: low bioavailability, improved by food intake. Drug Nutr Interact 1985;3:87-92.
5. Melander A, Danielson K, Hanson A, Rudell B, Scherstén B, Thulin T, Wåhlin E. Enhancement of hydralazine bioavailability by food. CLIN PHARMACOL THER 1977;22:104-7.
6. Shepherd AMM, Irvine NA, Ludden TM. Effect of food on blood hydralazine levels and response in hypertension. CLIN PHARMACOL THER 1984;36:14-8.
7. Liedholm H, Wåhlin-Boll E, Hanson A, Melander A. Influence of food on the bioavailability of "real" and "apparent" hydralazine from conventional and slow-release preparations. Drug Nutr Interact 1982;1:293-302.
8. Byrne AJ, McNeil J, Harrison PM, Louis W, Tonkin AM, McLean AJ. Stable oral availability of sustained release propranolol when coadministered with hydralazine or food: evidence implicating substrate delivery rate as a determinant of presystemic drug interactions. Br J Clin Pharmacol 1984;17(suppl 1):45S-50S.

Reply

To the Editor:

Melander et al. have made several points with regard to our recent article[1] in the JOURNAL on the effect of food on blood hydralazine levels after oral administration. I will deal with them in turn.

The oral bioavailability of hydralazine was stated to be increased by concomitant food administration. This study by Melander et al.[2] in 1977 used the method of Jack et al.[3] to measure plasma hydralazine levels. This method is nonspecific, measuring not only hydralazine but the acid-labile metabolites, of which the hydralazine pyruvic acid hydrazone (HPH) is a major component. More than 90% of the hydralazine measured by this assay is in fact HPH.[3] There is between 50 and 100 times as much HPH in plasma as there is hydralazine by 3 hours after single and repeated oral doses of hydralazine.[4] A more recent study by Liedholm et al.[5] also examines the oral bioavailability of hydralazine through the use of the assay of Zak et al.[6] This assay is likely to be less nonspecific than the method used in their previous study, but there is probably also acid hydrolysis of HPH at the acid pH used in this assay.[7] At the blood levels of hydralazine and HPH found in this study, detection of only 3% of the HPH as hydralazine will eliminate the finding of increased availability of hydralazine with food. Indeed, in this study there were no significant differences (paired and unpaired t test, one- and two-tailed; paired Wilcoxon test) in any of the plasma hydralazine parameters measured by the more specific hydralazine assay[6] between the subjects given hydralazine with or without food unless log transformation of the data was carried out. The hydralazine levels after slow-release hydralazine could not be measured by the more specific method as the levels were too low. Therefore, they were measured by the very nonspecific method of Jack et al.[3] It is clear that published data[2,5] regarding the effect of concomitant food on oral hydralazine bioavailability must be interpreted with great caution.

Melander et al. also state that the food effect is very transient and may have waned in 45 minutes. The effect of food on tablet dissolution and disintegration and on gastric emptying may indeed have waned by 45 minutes. However, the effect of food on the parameters examined in our study was still present. This is obviously true since we found not only a marked difference in blood hydralazine levels (mean [± SE] peak hydralazine level: food, 0.69 ± 0.22 μmol/L; fasted, 1.18 ± 0.23 μmol/L [$P < 0.02$]; AUC: food, 18.40 ± 5.06 μmol/L min; fasted, 31.25 ± 6.13 μmol/L min [$P < 0.02$]) but also a parallel reduction in vasodepressor response (fall in mean arterial pressure: food, 11 ± 2 mm Hg; fasted, 18 ± 3 mm Hg [$P < 0.001$]).

Melander et al. also state that heart rate was increased when hydralazine was given with food compared with when it was given without food. We too found this inappropriate tachycardia and postulated that it could be due to higher blood levels of HPH, which has been shown to induce tachycardia in dogs.[8]

In conclusion, there were differences in study design between our study (designed to examine the bioavailability of an oral solution) and those of Liedholm et al.[5] (designed in part to examine the effect of food on hydralazine passage to the absorptive area of the gut). However, in the absence of definitive data from the previous studies, there can be no basic disagreement between the information presented in any of the studies. We are presently performing a study to examine the effect of food on the oral bioavailability of conventional hydralazine tablets and of slow-release hydralazine through the use of a specific assay for blood hydralazine levels.

Alexander M. M. Shepherd, M.D., Ph.D.
Thomas M. Ludden, Ph.D.
Divisions of Clinical Pharmacology and Pharmacy,
Departments of Pharmacology and Medicine
University of Texas Health Sciences Center
7103 Floyd Curl Dr.
San Antonio, TX 78284

References

1. Shepherd AMM, Irvine NA, Ludden TM. Effect of food on blood hydralazine levels and response in hypertension. CLIN PHARMACOL THER 1984;36:14-8.
2. Melander A, Danielson K, Hanson A, Rudell B, Scherstén B, Thulin T, Wåhlin E. Enhancement of hydralazine bioavailability by food. CLIN PHARMACOL THER 1977;22:104-7.
3. Jack DB, Brechbuhler S, Degen PH, Zbinden P, Riess W. The determination of hydralazine in plasma by gas-liquid chromatography. J Chromatogr 1975;115:87-92.
4. Shepherd AMM, Ludden T, McNay JL, Lin M-S. Hydralazine kinetics after single and repeated oral doses. CLIN PHARMACOL THER 1980;28:804-11.
5. Liedholm H, Wåhlin-Boll E, Hanson A, Melander A. Influence of food on the bioavailabilty of "real" and "apparent" hydralazine from conventional and slow-release preparations. Drug Nutr Interact 1983;1:293-302.
6. Zak SB, Lukas G, Gilleran TG. Plasma levels of real and "apparent" hydralazine in man and rat. Drug Metab Dispos 1977;5:116-21.
7. Reece PA, Stanley PE, Zacest R. Interference in assays for hydralazine in humans by a major plasma metabolite, hydralazine pyruvic acid hydrazone. J Pharm Sci 1978;67: 1150-3.
8. Shepherd AMM, Musgrave GE, Badke FR, Walsh R. Tachycardia associated with hydralazine pyruvic acid hydrazone, the major plasma metabolite of hydralazine [Abstract]. Fed Proc 1980;39:1190.

LIST OF REVIEWERS

The Co-Editors wish to thank the following people who helped with the manuscript review process from Jan. 1 through June 30, 1985:

Abernethy, Darrell R., M.D., Ph.D.
Abrams, William B., M.D.
Affrime, Melton B., Pharm.D.
Albert, Kenneth S., Ph.D.
Ambre, John J., M.D., Ph.D.
Aogaichi, Keiko, M.D.
Aronoff, George R., M.D.
Bayliss, Celine Stahl, M.D.
Beaver, William T., M.D.
Becker, David, M.D.
Bennett, William M., M.D.
Benowitz, Neal L., M.D.
Berlin, Cheston M., Jr., M.D.
Bialer, Meir, Ph.D.
Bigger, John Thomas, Jr., M.D.
Bloomfield, Saul S., M.D.
Branch, Robert A., M.D.
Brater, Donald Craig, M.D.
Caruso, Frank S., Ph.D.
Case, David B., M.D.
Cody, Robert J., Jr., M.D.
Colburn, Wayne A., Ph.D.
Crout, J. Richard, M.D.
Cusack, Barry J., M.D.
Davies, R. O., M.D., Ph.D.
Desjardins, Robert E., M.D.
Drayer, Dennis E., Ph.D.
Drayer, Jan I., M.D.
Dujovne, Carlos A., M.D.
du Souich, Beltran P., M.D., Ph.D.
Dvorchik, Barry H., Ph.D.
Ehrlich, George E., M.D.
Ferguson, Roger K., M.D.
Finkel, Marion J., M.D.
Fleckenstein, Lawrence L., Pharm.D.
Freed, Curt R., M.D.
Freedman, Daniel X., M.D.
Gambertoglio, John G., Pharm.D.
Giacomini, Kathleen, Ph.D.
Gibson, Thomas P., M.D.
Gifford, Ray W., Jr., M.D.
Goldman, Peter, M.D.
Goredetsky, Charles W., M.D., Ph.D.
Greenblatt, David J., M.D.
Halushka, Perry V., M.D., Ph.D.
Hamilton, Bruce P., M.D.
Holtzman, Jordan L., M.D., Ph.D.
Hull, J. Heyward, Pharm.D.
Inaba, Ted, Ph.D.
Jaffe, Jerome H., M.D.
Jones, Brian, M.B.B.S.
Jones, Judith K., M.D., Ph.D.
Juan, David, M.D.
Jusko, William J., Ph.D.
Kadar, Dezso, Ph.D.
Kalow, Werner, M.D.
Kantor, Thomas G., M.D.
Karim, Aziz, Ph.D.
Kimura, Kazuo K., M.D., Ph.D.
Kreek, Mary Jeanne, M.D.
Kupersmith, Joel, M.D.
Lalka, David, Ph.D.
Laskin, Oscar, M.D.
Lasseter, Kenneth C., M.D.
Lertora, Juan J. L., M.D., Ph.D.
Levy, Micha, M.D.
Linday, Linda A., M.D.
Ludden, Thomas M., Ph.D.
Luderer, John R., M.D.
Manion, Carl V., M.D.
Martin, William R., M.D.
Martz, B. L., M.D.
McDonald, Robert H., Jr., M.D.
McMahon, F. Gilbert, M.D.
McNay, John L., M.D.
Mirkin, Bernard L., M.D., Ph.D.
Mitchell, Jerry, M.D., Ph.D.
Morgan, John Paul, M.D.
Murray, William J., M.D., Ph.D.
Naranjo, Claudio A., M.D.
Neiss, Edward S., M.D., Ph.D.
Nierenberg, David W., M.D.
Ogilvie, Richard Ian, M.D.
Okun, Ronald, M.D.
Olsen, George D., M.D.
O'Reilly, Robert A., M.D.
Peck, Carl C., M.D.
Perel, James M., Ph.D.
Potter, William Z., M.D., Ph.D.
Reele, Stots B., M.D.
Reuning, Richard H., Ph.D.
Rivlin, Richard, M.D.
Rollins, Douglas E., M.D., Ph.D.
Romankiewicz, John A., Pharm.D.
Ryan, Jerome R., M.D.
Schentag, Jerome J., Pharm.D.
Schneck, Dennis W., M.D., Ph.D.
Schrogie, John J., M.D.
Sellers, Edward M., M.D., Ph.D.
Shapiro, Alvin P., M.D.
Sheiner, Lewis B., M.D.
Shen, Danny D., Ph.D.
Shepherd, Alexander M. M., M.D., Ph.D.
Silver, Jonathan M., M.D.
Sitar, Daniel S., Ph.D.
Skelly, Jerome P., Ph.D.
Slattery, John T., Ph.D.
Smith, Cedric M., M.D.
Smith, Craig R., M.D.
Spielberg, Stephen P., M.D., Ph.D.
Stalker, Dennis J., Ph.D.
Stellman, Steven D., Ph.D.
Strom, Brian L., M.D.
Sunshine, Abraham, M.D.
Thompson, W. Leigh, M.D., Ph.D.
Ventura, Hector O., M.D.
Vestal, Robert E., M.D.
Walker, Barry R., M.D.
Wallenstein, Stanley L., M.S.
Wang, Richard I. H., M.D., Ph.D.
Weber, Michael A., M.D.
Weinberger, Miles M., M.D.
Weiner, Murray, M.D.
Weintraub, Michael, M.D.
Whitsett, Thomas L., M.D.
Wilkinson, Grant R., Ph.D.
Williams, Roger L., M.D.
Wilson, John T., M.D.
Winzelberg, Gary G., M.D.
Wolen, Robert L., Ph.D.
Yacobi, Avraham, Ph.D.

Notes of the American Society for Clinical Pharmacology and Therapeutics

The generosity of the following contributors in support of the annual meeting and the educational programs of the Society is sincerely appreciated.

Sponsoring donors

Ciba-Geigy Corporation, Pharmaceuticals Division
Hoffmann-La Roche Inc.
Eli Lilly and Company
Marion Laboratories, Inc.
Merck Sharp & Dohme Research Laboratories and Merck Sharp & Dohme Divison

Sustaining donors

Boehringer Ingelheim Corporation
Pfizer Pharmaceuticals and Pfizer Central Research

Contributing donors

Adria Laboratories Inc.
American Hoechst Corporation
McNeil Pharmaceutical
Ortho Pharmaceutical Corporation
Sandoz, Inc.
Schering Corporation
E. R. Squibb & Sons, Inc.
Stuart Pharmaceuticals, Division of ICI Americas Inc.
Syntex Research
Syva Company
Warner-Lambert Company
Wyeth Laboratories

Regular donors

Abbott Laboratories
American Cyanamid Company
Ayerst Laboratories
Beecham Laboratories
Berlex Laboratories, Inc.
Bristol-Myers Company
Du Pont Biomedical Products
Glaxo Inc.
Merrell Dow Research Institute
Revlon Health Care
Riker Laboratories, Inc./3M
Rorer Group Inc.
Searle Research and Development Division
Sterling Drug Inc.
The Upjohn Company
Wallace Laboratories

Program support

Allergan Pharmaceuticals, Inc.
Baxter Travenol Laboratories, Inc.
Biodecision Laboratories, Inc.
Fujisawa SmithKline Corporation
Harris Laboratories, Inc.
Ives Laboratories Inc.
Norwich Eaton Pharmaceuticals, Inc.
Pennwalt Pharmaceutical Division
Revlon Health Care Group, Ethical Products Division
A. H. Robins Company

USAN Council

List No. 265

New Names

The following nonproprietary names for the compounds described have been adopted by the United States Adopted Names (USAN) Council, which is sponsored by the American Medical Association, the American Pharmaceutical Association, and the US Pharmacopeial Convention, Inc., in cooperation with the respective pharmaceutical manufacturers. The designation USAN (United States Adopted Name) distinguishes these formally adopted nonproprietary names from other names. The information given under the category Therapeutic Claim is based on the manufacturer's claims at the time of publication. Adoption of USAN does not imply endorsement of the claims or products by the AMA, the US Pharmacopeia, or the APhA.

In some instances, the drugs listed are available only from the manufacturer to properly qualified investigators for clinical study.

USAN SURFILCON A

Pronunciation sŭr′ fĭl″ kŏn

Ingredient function contact lens material (hydrophilic)

Chemical names

(1) 1-ethenyl-2-pyrrolidinone polymer with methyl 2-methyl-2-propenoate and 2-propenyl 2-methyl-2-propenoate

(2) 1-vinyl-2-pyrrolidinone polymer with methyl methacrylate and allyl methacrylate

Structural formula

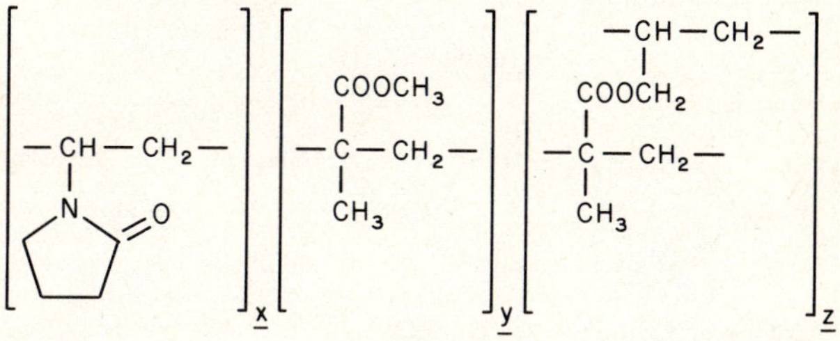

Molecular formula $(C_6H_9NO)x(C_5H_8O_2)y(C_7H_{10}O_2)z$

Trademark Permaflex

Manufacturer Coopervision Inc.

CAS registry No. 38809-73-3

USAN RECAINAM TOSYLATE

Pronunciation rĕ kān′ ăm

Therapeutic claim antiarrhythmic

Chemical names

(1) *N*-(2,6-dimethylphenyl)-*N*′-[3-[(1-methylethyl)amino]propyl]urea mono(4-methylbenzenesulfonate)

(2) 1-[3-(isopropylamino)propyl]-3-(2,6-xylyl)urea mono-*p*-toluenesulfonate

Structural formula

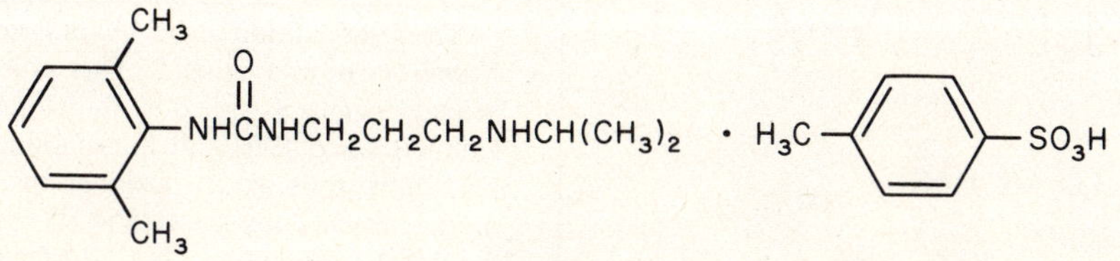

Molecular formula $C_{15}H_{25}N_3O \cdot C_7H_8O_3S$ or $C_{22}H_{33}N_3O_4S$

Molecular weight 435.57

Manufacturer Wyeth Laboratories Inc.

Code designation WY-42,362 tosylate

CAS registry No. 74752-08-2

USAN	ICOTIDINE
Pronunciation	ī kō′ tĭ dēn″
Therapeutic claim	H_2-receptor and H_1-receptor antagonist

Chemical names

(1) 2-[[4-(3-methoxy-2-pyridinyl)butyl]amino]-5-[(6-methyl-3-pyridinyl)methyl]-4(1*H*)-pyrimidinone

(2) 2-[[4-(3-methoxy-2-pyridyl)butyl]amino]-5-[(6-methyl-3-pyridyl)methyl]-4(1*H*)-pyrimidinone

Structural formula

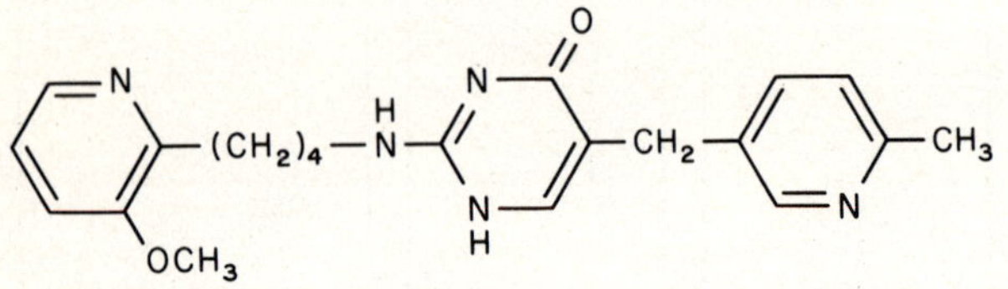

Molecular formula	$C_{21}H_{25}N_5O_2$
Molecular weight	379.46
Manufacturer	Smith Kline & French Laboratories
Code designation	SK&F 93319
CAS registry No.	71351-79-6

USAN	ASTIFILCON A
Pronunciation	ăs′ tĭ fĭl″ kŏn
Ingredient function	contact lens material (hydrophilic)

Chemical names

(1) methyl 2-methyl-2-propenoate polymer with 1-ethenyl-2-pyrrolidinone

(2) methyl methacrylate polymer with 1-vinyl-2-pyrrolidinone

Structural formula

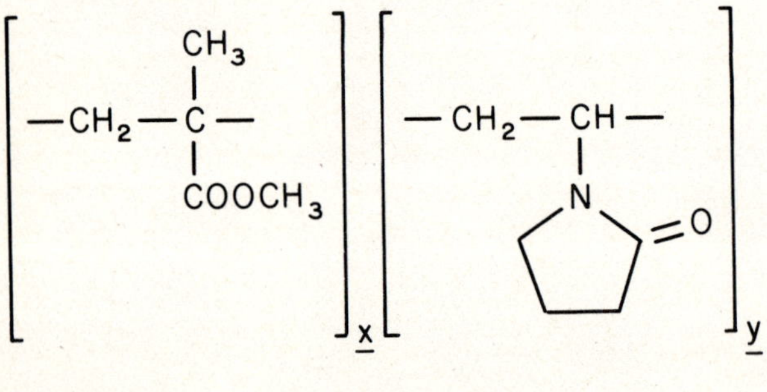

Molecular formula	$(C_5H_8O_2)x(C_6H_9NO)y$
Trademark	Breath-O
Manufacturer	Toray Industries, Inc. (Japan)
CAS registry No.	25655-01-0

USAN	INDOLAPRIL HYDROCHLORIDE
Pronunciation	ĭn dŏl′ ȧ prĭl″
Therapeutic claim	antihypertensive

Chemical names

(1) [2*S*-[1[*R**(*R**)],2α,3aβ,7aβ]]-1-[2-[[1-(ethoxycarbonyl)-3-phenylpropyl]amino]-1-oxopropyl]octahydro-1*H*-indole-2-carboxylic acid, monohydrochloride

(2) (2*S*,3a*S*,7a*S*)-1-[(*S*)-*N*-[(*S*)-1-carboxy-3-phenylpropyl]alanyl]hexahydro-2-indolinecarboxylic acid, 1-ethyl ester, monohydrochloride

Structural formula

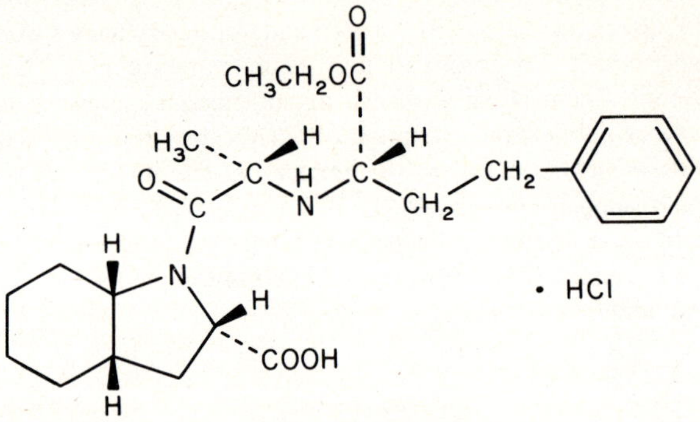

Molecular formula	$C_{24}H_{34}N_2O_5 \cdot HCl$
Molecular weight	467.01
Manufacturer	Parke-Davis
Code designation	CI-907
CAS registry No.	80828-32-6

NOTE: This statement provides new chemical information and supersedes previously published information (List No. 247).

New cumulative list of United States Adopted Names available

CLINICAL PHARMACOLOGY & THERAPEUTICS
VOLUME 38 NUMBER 5 NOVEMBER 1985

COMMENTARY

Premarketing observational studies of population pharmacokinetics of new drugs

Lewis B. Sheiner, M.D., and Leslie Z. Benet, Ph.D. *San Francisco, Calif.*

Recently, in a Food and Drug Administration (FDA) position paper, Dr. Robert Temple suggested, among other things, that a "pharmacokinetic screen" could be used to discover pharmacokinetic characteristics of new drugs in targeted patient populations, notably the elderly.[1] The reactions were considerable: The Pharmaceutical Manufacturers Association (PMA) responded negatively,* and at a workshop co-sponsored by the American Society for Clinical Pharmacology and Therapeutics and the FDA, considerable fear of the regulatory uses to which such data might be put was also expressed by industry spokespersons. Perhaps as a result, the recommendations for guidelines made to the FDA that evolved from that workshop do not mention the screen idea at all.[2]

From the Departments of Laboratory Medicine and Medicine, School of Medicine; Division of Clinical Pharmacology, Schools of Medicine and Pharmacy; and Department of Pharmacy, School of Pharmacy, University of California, San Francisco.

Supported in part by National Institutes of Health Grants No. GM 26676 and No. GM 26691.

Received for publication April 29, 1985; accepted July 25, 1985.

Reprint requests to: Lewis B. Sheiner, M.D., Professor of Laboratory Medicine and of Medicine, Clinics-255, University of California, San Francisco, CA 94143.

*Jennings J (on behalf of PMA): Personal communication (to Temple R), June 11, 1984.

We doubt whether the highly charged atmosphere engendered by discussions of new FDA requirements, regulations, or even guidelines is the proper one in which to debate the merits or demerits of a suggestion such as that of Dr. Temple. Herewith we take the opportunity to begin a less charged discussion of the pharmacokinetic screen idea as applied to new drug development. We discuss why premarketing studies of population pharmacokinetics of a new drug might be desirable, and how such studies might be conducted.

WHY STUDY POPULATION KINETICS?

In Dr. Temple's position paper, the means and ends of a pharmacokinetic screen are sketched, but not carefully defined. Basically, he advocates drawing (peak and) trough drug levels routinely during phase III studies and somehow using these to discover subgroups of patients with unusual kinetic characteristics. His suggestion amounts to performing therapeutic drug monitoring (TDM) of patients in phase III studies, but then, instead of using these data only clinically to adjust therapy for the individuals being studied, he proposes to draw inferences about population subgroups. When viewed in this light, the pharmacokinetic screen is seen to be an observational (i.e., nonexperimental) study of drug kinetics. Before we discuss the strengths and limitations of this type of study as compared with others, the questions to be addressed by any study of population kinetics should be stated.

Pathophysiologic effects. Certain pathophysiologic features of patients can regularly be shown to alter the dose-concentration relationship. For drugs eliminated largely by the kidney, renal failure usually causes steady-state drug levels to be greater than those of normal patients receiving the same drug dosage. A major quest of population kinetics is to discover which measurable pathophysiologic factors cause changes in the dose-concentration relationship and to estimate the degree to which they do so, so that appropriate dosage adjustment can be made. Because steady-state levels during chronic dosing are most often of primary therapeutic concern, influences on the two kinetic features determining these levels (bioavailability [F] and clearance [CL]) are of the greatest interest. Influences on the elimination $t_{1/2}$, which bears on choices of dosing interval, and volume of distribution (V_{area}), which bears on choice of loading dose, are of secondary interest. (Knowledge of CL plus either one of the two latter features suffices to determine the third.) One wishes to know about pathophysiologic effects on kinetics before a drug is marketed, so that appropriate a priori dosage adjustments can be made for population subgroups with altered kinetics.

Interindividual variability. A second feature of population kinetics that has received little attention, but is of considerable importance, is the magnitude of interindividual kinetic variability that is not explicable by (i.e., not correlated with) measurable pathophysiologic factors. An example is the degree of variability in CL values (from patient to patient) that remains after the influences of age, weight, renal function, and other known factors have been taken into account. The magnitude of such variability is important for several reasons. First, the safety and efficacy of a drug decreases as inexplicable variability increases. This is because drug levels outside the therapeutic range become more likely the greater the uncompensated variability in the relationship of dosage to steady-state drug level. Indeed, it is precisely because inexplicable interindividual variability tends to be so large in patients that TDM, in which measured drug levels are used to estimate the individuals' kinetics, has become popular. Sometimes the variability can be eliminated, for example, if it is due to large variability in F traceable to a defect in manufacture. Even when not correctable, a previously unrecognized pathophysiologic effect may be discovered to be partially accountable for the variability, and a priori dosage adjustment can be used. If neither correctable nor explicable, excess variability in certain subpopulations still alerts the practitioner to the necessity of careful observation or TDM in that population.

A final reason that knowledge of interindividual kinetic variability is important is so that optimal use can be made of measured drug levels when performing TDM. Such optimal use, involving an empiric Bayes approach, has been discussed elsewhere.[3,4]

Residual or intraindividual variability. Another population kinetic feature is the degree to which steady-state drug levels in individuals typically vary about their long-term average. They do vary (or appear to vary) due to inexplicable day-to-day kinetic variability and to drug level measurement error. Estimates of the magnitude of this kind of variability are important to the empiric Bayes TDM approach.

THE POPULATION OF INTEREST

Given that one wishes to learn about the population kinetics of new drugs before they are released, a general principle that should be obvious is that for a given drug, interest centers on its kinetics in the population(s) in which it is likely to be used. The kinetics in normal young men are largely irrelevant when treating most patients with most drugs. Certainly, basic kinetic features such as excretion vs. metabolism or a large vs. a small V_{area} will be common to all patient groups, but those population kinetic features of greatest immediate therapeutic concern can only be discovered by study of the relevant population. Thus drugs likely to be affected by pathophysiologic factors prevalent in the target population, and those with narrow therapeutic indices, are prime candidates for population kinetic studies. Criteria that might be used to identify drugs of particular concern in the elderly, for example, have been discussed elsewhere.[5]

HOW TO STUDY POPULATION PHARMACOKINETICS BEFORE MARKETING

Preliminary requirements. Before any study of population pharmacokinetics is undertaken, certain preliminary things must be known or available. First, one must have a sensitive and specific assay capable of measuring all species (parent drug and metabolites) of clinical relevance. This immediately suggests a second requirement: Preliminary studies must have demonstrated some correlation between drug or metabolite concentrations and clinically relevant effects (efficacy or toxicity). Clearly, a drug's kinetics are irrelevant if such correlations do not exist. A third requirement is also implied by the first: The drug's major metabolic pathways in man must be known. A fourth requirement is that preliminary kinetic studies must have established the basic model describing the drug's kinetics (e.g., linear vs. nonlinear). As will be seen shortly, several of the types of population kinetic studies to be suggested involve measuring only a few concentrations in each patient. Such data provide little information from which the basic kinetic model can be deduced. In short, observational population kinetic studies will add to, but will not replace, thorough preclinical evaluation of drug metabolism, kinetics, and dynamics.

The full study. To begin with the most elaborate, and most familiar, type of approach, a full pharmacokinetic study can be done in small groups of patients who exhibit potentially influential pathophysiologic features. These results can be compared with similar studies of patients not exhibiting such features.

Study requirements. These are well known and include a fixed and simple dosage regimen, possibly several separate studies (e.g., intravenous vs. oral dosing), multiple samples, meticulous data collection, and so on. This is an experimental study, not an observational one; therein lie both its strengths and weaknesses.

Strengths. (1) Such studies are well suited to estimating the magnitudes of pathophysiologic effects; (2) the study methodology is familiar and of proved validity; (3) standard data analysis techniques are applicable (e.g., weighted nonlinear least-squares regression); (4) distinct estimates of all pharmacokinetic features are obtained (i.e., individual kinetic parameters are all separately estimated), allowing influences on each to be separately quantified; and (5) inference is secure because independent variables are controlled by the experimentor.

Weaknesses. (1) Expense usually dictates that only a small number of individuals be studied. Estimates of interindividual variability will therefore be poor; (2) total expense may be quite high, as each study is costly and many studies may be required; (3) the ethics of extensively studying patients for speculative reasons when they, personally, will receive no benefit are questionable; (4) serendipity is not likely, since the magnitude of only those effects that are deliberately studied will be estimated; and (5) the requirements of the study design may, for ethical or other reasons, preclude the study of precisely those patients most likely to exhibit clinically significant differences in kinetics.

The single trough screen. At the other end of the spectrum, a very simple pharmacokinetic screen such as that suggested by Dr. Temple can be imagined. During open-label phase III studies, trough drug levels (one per patient) can be drawn. The status of the patient with respect to pathophysiologic features can be recorded, as well as the prescribed dosage regimen. Simple multiple linear regression may be used to explore the relationship of features to trough level (divided by daily dose) and important influences can be identified. Further, after all important factors have been accounted for in the regression, the residuals from the regression may be examined for outliers (exceptionally deviant levels or individuals), and further investigation of those patients' records can be undertaken in search of an explanation.

We would not suggest drawing peak levels as part of this design, as was proposed by Dr. Temple. Unless a drug is given intravenously (or as one of the newer sustained-release formulations), the absorption rate is highly variable from person to person. Furthermore, absorption and distribution rates are generally uninteresting in a therapeutic context, and are certainly less interesting than F or CL. Peak levels, however, are primarily determined by absorption and distribution rates. Consequently, sampling peak levels tells one virtually only about the variability of largely irrelevant kinetic processes and as a rule will contribute little to therapy. Moreover, should there be uncertainty as to timing of the last dose or when the level was measured (as is expected with this design), peak levels will be so noisy that whatever limited information they might otherwise have provided will be lost.

Requirements. Recognizing that the purpose of this type of study is simply to identify kinetically relevant factors and produce only a very approximate estimate of the size of their effects, data requirements can be quite lax. (1) Timing of drug levels need not be exact, but should be near trough; (2) it would be best if compliance with at least the last previous dose could be assured, but the patient's claim to this effect should be enough; (3) because of uncertain timing of doses and samples, the method can only reasonably apply to drugs dosed at intervals less than or equal to one $t_{1/2}$ (unless timing of dose and of level can be assured, as in inpatient studies); and (4) because the data will be noisy, the number of patients that must be studied will be relatively high. To provide a strong enough "signal," perhaps 20 to 40 patients will be needed for each pathophysiologic condition to be evaluated. This number will be less for conditions with greater effect magnitudes. Note, however, that an individual may have more than one condition, as long as the correlation between conditions is not too great. The single trough method, and all other methods to be discussed below, are observational. Their strengths and weaknesses flow primarily from this fact.

Strengths. (1) The method is quite simple, should

not interfere with the phase III trial, and should be practical; (2) simple and familiar data analysis techniques are used; (3) identification of outliers is semiobjective, as they can be defined in terms of multiples of the typical magnitude of a residual from the regression (standard deviation); and (4) since so little is demanded by the study design, all patients exposed to the drug in the parent study can be included; representativeness is thus assured.

Weaknesses. (1) This method is more qualitative than quantitative and cannot be expected to provide reliable quantitation of the magnitude of pathophysiologic effects due to uncertainties in the data (e.g., compliance, timing) and because the proportionality between trough level and steady-state average level will depend on CL/F itself. Thus inferences regarding this ratio based on relationships discovered between pathophysiology and trough levels may be biased; (2) no estimates of V_{area} or of $t_{1/2}$ are possible and effects on F and CL cannot be separated, as only their ratio is estimated; (3) no estimates whatever of inter- or intraindividual variability can be made (they are hopelessly confounded and a quantity that can be estimated, their "sum," is inflated by the uncertainties in the data); (4) a relatively large number (20 to 40) of patients must be studied for each "condition"; this, multiplied by five to 10 conditions, implies perhaps 400 patients; and (5) as an observational rather than experimental study, conclusions are tentative, not definitive, because independent variables are not controlled. If all the elderly patients happen to have renal impairment, and none of the younger ones do, the effects of renal impairment cannot be distinguished from those of age per se. Lesser degrees of correlation produce correspondingly lesser problems in inference, but the problems do not disappear.

The multiple trough screen. In this design, one attempts to obtain more than one trough level from each patient. Although single trough data need not be discarded, two or more trough values on separate occasions will allow estimation of some variance components. A simple linear model can still be used to relate trough levels (divided by daily dose) to factors, but now a random effects linear model is appropriate. Maximum likelihood is the most familiar approach to analyzing such data. The extended least-squares method, as implemented in NONMEM,[6] is in this case identical to the maximum likelihood approach.

Requirements. Relative to the single trough method, all that is additionally needed is several trough values from at least a sizeable fraction of the patients.

Strengths. This method has all the strengths of the single trough approach, plus (1) reasonable estimates of (total) interindividual variability in the ratio CL/F will be obtained, as will estimates of residual or intraindividual variability, and (2) fewer patients may be needed and greater precision of estimates of effect magnitude may be obtained because each patient is better studied.

Weaknesses. (1) Same as the first, second, and fifth weaknesses listed for the single trough method; (2) the estimates of both residual and interindividual variability may or may not be biased, but they will not be very precise unless the number of patients studied is quite large; and (3) NONMEM[6] or some program like it must be used and may be unfamiliar to the data analyst.

The full screen. In this method, an observational approach is still taken, which distinguishes this method from the full kinetic study, but more complete data are required. Several drug levels from each patient, each drawn at different times relative to the last dose, is the goal. To qualify as a full screen, many of the patients must have several levels sampled, and most of these must be sampled at different times relative to the last dose and to beginning therapy. Heterogeneity is the key to a successful study, as different routes, preparations, and other factors all add to the richness of the data set. The data are analyzed according to a pharmacokinetic population model with the use of NONMEM.[6]

Requirements. As listed for the multiple trough study, plus (1) data must be more secure; timing of dose and drug level must be, for the most part, within 0.1 to 0.2 $t_{1/2}$ of the true value; (2) NONMEM must be used; and (3) one must study about 10 to 20 individuals with each feature of interest.

Strengths. One may hope both to discover and quantify all of the major population kinetic features of interest. (1) With sufficient heterogeneity of data, separate estimates of two distinct population parameter combinations (V_{area}/F, CL/F) can be obtained. If the intravenous route is sometimes used, all three population values (CL, F, and V_{area}) can be distinguished; (2) separate components of interindividual kinetic variability can be estimated; (3) residual variability can be estimated; and (4) although more elaborate than the trough only methods, little interference with a phase III study will occur (one must only determine levels), so that the study continues to enjoy the advantages of low cost and a representative patient sample.

Weaknesses. (1) This is still an observational study and conclusions cannot be definitive; and (2) a more complex population model must be proposed (it is no longer linear), and NONMEM, which may be unfamiliar to the data analyst, is the only currently available software that can be used for the data analysis.

WHICH APPROACH TO USE?

Assuming for the moment that phase III population studies of some kind are deemed desirable, one must still choose which type of study (or studies) should be done.

The validity and practicality of a full kinetic study to answer focused questions about pathophysiologic effect magnitudes is well accepted. In cases in which such questions are sufficiently pressing, it is probably sound regulatory policy to require a full kinetic study.

The single trough approach has been widely used in the past, and many reports of the influence of factors such as obesity or renal failure on kinetics are based on this method. However, it has not been used in the new drug, phase III context, and has rarely been used in outpatients, so that certain practical questions about its use remain. Nonetheless, because the approach is so straightforward and the interpretation only semi-quantitative, there is little doubt that it will yield some information.

The multiple trough approach is similar to the single trough approach, and the same considerations apply, but now more information for very little more cost is available and more quantitative conclusions can be drawn.

The full screen has been studied through simulation[7,8] and has been applied in a number of studies.[9-14] It has been shown in the context of an already released drug in an inpatient setting to be a sensitive and precise method of estimating population kinetics. It has not, however, been used in a phase III context, and has been rarely used in outpatient studies. Several practical issues, therefore, remain to be explored if it is to be applied in a phase III context.

On the one hand, the one (experimental) method of proved value in the drug regulatory context (the full study) is expensive, limited, and ill suited for broadly screening and assessing population kinetics in phase III studies. On the other hand, observational methods, which are theoretically better suited to the task, have not previously been used in the phase III context. Among the several observational methods discussed, the multiple trough and full screen approaches seem to have a higher benefit:cost ratio than the single trough method. Whether to adopt any observational study design is the crucial question, and its answer depends on an assessment of the benefits and costs involved.

BENEFITS AND COSTS

What may be gained? Consider first the discovery and quantification of pathophysiologic factors peculiar to the target patient population that may or may not affect a drug's kinetics. For example, a screen may identify a group of patients whose plasma concentrations differ systematically from those expected from a study of apparently similar patients. All of the former may be found to be taking a particular other drug. In this case, serendipity will have identified (and quantified) a possible drug interaction. In contrast, a number of patients in phase III studies whose plasma concentrations are compatible with usual kinetics might also be taking other medications. If a sufficient number of patients are taking the same other drug, it may reasonably be concluded that a significant kinetic drug interaction does not occur. Such a scenario can be envisioned for many pathophysiologic factors identifiable in the target population. Thus we gain knowledge useful for therapeutic regulation: how to adjust dosage for patient subgroups to avoid excessive drug accumulation; for which groups to use TDM; and for such groups, how to apply a Bayesian dosage adjustment procedure. This is the major benefit to be gained from a pharmacokinetic screen.

A secondary benefit concerns the efficacy or toxicity of a drug. In any phase III study, a number of patients will exhibit aberrant responses. Generally, when such responses are observed, the patient's history as well as the experimental protocol followed in that patient are closely scrutinized to determine whether there is a valid reason for excluding the aberrant data. One obvious reason for an unusual pharmacodynamic response is that the patient exhibits unusual pharmacokinetics. At present this cause can only be guessed at. If a pharmacokinetic screen were included in the study design, the distinction between pharmacodynamic and pharmacokinetic abnormalities could be assessed. More broadly, the addition of a pharmacokinetic screen to phase III protocols would add significantly to the currently sparse information gathered on the relationship between pharmacodynamic response and plasma concentrations. One important consequence might be to find that despite significant differences in drug kinetics, patients still respond favorably to the administered dose. This hypothesis is often suggested based on subjective clinical evaluation; pharmacokinetic screen data might allow a more objective test of such a hypothesis.

Finally, the ability to estimate inter- and intraindividual variability from multiple trough or full screen data has additional benefits beyond those previously discussed. One might find, for example, that patients from a particular study site, or those evaluated on a particular study day from a specified site, or all assays performed in a particular laboratory were unusually disparate. The pharmacokinetic screen might then serve as a quality control device for evaluating a particular study site, investigator, or laboratory. It is generally recognized that a number of protocol errors, such as incorrect sampling times, inaccuracies in assessing patient dosing compliance, and errors in recording such information, often occur in clinical phase III trials. At present, our ability to identify such errors is limited; the pharmacokinetic screen would mitigate this limitation.

What are the problems? There are two major problem areas associated with adding an observational population pharmacokinetic study to phase III protocols. The first is practical. It might be argued, first, that phase III protocol compliance will decrease because of the added burden of plasma sampling during the phase III study. To the contrary, we argue that protocol compliance for phase III studies may improve with the addition of the monitoring made possible by the screen. We have heard a variety of other reasons why "it can't be done": patients won't cooperate; investigators won't cooperate; there is too much inaccuracy in the way phase III protocols are carried out to assure accurate sample collection; phase III investigators and their staffs are not familiar with the care that must be taken to obtain and handle drug plasma samples correctly; or that the addition of plasma sampling will compromise the pharmacodynamic results obtained. We believe that these problems are real, but that they can be overcome. Practical objections are often raised against new ideas, especially if there are other reasons to oppose them. We believe that the ingenuity of drug companies and investigators is more than equal to solving the practical problems posed by a pharmacokinetic screen, if only the resolve to do so be present.

The second potential problem area is mistrust. Its resolution will require a change in attitude on the part of the FDA and a belief in that change by the pharmaceutical industry. A valid concern of the industry is that identification of a factor possibly influencing kinetics during the phase III process will trigger an FDA request for a prospective study of that factor. Thus industry fears an intolerable prolongation of the drug approval process as the FDA requires investigation of each possible influence ad infinitum. Rarely, of course, the screen may suggest the presence of a potential interaction between kinetics and pathophysiology of such magnitude that it would be prudent to investigate the matter further before proceeding with release. This is always a hazard of gathering new information, but delay of release in such a case is in the manufacturer's interest (in terms of avoiding subsequent liability) as well as in the public's. For the most part, however, screen data will simply add to the store of information useful for planning and adjusting therapy with the new drug. The FDA's regulatory mandate and bureaucratic organization may make it poorly suited to deal with this essentially advisory, rather than regulatory, orientation, but if observational studies of new drugs are to become part of the regulatory context, then regulators must adapt to this new role and convince industry that they have.

CONCLUSION

Although it is apparent that certain practical issues must be addressed, and an adjustment in regulatory philosophy must be accomplished before observational population kinetic studies can be introduced as a routine part of premarketing new drug evaluation, the prospect is exciting and the effort seems worth undertaking. In doing so, industry and the FDA would agree jointly to accept a new responsibility: Not only to assure each patient about to receive a new drug that there is a reasonable probability of "safety and efficacy" for that person as a typical member of a target population, but also that the physician has the means to optimize therapy for the person as an individual.

References

1. Temple R. Discussion paper on the testing of drugs in the elderly. Washington, DC: Memorandum of the Food and Drug Administration of DHHS, Sept 30, 1983.
2. Reidenberg MM, Abrams WB. Report on "Workshop on Elderly" [Appendix V]. Sept 28, 1984.
3. Sheiner LB, Beal S, Rosenberg B, Marathe VV. Forecasting individual pharmacokinetics. CLIN PHARMACOL THER 1979;26:294-305.
4. Sheiner LB, Beal SL. Bayesian individualization of pharmacokinetics: simple implementation and comparison with nonBayesian methods. J Pharm Sci 1982;71:1344-8.
5. Report to the Royal College of Physicians. Medication for the elderly. J R Coll Phys London 1984;18:7.
6. Beal S, Sheiner LB. The NONMEM system. Am Stat 1980;34:118.
7. Sheiner LB, Beal SL. Evaluation of methods for estimating population pharmacokinetic parameters. I. Michaelis-Menten model: routine clinical pharmacokinetic data. J Pharmacokinet Biopharm 1980;8:553-71.
8. Sheiner LB, Beal SL. Evaluation of methods for estimating population pharmacokinetic parameters. III. Mono-exponential model: routine clinical pharmacokinetic data. J Pharmacokinet Biopharm 1983;11:303-19.
9. Sheiner LB, Rosenberg B, Melmon KL. Modelling of individual pharmacokinetics for computer-aided drug dosage. Comput Biomed Res 1972;5:441-59.
10. Sheiner LB, Rosenberg B, Marathe V. Estimation of

population characteristics of pharmacokinetic parameters from routine clinical data. J Pharmacokinet Biopharm 1977;5:445-79.

11. Ravenscroft P, Vozeh S, Weinstein M, Sheiner LB. Saliva lithium concentrations in the management of lithium therapy. Arch Gen Psychiatry 1978;35:1123-7.
12. Vozeh S, Katz G, Steimer J, Follath F. Population pharmacokinetic parameters in patients treated with oral mexiletine. Eur J Clin Pharmacol 1982;23:445-51.
13. Grasela TH, Sheiner LB, Rambeck B, et al. Steady-state pharmacokinetics of phenytoin from routinely collected patient data. Clin Pharmacokinet 1983;8:335-64.
14. Grasela TH, Sheiner LB. Population pharmacokinetics of procainamide from routine clinical data. Clin Pharmacokinet 1984;9:545-54.

ORIGINAL ARTICLES

Mephenytoin hydroxylation polymorphism: Characterization of the enzymatic deficiency in liver microsomes of poor metabolizers phenotyped in vivo

The rate of 4-hydroxylation and of *N*-demethylation of *S*- and *R*-mephenytoin was determined in liver microsomes of 13 extensive (EM) and two poor (PM) metabolizers of mephenytoin. Detailed kinetic studies were performed in microsomes of eight EMs and the two PMs. Microsomal mephenytoin metabolism in PMs was characterized by an increased Km (150.6 and 180.6 vs. a mean [±SD] 37.8 ± 9.6 µmol/L *S*-mephenytoin in 8 EMs), a decreased maximum rate of metabolism for *S*-mephenytoin hydroxylation (0.76 and 0.69 vs 4.85 ± 1.65 nmol 4-hydroxymephenytoin per milligram protein per hour), and loss of stereoselectivity for the hydroxylation of the *R*- and *S*-enantiomers of mephenytoin (*R/S* ratio: 1.10 and 0.76 vs. 0.11 ± 0.04 in 13 EMs). The formation of 4-OH-mephenytoin from *R*-mephenytoin and the demethylation reaction remained unaffected. These results support our hypothesis that the mephenytoin polymorphism is caused by a partial or complete absence or inactivity of a cytochrome P-450 isozyme with high affinity for *S*-mephenytoin. (Clin Pharmacol Ther 1985;38:488-94.)

U. Thomas Meier, M.Sc., Pierre Dayer, M.D., Pierre-Jean Malè, M.D., Thomas Kronbach, Ph.D., and Urs A. Meyer, M.D. *Basel, Switzerland*

A genetic polymorphism of deficient metabolism of mephenytoin (3-methyl-5-phenyl-5-ethylhydantoin) is observed in 2% to 5% of white subjects[1-3] and in 23% of Japanese subjects.[4] This deficiency, first described by Küpfer et al.[5] in 1979, appears to be inherited as an autosomal recessive trait and concerns one of the two major metabolic pathways of mephenytoin, namely aromatic hydroxylation. The other major pathway, *N*-demethylation, remains unaffected.

Mephenytoin has a center of asymmetry at the 5 position of the hydantoin ring, and its metabolism in man is highly stereoselective. Thus in normal subjects the *S*-enantiomer is almost completely hydroxylated in the *p* position of the phenyl ring and rapidly excreted as *S*-4-hydroxymephenytoin glucuronide, whereas the *R*-enantiomer is preferentially *N*-demethylated and slowly excreted as *R*-5-phenyl-5-ethylhydantoin (PEH, or nirvanol).[6,7] In subjects with deficient hydroxylation, the stereoselectivity of metabolite excretion after racemic mephenytoin dosing is virtually absent, suggesting that the deficiency affects only the 4-hydroxylation of *S*-mephenytoin. *S*- and *R*-metabolites are slowly excreted in equal amounts, predominantly as nirvanol.[8,9] The molecular mechanism responsible for the mephenytoin polymorphism has not been studied at the level of the hepatic enzymes catalyzing mephenytoin metabolism.

Our laboratory and others have provided recent evidence that another common polymorphism of drug metabolism that affects the oxidative metabolism of debrisoquin, sparteine, bufuralol, and several other drugs (debrisoquin/sparteine-type polymorphism) is caused by the deficiency of a specific hepatic cytochrome P-450 isozyme.[10-15] In population and family studies, intrasubject comparisons of the debrisoquin and mephenytoin hydroxylation phenotypes indicated that the two

From the Department of Pharmacology, Biocenter of the University.
Supported by Swiss National Science Foundation Grants No. 3.893.81 and No. 3.806.0.84.

Received for publication May 8, 1985; accepted Aug. 6, 1985.
Reprint requests to: Urs A. Meyer, M.D., Department of Pharmacology, Biocenter of the University, Klingelbergstr. 70, CH-4056 Basel, Switzerland.

Table I. In vivo metabolism of racemic mephenytoin and debrisoquin in 15 unrelated subjects

			Mephenytoin			*Debrisoquin*	
Subject	*Sex*	*Age (yr)*	*Urinary 4-OH-mephenytoin* (μmol)*	*Hydroxylation index*	*Phenotype*	*Urinary metabolic ratio**	*Phenotype*
V. A.†	F	56	1.8	127.3	PM	0.59	EM
R. E.†	F	41	4.3	53.4	PM	0.21	EM
G. M.†	M	64	114.2	2.0	EM	0.55	EM
B. R.	M	48	136.0	1.7	EM	22.80	PM
P. G.	F	67	50.1	4.6	EM	1.46	EM
P. J.†	F	53	121.6	1.9	EM	2.09	EM
W. N.	F	63	114.8	2.0	EM	0.28	EM
V. L.	F	26	115.4	2.0	EM	0.70	EM
M. C.†	F	85	35.7	6.4	EM	2.47	EM
L. P.†	M	55	28.7	8.0	EM	1.73	EM
P. C.	F	52	164.8	1.4	EM	12.60	PM
T. S.†	F	74	128.2	1.8	EM	1.47	EM
S. J.†	F	55	125.4	1.8	EM	1.20	EM
M. M.†	M	64	134.0	1.7	EM	2.79	EM
G. L.†	M	52	144.1	1.6	EM	0.26	EM

F = Female; M = male.
*Urine samples were collected for 8 to 12 hours after oral dosing with 100 mg (458 μmol) mephenytoin and 10 mg debrisoquin.
†Liver microsomes of these subjects were used for kinetic studies (Fig. 2).

polymorphisms occur independently.[1-3] This has been supported by the lack of inhibition of sparteine oxidation by mephenytoin in human liver preparations in vitro.[16] As both major reactions of mephenytoin (hydroxylation and demethylation) are catalyzed by cytochrome P-450–dependent monooxygenases,[17] we tested the hypothesis that in subjects with polymorphically deficient mephenytoin metabolism, a cytochrome P-450 isozyme catalyzing the 4-hydroxylation of *S*-mephenytoin is wholly or partly missing or inactive, while the cytochrome P-450 isozyme(s) for demethylation remain(s) intact. For this purpose we developed a sensitive assay for measurement of the metabolites of mephenytoin in urine and in human liver microsomes and investigated the metabolism of *S*- and *R*-mephenytoin in liver biopsy specimens of extensive (EM) and poor (PM) metabolizers of mephenytoin phenotyped in vivo.

METHODS

Our subjects were surgical patients, 26 to 85 years old, at the Geneva University Hospital who were undergoing laparotomy and liver biopsy for therapeutic or diagnostic reasons. Tissue from small wedge biopsy specimens (100 to 500 mg wet weight) not used for histologic examination was immediately frozen in liquid nitrogen and stored at −80° C. The project had the approval of the hospital clinical investigation review board.

Between 1 day and 1 week after surgery, the patients received a tablet containing 100 mg (458 μmol) racemic mephenytoin and 10 mg debrisoquin.* Urine was collected for the following 8 to 12 hours to determine simultaneously the hydroxylation phenotype of mephenytoin and debrisoquin. The subjects were classified according to their mephenytoin hydroxylation index (micromoles of *S*-mephenytoin administered/micromoles of 4-OH-mephenytoin in urine collected for 8 to 12 hours) and their urinary metabolic ratio of debrisoquin (debrisoquin/4-OH-debrisoquin) as EMs or PMs of the respective polymorphism by the criteria of Wedlund et al.[3] and Price Evans et al.[18] Urine samples were stored at −20° C until assayed.

Human liver microsomes were prepared by a micromethod as previously described,[15] with the modification that 0.15 mol/L potassium chloride containing 5 mmol/L EDTA was used instead of 25 mmol/L sucrose. Protein content was determined with the use of bovine serum albumin as standard.[19]

Microsomes (0.1 mg protein) were incubated in the presence of an NADPH-generating system[15] at 37° C for 1 hour in a total volume of 250 μl. The final substrate concentration was 1 mmol/L *R*- or *S*-mephenytoin in 1% propylene glycol (v/v) when used for determination of enantiomer ratios. A concentration range from 6.25 to 400 μmol/L *S*-mephenytoin in 0.25% propylene

*Formulation by Drs. Soliva and Büchi, School of Pharmacy, University of Berne, Switzerland.

Table II. Substrate stereoselectivity of in vitro metabolism in liver microsomes from EMs and PMs

	R-mephenytoin (nmol/mg protein/hr)		*S-mephenytoin (nmol/mg protein/hr)*		*R/S ratio*	
	4-OH-mephenytoin	*Nirvanol*	*4-OH-mephenytoin*	*Nirvanol*	*4-OH-mephenytoin*	*Nirvanol*
EMs						
P. G.	0.42	3.06	5.80	7.01	0.07	0.44
B. R.	0.44	2.37	3.57	4.55	0.12	0.52
P. J.*	0.43	4.30	3.85	7.13	0.11	0.60
W. N.	0.63	5.10	7.70	11.52	0.08	0.44
V. L.	0.16	0.99	1.30	2.42	0.12	0.41
M. C.*	0.42	4.73	5.44	8.88	0.08	0.53
L. P.*	0.26	1.85	3.71	4.65	0.07	0.40
P. C.	0.49	3.19	4.32	6.18	0.11	0.52
T. S.*	0.38	2.59	3.12	5.73	0.12	0.45
S. J.*	0.20	1.65	1.46	3.95	0.14	0.42
M. M.*	0.26	3.13	3.62	10.82	0.07	0.29
G. L.*	0.35	2.95	2.95	7.49	0.12	0.39
G. M.*	0.38	4.47	1.77	10.71	0.21	0.49
$\bar{X}$	0.37	3.11	3.74	7.00	0.11	0.45
±SD	± 0.13	± 1.26	± 1.81	± 2.84	± 0.04	± 0.08
PMs						
V. A.*	0.37	3.87	0.49	7.52	0.76	0.51
R. E.*	0.57	10.14	0.52	18.99	1.10	0.53

*Liver microsomes of these subjects were used in kinetic studies (Fig. 2).

glycol (v/v) was used for kinetic experiments. The reaction was stopped with 100 μl 2% sodium azide (w/v) containing 2.5 μmol/L phenobarbital as internal standard, and the mixture was extracted with 5 ml dichloromethane. After evaporation of the solvent, the residue was dissolved in 0.2 ml water and 100 μl was analyzed by reversed-phase HPLC. The enzymatic reaction showed the characteristics of a cytochrome P-450–catalyzed monooxygenase reaction, namely dependence on NADPH and inhibition by carbon monoxide. Product formation was linear with time and protein concentration. A detailed description and evaluation of the assay will be published elsewhere.[20]

After the addition of phenobarbital as internal standard, urine samples were treated by acid hydrolysis[6] and a 100 μl aliquot of the hydrolysate was extracted with 5 ml dichloromethane. The solvent was evaporated and the residue was dissolved in 1 ml water, of which 100 μl was injected into the HPLC. The chromatographic system consisted of a constant flow pump, a spectrophotometer set at 204 nm, and a model 7125 injector (Rheodyne Inc.). Columns (60 × 4.6 mm) were filled with Nucleosil-5-C-18 reversed-phase support (Macherey-Nagel). Chromatography was performed isocratically in 30% methanol/70% potassium phosphate buffer, 10 mmol/L at pH 7.0 (v/v) at a flow rate of 1 ml/min. The chromatograms were analyzed by the internal standard method. A linear calibration curve was obtained for 4-OH-mephenytoin over the range 1 to 250 μg/ml urine. The coefficient of variation at 5 μg/ml urine was 1.2% (n = 6). Retention times for 4-OH-mephenytoin and internal standard were 4.25 and 5.5 minutes, respectively.

R- and *S*-enantiomers of nirvanol and 4-OH-mephenytoin* were at least 96% pure[21] according to reported optical rotation values.[22] *R*- and *S*-mephenytoin were synthesized from the corresponding nirvanol enantiomers by methylation of the nitrogen in the 3 position of the hydantoin ring.[20,23]

RESULTS

Of 15 unrelated subjects, two (V. A. and R. E.) showed a mephenytoin hydroxylation index consistent with the PM phenotype (Table I). Both PMs of mephenytoin metabolized debrisoquin efficiently, with metabolic ratios reflecting the EM phenotype for this substrate. These results confirm the independence of the two polymorphisms.[1-3] An additional advantage of combined dosing with both drugs is that it allows judgment on subject compliance with mephenytoin dosing. As <2% of mephenytoin is excreted unchanged by both

*Provided by Drs. A. Küpfer and G. Karlaganis, Department of Clinical Pharmacology, University of Berne, Berne, Switzerland.

EMs and PMs,[3] the definition of a metabolic "ratio" is not possible. The age or sex of the subjects had no apparent influence on their phenotype (Table I).

Results of microsomal incubations with *R*- and *S*-mephenytoin are summarized in Table II. In liver microsomes of mephenytoin EMs phenotyped in vivo, *S*-mephenytoin was metabolized more efficiently than *R*-mephenytoin by both hydroxylation and demethylation, resulting in a mean (±SD) *R*/*S* ratio of 0.11 ± 0.04 (n = 13) and 0.45 ± 0.08 for 4-OH-mephenytoin and nirvanol, respectively. In microsomes of the first mephenytoin PM (V. A.), the expected marked decrease in the hydroxylation rate of *S*-mephenytoin resulted in an increased *R*/*S* ratio of 0.76, whereas the hydroxylation of *R*-mephenytoin and the nirvanol formation from both enantiomers were comparable with those of the EMs. The microsomal incubations of the second PM (R. E.) also formed metabolites with an increased *R*/*S* ratio (1.10), but had higher absolute demethylation rates for both enantiomers than those observed in all other subjects. Thus the two subjects with high mephenytoin hydroxylation indices as determined in vivo had lost the stereoselectivity for *S*-mephenytoin as manifested by *R*/*S* ratios of microsomal 4-hydroxylation activity near unity (Fig. 1). It must be realized that at substrate concentrations of 1 mmol/L, *R*-mephenytoin hydroxylation does not reflect conditions of maximal velocity of metabolism (V_{max}) because of the higher Michaelis-Menten constant (Km) of this reaction.[20]

The rate of 4-hydroxylation of *S*-mephenytoin in microsomes at different substrate concentrations resulted in apparent simple Michaelis-Menten kinetics for eight EMs and the two PMs (Fig. 2, *A*). The mean (±SD) apparent Km and V_{max} as determined by Eadie-Hofstee plots[24] in the eight EMs were 37.8 ± 9.6 (range 25.6 to 53.8) μmol/L *S*-mephenytoin and 4.85 ± 1.65 (range 2.49 to 7.55) nmol 4-OH-mephenytoin per milligram protein per hour, respectively. Compared with the EMs, the Km of the PMs was more than fourfold greater and the V_{max} was more than sixfold less (Fig. 2, *B*).

The substrate dependence of the demethylation of *S*-mephenytoin was almost linear in the concentration range measured (Fig. 2, *B*). Whereas the demethylation of one PM (V. A.) was within the range of the eight EMs, the other PM (R. E.) showed a two- to threefold increase in nirvanol formation over the entire concentration range (Fig. 2, *B*).

DISCUSSION

Our study demonstrates that mephenytoin polymorphism results from a deficiency of the hepatic micro-

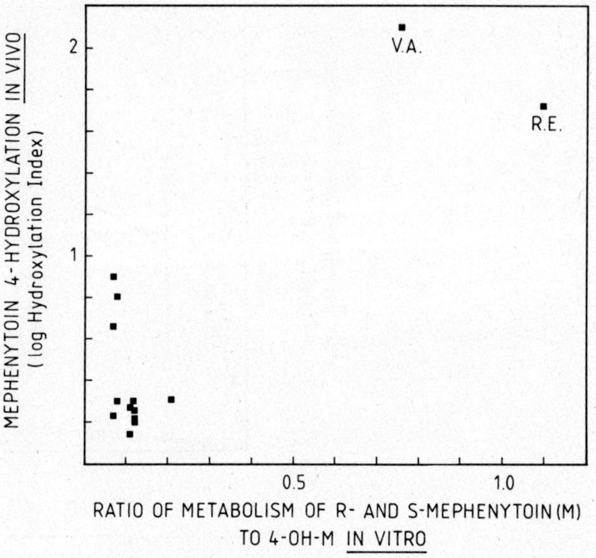

Fig. 1. In vivo hydroxylation index plotted against ratio of in vitro metabolism of *R*- and *S*-mephenytoin to 4-OH-mephenytoin of 15 unrelated subjects.

somal monooxygenase reaction that catalyzes the 4-hydroxylation of *S*-mephenytoin. In monooxygenase reactions, cytochrome P-450 isozymes are responsible for substrate binding and the stereo- and regioselectivity of the oxidation reactions. Our present findings are therefore consistent with the hypothesis that the absence or functional deficiency of a cytochrome P-450 isozyme with high affinity for this substrate causes the mephenytoin polymorphism. In hepatic microsomes of the two PMs of mephenytoin, there was an increased apparent Km and a decreased V_{max} for the 4-hydroxylation of *S*-mephenytoin and a striking loss of stereoselectivity for this reaction. These in vitro findings correlate well with the in vivo data of Wedlund et al.[3] Thus in EMs the mean (±SD) *S*/*R* ratio of mephenytoin measured in the 8-hour urine sample was 0.16 ± 0.12 (n = 152), indicating preferential metabolism of the *S*-enantiomer, whereas in PMs the ratio was near unity (0.99 ± 0.01; n = 4). Moreover, demethylation, the other major pathway of mephenytoin metabolism, was not affected in the PMs in vitro, consistent with the in vivo observation that demethylation is not affected by the polymorphism.[9] However, our observation of a preference of microsomal *S*-nirvanol production as compared with formation of the *R*-enantiomer (Table II) is not reflected in the urinary excretion pattern[8,9] or in the plasma concentration-time profiles[25] of either enantiomer. This discrepancy may be due to the fact that demethylation is determined at concentrations markedly below Km in vivo (serum concentrations of 70 to 140 μmol/L total

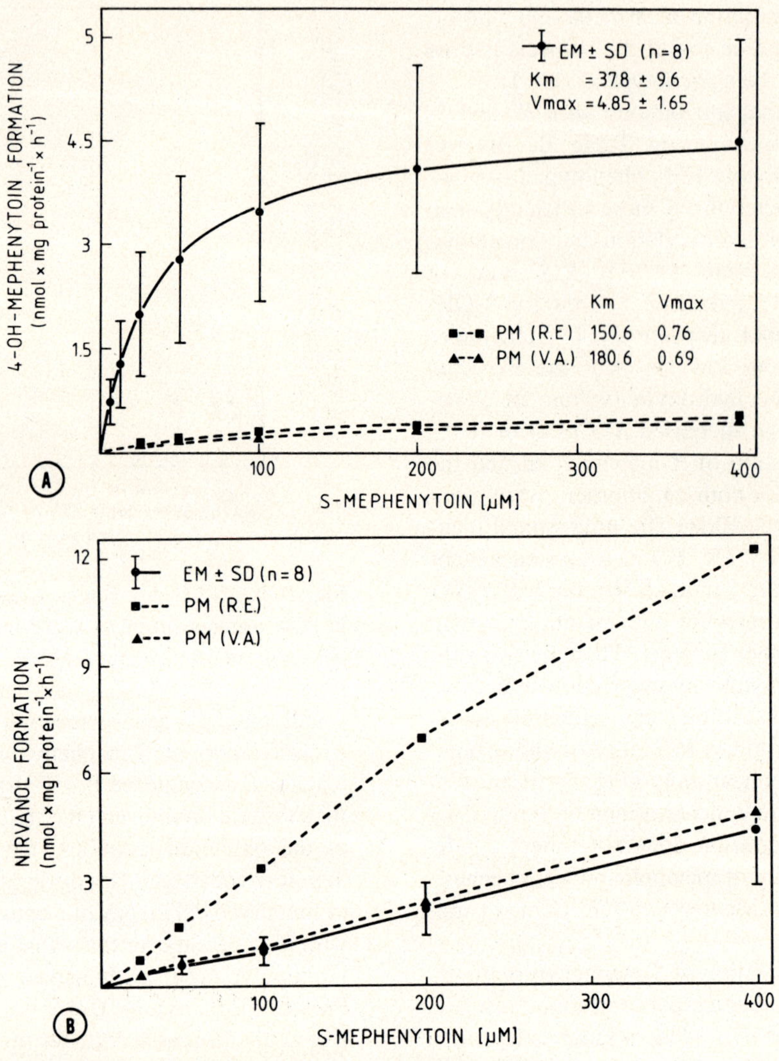

Fig. 2. Kinetics of *S*-mephenytoin 4-hydroxylation **(A)** and demethylation **(B)** in human liver microsomes from eight EMs and two PMs. Km values are given as μmol/L of *S*-mephenytoin, and V_{max} values are given as nanomoles of 4-OH-mephenytoin per milligram protein per hour.

hydantoin have been reported[26]) as well as in vitro (solubility limitations). Under these conditions comparisons of the stereospecificity of the reaction are of limited value.

Probably for similar reasons, the Eadie-Hofstee plots of the microsomal demethylation reaction indicate a complex kinetic pattern. While the mephenytoin demethylation rate of one PM (V. A.) was within the range of the eight EMs, as expected from in vivo findings,[9] the other PM (R. E.) showed increased nirvanol formation (Table II; Fig. 2, *B*). We presume that this subject had an increased activity of the enzyme(s) catalyzing demethylation because of induction by environmental factors. The probability of this induction is supported by the known inducibility of mephenytoin demethylation in rats*[,27] and by the suggested substrate induction of the reaction in man.[6,7] This is also reflected by the marked variation in nirvanol formation in the 13 EMs between 2.42 and 11.52 nmol nirvanol per milligram protein per hour (Table II). If the hydroxylation rate in this PM was only low because another metabolic pathway, i.e., demethylation, was increased and was not a result of a genetically determined deficiency, one would expect no change in the apparent Km and an even higher increase in demethylation compensating such low 4-OH-mephenytoin production in

*Meier UT. Unpublished observations, 1984.

vitro as well as in vivo. It is therefore reasonable to assume that this subject is a genetically determined PM of mephenytoin. Obviously, only family studies allow the unequivocal identification of a subject as a PM.

Because of the small amount of metabolites formed, the Km and V_{max} values for 4-OH-mephenytoin of the two PMs are based on determinations near the limit of detectability. This is because of the small size of the wedge biopsy specimen and the small concentration range of the substrate, which for reasons of limited solubility did not sufficiently exceed the Km. Nevertheless, data indicate that the PMs can clearly be distinguished from the EMs in vitro by their markedly increased Km and decreased V_{max} of hydroxylation (Fig. 2, *A*).

Interestingly, our findings are very similar to those characterizing the enzymatic deficiency in livers of subjects with the debrisoquin/sparteine-type polymorphism when (+)- and (−)-bufuralol are used as substrate.[13,15] The two independently occurring polymorphisms may thus be due to the same basic molecular mechanism(s) affecting two different genes.

In conclusion, the enzymatic data presented here support the hypothesis of the whole or partial loss or inactivity of a cytochrome P-450 isozyme with high affinity for the *S*-enantiomer of mephenytoin. Of several cytochrome P-450 isozymes recently purified from human liver,[*,13] one had a high activity for mephenytoin 4-hydroxylation. Preliminary studies with a rabbit antibody raised against this cytochrome P-450 isozyme indeed suggest that the presence of a functionally altered enzyme is the most probable cause of this polymorphism.

*Gut J, Meier UT, Catin T, Meyer UA. Manuscript in preparation.

We thank Drs. A. Küpfer, Berne, and J. Gut, Basel, for helpful suggestions and Drs. M. Jurima, T. Inaba, and W. Kalow, Toronto, for giving us insight in the preprints of the manuscripts cited as references 4 and 17.

References

1. Küpfer A, Preisig R. Pharmacogenetics of mephenytoin: a new drug hydroxylation polymorphism in man. Eur J Clin Pharmacol 1984;26:753-9.
2. Inaba T, Jurima M, Nakono M, Kalow W. Mephenytoin and sparteine pharmacogenetics in Canadian Caucasians. Clin Pharmacol Ther 1984;36:670-6.
3. Wedlund PJ, Aslanian WS, McAllister CB, Wilkinson GR, Branch RA. Mephenytoin hydroxylation deficiency in Caucasians: frequency of a new oxidative drug metabolism polymorphism. Clin Pharmacol Ther 1984; 36:773-80.
4. Jurima M, Inaba T, Kadar D, Kalow W. Genetic polymorphism of mephenytoin p(4′)-hydroxylation: difference between Orientals and Caucasians. Br J Clin Pharmacol 1985;19:483-7.
5. Küpfer A, Desmond P, Schenker S, Branch R. Family study of a genetically determined deficiency of mephenytoin hydroxylation in man. Pharmacologist 1979; 21:173.
6. Küpfer A, Roberts RK, Schenker S, Branch RA. Stereoselective metabolism of mephenytoin in man. J Pharmacol Exp Ther 1981;218:193-9.
7. Küpfer A, Desmond PV, Schenker S, Branch RA. Stereoselective metabolism and disposition of the enantiomers of mephenytoin during chronic oral administration of the racemic drug in man. J Pharmacol Exp Ther 1982;221:590-7.
8. Küpfer A, Desmond P, Schenker S, Branch RA. Pseudostereospecific R-mephenytoin demethylation in man. Clin Res 1980;28:239A.
9. Küpfer A, Desmond P, Patwardhan R, Schenker S, Branch RA. Mephenytoin hydroxylation deficiency: kinetics after repeated doses. Clin Pharmacol Ther 1984;35:33-9.
10. Davies DS, Kahn GC, Murray S, Brodie MJ, Boobis AR. Evidence for an enzymatic defect in the 4-hydroxylation of debrisoquine by human liver. Br J Clin Pharmacol 1981;11:89-91.
11. Meier PJ, Mueller HK, Dick B, Meyer UA. Hepatic monooxygenase activities in subjects with a genetic defect in drug oxidation. Gastroenterology 1983;85:682-92.
12. Minder EI, Meier PJ, Müller HK, Minder C, Meyer UA: Bufuralol metabolism in human liver: a sensitive probe for the debrisoquine-type polymorphism of drug oxidation. Eur J Clin Invest 1984;14:184-9.
13. Gut J, Gasser R, Dayer P, Kronbach T, Catin T, Meyer UA. Debrisoquine-type polymorphism of drug oxidation: purification from human liver of a cytochrome P450 isozyme with high activity for bufuralol hydroxylation. FEBS Lett 1984;173:287-90.
14. Distlerath LM, Guengerich FP. Characterization of human liver cytochrome P-450 involved in the oxidation of debrisoquine and other drugs by using antibodies raised to the analogous rat enzyme. Proc Natl Acad Sci USA 1984;81:7348-52.
15. Dayer P, Gasser R, Gut J, et al. Characterization of a common genetic defect of cytochrome P-450 function (debrisoquine-sparteine type polymorphism)—increased Michaelis constant (Km) and loss of stereoselectivity of bufuralol 1′-hydroxylation in poor metabolizers. Biochem Biophys Res Commun 1984;125:374-80.
16. Jurima M, Inaba T, Kalow W. Sparteine oxidation by the human liver: absence of inhibition by mephenytoin. Clin Pharmacol Ther 1984;35:426-8.
17. Jurima M, Inaba T, Kalow W. Mephenytoin metabolism *in vitro* by human liver. Drug Metab Dispos 1985;13: 151-5.

18. Price Evans DA, Mahgoub A, Sloan TP, Idle JR, Smith RL. A family and population study of the genetic polymorphism of debrisoquine oxidation in a white British population. J Med Genet 1980;17:153-5.
19. Lowry OH, Rosebrough NJ, Farr AL, Randall RJ. Protein measurement with the folin phenol reagent. J Biol Chem 1951;193:265-75.
20. Meier UT, Kronbach T, Meyer UA. Assay of mephenytoin metabolism in human liver microsomes by high performance liquid chromatography. Anal Biochem. (in press)
21. Butler TC. Metabolic demethylation of 3-methyl-5-ethyl-5-phenylhydantoin (Mesantoin). J Pharmacol Exp Ther 1952;104:299-308.
22. Sobotka H, Holzman MF, Kahn J. Optically active 5,5′disubstituted hydantoins. J Am Chem Soc 1932; 54:4697-702.
23. Chemische Fabrik vormals Sandoz: Verfahren zur Darstellung eines Derivates des 5,5-Phenyl-äthylhydantoins. Swiss Patent No 166,004, 1934.
24. Hofstee BHJ: On the evaluation of the constants Vm and Km in enzyme reactions. Science 1952;116:329-31.
25. Wedlund PJ, Aslanian WS, McAllister CB, Branch RA, Wilkinson GR. Stereoselective disposition of mephenytoin in genetically different populations [Abstract]. *In* Reidenberg MM, Lemberger L, eds. Proceedings of the Second World Conference on Clinical Pharmacology and Therapeutics. Washington, DC: July 30-Aug 5, 1983.
26. Troupin AS, Ojemann LM, Dodrill CB. Mephenytoin: a reappraisal. Epilepsia 1976;17:403-14.
27. Smith JA, Waddell WJ, Butler TC. Demethylation of N-methyl derivatives of barbituric acid, hydantoin and 2,4-oxazolidinedione by rat liver microsomes. Life Sci 1963;2:486-92.

Evaluation and application of the linear variable differential transformer technique for the assessment of human dorsal hand vein alpha-receptor activity

Diurnal, day-to-day, intrasubject, and intersubject variability of responsiveness of dorsal hand veins to norepinephrine has been investigated in healthy young subjects through the use of a novel technique in which a linear variable differential transformer (LVDT) is placed directly over the vein. Under constant operating conditions, control vein diameter remained consistent. There is log dose responsiveness to norepinephrine infused directly into the hand vein. There was little diurnal, day-to-day, or intrasubject variability in the dose of norepinephrine required to induce 50% constriction of hand vein diameter. The responsiveness to norepinephrine of different veins in either hand was also consistent. However, there was wide intersubject variability, apparently unrelated to age, gender, or other subject characteristics. We conclude that the LVDT method is reproducible and reliable and offers a relatively noninvasive means of assessing the effects of disease and drugs on the human dorsal hand vein in vivo. The LVDT technique has been applied to study the rate of onset, magnitude of effect, dose responsiveness, and duration of action of intravenous dihydroergotamine, 0.1, 0.2, and 0.4 mg, on human dorsal hand veins. Despite systemic intravenous administration, there was an average delay in maximum response of 30 minutes to 1 hour. Venoconstriction was incomplete, with a maximum reduction of approximately 50% of vein diameter after each of the larger doses. There was no significant difference between the effects produced by 0.2 or 0.4 mg, which persisted for 6 hours after dosing. (CLIN PHARMACOL THER 38:495-502, 1985.)

Assem O. Alradi, M.B., M.Sc.,* and S. George Carruthers, M.D.
London, Ontario, Canada

Knowledge of in vivo changes in human vascular α-receptors after drugs or disease remains relatively undeveloped. A major reason for this has been the lack of sensitive, safe, easily reproducible, and noninvasive techniques for measuring α-receptor function.

The linear variable differential transformer (LVDT) technique developed by Aellig[4] to measure compliance of superficial hand veins in man appears to overcome many of the problems faced with other techniques. Its major advantage is its relative simplicity of use. The amounts of drug infused are extremely small and systemic effects of such small doses are negligible. There is minimal risk to the subject and the tests can be repeated on many occasions. Aellig has reported his studies on a relatively small number of healthy men. There is little information on the temporal, intrasubject, or intersubject reproducibility of his method.

To determine if the LVDT technique provides a sensitive and easily reproducible means of assessing peripheral vein α-receptor responsiveness in man, we undertook the following investigations: Study 1—The evaluation of intrasubject variation in basal hand vein diameter in the same vein on repeated occasions; Study 2—the evaluation of intrasubject diurnal variation in hand vein α-receptor responsiveness during different times of the day (morning, afternoon, and evening); Study 3—the evaluation of intrasubject variation in

From the Divisions of Clinical Pharmacology and Cardiology, Departments of Medicine and Pharmacology and Toxicology, University Hospital and the University of Western Ontario.
Supported by the Medical Research Council of Canada (Grant No. MA-8624) and by Sandoz Canada Inc.
Presented in part at National Meeting of the American Federation of Clinical Research, Washington, D.C., May 1984 and at the Canadian Society for Clinical Investigation, Montreal, Quebec, September 1984.
Received for publication March 5, 1985; accepted Aug. 6, 1985.
Reprint requests to: Dr. S. G. Carruthers, Room 6-OF12, University Hospital, London, Ontario N6A 5A5, Canada.
*Trainee in Clinical Pharmacology from King Abdul-Aziz University, Jeddah, Saudi Arabia.

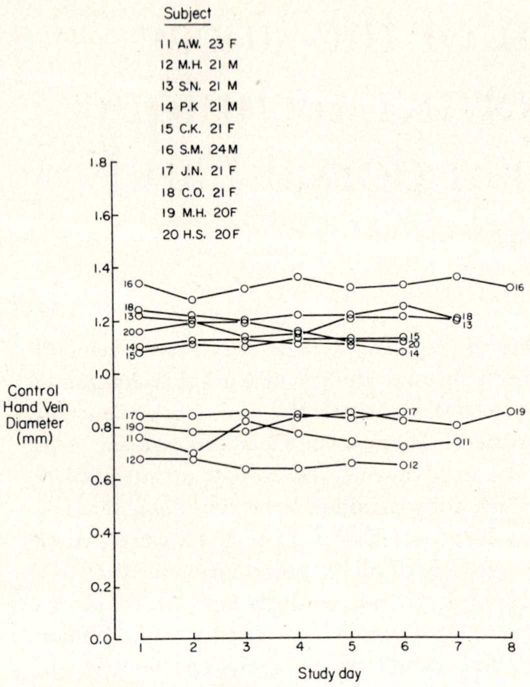

Fig. 1. Day-to-day reproducibility of hand vein diameter measurements during infusion of dextrose in saline solution in 10 subjects (age and sex are indicated). Measurements were made at the same point in the chosen vein on six or eight different occasions. F = Female; M = male.

hand vein α-receptor responsiveness on repeated occasions in the same vein; Study 4—the evaluation of intrasubject variation in hand vein α-receptor responsiveness on repeated occasions in different veins; Study 5—the evaluation of intersubject variability in hand vein α-receptor responsiveness; and Study 6—the application of the LVDT technique to the evaluation of onset, magnitude of effect, dose responsiveness, and duration of action of systemic intravenous dihydroergotamine (DHE), 0.1, 0.2, and 0.4 mg, on human dorsal hand veins.

METHODS

The LVDT[12] is an electromechanical device that produces an electrical output proportional to the displacement of a separate movable core. It consists of a primary coil and two secondary coils symmetrically spaced on a cylinder. A free-moving, rod-shaped magnetic core inside the coil assembly provides a path for the magnetic flux linking the coils. When the primary coil is energized by an external alternating current source, voltages are induced in the two secondary coils. These are connected series in opposition, such that the two voltages are of opposite polarity. Therefore, the net output of the transducer is the difference between these voltages, which is zero when the core is at the center or null position. When the core is moved from the null position, the induced voltage increases in the coil toward which the core is moved, while the induced voltage in the opposite coil decreases. The resultant voltage changes are linearly proportional to the displacement of the core.

An LVDT requires signal conditioning equipment and readout to function in a measurement system. The LVDT used in the present studies and a Schaevitz modular LVDT signal conditioner were manufactured by the Biomedical Engineering service at University Hospital with use of a Schaevitz type 025 MHR differential transformer and a Schaevitz type LPM 210 for the power supply, the amplification, and the conversion of the alternating current output to direct current output. The LVDT was calibrated such that a 1 mm displacement of the central core of the LVDT was equal to a deflection of 10 cm on the paper of the potentiometric recorder as measured on a Mitutoyo micrometer head model 197-101 (MTI Corporation) mounted on a support stand.

The subjects were healthy, adult, nonsmoking men and women. Each subject completed a brief medical history and underwent a physical examination. No subject had any history of asthma, hypertension, or heart failure. The studies were thoroughly discussed with the subjects and each was required to sign a consent form approved by the Health Sciences Standing Committee on Human Research of the University of Western Ontario. Subjects were requested not to take any aspirin or other nonsteroidal drugs for at least 12 days before each study and to avoid drinking coffee, alcohol, tea, cola, or other caffeine-containing beverages for at least 12 hours before entering a study. All subjects indicated compliance with these requests.

After emptying the urinary bladder, subjects rested in the supine position for at least 30 minutes in a quiet, temperature-controlled room at 20° C. Either forearm was placed on a rigid support sloping upwards at an angle of 30 degrees from the horizontal, a procedure that allowed complete emptying of the superficial hand veins. To reduce hand movement, the fingers and the forearm were secured by three loosely applied nylon straps. A sphygmomanometer cuff placed on the upper arm was then inflated to 45 mm Hg. A suitable large superficial vein with no apparent tributaries in the immediate area of examination was chosen and a 25-gauge butterfly needle was inserted into the vein. Continuous infusion of 5% dextrose in saline solution was started immediately at a constant rate of 0.1 ml/min through an infusion pump to prevent clotting in the needle and also to perform control measurements of venous diameter under the same conditions as during drug infusions.

The LVDT was placed over the summit of the chosen vein, 10 mm from the tip of the needle. The sphygmomanometer cuff was then deflated. Continuous recordings of the position of the core were made before and after inflation of the sphygmomanometer cuff to 45 mm Hg. The difference between the two positions of the core provided a measure of the control hand diameter vein under a congestion pressure of 45 mm hg (HVD^{45}). The dextrose in saline solution was then replaced by norepinephrine infused at the same rate of 0.1 ml/min. Norepinephrine was freshly prepared just before each experiment and administered in the following doses: 1, 4, 16, 64, and (if required) 256 ng/min. Each dose of the drug was infused for 5 minutes, with the cuff inflated for at least 2 minutes until a stable recording of maximum venous distension was obtained. Results are expressed as the $\overline{X} \pm SD$ and responses were compared by ANOVA.

RESULTS

Study 1. Day-to-day reproducibility of control measurements in the same vein. In each of 10 subjects the HVD^{45} was measured at the same point of the chosen vein on six or eight occasions in which the experiment was repeated during infusions of dextrose in saline solution.

The HVD^{45} varied by 0.02 to 0.12 mm. The mean difference amounted to 0.07 mm, which was about 7% of the mean diameter of the relaxed veins (Fig. 1). These results showed that the technique was highly reproducible in the measurements of the resulting vein on repeated occasions. Having established that it was feasible to expect a stable level of venous tone under our standard laboratory conditions, we progressed to studies of venous responsiveness to local infusion of norepinephrine.

Study 2. Intrasubject variation in hand vein α-receptor responsiveness during different times of the day. The experiment was conducted in 12 healthy subjects between the ages of 20 and 31 years (mean = 22.6 ± 3.4 years). In each subject two experiments in the morning, two in the afternoon, and two in the evening were conducted on different days with the chosen vein in exactly the same position.

All experiments showed log dose-response curves to norepinephrine. In subject 22 (K. K.), when the experiment was conducted twice in the morning, twice in the afternoon, and twice in the evening on different days, the doses of norepinephrine required to produce 50% constriction ($HVDR_{50}$) of hand vein diameter were

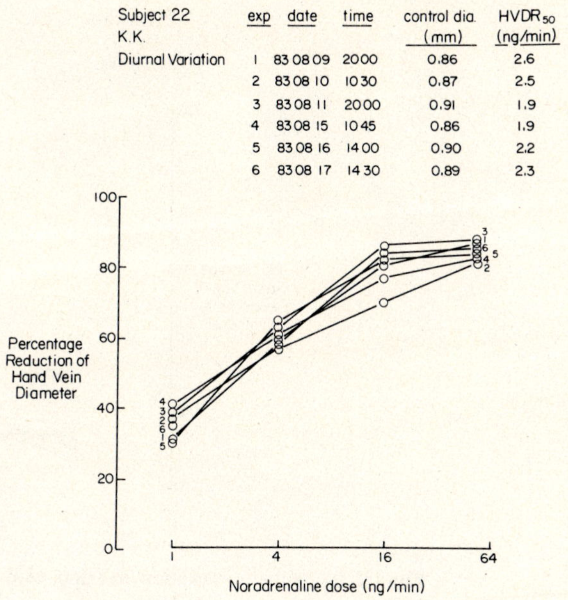

Fig. 2. Diurnal variation in hand vein α-receptor responsiveness to norepinephrine in a 21-year-old woman (subject 22).

similar; the mean dose for the morning was 2.2 ± 0.3 ng/min, for the afternoon it was 2.3 ± 0.1 ng/min, and for the evening it was 2.3 ± 0.4 ng/min (Fig. 2). Similar consistency was observed in the other 11 subjects.

Study 3. Intrasubject variability in α-receptor responsiveness in the same vein. In each of the 12 subjects reported in study 2, responsiveness to norepinephrine was measured at the same point on a vein on six different occasions. Because there was no evidence of diurnal variation, the results from each subject have been combined to assess intrasubject variability of α-receptor responsiveness in the same vein.

In subject 29 (J. B.) there was a consistent dose-response relationship with an $HVDR_{50}$ of 26 ± 2.8 ng/min (Fig. 3). The experiment was repeated six times in each of the 12 subjects at the same point in the vein, and the venoconstrictor response to norepinephrine was highly reproducible (Table I).

Study 4. Intrasubject variability in different veins. The experiment was conducted in another six healthy subjects between the ages of 20 and 31 years (mean = 22.1 ± 3.9). In each subject the experiment was repeated five times on separate occasions in different veins in either hand.

The experiment was repeated five times in subject 31 (L. H.) in different veins on either hand, and there was a consistent dose-response relationship, with an

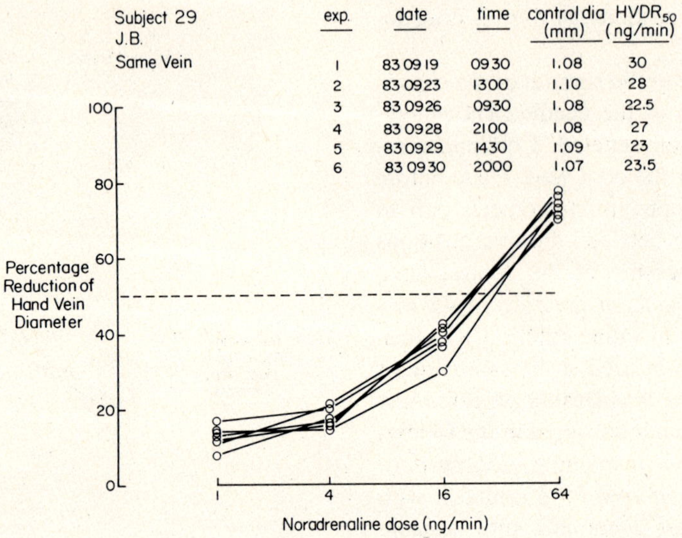

Fig. 3. Intrasubject variation in hand vein α-receptor responsiveness to norepinephrine in a 20-year-old woman (subject 29) in the same spot in a chosen vein on six different occasions.

Table I. Intrasubject variation in hand vein α-receptor responsiveness in the same vein

Subject No.	*Age (yr) and sex*	*Control diameter (mm)* Range	*Control diameter (mm)* $\bar{X} \pm SD$	*HVDR₅₀ (ng/min)* Range	*HVDR₅₀ (ng/min)* $\bar{X} \pm SD$	*Coefficient of variation*
21	23F	0.80-0.86	0.82 ± 0.02	152.0-170.0	160.0 ± 6.9	4.3%
22	21F	0.86-0.91	0.88 ± 0.02	1.9-2.6	2.2 ± 0.3	11.8%
23	31M	0.85-0.94	0.89 ± 3.00	5.0-7.8	6.4 ± 0.9	14.6%
24	21M	0.88-0.94	0.90 ± 0.02	44.0-49.0	46.0 ± 1.6	3.4%
25	21M	1.35-1.44	1.38 ± 0.03	15.5-21.0	18.5 ± 2.0	10.8%
26	24M	1.26-1.38	1.31 ± 0.04	98.0-130.0	114.0 ± 14.0	12.0%
27	22F	0.49-0.55	0.53 ± 0.03	38.0-47.0	44.0 ± 3.0	6.8%
28	28M	0.84-0.88	0.85 ± 0.01	28.0-36.0	32.0 ± 3.0	9.4%
29	20F	1.07-1.10	1.08 ± 0.01	22.5-30.0	26.0 ± 2.8	10.8%
30	20M	1.16-1.25	1.21 ± 0.03	27.0-31.5	29.6 ± 1.5	5.0%
31	20F	0.78-0.84	0.81 ± 0.02	93.0-110.0	102.0 ± 7.2	7.0%
32	20F	0.80-0.90	0.85 ± 0.04	1.5-2.2	1.8 ± 0.2	13.0%

F = Female; M = male.

$HVDR_{50}$ of 110 ± 11.7 ng/min (Fig. 4). Similar consistency was observed in the other five subjects in whom different veins were used (Table II). The coefficient of variation ranged from 4.6% to 15.9%.

Study 5. Intersubject variability in hand vein α-receptor responsiveness. The mean responses of individual subjects from studies 2 and 3 were compared (Fig. 5). There was wide intersubject variability in the norepinephrine $HVDR_{50}$, which ranged from 1.85 ng/min (C. H.) to 160 ng/min (A. W.), with a mean of 47.9 ± 46.8 ng/min.

Wide variation was observed within the six men, with $HVDR_{50}$ values ranging from 6.4 to 102 ng/min (mean = 43.6 ± 39.7 ng/min). Wide variation was also observed within the six women; the norepinephrine $HVDR_{50}$ ranged from 1.85 to 160 ng/min (mean = 53.2 ± 54.5 ng/min).

Study 6. Evaluation of onset, magnitude of effect, dose responsiveness, and duration of action of systemic intravenous DHE. Another group of eight healthy men aged 20 to 29 years (mean = 23.8 ± 3.3 years) received DHE, 0.1, 0.2, and 0.4 mg, in a double-blind, randomized manner. Each dose was infused in a total volume of 5 ml saline solution over 10 minutes on three separate occasions at least 2 days and no more than 6 days apart. Hand vein diameters were measured at −20, −15, and −10 minutes (controls) and at 0, 0.25, 0.5, 1, 2, 3, 4, 6, and 8 hours after the infusions.

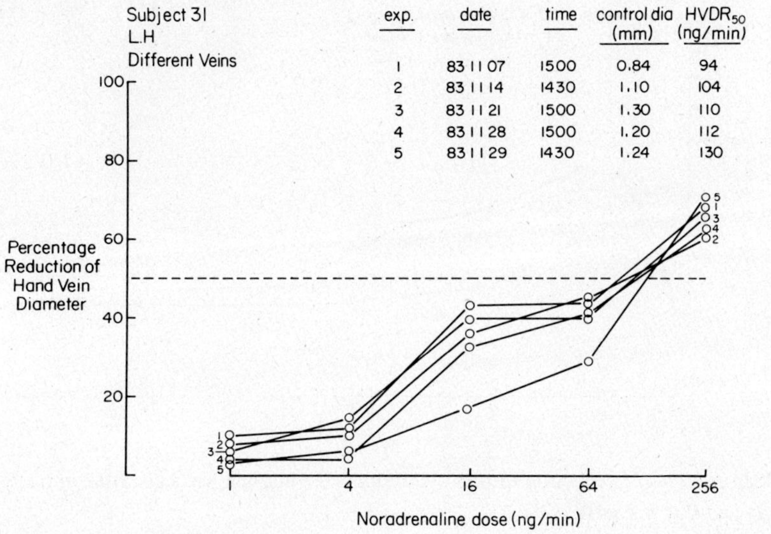

Fig. 4. Intrasubject variation in hand vein α-receptor responsiveness to norepinephrine in a 20-year-old woman (subject 31) in different veins.

Changes in hand vein diameters were calculated as percentage reductions in average control values for each subject.

The mean effects of the three doses of DHE are shown in Fig. 6. The venoconstrictor effect of each dose of DHE was evident at the end of the infusion. However, the mean maximum effects were not observed until 0.5 hours (for 0.1 mg) and 1 hour (for 0.2 mg and 0.4 mg). These average maximum effects were 25.9% ± 17.0% (0.1 mg), 43.2% ± 25.4% (0.2 mg), and 49.4% ± 22.9% (0.4 mg). There was dose responsiveness, with a flattening of the response curve between 0.2 and 0.4 mg, and venoconstriction was incomplete. There was no significant difference between the effects induced by 0.2 and 0.4 mg DHE, which persisted until 6 hours after dosing.

DISCUSSION

It is clear from our studies that the LVDT technique provides a simple, sensitive, and reproducible means of assessing α-receptor responsiveness of superficial hand veins in man. Using this method, Aellig[1-4] has shown the vasoconstrictor effect of direct infusions of 5-hydroxytryptamine, epinephrine, norepinephrine, and DHE.

The results of studies 2, 3, 4, and 5 confirm the log dose-response curve of norepinephrine infused locally into a superficial hand vein reported by other investigators who used the optical method[5, 11] and the LVDT.[1] The constrictor effect of norepinephrine appears to have been mediated locally, because the doses given were lower than the threshold doses for detectable systemic effects on heart rate or blood pressure in all cases. The venoconstrictor effect of norepinephrine can be completely antagonized by prior local infusion of the α-adrenoceptor blocker phentolamine,[5] indicating that the venoconstrictor effect of norepinephrine results from local α-adrenoceptor stimulation.

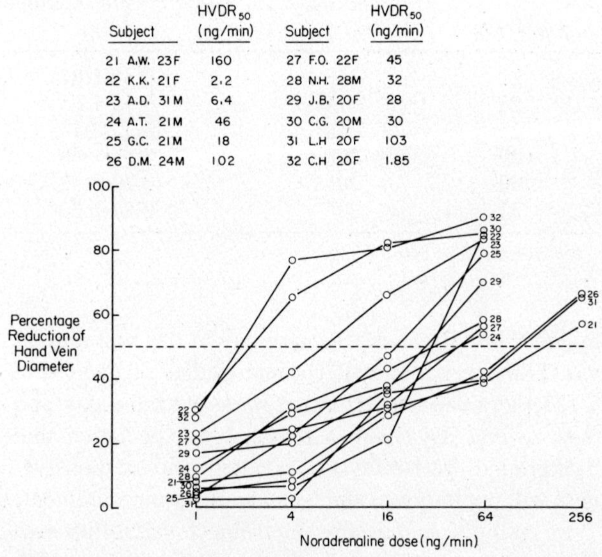

Fig. 5. Intersubject variation in hand vein α-receptor responsiveness to norepinephrine in 12 subjects (age and sex are indicated). F = Female; M = male.

Day-to-day and diurnal variations in hand vein α-receptor responsiveness in man have not been reported

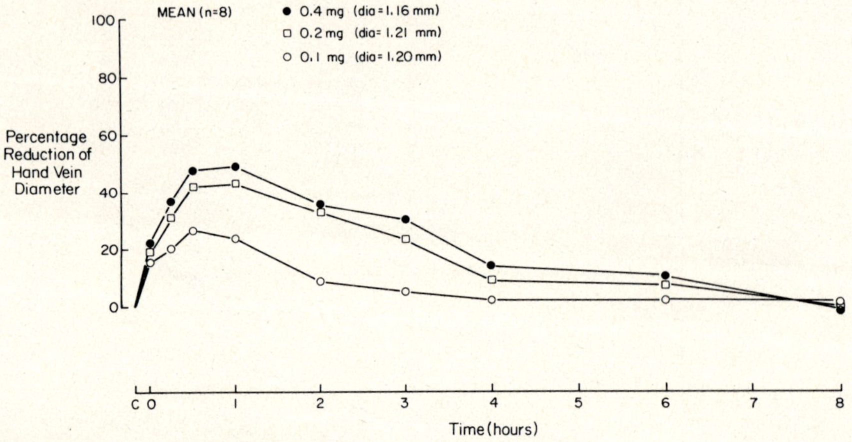

Fig. 6. Mean percentage reduction in hand vein diameter in eight subjects after intravenous doses of 0.1, 0.2, and 0.4 mg DHE.

Table II. Intrasubject variation of hand vein α-receptor responsiveness in different veins

Subject No.	*Age (yr) and sex (yr)*	*Range of control diameter (mm)*	*$HVDR_{50}$ (ng/min)* Range	*$HVDR_{50}$ (ng/min)* $\bar{X} \pm SD$	*Coefficient of variation*
22	21F	0.86-1.87	1.5-2.0	1.76 ± 0.19	10.7%
23	31M	0.65-1.65	5.8-7.5	6.62 ± 0.60	9.6%
25	21M	0.72-2.10	18.0-28.0	21.80 ± 3.40	15.9%
29	20F	0.87-1.68	23.5-32.0	25.90 ± 3.10	11.9%
30	20M	0.70-1.52	27.0-31.0	29.10 ± 1.35	4.6%
31	20F	0.84-1.30	94.0-130.0	110.00 ± 11.70	10.6%

F = Female; M = male.

by other investigators. Because day-to-day and diurnal variability was minimal, chronic studies of hand vein α-receptors can be performed throughout the day and over several days with a reasonable expectation that background variability in α-adrenergic responsiveness will not interfere with vein diameter measurement.

In Aellig's studies the intersubject variability was also moderately large.[4] In the region of 20% to 40% reduction in hand vein diameter, the standard error of the mean for five subjects was 7% to 9%, with a coefficient of variation of approximately 56%. The standard error of the mean concentration of phenylephrine required to halve cutaneous blood flow measured by radioactive xenon in 27 subjects was 7.5%, with a coefficient of variation of 119%.[8]

Our results did not show any apparent effect on dorsal hand vein α-receptor responsiveness of age, gender, or other physical characteristics such as resting heart rate, blood pressure, or race (all subjects were white except for three Orientals). The wide variability in dorsal hand vein α-receptor responsiveness between subjects is not readily explained. Larger numbers of subjects of differing age, race, and blood pressure status would be needed to assess this issue in a more critical manner to avoid the likelihood of a type II error.

It would be of interest to know how much variability exists in members of the same family and how much heredity and environmental factors independently influence α-receptor responses in peripheral hand veins. The wide variability between subjects may have important therapeutic implications in the variability between patients in terms of their responsiveness to drugs that stimulate or block α-adrenoceptors.

Because norepinephrine also stimulates β-adrenoceptors, its potential effects on β-adrenoceptors in peripheral veins must be considered. Sharpey-Schafer and Ginsburg[13] reported that isoprenaline caused dilation in the forearm veins in man, but Coupar[6] observed constriction of isolated saphenous veins in response to high concentrations of the drug (≥5 μg/ml). Eckstein et al.,[7] however, could not demonstrate any direct effect on the forearm veins and concluded that β-adrenoceptors were absent. Collier et al.[5] reported that isoprenaline had no effect when infused into the relaxed vein in doses of 4 to 256 ng/min, but isoprenaline had a dilator effect when it was infused over the same dose range into veins constricted by prior continuous infusion of either norepinephrine or 5-hydroxytryptamine. They also observed that propranolol infused at a dose of 1 μg/min for 10 minutes completely blocked the venodilator response to isoprenaline, and concluded that the superficial hand veins in man possess β-receptors that cause venous relaxation when stimulated. Because the superficial veins of subjects in a warm environment do not normally exhibit any tonic contraction, and because dose-response curves for isoprenaline can be demonstrated only in peripheral veins constricted by the prior administration of an agent such as norepinephrine, we have assumed that β-receptor stimulation was not of any significance in any of the studies described above.

With the use of an optical method for assessing venous tone, the venoconstrictor effect of DHE has been demonstrated after direct infusion of the drug into superficial hand veins in man.[1,2] Oral dosing of 10 mg DHE in 10 healthy volunteers reduced venous diameter by 30% ± 5% after 150 minutes.[1,2] Local infusion of phentolamine, an α-adrenoceptor–blocking drug, markedly inhibited the effect of DHE,[1,2] indicating that the venoconstrictor effect of DHE was also a result of α-adrenoceptor stimulation.

Mueller-Schweinitzer[9] has shown that only 30% of the venoconstrictor effect of DHE in spiral strips of canine saphenous veins could be inhibited by high concentrations of phentolamine, whereas about 60% was abolished by the addition of indomethacin. These results suggest that the venoconstrictor activity of DHE is mediated partially by the enhanced synthesis of a prostaglandin-like substance. Further investigation is necessary to show whether the quantitative difference between results reflect species differences or differences between in vivo and in vitro experiments.

Despite the systemic intravenous route we used, the mean maximum effects of DHE were not observed until 0.5 hours (for 0.1 mg) and 1 hour (for 0.2 and 0.4 mg). Aellig[4] recently studied the venoconstrictor effects of DHE and its main metabolite 8′hydroxy-DHE after direct local infusion of doses of 0.08 and 0.04 mg, respectively, into superficial hand veins. Aellig's data indicate that the pharmacologic activity of DHE may result not only from the unchanged drug but also from the 8′hydroxy metabolite, which is present in plasma in concentrations about five to seven times higher than those of DHE itself. However, these results do not explain why DHE or its 8′hydroxy metabolite should take from 30 to 60 minutes to achieve their maximum effects after direct local infusion. Other active metabolites of DHE may be formed, and the delay in their production might be responsible for the slow maximum effect. Alternatively, this latent period of onset may be related to a slow uptake of DHE or its metabolites from the blood to the tissue receptors.

Almost complete venoconstriction has been observed after locally infused norepinephrine, whereas the mean maximum venoconstrictor effect of DHE we observed was only 49.6%. It appears, therefore, that DHE or its metabolite(s) exhibit only partial agonist activity on α-receptors or that α-receptor stimulating activity is partially offset by the vasodilating activity of one or more DHE metabolites.

Certain details of the LVDT technique require comment. It is essential that the chosen vein have no subcutaneous tributaries in the immediate area of examination, because results can be affected if a leg of the tripod of the LVDT is placed over a vein. The influence of temperature is an important factor in interpretation of the results. Both local and environmental temperatures have been shown to have a profound effect on venous compliance.[10,14,15] It is important, therefore, that the room temperature remain essentially constant in different experiments. Time must be allowed for the subject to adjust to the laboratory temperature before the experiment is initiated. We appear to have avoided these problems because baseline observations and responses to norepinephrine in the same vein and in the same subject were extremely consistent.

The LVDT technique is simple and may be useful not only for experiments in healthy subjects but also in ill patients. It could be applied to study the regulation of α-receptors, to study alterations in hand vein α-receptor activity during aging or in disease states, to compare the efficacy and potency of various α-receptor agonists and antagonists, and to study the interactions between α-receptor agonists and antagonists.

Dr. Gordon Campbell was responsible for the construction of our equipment. We are grateful to Drs. David Freeman and Maurice Hirst for their helpful comments. We are especially thankful to Dr. Walter Aellig of Sandoz (Basle) for his very constructive advice.

Authors' note

Blueprints for the LVDT are available from Dr. Carruthers upon request.

References

1. Aellig WH: Venoconstrictor effect of dihydroergotamine in superficial hand veins. Eur J Clin Pharmacol **7**:137-139, 1974.

2. Aellig WH: Influence of ergot compounds on compliance of superficial hand veins in man. Postgrad Med J **52**(suppl 1):21-23, 1976.
3. Aellig WH: A new technique for recording compliance of human hand veins. Br J Clin Pharmacol **11**:237-343, 1981.
4. Aellig WH: Investigation of the venoconstrictor effect of 8-hydroxydihydroergotamine, the main metabolite of dihydroergotamine, in man. Eur J Clin Pharmacol **25**:239-242, 1984.
5. Collier JG, Nachev C, Robinson BF: Effect of catecholamines and other vasoactive substances on superficial hand veins in man. Clin Sci **43**:455-467, 1972.
6. Coupar IM: The effect of isoprenaline on adrenoceptors in human saphenous vein. Br J Pharmacol **39**:465-475, 1970.
7. Eckstein JW, Wendling MG, Abboud FM: Forearm venous responses to stimulation of adrenergic receptors. J Clin Invest **44**:1151-1159, 1965.
8. Henderson WR, Shelhamer JH, Reingold DB, Smith LJ, Evans R, Kaliner M: Alpha-adrenergic-responsiveness in asthma, analysis of vascular and pupillary responses. N Engl J Med **300**:642-647, 1979.
9. Mueller-Schweinitzer E: Studies on the peripheral mode of action of dihydroergotamine in human and canine veins. Eur J Pharmacol **27**:231-237, 1974.
10. Nachev C, Collier J, Robinson B: Simplified method for measuring compliance of superficial veins. Cardiovasc Res **5**:147-156, 1971.
11. Robinson BR: Assessment of the effect of drugs on the venous system in man. Br J Clin Pharmacol **6**:381-386, 1978.
12. Schaevitz H: A linear variable differential transformer. Cambridge, Mass., 1947, Proceedings of the Society for Experimental Stress, vol 4, pp 79-88.
13. Sharpey-Schafer EP, Ginsburg J: Humoral agents and venous tone: Effects of catecholamines, 5-hydroxytryptamine, histamine and nitrites. Lancet **2**:1337-1340, 1962.
14. Webb-Peploe MM, Shepherd JT: Response of dog's cutaneous veins to local and central temperature changes. Circ Res **23**:693-699, 1968.
15. Wood EJ, Eckstein JW: A tandem forearm plethysmograph for study of acute responses of the peripheral veins of man: The effect of environmental and local temperature change and the effect of pooling blood in the extremities. J Clin Invest **37**:41-50, 1958.

Pharmacodynamics of intravenous labetalol and follow-up therapy with oral labetalol

The effectiveness, safety, and pharmacodynamics of repeated doses of intravenous labetalol for rapid reduction of severe hypertension and of subsequent oral labetalol dosing were studied. Twelve patients with severe hypertension were admitted to the hospital after the withholding of antihypertensive therapy for 2 to 14 days. Thirty minutes after an injection of vehicle only, labetalol, 0.25 mg/kg body weight, was injected and followed by repeat injections of 0.5 mg/kg every 15 minutes until the supine diastolic blood pressure (BP) was reduced to <90 mm Hg or a total of 3.25 mg/kg had been administered. Twenty-four hours after the last injection, oral labetalol was started at an initial dosage of 100 or 200 mg b.i.d., then increased every 2 days until the standing diastolic BP was <90 mm Hg or a maximum daily dosage of 2400 mg was reached. The initial injection achieved mean falls in supine systolic/diastolic BPs of 11/7 mm Hg. Subsequent injections produced additional falls in a dose-related fashion; the mean falls after the last injection (total cumulative dose 2.7 mg/kg) were 40/20 mm Hg. The effect lasted for 12 hours or more in most patients and tended to be biphasic, with one peak at approximately 5 minutes and another much less pronounced peak at about 4 hours. There was no evidence of precipitous falls in BP. All patients were able to ambulate 6 hours after the last injection without symptoms of postural hypotension. Oral labetalol effectively and safely restored and maintained the BP reductions achieved with intravenous labetalol. (Clin Pharmacol Ther 38:503-508, 1985.)

Nicholas D. Vlachakis, M.D., Robert F. Maronde, M.D., James W. Maloy, Pharm.D., Milenko Medakovic, M.D., and Nadim Kassem, M.D.
Los Angeles, Calif.

Regardless of its cause, a marked elevation in blood pressure (BP) represents an immediate and long-term threat to life. Therefore, BP reduction in patients with severe hypertension is a primary therapeutic challenge. Marked and sudden reductions in BP may cause adverse effects related to decreased perfusion of vital organs.[9,16] Intravenous injection of currently available antihypertensive drugs has not proved to be an ideal approach for rapidly decreasing BP because the extent of the decrease is unpredictable.[1] Therefore, drugs that abruptly decrease BP must be administered by continuous intravenous infusion, which necessitates continuous monitoring of the effect and careful adjustment of dosage.[8]

Labetalol is an antihypertensive drug[3,4,13] that blocks β-adrenergic receptors and causes peripheral vascular vasodilation by blocking the α-adrenergic receptors and by stimulating β_2-receptors.[2] Bolus doses of 1.0 to 2.0 mg/kg[7,12,14,15] and intravenous infusions[6] of labetalol have been associated with steep falls in BP. This study was undertaken to assess the pharmacodynamics of a regimen of multiple bolus injections of labetalol beginning with a low initial dose (0.25 mg/kg) followed at 15-minute intervals by 0.5 mg/kg injections. The efficacy and safety of subsequent oral labetalol therapy were also studied.

From the Clinical Pharmacology Section, Department of Medicine, University of Southern California Medical Center.

Supported by a grant from Schering Corporation, Kenilworth, N. J., and Glaxo Inc., Research Triangle Park, N. C.

Received for publication March 20, 1985; accepted Aug. 8, 1985.

Reprint requests to: Nicholas D. Vlachakis, M.D., Department of Medicine, University of Southern California Medical Center, Los Angeles, CA 90033.

METHODS

Study design. This was an open-label study to evaluate intravenous labetalol followed by oral labetalol in patients with a standing diastolic BP between 115 and 130 mm Hg. The study was approved by the Institutional Review Board of the hospital.

The study was conducted in four phases. After giving informed consent, adult patients known to have moderate to severe essential hypertension entered a washout phase during which they took one placebo capsule twice a day and had their BP measured every 2 to 4 days. If the standing diastolic BP was >115 mm Hg after 2 weeks or >120 mm Hg at an earlier visit, the patient was admitted to the hospital and began a 2-day inpatient phase. On the next day beginning at 8 AM, the supine BP and heart rate were measured at 15-minute intervals for 1 hour. If the supine diastolic BP was >105 mm Hg at the last two of the four determinations, labetalol vehicle was injected intravenously over 2 minutes. Supine BP and heart rate were then measured at 5-minute intervals over 30 minutes. Thirty minutes after vehicle injection, 0.25 mg/kg labetalol was similarly administered and BP and heart rate were measured every 5 minutes. An additional 0.5 mg/kg labetalol was injected every 15 minutes until the supine diastolic BP was <90 mm Hg or had decreased by at least 25 mm Hg or a total of 3.25 mg/kg labetalol had been injected.

Patients were restricted to bed for 6 hours and were closely monitored and kept awake for 12 hours after the end of the intravenous injections. During this period, BP was measured at hourly intervals. Patients were discharged the following day.

Blood specimens were drawn before, 30 minutes after, and 3.5 hours after the start of intravenous labetalol therapy. Plasma levels of norepinephrine and epinephrine were determined with a radioenzymatic assay.[17]

Approximately 24 hours after the last injection, oral labetalol dosing began with either 100 mg b.i.d. (for patients who required ≤135 mg cumulative doses of intravenous labetalol) or 200 mg b.i.d. (for patients who required >135 mg cumulative doses of intravenous labetalol). At 2-day intervals, the dosage was increased until the standing diastolic BP was <90 mm Hg or had decreased by ≥30 mm Hg from the outpatient baseline level. The incremental dosages were 200, 400, 800, 1200, 1800, and 2400 mg/day. For dosages up to 1200 mg/day a twice-daily regimen was used and for dosages of 1800 and 2400 mg/day a three-times-daily regimen was used. If the above therapeutic goal was not achieved after labetalol, 2400 mg/day for 2 days, hydrochlorothiazide (HCTZ), 25 or 50 mg b.i.d., was added to the regimen.

The optimum labetalol dosage (with or without HCTZ) was administered during an additional 2-week maintenance period. Thereafter, patients were instructed to reduce the daily labetalol dose gradually over 1 to 2 weeks. The final visit of the study occurred after the withdrawal of labetalol was complete.

Evaluation of efficacy.

Intravenous labetalol. Supine BP recordings at 5, 10, and 15 minutes after each labetalol injection were averaged. These were used to evaluate the effect of the cumulative labetalol dose as compared with the effect of the vehicle. The average BPs recorded during the 24-hour period after the last labetalol injection were evaluated to determine the duration of the antihypertensive effect of intravenous labetalol.

Oral labetalol. The averages of three consecutive measurements after the patient was supine for 5 minutes and again after the patient was standing for 2 minutes were determined at each visit. The changes from baseline (i.e., the last visit of the placebo washout phase) in the systolic, diastolic, and mean BP [determined as: Diastolic BP + 0.33 (systolic BP − diastolic BP)] were used to evaluate efficacy.

Evaluation of safety. At the initial visit, each patient's medical history, physical examination, grading of retinopathy, 12-lead ECG, chest x-ray, and laboratory test results were obtained. The physical examination, ECG, and laboratory tests were repeated at the end of the oral labetalol phase. Any abnormalities and clinically significant changes were noted and evaluated. At each outpatient visit, supine and standing BPs were determined to assess any occurrences of orthostatic hypotension. Changes in heart rate and body weight and any reports of adverse experiences were also evaluated.

Patients. Twelve patients known to have severe hypertension were recruited from the Clinical Pharmacology–Hypertension Clinic. Patients with secondary or malignant hypertension, lung disease, advanced heart or renal failure, recent myocardial infarction or cerebrovascular accident, or significant hematologic, hepatic, or thyroid disease were excluded from the study. Of the 12 patients who participated, eight were men and four were women; there were nine blacks, two whites, and one American Indian. The median age was 47.5 years (range 31 to 64 years). The median duration of known hypertension was 8.5 years (range 1 to 30 years).

Statistical methods. Where appropriate, inferential analysis was used. Student's t test for matched pairs was used to compare the peak effects of labetalol with those of the vehicle. Changes from baseline in BP and heart rate were compared with zero by two-tailed paired t tests.

RESULTS

Intravenous labetalol. Seven of the 12 patients received seven injections (total cumulative dosage of labetalol was 3.25 mg/kg), two received five injections (total of 2.75 mg/kg), one received four injections (total of 2.25 mg/kg), and two received three injections (totals of 1.25 and 0.75 mg/kg, respectively). The mean cu-

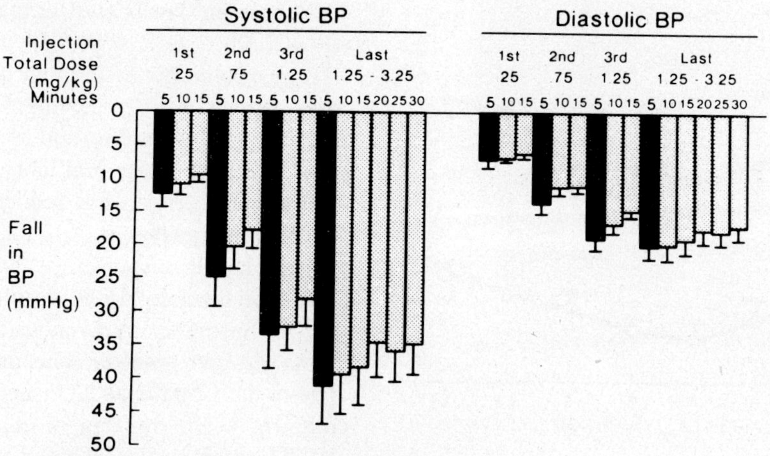

Fig. 1. Comparison of mean (± SE) reductions in supine BP at 5, 10, and 15 minutes after the first three and the last labetalol injections.

Table I. Patient listing of systolic/diastolic BPs (mm Hg) after repeated bolus injections

Patient No.	*Baseline*	*Cumulative labetalol dose (mg/kg)* 0.25	0.75	1.25	1.75	2.25	2.75	3.25
1	159/106	146/96	139/95*	129/89*	—	—	—	—
2	202/120	185/115	178/111	175/107	169/105	163/103	176/109	179/111
3	198/112	185/107	175/103	157/94	151/93	144/88	136/89	—
4	166/110	159/107	157/103	149/98	147/95	153/97	155/101	149/100
5	176/126	166/117	159/118	156/113	149/112	145/109	149/114	147/109
6	206/129	201/121	192/114	183/112	178/110	175/109	171/107	170/111
7	224/119	210/108	167/97	153/93	138/87	133/83	—	—
8	221/123	213/120	205/114	195/111	183/106	181/105	183/105	181/103
9	168/107	151/101	142/89	131/82	—	—	—	—
10	197/115	187/105	180/101	156/94	153/93	153/93	144/91	149/91
11	179/111	167/104	165/100	155/95	154/94	156/95	146/93	142/90
12	153/107	148/101	137/95	133/93	130/91	127/89	129/88	—

Values are the mean of the determinations at 5, 10, and 15 minutes after each injection. Baseline values are the average of the last three determinations after injection of vehicle.

*Patient 1 received cumulative doses of 0.25, 0.50, and 0.75 mg/kg.

mulative dose received was 2.7 mg/kg. The initial injection of 0.25 mg/kg caused supine BP reductions in all 12 patients. The mean decrease during the 15 minutes after injection was 11 mm Hg (range 5 to 17 mm Hg) in systolic BP and 7 mm Hg (range 3 to 11 mm Hg) in diastolic BP (Fig. 1; Table I). After the second injection the mean reductions from baseline were 21/12 mm Hg and they were 31/17 mm Hg after the third injection. During the 15 minutes after the last injection, the mean falls from baseline in supine BP were 40/20 mm Hg (range 17 to 91/9 to 36 mm Hg). Six of the 12 patients had average supine diastolic BPs reduced to ≤90 mm Hg (91 mm Hg in another). The remaining five patients had supine diastolic BPs of from 103 to 111 mm Hg; reductions in these five patients ranged from 9 to 20 mm Hg.

After each injection, the maximum mean reductions in systolic and diastolic BPs were achieved at 5 minutes, followed by a gradual slight increase over the next 10 minutes. Each subsequent injection achieved further BP falls. The dose-effect relationship was evaluated only for the first three injections, the minimum received by each patient. There was a significant ($P < 0.01$) linear dose-effect relationship for both the systolic and the diastolic BP. However, further BP reductions were achieved with additional injections in those patients who received cumulative doses >1.25 mg/kg. No relationship was found between the severity of hypertension at

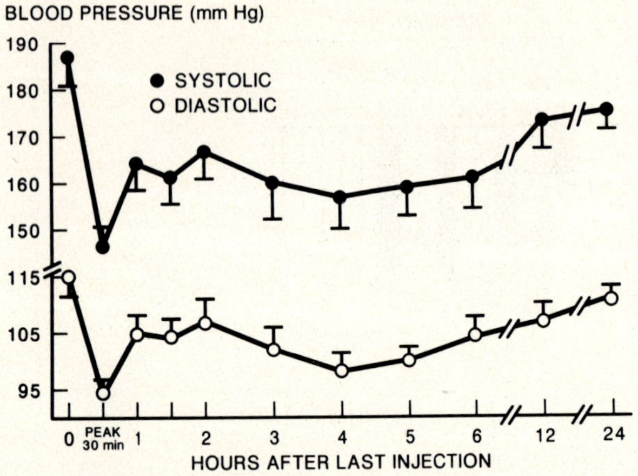

Fig. 2. Antihypertensive effect over 24 hours after last labetalol injection. Data are $\overline{X} \pm$ SE.

baseline and the BP reduction achieved after the 1.25 mg/kg cumulative dose.

After the last labetalol injection, the acute antihypertensive effect noted in the first few minutes was followed by a fading of the effect within the first 2 hours. This was followed by a secondary gradual decrease at approximately 3 to 4 hours that was less prominent than the initial decrease, then by a gradual recovery towards the baseline level (Fig. 2). Some effect was still seen in most patients 12 to 24 hours after the last labetalol injection; the mean fall at 12 hours was 14/8 mm Hg and at 24 hours it was 12/4 mm Hg.

The mean supine heart rate during the 12 hours after the last injection was 70 bpm, compared with a mean baseline heart rate of 77 bpm. The means of the lowest heart rates recorded for each patient during the first 30 minutes and the first 12 hours after the last injection were 66 and 62 bpm, respectively. Four patients had a minimum heart rate <60 bpm (50, 56, 56, and 58 bpm). The two former patients had baseline heart rates of 59 and 61 bpm, respectively.

One patient complained of mild headaches. Although patients were restricted to bed for 6 hours after the last injection, all were able to ambulate without evidence of orthostasis after this time.

Oral labetalol. The first oral dose of labetalol was taken approximately 24 hours after the last intravenous dose. Three patients received 100 mg and nine received 200 mg labetalol as the initial oral dose.

At 24 hours after the last intravenous labetalol injection, the mean systolic and diastolic BPs had not returned to the preinjection baseline levels. Within 2 hours of the initial oral dose, the supine systolic, diastolic, and mean BPs were significantly lower than baseline levels (last outpatient evaluation) by 16 ($P = 0.08$), 15 ($P < 0.005$), and 16 ($P = 0.011$) mm Hg, respectively. At the end of oral labetalol dosing, five patients were receiving 2400 mg/day, six were receiving 1800 mg/day, and one was receiving 800 mg/day. The mean daily oral labetalol dose was 1967 mg. At the end of oral dosing, reductions from baseline were 37/25 mm Hg ($P < 0.001$) for the supine BPs and 47/33 mm Hg ($P < 0.001$) for the standing BPs (Fig. 3). Thus oral labetalol dosing resulted in BP decreases similar to those after intravenous therapy.

At the end point of labetalol dosing alone, all but one of the 12 patients had standing diastolic BPs <100 mm Hg (<90 mm Hg in eight). Three patients had HCTZ added to the labetalol regimen, although labetalol alone had induced standing diastolic BP reductions of 21, 19, and 30 mm Hg, respectively. Standing diastolic BP was further reduced after HCTZ in two patients (from 100 to 83 mm Hg and from 98 to 87 mm Hg) but increased in the other (from 93 to 109 mm Hg).

At the end of oral labetalol dosing, the small physiologic postural diastolic BP increases (2.6 mm Hg) were transformed to small postural falls (5.7 mm Hg), and small postural systolic BP decreases (4.1 mm Hg) were augmented (13.7 mm Hg), resulting in an 8.4 mm Hg average postural decrease in mean BP. However, no symptoms of orthostatic hypotension were reported. Two patients reported mild fatigue during oral labetalol dosing at doses ≥1800 mg/day. The average weight gain from baseline to the end point of oral labetalol dosing was 1.6 kg. Results of laboratory tests, physical examinations, and ECGs indicated no significant adverse effects attributable to labetalol.

Effects of intravenous labetalol on plasma catecholamine levels. Plasma levels of norepinephrine were modestly but significantly higher at 30 minutes and 3.5 hours after the start of intravenous labetalol therapy. The increases in plasma epinephrine levels were less prominent but were also statistically significant (Table II).

DISCUSSION

Intravenous labetalol lowered the systolic and diastolic BPs in all patients in this study. The initial dose of 0.25 mg/kg iv lowered BP moderately without causing precipitous falls. Subsequent injections caused additional falls, but most of the total antihypertensive effect was achieved with cumulative doses of up to 1.25 mg/kg. This gradual and controlled lowering of the BP achieved by repeated bolus injections of labetalol is in contrast to the precipitous, excessive falls and hypo-

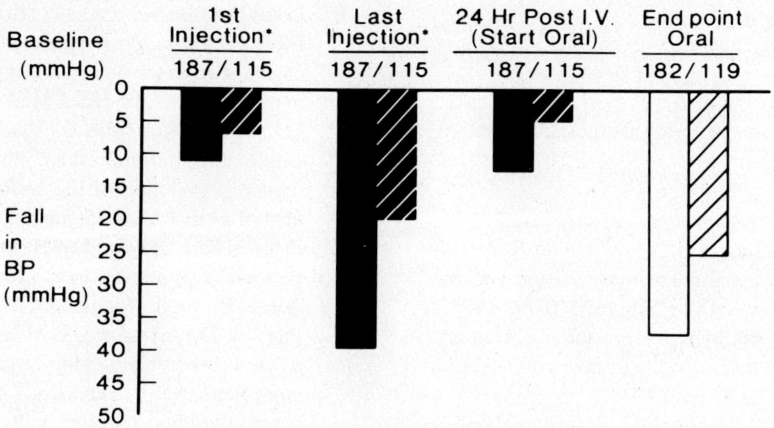

Fig. 3. Comparison of supine BP reductions achieved by oral labetalol with that of intravenous (*I.V.*) labetalol. *Average of readings 5, 10, and 15 minutes after injection.

tension described when high initial boluses of labetalol (1.0 to 2.0 mg/kg) were injected intravenously[7,12,14,15] or given by incremental infusion.[6]

A cumulative dose-effect relationship was demonstrated for the first three intravenous dose levels for which this relationship was evaluated. There was no evidence of any delay in effect or unpredictable abrupt BP fall. Six hours after the last injection, all patients were able to ambulate without evidence of orthostatic hypotension.

The duration of the antihypertensive effect after the last labetalol injection was relatively long; some effect was generally seen after 12 hours and in some cases after 24 hours. This is in contrast to drugs with a short duration of action for which dangerous increases in BP may follow an abrupt discontinuation of intravenous therapy.

Because the antihypertensive effect of intravenous labetalol was biphasic, with a transient partial loss of the initial effect followed by a modest secondary BP decrease, one might question when to initiate oral labetalol therapy. However, in another study oral labetalol therapy was begun when the BP started to rise after the reductions achieved with intravenous labetalol. No dramatic additional falls were associated with the initiation of oral dosing.[18]

The modest decrease in heart rate that is related to the β-adrenergic receptor blockade by labetalol is in contrast to the possibly deleterious reflex tachycardia that occurs with most of the available intravenously administered antihypertensive drugs.

With the intravenous regimen we used, no treatment-related adverse experiences were observed during the intravenous phase or during the subsequent 24-hour observation period. This is in contrast to the adverse

Table II. Effect of intravenous labetalol on plasma catecholamine levels (pg/ml)

	Pretreatment	*30 min after*	*3.5 hr after*
Norepinephrine	182 ± 22	361 ± 48*	367 ± 52*
Epinephrine	71 ± 10	81 ± 13†	86 ± 52†

Data are $\overline{X}$ ± SE.
*P < 0.001, †P < 0.05 compared with pretreatment value.

experiences (nausea, vomiting, faintness, hypotension) that occurred when a high dose of labetalol (1 to 2 mg/kg) was injected as a single bolus.[7,12,14,15] We found no clinically significant changes from placebo baseline in routine laboratory test results or ECGs measured at the end of the observation period. These findings indicate that the intravenous labetalol regimen we used is safe.

The first 200 mg oral dose of labetalol after the intravenous injection was well tolerated, and no symptomatic postural hypotension was reported. This is at variance with earlier observations that an initial 200 mg oral dose of labetalol not preceded by intravenous dosing caused symptomatic postural hypotension.[10,11]

The subsequent rapid titration of the oral labetalol dose in our study effectively restored the BP reductions attained earlier with intravenous labetalol. These reductions were effectively maintained by continuation of an oral labetalol regimen. Even in these patients with severe hypertension, oral labetalol alone was sufficient antihypertensive therapy in nine of 12 patients. Although three patients eventually required the addition of HCTZ, oral labetalol alone induced remarkable reductions in their BPs, albeit not quite to normotensive levels.

Intravenous labetalol was associated with a modest rise in plasma catecholamine concentrations, which is consistent with previous reports.[5]

We thank Lillian Mellars, Schering Corporation, for statistical analysis.

References

1. American Medical Association Committee on Hypertension: The treatment of malignant hypertension and hypertensive emergencies. JAMA **228:**1673-1679, 1974.
2. Baum T, Sybertz EJ: Antihypertensive actions of an isomer of labetalol and other vasodilator beta-adrenoceptor blockers. Fed Proc **42:**176-181, 1983.
3. Brogden RN, Heel RC, Speight TM, et al: Labetalol: A review of its pharmacology and therapeutic use in hypertension. Drugs **15:**251-270, 1978.
4. Brown JJ, Lever AF, Cumming AMM, et al: Labetalol in hypertension. Lancet **1:**1147, 1977.
5. Christensen NJ, Trap-Jensen J, Svendsen TL, et al: Effect of labetalol on plasma noradrenaline and adrenaline in hypertensive man. Eur J Clin Pharmacol **14:**227-230, 1978.
6. Cumming AMM, Brown JJ, Fraser R, et al: Blood pressure reduction by incremental infusion of labetalol in patients with severe hypertension. Br J Clin Pharmacol **8:**359-364, 1979.
7. Cumming AMM, Brown JJ, Lever AF, et al: Treatment of severe hypertension by repeated bolus injections of labetalol. Br J Clin Pharmacol **8**(suppl 2):199s-204s, 1979.
8. Finnerty FA: Malignant hypertension. Am Heart J **88:**265-268, 1974.
9. Graham DI: Ischemic brain damage of cerebral perfusion failure type after treatment of severe hypertension. Br Med J **4:**739, 1975.
10. Louis WJ, Christophidis N, Brignell M, et al: Labetalol: Bioavailability, drug plasma levels, plasma renin and catecholamines in acute and chronic treatment of resistant hypertension. Aust NZ J Med **8:**602-609, 1978.
11. Maronde R, Robinson D, Vlachakis ND, et al: Study of single and multiple dose pharmacokinetic/pharmacodynamic modeling of the antihypertensive effects of labetalol. Am J Med **75**(suppl 4A):40-46, 1983.
12. Pearson RM, Havard DWH: Intravenous labetalol in hypertensive patients treated with β-adrenoceptor blocking drugs. Br J Clin Pharmacol **3**(suppl 3):795-798, 1976.
13. Pugsley D, Armstrong B, Nassim M, et al: Combined α- and β-adrenoreceptor blockade in hypertension: A controlled trial of labetalol (AH 5158) compared with propranolol and placebo. Clin Sci Molec Med **51:**501s-503s, 1976.
14. Richards DA, Prichard BNC, Boakes AJ, et al: Pharmacological basis for antihypertensive effects of intravenous labetalol. Br Heart J **39:**99-106, 1977.
15. Rosei EA, Trust PM, Brown JJ, et al: Intravenous labetalol in severe hypertension. Lancet **2:**1093-1094, 1975.
16. Strandgaard S, Oleson J, Skinhoj E, et al: Autoregulation of brain circulation in severe arterial hypertension. Br Med J **1:**507-510, 1973.
17. Vlachakis ND, Alexander N, Velasquez MT, et al: A radioenzymatic microassay for simultaneous measurement of catecholamines and their deaminated metabolites. Biochem Med **22:**323-331, 1979.
18. Wilson DJ, Wallin JD, Vlachakis ND, et al: Intravenous labetalol in the treatment of severe hypertension and hypertensive emergencies. Am J Med **75**(suppl 4A):95-102, 1983.

Biologic determinants of propranolol disposition: Results from 1308 patients in the Beta-blocker Heart Attack Trial*

Our objective was to identify biologic determinants of propranolol serum levels in 1308 patients after myocardial infarction (MI). Patients had had their MI within the previous month. A steady-state propranolol dosage of 40 mg every 8 hours produced a mean trough concentration of 42 ng/ml with extremely great (fiftyfold) interindividual variability. Univariate and multivariate analyses suggested that this variability was the result of many biologic factors. Serum levels were higher in women, in older patients, and in patients receiving concomitant therapy with other antiarrhythmic drugs. Serum levels were also higher in patients with elevated serum creatinine and lactate dehydrogenase levels. Serum levels were lower in black patients than in white patients. Also, serum levels in smokers were lower than those in nonsmokers, but only markedly so in the outpatient setting (6 months after the MI). The influence of sex and race on drug disposition has not previously been reported for β-blocking drugs. Although a genetic deficiency in the oxidative metabolism of propranolol has been indicated, the frequency distribution of serum propranolol levels did not demonstrate a bimodal distribution for genetically distinct populations. (CLIN PHARMACOL THER 38:509-518, 1985.)

Thomas Walle, Ph.D., Robert P. Byington, Ph.D., Curt D. Furberg, M.D., Kevin M. McIntyre, M.D., and Pantel S. Vokonas, M.D.
Charleston, S. C., Houston, Tex., Bethesda, Md., and West Roxbury and Boston, Mass.

Great interindividual variability in the disposition of propranolol has long been of concern with respect to optimal therapy with this important cardiovascular drug. Thus a ten- to twentyfold difference in propranolol plasma levels between patients receiving identical oral doses has commonly been observed.[8,12,17,44,49,53,57,63,65,68] The reason for this variability is not well understood, although a number of factors have been identified that could affect the disposition of propranolol.[57] Rigorously controlled experimental conditions with regard to compliance, environmental factors, and analytic methodology have been suggested to minimize this variability.[72] However, since most studies have been carried out in rather small numbers of normal subjects or patients, it has not been possible to draw any clear conclusions regarding the magnitude of the interindividual variability in propranolol disposition and the factors contributing to it.

The Beta-Blocker Heart Attack Trial (BHAT)[6,9] has provided an opportunity to examine the disposition of propranolol in a large group of patients. Thus serum levels were measured in 1308 hospitalized patients receiving 40 mg propranolol every 8 hours under steady-state conditions. Univariate and multivariate analyses allowed correlational studies of propranolol levels with a variety of factors that may influence propranolol disposition, such as sex, race, age, smoking status, and use of other drugs.

METHODS

Study population. The patients studied in this analysis were the patients assigned to the propranolol therapy group of the BHAT.[6,9] The BHAT was a randomized, double-blind, placebo-controlled clinical trial de-

From the Department of Pharmacology, Medical University of South Carolina, Charleston; BHAT Coordinating Center, University of Texas Health Science Center, Houston; Clinical Application and Prevention Program, National Heart, Lung, and Blood Institute, Bethesda; Veterans Administration Hospital, West Roxbury; and Bostion University School of Medicine, Boston.

The research upon which this publication is based was performed pursuant to Contract No. N01-HV-7-2948 with the National Heart, Lung, and Blood Institute, National Institutes of Health, Department of Health and Human Services. Data analyses were supported in part by National Heart, Lung and Blood Institute Grant No. HL 29566.

Received for publication April 29, 1985; accepted May 26, 1985.

Reprint requests to: Thomas Walle, Ph.D., Department of Pharmacology, Medical University of South Carolina, 171 Ashley Ave., Charleston, SC 29425.

*A list of investigators may be found at the end of this article.

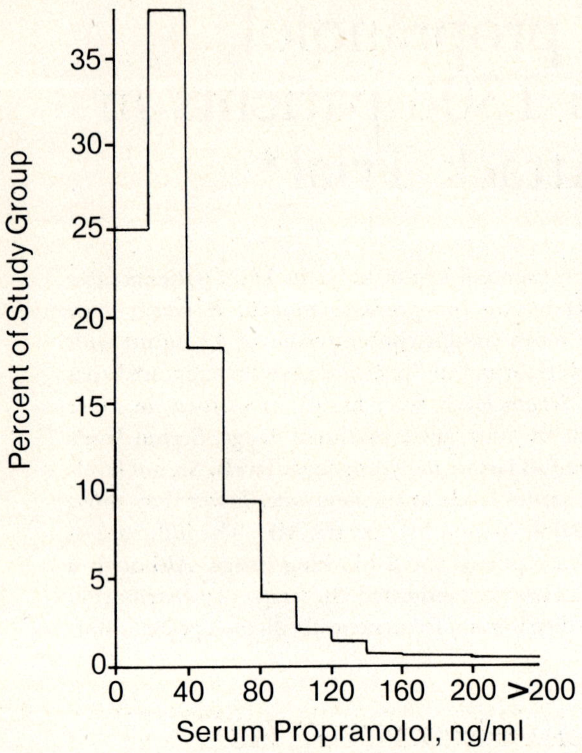

Fig. 1. Frequency distribution of serum propranolol levels in 1308 patients after a myocardial infarction. Serum levels were measured at 7 to 9 hours (trough) after at least six consecutive oral doses of propranolol, 40 mg every 8 hours, with most patients hospitalized. Levels in nine patients that exceeded 200 ng/ml (0.7% of the group) were 209, 221, 231, 253, 265, 310, 327, 332, and 415 ng/ml.

signed to test the efficacy of the long-term use of propranolol by patients immediately after (within 1 month) a myocardial infarction. Eligible men and women between the ages of 30 and 69 years were enrolled in the trial at 31 clinical centers throughout the United States and Canada. Eligibility criteria and study design are described elsewhere.[9]

The total number of patients enrolled in the trial was 3837; 1916 patients were assigned to the propranolol therapy group. Of the patients receiving propranolol, 264 were excluded from the present analysis either because they did not have their blood drawn (244 patients) or because their blood sample was lost (20 patients). One hundred seventy-nine patients were also excluded because they were not receiving a propranolol dosage of 40 mg every 8 hours. Finally, an additional 165 patients were excluded because they did not have their blood drawn 7 to 9 hours after dosing. Thus the present analyses were restricted to the 1308 patients (68.3% of all patients taking propranolol) who were taking 40 mg every 8 hours and who had their blood drawn 7 to 9 hours after the last dose. Of these, 889 (68.0%) were still in the hospital when they had their blood drawn; 419 (32.0%) were already discharged and had their blood drawn at home. The protocols for inpatients and outpatients were identical.

Protocol. Immediately after randomization (day 0) all patients were given a 20 mg oral dose of propranolol. If no adverse reactions were noted, the dose was increased to 40 mg every 8 hours. Blood samples for propranolol serum level determinations were drawn after a minimum of six consecutive doses of 40 mg within 7 to 9 hours after the last dose.

In a separate analysis, blood samples were also drawn at the 6-month follow-up visit in 836 patients who were seen as outpatients taking propranolol, 60 mg t.i.d. These samples were drawn at various times after the dose.

All blood samples (2.5 ml) were drawn by separate venipuncture into a Venoject evacuated tube system (Terumo Medical Corp.). Blood was allowed to clot between 30 minutes and 2 hours (preferably within 1 hour). Tubes were centrifuged at 1500 × g for 15 minutes. Immediately after centrifugation the serum was transferred from the evacuated tube into a polyethylene vial. The specimen was then placed in a freezer at an angled position until frozen, at which time it was stored in an upright position at −70° C. Specimens were shipped on a weekly basis in containers on dry ice to the Central Laboratory for analysis.

Serum propranolol determinations. All propranolol measurements were made by an HPLC method previously described.[64] Briefly, 1.0 ml serum was extracted at pH 12 with cyclohexane after addition of pronethalol as internal standard. The organic phase was evaporated and the residue was reconstituted in the mobile phase. Part of this was then chromatographed on a CN column (Applied Science Laboratories). The mobile phase was methanol:0.04 mol/L acetate buffer (55:45) at pH 4.5. A fluorescence detector was used.

Although it is possible to detect the presence of propranolol at levels <10 ng/ml, it is difficult to determine the exact concentration at these levels. Therefore, serum propranolol levels <10 ng/ml have been assigned the concentration of 5 ng/ml. The specificity of this method for propranolol was rigorously confirmed before the BHAT study by a molecularly specific gas chromatography-mass spectrometry assay.[74]

Statistical analysis. The mean and median serum propranolol levels were calculated at baseline for the

Table I. Multivariate relationship between the natural log of serum propranolol and 19 baseline patient characteristics that were univariately related to serum propranolol level (final step of stepwise multiple linear regression)

Patient characteristics	*β*	*Z of β*
Sex (men/women)	−0.488	−6.41
Age (yr)	0.008	2.47
Use of antiarrhythmics (yes/no)	0.231	3.29
Race (white/black)*	0.394	4.42
Serum creatinine level (mg/dl)	0.421	4.05
Elevated LDH level (yes/no)	0.110	1.97
Prior MI (yes/no)	0.111	1.55
Taking aspirin (yes/no)	0.173	1.63
Atrial fibrillation in hospital (yes/no)	0.162	1.45
Married (yes/no)	−0.090	−1.42
Time between admission and randomization (days)	0.008	1.13
Leisure activity (heavy/light)	−0.053	−0.97
Cardiomegaly (yes/no)	0.042	0.78
Taking β-blocker before hospitalization (yes/no)	0.075	0.72
Cigarette smoker (yes/no)	−0.029	−0.56
Taking digitalis (yes/no)	−0.040	−0.48
ST segment depression on ECG (present/absent)	0.017	0.29
Employed (yes/no)	−0.004	−0.07
High blood pressure history (yes/no)	0.002	0.04
Intercept	2.444	9.40

LDH = Lactate dehydrogenase; MI = myocardial infarction.
*Asians and other races are not included in this analysis.

Table II. Serum propranolol level by patient characteristics (subgroups shown are those independently related to serum propranolol level in the multivariate analysis [Table I])

	Serum propranolol level (ng/ml)		
Patient characteristics	$\bar{X}$	*Median*	*No. in group*
Sex			
Men	37.2	29.6	1110
Women	66.6	49.5	198
Age			
30-39 yr	29.3	25.0	73
40-49 yr	35.3	24.4	286
50-59 yr	40.4	31.9	547
60-69 yr	50.1	38.8	402
Taking antiarrhythmics			
Yes	53.5	42.0	192
No	39.6	30.2	1116
Race			
White	42.1	32.3	1167
Black	33.4	25.8	114
Asian	57.7	53.0	15
Other	56.3	27.5	12
Serum creatinine level			
≥Mean (1.01 mg/dl)	44.3	34.4	455
<Mean (1.01 mg/dl)	40.0	29.8	838
LDH level			
Elevated	43.7	33.2	923
Not elevated	37.4	28.7	329

LDH = Lactate dehydrogenase.

entire population of 1308 patients and for subgroups of this population. Differences in the means between subgroups were examined with an unpaired Z test on the mean of the natural log of the actual serum propranolol level. A $|Z|$ value ≥1.96 was used as the criterion to determine whether a patient characteristic correlated with serum propranolol level.

In a multivariate analysis, the natural log of the baseline serum propranolol level was regressed on those variables that were found to be univariately correlated with the serum propranolol level. A stepwise multiple linear regression model was used. Dichotomous variables were coded as "1,0" while continuous variables remained in their original units. Here also, a $|Z| \geq 1.96$ was used as the criterion to determine whether a patient characteristic independently correlated with serum propranolol level after adjustment for the other characteristics.

Because the patients were stratified by more than 50 variables and because so many of these subgroups are interrelated, the presentation of P values would have little meaning and may actually be misleading. Therefore, they will not be presented in this report.

RESULTS

The mean (±SD) trough serum propranolol level in 1308 patients with a recent myocardial infarction after steady-state oral doses of propranolol, 40 mg every 8 hours, was 41.6 ± 37.6 ng/ml (median = 31.7 ng/ml). A frequency distribution of serum propranolol levels is shown in Fig. 1. The skewness and wide variation of these values are evident from the figure. As many as 25% of the patients had quite low levels (<20 ng/ml), whereas 6% of the patients had quite high levels (>99 ng/ml). Values ranged from <10 to 415 ng/ml. The mean and distribution of the propranolol levels for inpatients and outpatients were similar (mean 41.0 and 42.9 ng/ml, respectively; Z = −0.94).

To examine the influence of biologic and demographic factors on these highly variable serum levels,

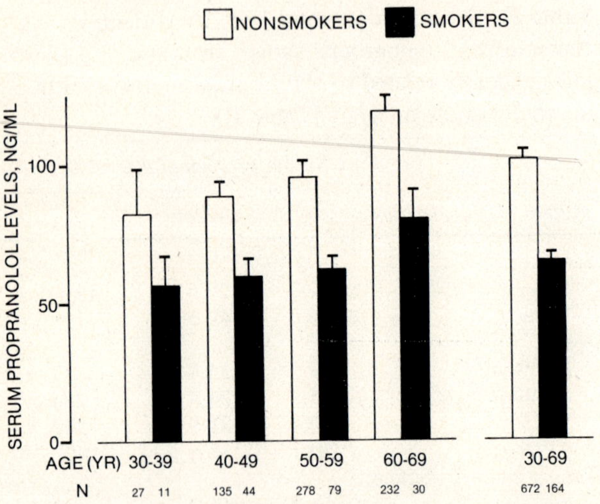

Fig. 2. Effects of smoking and age on serum propranolol levels in 836 patients at the 6-month visit: Mean (+SE) level of propranolol by age and smoking status. Data were restricted to those from patients given 60 mg propranolol three times a day. Blood samples were drawn at various times after the dose.

univariate and multivariate analyses were performed (Tables I and II). Of over 50 variables univariately examined, 19 were found to correlate univariately with the natural log of serum propranolol level. However, many of these variables were highly intercorrelated. Multivariate analysis, which included these 19 characteristics, indicated that the following six were independently related to higher serum propranolol levels after adjustment for the other characteristics (Table I): sex (female), age (older), use of antiarrhythmic drugs at entry, race (white), and elevated levels of serum creatinine and lactate dehydrogenase.

The mean and median serum propranolol levels for these six characteristics are listed in Table II. As noted in Table I, the most important biologic variable was sex. Univariately, the women had a mean level 79% higher than that for men (66.6 vs. 37.2 ng/ml). This difference was not dependent on a difference in weight (which was found not to be related even univariately to serum propranolol level). This is shown in Table III, which demonstrates 61% to 99% higher levels in women than in men at four different weight ranges. Moreover, when serum propranolol levels were examined with respect to body mass index (weight/height^2), the same sex difference was observed. There was also a significant increase in serum levels with age, from a mean of 29.3 ng/ml in the youngest group (30 to 39 years old) to 50.1 ng/ml (71% higher) in the oldest group (60 to 69 years old). This difference

Table III. Mean serum propranolol levels (ng/ml) by weight and sex

	Weight (lb)			
	101-130	*131-160*	*161-190*	*>190*
Men	41.2 (n = 37)	37.4 (n = 293)	37.3 (n = 488)	36.0 (n = 290)
Women	74.3 (n = 52)	60.1 (n = 74)	74.3 (n = 45)	61.4 (n = 24)

was also unrelated to the weight of the patients. Patients receiving concomitant therapy with other antiarrhythmic drugs had a higher mean serum propranolol level (53.5 ng/ml) than did those patients not taking antiarrhythmics (39.6 ng/ml). Also, race showed significant differences, with a lower mean level in blacks (33.4 ng/ml) than in whites (42.1 ng/ml). A tendency of higher levels in Asians (57.7 ng/ml) was noted, although the small sample of Asian patients prohibits firm conclusions. Finally, although elevated serum levels of creatinine and lactate dehydrogenase were significantly related to higher serum propranolol levels in the multivariate analysis (Table I), the magnitude of the univariate differences was very small (Table II).

Although smoking status at baseline had no independent effect on serum propranolol level in the multivariate analysis (Table I), nonsmokers univariately had a slightly higher serum propranolol level at baseline compared with cigarette smokers (43.8 vs. 40.0 ng/ml). Because it was believed that the smoking habits in the cigarette smokers during the initial hospitalization period were markedly reduced, the influence of smoking on serum propranolol levels was reanalyzed with respect to age in 836 patients at the 6-month visit (Fig. 2). The increased mean levels of propranolol with age (Table II) are still evident. In this outpatient setting there was now a more marked reduction (37%) in serum propranolol levels in smokers as compared with nonsmokers overall. Also, smokers had lower propranolol levels in each of the four age groups.

The combined effect of two patient characteristics that both lead to increased serum propranolol levels can, as expected, lead to greater differences between patients than either variable alone. This can be seen with regard to age and smoking at the 6-month visit in Fig. 2. Thus the nonsmoking older patients had a mean serum propranolol level that was more than double (119.0 ng/ml) the mean level in younger smoking patients (56.0 ng/ml). The combined effect of two patient characteristics is further emphasized in Table IV. Thus the older female patients had 125% higher levels (71.9 ng/ml) than the younger male patients (32.0 ng/ml), and the white patients taking antiarrhythmic drugs had 67% higher levels (53.9 ng/ml) than black patients receiving no antiarrhythmic drugs (32.1 ng/ml).

DISCUSSION

The most striking observation in the analysis of the serum propranolol levels in the BHAT study was the remarkably wide variation in these levels between patients, ranging from <10 to 415 ng/ml. This was seen despite the fact that all 1308 patients received an identical dose (40 mg every 8 hours) and had their blood samples drawn within a 2-hour period 7 to 9 hours after the last dose.

Before an attempt to examine the biologic determinants of this variability, it is important to discuss briefly other possible contributing factors. Obviously, of critical importance is adherence to the prescribed dosage regimen. As two thirds of the patients were hospitalized during this part of the study, adherence in this group must be judged as optimal. A lack of adherence could account for some of the very low levels, but could not explain the high levels observed in many patients. Furthermore, there was no statistical evidence that the distribution of propranolol levels in the inpatients and the outpatients differed. This would imply that if adherence was excellent in the hospitalized patients, it was comparable among the outpatients (who were following an identical protocol). Because serum levels will vary with time, blood sampling for all patients was done 7 to 9 hours (trough) after the previous dose. Also, blood samples were collected after at least six consecutive doses, a time that should be adequate for steady-state conditions to be reached.[18,72,80] Finally, the HPLC technique used to determine the serum levels was the same for all patients and was carried out by the BHAT Central Laboratory.[64] Possible interference from other drugs or from propranolol metabolites in this assay, leading to apparent higher propranolol levels, was adequately tested and does not seem to be a contributor.

The physiologic determinants of propranolol disposition have been thoroughly studied and reviewed by Wilkinson and Shand.[77] The most significant factor governing the plasma levels of propranolol after oral dosing is elimination by the liver before entry into the peripheral circulation. This depends on the ability of the liver to extract and metabolize the drug. Other factors that can contribute, although to a lesser extent, include the delivery of the drug to the liver (hepatic blood flow) and binding of the drug in the blood. Although several enzyme systems in the liver are involved in the metabolism of propranolol, the most important determinant of propranolol serum levels appears to be cytochrome P-450–mediated ring oxidation.[60,73] Thus the most important contributor to interindividual differences in propranolol serum levels appears to be differences in cytochrome P-450 activity.

Table IV. Mean serum propranolol levels (ng/ml) crosstabulated by selected baseline variables

(1) Age by sex

	Age (Yr)		
Sex	*30-49*	*50-59*	*60-69*
Men	32.0 (n = 326)	36.6 (n = 476)	43.5 (n = 308)
Women	53.8 (n = 33)	65.5 (n = 71)	71.9 (n = 94)

(2) Race by antiarrhythmic use

	*Race**	
Antiarrhythmic use	*Black*	*White*
Yes	46.2 (n = 11)	53.9 (n = 181)
No	32.1 (n = 103)	39.9 (n = 986)

*Asians and other races are not included in this table.

Analysis of the serum propranolol levels in individual patients with respect to biologic variables suggests several factors that contribute to the observed interindividual variations, some previously not noted (sex and race) and others previously demonstrated or suggested (age, smoking, and use of other drugs).

The finding of higher serum drug levels in women than in men has not previously been noted for any β-blocking drug, although data consistent with this observation can be deduced from a study of propranolol by Sotaniemi et al.[65] Sex differences in drug disposition, however, may be complicated by the use of oral contraceptives, which raise drug levels.[24,42,51] This does not appear to be a factor in the present study, in which the mean age of the female patients was 55 years. Also, differences in weight between women and men might have been expected to be a factor, but was not; weight was not even univariately related to the serum propranolol level. The influence of sex on drug metabolism in man has recently become of interest for several drugs. The clearance of some drugs including acetaminophen,[1] temazepam,[14] oxazepam,[28] lidocaine,[79] and several others[78] is clearly lower in women than in men, whereas there is no difference with other drugs such as phenytoin[13] and nitrazepam.[33] Such sex-related differences in the metabolism of propranolol and many other drugs are thought to be under androgen control[29,41] and may involve sex-specific cytochrome P-450 isoenzymes[36,43,76] as well as a sex-specific lipid environment.[5]

The observation that race may influence the disposition of propranolol also appears to be a novel observation for β-blocking drugs. Whereas the serum levels in blacks were significantly lower than those in whites, the levels in Asians tended to be higher. Although there are examples of differences in the disposition of drugs cleared mainly by oxidative metabolism between blacks and whites[7,25,81] and Asians and whites,[27,38,39,66] too little is known to rationalize any mechanism for our findings with propranolol. The influence of race on drug disposition appears to vary between drugs. Thus it has been shown that the clearance of antipyrine is lower in blacks than in whites,[7,25] which is in contrast to our findings with propranolol. Also, whereas the clearance of diazepam in Asians is lower than that in whites,[27] consistent with our observations for propranolol, the clearance of diphenhydramine is higher in Asians.[66] A greater deficiency in the oxidative metabolism of debrisoquin has been suggested in Asians as compared with whites.[38] It is clear that the mechanisms underlying ethnic differences in drug disposition are highly complex, presumably involving both genetic and environmental factors.[37]

The effect of age on the disposition of propranolol also appears complex and may be obscured by other factors, including smoking, although the multivariate analysis did suggest an independent effect for age. Higher serum levels of propranolol with increasing age, as observed in this study, have previously been noted in several investigations.[10,11,21] However, other studies[61,71] have not been able to demonstrate such an effect. It was suggested in one of these studies[71] that age has little or no influence on propranolol disposition per se, but that the effect of smoking, which leads to decreased propranolol levels,[21,26,71] was highly age related. Thus the increased clearance of propranolol in young smokers <35 years old was not observed in older smokers.[71] Our present data, however, clearly show that increasing age is associated with elevated serum propranolol levels in both smokers and nonsmokers (Fig. 2). Smoking per se had only a small absolute effect in our patients when hospitalized. This may likely be due to reduced smoking habits during this time. In contrast, there was a substantial reduction in propranolol levels in the smokers in all age groups at the 6-month visit (Fig. 2). Thus aging and smoking have opposite effects on propranolol disposition. Whereas the mechanism for the increasing propranolol levels with increasing age appears to be a combination of reduced cytochrome P-450 activity and hepatic blood flow,[10,71] the mechanism for the reduced propranolol levels in smokers appears to depend on induction of cytochrome P-450 activity.[35]

The observation that antiarrhythmic drugs increased the serum levels of propranolol is difficult to address specifically, since a number of drugs of this class were used. The most frequently used drug, quinidine, has in one recent study[30] been found to elevate propranolol levels by decreasing presystemic elimination, an observation consistent with our present findings. However, another study[23] showed no effect of quinidine on propranolol disposition. Although the finding of higher propranolol levels after the use of antiarrhythmic drugs does not have clear support in the literature, several other drugs are known to elevate propranolol levels by various mechanisms, including chlorpromazine,[70] hydralazine,[48] and cimetidine.[22,56]

Two factors not measured or controlled in the BHAT study are food intake and diet, both of which are known to alter propranolol levels. Thus when oral doses of propranolol are taken together with a high-protein meal, plasma levels increase significantly, presumably due to a transient increase in hepatic blood flow.[50] In contrast, chronic increases in the daily intake of protein and fat lead to reduced propranolol levels, whereas high-carbohydrate diets lead to elevated drug levels.[20] Similar observations have been made for other drugs.[3,40] These factors probably contribute to the large variations in propranolol levels in this study.

A factor not taken into consideration in our present evaluation of serum propranolol levels is serum binding. It is well known that levels of the main binding protein for propranolol, α_1-acid glycoprotein,[52,59] are elevated after a myocardial infarction,[4,34] as is the binding of propranolol.[58] Increased serum binding of propranolol would, however, not be expected to lead to major alterations in total serum levels of propranolol, as the hepatic elimination of propranolol is not restricted to the unbound fraction.[19]

Although a number of factors can influence the disposition of propranolol, each of these alone induces rather modest effects, leading to a maximum twofold variation in serum propranolol levels. The large interindividual variations in levels in our study are the result of many factors, as exemplified by the higher levels in older women compared with younger men or in white patients taking antiarrhythmic drugs compared with black patients receiving no antiarrhythmic drugs (Table IV).

The skewed frequency distribution of serum propranolol levels in Fig. 1, with very high levels in some patients, could also be due to a genetic deficiency in the metabolism of this drug, similar to what has been found in the oxidation of the antihypertensive drug debrisoquin[47,54,67] and the antiarrhythmic and oxytocic drug sparteine.[15,16] It has indeed been suggested that the oxidative metabolism of several β-blocking drugs, including metoprolol[2,46,62] and propranolol,[31,45,55,62] may be under the same genetic control as the oxidation of debrisoquin and sparteine. Based on the frequency of poor metabolizers of debrisoquin and sparteine,[15] 3% to 9% of poor metabolizers of propranolol would then have been expected among the BHAT patients. However, in this study there was no bimodal distribution of serum propranolol levels. A lack of bimodal distribution of plasma metoprolol levels has been used to argue against genetic polymorphism in the oxidative metabolism of this drug.[32] However, examination of the parent drug alone may result in significant overlapping between different genetic subgroups and may obscure bimodality in the frequency distribution. A better identification of a subgroup deficient in oxidation of propranolol as well as of other drugs should be based on metabolites or metabolic ratios rather than on measurements of parent drug alone. This was done in two recent studies.[45,55] In subjects who were poor metabolizers of debrisoquin, ring oxidation of propranolol appeared to be markedly suppressed. However, the plasma concentrations of propranolol were not elevated. This may be explained by the observation that the oral clearance of propranolol to 60% is dependent on other pathways than ring oxidation.[75] Further studies are clearly needed to answer the question about the importance of genetic polymorphism and propranolol disposition.

In summary, the great interindividual variation in the disposition of propranolol we observed depends on a combination of factors, including sex, race, age, smoking, and other drugs, probably also including diet. An additional factor may be genetic differences in oxidative metabolism not related to either sex or race. Although the BHAT was a seemingly well-controlled study, the analyses presented are post-hoc analyses and based only on a single determination of the serum propranolol level. As emphasized by Vesell and Penno,[69] it will be critically important to validate the present findings by a carefully controlled prospective study. The potential clinical significance of such marked variations in serum propranolol levels on outcome variables is currently being evaluated in the BHAT and a separate report is in preparation.

Study group investigators

Clinical centers

Baylor College of Medicine, Houston, Tex.
Craig M. Pratt, M.D., Principal Investigator
Boston University School of Medicine, Boston, Mass.
Pantel S. Vokonas, M.D., Principal Investigator
Brown University Affiliated Hospitals, Providence, R. I.
Robert J. Capone, M.D., Principal Investigator
Emory University, Atlanta, Ga.
Robert C. Schlant, M.D., Principal Investigator
Evanston Hospital, Evanston, Ill.
Gary N. Wilner, M.D., Principal Investigator
Geisinger Medical Center, Danville, Pa.
Charles A. Laubach, M.D., Principal Investigator
Greater Baltimore Medical Center, Baltimore, Md.
Thaddeus E. Prout, M.D., Principal Investigator
Henry Ford Hospital, Detroit, Mich.
Gerald M. Breneman, M.D., Principal Investigator
Kaiser Foundation Hospital, Portland, Ore.
John A. Grover, M.D., Principal Investigator
Lankenau Hospital, Philadelphia, Pa.
William L. Holmes, Ph.D., Principal Investigator
Long Island Jewish-Hillside Medical Center, New Hyde Park, N. Y.
Kul D. Chadda, M.D., Principal Investigator
Maimonides Medical Center, Brooklyn, N. Y.
Edgar Lichstein, M.D., Principal Investigator
Medical University of South Carolina, Charleston, S. C.
Peter C. Gazes, M.D., Principal Investigator
Medical College of Virginia, Richmond, Va.
David W. Richardson, M.D., Principal Investigator
Miami Heart Institute, Miami, Fla.
Frank L. Canosa, M.D., Principal Investigator
Montreal Heart Institute, Montreal, Quebec, Canada
Pierre A. Théroux, M.D., Principal Investigator
Mt. Sinai Hospital, Minneapolis, Minn.
Phillip J. Ranheim, M.D., Principal Investigator
Northwestern University Medical School, Chicago, Ill.
Olga M. Haring, M.D., Principal Investigator
Ogden Research Foundation, Ogden, Utah
C. Basil Williams, M.D., Principal Investigator
Overlook Hospital, Summit, N. J.
John J. Gregory, M.D., Principal Investigator
Pacific Health Research Institute, Honolulu, Hawaii
J. Judson McNamara, M.D., Principal Investigator
Providence Medical Center, Portland, Ore.
Gordon L. Maurice, M.D., Principal Investigator
Rush Presbyterian St. Lukes Medical Center, Chicago, Ill.
James A. Schoenberger, M.D., Principal Investigator
Rutgers Medical School Raritan Valley Hospital, New Brunswick, N. J.
Peter T. Kuo, M.D., Principal Investigator
Salt Lake Clinic Research Foundation, Salt Lake City, Utah
Allan H. Barker, M.D., Principal Investigator

State University of New York at Buffalo, Buffalo, N. Y.
Robert M. Kohn, M.D., Principal Investigator
University of California, Davis, Davis, Calif.
Nemat O. Borhani, M.D., Principal Investigator
University of California, San Francisco, San Francisco, Calif.
Mary Anne Warnowicz, D.O., Principal Investigator
University of Rochester School of Medicine, Rochester, N. Y.
Paul N. Yu, M.D., Principal Investigator
University of Southern California, Los Angeles, Los Angeles, Calif.
L. Julian Haywood, M.D., Principal Investigator
Veterans Administration Hospital, Little Rock, Ark.
Marvin L. Murphy, M.D., Principal Investigator
Veterans Administration Hospital, West Roxbury, Mass.
Kevin M. McIntyre, M.D., Principal Investigator

Coordinating Center
University of Texas, Houston, Tex.
C. Morton Hawkins, Sc.D., Director, Principal Investigator
J. David Curb, M.D., M.P.H.
Robert P. Byington, Ph.D.

Drug Distribution Center
Department of Health and Human Services, United States Public Health Service, Perry Point, Md.
James Grigdesby
Sydney H. Hamet
Patricia Murphy

ECG Reading Center
University of Minnesota, Minneapolis, Minn.
Richard S. Crow, M.D., Principal Investigator

24-hour Holter Ambulatory ECG Center
Anthropometrics Heart Clinic, Haddonfield, N. J.
Joel Morganroth, M.D., Principal Investigator

Central Laboratory
Bio-Science Laboratories, Van Nuys, Calif.
Frank Ibbott, Ph.D., Principal Investigator

National Heart, Lung, and Blood Institute
National Heart, Lung, and Blood Institute, Bethesda, Md.
Curt Furberg, M.D., Project Officer
Lawrence M. Friedman, M.D.
William T. Friedewald, M.D.

Steering Committee
Sidney Goldstein, M.D., Chairman

Policy/Data Monitoring Board
John Naughton, M.D., Chairman

References

1. Abernethy DR, Divoll M, Greenblatt DJ, Ameer B: Obesity, sex, and acetaminophen disposition. CLIN PHARMACOL THER **31:**783-790, 1982.
2. Alván F, von Bahr C, Seideman P, Sjöqvist F: High plasma concentrations of β-receptor blocking drugs and deficient debrisoquine hydroxylation. Lancet **1:**333, 1982.
3. Anderson DE, Conney AH, Kappas A: Nutrition and oxidative drug metabolism in man: Relative influence of dietary lipids, carbohydrate and protein. CLIN PHARMACOL THER **26:**493-501, 1979.
4. Bachmann GW, Weiss ME, Rapp W: Differenzierte quantitative Serumeiweissbestimmungen im Ablauf des Herzinfaktes. Schweiz W Med Wochenschr **98:**1825-1829, 1968.
5. Barr J, Skett P: The role of cytochrome P-450, NADPH-cytochrome P-450 reductase and lipids in sex differences in hepatic drug metabolism. Br J Pharmacol **83:**396P, 1984.
6. Beta-Blocker Heart Attack Trial Research Group: A randomized trial of propranolol in patients with acute myocardial infarction. I. Mortality results. JAMA **247:**1707-1714, 1982.
7. Branch RA, Salih SY, Homeida M: Racial differences in drug metabolizing ability: A study with antipyrine in the Sudan. CLIN PHARMACOL THER **24:**283-286, 1978.
8. Briggs WA, Lowenthal DT, Cirksena WJ, Price WE, Gibson TP, Flamenbaum W: Propranolol in hypertensive dialysis patients: Efficacy and compliance. CLIN PHARMACOL THER **18:**606-612, 1975.
9. Byington RP, Beta-Blocker Heart Attack Trial Research Group: Beta-Blocker Heart Attack Trial—Design, Methods, and Baseline Results. Cont Clin Trial **5:**382-437, 1984.
10. Castleden CM, George CF: The effect of aging on the hepatic clearance of propranolol. Br J Clin Pharmacol **7:**49-54, 1979.
11. Castleden CM, Kaye CM, Parsons RL: The effect of age on plasma levels of propranolol and practolol in man. Br J Clin Pharmacol **2:**303-306, 1975.
12. Chidsey CA, Morselli P, Bianchetti G, Morganti A, Leonetti G, Zanchetti A: Studies of the absorption and removal of propranolol in hypertensive patients during therapy. Circulation **52:**313-318, 1975.
13. De Leacy EA, McLeay CD, Eadie MJ, Tyrer JH: Effects of subjects' sex, and intake of tobacco, alcohol and oral contraceptives on plasma phenytoin levels. Br J Clin Pharmacol **8:**33-36, 1979.
14. Divoll M, Greenblatt DJ, Harmatz JS, Shader RI: Effect of age and gender on disposition of temazepam. J Pharm Sci **70:**1104-1107, 1981.
15. Eichelbaum M: Defective oxidation of drugs. Pharmacokinetic and therapeutic implications. Clin Pharmacokinet **7:**1-22, 1982.
16. Eichelbaum M, Spannbrucker N, Steincke B, Dengler HJ: Defective *N*-oxidation of sparteine in man. A new pharmacogenetic effect. Eur J Clin Pharmacol **16:**183-187, 1979.
17. Esler M, Zweifler A, Randall O, DeQuattro V: Pathophysiologic and pharmacokinetic determinants of the an-

tihypertensive response to propranolol. CLIN PHARMACOL THER **22**:299-308, 1977.
18. Evans GH, Shand DG: Disposition of propranolol. V. Drug accumulation and steady-state concentrations during chronic oral administration in man. CLIN PHARMACOL THER **14**:487-493, 1973.
19. Evans GH, Shand DG: Disposition of propranolol. VI. Independent variation in steady-state circulating drug concentrations and half-life as a result of plasma drug binding in man. CLIN PHARMACOL THER **14**:494-500, 1973.
20. Fagan TC, Walle T, Oexmann M-J, Walle UK, Bai SA: Long-term effects of high protein, high carbohydrate and high fat diets on the disposition of propranolol in man. Presented at the Second World Conference on Clinical Pharmacology and Therapeutics, Washington, DC, July 30-Aug. 5, 1983. (Abst. No. 23.)
21. Feely J, Crooks J, Stevenson IH: The influence of age, smoking and hyperthyroidism on plasma propranolol steady state concentration. Br J Clin Pharmacol **12**:73-78, 1981.
22. Feely J, Wilkinson GR, Wood AJJ: Reduction of liver blood flow and propranolol metabolism by cimetidine. N Engl J Med **304**:692-695, 1981.
23. Fenster P, Perrier D, Mayersohn M, Marcus FI: Kinetic evaluation of the propranolol-quinidine combination. CLIN PHARMACOL THER **27**:450-453, 1980.
24. Field B, Lu C, Hepner GW: Inhibition of hepatic drug metabolism by norethindrone. CLIN PHARMACOL THER **25**:196-198, 1979.
25. Fraser HS, Bulpitt CJ, Kahn C, Mould G, Mucklow JC, Dollery CT: Factors affecting antipyrine metabolism in West African villagers. CLIN PHARMACOL THER **20**:369-376, 1976.
26. Gardner SK, Cady WJ, Ong YS: Effect of smoking on the elimination of propranolol hydrochloride. Int J Clin Pharmacol Ther Toxicol **18**:421-424, 1980.
27. Ghoneim MM, Korttila K, Chiang C-K, Jacobs L, Schoenwald RD, Mewaldt SP, Kayaba K-O: Diazepam effects and kinetics in Caucasians and Orientals. CLIN PHARMACOL THER **29**:749-756, 1981.
28. Greenblatt DJ, Divoll M, Harmatz JS, Shader RI: Oxazepam kinetics: Effects of age and sex. J Pharmacol Exp Ther **215**:86-91, 1980.
29. Gustafsson J-Å, Mode A, Norstedt G, Skett P: Sex steroid induced changes in hepatic enzymes. Ann Rev Physiol **45**:51-60, 1983.
30. Hori R, Okumura K, Yasuhara M, Yatsuzuka A, Kawai C, Sakurai T: Alteration of propranolol pharmacokinetics by quinidine in man and rat. Presented at the Second World Conference on Clinical Pharmacology and Therapeutics, Washington, DC, July 30-Aug. 5, 1983. (Abst. No. 624.)
31. Inaba T, Nakano M, Otton SV, Mahon WA, Kalow W: A human cytochrome P-450 characterized by inhibition studies as the sparteine-debrisoquine monoxygenase. Rapid Commun **62**:860-862, 1984.
32. Jack DB, Wilkins M, Quarterman CP: Lack of evidence for polymorphism in metoprolol metabolism. Br J Clin Pharmacol **16**:188-190, 1983.
33. Jochemsen R, Van der Graaff M, Boeijinga JK, Breimer DD: Influence of sex, menstrual cycle and oral contraception on the disposition of nitrazepam. Br J Clin Pharmacol **13**:319-324, 1982.
34. Johansson BG, Kindmark CO, Trell EY, Wollheim FA: Sequential changes of plasma proteins after myocardial infarction. Scand J Clin Lab Invest **29**(suppl 124):117-126, 1972.
35. Jusko WJ: Role of tobacco smoking in pharmacokinetics. J Pharmacokinet Biopharm **6**:7-39, 1978.
36. Kamataki T, Maeda K, Yamazoe Y, Nagai T, Kato R: Sex difference of cytochrome P-450 in the rat: Purification, characterization and quantitation of constitutive forms of cytochrome P-450 from liver microsomes of male and female rats. Arch Biochem Biophys **225**:758-770, 1983.
37. Kalow W: Ethnic differences in drug metabolism. Clin Pharmacokinct **7**:373-400, 1982.
38. Kalow W, Otton SV, Kadar D, Endrenyi L, Inaba T: Ethnic differences in drug metabolism. Debrisoquine 4-hydroxylation in caucasians and orientals. Can J Physiol Pharmacol **58**:1142-1144, 1980.
39. Kalow W, Tang BK, Kadar D, Endrenyi L, Chan F-Y: A method for studying drug metabolism in populations: Racial differences in amobarbital metabolism. CLIN PHARMACOL THER **26**:766-776, 1979.
40. Kappas A, Anderson KE, Conney AH, Alvares AP: Influence of dietary protein and carbohydrate on antipyrine and theophylline metabolism in man. CLIN PHARMACOL THER **20**:643-653, 1976.
41. Kato R. Sex-related differences in drug metabolism. Drug Metab Rev **3**:1-32, 1974.
42. Kendall MJ, Quarterman CP, Jack DB, Beeley L: Metoprolol pharmacokinetics and the oral contraceptive pill. Br J Clin Pharmacol **14**:120-122, 1982.
43. Larrey D, Distlerath LM, Dannan GA, Wilkinson GR, Guengerich FP: Purification and characterization of the rat liver microsomal cytochrome P-450 involved in the 4-hydroxylation of debrisoquine, a prototype for genetic variation in oxidative drug metabolism. Biochemistry **23**:2787-2795, 1984.
44. Lehtonen A, Kanto J, Kleimola T: Plasma concentrations of propranolol in patients with essential hypertension. Eur J Clin Pharmacol **11**:155-157, 1977.
45. Lennard MS, Jackson PR, Freestone S, Tucker GT, Ramsay LE, Woods HF: The relationship between debrisoquine oxidation phenotype and the pharmacokinetics and pharmacodynamics of propranolol. Br J Clin Pharmacol **17**:679-685, 1984.
46. Lennard MS, Silas JH, Freestone S, Trevethick J: Defective metabolism of metoprolol in poor hydroxylators of debrisoquine. Br J Clin Pharmacol **14**: 301-303, 1982.
47. Mahgoub A, Idle JR, Dring LG, Lancaster R, Smith RL:

Polymorphic hydroxylation of debrisoquine in man. Lancet **2**:584-586, 1977.

48. McLean AJ, Skews H, Bobik A, Dudley FJ: Interaction between oral propranolol and hydralazine. CLIN PHARMACOL THER **27**:726-732, 1980.
49. Melander A, Danielson K, Scherstén B, Wåhlin E: Enhancement of the bioavailability of propranolol and metoprolol by food. CLIN PHARMACOL THER **22**:108-112, 1977.
50. Melander A, McLean A: Influence of food intake on presystemic clearance of drugs. Clin Pharmacokinet **8**:286-296, 1983.
51. O'Malley K, Stevenson IH, Crooks J: Impairment of human drug metabolism by oral contraceptive steroids. CLIN PHARMACOL THER **13**:552-557, 1972.
52. Piafsky KM, Borgå O, Odar-Cederlöf I, Johansson C, Sjöqvist F: Increased plasma protein binding of propranolol and chlorpromazine mediated by disease-induced elevations of plasma α_1 acid glycoprotein. N Engl J Med **299**:1435-1439, 1978.
53. Pine M, Favrot L, Smith S, McDonald K, Chidsey CA: Correlation of plasma propranolol concentration with therapeutic response in patients with angina pectoris. Circulation **52**:886-893, 1975.
54. Price Evans DA, Mahgoub A, Sloan TP, Idle JR, Smith RL: A family and population study of the genetic polymorphism of debrisoquine oxidation in a white British population. J Med Genet **17**:102-105, 1980.
55. Raghuram TC, Koshakji RP, Wilkinson GR, Wood AJJ: Polymorphic ability to metabolize propranolol alters 4-hydroxypropranolol levels but not beta blockade. CLIN PHARMACOL THER **36**:51-56, 1984.
56. Reimann IW, Klotz U, Siems B, Frölich JC: Cimetidine increases steady state plasma levels of propranolol. Br J Clin Pharmacol **12**:785-790, 1981.
57. Routledge PA, Shand DG: Clinical pharmacokinetics of propranolol. Clin Pharmacokinet **4**:73-90, 1979.
58. Routledge PA, Stargel WW, Wagner GS, Shand DG: Increased plasma propranolol binding in myocardial infarction. Br J Clin Pharmacol **9**:438-440, 1980.
59. Sager G, Nilsen OG, Jacobsen S: Variable binding of propranolol in human serum. Biochem Pharmacol **28**:905-911, 1979.
60. Schneck DW, Pritchard JF: The inhibitory effect of propranolol pretreatment on its own metabolism in the rat. J Pharmacol Exp Ther **218**:575-581, 1981.
61. Schneider RE, Bishop H, Yates RA, Quarterman CP, Kendall MJ: Effect of age on plasma propranolol levels. Br J Clin Pharmacol **10**:169-171, 1980.
62. Shah RR, Oates NS, Idle JR, Smith RL: Beta-blockers and drug oxidation status. Lancet **1**:508-509, 1982.
63. Shand DG: Individualization of propranolol therapy. Med Clin North Am **58**:1063-1069, 1974.
64. Simon M, Terry R: Propranolol in serum by high pressure liquid chromatography using nitrile (CN) bonded columns in reverse phase. Ther Drug Monitor **1**:265-276, 1979.
65. Sotaniemi EA, Anttila M, Pelkonen RO, Järvensivu P, Sundquist H: Plasma clearance of propranolol and sotalol and hepatic drug-metabolizing enzyme activity. CLIN PHARMACOL THER **26**:153-161, 1979.
66. Spector R, Choudhury AK, Chiang C-K, Goldberg MJ, Ghoneim MM: Diphenhydramine in Orientals and Caucasians. CLIN PHARMACOL THER **28**:229-234, 1980.
67. Tucker GT, Silas JH, Iyun AO, Lennard MS, Smith AJ: Polymorphic hydroxylation of debrisoquine. Lancet **2**:718, 1977.
68. Vervloet E, Pluym BFM, Cilissen J, Köhlen K, Merkus FWHM: Propranolol serum levels during twenty-four hours. CLIN PHARMACOL THER **22**:853-857, 1977.
69. Vesell ES, Penno MB: Assessment of methods to identify sources of interindividual pharmacokinetic variations. Clin Pharmacokinet **8**:378-409, 1983.
70. Vestal RE, Kornhauser DM, Hollifield JW, Shand DG: Inhibition of propranolol metabolism by chlorpromazine. CLIN PHARMACOL THER **25**:19-24, 1979.
71. Vestal RE, Wood AJJ, Branch RA, Shand DG, Wilkinson GR: Effects of age and cigarette smoking on propranolol disposition. CLIN PHARMACOL THER **26**:8-15, 1979.
72. Walle T, Conradi EC, Walle UK, Fagan TC, Gaffney TE: The predictable relationship between plasma levels and dose during chronic propranolol therapy. CLIN PHARMACOL THER **24**:668-677, 1978.
73. Walle T, Conradi EC, Walle UK, Fagan TC, Gaffney TE: 4-Hydroxypropranolol and its glucuronide after single and long-term doses of propranolol. CLIN PHARMACOL THER **27**:23-31, 1980.
74. Walle T, Morrison J, Walle UK, Conradi EC: Simultaneous determination of propranolol and 4-hydroxypropranolol in plasma by mass fragmentography. J Chromatogr **114**:351-359, 1975.
75. Walle T, Walle UK, Olanoff LS: Quantitative account of propranolol metabolism in urine of normal man. Drug Metab Dispos **13**:204-209, 1985.
76. Waxman DJ: Rat hepatic cytochrome P-450 isoenzyme 2c. J Biol Chem **259**:15481-15490, 1984.
77. Wilkinson GR, Shand DG: A physiological approach to hepatic drug clearance. CLIN PHARMACOL THER **18**:377-389, 1975.
78. Wilson K: Sex-related differences in drug disposition in man. Clin Pharmacokinet **9**:189-202, 1984.
79. Wing LMH, Miners JO, Birkett DJ, Foenander T, Lillywhite K, Wanwimolruk S: Lidocaine disposition—Sex differences and effects of cimetidine. CLIN PHARMACOL THER **35**:695-701, 1984.
80. Wood AJJ, Carr K, Vestal RE, Belcher S, Wilkinson GR, Shand DG: Direct measurement of propranolol bioavailability during accumulation to steady-state. Br J Clin Pharmacol **6**:345-350, 1978.
81. Woolhouse NM, Andoh B, Mahgoub A, Sloan TP, Idle JR, Smith RL: Debrisoquine hydroxylation polymorphism among Ghanaians and Caucasians. CLIN PHARMACOL THER **26**:584-591, 1979.

Pharmacologic reduction of sympathetic drive increases platelet alpha-2–receptor number

Several lines of evidence implicate sympathetic nervous system involvement in the pathophysiology of essential hypertension in man. Extrapolations are frequently made from in vitro measurements of plasma catecholamine levels to the physiologic role of the sympathetic system in hypertension. We assessed the utility and validity of such extrapolation from in vitro to in vivo measures of adrenergic function. Addition of guanadrel to diuretic therapy in 11 patients with essential hypertension reduced supine intra-arterial blood pressure from 135 ± 14/76 ± 9 to 127 ± 13/67 ± 5 mm Hg ($P < 0.02$). Supine heart rate was also reduced, from 77 ± 14 to 63 ± 13 bpm ($P < 0.001$). Plasma norepinephrine levels fell from 303 ± 107 to 170 ± 46 pg/ml ($P < 0.01$). Platelet α_2-receptor number ([^{3}H]yohimbine maximal binding) increased from 204 ± 77 to 301 ± 150 fmol/mg ($P < 0.02$). The pupillary mydriatic response to phenylephrine and the forearm arterial vasoconstrictor response to intra-arterial norepinephrine did not change. Thus guanadrel reduced blood pressure by decreasing sympathetic tone. In this milieu of low sympathetic activity the platelet α_2-receptor number increased, but physiologic responses to exogenous α-agonists did not change. Caution is therefore advised when extrapolating from in vitro measurement of plasma catecholamine levels and platelet α_2-receptor number to the in vivo physiologic significance.
(Clin Pharmacol Ther 1985;38:519-24.)

Brent Egan, M.D., Richard Neubig, M.D., Ph.D.* and Stevo Julius, M.D., Sc.D.
Ann Arbor, Mich.

A number of investigators have identified an important pathophysiologic role for the sympathetic nervous system in essential hypertension in man. Studies in our laboratory showed a crucial role for the adrenergic system in maintaining the elevated cardiac output and heart rate in borderline hypertension.[1] Despite normal cardiac output, patients with elevated plasma renin activity and either borderline or mild hypertension maintained a higher blood pressure through increased neurogenic vasoconstriction.[2,3] Other investigators reported increased pressor responsiveness to exogenous norepinephrine, but normal responses to angiotensin, in both borderline and established essential hypertension.[4,5] Studies evaluating local vascular responses also showed a similar heightened sensitivity to both exogenous and endogenous norepinephrine.[6,7]

Because of the potential importance of the adrenergic system in essential hypertension, methods for precise evaluation of sympathetic function would be useful. Plasma catecholamine levels are the most frequently measured index of sympathetic activity. Physiologic significance is then often extrapolated from measured catecholamine levels. We wished to evaluate the validity of extrapolating from the in vitro to the in vivo adrenergic environment. In this study, guanadrel sulfate (Hylorel; Pennwalt Pharmaceuticals), which inhibits noradrenaline storage in and release from the sympathetic nerve terminal, was added to diuretic monotherapy in patients with essential hypertension.[8] With this altered adrenergic environment we wanted to answer the following questions: (a) Would plasma catecholamine levels (a frequent index of sympathetic drive) fall during guanadrel therapy? (b) Would platelet α_2-receptor number change during therapy with a drug that reduces sympathetic drive? (c) Would sensitivity to exogenous catecholamines increase? (d) Would in vitro measures of sympathetic function (plasma catecholamines and

From the Division of Hypertension, Department of Internal Medicine, University of Michigan Medical Center.
Supported by Grant No. 1K08 HLO 1353 from the National Institutes of Health, by Grant No. 84-522-J1 from the American Heart Association (Michigan affiliate), and by Pennwalt Pharmaceuticals.
Received for publication March 25, 1985; accepted June 18, 1985.
Reprint requests to: Brent Egan, M.D., Division of Hypertension, R6669 Kresge Medical Research Bldg. #1, University of Michigan Medical Center, Ann Arbor, MI 48109-0010.
*Recipient of a Hartford Foundation Fellowship.

Table I. Comparison of supine baseline* hemodynamic and biochemical data before and after addition of guanadrel to diuretic monotherapy

	Study 1	*Study 2*	*P value*
HR (bpm)	77 ± 14	63 ± 13	<0.001
SBP (mm Hg)	135 ± 14	127 ± 13	<0.02
DBP (mm Hg)	76 ± 9	67 ± 5	<0.001
FABF (ml/100 ml forearm volume/min)	4.7 ± 2.2	4.3 ± 1.6	0.71
Plasma NE (pg/ml)	303 ± 107	170 ± 46	<0.01
Plasma E (pg/ml)	79 ± 25	60 ± 24	0.07
PRA (ng AI/ml/hr)	5.8 ± 3.9	4.6 ± 3.3	0.20
Platelet α_2-receptors (fmol/mg)	204 ± 77	301 ± 150	<0.02

HR = Heart rate; SBP = intra-arterial systolic blood pressure; DBP = intra-arterial diastolic blood pressure; FABF = forearm blood flow; NE = norepinephrine; E = epinephrine; PRA = plasma renin activity; AI = angiotensin I.
*After 30 minutes of rest.

platelet α_2-receptors) correlate with in vivo measurements of α-adrenergic physiologic responses in the forearm and pupil?

METHODS

Subjects. Eleven white patients (10 men and one woman) between 28 and 50 years old ($\bar{X} \pm SD$ = 36 ± 6 years) who were receiving diuretic monotherapy with suboptimally controlled casual blood pressure (>140 mm Hg systolic or >90 diastolic mm Hg in the office or >130 systolic or >85 diastolic at home) were enrolled. Subjects underwent complete history, physical, and routine laboratory examinations before entry into the study. All were healthy except for mild hypertension. They signed a written, informed consent form approved by the Hospital Committee for Human Research.

Study design. The guanadrel study was an open-label, nonrandomized evaluation of physiologic and biochemical variables before and again 3 weeks after the start of guanadrel sulfate therapy. After the first study, guanadrel was begun at 5 mg twice a day for the first 5 to 7 days. If blood pressures measured at home had not fallen to <130/85 mm Hg or by 10 mm Hg, the dosage was increased to 10 mg twice a day. Eight subjects achieved the target blood pressure level with guanadrel, 10 mg/day, in addition to their diuretic. Of the three remaining subjects, one received guanadrel, 5 mg twice a day, another took 15 mg twice a day, and a third took 30 mg twice a day. Subjects received the final dose of guanadrel 3 hours before each physiologic study.

Measurements. Blood pressure was measured first by mercury and cuff sphygmomanometry and subsequently in intra-arterial recordings.

Forearm blood flow was measured by venous occlusion, strain gauge plethysmography. The D. E. Hokanson, Inc. EC-3 plethysmograph and E-10 rapid cuff inflator were connected to the polygraph and recorder as described below.

The method for pupillary measurement has been described in detail.[9] In brief, pupil size was recorded with a binocular pupillograph for 30 seconds under standardized lighting conditions. Thirty measurements of pupil size during the final 3 seconds were averaged both before and 1 hour after phenylephrine dosing. The increase in size of the right pupil (1% phenylephrine was always instilled into the right eye) minus the change in the size of the control (left) pupil equalled the mydriatic response to 1% phenylephrine at 1 hour.

Plasma catecholamine[10] and plasma renin activity[11] assays were performed as previously described. To determine platelet membrane preparation and [^{3}H]yohimbine binding, 50 ml venous blood was immediately mixed with 1/9 volume of ACD (0.8 gm citric acid, 2.2 gm trisodium citrate, and 2.45 gm dextrose per 100 ml). After centrifugation for 7 minutes at 200 × g, the platelet-rich plasma was adjusted to pH 6.5 and centrifuged for 15 minutes at 2000 × g. The platelet pellet was resuspended in buffer (150 mmol/L NaCl, 1 mmol/L EDTA, and 20 mmol/L TrisCl at pH 7.6) and centrifuged again. The pellet was suspended in 10 ml homogenization buffer (10 mmol/L TrisCl at pH 7.6, 5 mmol/L EDTA, and 0.25 mol sucrose) and homogenized with five strokes of a "zero-clearance" homogenizer (Model K886030; Kontes Co.). The membrane fraction was collected by centrifugation for 20 minutes at 43,000 × g. The pellet was resuspended in 10 ml TME buffer (50 mmol/L TrisCl at pH 7.6, 10 mmol/L $MgCl_2$, and 1 mmol/L EGTA), then washed three times by pelleting and resuspending in TME buffer. [^{3}H]Yohimbine binding (1 to 20 nmol/L) was measured in triplicate as described.[12] Nonspecific binding was determined in the presence of 10^{-5} mol/L yohimbine. Scatchard plots of specific [^{3}H]yohimbine binding were prepared and maximum binding (B_{max}) and affinity (K_d) values were determined from linear least-squares fit of the data.

Protocol. Subjects came to the laboratory at 8 AM. Height, weight, baseline pupil size, and forearm volume were measured. Plastic catheters were placed in the left brachial artery and an adjacent vein. After 30 minutes of supine rest, venous blood for plasma catecholamine, plasma renin activity, and platelet α_2 receptor determinations was drawn. Arterial pressures

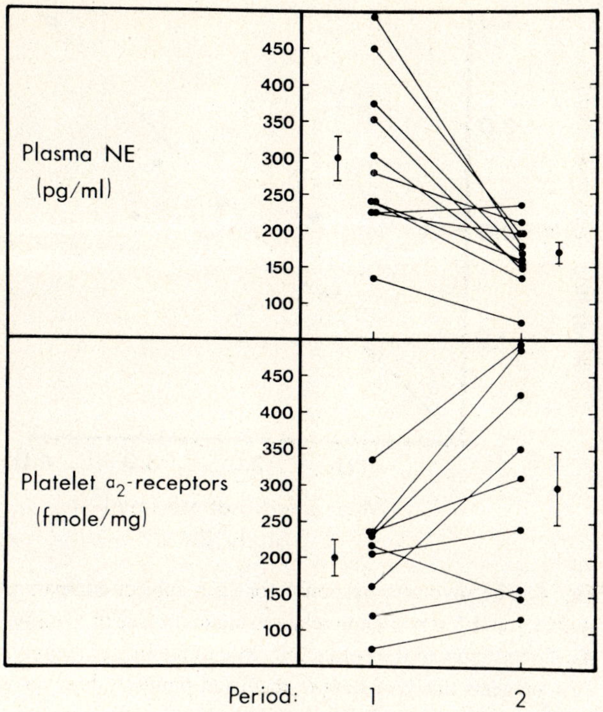

Fig. 1. Mean ($\pm$SE) and individual paired plasma norepinephrine *(NE)* and platelet α_2-receptor values ([^{3}H]yohimbine B_{max}) are shown for subjects in study 1 (diuretics) and study 1 (diuretic and guanadrel). Both the decrease in plasma norepinephrine level and the increase in platelet α_2-receptors were significant at $P < 0.05$.

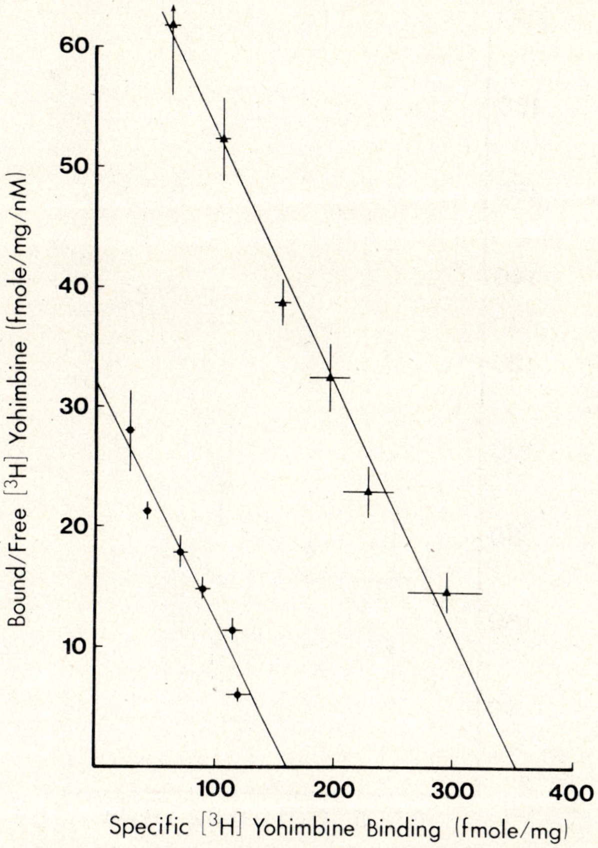

Fig. 2. Scatchard plot in one subject of [^{3}H]yohimbine binding to platelet membranes during the first study (diuretic alone; ●) and the second study (diuretic with guanadrel; ▲). The B_{max} (x-intercept) increased during guanadrel therapy from 160 to 353 fmol/mg protein, while the K_d (affinity = slope) did not change.

were monitored and measured by connecting the brachial cannula to a Hewlett-Packard Co. quartz transducer (1290 A), polygraph (4568 C), and oscilloscope (1308 A) and a Gould Inc. thermal recorder (TA 600).

After baseline supine measurements, a random order infusion of norepinephrine into the brachial artery was started at 0.005, 0.01, 0.02, 0.04, and 0.08 μg per 100 ml forearm volume per minute. Each norepinephrine infusion lasted 4 minutes and was followed by an 11-minute infusion of saline solution. Arterial pressure and forearm blood flow were measured during the last minute of each norepinephrine infusion and at each baseline saline solution infusion period. One hour before the completion of the hemodynamic measurements, 40 μl 1% phenylephrine was instilled into the lower conjunctival sac of the right eye. The study ended with recording of pupil size.

Statistical analysis. Data are reported as the $\overline{X} \pm$ SD. Comparisons of variables between the two studies were made by the paired t test. Statistical significance was defined by a P value <0.05.

RESULTS

In our 11 subjects, casual blood pressure at the first visit was 138 $\pm$ 13/89 $\pm$ 7 mm Hg, height was 180 $\pm$ 7 cm, and weight was 210 $\pm$ 37 lb. Values for heart rate, intra-arterial blood pressure, forearm blood flow, plasma catecholamine levels, plasma renin activity, and platelet α_2-receptors after 30 minutes supine rest are listed in Table I. Addition of guanadrel lowered supine heart rate and intra-arterial systolic and diastolic pressures. Forearm blood flow did not change, and plasma norepinephrine levels were reduced. Although plasma renin activity and plasma epinephrine levels tended to fall, the differences were not statistically significant.

Platelet α_2-receptor number increased as determined by Scatchard plots of [^{3}H]yohimbine binding. Because two specimens were lost, complete data on platelet α_2-

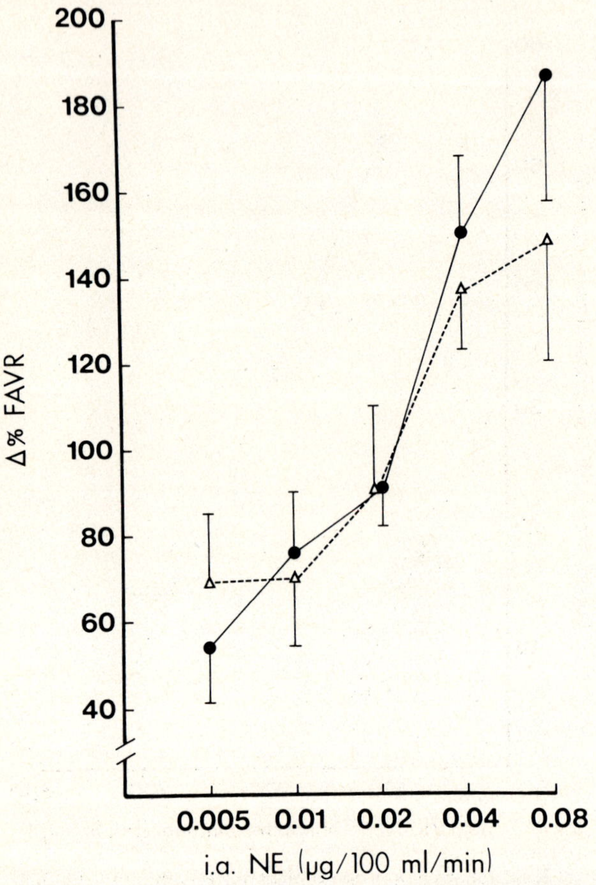

Fig. 3. Group $\overline{X} \pm$ SE of the percentage increase in forearm vascular resistance *(Δ% FAVR)* in response to five doses of intra-arterial norepinephrine *(i.a. NE)* given in random sequence in study 1 (diuretics; △) and study 2 (diuretic with guanadrel; ●). No significant differences were noted at any point on the dose-response curves when the two studies were compared.

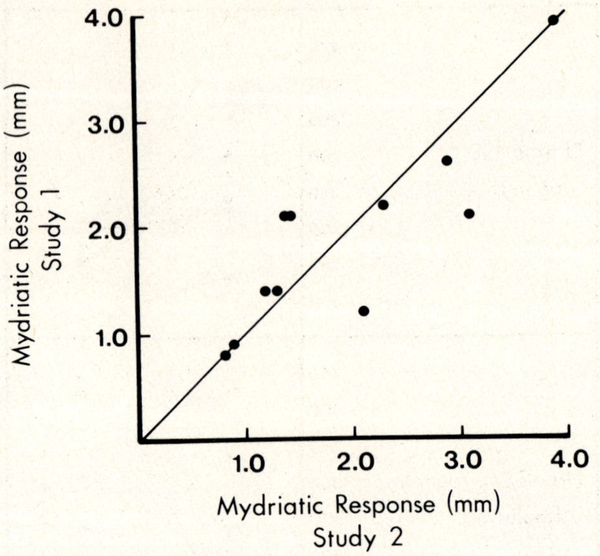

Fig. 4. The mydriatic response for each subject comparing studies 1 and 2 as shown in relationship to the line of identity. As shown, most of the points fell close to the line of identity. This suggests that α_1-receptor–mediated pupillary mydriasis did not change with addition of guanadrel.

receptors were available for only nine subjects. As shown in Fig. 1, eight of the nine subjects showed an increase in B_{max} ($P < 0.02$), while 10 of 11 had a reduction in norepinephrine levels ($P < 0.01$). The subject with a decreased B_{max} during the guanadrel trial received the lowest dose of the drug, 5 mg twice a day, and was the only subject without a reduction in the plasma norepinephrine level. However, in the whole group we found no significant correlation between either the absolute ($r = -0.39$) or percentage ($r = -0.31$) increase in α_2-receptors and the reduction in plasma norepinephrine level.

The amount of platelet protein recovered before and during guanadrel therapy was unchanged (3.2 ± 1.1 vs 2.8 ± 1.4 mg). This suggests that the increase in yohimbine binding was due to an increase in the number of binding sites rather than a decrease in the amount of protein recovered. While platelet α_2-receptor number increased, the K_d for yohimbine did not change during guanadrel therapy (5.4 ± 0.5 vs. 5.0 ± 0.8 nmol). Fig. 2 illustrates this increased B_{max} (x-intercept) without change in K_d (slope) in one subject. Guanadrel inhibited [^{3}H]yohimbine binding at high concentrations, with half-maximal inhibition at 50 mmol/L.

The percent forearm vasoconstrictor responses to locally infused norepinephrine (Fig. 3) and the pupillary mydriatic response to 1% ophthalmic phenylephrine (Fig. 4) did not change.

DISCUSSION

Addition of guanadrel to diuretic therapy reduced supine heart rate and intra-arterial blood pressure. Guanadrel also reduced the supine baseline plasma norepinephrine level. These declines are probably explained by the known ability of the drug to reduce noradrenaline storage in and release from the postganglionic sympathetic nerve terminal.[8] Platelet α_2-receptor number increased significantly, presumably in response to the reduced sympathetic drive. The effect of guanadrel on platelet α_2-receptor number is not likely to be due to a direct interaction with the α_2-receptors, because guanadrel inhibits [^{3}H]yohimbine binding only at very high concentrations (half-maximal inhibition at 50 mmol/L; data not shown). Pupillary mydriasis and forearm vasoconstriction in response to exogenous α-agonists did not change.

There are several salient findings of our study. First, plasma levels of norepinephrine, but not epinephrine, fell in response to a drug known to reduce sympathetic drive. The dissociation between the changes in the two measured catecholamines most likely reflects the postganglionic as opposed to central sympatholytic effects of guanadrel.[13] There is extensive interest in the utility of venous plasma catecholamine levels for the assessment of sympathetic nervous system activity.[14,15] It is evident that significant differences in regional release can occur without being reflected in the systemic venous catecholamine measurement.[16] It is also known that differences in reuptake between individuals may complicate interindividual comparisons.[17] However, our data further substantiate the value of plasma norepinephrine levels as an index of intraindividual changes in sympathetic drive.

Second, the increase in the number of platelet α_2-receptors during guanadrel therapy is of special interest. This is the first study in man to show a consistent increase in platelet α_2-receptors in response to a well-defined pharmacologic reduction of sympathetic drive and is in agreement with a similar study in rodents.[18] Patients with disease-related reduction in sympathetic drive such as idiopathic orthostatic hypotension have increased numbers of platelet α_2-receptors.[19,20] However, in other studies surgical reduction of sympathetic stimulation by ablation of pheochromocytoma tissue has produced conflicting results of either no change[21] or an increase[19] in platelet α_2-receptors. Administration of the pharmacologic α_2-agonists guanabenz and clonidine has also produced conflicting findings, showing either no change[22] or a decrease[23] in platelet α_2-receptor number. While it is not clear precisely which factors regulate platelet α_2-receptor number, it is not likely that circulating levels of plasma catecholamines are an overriding factor.[21,24]

Third, the functional measures of α-adrenergic responsiveness, norepinephrine-induced forearm vasoconstriction, and phenylephrine-induced pupillary mydriasis did not change during guanadrel therapy (Figs. 2 and 3). This is in contrast to the consistent decrease in plasma norepinephrine levels and increase in platelet α_2-receptor number. These observations indicate that caution is needed when extrapolating from differences in or changes of in vitro biochemical measurements of sympathetic activity to in vivo physiologic significance.

The possible explanations for these apparent discrepancies are many. However, we believe the most likely explanations are either that (1) the pupillary and vascular responses are largely α_1 effects and α_1-receptors may not upregulate as much as the platelet α_2-receptors,[18] or (2) the diuretics blunted physiologic responses to catecholamines,[25] perhaps by altering the intracellular environment.[26] Additional studies of responses to α_2-selective agonists in subjects not taking diuretics should answer these questions.

In summary, addition of guanadrel to diuretic monotherapy reduced blood pressure and heart rate in 11 patients with essential hypertension. This reduction was accompanied by a reduction in sympathetic drive (plasma norepinephrine level) and an increase in platelet α_2-receptors. Despite these changes, physiologic responses to exogenous α-agonists did not change. Consequently, extrapolations from in vitro measurements of sympathetic activity to in vivo physiologic significance may be incorrect. There are many potential explanations for this apparent dichotomy and they deserve further investigation.

We are indebted to our technical and data analysis staff of J. Mertens, M. Elkins, D. Rogers, D. Brant, M. Rapai, L. Vadnay, N. Schork, Olga Szamraj, and Mark Zamorski.

References

1. Julius S, Esler M. Autonomic nervous cardiovascular regulation in borderline hypertension. Am J Cardiol 1975;36:685-96.
2. Esler M, Julius S, Randall O, Ellis C, Kashima T. Relation of renin status to neurogenic vascular resistance in borderline hypertension. Am J Cardiol 1975;36:708-15.
3. Esler M, Julius S, Zweifler A, Randall O, Harburg E, Gardiner H, DeQuattro V. Mild high-renin essential hypertension. N Engl J Med 1977;296:405-11.
4. Meier A, Weidmann P, Grimm M, et al. Pressor factors and cardiovascular pressor responsiveness in borderline hypertension. Hypertension 1981;3:367-72.
5. Phillip TH, Distler A, Cordes U. Sympathetic nervous system and blood pressure control in essential hypertension. Lancet 1978;2:959-63.
6. Doyle A, Fraser J, Marshall R. Reactivity of forearm vessels to vasoconstrictor substance in hypertensive and normotensive subjects. Clin Sci 1959;18:441-53.
7. Amann FW, Bolli P, Kiowski W, et al. Enhanced alpha-adrenoreceptor–mediated vasoconstriction in essential hypertension. Hypertension 1981;3(suppl I):I119-23.
8. Freyburger WA, Peterson LJ, Kaiser DG, et al. Clinician's brochure on U 28,228 D (Cl-1388R). Kalamazoo, Mich: The Upjohn Company, 1968.
9. Egan B, Neubig R, Schneider R, Julius S. Methods for measuring vascular and nonvascular alpha-receptor sen-

sitivity in man. Proceedings of the Symposium on Adrenoceptors, Calcium and Exitation-Contraction Coupling: Mechanisms and Pharmacological Interference Satellite. J Cardiovasc Pharm. (in press)
10. Peuler JD, Johnson GA: Simultaneous single isotope radioenzymatic assay of plasma norepinephrine, epinephrine and dopamine. Life Sci 1977;21:625-36.
11. Haber E, Koerner T, Page LB, Kliman B, Purnode A. Application of a radioimmunoassay for angiotensin I to the physiologic measurement of plasma renin activity in normal healthy subjects. J Clin Endocrinol Metab 1969;29:1349-55.
12. Neubig RR, Brasier R, Szamraj O. Large-scale purification of $alpha_2$ adrenergic receptor enriched membranes from human platelets. Biochem Biophys Acta. (Submitted for publication)
13. Leveston SA, Shah SD, Cryer P. Cholinergic stimulation of norepinephrine release in man. J Clin Invest 1979;64:374-80.
14. Goldstein DS, McCarty R, Polinsky RJ, Kopin IJ. Relationship between plasma norepinephrine and sympathetic neural activity. Hypertension 1983;5:552-9.
15. Ibsen H, Julius S. Pharmacologic tools for assessment of adrenergic nerve activity in human hypertension. Fed Proc 1984;43:61-5.
16. Brown M, Jenner D, Allison D, Dollery C. Variations in individual organ release of noradrenaline measured by an improved radioenzymatic technique; limitations of peripheral venous measurements in the assessment of sympathetic nervous activity. Clin Sci 1981;61:585-90.
17. Esler M, Jackman G, Bobik A, et al. Norepinephrine kinetics in essential hypertension. Defective neuronal uptake of norepinephrine in some patients. Hypertension 1981;3:149-56.
18. Bylund D, Martinez J, Pierce D. Regulation of autonomic receptors in rat submandibular gland. Mol Pharmacol 1981;21:27-35.
19. Chobanian A, Tifft C, Sackel H, Pitruzella A. Alpha and beta-adrenergic receptor activity in circulating blood cells of patients with idiopathic orthostatic hypotension and pheochromocytoma. Clin Exp Hypertens [A] 1982; 4,5:793-806.
20. Kafka MS, Polinsky RJ, Williams A. Alpha-adrenergic receptors in orthostatic hypotension syndromes. Neurology (Cleveland) 1984;34:1121-5.
21. Pfeifer M, Ward K, Malpass T, et al. Variations in circulating catecholamines fail to alter human platelet alpha-2 adrenergic receptor number or affinity for [^{3}H]yohimbine or [^{3}H]dihydroergocryptine. J Clin Invest 1984; 74:1063-72.
22. Motulsky HJ, O'Connor DT, Insel PA. Platelet α_2-adrenergic receptors in treated and untreated essential hypertension. Clin Sci 1983;64:265-72.
23. Brodde OE, Anlauf M, Graben N, Bock KD. In vitro and in vivo downregulation of human platelet α_2-adrenoceptors by clonidine. Eur J Clin Pharmacol 1982; 23:403-9.
24. Snavely MD, Motulsky HJ, O'Connor DT, Ziegler MG, Insel PA. Adrenergic receptors in human and experimental pheochromocytoma. Clin Exp Hypertens [A] 1982;4,5:829-48.
25. Weidmann PM, Grimm M, Meier A, et al. Pathogenic and therapeutic significance of cardiovascular pressor reactivity as related to plasma catecholamines in borderline and established essential hypertension. Clin Exp Hypertens 1980;2:427-49.
26. Erne P, Bolli P, Burgisser E, et al. Correlation of platelet calcium with blood pressure. Effect of antihypertensive therapy. N Engl J Med 1984;310:1084-8.

Pharmacodynamic evaluation of the benzodiazepine–oral contraceptive interaction

The sedative, psychomotor, and memory effects of single oral doses of alprazolam (ALP), lorazepam (LOR), temazepam (TMP), and triazolam (TRZ) were evaluated in women taking oral contraceptives (OCs) and a comparable group of control women. Nine women taking OCs and 11 control women took doses of 1 mg ALP and 2 mg LOR and 10 OC users and 10 control women took 30 mg TMP and 0.5 mg TRZ on two occasions separated by 28 days. Minimal psychomotor impairment was noted after TMP. ALP, LOR, and TRZ produced greater performance impairment in the OC users. Correcting the maximum observed performance decrement for plasma concentration did not account for the differences between OC users and controls. After TMP, there was less sedation during the first 2 hours in OC users, who also had higher plasma TMP clearance. There were no differences in sedation between OC users and controls after ALP, LOR, and TRZ; however, there was <50% power to detect a 30% difference. Amnestic effects in OC users and controls did not differ after any of the four drugs. The observed patterns of anterograde amnesia were different, with the earliest and most pronounced recognition failure after TRZ (50% at 1.5 hours), while the LOR effect increased to a maximum (30%) 4 hours after dosing. Our data suggest that differences in benzodiazepine pharmacokinetics between OC users and control women do not account for observed differences in psychomotor impairment. Women taking OCs are more sensitive to the psychomotor effects of single oral doses of benzodiazepines. Statements about sensitivity of OC users to sedative and amnestic effects of benzodiazepines cannot be made with any degree of certainty. (Clin Pharmacol Ther 38:525-532, 1985.)

Patricia D. Kroboth, Ph.D., Randall B. Smith, Ph.D., Gary P. Stoehr, Pharm.D., and Randy P. Juhl, Ph.D. *Pittsburgh, Pa., and Kalamazoo, Mich.*

The pharmacokinetics of some benzodiazepines are altered in women who take oral contraceptives (OCs).[1,6,21,23] Although it is often assumed that changes in benzodiazepine pharmacokinetics will result in a parallel change in response, this hypothesis had not been tested. As part of a pharmacokinetic study[23] we evaluated the sedative, psychomotor, and memory effects of single doses of alprazolam (ALP), lorazepam (LOR), temazepam (TMP), and triazolam (TRZ) in women taking OCs and in control women who did not use OCs. The purpose of this study was to determine whether the magnitude of these effects differed between users of OCs and a comparable group of control women and whether differences in pharmacokinetics between the two groups were associated with differences in observed effects. In addition, we evaluated effects of these four drugs on pattern of memory impairment in the 4 hours after drug dosing.

From the Departments of Pharmacy Practice and Medicine, University of Pittsburgh, Pittsburgh, and The Upjohn Company, Kalamazoo.

Received for publication March 17, 1985; accepted July 16, 1985.

Reprint requests to: Patricia D. Kroboth, Ph.D., 239-B Victoria Building, University of Pittsburgh, Pittsburgh, PA 15261.

METHODS

Subjects and controls. Nineteen women 18 to 34 years old who had taken OCs for more than 3 months were selected. The control group consisted of 21 women who were similar in age, weight, and smoking history to the OC users. Participants were proved normal by history, physical examination, and biochemical screening profile and except for OCs they took no chronic medication. Alcohol and caffeine-containing beverages were not permitted for 24 hours before drug dosing and throughout the blood sampling periods. Participants were paid and gave written informed consent to participate. The study was approved by the Institu-

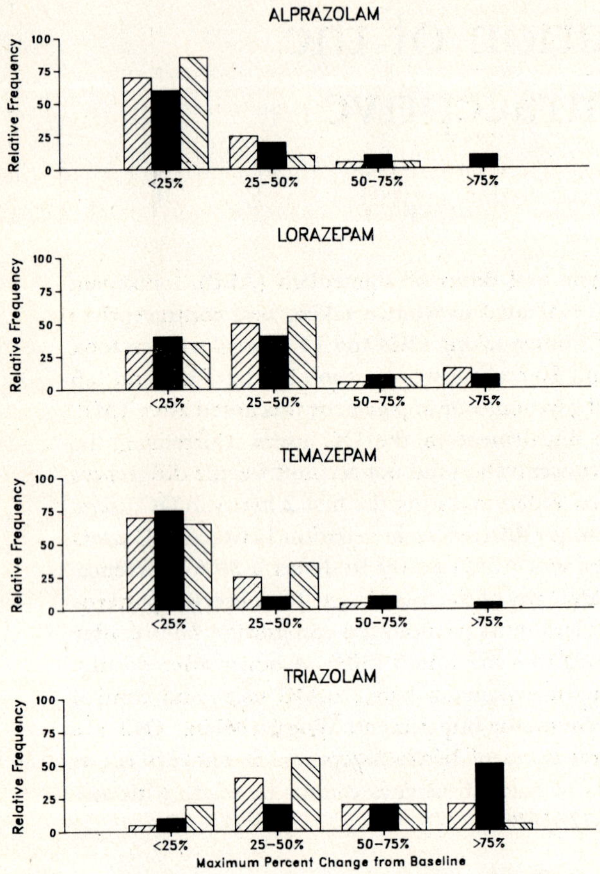

Fig. 1. Relative frequency of maximal percent change from baseline performance (E_{max}) on four psychomotor tests after single doses of four benzodiazepines in healthy women (OC users and controls combined). ▨ = AIM; ■ = ARRC; ▧ = DSS.

tional Review Board for Biomedical Sciences of the University of Pittsburgh.

Nine women taking OCs and 11 control women were assigned to take ALP and LOR in a crossover design; 10 OC users and 10 controls were assigned to receive TRZ and TMP. Treatments were separated by 28 days to control for intraindividual effects of menstrual cycle on benzodiazepine pharmacokinetics or pharmacodynamics. All OC users were taking combination OCs containing ≤35 μg ethinyl estradiol. Fifteen OC users were taking preparations with a progesterone equivalent of ≤0.6 mg norethindrone acetate; three women in the ALP-LOR group and one woman in the TRZ-TMP group took OCs containing 1.0 to 1.5 mg norethindrone acetate. There were no differences between OC users and controls in age, weight, or height.

After an overnight fast, a single oral dose of 1 mg ALP, 2 mg LOR, 30 mg TMP, or 0.5 mg TRZ was taken with 120 ml water. These doses correspond to those commonly prescribed. Blood samples were drawn at intervals for 24 hours after TRZ and for 36 hours after ALP, LOR, and TMP. The protocol for blood sampling and pharmacokinetic analysis has been reported.[23]

Pharmacodynamic evaluation. The Stanford Sleepiness Scale (SSS)[11] and a battery of four psychomotor tests were administered at time 0 (just before drug dosing) and at 1.25, 2.5, 5.0, and 8.25 hours thereafter. The battery consisted of digit symbol substitution (DSS), aiming (AIM), and a reaction test (Alpha Recognition Reaction Chronometry [ARRC]). The SSS was always administered first, with the other tests following in the same order each time. Subjects were familiarized with the tests at a practice session to minimize learning effects.

DSS and AIM[19,24] were scored for the number of correct responses in 90 seconds. ARRC is a computerized reaction test developed in our laboratory. Subjects were instructed to rest their right hand on the table surface in front of a computer keyboard. At varying intervals a randomly generated letter of the alphabet appeared in the center of the monitor. The time (in arbitrary units) required for the subject to press the corresponding key on the keyboard was the reaction time. After each letter was correctly identified, reaction time appeared on the screen, providing feedback to the subjects. Subjects then pressed a separate key to indicate readiness for the next random letter. After the screen cleared, another letter appeared at a random time to prevent a response rhythm from developing. The score for one test session was the mean of 20 timed reactions.

In addition to the SSS self evaluation of sedation, subject sedation was evaluated by the research nurse at each blood sampling. A four-point nurse-rated sedation (NRS) scale was used, in which 0 was "alert" and 3 was "unable to walk to the blood sample collection station."

Effects of the four drugs on memory were also evaluated. Before drug dosing a common object was shown to each subject. Then at 1.5, 2.5, and 4.0 hours after drug dosing, a picture of an object and a colored background was shown to each subject. Subjects were instructed to remember both the object in the picture and the color. The picture and color were different at each test time. However, neither the name of the object nor the color was verbally stated. Recall and then recognition were tested 10.5 hours after dosing. Subjects were asked to write the names of the objects and the colors on a piece of paper (recall). Subsequently, they

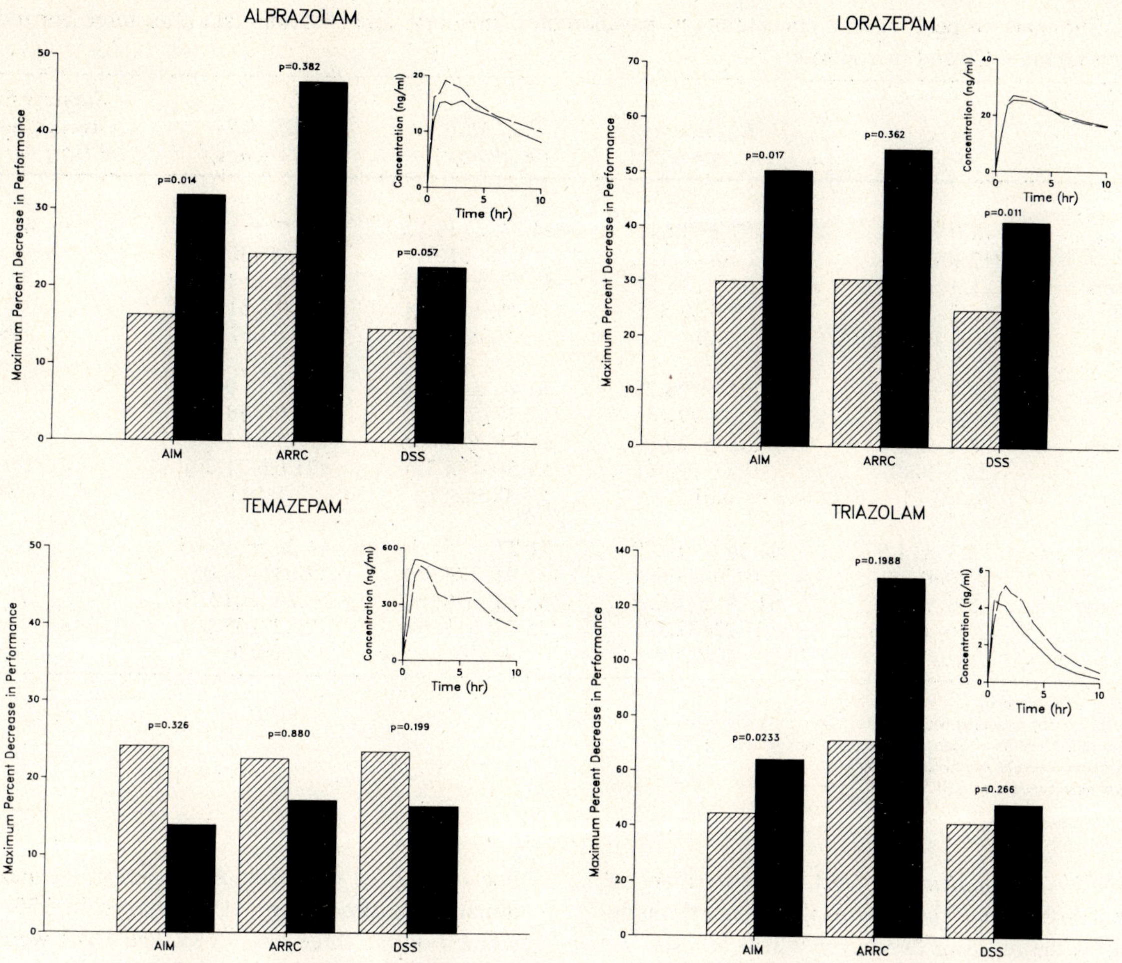

Fig. 2. Maximum percent decrease in performance after a single oral dose of benzodiazepine to control women *(hatched bars)* and women taking OCs *(solid bars)*. Note that the ordinate scales differ. Concentration-time plots are provided in the *insets* for controls *(solid lines)* and OC users *(dashed lines)*.

were asked to pick out the three pictures and colors they had seen previously from a group of six pictures and six colors (recognition).

Data analysis. To make all baseline scores equal to 0 and to express performance at subsequent times as the percent increase or decrease from baseline, the following equation was used: (Raw score − baseline)/baseline · 100%. The maximum observed decrement in performance (E_{max}) and an effect index was determined for each subject at each test. The effect index, which relates E_{max} to observed peak serum drug concentration (C_{max}), is defined as observed E_{max} divided by log C_{max} for each individual. E_{max} and effect index data for OC and control groups were tested for differences by the Mann-Whitney U two-sample test because of nonhomogeneity of variances. Subsequently, an effect ratio was calculated by dividing the mean effect index for the OC group (for each drug at each test) by the mean effect index for controls. This provides a means of comparing magnitude of effect adjusted for plasma concentrations in the two groups of women.

Performance and sedation scores from time 0 to 8.25 hours in OC users and controls were tested for differences by repeated-measures ANOVA.[4,25] This incorporates performance at 0, 1.25, 2.5, 5.0, and 8.25 hours as the repeated measure. Raw performance score was the dependent variable, while time was the independent variable. The Student-Newman-Keuls test was used subsequently to determine treatment differences and time of return to baseline.

The NRS score AUC was calculated as a measure of overall sedation. Differences were determined by one-

Table I. Summary of peak plasma concentration, psychomotor, memory, and sedation data after three benzodiazepines* in women taking OCs and in controls

	C_{max} *(ng/ml)*	E_{max} *AIM (% change)*†	E_{max} *ARRC (% change)*†	E_{max} *DSS (% change)*†	*Subjects failing recognition of at least one item*‡
ALP					
Controls	18.0 ± 4.2 (12.8–27.1)	16.37 ± 12.17 (2.56–47.41)	24.34 ± 18.75 (−3.28–61.64)	14.70 ± 7.99 (0.00–30.49)	4
OC users	21.3 ± 4.5 (16.3–30.3)	31.94 ± 18.27 (15.38–69.81)	46.77 ± 42.95 (13.46–134.38)	22.84 ± 12.90 (2.95–51.67)	5
P value	0.10 > P > 0.05	0.014	0.382	0.057	0.498
LOR					
Controls	26.7 ± 4.5 (20.0–33.5)	30.01 ± 25.23 (7.03–99.28)	30.48 ± 12.19 (17.31–53.33)	24.99 ± 9.71 (2.04–38.57)	7
OC users	28.4 ± 2.8 (26.5–32.0)	50.33 ± 20.04 (19.57–79.31)	54.31 ± 50.96 (15.58–176.79)	41.15 ± 14.82 (21.62–71.70)	8
P value	>0.15	0.017	0.362	0.011	0.194
TRZ					
Controls	5.3 ± 1.9 (2.20–9.38)	44.56 ± 17.70 (28.30–73.60)	71.27 ± 51.36 (23.91–178.85)	41.26 ± 19.05 (22.41–77.05)	5
OC users	5.6 ± 2.8 (2.66–11.30)	64.18 ± 19.38 (27.22–87.32)	130.83 ± 85.92 (35.71–313.70)	48.26 ± 12.76 (22.22–65.00)	7
P value	>0.35	0.023	0.199	0.226	0.361

Data are $\overline{X}$ ± SD (range).
*TMP data are not presented because effects were minimal.
†P values reflect results of Mann-Whitney two-sample test.
‡P values reflect results of chi-square analysis.
§P values reflect results of ANOVA.

way ANOVA, with Duncan's test for assessment of treatment differences. The level of significance throughout reflects the result of two-tailed statistical tests.

Effects of the drugs on memory in OC users and controls were compared by chi-square analysis. When no significant differences between groups was found after a drug, a protected chi-square analysis was done comparing recognition failure at the three times after drug dosing (1.5, 2.5, and 4.0 hours). Differences between individual time points were detected by multiple pairwise comparisons (chi-square) with Bonferroni's correction.[2]

RESULTS

Comparison of the raw scores for baseline performance showed no difference between OC users and controls. There were also no differences in baseline among the four drug treatments.

The distribution of E_{max} values after the four drugs is shown in Fig. 1. The trend for differences is readily noted. At the doses used, TMP produced the least impairment, with more than 60% of the subjects having <15% decrease in performance on AIM and ARRC; over 70% of the subjects had <25% change from baseline on any of the tests. ALP caused the next least impairment, producing <15% change in 35% of the women on the three tests. TRZ and LOR were at the opposite extreme, producing >25% impairment in 90% and 70% of the subjects, respectively.

E_{max} values for OC and control groups were compared for each drug and are presented with mean plasma concentration-time plots in Fig. 2. After TMP there were no differences between groups on any test. Table I provides additional information (including the range of observations) about psychomotor, sedative, and memory effects observed in OC users and controls.

Table II provides the mean effect index (E_{max}/log C_{max}) for each of the performance tests after the four drugs for OC users and controls. Effect ratios and statistical significance values are also provided.

Response to the four drugs over time was evaluated in OC users and controls by repeated-measures ANOVA. These results were similar to those obtained when E_{max} values were evaluated. However, repeated-measures ANOVA provided the additional ability to determine times at which performance scores differed from baseline. Post-hoc comparisons with the Student-Newman-Keuls test revealed that for each drug and test,

Total items not recognized‡	*NRS AUC 0 to 2 hr (sedation units · hr)§*
10	1.86 ± 1.14 (0.05–4.00)
11	2.11 ± 1.41 (0.0–3.75)
0.980	0.669
9	1.73 ± 1.38 (0.00–4.25)
14	2.06 ± 1.83 (0.00–4.75)
0.246	0.652
11	3.60 ± 1.08 (1.50–4.75)
20	3.68 ± 1.80 (1.25–6.50)
0.061	0.911

performance was impaired at 1.25 and 2.5 hours in OC users and controls. Performance had returned to the baseline level by 5 hours in all cases except for DSS after ALP (performance on this test returned to baseline by 8.25 hours).

When NRS score AUCs were compared, there were no differences between OC users and controls after TRZ, ALP, or LOR at any of the time intervals (0 to 1, 0 to 2, 0 to 3, or 0 to 4 hours) through 4 hours after dosing. During the first 2 hours after TMP, however, OC users were less sedated (2.1 ± 1.5 sedation unit · hr) than controls (3.6 ± 1.3 sedation units · hr; P = 0.04).

All subjects were able to recall the object presented before ingestion of the study drug. By chi-square analysis there were no differences between OC and control groups in the number of subjects who failed to recognize items or in the number of items not recognized. Fig. 3 summarizes the percent frequency of recognition failure for each drug at 10.5 hours for pictures and colors presented at 1.5, 2.5, and 4.0 hours. Each drug was evaluated separately for differences in memory at the three times. Because three pairwise comparisons were done (1.5 vs. 2.5 hours, 1.5 vs. 4.0 hours, and 2.5 vs. 4.0 hours), a $P < 0.016$ was the critical value for significance. After TRZ, memory impairment was greater at 1.5 hours than at 2.5 hours (P = 0.002) and 4.0 hours ($P < 0.001$). After TMP, there were more recognition failures at 1.5 than at 2.5 hours (P = 0.013). After LOR, memory loss was greater at 4.0 hours than at 1.5 hours (P = 0.01). There were no differences in recognition failure at the three times after ALP dosing.

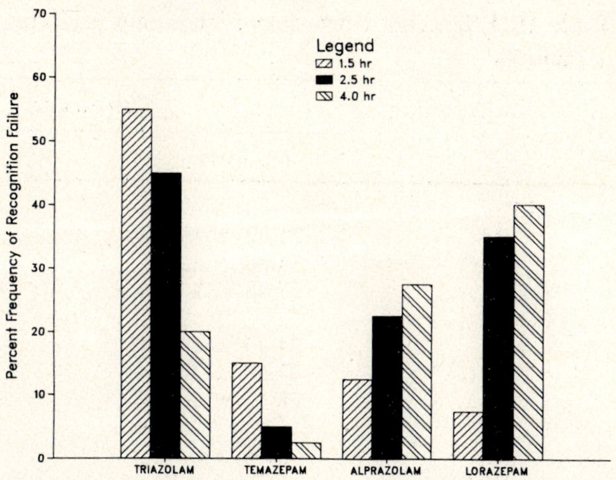

Fig. 3. Relative frequency of failure to recognize colors and objects presented at 1.5, 2.5, and 4.0 hours after drug dosing. The test of recognition was at 10.5 hours after dosing. Data for controls and OC users are combined.

DISCUSSION

In this study, differences in benzodiazepine pharmacokinetics were noted between users of OCs and a comparable group of control women. Our evaluation of psychomotor performance suggests that differences in kinetics do not explain the difference in observed degree of impairment. Women who take OCs appear to be more sensitive to the psychomotor effects of single oral doses than are control women.

Inspection of Fig. 2 makes this more clear. After single-dose administration, ALP and TRZ clearance is about 20% lower in women taking OCs than in control women.[23] Correspondingly, women taking OCs experience greater psychomotor impairment after a single dose of either ALP or TRZ. This suggests that decreased drug clearance (increased AUC) accounts for the increased psychomotor impairment. However, closer inspection reveals disparity between the kinetic and dynamic changes. With regard to LOR, OC users experienced greater impairment than controls despite similar pharmacokinetics. TMP induced such a small effect on psychomotor performance that information from this drug cannot be used to draw meaningful conclusions.

To evaluate more carefully the contribution of peak plasma concentration to magnitude of psychomotor im-

Table II. Effect index data for psychomotor performance after four benzodiazepines in women taking OCs and in controls

	*Effect index**			
	OC users	*Controls*	*P value†*	*Effect ratio‡*
ALP				
AIM	−24.42 ± 13.94	−13.19 ± 10.03	0.025	1.85
ARRC	34.86 ± 30.85	19.26 ± 14.78	0.470	1.81
DSS	−17.48 ± 9.62	−11.96 ± 6.54	0.087	1.46
LOR				
AIM	−34.74 ± 14.04	−21.31 ± 18.40	0.017	1.63
ARRC	37.88 ± 36.21	21.52 ± 8.79	0.518	1.76
DSS	−28.42 ± 10.53	−17.59 ± 6.83	0.014	1.62
TMP				
AIM	−5.06 ± 6.53	−8.58 ± 8.04	0.326	.59
ARRC	6.31 ± 8.18	8.06 ± 9.23	0.940	.78
DSS	−5.99 ± 4.23	−8.38 ± 3.44	0.174	.71
TRZ				
AIM	−92.49 ± 23.22	−68.12 ± 24.05	0.060	1.36
ARRC	175.80 ± 87.35	102.20 ± 62.74	0.028	1.72
DSS	−71.27 ± 21.97	−62.32 ± 22.81	0.514	1.14

Data are $\overline{X}$ ± SD.
*E_{max}/log C_{max} for each subject.
†P value reflects the results of Mann-Whitney two-sample test.
‡Effect ratio is the mean effect index for the OC group divided by the mean value for the controls.

pairment, effect ratios were calculated. These provide a means of comparing magnitude of response adjusted for plasma concentration, and indicate whether OC users or controls experienced a greater drug effect. The ratios of >1.0 for ALP, LOR, and TRZ indicate that women taking OCs had 14% to 85% more psychomotor impairment than their counterparts who did not take OCs (Table II).

The explanation for increased sensitivity of women taking OCs is not clear. Increases in receptor sensitivity or permeability of biologic membranes, decreased protein binding, and additive depressive central nervous system effects of OCs are possibilities. Of these, we can only comment on protein binding. The percent free TRZ did not differ between OC users (8.4% ± 1.5%) and controls (8.5% ± 1.6%); protein binding of the other drugs was not evaluated.

The psychomotor tests we used are not specific for a single brain center, but are global measures of central nervous system function. They depend on the ability to recognize and ultimately respond to a stimulus. Once the stimulus is presented, a number of brain centers become involved in the recognition and processing of the information. Level of alertness, motivation of the subject, learning and memory from previous exposures to the stimulus, underlying personality of the subject, and motor function all affect the observed response.[9] Although the tests are global in nature, DSS tends to measure predominantly sensory function. AIM measures motor function, particularly coordination, while ARRC assesses both sensory and motor ability.[10] In our present study we observed fairly good agreement between the degree of impairment in AIM and DSS, which suggests that sensory and motor centers are affected similarly by the doses of the benzodiazepines evaluated.

Based on our sedation data, differences between OC users and controls are less clear. In contrast to the psychomotor data, there were no differences in degree of sedation between OC users and controls after ALP, LOR, and TRZ. After TMP, however, less sedation was observed in the OC users, who also cleared the drug more rapidly from plasma. The overall lack of difference may not be real, however, because there was <50% power to detect a 30% difference in level of sedation with all four sets of data (ALP, LOR, TMP, and TRZ).

There are no published studies of OC-benzodiazepine pharmacodynamic interactions with which to compare our results. However, other investigators have evaluated effect of menstrual cycle phase on memory and psychomotor impairment induced by alcohol and diazepam, respectively. Jones and Jones[13] reported that amnesic effects of alcohol were not affected by menstrual cycle phase, but that they did differ between men and women. In our study we noted no consistent differences in memory effects between OC users and controls.

Hence conclusions regarding the role of hormonal variations in women or exogenously administered hormones in influencing recall ability seem premature.

Conversely, the work by Ellinwood et al.[5] demonstrated a trend for greater diazepam-induced psychomotor impairment on day 28 than on day 10 in women taking OCs. Our data, which demonstrate greater psychomotor impairment in women taking OCs, strengthens the hypothesis that hormonal variations (or exogenously administered hormones) influence the degree of psychomotor impairment caused by benzodiazepines. The role of the dose of exogenous progesterone on pharmacokinetics or response cannot be determined, since only three women took OCs with a high progesterone content. We are not able to make a statement about effect of day of menstrual cycle based on our data because we did not control for this, and there was scatter over days of the cycle in both OC and control groups.

Although there were no differences between OC users and controls with regard to the anterograde amnesia, Fig. 3 demonstrates different patterns of recognition failure after the four benzodiazepines. Differences in potencies of the doses administered, pharmacokinetic profiles, or receptor affinities of the individual agents are possible explanations for this. Although a combination of these factors may be involved, benzodiazepine concentrations in the brain and binding affinity to benzodiazepine receptors are the most likely explanations for the differences.[12] TRZ, 0.5 mg, caused the earliest and highest frequency of recognition failure (50% at 1.5 hours). In contrast, amnesia was relatively infrequent (7.5%) at 1.5 hours after LOR, but increased to peak frequency (30%) at 4 hours. Our observed time course for LOR is similar to that reported by Brown et al.,[3] who administered 3 mg iv doses of LOR and found the peak frequency of impaired delayed recall (about 90%) at approximately 4 hours after dosing. Comparison with our data also suggest that there is a dose-response relationship for frequency of memory impairment. In contrast, Kothary et al.[15] evaluated 2 mg LOR and reported a similar maximum frequency of recognition failure (30%), but at an earlier time (2 hours). Others have evaluated memory loss after benzodiazepines,[14,18,22] but to our knowledge the time course of impairment after TRZ, ALP, and TMP has not previously been reported.

Pharmacokinetic interactions of OCs with other drugs have been described. However, none of these interactions have been evaluated for concomitant changes in pharmacodynamics. For only a few other drug-benzodiazepine interactions has response been evaluated. Benzodiazepine interactions with alcohol[17] and diazepam interactions with cimetidine[7] and theophylline[8] are notable exceptions. Our study provides an important first step in evaluating the clinical significance of OC-induced changes in the pharmacokinetics of other drugs.

Results of interactions of ALP, TRZ, and LOR with OCs seem to indicate that women taking OCs are more sensitive than control women to the psychomotor effects of single oral doses of benzodiazepines. Statements about differences in sensitivity to sedative and amnesic effects of the benzodiazepines cannot be made with any degree of certainty. Establishing the true clinical significance of our findings is difficult because tolerance to psychomotor impairment may develop during chronic benzodiazepine dosing. In addition, psychomotor impairment in women with anxiety may be less than that in normal volunteers[16,20]; however, even anxious patients will most likely experience psychomotor impairment during chronic therapy with high doses.[16] Further examination of the question of OC-induced changes in benzodiazepine pharmacokinetics and pharmacodynamics is needed. To provide a better assessment of the clinical implications, this interaction should be examined in a multiple-dose benzodiazepine study of pharmacokinetics and dynamics in OC users and in control women on specific days of the menstrual cycle.

References

1. Abernethy DR, Greenblatt DJ, Divoll M, Arendt R, Ochs HR, Shader RI: Impairment of diazepam metabolism by low-dose estrogen-containing oral-contraceptive steroids. N Engl J Med **306**:791-792, 1982.
2. Abt K: Significance testing of many variables. Neuropsychobiologia **9**:47-50, 1983.
3. Brown J, Lewis V, Brown M, Horn G, Bowes JB: A comparison between transient amnesias induced by two drugs (diazepam or lorazepam) and amnesia of organic origin. Neuropsychobiologia **20**:55-70, 1982.
4. Dixon WJ, editor: BMDP Statistical Software. Los Angeles, 1983, University of California Press.
5. Ellinwood EH, Easler ME, Linnoila M, Molter DW, Heatherly DG, Bjornsson TD: Effects of oral contraceptives on diazepam-induced psychomotor impairment. CLIN PHARMACOL THER **35**:360-366, 1984.
6. Giles HG, Sellers EM, Naranjo CA, Frecker RC, Greenblatt DJ: Disposition of intravenous diazepam in young men and women. Eur J Clin Pharmacol **20**:207-213, 1981.
7. Greenblatt DJ, Abernethy DR, Morse DS, Harmatz JS, Shader RI: Clinical importance of the interaction of diazepam and cimetidine. N Engl J Med **310**:1639-1643, 1984.
8. Henauer SA, Hollister LE, Gillespie HK, Moore F: Theophylline antagonizes diazepam-induced psychomotor impairment. Eur J Clin Pharmacol **25**:743-747, 1983.

9. Hindmarch I: Psychomotor function and psychoactive drugs. Br J Clin Pharmacol **10:**189-209, 1980.
10. Hindmarch I: Psychological performance models as indicators of hypnotic effects. *In* Hindmarch I, Ott H, Roth T, editors: Sleep, benzodiazepines and performance. Experimental methodologies and research prospects. New York, 1984, Springer-Verlag.
11. Hoddes E, Zarcone V, Smythe H, Phillips R. Dement WC: Quantification of sleepiness: A new approach. Psychophysiology **10:**431-436, 1973.
12. Jack ML, Colburn WA, Sprit NM, Bautz G, Zanko M, Horst WD, O'Brien RA: A pharmacokinetic/pharmacodynamic/receptor binding model to predict the onset and duration of phamacological activity of the benzodiazepines. Prog Neuropsychopharmacol Biol Psychiatry **7:**629-635, 1983.
13. Jones BM, Jones MK: Alcohol effects in women during the menstrual cycle. Ann NY Acad Sci **273:**576-587, 1976.
14. Juhl RP, Daugherty VM, Kroboth PD: Incidence of next-day anterograde amnesia caused by flurazepam hydrochloride and triazolam. Clin Pharm **3:**622-625, 1984.
15. Kothary SP, Brown ACD, Pandit UA, Samra SK, Pandit JK: Time course of antirecall effect of diazepam and lorazepam following oral administration. Anesthesiology **55:**641-644, 1981.
16. Linnoila M, Erwin CW, Brendle A, Simpson D: Psychomotor effects of diazepam in anxious patients and healthy volunteers. J Clin Psychopharmacol **3:**88-96, 1983.
17. Mattila MJ: Interactions of benzodiazepines on psychomotor skills. Br J Clin Pharmacol **18:**21S-26S, 1984.
18. McKay AC, Dundee JW: Effect of oral benzodiazepines on memory. Br J Anaesth **52:**1247-1257, 1980.
19. Moran LJ, Mefferd RB: Repetitive psychometric measures. Psychol Rep **5:**269-275, 1959.
20. Oblowitz H, Robins AH: The effect of clobazam and lorazepam on the psychomotor performance of anxious patients. Br J Clin Pharmacol **16:**95-99, 1983.
21. Patwardan RV, Mitchell MC, Johnson RF, Schenker S: Differential effects of oral contraceptive steroids on the metabolism of benzodiazepines. Hepatology **3:**248-253, 1983.
22. Roehrs T, Zorick FJ, Sicklesteel JM, Wittig RM, Hartse KM, Roth T: Effects of hypnotics on memory. J Clin Psychopharmacol **3:**310-313, 1983.
23. Stoehr GP, Kroboth PD, Juhl RP, Wender DB, Phillips JP, Smith RB: Effect of oral contraceptives on triazolam, temazepam, alprazolam, and lorazepam kinetics. CLIN PHARMACOL THER **36:**683-690, 1984.
24. Wechsler D: A manual for the Wechsler Adult Intelligence Scale. New York, 1955, Psychological Corporation.
25. Winer BJ: Statistical principles in experimental design, ed 2. New York, 1971, McGraw-Hill Book Company.

Fecal blood loss during isoxicam and piroxicam administration for 28 days

After an 11-day baseline period, groups of eight healthy men received isoxicam, 200 mg once a day, or piroxicam, 20 mg once a day, for 28 days. Fecal blood loss (FBL) was quantitated by the ^{51}Cr-labeled erythrocyte method. FBLs for both isoxicam and piroxicam were only slightly higher than baseline for the first 3 drug dosing days, confirming the results of a previously published 4-day study of piroxicam, but FBL subsequently steadily increased, with maxima occurring for most subjects receiving isoxicam in 2 or 3 weeks and for most subjects receiving piroxicam in 3 or 4 weeks. This implies that dosing for 7 days or less, as is frequent in FBL studies of nonsteroidal anti-inflammatory drugs, may be insufficient to detect the peak drug-induced FBL. In week 4, FBL for both drugs was elevated approximately 0.6 ml/day over baseline. FBLs in week 4 were comparable to those reported for naproxen and less than those reported for indomethacin and acetylsalicylic acid. Statistical analyses of weekly plasma drug minimum concentrations suggest steady state was reached at week 2 for isoxicam and week 3 for piroxicam. There were large between-subject variations in steady-state plasma drug concentrations for both drugs. One subject in each drug group indulged in excessive alcohol consumption during the medication period, with a concomitant significant increase in FBL, which suggests exacerbation of the drug effect. (Clin Pharmacol Ther 1985;38:533-7.)

John W. Hooper, Ph.D., June A. Anslow, B.Sc., William S. Martin, M.D., Pedro Araujo, B.Sc., and Andrew Darke, Ph.D.
Montreal, Quebec, and Toronto, Ontario, Canada

Nonsteroidal anti-inflammatory drugs (NSAIDs) are associated with varying degrees of gastrointestinal intolerance. A new chemical class of these drugs based on the oxicam nucleus, of which piroxicam is the progenitor, has been developed. A new member of the oxicam class, isoxicam, has been extensively studied in rheumatoid arthritis and osteoarthritis.[1,2] The usually recommended doses are 200 mg/day for isoxicam[1] and 20 mg/day for piroxicam.[2] Both drugs have plasma $t_{1/2}$ values >24 hours, allowing once-daily dosing. Assessment of drug-induced fecal blood loss (FBL) by measurement of fecal radioactivity after radiolabeling of erythrocytes with chromium 51 is a common method of assessing gastrointestinal tolerance of NSAIDs.[3-9] A previous study[3] of piroxicam, 20 mg once a day, in 10 healthy subjects reported no change in FBL over baseline levels during 4 days of dosing. However, it is unlikely that steady state was reached in this time, and thus the effect of the drug on FBL may not have had time to develop.

Our objective was to compare the FBL induced by equipotent once-daily doses of isoxicam and piroxicam over a period of 28 days in healthy subjects.

METHODS

Our subjects were 16 healthy men between 18 and 40 years old ($\overline{X}$ = 24 years) and weighing between 64 and 92 kg ($\overline{X}$ = 74 kg). Pre- and posttreatment health screenings included a medical history (pretreatment only), a complete physical examination, and hematology, serum chemistry, and urinalysis evaluations. Subjects with a history or current evidence of cardiovascular, hepatic, renal, allergic, or significant gastrointestinal disease, including hemorrhoids, spontaneous nosebleeds, gingival disease, or any other gastrointestinal bleeding disorder; who smoked >4 cigarettes a day; who used excessive seasoning; or who had used any prescription or over-the-counter drug in the 14 days before the study were excluded. Subjects were prohibited from taking medication other than isoxicam or piroxicam and from using excessive seasoning. Dental flossing was prohibited and subjects were provided with

From Bio-Research Laboratories, Montreal, and Warner Lambert, Toronto.
Received for publication June 6, 1984; accepted June 10, 1985.
Reprint requests to: John W. Hooper, Vice-President, Scientific Affairs, Bio-Research Laboratories, 87 Senneville Rd., Montreal, Quebec H9X 3R3, Canada.

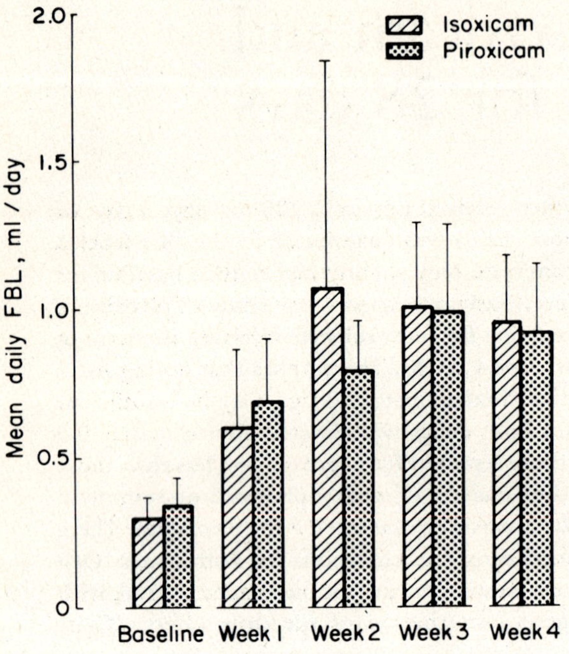

Fig. 1. Mean (±SD) daily FBL in subjects receiving isoxicam or piroxicam.

a soft toothbrush and instructed to use only this instrument, to minimize the possibility of self-induced gum bleeding. Because there is evidence that excessive consumption of alcohol exacerbates drug-induced FBL with acetylsalicylic acid (ASA),[6] subjects were instructed to avoid alcohol and in any event to limit their intake to no more than 2 to 3 drinks on no more than 2 to 3 occasions per week.

Labeling of erythrocytes was achieved through the drawing of 25 ml blood, the addition of 200 μCi USP sodium chromate Cr-51 injection solution by standard techniques, and the reinjection of the labeled blood. After 11 drug-free days (baseline period) subjects were randomly assigned to therapy with isoxicam, 200 mg once a day, or piroxicam, 20 mg once a day, for 28 days. The daily dose was to be taken with breakfast. Feces, free of urine contamination, were collected daily throughout the baseline and drug dosing periods. The samples were pooled for alternating 3- and 4-day periods to smooth day-to-day variations in FBL.

Pooled fecal specimens were homogenized with paint solvent to facilitate stool disintegration, an antifoaming agent to minimize bubble formation that could produce spuriously low ^{51}Cr counts, and hydroxymethyl cellulose/ammonium hydroxide to produce a stable suspension/gel, since settling could also affect the ^{51}Cr count. Homogeneity studies on aliquots taken from the top, middle, and bottom of the left and right sides of the homogenization container for two clinical samples gave results within ±5% of each other (95% confidence). Stability data on the same samples indicated no significant change in ^{51}Cr counts, adjusted for radioactive decay, over a period of 16 days. To maximize counting efficiency for the anticipated low counts at the end of the study, a counter with a large crystal and well diameter was used for counting duplicate 30 ml aliquots of the homogenized samples. The counter was surrounded with lead shielding to minimize background counts (20 to 24 cpm) and thus to increase sensitivity. Calibration and quality control samples were run with each batch of study samples. Counting was conducted for a minimum of 10 minutes and until at least 750 counts had accumulated. Blood samples were collected at regular intervals and counted for ^{51}Cr, and erythrocyte decay curves were constructed from the corrected (for radioactive decay and background) data. Blood radioactivity concentrations were calculated from these curves for the beginning of each fecal pooling period and used in the calculation of FBL for the period. For feces, counts were corrected for background count, and corrections were made for both feces and blood for ^{51}Cr decay back to the time of erythrocyte labeling with data from the daily calibration standards. Quality control samples with mean corrected counts of 36 and 136 cpm were counted with each batch of study samples. The coefficients of variation for these samples were 6.0% and 2.9%, respectively. Of the 176 fecal samples counted in the study, 72% had (corrected) counts >36 cpm and 96% had counts >20 cpm.

To assess compliance, subjects completed drug diaries and pill counts were conducted. To assess compliance further and to estimate when steady state was reached, blood samples were collected for drug level determinations at the end of the baseline period and just before drug dosing on the last day of each week. Blood samples were centrifuged as soon as possible after collection and the resulting plasma samples were stored at −15° ± 3° C pending HPLC analysis. For analysis, plasma samples were diluted with acetonitrile containing the internal standard indomethacin and centrifuged to remove precipitated proteins. The supernatant was chromatographed on a μ-Bondapak CN column (Waters Associates, Inc.) with a mixture of pH 4.0 aqueous acetate buffer (65%) and acetonitrile (35%) as the mobile phase. Isoxicam and piroxicam were quantitated by peak height ratios to the internal standard with ultraviolet detection at 352 nm. A plasma blank, six or seven standards (0.2 to 8.0 μg/ml for

Table I. Mean FBL (ml/day)

	Subject No.	*Baseline*	*Wk 1*	*Wk 2*	*Wk 3*	*Wk 4*
Isoxicam	1	0.30	0.36	0.50	1.06	(4.36)
	2	0.25	0.58	0.81	1.27	0.90
	4	0.31	0.89	2.86	0.80	0.94
	6	0.27	0.55	0.88	1.04	0.71
	9	0.27	0.44	0.66	0.92	0.88
	10	0.41	1.07	1.21	0.99	1.15
	12	0.41	0.64	1.23	1.49	1.35
	15	0.20	0.29	0.45	0.57	0.80
$\bar{X} \pm SD$		0.30 ±0.07	0.60 ±0.26	1.08* ±0.78	1.02* ±0.28	0.96† ±0.22
Piroxicam	3	0.36	0.99	1.02	1.15	1.17
	5	0.51	0.69	0.92	1.39	0.82
	7	0.35	0.51	0.62	0.90	0.73
	8	0.28	0.56	0.91	1.14	1.24
	11	0.28	0.93	0.74	0.82	0.86
	13	(0.54)	(0.61)	(3.87)	(0.91)	(1.30)
	14	0.28	0.51	0.58	0.56	0.70
	16	(1.23)	(1.99)	(0.72)	(13.64)	(1.15)
$\bar{X} \pm SD$		0.34 ±0.09	0.70† ±0.21	0.80† ±0.18	0.99* ±0.29	0.92* ±0.23

Numbers in parentheses are not included in the determination of the mean or in the statistical analyses (see text).
*Significantly different from baseline ($P < 0.01$) and from week 1 ($P < 0.05$).
†Significantly different ($P < 0.01$) from baseline.

piroxicam and 1.0 to 20.0 μg/ml for isoxicam), and two quality control samples were run with each batch of study samples.

Data for the 3- and 4-day fecal pooling periods in each week were combined and the mean daily FBLs during each week were evaluated for differences between drug groups within weeks and for differences between weeks within drug groups by the SAS general linear models repeated-measures test. Significant differences ($P < 0.05$) were examined by two-way ANOVA and Duncan's multiple range test.

RESULTS

All 16 subjects completed the study and all blood and fecal samples were successfully counted for ^{51}Cr. Mean (±SD) daily FBLs for the two drug groups are shown in Table I and Fig. 1. Data for the baseline period exclude the first 4 days after erythrocyte labeling, because biliary excretion of free ^{51}Cr or slow gastrointestinal transit times could have affected the values for this period. Subject 16 (taking piroxicam) had a mean daily FBL of 1.23 ml in the baseline period (compared with 0.32 ± 0.08 ml for the other 15 subjects) and FBL "spikes" throughout the study, suggestive of a preexisting gastrointestinal tract lesion. This subject was excluded from the evaluation. Subject 13 (taking piroxicam) admitted to several episodes of "excessive" alcohol consumption and subject 1 (taking isoxicam) also drank alcohol to excess 5 days before the end of the study. Because excessive alcohol consumption could exacerbate drug-induced FBL, data for the entire study for subject 13, and those for the last week of the study for subject 1, were excluded from the determinations of the means and the statistical analyses.

Differences between drug regimens in each week were not significant, but most of the means during the dosing period were significantly higher than those at baseline (Table I). The mean FBLs for weeks 2 and 3 for isoxicam and for weeks 3 and 4 for piroxicam were higher than those in week 1. There were no significant differences among weeks 2, 3, and 4 for either drug.

Mean (±SD) minimum plasma steady-state drug concentrations at the end of each week are listed in Table II. For the isoxicam group the only significant difference was between weeks 1 and 3. For piroxicam, plasma concentrations for weeks 2, 3, and 4 were all higher than those at the end of week 1. Those at the end of weeks 3 and 4 were also higher than those at the end of week 2. There was considerable between-subject variation in steady-state plasma concentrations within drug groups, with threefold differences for piroxicam and sixfold differences for isoxicam in week 4

Table II. Mean (+SD) minimum plasma concentrations (mg/ml)

	Pretreatment	*End of wk 1*	*End of wk 2*	*End of wk 3*	*End of wk 4*
Isoxicam (n = 8)	0.0	31.3 ± 12.9	37.5 ± 15.4	40.7 ± 18.2*	38.6 ± 20.5
Piroxicam (n = 8)	0.0	3.85 ± 1.31	4.81 ± 1.82*	5.54 ± 1.68†	6.09 ± 2.33†

*Significantly higher ($P < 0.05$) than week 1.
†Significantly higher ($P < 0.05$) than weeks 1 and 2.

Table III. Daily FBL

Drug and study	*Daily dose (mg)*	*Duration of dosing (days)*	*No. of subjects*	*Mean FBL at end of study (ml/day)*
Isoxicam*	200	28	7	0.96
Piroxicam*	20	28	6	0.92
Piroxicam[1]	20	4	10	0.23
Piroxicam[1]	40	4	9	0.21
Ibuprofen[2]	900	5	3	0.86
Indoprofen[2]	600	5	4	1.11
Tolmetin[3]	1200	4-6	10	1.2
Indomethacin[3]	200	4-6	10	2.1
Diflunisal[4]	500	5	5	0.48
Oxaprozin[5]	1200	14	10	2.3
Fenoprofen[6]	2400	7	14	2.2
Naproxen[7]	750	14	6	1.09
ASA (uncoated)[5]	3900	14	11	8.8
ASA (uncoated)†	3900	10	11	7.41
ASA (coated)†	3900	8	10	3.26

*This study.
†Bio-Research Laboratories: Unpublished data, 1983.

between the highest and the lowest concentrations. Except for subject 4 in the isoxicam group, whose plasma concentrations declined steadily over the course of the 4 weeks, plasma concentration data revealed no evidence of poor subject compliance with the dosing regimen. However, pill counts, drug diaries, and close questioning of subject 4 failed to provide any other evidence of noncompliance for this (or any other) subject, and thus this subject's data were included in the statistical evaluations.

Adverse experiences judged possibly drug related were limited to stomach cramps and diarrhea for 6 days during week 2 for subject 4 (taking isoxicam), a "dull stomach ache" in the week after excessive alcohol consumption for subject 1 (taking isoxicam), stomach cramps on the last day of the study for subject 16 (taking piroxicam), and "red blood in the stool" reported on several occasions by subject 13 (taking piroxicam). Abnormalities after the study consisted of very slight elevations in BUN in two subjects in each drug group (nos. 1, 6, 8, 11), a mildly elevated SGPT for subject 12 (taking isoxicam), and mildly elevated SGOT, SGPT, and lactate dehydrogenase levels for subject 3 (taking piroxicam). Most abnormal laboratory values returned to normal 8 days after the end of therapy and all were normal after a further 17 days.

DISCUSSION

After 3 days of drug therapy, the mean (±SD) increases in FBL over baseline for isoxicam and piroxicam were 0.07 ± 0.12 and 0.17 ± 0.20 ml/day. This confirms the findings of Bianchine et al.[3] that piroxicam induces no significant change in FBL over a 4-day dosing period. However, in our study FBL steadily increased after the initial 3-day period, reaching a mean plateau of approximately 1.0 ml/day for both drugs with maximal FBL during weeks 2 or 3 for seven of the eight subjects receiving isoxicam and during weeks 3 or 4 for five of the six subjects receiving piroxicam. Results of statistical analyses of the plasma concentration data suggest that steady state was reached during week 2 for isoxicam and week 3 for piroxicam. It seems possible that the effect of NSAIDs on FBL could be at least partially systemically mediated, and thus the time of maximal FBL we report could be partially dependent on the time steady-state levels were reached. Nevertheless, our results suggest that dosing periods of 7 days or less, as have been used in many studies of FBL induced by NSAIDs with shorter $t_{1/2}$ values, may have been inadequate to detect maximal FBL. This tends to be corroborated by data from FBL studies of both coated and uncoated ASA formulations (3.9 gm/day) performed in our laboratory in which, with methods essentially identical to that described above, FBL was on the average still rising on the last day of an 8-day study.

Isoxicam and piroxicam induced similar and minimal increases in FBL. These results are compared in Table III, with some representative data from the literature for other NSAIDs and with data from ASA studies carried out in our laboratory. The FBL induced by isoxicam and piroxicam in week 4 was of the order of that induced by naproxen in 14 days and less than that induced by indomethacin in 4 to 6 days and by ASA in 8 to 14 days. Meaningful comparisons with the FBL induced by the other drugs in Table III are difficult because of the possibility that their short duration may have underestimated the true FBL.

Isoxicam and piroxicam were well tolerated, and the minor elevations in BUN and liver enzymes levels we saw have been reported with the oxicam and other classes of NSAIDs. Both subjects who indulged in excessive alcohol consumption (nos. 1 and 13, one taking isoxicam and one taking piroxicam) had rises in FBL averaging 5 to 6 ml/day over the following 3- or 4-day period. For subject 1 (taking isoxicam) the rise in FBL was accompanied by an intermittent dull stomach ache for 7 days. This suggests that the exacerbating effect of excessive alcohol consumption on ASA-induced FBL[6] may well extend to the other intrinsically less ''irritating'' drugs of this class.

References

1. Downie WW, Gluckman MI, Ziehmer BA, Boyle JA. Isoxicam. Clin Rheum Dis 1984;10:385-99.
2. Physicians Desk Reference, ed 39. Oradel, NJ: Medical Economics Company, Inc, 1985.
3. Bianchine JR, Procter RR, Thomas FB. Piroxicam, aspirin and gastrointestinal blood loss. CLIN PHARMACOL THER 1982;32:247.
4. Porro GB, Corvi G, Fucella LM, Goldaniga GC, Valzelli G. Gastrointestinal blood loss during administration of indoprofen, aspirin and ibuprofen. J Int Med Res 1977;5:155.
5. Beirne JA, Bianchine JR, Johnson PC, Wortham GF. Gastrointestinal blood loss caused by tolmetin, aspirin and indomethacin. CLIN PHARMACOL THER 1975;16:821.
6. Deschepper PJ, Tjandrarraga TB, De Room M, Verhaest L, Daurio C, Steelman SL, Tempero KF. Gastrointestinal blood loss after diflunisal and after aspirin: effect of alcohol. CLIN PHARMACOL THER 1978;23:669.
7. Lussier A, LeBel E, Tetrault L. Gastrointestinal blood loss of oxaprozin and aspirin with placebo control. J Clin Pharmacol 1982;22:173.
8. Loebl DH, Craig RM, Culic DD, Ridolfo AS, Falk J, Schmid FR. Effect of aspirin, fenoprofen and acetaminophen in rheumatoid arthritis as determined by sequential gastroscopy and radioactive fecal markers. JAMA 1977;237:976.
9. Lussier A, Arsenault A, Varady J. Gastrointestinal microbleeding after aspirin and naproxen. CLIN PHARMACOL THER 1978;23:402.

Determinants of systemic availability of oral hydralazine in heart failure

Short-term therapy with oral hydralazine can favorably affect abnormal hemodynamics in patients with congestive heart failure, but the range of dosage is large. To investigate whether this variability in effective dose is a result of altered systemic availability, we studied 10 patients with congestive heart failure. Bioavailability (F) was calculated as the ratio of the blood AUC for a single 75 mg oral dose to the AUC of a 0.3 mg/kg iv dose. Acetylation capability was determined by sulfamethazine metabolic clearance (CL_{smz}). The F value in six subjects with CL_{smz} >100 ml/min was 9.9% ± 6.0% ($\bar{X}$ ± SD) and was lower than the value of 26.2% ± 13.0% ($P < 0.05$) in the four patients with CL_{smz} <60 ml/min. Thus acetylation ability is an important consideration during low-dose hydralazine therapy (≤225 mg/day). The clearance of the single intravenous dose of hydralazine averaged 29.5 ± 8.0 ml/min/kg, which is not different than that reported in populations without heart failure. After oral dosage titration to induce maximum hemodynamic changes, the dose-normalized hydralazine AUC rose from 53.5 ± 50.5 to 247.2 ± 213.4 min/L × 10^3. Thus large oral doses of hydralazine result in disproportionate increases in systemic availability compatible with saturation of the first-pass effect or systemic clearance. In the doses required for maximum hemodynamic effects in our patients (225 to 3000 mg/day), this saturation phenomenon was a prominent determinant of systemic availability. (Clin Pharmacol Ther 38:538-543, 1985.)

Michael H. Crawford, M.D., Thomas M. Ludden, Ph.D., and Gemma T. Kennedy, M.S.N. *San Antonio and Austin, Tex.*

Pharmacologically induced afterload reduction is regarded as a valuable option in the therapy of patients with congestive heart failure. Studies with oral hydralazine have demonstrated beneficial hemodynamic effects in congestive heart failure, but the effective dosage range has been wide (150 to 3000 mg/day).[14,15] This large dosage range has obstructed clinical use of this drug. Several explanations for the variability in effective dose are possible. First, bioavailability may be altered in patients with organ congestion due to heart failure. Hydralazine is extensively metabolized by the liver and intestinal wall after oral dosing. A major pathway for hydralazine metabolism is acetylation, which is genetically determined.[17,19,20] People can usually be divided into rapid or slow acetylator phenotypes, but information about the importance of acetylator phenotype in determining hydralazine dosage in congestive heart failure is not available. Vascular congestion of the viscera may lead to malabsorption of hydralazine in patients with congestive heart failure. There may also be alterations in the formation of hydralazine hydrazones in the systemic circulation of patients with congestive heart failure. It therefore seems likely that congestive heart failure could result in altered plasma concentrations of hydralazine, which may lead to variability in dosing.

The second possibility for the wide effective dosage range of oral hydralazine in congestive heart failure is alterations in vascular responsiveness or other undefined changes in pharmacodynamics. There are currently no techniques for measuring hydralazine pharmacodynamics in patients with congestive heart failure, but altered pharmacokinetics can be readily investigated. Accordingly, our purpose was to evaluate the systemic availability of oral hydralazine in patients with congestive heart disease.

METHODS

Our subjects were 10 men 49 to 70 years old ($\bar{X}$ = 60 years) with chronic congestive heart failure who were

From the Departments of Medicine and Pharmacology, University of Texas Health Science Center and Veterans Administration Hospital, San Antonio, and College of Pharmacy, University of Texas, Austin.

Supported by a grant-in-aid from The American Heart Association (Texas affiliate) and National Institutes of Health Grant No. RR-01346 to the General Clinical Research Center.

Received for publication Dec. 4, 1984; accepted June 17, 1985.

Reprint requests to: Michael H. Crawford, M.D., Department of Medicine, University of Texas Health Science Center, 7703 Floyd Curl Dr., San Antonio, TX 78284.

being considered for vasodilator therapy because they remained symptomatic (New York Heart Association class III) while receiving therapeutic serum levels of digoxin (range 0.8 to 1.7 ng/ml) and large doses of furosemide (>200 mg/day). Patients with evidence of hepatic impairment after serum chemistry analysis and those with more than mild renal functional abnormalities were excluded. Serum creatinine levels ranged from 0.8 to 2.7 mg/dl and BUN levels ranged from 15 to 36 mg/dl. The diagnosis was primary cardiomyopathy in three patients, ischemic heart disease in six, and hypertensive heart disease in one. None had primary valvular heart disease.

Subjects were admitted to the Special Diagnosis and Treatment Unit and were interviewed by a dietition to estimate the sodium content of their usual diet. This diet was maintained in the hospital, as was the dose of digoxin and diuretics they had been taking before the study. Subjects were observed for 3 or more days while following their usual regimen to ensure that their weights were stable, that they had therapeutic digoxin levels, that their serum potassium level was normal, and that they were not having arrhythmias. On the first study day acetylation ability was assessed by determining the metabolic clearance of oral sulfamethazine. This was accomplished by administering sulfamethazine, 10 mg/kg po, and drawing blood samples before and 0.5, 1, 1.5, 2, 3, 4, 6, 8, 12, 16, 20, and 24 hours after the dose. Each sample was assayed for sulfamethazine and *N*-acetyl sulfamethazine by the method of Olson et al.[13] A twenty-four hour urine sample was also assayed for sulfamethazine and its acetyl derivative to determine renal clearances. Sulfamethazine total clearance was estimated as the dose administered divided by the plasma AUC. Renal clearance was calculated as amount excreted in 24 hours divided by the corresponding AUC. Apparent metabolic clearance (CL_{smz}) was calculated as total clearance minus renal clearance. The low dose of sulfamethazine (10 mg/kg) was used to minimize the influence of factors causing its nonlinear kinetic behavior.[3]

On the second and third study days indocyanine green (ICG), 0.5 mg/kg iv, was injected and blood samples were drawn at 2, 5, 8, 10, 12, and 15 minutes after dosing and were assayed spectrophotometrically for ICG content. Clearance of ICG was estimated by dividing the intravenous dose by the AUC extrapolated to infinity. Clearance of ICG was used as an index of hepatic blood flow.

After the determination of ICG clearance, hydralazine was either injected intravenously (0.3 mg/kg over 100 seconds) or taken by mouth (75 mg tablet). The sequence of intravenous and oral hydralazine dosing was randomized between days 2 and 3. Blood samples were drawn 2, 5, 10, 15, 20, 30, 45, 60, 75, 90, 105, 120, 150, 180, 210, and 240 minutes after hydralazine dosing. The samples were assayed for hydralazine by a specific HPLC technique.[8]

On the fourth study day a balloon-tipped, flow-directed right heart catheter was inserted percutaneously into the pulmonary artery to measure pulmonary artery and right atrial pressures and to determine cardiac output by the thermodilution technique. After control measurements, oral hydralazine dosing began, progressively increasing in dose every 8 hours according to the following schedule: 75, 100, 150, 225, 300, 400, 550, 750, and 1000 mg. During the course of therapeutic hydralazine dosing, heart rate and systemic blood pressure (cuff sphygmomanometer) were determined as necessary for optimal patient care, but heart rate, blood pressure, pulmonary artery pressure and cardiac output were also determined for purposes of our study every 8 hours just before the next hydralazine dose. The hydralazine dose was not increased further if cardiac output did not rise >10% compared with the last determination and if the pulmonary artery wedge pressure was <18 mm Hg. Four subjects met the latter criterion and five achieved the maximum dose of hydralazine. One subject did not complete the study because the initial 75 mg oral dose of hydralazine induced angina pectoris. Thus only initial bioavailability data is available on this subject (no. 6).

Subsequently, the pulmonary artery catheter was removed and the subjects were stabilized on their final dose of hydralazine for at least three dosing intervals (24 hours). In three subjects this dosage stabilizing period required a decrease in the maximum dose of hydralazine because of gastrointestinal side effects. The furosemide dose in all subjects had to be reduced during hydralazine dosing because of marked diuresis. The digoxin dose was kept constant in all subjects. On the final study day ICG clearance was measured and the hydralazine AUC was determined after the final dose.

The hydralazine blood concentration-time data after intravenous injection were fit to equations describing two- and three-compartment open kinetic models with zero-order input into and first-order elimination from the central compartment.[5,6] Curve fitting was by the nonlinear regression analysis program NONLIN[12] with iteration of physiologic kinetic parameters, i.e., clearances and volumes. Each data point was weighted by the reciprocal of the concentration squared. The appro-

Table I. Hydralazine pharmacokinetics

Subject No.	CL_{smz} (ml/min)	CL_{hyd} (ml/min/kg)	V_{ss} (L/kg)	$t_{1/2}$ (min)	F (%)	Dose-normalized AUC (min/L × 10^3) Initial	Dose-normalized AUC (min/L × 10^3) Final	ICG Clearance (ml/min) Initial	ICG Clearance (ml/min) Final
1	239	37.9	2.060	158	2.4	5.1	10.2	632	667
2	54	25.6	0.656	102	12.2	47.4	303.0	403	471
3	224	26.1	0.912	135	8.2	27.9	115.0	322	255
4	22	21.6	0.797	102	28.7	139.0	443.0	276	532
5	106	40.5	2.470	89	19.8	30.8	200.0	182	260
6	10	36.5	0.766	57	42.9	—	—	1166	—
7	116	37.9	2.030	112	13.4	31.6	370.0	100	100
8	110	17.7	0.442	94	9.2	39.7	100.0	283	366
9	220	26.4	0.904	109	6.6	18.8	31.6	720	1281
10	42	25.1	2.380	241	21.0	141.0	652.0	228	198
$\overline{X}$	114.3	29.5	1.340	105*	16.4	53.5	247.2	305	459
SD	86.4	8.0	0.791		12.1	50.5	213.4	233	356

CL_{hyd} = Clearance of hydralazine; V_{ss} = volume of distribution at steady state.
*Harmonic mean.

priate model for each data set was determined according to the criteria of Boxenbaum et al.[1] The three-compartment model was found to be appropriate for nine of the 10 subjects. Hydralazine clearance was related to ICG clearance to determine if hepatic blood flow influenced the former.

The blood AUC after oral dosing was determined by the trapezoid method and corrected to time infinity. For pharmacokinetic calculations the AUC value was corrected for the predose concentration, even though this resulted in <5% difference in AUC values. The fraction of dose that was bioavailable (F) was calculated as the ratio of the AUC for the single 75 mg oral dose to the AUC for the 0.3 mg/kg iv dose with correction for differences in dose size. F was compared between rapid and slow acetylator phenotypes to determine if the relationship to phenotype was preserved in patients with heart failure. The AUCs for the single 75 mg oral dose and the final oral dose of hydralazine were normalized for dose and compared to determine the effects of multiple dosing on systemic availability.

All right heart pressures were recorded. Mean pulmonary artery wedge and right atrial pressures were obtained from the phasic waveforms. Mean aortic pressure was estimated by adding the cuff sphygmomanometer–derived systolic pressure to twice the diastolic pressure and dividing this sum by 3. Systemic vascular resistance was estimated by subtracting the mean right atrial pressure from the mean aortic pressure, dividing by the cardiac output, and multiplying by the correction factor 80, to convert mm Hg · min/L to dyne · sec/cm.[5]

Statistical comparison between control values and those after hydralazine dosing were analyzed by Student's paired t tests. All values are expressed as the $\overline{X}$ ± SD. Correlations were performed by linear regression analysis (Pearson's method).

RESULTS

Initial pharmacokinetic studies (Table I). CL_{smz} ranged from 10 to 239 ml/min ($\overline{X}$ = 114.3 ± 86.4 ml/min). Six subjects had values >100 ml/min and in the remaining four subjects the CL_{smz} was <60 ml/min. The clearance of a single intravenous dose of hydralazine averaged 29.5 ± 8.0 ml/min/kg (range 17.7 to 40.5 ml/min/kg). The corresponding steady-state volume of distribution was 1.34 ± 0.791 L/kg and the terminal $t_{1/2}$ was 105 minutes (range 57 to 241 minutes).

Hydralazine F ranged from 2.4% to 42.9% ($\overline{X}$ = 16.4% ± 12.1%) and was exponentially related to CL_{smz} (Fig. 1). The value of 9.9% ± 6.0% in the six subjects with CL_{smz} >100 ml/min was lower ($P < 0.05$) than the value of 26.2% ± 13.0% in the four subjects with CL_{smz} <60 ml/min. Thus the bioavailability of a small oral dose (75 mg) was influenced by acetylation ability in these subjects with heart failure.

ICG clearance before intravenous hydralazine averaged 329 ± 208 ml/min and the value before the first oral dose was 305 ± 233 ml/min. These two control values (days 2 and 3) did not differ significantly. ICG clearance was not related to hydralazine clearance ($r = -0.07$).

Effects of multiple doses. The AUC for the final dose

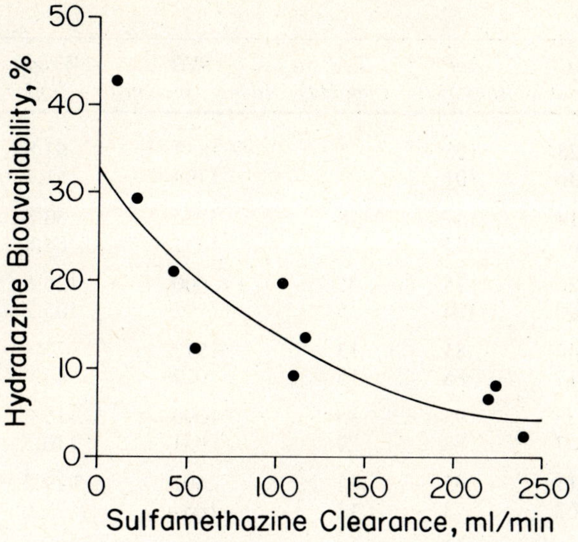

Fig. 1. Hydralazine bioavailability is exponentially related to CL_{smz} (r = 0.88).

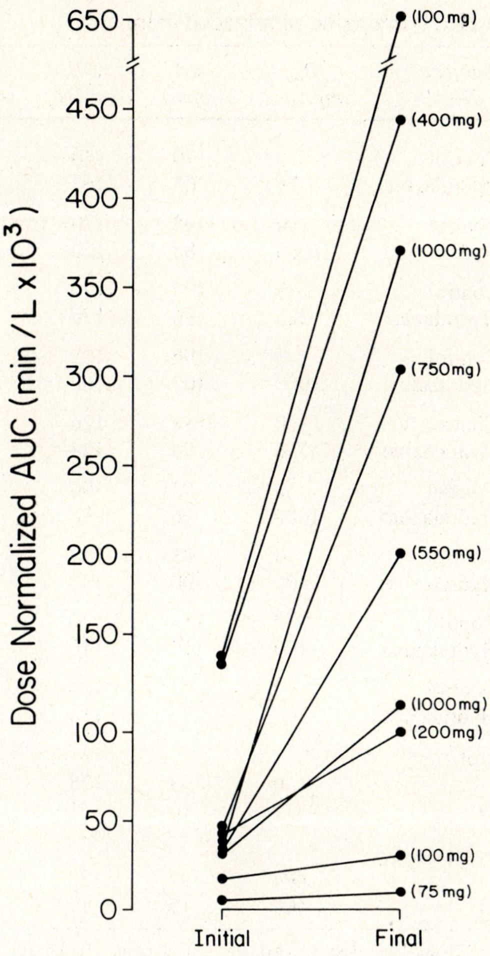

Fig. 2. Dose-normalized AUC after the first and final oral doses of hydralazine in each subject.

of hydralazine was always larger than the AUC derived from the first dose of drug; this phenomenon persisted when the AUCs were normalized for dose (Fig. 2). Thus the AUC increased out of proportion to the dose. ICG clearance rose to 459 ± 356 ml/min, which was not significantly different from either control value. Thus changes in hepatic blood flow do not explain the marked increases in AUC after multiple dosing.

The maximum hemodynamic effect occurred at hydralazine doses of 75 to 1000 mg t.i.d. ($\overline{X}$ = 494 mg every 8 hours; Table II). Heart rate, systolic blood pressure, and mean aortic pressure did not change at the maximum dose as compared with control. Pulmonary artery wedge pressure fell from a control value of 30 ± 11 to 22 ± 10 mm Hg ($P < 0.005$) and cardiac output rose from 4.03 ± 1.50 to 5.60 ± 1.90 L/min ($P < 0.005$). Systemic vascular resistance fell from 1846 ± 839 to 1202 ± 385 dyne · sec/cm^5 ($P < 0.05$). These hemodynamic changes were accompanied by diuresis in all subjects, resulting in a decrease in weight from 86.9 ± 23.0 to 79.1 ± 19.8 kg on the last day of the study ($P < 0.01$). Thus oral hydralazine was effective short-term therapy for these subjects with congestive heart failure.

DISCUSSION

The mean blood clearance value we measured after a single intravenous dose of hydralazine was somewhat lower than that found in patients with hypertension of a similar age who did not have heart failure.[9,10] Bioavailability was higher in our slow acetylators than in the rapid acetylators, but was of the order of that reported in the group of patients with hypertension studied by Shepperd et al.[18] Therefore, bioavailability is related to acetylation ability at the modest oral dose used for this determination, but because bioavailability is not markedly different and systemic clearance is only somewhat less than that found in patients with hypertension, it would appear that congestive heart failure per se has only a modest total effect on hydralazine concentrations after a single small oral dose.

The disproportionate rise in the dose-normalized AUC from the first to the final oral doses of hydralazine suggests that there is saturation of the first-pass effect or of systemic clearance. However, an influence on absorption cannot be excluded. Another question that arises is whether multiple dosing alone increases AUC. No such evidence of this phenomenon was observed in patients with hypertension, but they were given the same dose on many occasions.[18] In our study multiple dosing involved increasing doses; therefore, it is dif-

Table II. Hydralazine pharmacodynamics

Subject No.	D_{max} (mg t.i.d.)	HR (bpm)	SBP (mm Hg)	PAWP (mm Hg)	CO (L/min)	AoP (mm Hg)	RAP (mm Hg)	SVR (dyne · sec/cm⁵)	Weight (kg)
1 Control	0	70	140	16	4.28	103	5	1832	63.8
Hydralazine	75	65	162	11	4.36	101	2	1798	61.2
2 Control	0	108	170	47	3.14	137	8	3286	80.8
Hydralazine	1000	88	120	29	5.01	93	7	1381	68.8
3 Control	0	104	120	34	7.20	75	21	600	126.6
Hydralazine	225	96	136	18	9.90	104	6	792	105.2
4 Control	0	106	108	35	3.47	81	13	1579	75.4
Hydralazine	1000	103	108	32	6.14	85	15	912	64.7
5 Control	0	88	126	45	4.38	95	35	1096	116.0
Hydralazine	550	94	124	42	5.07	88	29	931	110.3
7 Control	0	92	100	28	2.11	85	14	2692	79.2
Hydralazine	1000	96	98	24	4.63	73	12	1054	72.6
8 Control	0	83	148	27	4.27	107	17	1686	85.3
Hydralazine	400	100	130	17	5.59	97	10	1245	80.2
9 Control	0	114	120	22	4.73	93	12	1370	98.2
Hydralazine	100	110	110	13	6.74	82	6	902	94.3
10 Control	0	72	124	17	2.73	88	4	2476	56.5
Hydralazine	100	72	114	15	3.15	81	10	1803	54.9
Control									
$\overline{X}$	0	93	128	30	4.03	96	12	1846	86.9
SD		16	21	11	1.50	18	10	839	23.0
Hydralazine									
$\overline{X}$	494	92	122	22*	5.60*	89	10†	1202†	79.1‡
SD	409	15	19	10	1.90	10	9	385	19.8

D_{max} = Hydralazine dose at maximum hemodynamic effects; HR = heart rate; SBP = systolic blood pressure; PAWP = pulmonary artery wedge pressure; CO = cardiac output; AoP = mean aortic pressure; RAP = mean right atrial pressure; SVR = systemic vascular resistance.
*P < 0.005, †P < 0.05, ‡P < 0.01 compared with control value.

ficult to assess the role of multiple dosing. However, one subject (no. 1) whose initial and final dose was the same (75 mg) did have an increase in the AUC, from 2.0 to 3.9 mol/min. Therefore, we cannot exclude this possibility based on our study.

Packer et al.[14] noted in their 45 patients with congestive heart failure who were taking hydralazine that those requiring >100 mg/day had higher mean right atrial pressures than those who responded to a smaller dose. One interpretation is that liver congestion and reduced hepatic blood flow may be important in the increased dosage requirements of some patients. Several studies have shown that renal blood flow is increased by hydralazine in patients with congestive heart failure, but the effects on hepatic blood flow have been more variable.[2,7,11] There were similar results when hepatic blood flow increased in some of our patients, but the increase was small and overall there was no significant change in hepatic blood flow during hydralazine therapy. Also, no relationship was found between ICG and hydralazine clearances. Therefore, the small changes in hepatic blood flow observed in some patients do not explain the marked increases in AUC during therapy as compared with the potential effects of saturation of the first-pass phenomenon or of systemic clearance.

Our results may have implications for the long-term therapy of patients with congestive heart failure. If low doses of hydralazine are used to avoid the development of the side effect of a systemic lupus erythematosus–like state, rapid acetylators may receive inadequate therapy. This may explain why a recent randomized, double-blind, placebo-controlled, multicenter trial of hydralazine, 200 mg/day, found no significant improvement in patients with chronic congestive heart failure after an average follow-up of 20 weeks.[4] When large oral doses are required for therapeutic effect, acetylator phenotype is of less consequence, as is supported by the disproportionate increases in hydralazine concentrations in our study. Despite this increase in concentration, the maximum short-term response to hydralazine occurred at an average dosage of 494 mg every 8 hours, with five subjects requiring a dosage of 1000 mg every 8 hours. Thus increased dosage requirements in some patients with congestive heart failure may be due to alterations in pharmacodynamics rather than alterations in pharmacokinetics. With the realization that high doses may be required for maximum pharmacologic effects, the dose of hydralazine must be based on individual patient responses. However, the frequency of the systemic lupus erythematosus reaction increases with dosage and duration of exposure to hydralazine, appearing in up to 20% of patients receiving ≥400 mg/day.[16] Because this drug was very effective in all our subjects, short-term high-dose oral hydralazine therapy should be considered in patients with congestive heart failure who do not respond to other drugs.

The advice of John L. McNay, M.D., and Robert A. O'Rourke, M.D., are greatly appreciated. The nursing and dietetic care provided by the staff of the Audie Murphy Memorial Veterans Administration Hospital Special Diagnosis and Treatment Unit (General Clinical Research Center) is also appreciated.

References

1. Boxenbaum HG, Reigelman S, Elashoff RM: Statistical estimations of pharmacokinetics. J Pharmacokinet Biopharm **2**:123-148, 1974.
2. Cogan JJ, Humphreys MH, Carlson CJ, Rapaport E: Renal effects of nitroprusside and hydralazine in patients with congestive heart failure. Circulation **61**:316-322, 1980.
3. duSouich P, Lalka D, Slaughter R, Elvin AT, McLean AJ: Mechanisms of nonlinear disposition kinetics of sulfamethazine. CLIN PHARMACOL THER **25**:172-182, 1979.
4. Franciosa JA, Weber KT, Levine B, Kinasewitz GT, Janicki JS, West J, Henis MMJ, Cohn JN: Hydralazine in the long-term treatment of chronic heart failure: Lack of difference from placebo. Am Heart J **104**:587-594, 1982.
5. Gibaldi M, Perrier D: Pharmacokinetics. New York, 1975, Marcel Dekker, Inc.
6. Kramer WG, Lewis RG, Cobb TC, Forester WF, Visconti JA, Wonke LA, Boxenbaum HG, Reuning RH: Pharmacokinetics of digoxin: Comparison of a two and three compartmental model in man. J Pharmacokinet Biopharm **2**:299-321, 1974.
7. Leier CV, Magorien RD, Desch CE, Thompson MJ, Unverferth DV: Hydralazine and isosorbide dinitrate: Comparative central and regional hemodynamic effects when administered alone or in combination. Circulation **63**:102-109, 1981.
8. Ludden TM, Ludden LK, Wade KE, Allerheiligen SRB: Determination of hydralazine in human whole blood. J Pharm Sci **72**:693-695, 1983.
9. Ludden TM, Shepherd AMM, McNay JL, Lin MS: Effect of intravenous dose on hydralazine kinetics after administration. CLIN PHARMACOL THER **34**:148-152, 1983.
10. Ludden TM, Shepherd AMM, McNay JL, Lin MS: Hydralazine kinetics in hypertensive patients after intravenous administration. CLIN PHARMACOL THER **28**:736-742, 1980.
11. Magorien RD, Triffon DW, Desch CE, Bay WH, Unverferth DV, Leier CV: Prazosin and hydralazine in congestive heart failure. Ann Intern Med **95**:5-13, 1981.
12. Metzler CM, Elfring GL, McEwen AJ: A users manual for NONLIN and associated programs. Kalamazoo, Mich, 1974, The Upjohn Co.
13. Olsen W, Miceli J, Weber W: Dose-dependent changes in sulfamethazine kinetics in rapid and slow isoniazid acetylators. CLIN PHARMACOL THER **23**:204-211, 1978.
14. Packer M, Meller J, Medina N, Gorlin R, Herman MV: Dose requirements of hydralazine in patients with severe chronic congestive heart failure. Am J Cardiol **45**:655-660, 1980.
15. Packer M, Meller J, Medina N, Gorlin R, Herman MV: Importance of left ventricular chamber size in determining the response to hydralazine in severe chronic heart failure. N Engl J Med **303**:250-255, 1980.
16. Perry HM Jr: Late toxicity to hydralazine resembling systemic lupus erythematosus or rheumatoid arthritis. Am J Med **54**:58-72, 1973.
17. Reidenberg MM, Drayer D, DeMarco AL, Bello CT: Hydralazine elimination in man. CLIN PHARMACOL THER **14**:970-977, 1973.
18. Shepherd AMM, Ludden TM, McNay JL, Lin MS: Hydralazine kinetics after single and repeated oral doses. CLIN PHARMACOL THER **28**:804-811, 1980.
19. Talseth T: Studies on hydralazine. III. Bioavailability of hydralazine in man. Eur J Clin Pharmacol **10**:395-401, 1976.
20. Zacest R, Koch-Weser J: Relation of hydralazine plasma concentration to dosage and hypotensive action. CLIN PHARMACOL THER **13**:420-425, 1972.

Assessment of dezocine for morphine-like subjective effects and miosis

Dezocine is an analgesic soon to be marketed in the United States. In this study we examined the abuse potential of dezocine. Subjective and miotic effects of single subcutaneous doses of dezocine, morphine, and placebo were assessed under double-blind conditions in 10 adult male nondependent drug abusers. Dezocine and morphine were equipotent in inducing a constellation of effects typical of opioid agonists, including miosis and increases in opioid signs and symptoms, liking, and euphoria. Both drugs were consistently identified by subjects as being "dope" (opiates). Thus the profile of effects of single doses of dezocine indicate that the drug has the potential to be abused. However, the agonist-antagonist activities of dezocine demonstrated by others suggest that its abuse potential is less than that of morphine. (CLIN PHARMACOL THER 38:544-548, 1985.)

Donald R. Jasinski, M.D., and Kenzie L. Preston, Ph.D. *Baltimore, Md.*

Dezocine (Wy-16,225) is a bridged aminotetralin classed as a mixed agonist-antagonist opioid. In man dezocine is equipotent or slightly more potent than morphine in inducing analgesia.[1,3] This drug will soon be marketed as an injectable analgesic in the United States.

The dependence potential of dezocine has been studied in monkeys, with conflicting results. Initially, Malis et al.[9] concluded that dezocine differed from narcotic analgesics such as morphine in that it lacked physical dependence liability and, therefore, might also lack addiction liability in man. No physical dependence resulted from chronic administration, nor did dezocine suppress abstinence in monkeys exhibiting morphine withdrawal.[9] Subsequently, however, studies involving behavioral pharmacologic techniques demonstrated that dezocine had morphine-like stimulus and reinforcing properties in nondependent monkeys.[11,13] These studies suggest that dezocine does have the potential to be abused.

To assess the abuse potential of dezocine, we evaluated its ability to produce miosis and morphine-like subjective effects and euphoria in an addict population.

METHODS

Subjects were male federal prisoners with long-term histories of opiate abuse. At the time of our studies they were incarcerated at the Addiction Research Center at Lexington, Ky., and were not physically dependent on opiates. Subjects were in good health with no serious psychiatric disorders, either past or present, other than their opiate abuse.

Drugs were weighed as the salts; dezocine hydrobromide was dissolved in water and morphine sulfate was dissolved in normal saline solution. Doses were administered in a constant volume of 2 ml. Two milliliters of normal saline solution served as the placebo.

Ten subjects were each given the six following treatments under double-blind conditions: dezocine hydrobromide (15, 30, and 60 mg), morphine sulfate (15 and 30 mg), and placebo. Drugs were administered subcutaneously in random order at weekly intervals.

Miosis, subjective effects, and euphoria were measured by standard procedures.[5] Pupils were photographed at 0.5 and 1 hour before and at 0.5, 1, 2, 3, 4, 5, 6 and 12 hours after drug dosing. At the same intervals after dosing subjects completed the single-dose questionnaire and a questionnaire containing items from the Morphine-Benzedrine Group (MBG) to measure euphoria, the Pentobarbital-Chlorpromazine-Alcohol Group (PCAG) to measure apathetic sedation, and the Lysergic acid diethylamide–Specific Group (LSD) to measure dysphoria. At the same times that subjects completed questionnaires, trained observers recorded the behavioral effects of the test drugs by completing an observer version of the single-dose questionnaire for opiate signs and liking.

RESULTS

Both morphine and dezocine constricted pupils and produced increased responses on the MBG (euphoria), opiate signs and symptoms, and liking scales. Com-

From the Department of Health and Human Services, Public Health Service, Alcohol, Drug Abuse and Mental Health Administration, National Institute on Drug Abuse Addiction Research Center.
Received for publication March 14, 1985; accepted June 17, 1985.
Reprint requests to: Donald R. Jasinski, M.D., NIDA Addiction Research Center, P. O. Box 5180, Baltimore, MD 21224.

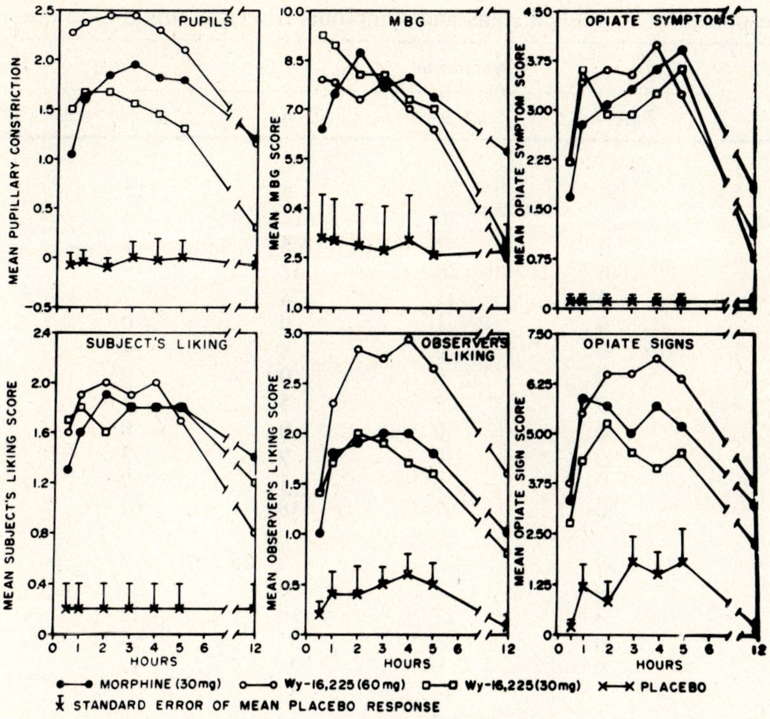

Fig. 1. Time action curves for the comparison of dezocine *(Wy-16,225)*, morphine, and placebo. For pupils, each *point* represents the mean change in pupil diameter from predrug control. For signs and symptoms, liking, and MBG scales, each *point* represents the mean response. The responses to 15 mg morphine and 15 mg dezocine were omitted.

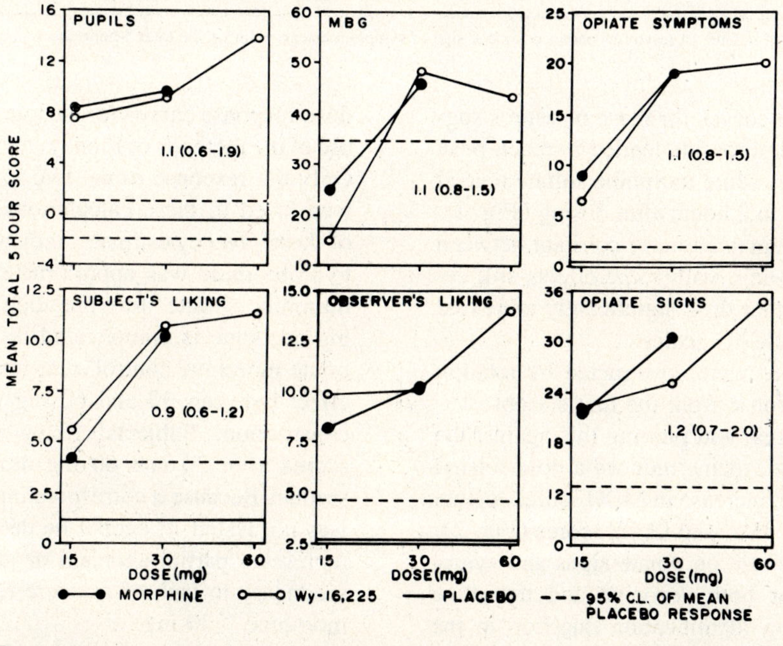

Fig. 2. Dose-response curves from 10 subjects for the comparison of dezocine *(Wy-16,225)*, morphine, and placebo. For pupils, each *point* represents the mean total 5-hour change in diameter from predrug control. For signs and symptoms, liking, and MBG scales, each *point* represents mean total 5-hour scores. *Numbers* represent relative potencies and 95% confidence limits expressed as milligrams of dezocine equivalent to 1 mg morphine.

Table I. Cumulative responses of individual signs and symptoms from the single-dose questionnaire*

		Morphine		*Dezocine*		
	Placebo	*15 mg*	*30 mg*	*15 mg*	*30 mg*	*60 mg*
Opiate symptoms						
Normal	54	26	5	15	8	3
Turning of stomach	0	20	22	3	10	15
Skin itchy	0	7	28	9	26	27
Relaxed	6	20	32	19	40	31
Coasting	0	11	28	7	29	31
Soap box	0	1	0	0	6	0
Pleasant sick	0	0	8	4	2	11
Drive	0	0	0	0	1	2
Sleepy	0	3	5	1	3	0
Drunk	0	0	0	0	0	0
Nervous	0	9	9	3	11	11
Other	0	0	1	2	0	11
Total	60	97	138	63	136	142
Opiate signs						
Normal	39	5	2	3	0	2
Scratching	9	27	48	37	39	55
Red eyes	3	27	30	12	19	38
Relaxed	20	55	57	57	60	56
Coasting	9	9	24	12	21	27
Soap box	1	30	33	27	22	30
Vomiting	0	3	4	1	2	11
Nodding	0	1	0	2	0	2
Sleepy	8	2	5	5	8	5
Nervous	0	9	13	6	10	8
Drunk	1	1	3	1	1	7
Other	4	22	17	19	11	26
Total	94	191	236	182	193	267

*Each value represents the total number of responses obtained for that sign or symptom category during the total 5-hour observation period (maximum = 60).

parisons of time-action curves for these measures suggest that dezocine hydrobromide tended to reach peak effects in 0.5 to 1 hour, while morphine sulfate tended to reach peak effects 1 to 2 hours after dosing (Fig. 1). Effects of both drugs remained fairly constant between 1 and 5 hours after dosing, with some effects still evident at 12 hours. Neither drug significantly increased scores on the LSD or PCAG scales.

Dose-response curves were constructed by totaling and averaging the response from the first six observations (total 5-hour scores) and plotting this against the dose. Like morphine, dezocine induced a dose-related miosis and dose-related increase in MBG scores, opiate signs and symptoms scores, and liking scores (Fig. 2).

The profiles of response on opiate signs and symptoms were similar for both dezocine and morphine (Table I). On the drug identification question in the single-dose questionnaire, dezocine was consistently identified as an opiate (''dope'') by both subjects and observers (Table II).

Relative potencies (Fig. 2) were calculated from dose-response curves for the total 5-hour responses with use of the methods of Finney[2] for parallel line bioassays. Only the response to the two lower doses of dezocine were used in these calculations. The geometric mean of these potency estimates indicated that 1 mg dezocine hydrobromide was approximately equivalent to 1 mg morphine sulfate. Interpretation of the response to 60 mg dezocine is complicated by the lack of an appropriate morphine control. Our results showed no ceiling effect between 30 and 60 mg dezocine for pupillary constriction. Subjects' liking and opiate symptoms scores after 30 and 60 mg dezocine, however, were similar. Because a corresponding 60 mg morphine dose was not tested, it cannot be determined if this plateau represents partial agonism or an experimental artifact secondary to lack of measure responsivity to doses of morphine >30 mg.

DISCUSSION

In our subjects, single doses of subcutaneous dezocine induced a typical morphine-like profile of effects.

Table II. Cumulative drug identifications from the single-dose questionnaire*

Identification	Placebo	Morphine 15 mg	Morphine 30 mg	Dezocine 15 mg	Dezocine 30 mg	Dezocine 60 mg
By subjects						
Blank	54	27	3	28	8	3
Dope	0	27	54	23	43	44
Cocaine	6	6	0	0	0	0
Marijuana	0	0	0	0	0	6
Meprobamate	0	0	0	4	0	0
Other	0	0	3	6	3	13
By observers						
Blank	39	5	2	3	0	2
Dope	21	55	58	57	60	55
Cocaine	0	0	0	0	0	0
Other	0	0	5	2	3	0

*Each value represents the total number of responses obtained for that drug category during the total 5-hour observation period (maximum = 60). Barbiturate, alcohol, amphetamine, LSD, or chlorpromazine HCl identifications were not reported by subjects or observers.

Dezocine constricted pupils, produced morphine-like signs and symptoms, and increased scores on the MBG (euphoria) scale. Subjects liked dezocine and identified the drug as an opiate. Dezocine and morphine were approximately equipotent in inducing miosis and euphoria. Dezocine, however, had a more rapid onset and a shorter duration of action than morphine.

This profile of effects for single doses of dezocine in substance abusers is unlike that of agonist-antagonists such as nalorphine, cyclazocine, and pentazocine. Under similar conditions these drugs are not identified as opiates, induce a profile of symptoms and signs different from those of morphine, and induce increased LSD and PCAG scores.[5,6]

Findings in both animals and man indicate that dezocine is an opioid agonist/antagonist that can induce morphine-like agonist effects under certain experimental conditions. At therapeutic doses, dezocine is equipotent or slightly more potent than morphine in inducing analgesia and respiratory depression in man.[1,3] In drug discrimination paradigms, dezocine induced morphine-like stimulus effects in monkeys.[11,13] These results are compatible with our findings that dezocine and morphine were equipotent in inducing miosis and morphine-like subjective effects in an addict population.

In our opinion, the observation that dezocine is a euphoriant with a profile of subjective effects similar to that of morphine in substance abusers indicates that the drug has the potential to be abused.[7,8] The antagonist activity,[9] limited respiratory depressant activity,[3,10] and the lack of physical dependence capacity[4,9,12] in animals suggests that the abuse potential of dezocine may be less than that of morphine-like agonists.

References

1. Downing JW, Brock-Utne JG, Barclay A, Schwegmann IL: WY-16225 (dezocine), a new synthetic opiate agonist-antagonist and potent analgesic: Comparison with morphine for relief of pain after lower abdominal surgery. Br J Anaesth **53**:59-64, 1981.
2. Finney DK: Statistical method in biological assay, ed 2. New York, 1964, Hofner Publishing Company.
3. Gal TJ, Difazio CA: Ventilatory and analgesic effects of dezocine in man. Anesthesiology **61**:716-722, 1984.
4. Greenberg R, Ippersiel R: Lack of dependence liability of dezocine (WY-16225) in the myenteric plexus-longitudinal muscle strip of the guinea pig ileum. *In* Way EL, editor: Endogenous and exogenous opiate agonists and antagonists. Elmsford, NY, 1980, Pergamon Press, pp 505-508.
5. Jasinski, DR: Assessment of the abuse potential of morphine-like drugs (methods used in man). *In* Martin WR, editor: Handbook of experimental pharmacology, vol 45/1. Heidelberg, West Germany, 1977, Springer-Verlag, pp 197-258.
6. Jasinski DR: Human pharmacology of narcotic antagonists. Br J Pharmacol **7**:287s-290s, 1979.
7. Jasinski DR, Johnson RE, Henningfield JE: Abuse liability assessment in human subjects. Trends Pharmacol Sci **5**:196-200, 1984.
8. Jasinski DR, Pevnick JS, Griffith JD: Human pharmacology and abuse potential of the analgesic buprenorphine: A potential agent for treating narcotic addiction. Arch Gen Psychiatr **35**:501-516, 1978.
9. Malis JL, Rosenthale MR, Gluckman MI: Animal pharmacology of WY-16225, a new analgesic agent. J Pharmacol Exp Ther **194**:488-498, 1975.
10. Romagnoli A, Keats AS: Ceiling respiratory depression by dezocine. CLIN PHARMACOL THER **35**:367-373, 1984.
11. Schaefer GJ, Holtman SG: Morphine-like stimulus ef-

fects in the monkey: Opioids with antagonist properties. Pharmacol Biochem Behav **14:**241-245, 1981.

12. Swaine HH, Seevers MH: Addendum 1. *In* Report of the Committee on Problems of Drug Dependence, Thirty-sixth meeting, Mexico City, D.F., March 10-14, 1974, pp 27-28.

13. Young AM, Stephens KR, Hein DW, Woods JH: Reinforcing and discriminative stimulus properties of mixed agonist-antagonist opioids. J Pharmacol Exp Ther **229:**118-126, 1984.

Prilocaine in arthroscopy: Clinical pharmacokinetics and rational use

Prilocaine pharmacokinetics were determined in 60 patients receiving the drug by two different routes of administration (intra-articular and subcutaneous) during arthroscopy under local anesthesia with controlled pressure irrigation. Resorption of prilocaine by subcutaneous tissues was slow and did not lead to high serum levels. On the contrary, prilocaine resorption by the synovium was fast and induced a sharp serum peak (265.8 ± 163.5 ng/ml) in the hour after the end of the examination. The drug was completely eliminated from the blood after 24 hours, as the prilocaine $t_{1/2}$ is about 5 hours. The first procedure was perfected to reduce the risk of methemoglobinemia, which occurred in four of 105 patients. Applied pressure was lowered to 100 mm Hg to prevent the escape of anesthetic solution into the soft tissue of the leg, the prilocaine concentration was reduced to 1 gm/L, and the arthroscope was only set up after a delay to allow the intra-articular anesthetic effect of prilocaine to become established. So far, 200 arthroscopies have been performed with this improved protocol without any problem. (Clin Pharmacol Ther 38:549-553, 1985.)

Danièle Debruyne, D.Chem., Maurice Moulin, M.D., Claude Thomassin, M.D., Bruno Locker, M.D., Jack Tartiere, M.D., Marie-Claire Bigot, B.S., Michel Besnard, M.D., Catherine Berthelin, M.D., and Jacques Beguin, M.D.
Caen, France

For some years we have used arthroscopy as a diagnostic or surgical technique,[3] first under general anesthesia, then under local anesthesia, and now under local anesthesia with controlled pressure irrigation. This study was initially designed to investigate the pharmacokinetics of prilocaine for 24 hours after dosing in 60 patients undergoing arthroscopy according to the anesthesia procedure of Wredmark and Lundh.[13] As methemoglobinemia occurred in four of 105 patients clinically examined (including the 60 subjects undergoing pharmacokinetic study), the procedure was perfected to avoid these systemic accidents. Serum levels and pharmacokinetics were then determined in 10 patients. The reliability of the new improved method has so far been tested in 200 patients.

METHODS

Seventy patients (21 women and 49 men; mean [±SD] age 29.3 ± 13.4 years [only six patients were >50 years old]) with symptoms of internal derangement of the knee were examined with an arthroscope (4 mm in diameter) under local anesthesia through the use of controlled pressure irrigation. No patient had hepatic or renal insufficiency.

According to the first anesthesia procedure A, upon admission to the operating room, patients (n = 43) were given subcutaneous injections of prilocaine with epinephrine (either 100, 150, 200, or 300 mg as directed by the physician) around the spots of introduction of the surgical instruments at the arthroscopic site. Ten to fifteen minutes later, at time = 0, a continuous pressure irrigation system connected to an arthroscope was set up and 1 or 2 L of isotonic saline solution with 2 gm/L prilocaine flowed through the knee joint throughout the examination under a constant applied pressure of approximately 150 mm Hg. For the pharmacokinetic study, some patients (n = 12) received subcutaneous injections of lidocaine and an irrigation of prilocaine and others (n = 5) were given subcutaneous injections of prilocaine and an irrigation of isotonic saline solution. Patients received hydroxyzine and atropine sulfate 1 hour before the examination, and during the operation diazepam or fentanyl were given when required to quiet the patient and allay anxiety or to relieve pain.

According to our second improved procedure B, patients (n = 10) were first given a subcutaneous injec-

From the Laboratory of Pharmacology, Department of Anaesthesia, and Units of Orthopaedia B and Rhumatology, University Hospital Center of Caen.

Received for publication Feb. 26, 1985; accepted June 19, 1985.

Reprint requests to: Danièle Debruyne, Laboratory of Pharmacology, University Hospital Center of Caen, 14032 Caen CEDEX, France.

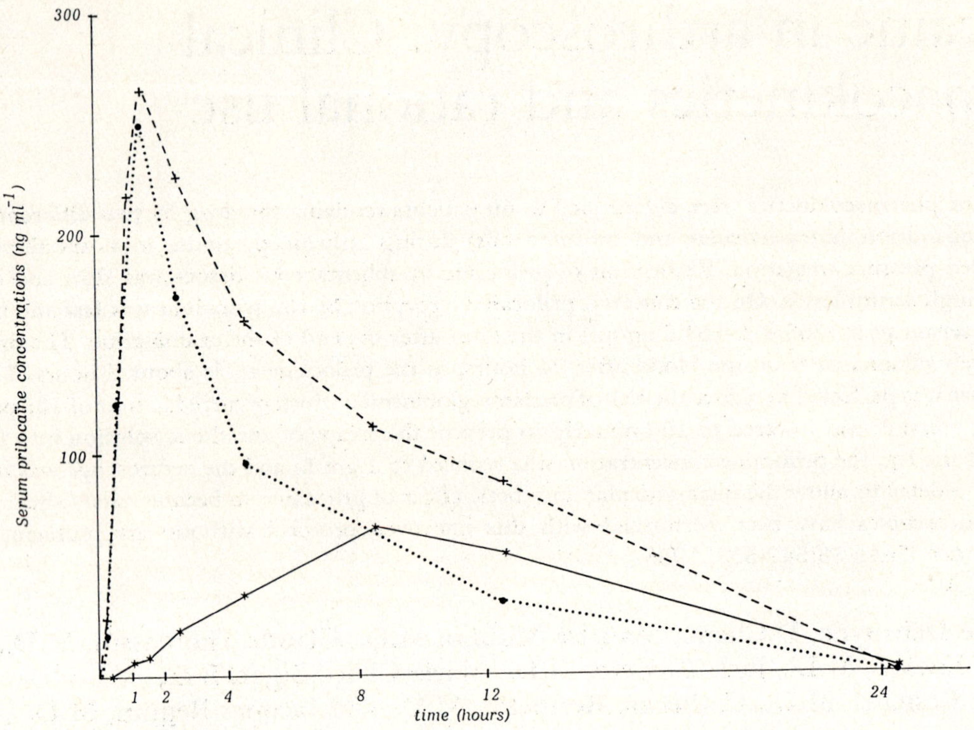

Fig. 1. Mean serum prilocaine concentration-time curve in patients given prilocaine by subcutaneous injection and irrigation (+), irrigation alone (●), and subcutaneous injection alone (*) for arthroscopy (procedure A).

Table I. Mean serum concentrations in 10 patients given a subcutaneous injection of lidocaine followed by irrigation with 1 gm prilocaine over 30 minutes (procedure B)

Time after start of irrigation (hr)	*Prilocaine serum levels (ng/ml)*	*Lidocaine serum levels (ng/ml)*
0.08	19.8 ± 27.4	49.4 ± 38.6
0.25	28.0 ± 32.5	62.2 ± 38.1
0.50	53.3 ± 84.0	85.8 ± 58.0
1	137.1 ± 220.2	140.6 ± 117.2
2	167.5 ± 148.3	164.7 ± 121.0
4	94.7 ± 61.3	146.0 ± 86.7
8	46.6 ± 31.4	145.9 ± 104.2
12	32.9 ± 22.9	146.7 ± 109.5
24	ND	73.5 ± 47.3

Data are $\overline{X}$ ± SD.
ND = Not detectable.

tion of 1% lidocaine with epinephrine (100 mg) at the arthroscopic site. Then 100 to 150 ml isotonic saline solution with 1 gm/L prilocaine were introduced into the knee joint cavity with a long needle (18-gauge) connected to the pressure system to distend the knee. The arthroscope was set up only when both superficial and deep anesthesia were considered to be sufficient (after 10 to 15 minutes). The prilocaine solution within the joint was evacuated when it was too soiled and replaced by a clean anesthetic solution. This exchange was performed as often as required. The total volume of 1 gm/L prilocaine solution used in this procedure was 1 L. The pressure irrigation system was set at a pressure of only 100 mm Hg. Additional subcutaneous injections (50 mg) of lidocaine were given when more surgical instruments were introduced. No premedication was given before patients entered the operating ward and no sedative or analgesic was required during arthroscopy.

Blood samples were drawn 5, 15, and 30 minutes after the start of irrigation, at the end of irrigation, and 0.5, 1, 2, 4, 8, 12 and 24 hours thereafter. All samples were immediately centrifuged and serum samples were frozen until analyzed. The intensity of analgesia was scored as none (0), low (1), moderate (2), good (3), and excellent (4).

Serum prilocaine and lidocaine were assayed by gas chromatography. The drugs were extracted with chloroform in phosphate buffer (pH 11) from a 500 μl serum

Table II. Pharmacokinetic parameters for prilocaine in patients undergoing arthroscopy

	Procedure A			*Procedure B (intra-articular instillation)*
	Subcutaneous injection	*Intra-articular irrigation*	*Subcutaneous injection and intra-articular irrigation*	
$t_{1/2}$ (hr) from 2 to 3 hr	—	2.18 ± 1.65	3.17 ± 3.13	2.33 ± 0.74
$t_{1/2}$ (hr) from 9 to 15 hr	7.50 ± 3.12	5.32 ± 4.06	4.69 ± 2.84	5.66 ± 4.05
k_a (hr^{-1})	0.33 ± 0.14	2.57 ± 2.17	2.17 ± 0.97	0.88 ± 0.41
t_{max} (hr)	7.61 ± 1.99	1.22 ± 0.41	1.43 ± 0.54	1.96 ± 0.78
t_{lag} (hr)	1.89 ± 1.30	0.29 ± 0.13	0.30 ± 0.16	0.20 ± 0.22
$AUC_{(0\rightarrow24)}$(ng/ml · hr)	864 ± 807	1411 ± 974	2638 ± 1516	1159 ± 790

Data are $\overline{X}$ ± SD.
k_a = Absorption constant; t_{max} = time to maximum concentration; t_{lag} = lag time.

sample spiked with procaine as internal standard. After mixing and centrifugation, an aliquot (5 μl) of the organic layer was injected into the chromatograph under the following conditions: solid injector temperature, 275° C; methylsilicone fused silica capillary column (25 m × 0.31 mm) temperature, 200° C; nitrogen-selective detector temperature, 290° C; and carrier gas (nitrogen U) pressure, 5.6 psig.

The apparent $t_{1/2}$ values were calculated by linear-log regression analysis of data from 2 to 3 and from 9 to 15 hours after the start of irrigation. Pharmacokinetic parameters for each patient were calculated according to Gibaldi and Perrier.[7] The prilocaine plasma AUC was determined by the trapezoidal rule during the period 0 to 24 hours. Results are expressed as the $\overline{X}$ ± SD. Data were analyzed by Student's t test and linear regression analysis was performed to evaluate the correlation between various parameters. A value of $P < 0.05$ was considered statistically significant.

RESULTS

Fig. 1 illustrates the serum prilocaine concentration-time profiles of patients who were given this anesthetic by subcutaneous injection (n = 5), by irrigation (n = 12), and by both subcutaneous injection and irrigation (n = 39) during arthroscopy of mean duration 0.69 ± 0.30 hour according to procedure A. Four patients whose serum concentrations produced toxic symptoms were not included in the calculation of the average.

Serum levels determined in 10 patients receiving 1 L isotonic saline solution with 1 gm prilocaine during a 0.5-hour arthroscopy after a subcutaneous injection of lidocaine (procedure B) are listed in Table I. Table II groups together the calculated pharmacokinetic parameters. The AUC(0-24) did not correlate with age, weight, duration of irrigation, or intensity of anesthesia. There was no appreciable difference between the AUC(0-24) in men and women. The maximum concentrations observed with procedure A (265.8 ± 163.5 ng/ml) were significantly higher than those (167.5 ± 148.3 ng/ml) observed with procedure B. The side effect related to high serum prilocaine levels in four patients who experienced accidental subcutaneous escape of irrigating solution during arthroscopy are listed in Table III.

DISCUSSION

At first arthroscopies were performed according to Wredmark and Lundh (procedure A). Our objectives were to determine the time of complete elimination of prilocaine from systemic circulation, to distinguish between the drug fraction absorbed by the synovium from that drained by the subcutaneous tissues, and to calculate the pharmacokinetics for the two resorption routes. As these routes were inbricated in 39 patients, data fitting to a two-compartment model was not effected. Apparent $t_{1/2}$ values were then determined to compare prilocaine elimination in the different conditions.

For most patients prilocaine was not detectable in the serum after 24 hours. Moreover, in the five patients from whom blood samples were also drawn at 10, 13, 16, and 19 hours, no drug was found at 19 hours (all cases) or at 16 hours (three cases). The resorption of prilocaine administered by the subcutaneous route was slow and did not lead to high serum levels. On the contrary, prilocaine was rapidly resorbed by the synovium and there was a sharp serum peak.

The exchanges across the synovial membrane are ensured by a number of physical mechanisms such as diffusion, filtration, and lymphatic drainage. They depend on the chemical properties of the drugs (lipophilia, pKa, protein binding) and such complex physiologic conditions as the degree of inflammation of the joint.[12] Thus drug absorption from the synovium varies

Table III. Side effects and serum levels of prilocaine in four patients with accidental subcutaneous escape of irrigating solution during arthroscopy

Patient No.	*Sex/age (yr)*	*Symptoms*	*Associated factors*	*Prilocaine serum levels (ng/ml)*	*Methemoglobinemia*
1	F/17	Pallor Cyanosed lips, hands, and feet (4 hr)	Small subcutaneous escape of anesthetic solution into the leg during irrigation	825.4 (0 hr) 923.7 (1 hr) 1256.9 (2 hr) 870.0 (4 hr) 262.0 (8 hr) 167.0 (12 hr) 0 (24 hr)	0% (4 hr) 0% (12 hr)
2	F/16	Pallor Cyanosed lips, hands, and feet resistant to oxygen (4 hr)	Discrete subcutaneous escape of prilocaine	1251.9 (4 hr) 132.1 (20 hr)	<5% (4 hr) 0% (20 hr)
3	F/36	Generalized tingling, slight drowsiness (1.5 hr) Cyanosed lips, nails, livid face (2 hr)	Considerable escape of anesthetic filtering in anterior side of thigh	975.9 (0 hr) 2293.6 (0.5 hr) 2800.4 (1 hr) 1910.1 (2 hr) 473.4 (4 hr) 233.5 (8 hr) 77.8 (12 hr) 0 (24 hr)	30% (2.5 hr) 28% (4 hr) 23% (8 hr) 0% (12 hr)
4	F/26	Cyanosed hands and lips (3.5 hr)	Subcutaneous escape of anesthetic solution	334.5 (8 hr) 202.5 (10 hr)	15% (3.5 hr) 12% (8 hr) 0% (10 hr)

The time after the end of irrigation is given in parentheses.

and pharmacokinetics must be determined for each drug.[5]

The serum levels obtained when both routes were used concomitantly were the sum of the serum levels obtained when the two routes were used separately. Apart from the first peak at a mean time of 1.4 hour corresponding to maximal synovial absorption, a second distinct peak was also observed in nine patients at a mean time of 5 hours (group of 43 patients with procedure A). This second peak probably corresponds to the absorption of the previous subcutaneous injection. In addition, a third peak was recorded in five patients. This was believed to be caused by movement of the patient after the examination (articular movement may provoke increased absorption by systemic circulation).

Procedure A was used in 105 patients. When the operating cloth was removed, four patients exhibited temporary distension of the leg, a sign of the accidental subcutaneous escape of irrigating solution into the periarticular soft tissues. During the following 4 hours these patients presented symptoms such as cyanosis and pallor. Prilocaine was presumed to be responsible for these side effects, which were associated with high serum prilocaine levels and have been reported previously.[1,6,11] The *O*-toluidine compound, which is an intermediate in the metabolism of prilocaine, is regarded as the real entity responsible for methemoglobinemia.[8] We therefore decided to modify the anesthesia procedure to avoid such accidents and at the same time to improve patient comfort. First, subcutaneous lidocaine, which has a short delay in action,[4] was injected in place of prilocaine and the prilocaine concentration in the irrigating solution was reduced to 1 gm/L. Despite the fact that the toxicity observed in procedure A was certainly not related to the subcutaneous administration of prilocaine, it was preferable in our opinion not to overload prilocaine levels with delayed subcutaneous absorption. Second, the pressure applied to the irrigation system was lowered to 100 mm Hg to lessen the risk of subcutaneous escape of anesthetic solution. It should be pointed out that sufficient pressure must be maintained to give the following four benefits: better visualization because of increased distention; improved endurance especially at the end of examination; more effective and swift washing; and opposition to bleeding (pressure higher than blood pressure). At the same time the anesthetic must be added to irrigating solution such that patients are able to endure the applied pressure. We continued to use prilocaine because of its rapid elimination.[2] Finally, prilocaine was administered in the knee

Treatment	*Evolution*
Oxygen	Side effects disappeared in about 8 hr
—	Symptoms disappeared after about 9 hr
Methylene blue, 200 mg iv (2 hr), 1 gm during 1 hr (8 hr)	Complete disappearance of cyanosis (9 hr)
Methylene blue, 1 gm (8 hr)	Favorable

socket 10 to 15 minutes before setting up the arthroscope to give the intra-articular anesthesia time to become established. This improved patient comfort and made it unnecessary to give adjuvant sedatives and analgesics during the examination.

The lidocaine and prilocaine concentrations determined in 10 patients undergoing examination with anesthesia procedure B were much lower than toxic concentrations[10] while the calculated pharmacokinetic parameters were roughly the same. Using this new protocol we have so far carried out 200 arthroscopies. No toxic effects on the central nervous or cardiovascular systems[9] and no methemoglobinemia have been observed, and no patient has complained of any other symptom.

It should be noted, however, that the use of this technique (arthroscopy under local anesthesia with controlled pressure irrigation) may be limited and general anesthesia unavoidable in patients with painful knees (arthrosynovitis or osteoarthritis) and trauma of recent date requiring muscular relaxation for precise ligament testing.

We thank H. Fusibet for technical assistance.

References

1. Arens JF, Carrera AE: Methemoglobin levels following epidural anaesthesia with prilocaine for vaginal deliveries. Anesth Anal **49:**219-222, 1970.
2. Arthur GR, Scott DHT, Boyes RN, Scott DB: Pharmacokinetic and clinical pharmacological studies with mepivacaine and prilocaine. Br J Anaesth **51:**481-485, 1979.
3. Beguin JA, Heron JF, Sabathier JP, Locker B, Soucquieres G: Arthroscopie du genou. Nouv Presse Med **11:**3619-3621, 1982.
4. Benowitz NL, Meister W: Clinical pharmacokinetics of lignocaine. Clin Pharmacokinet **3:**177-201, 1978.
5. Debruyne D, Moulin MA, Carmes C, Beguin JA, Locker B: Monitoring serum bupivacaine levels during arthroscopy. Eur J Clin Pharmacol **27:**733-735, 1985.
6. Ford GR, Agnew TM: Methaemoglobinemia following prilocaine local anaesthesia. N Engl Med J **76:**104-105, 1972.
7. Gibaldi M, Perrier D: Pharmacokinetics. New York, 1976, Marcel Dekker, Inc.
8. Hjelm M, Holmdhal MH: Biochemical effects of aromatic amines. II. Cyanosis, methemoglobinemia and Heinz-body formation induced by a local anaesthetic agent (prilocaine). Acta Anaesth Scand **9:**99-104, 1965.
9. Moore DC: Local anesthetic drugs: Tissue and systemic toxicity. Acta Anaesthesiol Belg **4:**283-300, 1981.
10. Scott DB: Evaluation of the toxicity of local anaesthetic agents in man. Br J Anaesth **47:**56-60, 1975.
11. Scott DA, Owen JA, Richmond J: Methaemoglobinemia due to prilocaine. Lancet **2:**728-729, 1964.
12. Simkin PA, Nilson KL: Trans-synovial exchange of large and small molecules. Clin Rheum Dis **7:**99-129, 1981.
13. Wredmark T, Lundh R: Arthroscopy under local anaesthesia using controlled pressure-irrigation with prilocaine. J Bone Joint Surg **64:**583-585, 1982.

Effects of betaxolol, propranolol, and atenolol on isoproterenol-induced beta-adrenoceptor responses

Five healthy young men received, in a double-blind fashion, single oral doses of 10 mg betaxolol, 40 mg betaxolol, 50 mg atenolol, 40 mg propranolol, and placebo. After the dose each received serial 12-minute infusions of isoproterenol sulfate through the dose range 0.5 to 32 μg/min until the heart rate rose by 40 bpm or the subject could not tolerate the effects of the infusion. Heart rate, finger tremor, blood pressure, and forearm blood flow were measured after each infusion. Dose-response curves were constructed for the changes in these parameters with increasing doses of isoproterenol. The ascending order of potency of the drugs in preventing the changes in heart rate, finger tremor, diastolic blood pressure, forearm blood flow, and forearm vascular resistance induced by isoproterenol was placebo, 10 mg betaxolol, 50 mg atenolol, 40 mg betaxolol, and 40 mg propranolol. The ascending order of potency of the drugs in preventing the change in systolic blood pressure induced by isoproterenol was placebo, 10 mg betaxolol, 50 mg atenolol, 40 mg propranolol, and 40 mg betaxolol. Betaxolol, 10 mg, is equally cardioselective to 50 mg atenolol and at a dose of 40 mg betaxolol also exhibits cardioselectivity. (CLIN PHARMACOL THER 38:554-559, 1985.)

James G. Riddell, M.D., and Robin G. Shanks, D.Sc., M.D. *Belfast, Northern Ireland*

Betaxolol is a potent long-acting β-adrenoceptor–blocking drug that in animals is cardioselective, has weak membrane stabilizing activity, and no partial agonist activity.[3] In man, betaxolol induces a dose-dependent reduction in exercise tachycardia and has a plasma elimination $t_{1/2}$ of 24 hours.[2]

β-Adrenoceptor–blocking drugs are cardioselective if they reduce the increase in heart rate caused by the intravenous infusion of isoproterenol while having lesser effects on other β-adrenoceptor–mediated responses such as vasodilation, bronchodilation, or increase in finger termor.[1,6] In this study we compared the effect of betaxolol with atenolol, a widely used cardioselective β-blocking drug; propranolol, a noncardioselective drug; and placebo on the changes in heart rate, finger tremor, blood pressure, and forearm blood flow caused by serial 12-minute infusions of isoproterenol and on exercise-induced tachycardia.

From the Department of Therapeutics and Pharmacology, The Queen's University of Belfast.

Supported in part by Laboratoire d'Etudes et de Recherches Synthélabo.

Received for publication Nov. 24, 1984; accepted June 27, 1985.

Reprint requests to: Professor R. G. Shanks, Department of Therapeutics and Pharmacology, The Whitla Medical Building, 97 Lisburn Rd., Belfast BT9 7BL, Northern Ireland.

METHODS

At weekly intervals in a double-blind, Latin square design, five healthy men (mean age 22 ± 3.1 years; mean weight 73 ± 7.6 kg) received, on separate occasions, single oral doses of 10 and 40 mg betaxolol, 40 mg propranolol, 50 mg atenolol, and placebo. At about 8 AM after a light breakfast containing no caffeine, subjects came to the temperature-controlled room (23° to 24° C) in which the study was performed and received their doses. One hour later a slow intravenous saline solution infusion was started in a dorsal foot vein. Heart rate was monitored continuously from chest ECG leads attached to a Minigraph (Cardiac Recorders, Ltd.) and heart rate was calculated from five R-R intervals on lead II of the ECG. Blood pressure was measured as the mean of two observations with a random zero sphygmomanometer on the left arm. Systolic and diastolic blood pressures were taken as the Korotkoff phases I and V, respectively. Finger tremor was measured with a piezoelectric accelerometer taped to the dorsum of the middle phalanx of the middle finger of the left hand. The fingers and hand were outstretched horizontally in the same plane as the left forearm, which was comfortably supported to the wrist on a wooden rest. The output of the accelerometer was displayed directly through a preamplifier by a pen recorder and

Table I. Mean (±SD) values during saline solution infusion in five subjects

	Placebo	*Betaxolol, 10 mg*	*Betaxolol, 40 mg*	*Atenolol, 50 mg*	*Propranolol, 40 mg*
Heart rate (bpm)	60.2 ± 7.5	54.2 ± 7.3	50.0 ± 7.0	52.4 ± 10.1	54.0 ± 15.1
Systolic blood pressure (mm Hg)	123.8 ± 5.0	120.0 ± 9.7	114.0 ± 7.8*	115.2 ± 6.3*	109.8 ± 5.1*
Diastolic blood pressure (mm Hg)	65.6 ± 12.9	70.2 ± 13.4	70.4 ± 8.6	69.8 ± 7.1	69.6 ± 11.5
Finger tremor (arbitrary units)	84.8 ± 33.3	97.6 ± 54.4	77.6 ± 33.1	180.0 ± 44.1	71.0 ± 35.5
Forearm blood flow (ml/dl/min)	3.61 ± 1.10	2.65 ± 0.38	2.22 ± 0.23	2.67 ± 0.59	2.73 ± 0.41
Forearm vascular resistance (arbitrary units)	25.6 ± 9.2	33.4 ± 6.1	36.8 ± 2.2	32.8 ± 6.1	30.8 ± 4.1

*P < 0.05 compared with placebo.

Table II. Mean (±SD) heart rate increases (bpm) induced by isoproterenol sulfate infusion

	0.5 μg/min (n = 5)	*1.0 μg/min (n = 5)*	*2.0 μg/min (n = 4)*
Placebo	12.2 ± 7.2	20.2 ± 6.8	39.8 ± 7.5
Betaxolol, 10 mg	1.8 ± 2.7	10.4 ± 7.1*†	18.4 ± 12.9*†
Betaxolol, 40 mg	0.0 ± 3.4	6.2 ± 5.2*	8.0 ± 6.3*
Atenolol, 50 mg	4.6 ± 4.5	10.0 ± 9.3*†	12.0 ± 7.6*†
Propranolol, 40 mg	0.2 ± 4.7	0.2 ± 8.6*	1.2 ± 8.3*

*P < 0.05 compared with placebo.
†P < 0.05 compared with propranolol, 40 mg.

was also integrated and displayed on the same recorder. Tremor was measured as the sum of the integrated signal over the third minute of recording.[1] Right forearm blood flow was measured by venous occlusion plethysmography[5] with a mercury-in-rubber strain gauge. The venous cuff was inflated to 70 mm Hg for 10 seconds, then deflated for 5 seconds. Ten flow measurements were recorded and the mean was calculated.

Isoproterenol sulfate was infused at 0.5 μg/min for 12 minutes and heart rate, finger tremor, blood pressures, and forearm blood flow were determined during the final 4 minutes of the infusion. The rate of isoproterenol infusion was doubled and after a further 8 minutes the same measurements were repeated. Serial 12-minute infusions of isoproterenol were made through the range 0.5, 1.0, 2.0, 4.0, 8.0, 16.0, and 32.0 μg/min until the heart rate had increased by 40 bpm or the subject could no longer tolerate the effects of the isoproterenol. After 30 minutes of rest, the exercise heart rate was determined immediately after the subject stepped on and off a box 46 cm high, 32 steps per minute for 3 minutes.

Results are expressed as the $\overline{X}$ ± SD and were assessed by the SPSS programs for ANOVA. Because the variances were not equal, a nonparametric method was used to assess whether any differences were significant and the parametric analysis was used to suggest where the differences lay. A P value <0.05 was considered significant.

RESULTS

The mean resting heart rate, blood pressure, finger tremor, forearm blood flow, and forearm vascular resistance for the five subjects while receiving the saline solution infusion 1.5 hours after drug dosing and before the isoproterenol infusions are listed in Table I. There are no significant differences between the resting heart rate, tremor, diastolic blood pressure, forearm blood flow, and forearm vascular resistance after any drug, but the systolic blood pressure was reduced after each of the β-adrenoceptor blockers except betaxolol, 10 mg. There are no differences beween effects of the individual drugs.

The increase in heart rate induced by the infusions of isoproterenol sulfate, 0.5, 1.0, and 2.0 μg/min, are listed in Table II and the complete log dose-response curve is shown in Fig. 1. None of the drugs had a significant effect on heart rate after isoproterenol, 0.5 μg/min. All the drugs reduced the increase in heart rate after isoproterenol, 1.0 and 2.0 μg/min, but 10 mg betaxolol (10.4 ± 7.1 and 18.4 ± 12.9 bpm) and 50 mg atenolol (10.0 ± 9.3 and 12.0 ± 7.6 bpm) had significantly less effect than 40 mg propranolol (−0.2 ± 8.6 and 1.2 ± 8.3 bpm). The increasing order of potency on the dose-response curve is placebo, 10 mg betaxolol, 50 mg atenolol, 40 mg betaxolol, and 40 mg propranolol.

None of the drugs had a significant effect on the percentage increase in tremor (Table III) induced by

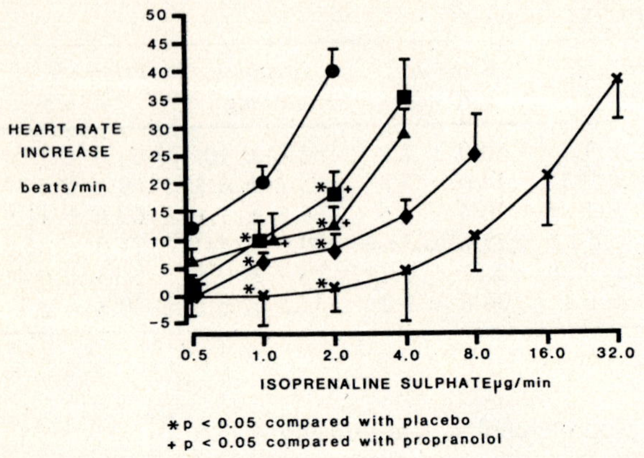

Fig. 1. Mean (±SE) effects of 10 mg betaxolol (■), 40 mg betaxolol (◆), 50 mg atenolol (▲), 40 mg propranolol (×), and placebo (●) on the increase in heart rate after serial 12-minute infusions of isoproterenol in five normal men.

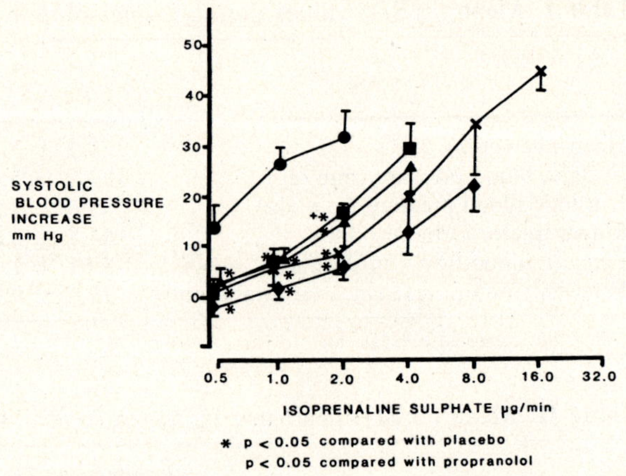

Fig. 3. Mean (±SE) effects of 10 mg betaxolol (■), 40 mg betaxolol (◆), 50 mg atenolol (▲), 40 mg propranolol (×), and placebo (●) on the increase in systolic blood pressure after serial 12-minute infusions of isoproterenol in five normal men.

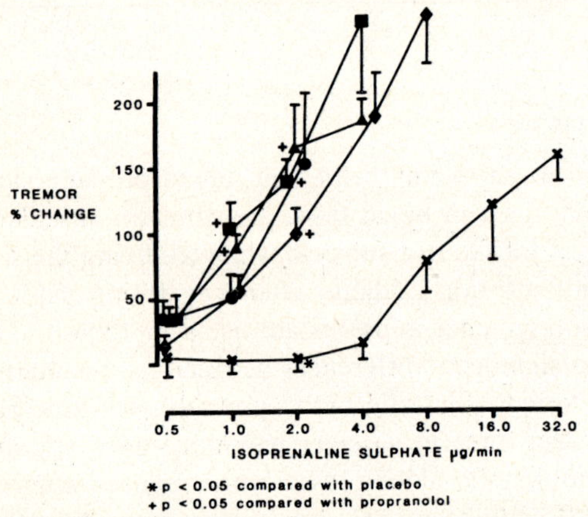

Fig. 2. Mean (±SE) effects of 10 mg betaxolol (■), 40 mg betaxolol (◆), 50 mg atenolol (▲), 40 mg propranolol (×), and placebo (●) on the percentage increase in finger tremor after serial 12-minute infusions of isoproterenol in five normal men.

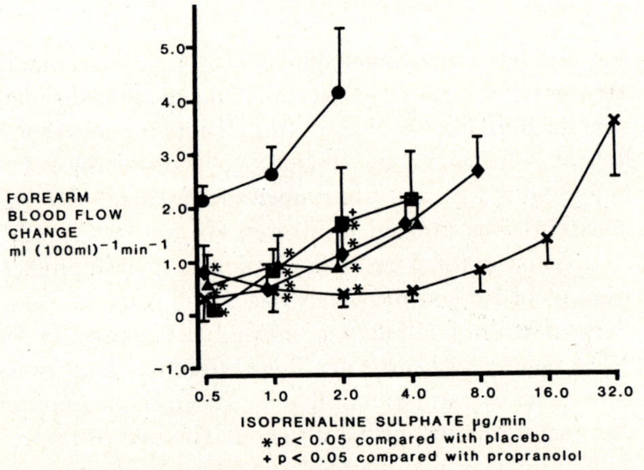

Fig. 4. Mean (±SE) effects of 10 mg betaxolol (■), 40 mg betaxolol (◆), 50 mg atenolol (▲), 40 mg propranolol (×), and placebo (●) on the increase in forearm blood flow after serial 12-minute infusions of isoproterenol in five normal men.

isoproterenol, 0.5 μg/min, but at an isoproterenol infusion rate of 1.0 μg/min 40 mg propranolol (3.6% ± 10.3%) was significantly more effective than 10 mg betaxolol (104.6% ± 42.5%) and 50 mg atenolol (88.2% ± 24.8%), which did not differ from placebo (50.4% ± 36.0%). At isoproterenol, 2.0 μg/min, 40 mg propranolol (4.6% ± 13.8%) reduced the percentage increase in tremor more than did placebo (154.3% ± 124.2%), 10 mg betaxolol (140.6% ± 37.7%), 40 mg betaxolol (98.0% ± 46.5%), and 50 mg atenolol (167.0% ± 64.5%). The effects of both doses of betaxolol and 50 mg atenolol did not differ from placebo. The full dose-response curves are shown in Fig. 2.

As shown in Table IV, all doses of all drugs reduced the increase in systolic blood pressure induced by the three isoproterenol infusions. The increase after 10 mg betaxolol (17.4 ± 4.0 mm Hg) was greater than that after 40 mg propranolol (9.0 ± 8.8 mm Hg) but did not differ from that after 50 mg atenolol (14.6 ± 9.8

Table III. Mean (±SD) percentage increases in finger tremor after isoproterenol sulfate infusion

	0.5 μg/min (n = 5)	*1.0 μg/min (n = 5)*	*2.0 μg/min (n = 4)*
Placebo	34.6 ± 32.0	50.4 ± 36.0	154.3 ± 124.2
Betaxolol, 10 mg	36.2 ± 41.3	104.6 ± 42.5*	140.6 ± 37.7*
Betaxolol, 40 mg	14.2 ± 17.7	56.2 ± 26.0	98.0 ± 46.5*
Atenolol, 50 mg	31.6 ± 27.8	88.2 ± 24.8*	167.0 ± 64.5*
Propranolol, 40 mg	5.6 ± 29.1	3.6 ± 10.3	4.6 ± 13.8†

*P < 0.05 compared with propranolol, 40 mg.
†P < 0.05 compared with placebo.

Table IV. Mean (±SD) increases in systolic blood pressure (mm Hg) induced by isoproterenol sulfate infusion

	0.5 μg/min (n = 5)	*1.0 μg/min (n = 5)*	*2.0 μg/min (n = 4)*
Placebo	13.8 ± 9.7	27.0 ± 6.4	32.0 ± 10.5
Betaxolol, 10 mg	1.8 ± 2.9*	7.2 ± 5.7*	17.4 ± 4.0*†
Betaxolol, 40 mg	−1.8 ± 2.5*	1.6 ± 4.8*	5.6 ± 4.0*
Atenolol, 50 mg	2.4 ± 6.3*	7.4 ± 5.6*	14.6 ± 9.8*
Propranolol, 40 mg	0.4 ± 1.5*	3.6 ± 5.9*	9.0 ± 8.8*

*P < 0.05 compared with placebo.
†P < 0.05 compared with propranolol, 40 mg.

Table V. Mean (±SD) decreases in diastolic blood pressure (mm Hg) induced by isoproterenol sulfate infusion

	0.5 μg/min (n = 5)	*1.0 μg/min (n = 5)*	*2.0 μg/min (n = 4)*
Placebo	21.0 ± 10.2	41.0 ± 14.5	61.8 ± 11.1
Betaxolol, 10 mg	6.8 ± 5.4	6.6 ± 3.8*	32.8 ± 24.3*†
Betaxolol, 40 mg	2.8 ± 4.6*	2.2 ± 8.8*	9.6 ± 12.8*
Atenolol, 50 mg	0.2 ± 1.9*	9.0 ± 4.9*	24.6 ± 14.6*†
Propranolol, 40 mg	−1.0 ± 1.7*	−0.8 ± 7.6*	−1.8 ± 9.7*

*P < 0.05 compared with placebo.
†P < 0.05 compared with propranolol, 40 mg.

mm Hg) at an isoproterenol infusion of 2.0 μg/min. The systolic blood pressure dose-response curves are shown in Fig. 3; the ascending order of potency is placebo, 10 mg betaxolol, 50 mg atenolol, 40 mg propranolol, and 40 mg betaxolol.

All the drugs (except 10 mg betaxolol after isoproterenol, 0.5 μg/min) significantly attenuated the fall in diastolic blood pressure induced by isoproterenol (Table V), but the fall in pressure after 10 mg betaxolol (32.8 ± 24.3 mm Hg) and 50 mg atenolol (24.6 ± 14.6 mm Hg) was greater than that after 40 mg propranolol (−1.8 ± 9.7 mm Hg) during the 2.0 μg/min infusion of isoproterenol. The dose-response curves are similar to those in Fig. 1, with the same order of potency.

Compared with placebo, all the drugs reduced the increase in forearm blood flow induced by all three infusion rates of isoproterenol (Table VI). With placebo the forearm blood flow increased from 2.13 ± 0.63 to 4.12 ± 2.38 ml/dl/min with isoproterenol, 0.5 to 2.0 μg/min. After isoproterenol, 2.0 μg/min, 10 mg betaxolol had less of an effect on the increase in forearm blood flow (1.74 ± 2.16 ml/dl/min) than 40 mg propranolol (0.37 ± 0.53 ml/dl/min). The full dose-response curves are shown in Fig. 4; the increasing order of potency is placebo, 10 mg betaxolol, 50 mg atenolol, 40 mg betaxolol, and 40 mg propranolol.

None of the drugs prevented the decrease in forearm vascular resistance (Table VII) induced by isoproterenol, 0.5 μg/min, but at 1.0 μg/min 40 mg propranolol (1.9 ± 6.2 arbitrary units [U]) was more effective than 10 mg betaxolol (8.0 ± 8.2 U), which did not differ from placebo (11.2 ± 3.4 U). At this infusion rate, 40 mg betaxolol (0.2 ± 9.1 U) and 50 mg atenolol

Table VI. Mean (±SD) changes in forearm blood flow (ml/dl/min) induced by isoproterenol sulfate infusion

	0.5 μg/min (n = 5)	*1.0 μg/min (n = 5)*	*2.0 μg/min (n = 4)*
Placebo	2.13 ± 0.63	3.16 ± 1.18	4.12 ± 2.38
Betaxolol, 10 mg	0.07 ± 0.24*	0.82 ± 0.93*	1.74 ± 2.16*†
Betaxolol, 40 mg	0.66 ± 0.95*	0.52 ± 1.03*	1.14 ± 0.96*
Atenolol, 50 mg	0.45 ± 1.04*	0.93 ± 1.24*	0.89 ± 1.45*
Propranolol, 40 mg	0.20 ± 0.59*	0.29 ± 0.58*	0.37 ± 0.53*

*P < 0.05 compared with placebo.
†P < 0.05 compared with propranolol, 40 mg.

Table VII. Mean (±SD) decreases in forearm vascular resistance (arbitrary units) induced by isoproterenol sulfate infusion

	0.5 μg/min (n = 5)	*1.0 μg/min (n = 5)*	*2.0 μg/min (n = 4)*
Placebo	5.4 ± 3.7	11.2 ± 3.4	14.0 ± 3.8
Betaxolol, 10 mg	2.0 ± 3.0	8.0 ± 8.2*	15.4 ± 10.4*
Betaxolol, 40 mg	2.0 ± 2.4	0.2 ± 9.1†	7.8 ± 6.5†
Atenolol, 50 mg	−1.8 ± 4.5	3.0 ± 4.4†	7.4 ± 2.6†
Propranolol, 40 mg	3.1 ± 6.6	1.9 ± 6.2†	1.2 ± 3.9†

*P < 0.05 compared with propranolol, 40 mg.
†P < 0.05 compared with placebo.

Table VIII. Mean (±SD) exercise heart rates 30 minutes after the last isoproterenol sulfate infusion

	Heart rate (bpm)
Placebo	156.6 ± 8.5
Betaxolol, 10 mg	120.4 ± 12.7*
Betaxolol, 40 mg	107.2 ± 10.5*†
Atenolol, 50 mg	116.6 ± 4.7*
Propranolol, 40 mg	126.2 ± 4.9*

*P < 0.05 compared with placebo.
†P < 0.05 compared with propranolol, 40 mg.

(3.0 ± 4.4 U) had a greater effect than placebo. At 2.0 μg/min isoproterenol, 40 mg propranolol (1.2 ± 3.9 U) prevented the decrease in forearm vascular resistance better than did placebo (14.0 ± 3.8 U) and 10 mg betaxolol (15.4 ± 10.4 U), whose effects did not differ. Betaxolol, 40 mg (7.8 ± 6.5 U), and 50 mg atenolol (7.4 ± 2.6 U) had a greater effect than placebo.

The mean exercise heart rates for the five subjects 30 minutes after the last infusion of isoproterenol are listed in Table VIII. All the drugs reduced the exercise tachycardia and the only difference between drugs was that 40 mg betaxolol (107.2 ± 10.5 bpm) had a greater effect than 40 mg propranolol (126.2 ± 4.9 bpm).

DISCUSSION

Cardioselectivity is assessed by comparing the effects of infused isoproterenol on heart rate and other β-adrenoceptor–mediated responses.[6] To ensure comparability between drugs it is necessary to choose doses that are equipotent at the β_1-receptor, which can be assessed by exercise tachycardia monitoring. In our study there were no significant differences between the effects of 10 mg betaxolol, 40 mg propranolol, and 50 mg atenolol, on exercise tachycardia 30 minutes after the last isoproterenol infusion. The greater exercise tachycardia after 40 mg propranolol (126.2 ± 4.9 bpm) than after 50 mg atenolol (116.6 ± 4.7 bpm) and 10 mg betaxolol (120.4 ± 12.7 bpm) may be due to the longer time after dosing before the exercise heart rate was measured. After propranolol at least two further infusions of isoproterenol were usually necessary to raise the heart rate by >40 bpm, thus postponing the measurement of the exercise heart rate by nearly an hour, during which time the plasma propranolol concentration would have started to fall.

The β_1-adrenoceptor blockade of a drug may also be assessed by its effect on the rise in systolic blood pressure caused by isoproterenol infusion. With this criterion, which unlike exercise tachycardia was measured during the study, 40 mg propranolol and 40 mg betaxolol were approximately equipotent, as were 10 mg betaxolol and 50 mg atenolol.

The cardioselective β-adrenoceptor–blocking drugs are less effective than the nonselective drugs in preventing the increase in heart rate after isoproterenol infusion. This is due to both a reflex component of the tachycardia arising from the fall in mean arterial pressure[6] and the presence of β_2-receptors in the heart[4] that are not enervated. In our study both 10 mg betaxolol and 50 mg atenolol had less of an effect than 40 mg propranolol on the increase in heart rate caused by isoproterenol but were equally effective in reducing exercise tachycardia. It would appear that at these doses atenolol and betaxolol are equally cardioselective.

The decreased diastolic blood pressure and forearm vascular resistance and the increased forearm blood flow and finger tremor induced by isoproterenol infusions are mediated through the β_2-receptor.[1,6] The changes in diastolic blood pressure with the serial infusions of isoproterenol were greater after 10 mg betaxolol and 50 mg atenolol than after 40 mg propranolol, suggesting that the β_2-receptor was affected less by the former two drugs than by the latter drug. Similar effects were noted for forearm vascular resistance, forearm blood flow, and finger tremor. This again suggests that the two drugs at these doses are equally cardioselective. However, both induce greater effects than placebo, confirming that they are exerting some blockade at the β_2-receptor.

Cardioselectivity is a dose-dependent phenomenon.[6] While 40 mg betaxolol exerted a greater effect on exercise tachycardia than did 40 mg propranolol, the isoproterenol dose-response curves for the changes in heart rate, finger tremor, diastolic blood pressure, forearm blood flow, and forearm vascular resistance after this dose of betaxolol lie to the left of those after propranolol. Thus even at the higher dose betaxolol exhibited cardioselectivity.

We are grateful to Dr. J. D. Merrett for statistical advice.

References

1. Arnold JMO, McDevitt DG: An assessment of physiological finger tremor as an indicator of beta-adrenoceptor function. Br J Clin Pharmacol **16:**167-174, 1983.
2. Balnave K, Neill JD, Russell CJ, Harron DWG, Leahey WJ, Wilson R, Shanks RG: Observations on the efficacy and pharmacokinetics of betaxolol (SL 75212), a cardioselective beta-adrenoceptor blocking drug. Br J Clin Pharmacol **11:**171-180, 1981.
3. Boudot JP, Cavero I, Fenard S, LeFevre-Borg F, Manoury P, Roach AG: Preliminary studies on SL 75212, a potent cardioselective beta adrenoceptor antagonist. Br J Clin Pharmacol **66:**445P, 1979.
4. Brown JE, McLeod AA, Shand DG: Evidence for cardiac beta-2-adrenoceptors in man. CLIN PHARM THER **33:**424-428, 1982.
5. Greenfield ADM: Venous occlusion plethysmography. Methods Med Res **8:**293-301, 1960.
6. McDevitt DG: The assessment of beta-adrenoceptor blocking drugs in man. Br J Clin Pharmacol **4:**413-425, 1977.

Effect of naloxone on the actions of captopril

Captopril inhibits the metabolism of endogenous opioids in vitro and potentiates their effects in vivo. We examined the hypothesis that endogenous opioids contribute to the actions of captopril in man. The acute cardiovascular and autonomic effects of oral captopril, intravenous naloxone, and their combination were examined in eight healthy men with normotension in a double-blind, placebo-controlled study of a Latin squares design. Naloxone altered neither blood pressure nor heart rate. There were significant falls in systolic blood pressure during captopril dosing alone, but there was no fall in blood pressure during combination therapy. Heart rates were higher during the combination than during captopril alone. The combination caused sedation, but neither captopril nor naloxone alone had any behavioral effects. Modification of the acute circulatory effects of captopril by naloxone suggests a role for endogenous opioids in the responses to converting enzyme inhibition. The sedation caused by the combination raises the possibility that captopril may exert central nervous actions in man. (CLIN PHARMACOL THER 38:560-565, 1985.)

Adesuyi A. Ajayi, B.Sc., M.B.Ch.B.,* Brian C. Campbell, M.D., Peter C. Rubin, D.M., and John L. Reid, D.M.** *Glasgow, United Kingdom*

The angiotensin converting enzyme inhibitor captopril is valuable in the management of hypertension and as an off-loading agent in congestive heart failure. Its efficacy in these conditions may result from arteriolar dilatation[15,36] after withdrawal of the vasopressor role of angiotensin II.[14,15] While this action may not be confined to plasma,[37] the original proposal that it reflects the sole hypotensive mechanism has been questioned.[20] Arteriolar dilation induced by captopril would be expected to give rise to a baroreflex-mediated tachycardia that is normally associated with a vasodilator drug.[24] Absence of reflex tachycardia despite blood pressure reduction with captopril is therefore an unexpected yet consistent finding in normal subjects[5,33] and in patients with hypertension.[35] Several explanations for this have been proposed, including parasympathetic activation[1,5,35] after discontinuance of angiotensin II–mediated vagal inhibition,[21,31] a selective venodilator action,[7] or a modification of baroreflexes.[16]

Opioid receptor agonists have also been shown to reduce blood pressure without tachycardia in animals[25] and in man,[28] a hemodynamic profile similar to that of captopril. It is established that endogenous opioids modulate blood pressure and cardiovascular homeostasis at the level of the brainstem by reducing baroreflex sensitivity.[27,30]

In vitro, captopril inhibits enkephalinase, a carboxypeptidase involved in the catabolism of endogenous opioids,[3] and potentiates the vasodepressor response to[10] and the analgesic action of[34] metenkephalin. Thus another possible explanation for the absence of tachycardia after captopril-induced hypotension is that captopril reduces baroreflex sensitivity by enhancing effects of endogenous opioids by inhibiting their metabolism. If this hypothesis were correct, then concomitant administration of the opiate antagonist naloxone with captopril would be expected to elicit tachycardia and might interfere with the fall in blood pressure. In a preliminary pilot study in man, naloxone was shown to modify the effect of captopril.[29] Our present study examines in greater detail the actions of naloxone on the cardiovascular and autonomic responses to captopril and explores central and peripheral mechanisms of the interaction.

METHODS

Eight men with normotension aged 25 ± 5 years and weighing 69 ± 5 kg gave written informed con-

From the University Department of Materia Medica, Stobhill General Hospital.

Presented in part at the meeting of the British Pharmacology Society, Cardiff, April 11, 1985.

Received for publication April 15, 1985; accepted July 5, 1985.

Reprint requests to: Dr. A. A. Ajayi, University Department of Materia Medica, Stobhill General Hospital, Glasgow G21 3UW, United Kingdom.

*Recipient of ORS and University of Glasgow postgraduate awards.

**Wellcome Trust Senior Fellow in Clinical Science.

sent to participate in the study, which was approved by the local Ethical Review Committee. They were judged healthy by history, clinical examination, biochemical screening (SMA-12), hematology testing, 12-lead ECGs, and urinalysis. The subjects were salt replete as assessed by 24-hour urinary sodium excretion (129 ± 43 mmol) measured before the study. Diet was maintained unchanged throughout the study. The study was of a randomized, placebo-controlled, double-blind, double-dummy, crossover design. Subjects were studied on four occasions at least 1 week apart. Treatment order was allocated according to a balanced (4 × 4) Latin squares design. Subjects received captopril with naloxone, captopril with 0.9% saline solution vehicle, naloxone with a placebo tablet (identical in appearance to captopril), and 0.9% saline solution vehicle with placebo tablet.

On each study day subjects arrived at the clinical investigation unit at 8:30 AM after an overnight fast. They avoided coffee, tea, alcohol, and cigarettes from 10 PM on the night before the study day and all prescription medicines in the 2 weeks before the study. They lay supine in a bed while a venous cannula was inserted into an arm vein. Blood pressure and heart rate were measured by a semiautomatic sphygmomanometer. ECG electrodes were attached onto the precordium for measurement of heart period and heart rate on a Grass Instruments Co. polygraph 7B1B. Naloxone HCl (Narcan; Endo Laboratories, Inc.), 10 mg bolus followed by 0.041 mg/min (total 10 mg), or 0.9% saline solution vehicle was given as a continuous intravenous infusion that continued throughout the study. A 50 mg captopril tablet or an identical-appearing placebo was taken with 200 ml water 60 minutes after the start of the naloxone or saline solution infusion. Supine and erect blood pressures and heart rate were recorded at 0, 15, 30, 60, 90, 120, and 180 minutes. Because of the short duration of action of naloxone[11] due to rapid distribution,[23] we chose a dosing schedule to cause adequate and maintained blockade of opiate receptors and to administer captopril while continuing the naloxone infusion.

Tests of autonomic reflex function, dynamic exercise, and the Valsalva maneuver were undertaken 90 minutes after oral captopril dosing. Dynamic exercise by bicycle ergometry at 0.75 of maximum work capacity (150W to 175W) was undertaken for 2 minutes. Blood pressure and heart rate were measured before and after the test. The Valsalva maneuver was performed in duplicate. Subjects exhaled to hold a column of mercury in a modified sphygmomanometer at 50 mm Hg for 15 seconds. Blood pressure was recorded before and 5 to 7 seconds after termination of the procedure, which coincides with the period of the systolic blood pressure overshoot.[32] The ECG was recorded continuously.

Behavioral effects of the treatments were assessed by a self-rating 100 mm visual analog scale[4] and questionnaire. The visual analog scale was presented on each day at 120 minutes and subjects were asked to consider their state of sedation from "wide awake" (0 mm) to "almost asleep" (100 mm). They also responded to a checklist with responses, "I can hardly stay awake," "I feel drowsy," "I don't feel different from usual," "I feel more alert than usual," and "I feel very alert."

Blood samples for plasma angiotensin converting enzyme activity were collected through an indwelling venous cannula at 1 hour before and at 180 minutes after captopril or placebo treatment. Samples were measured by the method of Cushman and Cheung[9] as modified by Chiknas.[6] One enzyme unit generates 1 mmol hippuric acid per minute from the tripeptide substrate hippuryl-histidyl leucine. Samples were analyzed within 2 to 4 hours of collection, to minimize the reversal of angiotensin converting enzyme inhibition that occurs with storage of plasma samples containing captopril.[26]

Data are expressed as the $\overline{X}$ ± SD. Changes in blood pressure and heart rate during autonomic testing and in visual analog scores were evaluated by Latin squares analyses, which included assessment of treatment effect, day effect, and time-treatment interaction. Blood pressure and heart rate measurements were subjected to repeated-measures ANOVA followed by pairwise comparisons. Blood pressure and heart rate changes have been corrected for individual changes on the placebo treatment day. The blood pressure AUC was obtained by computer-assisted analysis over time.

RESULTS

Captopril and naloxone were generally well tolerated. Two subjects experienced mild symptoms of postural dizziness while taking captopril and three subjects (one of whom was dizzy) were drowsy and sedated after captopril together with naloxone.

Plasma angiotensin converting enzyme activity was inhibited to the same extent after captopril alone ($P < 0.01$) and captopril with naloxone ($P < 0.01$). Neither naloxone alone nor placebo affected plasma angiotensin converting enzyme activity (Table I).

The erect systolic blood pressure fell after captopril but not after the combination of captopril and naloxone ($P < 0.05$ [ANOVA]; Fig. 1). Diastolic blood pressure was influenced neither by captopril alone nor in combination with naloxone. Naloxone alone had no effect on erect or supine blood pressure (Table II). Heart rate

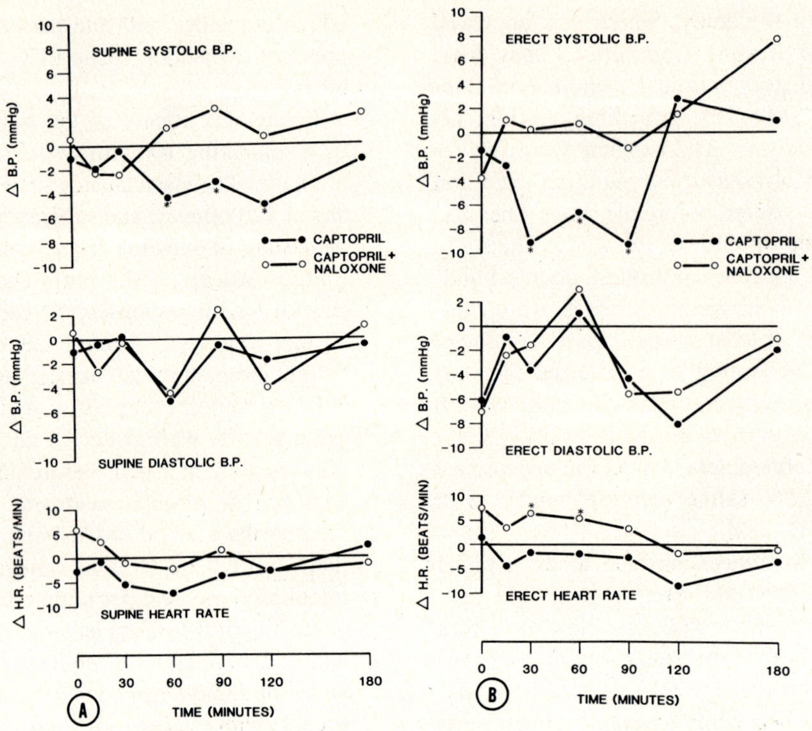

Fig. 1. Mean (n = 8) supine **(A)** and erect **(B)** blood pressure *(B.P.)* and heart rate *(H.R.)* corrected for changes on the placebo treatment day. *P < 0.05 (ANOVA).

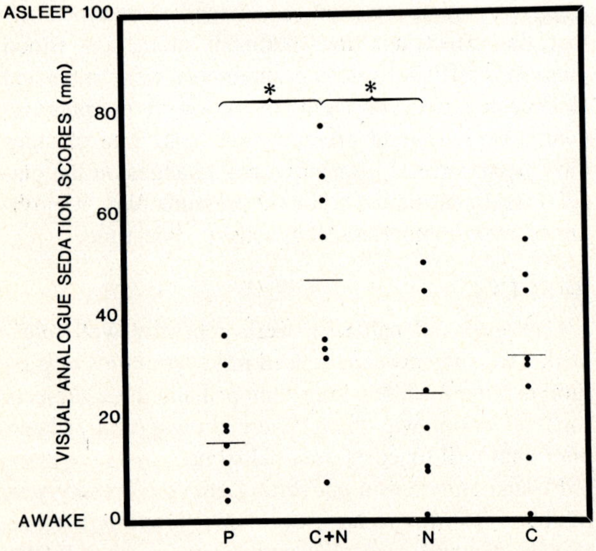

Fig. 2. Individual and mean sedation scores during placebo *(P)*, captopril and naloxone *(C + N)*, naloxone alone *(N)*, and captopril alone *(C)* dosing. *P < 0.05 (ANOVA).

in the erect position was higher during captopril and naloxone dosing than during dosing with captopril alone (P < 0.02 [ANOVA]; Fig. 1). Naloxone alone had no effect on supine or erect heart rate.

Baseline blood pressure during autonomic testing tended to be higher during the combination than during captopril alone. Bicycle ergometry (a test of sympathetic function) significantly increased (P < 0.01) blood pressure and heart rate, but there were no differences in the blood pressure or heart rate increments during the different treatments. The 95% confidence limits for a difference in the blood pressure rise and the exercise-induced tachycardia were 21.5 and 19.9, respectively. There was a consistent systolic blood pressure overshoot after the Valsalva maneuver, which is a noninvasive test of baroreceptor reflex function. No significant treatment effects were detected. The 95% confidence limits for a difference between treatments in the systolic blood pressure overshoot and Valsalva ratio were 22 and 0.34, respectively. Pressor and chronotropic responses during autonomic testing are summarized in Table III.

Sedation scores assessed by visual analog scales were increased by the combination of captopril and naloxone (P < 0.05 [ANOVA]) but not by captopril alone or naloxone alone (Fig. 2). The scores at 2 hours were 47 ± 23 mm after captopril and naloxone, 17 ± 14 mm after placebo, 32 ± 23 mm after captopril alone, and 25 ± 17 mm after naloxone alone, with a 95% confidence interval for a difference of 22.06. Three

Table I. The effect of captopril, naloxone, and their combination on plasma angiotensin converting enzyme activity.

Angiotensin converting enzyme activity (EU/ml)	*Captopril with naloxone*	*Captopril alone*	*Naloxone alone*	*Placebo*
60 min before treatment	22.7 ± 9.8	21.4 ± 8.5	23.6 ± 9.6	19.6 ± 10.2
180 min after treatment	14.4 ± 5.6*	14.4 ± 7.2*	17.2 ± 9.3	16.5 ± 6.5

Data are $\overline{X}$ ± SD (n = 8).
EU = Enzyme unit.
*P < 0.01 compared with baseline (paired t test with Bonferroni correction).

Table II. AUC of systolic blood pressure corrected for placebo

AUC (mm Hg · min)	*Captopril with naloxone*	*Captopril alone*	*Naloxone alone*
Erect	284 ± 800	−830 ± 982*	141 ± 887
Supine	166 ± 1085	−520 ± 871†	391 ± 1407

Data are $\overline{X}$ ± SD (n = 8). The negative signs denote a hypotensive effect compared with placebo.
*P < 0.02 compared with naloxone alone and captopril with naloxone.
†P < 0.05 compared with naloxone (paired test with Bonferroni correction).

Table III. Response to autonomic tests

	Captopril with naloxone	*Captopril alone*	*Naloxone alone*	*Placebo*
Dynamic exercise				
Pretest systolic BP (mm Hg)	118.5 ± 9.4	117 ± 10.5	121.6 ± 11	118 ± 6.5
Change (mm Hg)	25.9 ± 15.0	36.8 ± 21	25.9 ± 15.6	33.8 ± 9.8
Pretest heart rate (bpm)	76.5 ± 8.7	72.6 ± 10.1	71.1 ± 16.1	76.1 ± 8.3
Change (bpm)	75.1 ± 6.6	65.3 ± 19.6	84.1 ± 15.2	73.1 ± 14.5
Valsalva maneuver				
Pretest systolic BP (mm Hg)	114.3 ± 7.1	111 ± 10.5	117.6 ± 8.2	115.3 ± 6.9
Systolic BP overshoot (mm Hg)	10.5 ± 10.9	8.0 ± 6.7	8.8 ± 9.7	8.9 ± 10.8
Valsalva ratio	1.90 ± 0.52	1.87 ± 0.35	1.90 ± 0.39	1.99 ± 0.42

Data are $\overline{X}$ ± SD (n = 8).
BP = Blood pressure.

subjects, one of whom exhibited postural dizziness during dosing with captopril alone, were drowsy for up to 2 hours after the combination but not during captopril or naloxone alone (Fig. 2). Drowsiness after captopril and naloxone was confirmed by direct questions and clinical observations and correlated with an increased sedation score on the visual analog scales.

DISCUSSION

Our results confirm earlier findings that captopril causes modest falls in blood pressure in salt-replete subjects with normotension without compensatory tachycardia. Our findings of an attenuation of the acute hypotensive effect of captopril when given in combination with naloxone confirm the earlier observations of Rubin et al.[29] and are consistent with the concept that endogenous opioids may be involved in some of the actions of captopril in man. Coadministration of captopril and naloxone resulted in heart rates that were higher than those after captopril alone or placebo or naloxone alone. This observation is in keeping with our initial hypothesis. Opioid agonists have been shown to reduce baroreflex sensitivity, while the opiate antagonist naloxone increases baroreflex sensitivity in man.[28] The increased heart rate after combined captopril and naloxone may then reflect a release of baroreflex activity caused by a captopril-induced increase in endogenous opioid concentration. A contribution of endogenous opioids to the circulatory actions of captopril in man is consistent with the finding of naloxone reversal of captopril-induced hypotension and bradycardia in the dog.[19,22] Similar observations of naloxone-reversible hypotension have been made with the nonthiol converting enzyme inhibitors enalapril and enalaprilat in the dog.*

*Montastruc JL: Personal communication, 1985.

Our hypothesis assumes a high specificity of action for naloxone as an opiate antagonist and an action in the central nervous system at sites relevant to blood pressure homeostasis. We therefore assessed the relative importance of central and peripheral sites of action by visual analog scale for sedation and autonomic reflexes. Neither captopril nor naloxone had separate behavioral effects. An increased sedation score during combined captopril and naloxone dosing coupled with drowsiness in some subjects raises the possibility that captopril influences the central nervous system in man. The possible mechanisms involved in this effect are not clear. This finding was somewhat unexpected, since it has been claimed in autoradiographic studies that captopril does not cross the blood-brain barrier in rats.[17] It is known, however, that certain brain stem and hypothalamic sites with opioidergic neurons involved in cardiovascular regulation are not "protected" by the barrier.[2] In addition, systemically administered captopril may modify the endogenous brain renin-angiotensin system.[8,12,13]

The observation that captopril does not alter baroreflex function in subjects with hypertension[38] may argue against a central effect, and our observation of unchanged autonomic reflexes does not permit a clear conclusion. It is possible, however, that captopril and naloxone may interact outside the brain on opioid mechanisms, contributing to presynaptic sympathetic transmission in the heart.[18]

In conclusion, naloxone modified both systolic blood pressure and heart rate responses to captopril. These findings suggest that endogenous opioids may contribute to the acute hemodynamic effects of captopril in man. The mechanism of the sedative effect of the combination is not clear, but it raises the possibility that captopril may exert an effect on the central nervous system in man. Further evaluation of the influence of naloxone on the effects of chronic captopril therapy in patients with hypertension is required.

We thank Dr. D. J. Sumner for advice on statistical analysis.

References

1. Ajayi AA, Campbell BC, Howie CA, Reid JL: Acute and chronic effects of converting enzyme inhibitors enalapril and lisinopril on reflex control of heart rate in normotensive man. J Hypertens **3**:47-53, 1985.
2. Arnold MA, Carr DB, Togasaki DM, Plan MC, Martin JB: Caffeine stimulates endorphin release in blood, but not in cerebrospinal fluid. Life Sci **31**:1017-1024, 1982.
3. Arregiu A, Lee CM, Emson PC, Iversen LL: Separation of human brain angiotensin converting enzyme from enkephalin degrading activity. Eur J Pharmacol **59**:141-144, 1979.
4. Bond A, Lader M: The use of analogue scales in rating subjects' feelings. Br J Med Psychol **47**:211-218, 1974.
5. Campbell BC, Sturani A, Reid JL: Evidence of parasympathetic activity of the angiotensin converting enzyme inhibitor, captopril, in normotensive man. Clin Sci **68**:49-56, 1985.
6. Chiknas SG: A liquid chromatography assisted assay for converting enzyme (peptidyl dipeptidase) in serum. Clin Chem **25**:1254-1262, 1979.
7. Cody RJ, Tarazi RC, Bravo EL, Fouad FM: Haemodynamics of orally active converting enzyme inhibitor (SQ 14225) in hypertensive patients. Clin Sci Mol Med **55**:453-459, 1978.
8. Cohen ML, Kurz KD: Angiotensin converting enzyme inhibition in tissues from spontaneously hypertensive rats after treatment with captopril or MK 421. J Pharmacol Exp Ther **220**:63-69, 1982.
9. Cushman DW, Cheung HS: Spectrophotometric assay and properties of the angiotensin converting enzyme of rabbit lung. Biochem Pharmacol **20**:1637-1648, 1971.
10. Di Nicolantonio R, Hutchison JS, Takata Y, Veroni M: Captopril potentiates the vasodepressor action of metenkephalin in anaesthetised rats. Br J Pharmacol **80**:405-408, 1983.
11. Evans JM, Hogg MJ, Lunn JN, Rosen M: Degree and duration of reversal by naloxone of effects of morphine in conscious subjects. Br Med J **2**:589-591, 1974.
12. Evered MD, Robinson MM, Richardson MA: Captopril given intracerebroventricularly, subcutaneousy or by lavage inhibits angiotensin-converting enzyme activity in the rat brain. Eur J Pharmacol **68**:443-449, 1980.
13. Felix D, Schelling P: Angiotensin converting enzyme blockade by captopril changes angiotensin II receptors and angiotensin concentrations in the brain of SHR-SP and WKY rats. Neurosci Lett **34**:45-50, 1982.
14. Fergusson H, Brunner HR, Turini CA, Gavras H: A specific orally active inhibitor of angiotensin converting enzyme in man. Lancet **1**:775-778, 1977.
15. Gavras H, Brunner HR, Laragh JH, Sealy JE, Gavras I, Vucovich RA: An angiotensin converting enzyme inhibitor to identify and treat vasoconstrictor and volume factors in hypertensive patients. N Engl J Med **291**:817-821, 1974.
16. Hatton R, Clough D, Faulkner K, Conway J: Angiotensin converting enzyme inhibitor resets baroreceptor reflexes in conscious dogs. Hypertension **3**:676-681, 1981.
17. Heald AF, Ita CE: Distribution in rats of an inhibitor of angiotensin converting enzyme (SQ14225) as studied by whole body autoradiography and liquid scintillation counting. Pharmacologist **19**:129, 1977.
18. Konishi S, Tsuno A, Otsoka M: Enkephalin as a transmitter for presynaptic inhibition in sympathetic ganglia. Nature **294**:80-82, 1981.
19. Laubie M, Schmitt HH: Indication for central vagal endorphinergic control of heart rate in dogs. Eur J Pharmacol **71**:401-409, 1981.
20. Lazar JD: Angiotensin converting enzyme inhibitors. *In*

Turner P, Shand G, editors: Recent advances in clinical pharmacology, ed 3. London, 1983, Churchill Livingstone.
21. Lumbers ER, McCloskey DI, Potter EK: Angiotensin II of baroreceptor evoked activity in cardiac inhibition by vagal efferent nerves in the dog. J Physiol **194:**69-80, 1979.
22. Montastruc P, Montastruc JL, Gillard-Plaza G: Influence of naloxone on the captopril-induced decrease in vagal pressor reflexes. J Pharmacol (Paris) **15:**421-426, 1984.
23. Ngai SH, Berkowitz BA, Yang JC, Hempstead J, Spector S: Pharmacokinetics of naloxone in rats and in man. Basis for its potency and short duration of action. Anesthesiology **44:**398-401, 1976.
24. Oates HF, Graham RM, Stokes GS: Mechanism of the hypotensive action of prazosin. Arch Int Pharmacodyn Ther **227:**41-58, 1977.
25. Petty MA, Reid JL: The effect of opiates on arterial baroreceptor reflex function in the rabbit. Naunyn Schmiedebergs Arch Pharmacol **319:**206-211, 1982.
26. Roulston JE, MacGregor GA, Bird R: The measurement of angiotensin converting enzyme in subjects receiving ceptopril. N Engl J Med **303:**397, 1980.
27. Rubin PC, Blaschke TF, Guilleminault C: Effects of naloxone, a specific opioid inhibitor, on blood pressure fall during sleep. Circulation **63:**117-121, 1981.
28. Rubin PC, McLean K, Reid JL: Endogenous opioids and baroreflex control in humans. Hypertension **5:**535-538, 1983.
29. Rubin PC, Millar JA, Sturani S, Lawrie C, Reid JL: The influence of naloxone on the circulatory effects of captopril. Br J Clin Pharmacol **17:**713-717, 1984.
30. Rubin PC: Opioid peptides in blood pressure regulation in man. Clin Sci **66:**625-630, 1984.
31. Scroop GC, Lowe RD: Central pressor effect of angiotensin mediated by the parasympathetic nervous system. Nature **220:**1331-1332, 1968.
32. Sharpey-Schafer EP: Effects of Valsalva manoeuvre on normal and failing circulation. Br Med J **1:**693, 1955.
33. Shepherd AN, Campbell BC, Reid JL: Effects of captopril on angiotensin converting inhibitors in normotensive sodium replete volunteers. J Cardiovasc Pharmacol **4:**381-387, 1982.
34. Stine SM, Yang HY, Costa E: Inhibition of in situ metabolism of ^{3}H-Met^{5}-enkephalin and the potentiation of metenkephalin analgesia by captopril. Brain Res **188:** 295-299, 1979.
35. Sturani A, Chiarini C, Degli Esposti E, Santoro A, Zuccala A, Zuchelli P: Heart rate control in hypertensive patients treated by captopril. Br J Clin Pharmacol **14:**849-855, 1982.
36. Turini GA, Brunner HR, Grilac M, Waeber B, Gavras H: Improvement of chronic congestive heart failure by oral captopril. Lancet **1:**1213-1215, 1979.
37. Unger T, Ganten D, Lang RE, Scholkens BA: Is tissue converting enzyme inhibition a determinant of antihypertensive efficacy of converting enzyme inhibitors? Studies with the two different compounds HOE 498 and MK 421, in spontaneously hypertensive rats. J Cardiovasc Pharmacol **6:**840-843, 1984.
38. Warren SE, O'Connor DT, Cohen IM: Autonomic and baroreflex function after captopril in hypertension. Am Heart J **105:**1002-1008, 1983.

Oxidation of hydrazine metabolites formed from isoniazid

Studies in rats indicate that the metabolic activation of acetylhydrazine, a metabolite of isoniazid, is a critical determinant of the hepatotoxicity of isoniazid. As demonstrated in that model, the formation of $^{14}CO_2$ after the administration of ^{14}C-acetylisoniazid reflects the activity of the toxic pathway. A similar approach in man should make it possible to demonstrate the presence and to assess the quantitative importance of this toxifying pathway, and thus to evaluate its role in the pathogenesis of isoniazid hepatitis. We gave 300 mg isoniazid together with 10 μCi ^{14}C-acetylisoniazid (12 mg) to 17 healthy subjects and determined the time course of the plasma concentrations of isoniazid, acetylisoniazid, acetylhydrazine, and diacetylhydrazine and of the exhalation of $^{14}CO_2$. The time course of $^{14}CO_2$ in breath closely paralleled the plasma concentration-time curve of acetylhydrazine but not those of acetylisoniazid or diacetylhydrazine, indicating that the $^{14}CO_2$ originated directly from the metabolism of acetylhydrazine. The cumulative exhalation of $^{14}CO_2$ increased with decreasing rate of acetylation of isoniazid, such that slow acetylators generated more $^{14}CO_2$ than rapid acetylators. Simulation studies demonstrated that even if the data are corrected for the different formation of acetylisoniazid from isoniazid in slow and rapid acetylators, the slow acetylators still generated more $^{14}CO_2$. The data therefore indicate that a substantial fraction of the acetylhydrazine formed from isoniazid passes through a pathway that has been shown in animals to generate highly reactive and hepatotoxic intermediates. The observation that slow acetylators metabolize more isoniazid via the toxic pathway, together with recent data showing an exceptionally high incidence of hepatitis in slow acetylators receiving large therapeutic doses of isoniazid, further support the hypothesis that the metabolic activation of acetylhydrazine from isoniazid is an important determinant of the hepatotoxicity of isoniazid in man. (CLIN PHARMACOL THER 38:566-571, 1985.)

Bernhard H. Lauterburg, M.D., Charles V. Smith, Ph.D., Elizabeth L. Todd, Ph.D., and Jerry R. Mitchell, M.D., Ph.D. *Houston, Tex.*

The treatment of tuberculosis with isoniazid is associated with a high incidence of hepatotoxicity,[1,3,7,8,14] but the pathogenesis of isoniazid-induced liver injury in man is uncertain. In only a few patients has the hepatitis resulting from isoniazid been accompanied by clinical features commonly associated with a hypersensitivity reaction.[11,14] On the other hand, evidence for a direct toxic reaction as suggested by experiments in animals is also not conclusive. Based on earlier animal studies, a critical determinant of isoniazid toxicity appears to be the fraction of isoniazid converted to acetylhydrazine, which is then activated in the liver by the cytochrome P-450 monooxygenase system to a chemically reactive hepatotoxic metabolite.[14,17]

Acetylhydrazine is a metabolite of isoniazid in man also,[22] and metabolic activation of acetylhydrazine by hepatic monooxygenases occurs with human liver microsomes.[17] However, a relationship between exposure to acetylhydrazine and liver injury has not been established, and it is not known whether metabolic activation of acetylhydrazine accounts for isoniazid hepatotoxicity. In animal models the toxic pathway can be assessed by following the covalent binding of the toxic radical metabolite to hepatic macromolecules and correlating covalent binding with hepatocellular necrosis.[21] Such an approach is not feasible in man. However, the toxic metabolite also yields acetate, which is further metabolized to CO_2.[21] After the administration of ^{14}C-acetylhydrazine or ^{14}C-acetylisoniazid labeled in the acetyl moiety, $^{14}CO_2$ will appear in breath and the amount of $^{14}CO_2$ exhaled will reflect the fraction of the dose passing through the toxic pathway.[21]

A similar approach should make it possible to demonstrate the presence and to assess the quantitative importance of this toxifying pathway in man. We have

From the Department of Internal Medicine and Institute for Lipid Research, Baylor College of Medicine.
Received for publication Nov. 19, 1984; accepted July 16, 1985.
Reprint requests to: Bernhard H. Lauterburg, M.D., Baylor College of Medicine, One Baylor Plaza, Room 826E, Houston, TX 77030.

tested this hypothesis by administering a tracer dose of ^{14}C-acetylisoniazid together with 300 mg isoniazid to normal healthy subjects. Our data demonstrate that a substantial fraction of an acetylisoniazid dose is metabolized to CO_2 and that very slow acetylators, who may be at a high risk of incurring liver injury from isoniazid,[15] metabolize a larger fraction of this metabolite to CO_2 than do rapid acetylators.

METHODS

Seventeen subjects (seven women and 10 men) between 19 and 28 years old gave informed consent to participate in the study, which had been approved by the Baylor Institutional Review Board for Human Research. Subjects had normal hepatic and renal function as judged from their levels of serum transaminase, alkaline phosphatase, bilirubin, albumin, and creatinine and BUN. They had not taken any other medication during the 10 days before the study and none of the subjects was overweight.

After an overnight fast they took 300 mg isoniazid dissolved in water together with 10 μCi ^{14}C-acetylisoniazid (12 mg). The labeled compound (specific activity 0.15 mCi/mmol) was synthesized as described previously,[21] and its purity exceeded 98% as verified by TLC on silica gel with propanol:methanol (70:30) as the mobile phase and zonal scanning. Blood was drawn from an antecubital vein at intervals for 4 hours for the determination of the rate of disappearance of isoniazid. In six subjects blood was drawn at intervals for 36 hours for the determination of the time course of the plasma concentrations of isoniazid, acetylisoniazid, acetylhydrazine, and diacetylhydrazine. Expired CO_2 was collected by blowing exhaled air through a glass tube into a scintillation vial containing 2 ml 1N Hyamine 10X (Rohm & Haas Co.), a base, and 2 ml ethanol plus one drop phenolphthalein until neutralization was achieved by the trapping of 2 mmol CO_2 (indicated by the loss of color of the indicator). Subjects remained bedridden for the duration of the study to minimize variations in the endogenous production of CO_2. They received their first meal 3 hours after drug dosing and then followed a regular diet.

After this initial study, six subjects took phenobarbital, 2 mg/kg/day, in two divided doses for 5 days. Thereafter, they underwent a repeat study of isoniazid metabolism 24 hours after the last dose of phenobarbital.

The specific activity of the exhaled CO_2 was calculated from the known amount of CO_2 trapped in each vial (2 mmol) and the radioactivity contained in the 4 ml of neutralized trapping solution. Radioactivity was measured by liquid scintillation spectrometry with the

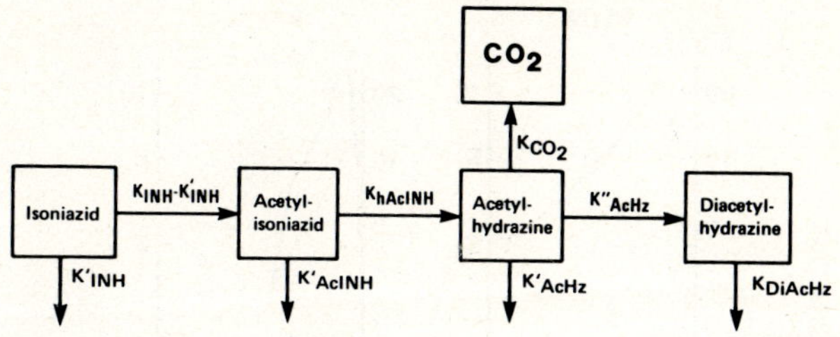

Fig. 1. Kinetic model describing the formation of CO_2 from isoniazid.

channels ratio technique for quench correction. The cumulative expiration of labeled CO_2 was estimated from these intermittently measured specific activities as the product of the AUC of $^{14}CO_2$ in breath and endogenous CO_2 production, which was assumed to be 9 mmol/kg · hr.[23]

Plasma concentrations of isoniazid, acetylisoniazid, acetylhydrazine, and diacetylhydrazine were measured by GC-MS with deuterated analogs as internal standards.[9] The fractional rate of disappearance of isoniazid from the circulation and of $^{14}CO_2$ from breath was calculated by least-squares regression analysis after logarithmic transformation of the data. The data points following the peak value were used in the calculations.

The acetyl moiety of acetylhydrazine giving rise to the exhaled $^{14}CO_2$ is not present in the parent compound isoniazid, which is why labeled acetylisoniazid and not labeled isoniazid was used. Our experimental data therefore do not take into account the influence of the first metabolic step, i.e., the acetylation of isoniazid to acetylisoniazid, on the fraction of a dose of isoniazid passing through the toxic pathway. To study the effect of this first metabolic step on the generation of CO_2 from isoniazid, we simulated the production of CO_2 from isoniazid for a slow and a rapid acetylator using the model shown in Fig. 1. The two simulations differ only in the rates of acetylation of isoniazid ($k_{INH} - k'_{INH}$ = 0.55 in the rapid and 0.1 in the slow acetylator) and of acetylhydrazine (k''_{AcHz}), which was assumed to be half the rate of isoniazid acetylation,[4] i.e., 0.275 for the rapid and 0.05 for the slow acetylator. The rates of urinary excretion of isoniazid (k'_{INH} = 0.025) and the rate of hydrolysis of acetylisoniazid to acetylhydrazine (k_{hAcINH} = 0.09) are assumed to be identical in the slow and rapid acetylators, and the parameter estimates are based on published data.[4,13] The rate of formation of CO_2 from acetylhydrazine (k_{CO_2}) was assumed to be 0.02 in both the rapid and the slow acetylators. For the simulation, the system of differential equations describing the model was integrated numerically by the computer program DIFFEQ of PROPHET,[18] which uses the algorithm of MLAB.

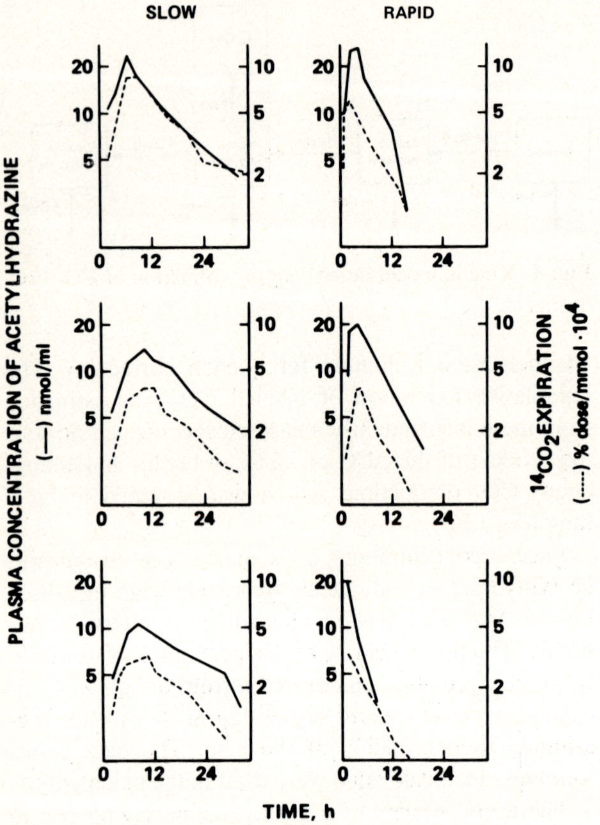

Fig. 2. Time course of the plasma concentration of acetylhydrazine and $^{14}CO_2$ in breath after 300 mg isoniazid and 10 μCi ^{14}C-acetylisoniazid by mouth to three slow and three rapid acetylators.

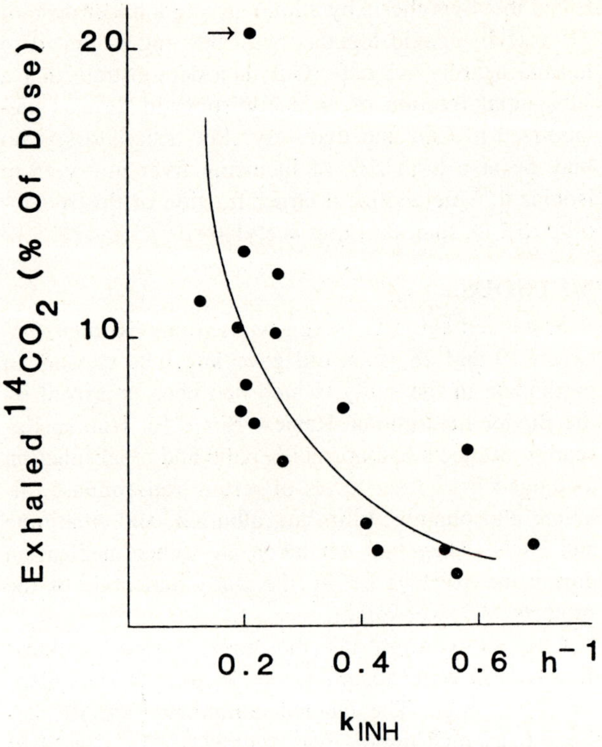

Fig. 3. Cumulative exhalation of $^{14}CO_2$ as a function of the rate of disappearance of isoniazid. *Arrow* denotes the subject who metabolized much of the ^{14}C-isoniazid to $^{14}CO_2$ even before phenobarbital dosing.

RESULTS

After the oral administration of isoniazid and ^{14}C-acetylisoniazid, the specific activity of exhaled $^{14}CO_2$ rose rapidly and then declined, with an apparent $t_{1/2}$ ranging from 3.9 to 14 hours. The rate of disappearance of $^{14}CO_2$ from breath was much slower than, but increased with, the increasing rate of disappearance of isoniazid; the latter is determined mainly by the rate of acetylation. Like the apparent plasma $t_{1/2}$ of acetylhydrazine, the proposed precursor of the $^{14}CO_2$, the $t_{1/2}$ of $^{14}CO_2$ in breath was on the average four times longer than that of isoniazid. Indeed, the time course of $^{14}CO_2$ in breath paralleled the simultaneously determined plasma concentrations of acetylhydrazine, further supporting the contention that the measured $^{14}CO_2$ originated from the metabolism of acetylhydrazine (Fig. 2).

The estimated cumulative exhalation of $^{14}CO_2$ ranged from 1.8% to 20.5% of the administered radioactivity and decreased as the rate of disappearance of isoniazid (and thus the rate of acetylation) increased (Fig. 3). The fraction of the administered radioactivity appearing in breath was related closely to the plasma acetylhydrazine AUC as measured in six subjects (r = 0.92; Table I). In contrast, the plasma AUCs of acetylisoniazid and diacetylhydrazine tended to increase as the rate of acetylation increased (Table I). Consequently, there was a negative correlation between the fraction of the administered radioactivity appearing in breath and the plasma AUCs of acetylisoniazid (r = 0.74) and diacetylhydrazine (r = 0.81), making these metabolites unlikely sources for the exhaled $^{14}CO_2$.

The production of $^{14}CO_2$ increased in five of the six subjects after phenobarbital pretreatment (Table II). The subject in whom the exhalation of $^{14}CO_2$ decreased slightly after phenobarbital metabolized an extraordinarily high percentage of the administered radioactivity to $^{14}CO_2$ before phenobarbital, suggesting that his drug metabolizing enzyme system might have been induced even before phenobarbital treatment. The rates of disappearance of isoniazid from plasma did not change after phenobarbital.

In these studies all subjects received an identical dose of labeled acetylisoniazid from which they generated

Table I. Formation of $^{14}CO_2$ from ^{14}C-acetylisoniazid and plasma AUCs of acetylisoniazid, acetylhydrazine, and diacetylhydrazine

Subject No.	k_{INH}* *(hr^{-1})*	*Acetylisoniazid AUC (nmol/ml · hr)*	*Acetylhydrazine AUC (nmol/ml · hr)*	*Diacetylhydrazine AUC (nmol/ml · hr)*	$^{14}CO_2$ *(% dose)*
1	0.198	34	328	25	7.4
2	0.218	51	380	31	7.0
3	0.273	100	379	19	5.6
4	0.422	100	197	75	2.5
5	0.545	65	150	143	2.6
6	0.572	122	103	248	1.8

*Fractional rate of isoniazid disappearance from circulation.

similar amounts of labeled acetylhydrazine, because the rate of hydrolysis of acetylisoniazid to acetylhydrazine is much the same in all individuals and is independent of the acetylator status.[13] If acetylisoniazid is formed in vivo, however, not all subjects will be exposed to the same amount, because rapid acetylators will form more acetylisoniazid and thus generate more acetylhydrazine than will slow acetylators.

To assess the influence of this first acetylation step, which is missing in the experimental data, we therefore simulated the formation of CO_2 from isoniazid for a rapid and a slow rate of acetylation. The simulations predict that 9.8% and 3.1% of a dose of acetylisoniazid are metabolized to CO_2 if the rates of acetylation are 0.10 and 0.55 hours^{-1}, respectively. These values agree well with the experimentally determined fractions (Fig. 4). The simulations further demonstrate that the fraction of a dose of isoniazid metabolized to CO_2 via acetylhydrazine is smaller than that of acetylisoniazid. However, because rapid acetylators metabolize most of the isoniazid to acetylisoniazid, only a minimally smaller fraction (2.9%) appears in breath if the formation of CO_2 from isoniazid via acetylisoniazid and acetylhydrazine is simulated (Fig. 4). In contrast, the fraction decreases from 9.8% to 6.0% if the rate of acetylation is slow, because slow acetylators excrete approximately one third of a dose of isoniazid unchanged (Fig. 5). Nevertheless, the fraction of a dose of isoniazid metabolized to CO_2 will still be twice as high in slow acetylators.

DISCUSSION

The formation of $^{14}CO_2$ from ^{14}C-acetylisoniazid demonstrates that the acetyl moiety of acetylisoniazid is metabolized in man as it is in experimental animals. In animal models in which the metabolic activation of the acetyl moiety to a toxic metabolite can be correlated with toxicity by comparing covalent binding of the metabolite with the extent of hepatic damage observed histologically, the metabolism of the acetyl moiety to

Table II. Effect of phenobarbital, 2 mg/kg, for 5 days of the formation of $^{14}CO_2$ from ^{14}C-acetylisoniazid

Subject No.	*Before phenobarbital (% dose)*	*After phenobarbital (% dose)*
6	1.8	4.2
7	6.2	7.2
8	8.6	10.0
9	9.2	10.9
10	11.2	13.8
11	20.5	19.2

CO_2 reflects the activity of the toxifying pathway.[21] It is not possible in man to examine for a similar correlation between the formation of CO_2 and the hepatotoxicity of isoniazid, but indirect evidence suggests that the exhalation of $^{14}CO_2$ also reflects the toxic pathway in man.

First, the time course of the specific activity of $^{14}CO_2$ in breath closely paralleled the plasma concentration of acetylhydrazine, which is the substrate for the metabolic step leading to the formation of the toxic metabolite.[17,21] The measured $^{14}CO_2$ could conceivably result from the metabolism of acetate originating from hydrolysis of ^{14}C-acetylisoniazid and ^{14}C-diacetylhydrazine. Because the clearance of acetylisoniazid is similar in slow and rapid acetylators[13] and more diacetylhydrazine is formed in rapid than in slow acetylators,[10,15,22] rapid acetylators would be expected to metabolize at least an equal if not a larger fraction of the administered radioactivity to $^{14}CO_2$ if such hydrolysis contributed significantly to the exhaled $^{14}CO_2$. However, rapid acetylators metabolized a much smaller fraction of the ingested dose to $^{14}CO_2$ than did slow acetylators.

Secondly, hydrolysis of the acetylated hydrazine metabolites of isoniazid would not be expected to increase after pretreatment with phenobarbital. Nonetheless, the exhalation of $^{14}CO_2$ increased somewhat after enzyme

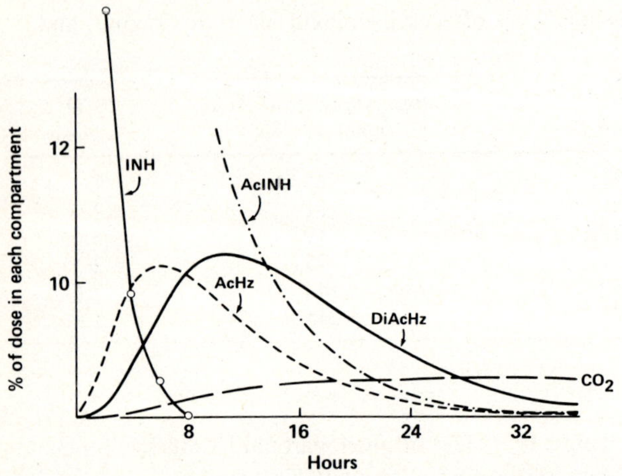

Fig. 4. Calculated time course of the plasma concentrations of isoniazid *(INH)*, acetylisoniazid *(AcINH)*, acetylhydrazine *(AcHz)*, and diacetylhydrazine *(DiAcHz)* and estimated cumulative appearance of CO_2 in breath generated from isoniazid in a rapid acetylator.

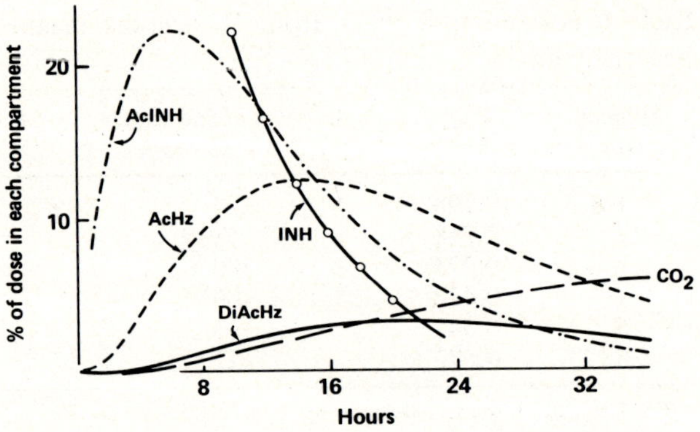

Fig. 5. Calculated time course of the plasma concentrations of isoniazid *(INH)*, acetylisoniazid *(AcINH)*, acetylhydrazine *(AcHz)*, and diacetylhydrazine *(DiAcHz)* and estimated cumulative appearance of CO_2 in breath generated from isoniazid in a slow acetylator.

induction in all but one subject. Even in rats, in which enzyme induction can be accomplished under better-controlled conditions and with relatively higher doses of inducer, pretreatment with phenobarbital increases the formation of $^{14}CO_2$ from ^{14}C-acetylhydrazine by only 24% (from 9.8% to 12.2% of the administered dose in 6 hours).[21]

Finally, our findings are in agreement with recent observations of an increased susceptibility of slow acetylators to the hepatotoxic effects of isoniazid.[3,16] In our studies the rate of acetylation was a major determinant of the fraction of acetylisoniazid metabolized to $^{14}CO_2$. Even when the initial metabolic step, the acetylation of isoniazid to acetylisoniazid, is taken into account, slow acetylators metabolize a larger fraction of a dose of isoniazid to CO_2. Intuitively, slow acetylators ($k_{INH} < 0.3$)[15] might be expected to be exposed to less acetylhydrazine than are rapid acetylators. Although slow acetylators do generate less acetylhydrazine from a given dose of isoniazid, the rate of acetylation of acetylhydrazine to the relatively nontoxic diacetylhydrazine is so much slower in slow acetylators that more acetylhydrazine will be available to the toxifying pathway. The balance between formation and further acetylation of acetylhydrazine leads to a marked increase in the metabolism of acetylhydrazine through the cytochrome P-450 pathway, particularly in very slow acetylators who would therefore be expected to be at greater risk of developing liver injury from isoniazid. In a recent prospective study of 56 slow and 56 rapid acetylators, clinically overt hepatitis occurred in three patients who were very slow acetylators (acetylation index <1.3).[15]

As suggested by our observations on the effect of phenobarbital pretreatment, enzyme induction will increase the fraction of a dose of isoniazid metabolized through the toxifying pathway. This fraction further increases after larger doses of isoniazid, leading to saturation of the acetylation steps.[19] These effects of enzyme induction and dose could explain the exceptionally high incidence of clinically significant liver injury in slow acetylators when isoniazid, 10 mg/kg, is taken with rifampin, a known enzyme inducer, and ethambutol.[16]

In other studies with high doses of isoniazid taken once to twice a week, mean serum transaminase values were similar in slow and rapid acetylators.[5,12,20] One possible explanation for the low incidence of significant liver injury is that cumulation of acetylhydrazine may be a critical determinant of the toxicity of isoniazid and is not likely to occur during intermittent therapy.[9,10] Moreover, the slow acetylator phenotype is but one of the risk factors for the development of liver injury from isoniazid. Increasing age leads to a striking increase in the incidence of hepatic injury from isoniazid,[2,3,7,8,14] although the rate of acetylation does not appear to decrease with age.[6] Chronic alcohol consumption also increases the risk of liver damage with isoniazid,[3,7,8] possibly by induction of the drug metabolizing enzyme system. Indeed, the high use of alcohol in the study population may have contributed to the high incidence of isoniazid hepatitis in rapid acetylators reported in a small group of patients in an earlier study.[13] It is not yet clear how increasing age and chronic alcohol consumption alter the disposition of the potentially toxic hydrazine metabolites of isoniazid.

Our data do not resolve the mechanism of isoniazid toxicity in man. Clearly, factors other than acetylator phenotype and exposure to acetylhydrazine are involved in the hepatotoxicity of isoniazid. Nevertheless, our observation that very slow acetylators are exposed to more acetylhydrazine, together with recent data showing an increased incidence of liver injury among slow acetylators, particularly if they receive high doses of isoniazid plus rifampin,[16] are consistent with the hypothesis that liver damage by isoniazid may result from the metabolic activation of acetylhydrazine to a toxic metabolite.

In conclusion, a substantial fraction of a dose of acetylisoniazid is metabolized to CO_2 in man. The analysis of the formation of CO_2 in relation to the time course of the plasma concentrations of the hydrazine metabolites of isoniazid, together with the effect of enzyme induction, indicate that the formation of CO_2 in man apparently reflects the amount of isoniazid-derived acetylhydrazine passing through the toxic monooxygenase pathway, which is in agreement with data from animal studies.[21]

References

1. Bailey WC, Taylor SL, Dascomb HE, Greenberg HG, Ziskind MM: Disturbed hepatic function during isoniazid chemoprophylaxis. Am Rev Respir Dis **107:**523-529, 1973.
2. Black M, Mitchell JR, Zimmerman HJ, Ishak KG, Epler GR: Isoniazid-associated hepatitis in 114 patients. Gastroenterology **69:**289-302, 1975.
3. Dickinson DS, Bailey WC, Hirschowitz BI, Soong SJ, Eidus L, Hodgkin MM: Risk factors for isoniazid (INH)-induced liver dysfunction. J Clin Gastroenterol **3:**271-279, 1981.
4. Ellard GA, Gammon PT: Pharmacokinetics of isoniazid metabolism in man. J Pharmacokinet Biopharm **4:**83-113, 1976.
5. Ellard GA, Mitchison DA, Girling DJ, Nunn AJ, Fox W: The hepatic toxicity of isoniazid among rapid and slow acetylators of the drug. Am Rev Respir Dis **118:** 628-629, 1978.
6. Farah F, Taylor W, Rawlins MD, James O: Hepatic drug acetylation and oxidation: Effects of aging in man. Br Med J **2:**155-156, 1978.
7. Groenhagen-Riska C, Hellstrom PE, Froeseth B: Predisposing factors in hepatitis induced by isoniazid-rifampin treatment of tuberculosis. Am Rev Respir Dis **118:**461-466, 1978.
8. Kopanoff DE, Snider DE, Carss GJ: Isoniazid-related hepatitis. A U.S. Public Health Service Cooperative Surveillance Study. Am Rev Respir Dis **117:**991-1001, 1978.
9. Lauterburg BH, Smith CV, Mitchell JR: Determination of isoniazid and its hydrazino metabolites acetylisoniazid, acetylhydrazine, and diacetylhydrazine in human plasma by gas chromatography-mass spectrometry. J Chromatogr **224:**431-438, 1981.
10. Lauterburg BH, Smith CV, Todd EL, Mitchell JR: Pharmacokinetics of the toxic hydrazino metabolites formed from isoniazid in man. J Pharmacol Exp Ther. (In press.)
11. Maddrey WC, Boitnott JK: Isoniazid hepatitis. Ann Intern Med **79:**1-12, 1973.
12. Mitchell JR, Long MW, Thorgeirsson UP, Jollow DJ: Acetylation rates and monthly liver function tests during one year of isoniazid preventive therapy. Chest **68:**181-190, 1975.
13. Mitchell JR, Thorgeirsson UP, Black M, Timbrell JA, Snodgrass WR, Potter WZ, Jollow DJ, Keiser HR: Increased incidence of isoniazid hepatitis in rapid acetylators: Possible relation to hydrazine metabolites. CLIN PHARMACOL THER **18:**70-79, 1975.
14. Mitchell JR, Zimmerman HJ, Ishak KG, Thorgeirsson UP, Timbrell JA, Snodgrass WR, Nelson SD: Isoniazid liver injury: Clinical spectrum, pathology and probable pathogenesis. Ann Intern Med **84:**181-192, 1976.
15. Musch E, Eichelbaum M, Sassen WB, Castro-Parra M, Wang JK, Brestowski U, Baur MP, Dengler HJ: Beziehung Zwischen INH-Metabolismus und INH-Hepatotoxizitaet unter tuberkulostatischer Kombinationbehandlung. Verh Dtsch Ges Inn Med **87:**224-228, 1981.
16. Musch E, Eichelbaum M, Wang JKV, Sassen W, Castro-Parra M, Dengler HJ: Die Haeufigkeit hepatotoxischer Nebenwirkungen der tuberkulostatischen Kombinations therapie (INH, RMP, EMB) in Abhaengigkeit vom Acetyliererphaenotyp. Klin Wochenschr **60:**513-519, 1982.
17. Nelson SD, Mitchell JR, Timbrell JA, Snodgrass WR, Corcoran GB: Isoniazid and iproniazid: Activation of metabolites to toxic intermediates in man and rat. Science **193:**901-903, 1976.
18. Perry HM: DIFFEQ. *In* Perry HM, editor: PROPHET public procedures notebook. Cambridge, Mass., 1982, Bolt, Beranek and Newman, Inc.
19. Peters JH, Miller KW, Brown P: Studies on the metabolic basis for isoniazid inactivation in man. J Pharmacol Exp Ther **150:**298-304, 1965.
20. Singapore Tuberculosis Service/British Medical Research Council: Controlled trial of intermittent regimens of rifampin plus isoniazid for pulmonary tuberculosis in Singapore. Am Rev Respir Dis **116:**807, 1977.
21. Timbrell JA, Mitchell JR, Snodgrass WR, Nelson SD: Isoniazid hepatotoxicity: The relationship between covalent binding and metabolism in vivo. J Pharmacol Exp Ther **213:**364-369, 1980.
22. Timbrell JA, Wright JM, Baillie TA: Monoacetylhydrazine as a metabolite of isoniazid in man. CLIN PHARMACOL THER **22:**602-608, 1977.
23. Winchell HS, Stahelin H, Kusubov N, Slanger B, Fish M, Pollycove M, Lawrence JH: Kinetics of CO_2-HCO_3 in normal adult males. J Nucl Med **12:**711-715, 1970.

Excretion patterns of cannabinoid metabolites after last use in a group of chronic users

The urinary excretion patterns of 86 chronic cannabis users were examined after their last cannabis use by two common screening methods, the semiquantitative EMIT-d.a.u. and the qualitative EMIT-st (Syva Company). We demonstrated that under very strictly supervised abstinence, chronic users can have positive results for cannabinoids in urine at 20 ng/ml or above on the EMIT-d.a.u. assay for as many as 46 consecutive days from admission, and can take as many as 77 days to drop below the cutoff calibrator for 10 consecutive days. For all subjects, the mean excretion time was 27 days. Subject excretion patterns were clearly biphasic, with initial higher rates of excretion not sustained. During the subsequent period of leveling off, most subjects had one or more separate sequences of cannabinoid-negative urine test results, lasting a mean of 3 days each and followed by at least one positive result. Demographic, body type, and drug history variables proved to be only moderate predictors of excretion patterns. Findings were discussed in the context of potential clinical and forensic application. (CLIN PHARMACOL THER 1985;38:572-8.)

George M. Ellis, Jr., B.A., Marian A. Mann, B.A., Barbara A. Judson, M.S., N. Ted Schramm, M.A., and Agop Tashchian, CPT MC, USNR *San Diego, Calif.*

Although it is generally agreed that delta-9-tetrahydrocannabinol (Δ9-THC) is the major psychoactive component of the cannabis (marijuana) plant, there are other cannabinoid constituents, as well as metabolites, that have psychoactive effects. One area of scientific interest is the lengthy retention time of the major metabolites, which seem to persist in the system for up to several weeks after repeated exposure. Very few studies have been made of the actual parameters and profiles of cannabis excretion. Lemberger et al.[1,2] reported that after intravenous injection, cannabis metabolites are excreted in the urine and feces for more than a week in both nonusers and chronic users. Hollister and Kanter[3] reported that a metabolite was found in the urine of nonusers for 72 hours after a single exposure. In the most extensive study to date, Dackis et al.[4] used the EMIT-d.a.u. (Syva Company) methodology in a locked ward setting and reported on seven heavy users who had positive urinalysis results from 14 to 36 days after their last known cannabis use.

We examined the urinary excretion patterns of chronic (regular) cannabis abusers after their last use. This investigation will provide data on the number of days that urine samples of chronic users produce cannabinoid-positive results and examine the various data elements that help establish the subjects' urine excretion patterns.

From the Treatment Department, Naval Drug Rehabilitation Center.
Received for publication March 14, 1985; accepted July 25, 1985.
Reprint requests to: George M. Ellis, Jr., Director of Drug Abuse Services, Behavior Research Incorporated, 3456 Camino del Rio North, Suite 101, San Diego, CA 92108.

METHODS

Subjects. Our subjects were 86 male and female enlisted service personnel undergoing residential treatment for drug and alcohol dependence at the Naval Drug Rehabilitation Center in San Diego. Included in the study were arriving personnel with cannabinoid-positive urine samples for a minimum of the first 3 days after admission, drawn from a sample of 274 entering personnel that were tested over a 5-month period. Subjects were predominantly male (97.7%) and Caucasian (72.1%) and ranged in age from 18 to 34 years ($\overline{X}$ = 22.8 years). They had a history of marijuana use from 2 to 21 years ($\overline{X}$ = 8.9 years) and most (60.5%) used the drug once a day or more often. Over half (55.8%) were abusers of more than one drug, and almost one third (30.2%) were considered heavy users of one or more drugs besides marijuana.

Procedure. Subjects provided first morning voids under direct observation and precise chain-of-custody collection procedures. All urine samples were tested by

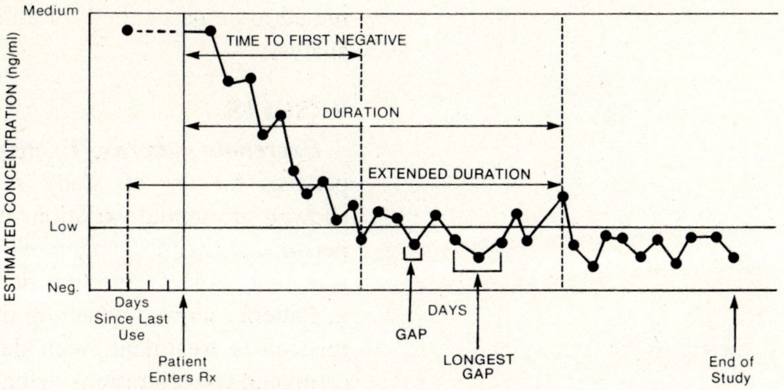

Fig. 1. Urine excretion pattern components: time to first negative result, duration, extended duration, negative gaps, and longest negative gap.

both the semiquantitative EMIT-d.a.u. and the qualitative EMIT-st (Syva Company) cannabinoid assays. Specific gravities, void order, and any prescribed medications were noted. Urine was collected daily until subjects had 10 consecutive cannabinoid-negative tests as determined by EMIT-d.a.u. Within the first week after arrival, data were collected in personal interviews for subject age, sex, body type (lean, average, obese), weight, and a height-weight integrated index (adapted from U.S. Navy combined standards). Self-reported data were also obtained on length of time since last use of cannabis before treatment entry; route of cannabis administration; amount administered during each use; history of cannabis use for lifetime, 6 months, 1 month, and 1 week before treatment entry; and history of alcohol and other drug use.

While it is impossible to state categorically that no marijuana could have been used by subjects while in the Center, the closely supervised conditions made this extremely unlikely. Subjects were never allowed to leave the facility for any reason without staff escort (total Center staff size was 150). Subjects were monitored by staff members 24 hours a day, 7 days a week, including every 15 minutes throughout the night. Subjects were singled out for special staff attention and urine results were carefully scrutinized each testing day and matched with staff clinical observations to reaffirm subject abstinence.

EMIT methodologies and equipment. According to the product literature, EMIT homogeneous enzyme immunoassays for cannabinoids are designed to detect a major urinary metabolite of Δ9-THC, 11-nor-Δ9-THC-9-carboxcylic acid, or a combination of one or more analyte equivalents such as 11-hydroxy-Δ9-THC, 8,β-hydroxy-Δ9-THC, or 8,β-11-hydroxy-Δ9-THC. The semiquantitative EMIT-d.a.u. assay system estimates metabolite concentration with a low or cutoff calibration of 20 ng/ml, a 95% detection level of 50 ng/ml, a medium calibrator of 75 ng/ml, and a detection range to 82.5 ng/ml (all results estimated to be ≥82.5 ng/ml are reported as 82.5 ng/ml). The amount of cannabinoids read from the calibration curve is approximate and expressed as analyte equivalents. The qualitative EMIT-st drug detection system identifies metabolite presence with a low or cutoff calibration of 100 ng/ml and a 95% detection level of 200 ng/ml.

Definitions. The cannabinoid excretion pattern was broken into five basic components: time to first negative result, duration, extended duration, number of negative "gaps," and length of the longest negative "gap" (Fig. 1). The time to the first negative result was defined as the number of cannabinoid-positive days after admission until a subject first produced a cannabinoid-negative urine sample. Duration was the number of days after admission, negative or positive, until the subject provided the last positive urine sample. Extended duration was the number of days in the subject's duration added to the number of days of claimed abstinence before admission to treatment. Number of negative gaps was defined as the number of times a pattern of cannabinoid-positive urine tests turned negative then returned positive. Length of the longest negative gap was the greatest number of days such a negative sequence lasted.

Data analyses. The excretion pattern for each subject was graphed for each method. Excretion outcome data were analyzed for the whole sample and for a by-group categorization based on self-reported light, moderate, or heavy cannabis use over the last month and last 6 months before admission. Wilcoxon two-sample rank tests were done to determine differences between the groups on urine test, demographic, and history vari-

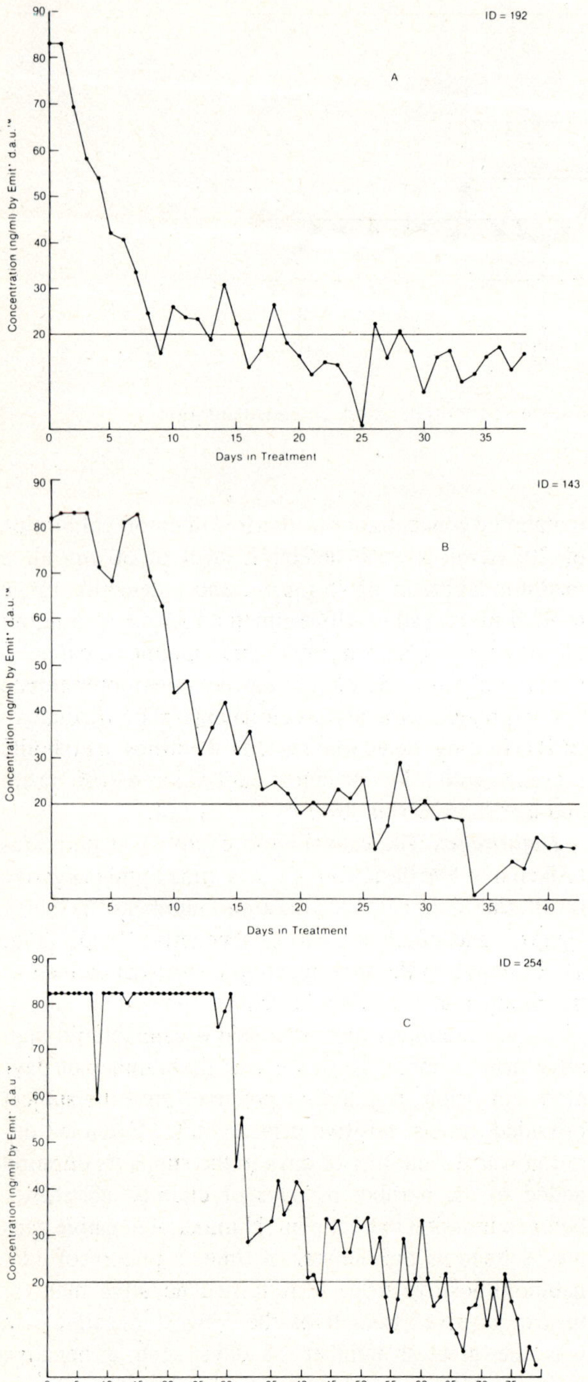

Fig. 2. Estimated daily urine level equivalents for three cannabis users. **A,** Light user; **B,** heavy user; **C,** heavy user.

ables. Pearson product-moment correlations were calculated to examine statistical relationships between variables. Because of the complexity of the study components, a stepwise regression procedure was determined to be best suited for an exploratory multivariate analysis.

RESULTS

Excretion patterns. Examination of the excretion patterns for the 86 study subjects by EMIT-d.a.u. showed substantial variations in form, slope, and number of days with cannabinoid-positive results. Representative subject excretion patterns are shown in Fig. 2. Patterns showed generally declining values after admission to treatment, with day-to-day fluctuations in estimated concentrations evident in most cases. Nonetheless, there were no obvious large peaks in the excretion patterns that suggested continued use during the Center stay. Inspection of the excretion graphs revealed a biphasic pattern. After a fairly steep drop in excretion levels, metabolite concentrations often fluctuated around the low or cutoff calibration level (20 ng/ml), causing prominent negative gaps in the graphs of both the EMIT-d.a.u. and EMIT-st results. There seemed to be no relationship between special events (i.e., extra physical exercise), medications taken, or weight loss and major shifts in excreted cannabinoid concentration.

Data were obtained primarily (91.2%) from the first void of the morning. Of the five subjects who provided two urine samples in the same morning, one showed an increase in estimated concentration between successive voids; the others showed estimated decreases of from 5 to 42 ng/ml as determined by EMIT-d.a.u.

Time to first negative result, duration, and extended duration. Table I shows descriptive statistics for the excretion pattern outcome variables for all subjects. For both testing methods, and especially for the more sensitive EMIT-d.a.u. procedures, subjects showed broader ranges and greater means than previously described in anecdotal reports or in the literature. When subjects were divided into light, moderate, and heavy use categories (Table I), the expected directional increases in these outcome variables were observed in most cases. However, there was substantial overlap in the ranges observed. Wilcoxon two-sample rank tests between groups showed significant differences for both methods in time to first negative result and in duration for only the light/heavy and moderate/heavy user comparisons. Extended duration was significantly different only for the light/heavy user comparison determined by EMIT-d.a.u.

Table II shows the frequency of duration of cannabinoid excretion patterns for both testing methods. When one considers the time it took to maintain negative results for 10 consecutive days, almost one third (32.6%) of the subjects (most of them heavy users)

Table I. Cannabinoid excretion patterns by EMIT-d.a.u. and EMIT-st methods: Overall and by intensity of use (light/moderate/heavy) in last month and last 6 months before treatment admission

	Time to first negative result (days)	*Duration (days)*	*Extended duration (days)*	*No. of negative gaps*	*Length of longest negative gap (days)*
All subjects (n = 86)					
EMIT-d.a.u.					
$\overline{X}$	16.0	27.1	32.0	2.6	3.4
SD	10.7	16.6	18.1	1.8	2.7
Range	3-46	3-77	6-81	0-8	0-10*
EMIT-st					
$\overline{X}$	4.3	9.2	14.1	1.0	2.7
SD	4.5	10.3	12.8	1.5	4.8
Range	0-22	0-45	1-55	0-8	0-26
Group 1: Light users (n = 8)					
EMIT-d.a.u					
$\overline{X}$	8.5	12.9	18.2	1.2	2.0
SD	5.2	10.3	10.3	1.8	2.7
Range	3-18	3-29	7-34	0-5	0-7*
EMIT-st					
$\overline{X}$	1.0	3.4	8.7	0.6	1.6
SD	1.5	4.2	5.1	0.9	2.4
Range	0-3	0-11	4-18	0-2	0-6
Group 2: Moderate users (n = 26)					
EMIT-d.a.u.					
$\overline{X}$	11.8	22.7	32.5	2.2	3.9
SD	7.4	13.0	19.2	1.5	3.3
Range	3-33	3-63	8-70	0-6	0-10*
EMIT-st					
$\overline{X}$	3.3	6.1	15.9	0.4	2.8
SD	3.2	8.9	17.1	0.8	6.4
Range	0-14	0-34	2-55	0-4	0-26
Group 3: Heavy users (n = 52)					
EMIT-d.a.u.					
$\overline{X}$	19.1	31.5	33.9	2.9	3.4
SD	11.5	17.4	17.7	1.9	2.3
Range	3-46	4-77	6-81	0-8	0-9*
EMIT-st					
$\overline{X}$	5.3	11.6	14.1	1.4	2.9
SD	5.0	10.9	10.9	1.7	4.1
Range	0-22	0-45	1-47	0-8	0-21

Light use is defined as cannabis use weekly or less often over the last month and six months preceding admission. Moderate use is defined as use two to six times per week in either time frame or averaged over the last month and 6 months. Heavy use is defined as use daily or more often in either the last month or 6 months.
*By operational procedures (see text), subjects were automatically terminated from the study after 10 days of negative EMIT-d.a.u. results.

remained positive by the EMIT-d.a.u. at 20 ng/ml for more than a month, with four subjects remaining positive for >2 months.

Number of negative gaps and length of longest negative gap. For both testing methods, there was a similarly wide range in the number of negative gaps (Table I). Negative gaps were noted in 87.2% of our subjects by EMIT-d.a.u. testing (75 of 86 cases) and in 47.7% of our subjects by EMIT-st testing (41 of 86 cases). Only a few of the demographic and history variables correlated with the number of negative gaps.

There was a wide range in the longest negative gap observed (Table I), with the Emit-st range of particular note. The length of the longest negative gap extended >3 days in 39.5% of our subjects as determined by EMIT-d.a.u. testing (34 of 86 cases) and in 24.4% of our subjects as determined by EMIT-st testing (21 of 86 cases). Of particular interest is that six subjects (7.0%) had a longest negative gap as determined by EMIT-st >10 days. It should be remembered that the length of the longest gap in EMIT-d.a.u. testing was limited by operational definition to only 10 days, the criterion for termination from the study.

Wilcoxon two-sample rank tests showed little con-

Table II. Frequency distribution of the duration of excretion patterns as determined by EMIT-d.a.u. and EMIT-st

	EMIT-d.a.u.		*EMIT-st*	
Days	*No.*	*%*	*No.*	*%*
0	0	0.0	13	15.1
1-10	12	14.0	47	54.7
11-20	22	25.6	15	17.4
21-30	24	27.9	5	5.8
31-40	9	10.5	5	5.8
41-50	14	16.3	1	1.2
51-60	1	1.2	0	0.0
61-70	1	1.2	0	0.0
71-80	3	3.5	0	0.0

sistency in significant differences between groups in either the number of negative gaps or the length of the longest negative gap.

As expected, excretion variables correlated most highly with the other excretion variables (with r values ranging up to 0.89). Many of the history and demographic variables were also significantly related to the excretion variables, but the correlation coefficients were considerably smaller (with r values ranging up to 0.44) than those observed between the excretion variables themselves.

When all variables were placed in the stepwise regression procedure with time to first negative result, duration, and extended duration, the excretion outcome variables proved to the greatest predictors, accounting for between 72.1% and 100.0% of the variability. When the excretion outcome variables were removed, the 12 demographic and history variables selected for evaluation were only modest contributors to a predictive model, either singly or in complement (Table III). For the EMIT-d.a.u., although the overall hypothetic models were significant ($P < 0.001$), the percent of variability accounted for by variables in the time to first negative result, duration, and extended duration regressions were relatively slight (35.7%, 42.7%, and 48.3%, respectively). Similar results were seen in the EMIT-st analyses, with the variables in the time to first negative result, duration, and extended duration regressions accounting for 41.4%, 31.8%, and 59.2% of the variability, respectively, despite overall significant models ($P < 0.001$). Three of the demographic and history variables (age, weight, and having a history of cannabis use more than once a day) seemed to be the most prominent, but their overall predictive value could only be judged as moderate.

DISCUSSION

Despite considerable clinical and forensic interest, there have been surprisingly few published data on the length of cannabinoid excretion in the urine of chronic users after last use. Important data were provided by Dackis et al.,[4] whose seven subjects had a mean of 24 days with cannabinoid-positive results (with an upward range of 36 days) before a first negative result was observed. A published case study[5] gave data on a chronic smoker who provided cannabinoid-positive urine samples for 15 consecutive days after reportedly ceasing use, and who was still positive after 20 days of testing. (Both of these studies used EMIT-d.a.u. testing with a 20 ng/ml cutoff.) Our results are in general agreement with those data and substantially extend the published findings. Urine samples from our 86 chronic users were still cannabinoid positive up to 46 days ($\bar{X}$ = 16 days) as determined by EMIT-d.a.u. before the first negative result, and took up to 77 days ($\bar{X}$ = 27 days) to drop below the 20 ng/ml cutoff for 10 consecutive days (Table I). Both the extended range of positive days and the variations in the excretion outcome variables for both EMIT-d.a.u. and EMIT-st were unexpected and not previously reported.

Our study validates the reliability and usefulness of the EMIT-d.a.u. method for determining urinary excretion patterns after chronic cannabinoid use. Our results also provide new information that should be taken into account in the interpretation of urine test results for cannabinoids, regardless of the method used. Current applications of urinalysis, such as in surveillance of identified users, should be reevaluated in light of our data.

Our data generally confirm previous research that chronic users can take, on the average, about a month to achieve consistently negative urine samples as determined by a sensitive urine assay such as the EMIT-d.a.u. that uses a 20 ng/ml cutoff calibration (Table I).

In terms of the duration of positive results, well over half (60.6%) of our chronic users had cannabinoid-positive results for ≥21 days after last use, almost one third (32.7%) had positive results for >30 days, and 4.7% had positive results for >60 days before dropping below the EMIT-d.a.u. 20 ng/ml cutoff for 10 consecutive days (Table II). There was a natural break observed in the distribution at 50 days, which based on these data seems to be a reasonable upward limit for the evaluation of most chronic users (Table II). The five subjects who had positive results for >50 days had been heavy users for at least 12 years; however, there were

Table III. Contribution of index history variables to predicting excretion pattern outcomes*

EMIT-d.a.u.				*EMIT-st*			
Index variable	*Cumulative r^2*	*Contribution to outcome (F value)*	*P value*	*Index variable*	*Cumulative r^2*	*Contribution to outcome (F value)*	*P value*
Time to first negative result							
MJ use in last week†	0.183	7.63	0.008	MJ use in last week	0.186‡		
Age	0.268	6.02	0.017	Age	0.292	11.54	0.001
History of MJ use more than daily	0.321	5.48	0.023	History of MJ use more than daily	0.339	6.35	0.015
Weight	0.357	3.17	NS	MJ use in last month†	0.369	13.18	0.001
				Weight	0.414	6.54	0.013
Duration							
History of MJ use more than daily	0.184	8.14	0.006	Weight	0.141	12.29	0.001
Weight	0.305	13.29	0.001	History of MJ use more than daily	0.274	11.06	0.002
MJ use in last 6 months†	0.346	6.54	0.013	Age	0.318	3.73	NS
Age	0.396	6.42	0.014				
Days since last use†	0.427	2.97	NS				
Extended duration							
Days since last use	0.120	10.23	0.002	Days since last use	0.375	43.66	0.001
History of MJ use more than daily	0.273	8.14	0.006	Weight	0.464	13.56	0.001
Weight	0.381	13.29	0.001	History of MJ use more than daily	0.543	5.92	0.020
MJ use in last 6 months	0.423	6.54	0.013	Age	0.575	5.43	0.020
Age	0.483	6.42	0.014	MJ use in last 6 months	0.592	2.30	NS

MJ = Marijuana; NS = not significant.
*Stepwise multiple regression evaluating 12 index history variables including age, physical characteristics (weight, height-weight index, body type), and recent and long-term patterns of marijuana use (n = 61).
†Before admission to treatment.
‡Contribution of variable before being removed by stepwise regression procedure.

other subjects with similar cannabis histories who had cannabinoid-positive results for <50 days.

Of those chronic users who had a cannabinoid-positive result on the EMIT-st, only a few (15.1%) had positive results on the EMIT-st for ≥21 days, while a majority (64.4%) had positive results for ≤10 days before returning to a consistently negative pattern (Table II).

Although there were statistically significant differences in the means of many of the excretion variables between subjects grouped by self-reported light, moderate, and heavy use, the amount of overlap in the ranges was noteworthy. While it is not clear how individual data points would be affected by urine samples collected randomly during the day, the outside ranges could aid in the interpretation of test results. Thus if a subject claimed to be a light user, one would expect to see a first negative test result on the EMIT-d.a.u. within approximately 18 days after ceasing use and the daily test results to start being consistently negative no more than a month after last use.

Although many were statistically significant, few of the demographic and history variables showed substantial correlative relationships with the excretion pattern components. Based on the stepwise regression analysis, demographic and history variables showed little usefulness as predictors of excretion patterns (Table III). There was a lack of real predictive prominence of body type, weight, and height-weight index, despite suggestions of previous research in animals.[6] Weight alone seemed to show the most promise. Age was evident in almost every regression; however, its overall importance appeared relatively small. Also demonstrating little impact were the various cannabis history variables.

Although expected, the identification of a clear biphasic pattern in urine has not been previously reported in the literature on cannabinoid excretion. Also of interest is the fluctuating effect in the day-to-day EMIT-d.a.u. determinations, especially around the cutoff level that created the strings of negative gaps. This phenomenon is not too surprising for a long-persisting analyte, but might tend to confuse the proper interpretation of results for those not familiar with this phenomenon. This can be partly attributed to the semiquantitative nature of the assay and the differing reactivity with the metabolites, to differing amounts of the metabolites being released in the body, and to increased test variability when measuring values at the extreme end of the calibration curve. Once a subject had a urine test result that went below the 20 ng/ml cutoff, no subsequent test ever went above the medium calibrator (75 ng/ml) and only five subjects (6.7% of the subjects with negative EMIT-d.a.u. gaps) had positive urine samples >50 ng/ml.

Estimates of time since last use derived from a single urine test result or even a spaced series of results would seem to have limited forensic value. Our study reaffirms that a positive urine test result from a chronic user does not necessarily indicate recent or continued use. Because of large individual variability, a positive test result may reflect use within the past few hours, days, weeks, or even months, depending on the cutoff calibration level selected. Because of the special sensitivity demonstrated by the EMIT assay, which cross-reacts with a broad metabolite mix rather than a single prominent metabolite such as the 9-carboxy-THC (COOH-THC), it is clear from previous comparative research that the duration of positive results would also be affected when an alternate method is used.[7,8] Additionally, some urine specimens have been found to have lower concentrations of free COOH-THC than expected based on unpredictable rates of metabolization to its glucuronide ester.[9-11] Even EMIT results must be interpreted with some small amount of caution because assay response may vary slightly with the relative ratio of free COOH-THC and this unstable glucuronide conjugate.* Finally, the impact of the differences of drug potency (plant genetics), the potential interactive effect of previous alcohol and other drug abuse, and the differences in bioavailability of Δ9-THC in the route and pattern of administration due to the experience of the user would seem important, but such studies were beyond the scope of our investigation.

*Willette RE: Personal communication, 1985.

Donald Avoy, M.D., and David Himmelberger, M.S., of Syva Company, Palo Alto, Calif., provided operational support and technical assistance in the project. Avram Goldstein, M.D., Addiction Research Foundation, Palo Alto, Calif.; Robert Willette, Ph.D., Research Design, Annapolis, Md.; and John Irving, CDR MSC, USN, Naval Medical Command, Washington, D. C., provided helpful guidance in the draft review. Lyn Chilcote of the Naval Drug Rehabilitation Center provided technical review of project materials. Hospital Corpsmen Phillip Mucha, Rande Stanvitch, and F. Lincoln Merritt of the Naval Drug Rehabilitation Center conducted most of the urinalyses.

References

1. Lemberger L, Silberstein SD, Axelrod J, Kopin IJ. Marijuana: Studies on the disposition and metabolism of delta-9-tetrahydrocannabinol in man. Science 1970;170:1320-2.
2. Lemberger L, Tamarkin NR, Axelrod J, Kopin IJ. Delta-9-tetrahydrocannabinol: Metabolism and disposition in long-term marihuana smokers. Science 1971;173:72-4.
3. Hollister LE, Kanter SL. Laboratory verification of "heavy" and "light" users of cannabis. Drug Alcohol Depend 1980;5:151-2.
4. Dackis CA, Pottash ALC, Annitto W, Gold MS. Persistence of urinary marijuana levels after supervised abstinence. Am J Psychiatry 1982;139:1196-8.
5. Clinical summary addendum, EMIT-d.a.u. and EMIT-st urine cannabinoid assays. Palo Alto, Calif: Syva Company, 1982:40-4.
6. Garrett ER, Hunt CA. Pharmacokinetics of Δ9-tetrahydrocannabinol in dogs. J Pharm Sci 1977;66:395-407.
7. Jones AB, ElSholy HW, Arafat ES, ElSohly MA. Analysis of the major metabolite of Δ9-tetrahydrocannabinol in urine. IV. A comparison of five methods. J Anal Toxicol 1984;8:249-51.
8. Irving J, Leeb B, Foltz RL, Cook CE, Bursey JT, Willette RE. Evaluation of immunoassays for cannabinoids in urine. J Anal Toxicol 1984;8:192-6.
9. Peat MA, Finkle BS, Deyman ME. Laboratory evaluation of immunoassay kits for the detection of cannabinoids in biological fluids. In: Hawks RL, ed. The analysis of cannabinoids in biological fluids. Rockville, Md: National Institute on Drug Abuse 1982:85-98; NIDA Research Monograph 42.
10. Foltz RL. Analysis of cannabinoids in physiological specimens by gas chromatography/mass spectrometry. In: Baselt RC, ed. Advances in analytical toxicology, vol I. Foster City, Calif: Biomedical Publications, 1984:125-57.
11. Williams PL, Moffat AC. Identification in human urine of Δ9-tetrahydrocannabinol-11-oic acid glucuronide: A tetrahydrocannabinol metabolite. J Pharm Pharmacol 1980;32:445-8.

Ultra-short-acting beta-blockade: A comparison with conventional beta-blockade

Esmolol is a β_1-selective adrenoceptor blocker that is rapidly metabolized by blood and liver esterases. The β-receptor and hemodynamic effects of esmolol were determined in a group of 12 healthy men and were compared with those induced by both oral and intravenous propranolol. Esmolol was rapidly effective in inducing at least 90% of steady-state β-blockade within 5 minutes of either initiating or changing the esmolol infusion rate. More importantly, when esmolol infusion was discontinued the β-blockade had totally disappeared by 18 minutes after esmolol, 300 μg/kg/min, and had been reduced by 50% after 750 μg/kg/min. In contrast, 30 minutes after discontinuation of a propranolol infusion, there was no change in the level of β-blockade. Propranolol was much more potent at blocking isoproterenol-induced tachycardia (dose ratio 33.5 ± 2.5) than was even the highest dose (750 μg/kg/min) of esmolol (dose ratio 13.1 ± 1.0). The same dose of intravenous propranolol was approximately equipotent to oral propranolol, 40 mg every 8 hours (dose ratio 33.5 ± 2.5 and 34.5 ± 3.6, respectively). In contrast, propranolol, 40 mg every 8 hours, and esmolol, 300 μg/kg/min, were equipotent in antagonizing exercise-induced tachycardia (40.1% ± 2.3% and 42.7% ± 3.2%, respectively). Esmolol had striking hypotensive effects. Systolic blood pressure fell by 20 mm Hg during esmolol infusions of 750 μg/kg/min. Esmolol appears to be a potent β_1-selective adrenoceptor antagonist with a particularly strong hypotensive effect. It is likely to be very useful in the treatment of hemodynamically unstable patients and may be useful in the emergency treatment of hypertension. (CLIN PHARMACOL THER 1985;38:579-85.)

Charles S. Reilly, M.D.,* Margaret Wood, M.D., Richard P. Koshakji, Ph.D., and Alastair J. J. Wood, M.D. *Nashville, Tenn.*

β-Adrenoceptor–blocking agents are among the most widely prescribed groups of drugs and are used in the treatment of hypertension, angina, and cardiac arrhythmias and in the symptomatic treatment of thyrotoxicosis. An important recent indication for β-blockers is in the therapy of patients after a myocardial infarction.[1-3] Although it is not clear how soon β-blocker therapy should be started after a myocardial infarction, there is increasing evidence to suggest that patients benefit from β-blockade instituted as early as possible in the postinfarct period.[3] Recent studies have demonstrated the benefits of β-blockade during anesthesia and coronary artery bypass surgery.[4] Thus there are increasing demands to administer β-blockade to potentially hemodynamically unstable patients.

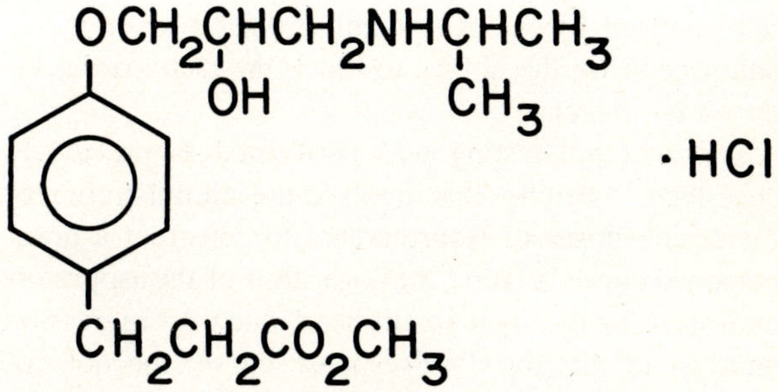

Esmolol

Physicians frequently feel reluctant to administer a β-blocker intravenously to patients in a critical care setting, because if β-blockade is induced by conventional drugs and an adverse effect occurs, it takes considerable time for the effects to wear off because of the

From the Departments of Pharmacology, Medicine, and Anesthesiology, Vanderbilt University School of Medicine.

Supported in part by United States Public Health Service Grants No. RR95 and No. HL14192 and by a grant from American Critical Care, Inc.

Received for publication May 8, 1985; accepted July 25, 1985.

Reprint requests to: Dr. Alastair J. J. Wood, Department of Pharmacology, Vanderbilt University School of Medicine, Nashville, TN 37232.

*Present address: Department of Anaesthesia, Royal Hallamshire Hospital, Sheffield, United Kingdom.

relatively long $t_{1/2}$ of the currently available β-blockers. Also, should the patient's condition change such that β-receptor agonists are required to maintain cardiac output, such as after cardiac surgery, then conventional doses of β-receptor stimulants will produce no effect. Because of the concerns about administering conventional β-blockers to unstable patients, attempts have been made to develop drugs with an ultra-short duration of action.[5] Esmolol (see structure) is an ultra-short-acting β_1-selective adrenoceptor antagonist that is rapidly metabolized by both blood and liver esterases such that its $t_{1/2}$ in man is <10 minutes.[6]

We evaluated the potency and hemodynamic effects of esmolol in man and compared the effects of esmolol with those of the conventional β-blocker propranolol after oral or intravenous dosing to determine the appropriate dose of propranolol for continuing oral β-blockade after the end of esmolol dosing.

METHODS

Subjects. With the approval of the Institutional Review Board, 12 healthy men with a mean (±SE) age of 25.5 ± 1.2 years and weight of 75.7 ± 2.6 kg were studied. Each subject received both esmolol and propranolol in random order. There was at least a 48-hour washout between propranolol and esmolol dosing when propranolol was given first and at least a 24-hour washout between drugs when esmolol was given first.

Measurement of β-blockade. The extent of β-blockade was measured by determining the ability of the β-adrenoceptor antagonist to block first the increased heart rate induced by the β-receptor agonist isoproterenol, and second by the ability to block the tachycardia induced by exercise.

Isoproterenol testing was performed as previously described.[7-9] Briefly, this involved the administration of increasing doses of isoproterenol to construct a dose-response curve relating the logarithm of the isoproterenol dose to the increase in heart rate. By regression analysis of this log dose-response curve, the dose of isoproterenol required to raise the heart rate by 25 bpm (I_{25}) was calculated. The extent of β-blockade was expressed as the ratio of the I_{25} required after β-blockade to that required before β-blockade (dose ratio).[7,8]

Esmolol phase. Seven of the subjects received a placebo infusion followed by 100, 200, and 300 μg/kg/min esmolol after loading doses, while six subjects received a placebo infusion followed by 100, 250, 500, and 750 μg/kg/min esmolol after loading doses (one subject received both regimens on separate days). Each infusion rate was administered for 1 hour and then stepped up to the next dose. A loading dose of 500 μg/kg/min for 1.0, 1.25, and 1.5 minutes was given before the 100, 200, and 300 μg/kg/min infusions, respectively, while 1250 μg/kg/min was given for 1.0, 1.25, and 1.5 minutes before the 250, 500, and 750 μg/kg/min infusions, respectively.

The I_{25} was determined as described above during the placebo infusion and after 30 minutes at each dose level of esmolol. In addition, to determine the speed of onset of additional β-blockade after each dosage change, the I_{25} estimated at the previous esmolol dose was readministered and the increase in heart rate was measured 5 and 25 minutes after each increase of the esmolol infusion rate. A blood sample was drawn during the isoproterenol study for measurement of esmolol concentrations.

After the esmolol infusion was stopped, the I_{25} during the placebo infusion was readministered 2, 6, 10, 14, and 18 minutes afterwards to determine the time to full recovery from β-blockade. Blood pressure and heart rate were measured 10, 20, and 30 minutes after each dosage change and during the period after the esmolol infusion was terminated.

Intravenous propranolol phase. All twelve subjects received a placebo infusion followed by a loading dose of 9.9 mg propranolol administered over 9 minutes and a maintenance infusion of 55 μg/min propranolol. Blood pressure and heart rate were measured during the placebo infusion and at 10, 20, and 30 minutes after the start of the propranolol infusion. Plasma samples were drawn for measurement of propranolol by HPLC[10] 50 minutes after the start of the propranolol infusion, which was approximately the midpoint of the isoproterenol test. The I_{25} was determined during the placebo infusion and 30 minutes after the start of the propranolol infusion. The dose ratio was calculated as described above.

Oral propranolol phase. After completing the intravenous propranolol study, all 12 subjects then received oral propranolol, 10 mg every 8 hours, for 4 days. On day 5, 2 hours after the morning dose of propranolol, isoproterenol testing was repeated. The propranolol dose was then increased to 20 mg every 8 hours for 2 days, then 40 mg every 8 hours for 2 days. On day 2 at each dose level, 2 hours after the morning dose, isoproterenol testing was repeated and plasma was drawn at the beginning and end of the isoproterenol test for measurement of the mean propranolol concentration.

Exercise testing. In six of the subjects the effects of esmolol, 300 μg/kg/min, and propranolol, 40 mg po every 8 hours, on exercise-induced tachycardia were compared. The subjects, who had been familiarized with the procedure on previous days, exercised on a

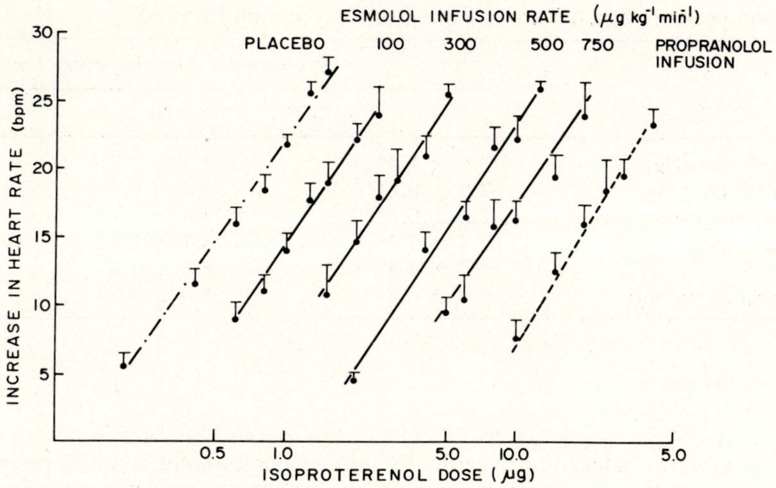

Fig. 1. Mean (± SE) log dose-response curves to isoproterenol during infusions of placebo, esmolol, or propranolol.

Table I. Dose ratios during esmolol and propranolol infusions and during propranolol, 40 mg po every 8 hours

	Esmolol infusion (μg/kg/min)					
	100	*300*	*500*	*750*	*Intravenous propranolol*	*Oral propranolol*
Dose ratio	2.02 ± 0.08	3.95 ± 0.17	7.77 ± 0.38	13.11 ± 1.0	33.52 ± 2.52	34.46 ± 3.6
Concentration (ng/ml)	330 ± 0.05	820 ± 0.12	2600 ± 580	4310 ± 860	43.8 ± 3.3	64.4 ± 8.9

Data are $\overline{X}$ ± SE.

treadmill for 3 minutes at each of four grades of exercise. The gradients and speed of the treadmill at each stage of exercise were 10%/1.7 mph, 12%/2.5 mph, 14%/3.4 mph, and 16%/4.2 mph. ECG monitoring was performed throughout the procedure and the heart rate was determined from the ECG for the final 30 seconds at each exercise grade. The heart rate increase induced by exercise was calculated as the difference between the maximum heart rate during the final 30 seconds of exercise and the maximum heart rate during a similar period after stabilization immediately before exercise. During propranolol dosing the exercise test was performed approximately 2 hours after the last dose of propranolol, 40 mg po every 8 hours.

To determine the effects of esmolol on exercise tachycardia, subjects also exercised after a loading dose of 500 μg/kg/min esmolol for 1.5 minutes, followed by an infusion of 300 μg/kg/min esmolol for 30 minutes. The esmolol infusion continued during exercise.

The increase in heart rate was also determined after the subjects had exercised on a separate occasion when they had not received β-receptor antagonists for at least 48 hours. The extent of β-blockade was expressed as: Degree of suppression of exercise-induced tachycardia = (Rise in heart rate without β-blocker − rise in heart rate during β-blockade)/rise in heart rate without β-blocker.

Statistical analysis was by ANOVA and Student's t test for paired and unpaired values where appropriate. $P < 0.05$ was taken as the minimum level of significance.

RESULTS

The I_{25} values measured during the placebo infusion that preceded both the propranolol and esmolol phases were virtually identical (1.21 ± 0.08 and 1.27 ± 0.08 μg, respectively). The mean dose-response curves relating the increase in heart rate to the logarithm of the isoproterenol dose during infusions of placebo, esmolol, and propranolol are shown in Fig. 1. The propranolol infusion was more potent at inhibiting the isoproterenol-induced rise in heart rate than the highest dose of esmolol. The mean dose ratio during the four infusion rates of esmolol ranged from 2.02 to 13.1. The intravenous propranolol infusion and propranolol, 40 mg po every 8 hours, were equally effective in antagonizing isoproterenol-induced tachycardia, resulting in dose ratios of 33.5 and 34.5, respectively, although the pro-

Table II. Change in blood pressure and heart rate during oral propranolol dosing

	Propranolol dose (mg every 8 hr)		
	10	*20*	*40*
Change in systolic BP (mm Hg)	3.3 ± 1.4*	4.5 ± 1.2†	6.83 ± 1.2†
Change in diastolic BP (mm Hg)	2.9 ± 0.8*	3.5 ± 0.7*	5.6 ± 1.0†
Change in mean BP (mm Hg)	2.6 ± 0.81*	3.8 ± 0.7†	5.8 ± 0.9†
Change in heart rate (bpm)	3.4 ± 2.2	3.1 ± 2.9	5.6 ± 2.0*
Dose ratio	9.4 ± 0.8	18.5 ± 1.5	34.5 ± 3.7
Propranolol concentration (ng/ml)	9.6 ± 0.8	28.0 ± 3.5	64.4 ± 8.9

Data are $\bar{X}$ ± SE.
BP = Blood pressure.
*P < 0.05, †P < 0.005 compared with baseline.

Table III. Suppression of exercise-induced tachycardia by intravenous esmolol and oral propranolol

	Propranolol (40 mg every 8 hr)	*Esmolol (300 μg/kg/min)*
Suppression of exercise-induced tachycardia (%)	40.1% ± 2.3%	42.7% ± 3.2%

Data are $\bar{X}$ ± SE.

Table IV. Change in blood pressure and heart rate during esmolol and propranolol infusions

	Esmolol infusion (μg/kg/min)					*Intravenous propranolol*
	100	*200*	*300*	*500*	*750*	
Change in systolic BP (mm Hg)	−3.92 ± 0.7*	−8.0 ± 1.2*	−8.4 ± 1.6*	−15.8 ± 2.3*	−19.4 ± 1.8*	−6.08 ± 0.8*
Change in diastolic BP (mm Hg)	−1.0 ± 0.6	−2.9 ± 1.1†	−2.3 ± 0.9†	−2.3 ± 1.8	−4.0 ± 0.9†	−1.3 ± 0.8
Change in mean arterial pressure (mm Hg)	−2.0 ± 0.5*	−4.6 ± 1.0*	−4.3 ± 1.1†	−8.2 ± 1.9†	−10.0 ± 1.7*	−2.8 ± 0.7*
Change in heart rate (bpm)	−2.4 ± 1.3	−6.1 ± 2.2†	−4.9 ± 2.5	+2 ± 2.3	+5.6 ± 4.0	−5.1 ± 1.0*

Data are $\bar{X}$ ± SE.
BP = Blood pressure; − = decrease from baseline; + = increase from baseline.
*P < 0.005, †P < 0.05 compared with pretreatment value.

pranolol concentrations were slightly higher after oral dosing (Table I). The isoproterenol dose ratios after oral propranolol are listed in Table II.

The comparison between the ability of intravenous esmolol and oral propranolol to suppress exercise-induced tachycardia is shown in Table III. Esmolol, 300 μg/kg/min, and propranolol, 40 mg every 8 hours, were equipotent in suppressing exercise-induced tachycardia.

Infusion of esmolol was associated with a dose-related fall in blood pressure (Table IV; Fig. 2). This was most striking for systolic blood pressure, which fell by almost 20 mm Hg ($P < 0.005$) during the 750 μg/kg/min infusion (Fig. 2). In one subject the esmolol infusion was terminated after the 500 μg/kg/min dose because systolic blood pressure had fallen from 117 to 90 mm Hg during the 500 μg/kg/min infusion. During the propranolol infusion, however, the fall in blood pressure was much less than that after the highest esmolol dose (Table IV). Blood pressures and isoproterenol dose ratios during oral propranolol dosing are listed in Table II.

During both oral and intravenous propranolol (Tables II and III) the heart rate showed the expected fall. The change in heart rate during the esmolol infusion is shown in Fig. 3. Although the heart rate fell significantly during the infusions of 200 and 250 μg/kg/min esmolol, this fall was reversed at the higher doses of esmolol, such that the heart rate was actually nonsignificantly above the baseline value during the 500 and 750 μg/kg/min infusions. This happened when there was a considerable reduction in blood pressure and may reflect reflex cardiac stimulation due to the esmolol-induced hypotension.

To determine how rapidly a constant level of β-blockade was achieved with esmolol, the I_{25} during the previous esmolol dosing was administered 5 and 25 min-

Table V. Speed of achieving new steady-state β-blockade with esmolol*

Esmolol dose (μg/kg/min)	*5 min after dose increase (% predicted)*	*25 min after dose increase (% predicted)*
100	101.5 ± 4.1	112.5 ± 5.1
200	89.6 ± 2.4	96.4 ± 2.5
300	94.0 ± 5.1	98.2 ± 5.8

Results are shown as the percentage of the predicted response based on the subsequently calculated dose-response curve.

utes after each increase in esmolol infusion rate during the 100, 200, and 300 μg/kg/min infusions. Heart rate responses to these doses of isoproterenol are listed in Table V. The response to this dose of isoproterenol was at least 90% of the response determined from the subsequent isoproterenol dose-response curve, implying that at least 90% of the eventual new steady-state level of β-blockade was reached within 5 minutes of either starting the esmolol infusion or altering the esmolol infusion rate.

Because of esmolol's rapid metabolism, the speed of reversal of esmolol's effects was studied after the end of both the 300 and 750 μg/kg/min infusions (Table VI). After the 300 μg/kg/min esmolol infusion there was a rapid return of both heart rate and blood pressure to preinfusion levels. However, at the higher (750 μg/kg/min) rate, blood pressure rose after the infusion stopped but it had not fully recovered by 18 minutes after the infusion. After the 750 μg/kg/min infusion, the heart rate, which during the infusion was already above the values before esmolol dosing, rose even higher. There was no significant change in either heart rate or systolic blood pressure 15 or 30 minutes after the propranolol infusion was stopped.

To assess the time to recover from β-blockade after the esmolol infusion was stopped, the estimated I_{25} during the placebo infusion was readministered at the end of the infusion and then on multiple occasions up to 18 minutes after the infusion was stopped (Table VII). Because the I_{25} during placebo infusion had to be estimated during the experiment and was therefore slightly different than that measured from the subsequent linear regression analysis, the heart rate increase that this dose would actually have induced as determined from log-linear regression analysis of the isoproterenol dose-response curve was calculated and is listed in Table VII for consistency. Although the I_{25} induced only a mean increase in heart rate of 5 bpm during the 300 μg/kg/min esmolol infusion, this had more than doubled 2 minutes after the infusion was stopped, and full recovery had occurred by 18 minutes. During the higher 750 μg/kg/min infusion rate, the baseline I_{25} dose induced no change in heart rate; however, even at this dose recovery was rapid, although less complete than at the lower dose. Administration of the I_{25} from the placebo infusion produced no change in heart rate at the end of the propranolol infusion, and there was no response to this dose during the recovery period of up to 30 minutes. In addition, the study was stopped in one subject after the 500 μg/kg/min esmolol dose because of hypotension and a feeling of malaise. During the infusion of the highest dose of esmolol, five of the subjects developed headaches lasting 1 to 6 hours, and in two subjects the headaches were severe. In one of the five subjects the headache began at the 250 μg/kg/min dose. Nausea also accompanied headache in two subjects (one of whom vomited) at the highest dose of esmolol. One subject developed diarrhea during oral propranolol dosing.

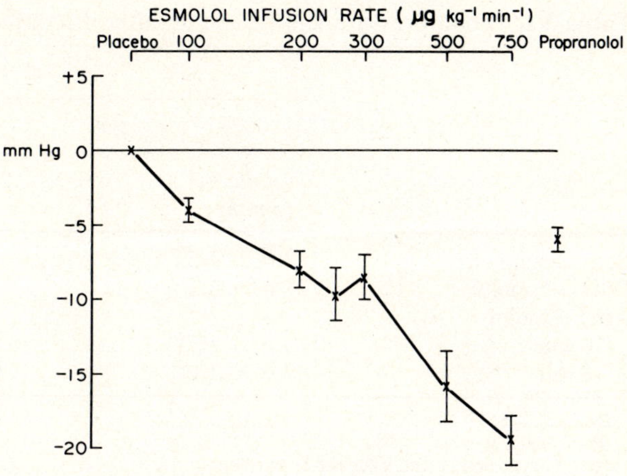

Fig. 2. Mean (±SE) changes in systolic blood pressure during infusions of esmolol and propranolol.

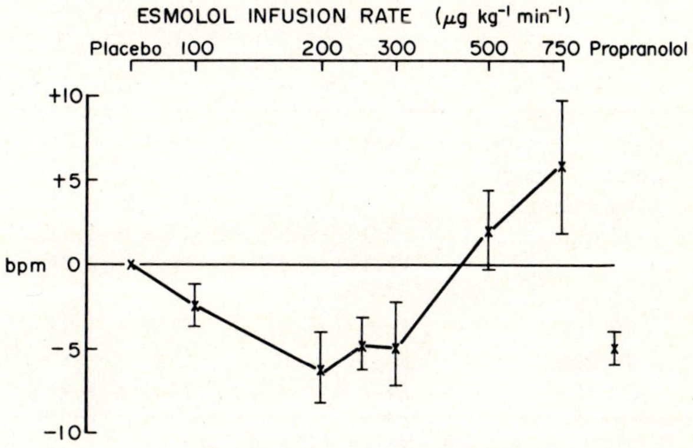

Fig. 3. Mean (±SE) changes in heart rate during infusions of esmolol and propranolol.

Table VI. Blood pressure and heart rate after discontinuation of esmolol infusion

	Infusion rate (μg/min/kg)			
	300		*750*	
	Systolic BP (mm hg)	*Heart rate (bpm)*	*Systolic BP (mm Hg)*	*Heart rate (bpm)*
Before esmolol	117.0 ± 1.5	62.3 ± 2.9	116.3 ± 1.9	69.3 ± 2.4
During esmolol	108.6 ± 2.1*	56.0 ± 2.2*	95.7 ± 1.4	75.5 ± 2.5
After esmolol				
10 min	113.6 ± 1.7†	63.6 ± 2.5†	106.5 ± 2.0†	82.2 ± 1.6†
18 min	117.6 ± 1.6†	63.4 ± 3.1†	110.5 ± 1.6†	79.3 ± 2.6†

Data are $\overline{X}$ ± SE.
BP = Blood pressure.
*P < 0.05 compared with value before esmolol.
†P < 0.05 compared with value at end of infusion.

Table VII. Heart rate response to baseline I_{25} after the end of the esmolol infusion

	Esmolol (μg/kg/min)	
Time	*300*	*750*
Before esmolol	24.2 ± 0.6	23.9 ± 0.8
End of infusion	5.5 ± 1.3*	0*
After esmolol		
2 min	13.9 ± 0.6*	7.8 ± 1.5*
	17.3 ± 0.8*	11.2 ± 1.6*
6 min		
10 min	18.6 ± 0.8*	11.8 ± 1.3*
14 min	20.3 ± 1.3*	—
18 min	24.7 ± 0.7	14.0 ± 1.4*

*P < 0.05 compared with value before esmolol.

DISCUSSION

Clinicians have frequently been inhibited from instituting β-blockade in the acute care setting for fear that should adverse effects develop, the pharmacokinetic characteristics of the drug would prevent their rapid reversal, with potentially disastrous results. Our study has shown that in man, esmolol is an ultra-short-acting β-adrenoceptor antagonist that can rapidly induce effective β-blockade and that, in keeping with its extremely short $t_{1/2}$, steady state is reached very rapidly. When the infusion of esmolol was terminated, the β-blocking effect wore off very rapidly, so that after the 300 μg/kg/min infusion substantial recovery had occurred by 2 minutes and full recovery had occurred by 18 minutes. This was in marked contrast to the persistence of the changes after propranolol, with which there was no loss of β-blockade over the first 30 minutes after the propranolol infusion was stopped.

The relative β-blocking potency of esmolol and propranolol differ depending on whether the extent of β-blockade is determined by suppression of exercise- or of isoproterenol-induced tachycardia. This discrepancy is seen with other β_1-selective antagonists.[11] At doses that produce equal suppression of exercise-induced tachycardia, nonselective β-blockers are more effective in blocking the rise in heart rate induced by isoproterenol than are β_1-selective drugs. The explanation for this discrepancy is not completely clear. Isoproterenol is a nonselective β-receptor stimulant, and it stimulates both β_1- and β_2-receptors. Stimulation of vascular β_2-receptors causes a reduction in blood pressure, which might reflexly increase heart rate. When a nonselective β-blocker such as propranolol is administered, β_2-receptor–mediated vasodilation is blocked; however, a β_1-selective blocker is less effective in antagonizing this β_2-induced vasodilation. In contrast, during exercise the sympathetic component of tachycardia is thought to be produced by the adrenergic neurotransmitter norepinephrine, which is relatively β_1-selective, so that selective and nonselective drugs are equally effective.[11] However, recent studies have suggested that the reduced effect of selective β-blockers in antagonizing isoproterenol-induced tachycardia is not simply due to lack of effects on the vascular receptors.[11] The recognition that cardiac β-receptors are of both the β_1 and β_2 type[12] has resulted in the suggestion that the differences between selective and nonselective β-blockers in antagonizing the effects of isoproterenol on the heart may be due to the inability of the selective β-blockers to antagonize the effects of isoproterenol on the cardiac β_2-receptors.[11]

One of the striking effects of esmolol we demonstrated was the dose-related depression of blood pressure, which was reduced by about 20 mm Hg (systolic) at an esmolol infusion rate of 750 μg/kg/min. Although this dose is higher than those that are likely to be used therapeutically, in a previous study[15] five of 16 patients receving esmolol therapy had a dose-dependent fall in systolic blood pressure to <100 mm Hg. The fall in systolic blood pressure in the present study was about fourfold to fivefold greater than the fall in diastolic blood pressure and was greater than that induced by propranolol infusion at the dosage used. The explanation for this hypotensive effect is not clear. A direct stimulant effect on vascular β_2-receptors is one possible explanation, but studies in animals have not demonstrated any intrinsic sympathomimetic activity.[5] It is also possible that esmolol or one of its metabolites has direct vasodilating effects, or that some other unrecognized property of esmolol accounts for the fall in blood pressure.

It was also of interest that although the lower doses of esmolol induced the fall in heart rate expected from a β-adrenergic antagonist, higher doses of esmolol were associated with an increased heart rate. This increased heart rate at the higher esmolol doses may have been caused by reflex cardiac stimulation in response to the fall in blood pressure. An alternative explanation is that high doses of esmolol have a direct stimulant effect on the heart.

The hypotensive effect of esmolol is of interest and seems to be much greater than can be accounted for simply by β-blockade. This property may have therapeutic value, as esmolol may be useful in hypertensive emergencies in which its rapid rate of onset and offset would allow easy dose titration in a fashion analogous to nitroprusside, but without the risks of toxicity produced by the breakdown products of nitroprusside.

The rise in heart rate after esmolol discontinuation might be explained by the occurrence of the so-called β-blocker withdrawal syndrome. Such a syndrome has been described after the withdrawal of a number of other β-blockers.[13,14] It will be important in further studies to determine if this is the explanation, as the patient group for whom ultra-short-acting β-blockers will be used would be particularly at risk from the increased myocardial oxygen demands caused by a β-blocker withdrawal syndrome.

Our data demonstrate that esmolol rapidly achieves steady-state β-blockade in man and that this blockade is very rapidly reversible when esmolol infusion is stopped. The rapidity of disappearance of β-blockade after the esmolol infusion is stopped will extend the group of patients to whom intravenous β-blockade can be administered by giving the clinician confidence in his or her ability to reverse rapidly any adverse effect of β-blockade simply by discontinuing the infusion.

References

1. The Norwegian Multicenter Study Group. Timolol-induced reduction in mortality and reinfarction in patients surviving acute myocardial infarction. N Engl J Med 1981;304:801-7.
2. β-Blocker Heart Attack Trial Research Group. A randomized trial of propranolol in patients with acute myocardial infarction. I. Mortality results. JAMA 1982; 247:1707-14.
3. Hjalmarson Å, Herlitz J, Mäek I, et al. Effect on mortality of metoprolol in acute myocardial infarction. A double-blind randomized trial. Lancet 1981;2:823-7.
4. Hammon JW Jr, Wood AJJ, Prager RL, Wood M, Muirhead J, Bender HW Jr. Perioperative beta blockade with propranolol: reduction in myocardial oxygen demands and incidence of atrial and ventricular arrhythmias. Ann Thorac Surg 1984;38:363-7.
5. Zarolinski J, Borgman RJ, O'Connell JP, et al. Ultrashort acting beta-blockers: a proposal for the treatment of the critically ill patient. Life Sci 1982;31:899-907.
6. Sum CY, Yacobi A, Kartzinel R, Stampfli H, Davis CS, Lai CM. Kinetics of esmolol, an ultra-short-acting beta blocker, and of its major metabolite. CLIN PHARMACOL THER 1983;34:427-34.
7. Vestal RE, Wood AJJ, Shand DG. Reduced β-adrenoceptor sensitivity in the elderly. CLIN PHARMACOL THER 1979;26:181-6.
8. Cleveland CR, Rangno RE, Shand DG. A standardized isoproterenol sensitivity test. The effects of sinus arrhythmia, atropine, and propranolol. Arch Intern Med 1972;130:47.
9. Fraser J, Nadeau J, Robertson D, Wood AJJ. Regulation of human leukocyte beta receptors by endogenous catecholamines. Relationship of leukocyte beta receptor density to the cardiac sensitivity to isoproterenol. J Clin Invest 1981;67:1777-84.
10. Wood AJJ, Carr K, Vestal RE, Belcher S, Wilkinson GR, Shand DG. Direct measurement of propranolol bioavailability during accumulation to steady-state. Br J Clin Pharmacol 1978;6:345-50.
11. Brown JE, McLeod AA, Shand DG. Evidence for cardiac β_2-adrenoceptors in man. CLIN PHARMACOL THER 1983; 33:424-8.
12. Robberecht P, Delhaye M, Taton G, et al. The human heart beta-adrenergic receptors. I. Heterogeneity of the binding sites: presence of 50% $beta_1$- and 50% $beta_2$-adrenergic receptors. Mol Pharmacol 1983;24:169-73.
13. Shand DG, Wood AJ: Propranolol withdrawal syndrome—why? Circulation 1978;58:202-3.
14. Wood AJJ. β-Blocker withdrawal. Drugs 1983;25(suppl 2):318-21.
15. Byrd RC, Sung RJ, Marks J, Parmley WW. Safety and efficacy of esmolol (ASL-8052: an ultrashort-acting beta-adrenergic blocking agent) for control of ventricular rate in supraventricular tachycardias. J Am Coll Cardiol 1984;3:394-9.

Pharmacokinetics of bupropion and its major basic metabolites in normal subjects after a single dose

The pharmacokinetics of bupropion (BUP) and its three major basic metabolites (the erythroamino alcohol [EB], the threoamino alcohol [TB], and the hydroxy [HB] metabolites) were characterized after a single, oral, 200 mg dose of BUP in six healthy men. Twenty-one sequential plasma samples for analysis by HPLC were drawn from each subject over the 56-hour period after dosing. Pharmacokinetic analyses were by noncompartmental methods. The mean elimination $t_{1/2}$ values of BUP, TB, EB, and HB were 9.8, 19.8, 26.8, and 22.2 hours, respectively. The mean plasma AUCs of TB and HB were 2.4 and 10.3 times greater, respectively, than that for BUP. Because of the substantial presence of these metabolites in systemic circulation, further studies are recommended to understand further their roles in the clinical profile of this new antidepressant. (CLIN PHARMACOL THER 38:586-589, 1985.)

S. Casey Laizure, Pharm.D., C. Lindsay DeVane, Pharm.D., Jonathan T. Stewart, M.D., Cynthia S. Dommisse, Pharm.D., and Allen A. Lai, Ph.D. *Gainesville, Fla., and Research Triangle Park, N. C.*

Bupropion hydrochloride (BUP) is a structurally novel nontricyclic antidepressant (Fig. 1). It is not a monamine oxidase inhibitor and exerts little or no inhibition of reuptake of norepinephrine or serotonin in rat brain synaptosomes.[5] Its antidepressant efficacy has been established in open and double-blind, placebo-controlled studies.[2,3,7] Investigations of its autonomic and cardiovascular pharmacology show BUP to be free of any significant sympathomimetic, sympatholytic, anticholinergic, or cardiovascular effects, thereby suggesting that it will have important clinical advantages over the widely used tricyclic antidepressants.[4,8]

BUP is highly metabolized in both rats and man. In rats, its metabolism appeared to be predominantly by side-chain oxidative cleavage, while reduction of the intact parent aminoketone to an aminoalcohol was an additional pathway in man.[11] The major metabolites are the erythroamino alcohol (EB), the threoamino alcohol (TB), and the hydroxy (HB) metabolite (Fig. 1). These metabolites exhibit some pharmacologic activity in the antitetrabenzine rodent model,[11] yet very little has been published concerning their pharmacokinetics. Our purpose was to investigate the kinetics of BUP and its major basic metabolites after a single oral dose of BUP in normal subjects.

From the Colleges of Pharmacy and Medicine, University of Florida, Gainesville, and Wellcome Research Laboratories, Research Triangle Park.

Supported in part by a grant from the Burroughs Wellcome Co.
Received for publication April 9, 1985; accepted July 30, 1985.

Reprint requests to: C. Lindsay DeVane, Pharm.D., Departments of Pharmacy Practice and Psychiatry, Box J-4, JHMHC, Gainesville, FL 32610.

METHODS

Our subjects were six healthy adult men with no history of cardiovascular, gastrointestinal, renal, hepatic, or endocrine disease. All were judged to be in good health based on their previous medical history, a complete physical examination, evaluation of ECGs, and routine clinical laboratory test results. All studies were performed in the Clinical Research Center of the J. Hillis Miller Health Center at the University of Florida and were approved by human investigation committees. Written informed consent was obtained from each subject before the study.

After an overnight fast, subjects took a single, oral 200 mg dose of BUP HCl as two 100 mg tablets. Blood samples for drug assay were drawn by venipuncture or through an indwelling cannula in an antecubital vein and placed in tubes containing sodium heparin as anticoagulant. Plasma was separated within 30 minutes and frozen at $-17°$ C until assayed. Twenty-one samples were drawn beginning immediately before drug dosing and 10, 20, 30, 40, 60, 80, and 100 minutes and 2, 2.5, 3, 4, 6, 8, 12, 16, 24, 32, 40, 48, and 56 hours thereafter. Each subject was monitored for side effects throughout the study.

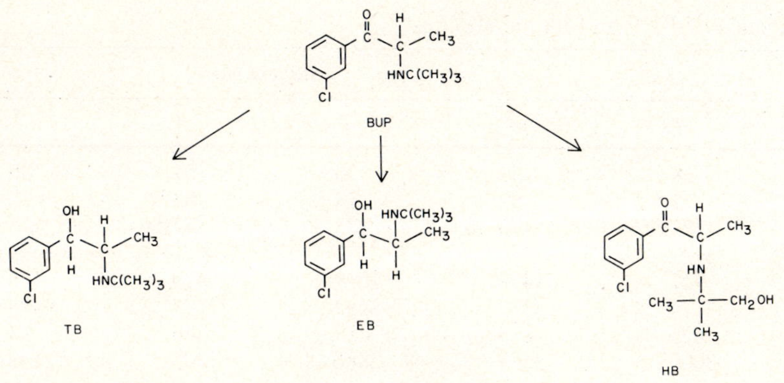

Fig. 1. Chemical structures of bupropion *(BUP)* and its basic metabolites. *TB* = Threoamino alcohol; *EB* = erythroamino alcohol; *HB* = hydroxybupropion.

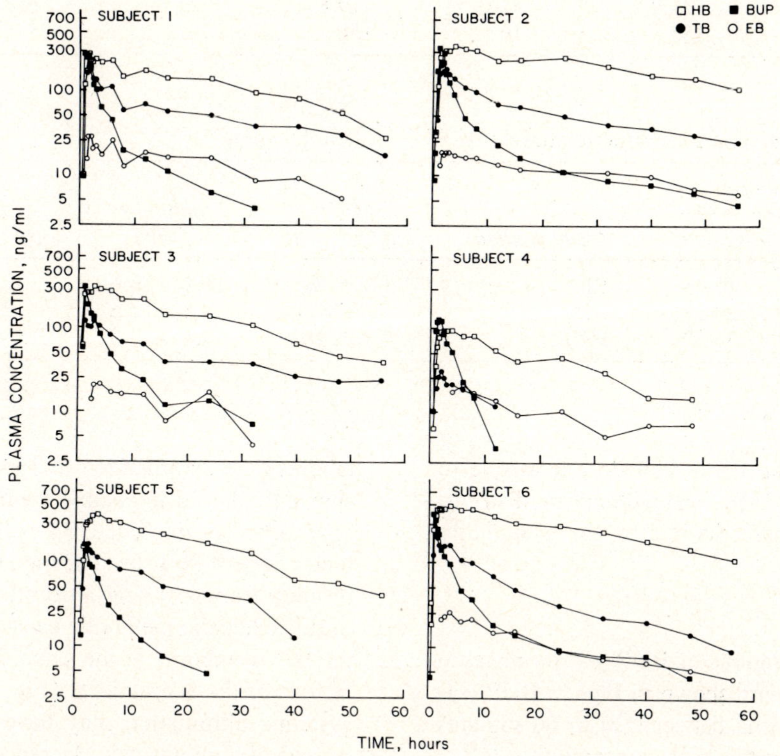

Fig. 2. Concentration-time course of BUP and its major metabolites in six healthy men.

The concentration of BUP and its three major metabolites in plasma was determined by HPLC according to the ion-pairing method developed by Cooper et al.[1] The within-day coefficient of variation at ≥10 ng/ml did not exceed 5% and the between-day coefficient of variation did not exceed 10%.

Kinetic analyses were by noncompartmental methods. However, nonlinear least-squares regression[9] was also used to fit the concentration-time course data, based on each subject's BUP plasma data, to a three-term exponential equation to determine additional pharmacokinetic parameters. For BUP and the metabolites, the partial AUC was determined by the Lagrange method.[12] The terminal slopes were obtained from nonlinear regression and used to extrapolate for total AUC from the last measured time point to infinity.

The pharmacokinetic parameters were calculated by standard methods and included elimination $t_{1/2}$, plasma

Table I. Single-dose kinetics of BUP and its metabolites

	Subject No.					
	1	*2*	*3*	*4*	*5*	*6*
Age (yr)	38	59	36	51	36	39
Weight (kg)	72.5	82.2	79.8	82.9	82.3	82.2
Dose (mg free base)	173.56	173.56	173.56	173.56	173.56	173.56
AUC (ng/ml · hr)						
BUP	927	1498	1099	479	626	1349
HB	7174	15303	8152	2207	9498	19465
EB	675	835	457	446	*	605
TB	3000	3597	2886	305	2148	2363
Elimination $t_{1/2}$ (hr)						
BUP	8.6	23.1	6.9	3.9	6.9	9.5
HB	22.2	25.7	21.6	15.4	17.5	30.8
EB	22.8	43.4	22.5	24.8	*	20.5
TB	26.3	27.5	27.3	9.0	14.4	14.4
V_{area}/F (L/kg)	31.9	47.0	19.8	24.8	33.7	21.4
CL/F (L/hr)	187	116	158	362	277	128

*Unable to quantitate.

Table II. Comparison of pharmacokinetic studies of BUP in healthy men

	Subjects						
	n	*Age (yr)*	*Assay method*	*AUC (ng/ml · hr)*	*Elimination $t_{1/2}$ (hr)*	*CL/F (L/hr/kg)*	*V_{area}/F (L/kg)*
Findlay et al.[7]	12	19-43	RIA	1206 ± 81	11.2 ± 0.6	2.2	35.7
Posner et al.[11]	8	20-35	RIA	1417*	18.8 ± 2.5	1.3	33.1 ± 3.3
Present study	6	36-59	HPLC	996 ± 163	9.8 ± 2.8	2.5 ± 0.5	29.8 ± 4.1

Data are $\overline{X}$ ± SE.
*Normalized to dose used in present study.

clearance divided by the fraction of dose available to systemic circulation (CL/F), and volume of distribution in the terminal phase divided by the availability (V_{area}/F).

RESULTS

The plasma concentrations of BUP and its metabolites in the six subjects are shown in Fig. 2. BUP was first measurable in plasma between 20 to 60 minutes after dosing. Values for the peak concentration (C_{max}) of bupropion ranged from 126 to 388 ng/ml and occurred (t_{max}) within 100 minutes.

The three metabolites generally appeared later in plasma and were present in all subjects (Fig. 2). Quantitation of EB was not possible for subject 5 because of technical difficulties. The C_{max} of HB and TB ranged from 94 to 486 ng/ml and from 27 to 213 ng/ml, respectively, and usually exceeded the C_{max} of BUP. The C_{max} of EB was lower than that of BUP in all subjects. C_{max} of the metabolites usually occurred later than that for BUP, and t_{max} ranged from 80 minutes to 6 hours.

The pharmacokinetic parameters for BUP and its metabolites are summarized in Table I. The CL/F values showed 3.1-fold intersubject variability and all values approached or exceeded the estimated average hepatic blood flow of 90 L/hr. The high CL/F values may have resulted from low oral absorption or a high degree of intrinsic hepatic metabolic capacity. The appearance of the HB metabolite at the same time in plasma as BUP in four of the six subjects (Fig. 2) suggested that presystemic elimination may have occurred as a consequence of high intrinsic clearance. The V_{area}/F is a measure of the distribution and bioavailability of BUP. The high values are in keeping with a lipophilic compound with extensive tissue uptake.

There have been no reports on the disposition of these major metabolites after a single dose. With BUP elimination $t_{1/2}$ values in the range of 4 to 23 hours (Table I), the time required for BUP to reach steady state should not exceed 4 days. However, with metabolite $t_{1/2}$ values as long as 43.4 hours (Table I), the steady state for drug plus metabolites of interest may not be reached for 6 days or longer, until four to five $t_{1/2}$s elapse.

DISCUSSION

BUP is expected to be a widely used antidepressant. Its metabolism and pharmacokinetic profile have been well described.[6,10,11] Results from previous single-dose studies of BUP pharmacokinetics are compared with those from our present study in Table II. We used a highly sensitive and specific analytic method,[1] and the major pharmacokinetic parameters are comparable for all three studies. This serves to validate the use of either assay for determination of BUP kinetics. While our subjects were older than have been previously studied, clearance values are very similar to those reported by Findlay et al.[6] Thus the kinetic profiles of BUP metabolites appear valid based on previous data for BUP in younger subjects.

The mean AUCs of TB and HB were 2.4 and 10.3 times greater, respectively, than that for BUP (Table I). The extended $t_{1/2}$ of the metabolites and their larger AUC values compared with BUP imply that substantial plasma accumulation should occur at steady state after chronic BUP dosing. Cooper et al.[1] reported much greater plasma concentrations of all three metabolites at steady state compared with BUP in eight patients taking daily BUP doses from 100 to 450 mg.

Inclusion of the major basic metabolites of BUP in pharmacokinetic studies is important because of their potential contributions to therapeutic or adverse effects. The need remains to assess further their kinetics at steady state and the influence of factors such as drug interactions and disease states. Because of the substantial presence of the metabolites in systemic circulation, further studies are recommended to understand further their roles in the clinical profile of this new antidepressant.

References

1. Cooper TB, Suckow RF, Glassman A: Determination of bupropion and its major basic metabolites in plasma by liquid chromatography with dual-wavelength ultraviolet detection. J Pharm Sci **73:**1104-1107, 1984.
2. Fabre LF, McLendon D: Double-blind placebo controlled study of bupropion hydrochloride (Wellbutrin) in the treatment of depressed in-patients. Curr Ther Res **23:**393-402, 1978.
3. Fann WE, Schroeder DH, Mehta NP, Soroko FE, Maxwell RA: Clinical trial of bupropion HCl in treatment of depression. Curr Ther Res **23:**222-229, 1978.
4. Farid FF, Wenger TL, Tsai SY, Singh BN, Stern WC: Use of bupropion in patients who exhibit orthostatic hypotension on tricyclic antidepressants. J Clin Psychiatry **44**(suppl 5):170-173, 1983.
5. Ferris RM, Beaman OJ: Bupropion: A new antidepressant drug, the mechanism of action of which is not associated with down-regulation of postsynaptic β-adrenergic, serotonergic (5-HT-2), α-adrenergic, imipramine and dopaminergic receptors in brain. Neuropharmacology **22:**1257-1262, 1983.
6. Findlay JWA, Rogers JZ, Smith PG, et al: Pharmacokinetics of bupropion, a novel antidepressant agent, following oral administration to healthy subjects. Eur J Clin Pharmacol **21:**127-135, 1981.
7. Halaris AE, Stern WC, Harto-Traux N: Clinical efficacy of the new antidepressant bupropion (Wellbutrin). Psychopharmacol Bull **17:**140-142, 1981.
8. Halaris AE, Stern WC, van Wyck Fleet J, Rochelle MR: Evaluation of the safety and efficacy of bupropion in depression. J Clin Psychiatry **44**(suppl 5):101-103, 1983.
9. Metzler CM, Elfring GL, McEwen AJ: A package of computer programs for pharmacokinetic modeling. Biometrics **30:**562, 1974.
10. Posner J, Bye A, Jeal S, Peck AW, Whiteman P: Alcohol and bupropion pharmacokinetics in healthy male volunteers. Eur J Clin Pharmacol **26:**627-630, 1984.
11. Schroeder DH: Metabolism and kinetics of bupropion. J Clin Psychiatry **44**(suppl 5):79-81, 1983.
12. Yeh KC, Kwan KC: A comparison of numerical integrating algorithms by trapezoidal, Lagrange, and spline approximation. J Pharmacokinet Biopharm **6:**79-97, 1978.

The pharmacokinetic and bactericidal characteristics of oral cefixime

The pharmacokinetics of cefixime (FK 027), a broad-spectrum cephalosporin, were assessed in 12 normal subjects after single oral doses of 50, 100, 200, and 400 mg. Mean peak serum concentrations were 1.02, 1.46, 2.63, and 3.85 μg/ml after the four respective doses. Respective mean serum levels at 12 hours were 0.16, 0.33, 0.72, and 1.13 μg/ml. Volumes of distribution averaged 0.1 L/kg body weight, and the elimination $t_{1/2}$ was 3 hours for all doses. The AUC was 7.01, 11.4, 22.5, and 36.4 μg · hr/ml for the four doses, respectively. Serum clearance averaged 0.4 mg/min/kg and mean 24-hour urinary recovery was 21%, 19%, 20%, and 16% for the four respective doses. Serum bactericidal titers at 4 hours exceeded 1:16 for *Streptococcus pneumoniae, S. pyogenes, Hemophilus influenzae,* and *Branhamella catarrhalis.* Urine bactericidal titers exceeded 1:8 for *Escherichia coli, Klebsiella pneumoniae,* and *Enterobacter cloacae* resistant to the available oral cephalosporins. (CLIN PHARMACOL THER 38:590-594, 1985.)

David C. Brittain, Brian E. Scully, Toshiharu Hirose, and Harold C. Neu
New York, N. Y.

Cefixime is a new cephalosporin antibiotic that can be taken by mouth.[2] It inhibits a wide variety of gram-positive and gram-negative aerobic bacteria, including *Hemophilus influenzae, Neisseria gonorrhoeae, Escherichia coli,* and *Klebsiella pneumoniae* resistant to ampicillin, cephalexin, cefaclor, and trimethoprimsulfamethoxazole. Cefixime is not hydrolyzed by the common plasmid or by chromosomal β-lactamases that inactivate the currently available oral penicillins and cephalosporins.[2] These in vitro advantages over currently available oral cephalosporins such as cephalexin and cefaclor may provide an oral cephalosporin that could be used to treat some of the more difficult respiratory and urinary tract infections in an outpatient setting.

To evaluate this potential, we studied the pharmacokinetic characteristics of cefixime after four different oral doses. In addition, serum bactericidal titers were determined against four important respiratory pathogens and urine bactericidal titers were determined against three urinary pathogens, *E. coli, K. pneumoniae,* and *Enterobacter cloacae,* that are resistant to ampicillin and cephalexin.

From the Division of Infectious Diseases, Departments of Medicine and Pharmacology, College of Physicians and Surgeons, Columbia University.

Supported by a grant from Fujisawa Pharmaceutical Co., Ltd., Osaka, Japan.

Received for publication April 29, 1985; accepted Aug. 6, 1985.

Reprint requests to: Harold C. Neu, Department of Medicine, 630 W. 168th St., New York, NY 10032.

METHODS

Subjects. Twelve men were studied after giving informed consent. All were healthy and none had taken any drugs within 14 days of the study. The mean age of the subjects was 27 years (range 24 to 31 years) and the mean weight was 74.0 kg (range 64.0 to 85.0 kg). General physical examination results were normal. Laboratory tests (complete blood counts, SMAC-20 blood chemistry tests, and urine analysis) were made before entry into the study. Physical examinations and laboratory tests were repeated at the end of the study.

Drug dosing and sampling procedure. Each of the 12 subjects received four doses of drug (50, 100, 200, and 400 mg) in a fasting state. The four doses were taken in random order in a double-blind fashion with a 1-week interval between each dose.

After an overnight fast, cefixime was given with 240 ml water. An identical volume of water was given at 2 hours and again at 4 hours with lunch. Another 240 ml water was given at 6 hours, followed by resumption of regular eating habits.

Blood samples were drawn through a heparin reservoir. Samples were collected just before each drug dose (t = 0) and 0.5, 1, 1.5, 2, 3, 4, 5, 6, 8, and 12 hours thereafter. Serum was separated by centrifugation and stored at −24° C until assayed.

Urine specimens were also obtained just before each weekly drug dose. Subsequent urine specimens were collected in timed intervals from 0 to 2, 2 to 4, 4 to 6, 6 to 8, 8 to 12, and 12 to 24 hours after dosing and aliquots were frozen at −24° C until assayed.

Antibiotic assay. Concentrations of drug in serum and urine were determined with disc diffusion bioassay. Filter paper discs (8 mm) were dipped into standard solutions of cefixime and placed on filter paper blotters for 1 minute to absorb excess moisture. The discs (containing 20 to 25 μl standard solution) were placed on nutrient agar plates (Difco Laboratories) containing assay organisms and incubated at 37° C for 18 hours. The zones of inhibition diameters for each of three discs for each dilution of the standard solutions were measured, averaged, and plotted on semilogarithmic paper as a function of known drug concentration. Best-fit standard curves were created and programmed into a computer. Samples from the subjects were plated in triplicate in a similar manner and incubated simultaneous with the standard solutions. The zones of inhibition were converted to antibiotic concentrations through use of the computer-derived standard curves.

The test organism used for serum determinations was *E. coli* ATCC 39188, which will detect active drug in a medium of Difco nutrient agar. Standard solutions of drug were prepared daily in pooled human serum possessing no activity against the test organism. The lower limit of antibiotic detection was 0.1 μg/ml for serum. The coefficient of variation of replicate samples was 4% to 6%.

The test organism used for urine determinations was *Bacillus subtilis* ATCC 6633 in a medium containing agar (10 μg/L), trisodium citrate (10 μg/L), polypeptone (5 μg/L), and beef extract (3 μg/L). This will detect only active drug. Standard solutions of antibiotics were prepared in 0.067 mol/L phosphate buffer at pH 7.0. Urinary antibiotic levels of 2 μg/ml could be detected with this technique. Samples containing lower concentrations were assayed with an *E. coli* system similar to that used for serum samples.

Bactericidal levels. Bactericidal activity in serum and urine was determined for the 200 and 400 mg doses. Serial twofold tube dilutions were prepared in liquid medium with 5×10^5 bacteria per milliliter (final concentration) added to each 1 ml tube and incubated overnight. Samples (0.01 ml) were streaked on agar plates and incubated for 24 hours at 35° C. The bactericidal level was taken as the dilution at which there was no growth.

Serum samples drawn 4 hours after drug dosing were tested against four respiratory pathogens. The organisms used were a mucoid strain of *Streptococcus pneumoniae* type 3; a trimethoprim-sulfamethoxazole–resistant, β-lactamase–producing *H. influenzae;* a β-lactamase–producing *Branhamella catarrhalis;* and a penicillin-susceptible *S. pyogenes*. The cefixime minimum bactericidal concentrations (MBCs) for these bacteria were 0.125, 0.25, 0.5, and 0.125 μg/ml, respectively.

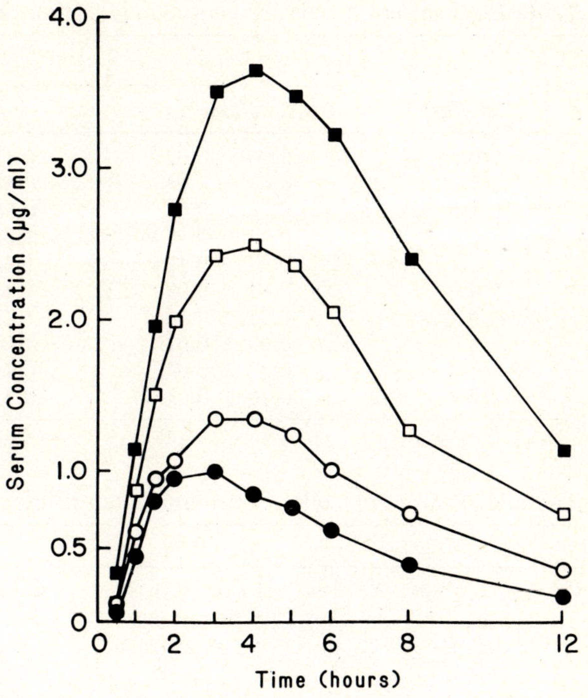

Fig. 1. Serum concentrations of cefixime after oral doses of 50 (●), 100 (○), 200 (□), and 400 (■) mg.

The streptococcal species were grown in Schaedler's broth with 5% human blood and plated on blood agar. The *H. influenzae* and *B. catarrhalis* were grown in Schaedler's broth (with the addition of 5% human blood with the latter organism) and plated on chocolate agar.

Urine samples collected between 2 and 4 and between 12 and 24 hours after drug dosing were tested against three urinary pathogens: *E. coli, K. pneumoniae,* and *En. cloacae*. All were resistant to ampicillin and cephalexin, and the first two were also resistant to tetracycline, carbenicillin, cefoperazone, and trimethoprim-sulfamethoxazole. The cefixime MBCs were 0.5, 0.125, and 4.0 μg/ml, respectively.

Data analysis. Pharmacokinetic parameters were generated by a NONLIN computer program.[1] A one-compartment open model was used and best-fit serum concentration-time curves were formed by a weighted nonlinear least-squares regression analysis. The equations used was:

$$C = \frac{k_a \cdot C_0}{k_a - k_e} \left(e^{-ke(t-\tau)} - e^{-ka(t-\tau)}\right)$$

where C is the serum concentration at time t, C_0 is the

Table I. Mean serum cefixime concentrations after oral dosing

	Cefixime concentration (μg/ml)			
Time (hr)	*50 mg*	*100 mg*	*200 mg*	*400 mg*
0.5	0.06 ± 0.02	0.12 ± 0.04	0.15 ± 0.03	0.33 ± 0.07
1	0.43 ± 0.03	0.58 ± 0.08	0.86 ± 0.10	1.23 ± 0.14
1.5	0.78 ± 0.08	0.94 ± 0.06	1.50 ± 0.14	1.95 ± 0.18
2	0.94 ± 0.11	1.06 ± 0.05	1.97 ± 0.16	2.72 ± 0.17
3	0.97 ± 0.12	1.33 ± 0.07	2.42 ± 0.17	3.51 ± 0.22
4	0.84 ± 0.09	1.33 ± 0.08	2.48 ± 0.20	3.63 ± 0.24
5	0.75 ± 0.10	1.23 ± 0.10	2.35 ± 0.17	3.47 ± 0.24
6	0.60 ± 0.07	1.00 ± 0.10	2.04 ± 0.15	3.22 ± 0.26
8	0.37 ± 0.04	0.71 ± 0.07	1.31 ± 0.16	2.39 ± 0.23
12	0.16 ± 0.03	0.33 ± 0.05	0.72 ± 0.07	1.13 ± 0.13

Data are $\bar{X}$ ± SE.

Table II. Pharmacokinetics of cefixime after different doses

	50 mg	*100 mg*	*200 mg*	*400 mg*
C_{max} (μg/ml)	1.02 ± 0.12	1.46 ± 0.09	2.63 ± 0.20	3.85 ± 0.23
t_{max} (hr)	2.7 ± 0.2	3.4 ± 0.2	3.9 ± 0.2	4.3 ± 0.3
k_a (hr^{-1})	0.88 ± 0.17	0.55 ± 0.07	0.46 ± 0.07	0.35 ± 0.04
k_e				
hr^{-1}	0.28 ± 0.03	0.25 ± 0.02	0.24 ± 0.02	0.25 ± 0.02
hr	0.50 ± 0.06	0.47 ± 0.07	0.54 ± 0.06	0.40 ± 0.04
C_0 (μg/ml)	1.91 ± 0.28	2.72 ± 0.19	5.47 ± 0.54	8.48 ± 0.57
V_{area}				
L	7.00 ± 0.95	7.47 ± 0.50	8.40 ± 1.04	8.02 ± 0.58
L/kg	0.095 ± 0.013	0.10 ± 0.01	0.11 ± 0.01	0.11 ± 0.01
$t_{1/2\alpha}$ (hr)	1.06 ± 0.15	1.44 ± 0.16	1.73 ± 0.16	2.16 ± 0.17
$t_{1/2\beta}$ (hr)	3.02 ± 0.53	2.98 ± 0.26	3.07 ± 0.28	3.05 ± 0.33
AUC (μg · hr/ml)	7.01 ± 0.75	11.4 ± 1.0	22.5 ± 1.6	36.4 ± 3.3
CL_S (ml/min/kg)	0.39 ± 0.16	0.41 ± 0.11	0.43 ± 0.13	0.45 ± 0.16
CL_R (ml/min/kg)	0.083 ± 0.035	0.079 ± 0.022	0.086 ± 0.026	0.072 ± 0.026

Data are $\bar{X}$ ± SE.
CL_R = Renal clearance.

fictive serum concentration at t = 0, k_a is the absorption constant, k_e is the elimination constant, and τ is the time between drug dosing and the beginning of drug absorption. The apparent volume of distribution (V_{area}) was defined as: $V_{area} = (f \cdot D)/C_0$, where f is the bioavailability constant (urinary recovery/administered dose) and D is the administered dose. Serum $t_{1/2}$ values were calculated for the absorption ($t_{1/2\alpha} = \ln 2/k_a$) and elimination ($t_{1/2\beta} = \ln 2/k_e$) phases.

Serum clearance (CL_S) was calculated as: $CL_S = V_{area} \cdot k_e$, and urine clearance was calculated as $CL_S \cdot f$. The AUC was determined as: AUC = C_0/k_e. Mean peak serum concentrations (C_{max}) and time to peak concentrations (t_{max}) were calculated directly.

Repeated-measures ANOVA with the dose as the variable was used to compare results at different doses. Bactericidal titers shown are geometric means of the titers of the individual subjects. The geometric mean titer was defined as the antilog$_2$ of the mean of the log$_2$ of the reciprocal of the titer dilutions.

RESULTS

Mean serum concentrations of cefixime after oral doses of 50, 100, 200, and 400 mg are listed in Table I. Concentration-time curves based on these data are shown in Fig. 1. Mean C_{max} ranged from 1.02 μg/ml for the 50 mg dose to 3.85 μg/ml for the 400 mg dose. The t_{max} was dose dependent and was 2.7 hours for the 50 mg dose, 3.4 hours for the 100 mg dose, 3.9 hours for the 200 mg dose, and 4.3 hours for the 400 mg dose. Twelve hours after drug dosing, serum concentrations averaged 0.16 μg/ml for the 50 mg dose, 0.33 μg/ml for the 100 mg dose, 0.72 μg/ml for the 200 mg dose, and 1.13 μg/ml for the 400 mg dose. The

Table III. Mean percent urinary recovery of cefixime after different doses

	Percent recovery			
Time (hr)	*50 mg*	*100 mg*	*200 mg*	*400 mg*
0-2	2.33 ± 0.55	2.20 ± 0.43	1.59 ± 0.42	0.98 ± 0.15
2-4	6.24 ± 0.86	4.86 ± 0.59	5.08 ± 0.50	3.61 ± 0.42
4-6	4.82 ± 0.70	4.28 ± 0.60	5.02 ± 0.59	4.05 ± 0.49
6-8	3.12 ± 0.60	3.56 ± 0.57	3.56 ± 0.56	2.75 ± 0.29
8-12	2.88 ± 0.53	2.69 ± 0.48	3.03 ± 0.43	2.88 ± 0.35
12-24	1.82 ± 0.32	1.73 ± 0.32	1.71 ± 0.21	1.59 ± 0.32
Total	21.2 ± 2.87	19.3 ± 2.09	20.0 ± 1.82	16.1 ± 1.32

Data are $\bar{X}$ ± SE.

Table IV. Urinary cefixime concentrations after oral dosing

	Cefixime concentration (μg/ml)			
Time (hr)	*50 mg*	*100 mg*	*200 mg*	*400 mg*
0-2	16.9 (1.8-76.8)	24.2 (3.8-68.1)	34.1 (2.2-103)	43.5 (4.2-89.2)
2-4	36.8 (2.5-121)	56.3 (6.9-143)	107 (13.2-397)	127 (24.7-230)
4-6	33.7 (3.3-112)	72.8 (13.0-224)	107 (41.1-338)	164 (29.2-345)
6-8	19.0 (5.5-60.9)	36.1 (6.2-124)	62.7 (15.7-198)	136 (17.3-305)
8-12	8.3 (2.2-28.5)	15.4 (2.9-40.0)	32.0 (6.8-76.8)	68.8 (13.5-194)
12-24	2.01 (0.4-5.21)	3.88 (1.5-8.8)	6.70 (3.1-15.2)	10.8 (1.6-44.4)

Data are $\bar{X}$ (range).

Table V. Geometric mean 4-hour serum cefixime bactericidal titers after 200 and 400 mg

Dose (mg)	*S. pneumoniae*	*S. pyogenes*	*H. influenzae*	*B. catarrhalis*
200	1:20 (1:16-1:32)	1:51 (1:32-1:64)	1:14 (1:2-1:64)	1:13 (1:8-1:16)
400	1:32 (1:32)	1:72 (1:64-1:128)	1:15 (1:2-1:64)	1:16 (1:8-1:32)

Data are $\bar{X}$ (range).

V_{area} averaged 0.1 L/kg body weight (Table II). An elimination $t_{1/2}$ of 3 hours was remarkably consistent from dose to dose. The calculated C_{max} values were dose dependent and the AUCs increased linearly.

Urinary recovery of the drug as a percent of the administered dose is listed in Table III. The highest excretion was in the 2 to 4 and the 4 to 6–hour periods. Total 24-hour recovery ranged from 16% to 21% of the administered dose. Urine concentrations were a function of urine volumes. The mean urine concentrations and ranges for the 12 subjects are listed in Table IV.

Mean serum bactericidal titers against four respiratory pathogens are listed in Table V. At 4 hours after dosing, bactericidal activity was >1:8 dilution against all four organisms for both the 200 and 400 mg doses, with a titer of 1:32 for the *S. pneumoniae* and 1:72 for the *S. pyogenes* 4 hours after the 400 mg dose.

Urine collected during the 2-to-4–hour "peak" period showed greater killing activity than urine collected during the 12-to-24–hour "trough" period (Table VI). However, even during the trough period, urine collected after the 200 mg dose was bactericidal in a dilution of at least 1:5 for all three pathogens.

Cefixime was tolerated at all four doses without adverse effect by all 12 subjects. No gastrointestinal symptoms, abnormal physical findings, or laboratory abnormalities were noted.

DISCUSSION

The pharmacokinetics of cefixime are quite different from those of currently available cephalosporins

Table VI. Geometric mean urine cefixime bactericidal titers after 200 and 400 mg

Dose (mg)	*Period (hr)*	*E. coli*	*K. pneumoniae*	*En. cloacae*
200	2-4	1:81 (1:64-1:128)	1:102 (1:64->1:256)	1:8 (1:4-1:32)
	12-24	1:18 (1:8-1:64)	1:64 (1:8-1:64)	1:5 (1:2-1:8)
400	2-4	1:144 (1:32->1:256)	1:114 (1:16->1:256)	1:18 (1:4-1:64)
	12-24	1:23 (1:8-1:32)	1:64 (1:64-1:128)	1:4 (1:2-1:16)

Data are $\overline{X}$ (range).

such as cephalexin, cephradine, and cefaclor, which have a serum $t_{1/2}$ of <1 hour, and cefadroxil, which has a $t_{1/2}$ of approximately 1.2 hours.[3,4] Cefixime also differs from the aforementioned oral cephalosporins because urinary recovery of cephalexin, cephradine, and cefadroxil ranges from 80% to 100% compared with only 20% for cefixime. The AUC for 400 mg cefixime (36.4 μg · hr/ml) is greater than that reported for 500 mg cephradine (27.5 μg · hr/ml) or for cephalexin (29 μg · hr/ml).[3,4] In contrast to the aforementioned drugs, only 20% of cefixime was recovered in the urine. It is suggested that an appreciable amount of cefixime is not absorbed and that there is biliary secretion of the drug. Studies are in progress to establish the precise reasons for this low urinary excretion.

Cefixime has an antibacterial spectrum sufficiently broad to suggest a potentially important clinical future. We had found minimal inhibition concentrations at 90% (MIC_{90}) values to be ≤0.2 μg/ml for group A and B streptococci, *S. pneumoniae, Neisseria* species, *H. influenzae, B. catarrhalis, K. pneumoniae, K. oxytoca,* and *Proteus mirabilis*. The MIC_{90}s are ≤2 μg/ml for *E. coli, Providencia* species, *Citrobacter diversus, P. vulgaris,* and *Salmonella, Shigella,* and *Campylobacter* species. These MIC_{90} values are much lower than those of currently available cephalosporins for *Enterobacteriaceae,* and cefixime has activity comparable with that of cephalexin and cefaclor against streptococcal species. Bacteria with MICs above attainable serum levels include staphylococci, *Listeria monocytogenes,* enterococci, *Pseudomonas aeruginosa,* and *Acinetobacter anitratus*. Approximately 50% of *Enterobacter, Serratia,* and *Citrobacter* species, which are a cause of nosocomial urinary tract infections, would be inhibited by the serum concentrations we found, and most would be inhibited by the higher urinary concentrations.

Because serum levels >1 μg/ml are maintained for 8 hours after a 200 mg dose of cefixime, a twice-daily dosing program for respiratory pathogens such as *H. influenzae, B. catarrhalis, S. pyogenes,* and *S. pneumoniae* should be possible. The serum bactericidal titers at 4 hours also support such a program. Once-daily dosing would provide adequate urine concentrations for the most common urinary pathogens, with the exception of *P. aeruginosa* and enterococci. Of particular note is the urinary activity against the cephalexin, ampicillin, and trimethoprim-sulfamethoxazole–resistant *E. coli* and *K. pneumoniae*. The possibility of a single 400 mg dose in the treatment of simple cystitis could be clinically investigated. In view of the serum levels of cefixime achieved with these doses, it would not be appropriate to use in the treatment of staphylococcal infections, because the MIC_{90} values of staphylococci are ≥25 μg/ml.[2] Clinical studies are in progress to determine if the pharmacokinetic properties can be translated into clinical practice.

We thank Fujisawa Pharmaceutical Co., Ltd., for the supply of cefvixime.

References

1. Metzler CM, Elfring GL, McElwen AJ: A user's manual for NONLIN and associated programs. Kalamazoo, Mich., 1974, The Upjohn Co.
2. Neu HC, Chin NX, Labthavikul P: Comparative in vitro activity and beta-lactamase stability of FR 17027, a new orally active cephalosporin. Antimicrob Agents Chemother **26:**174-180, 1984.
3. Pfeffer M, Jackson A, Ximenes J, Perche de Menezes J: Comparative human oral clinical pharmacology of cefadroxil, cephalexin and cephradine. Antimicrob Agents Chemother **11:**331-338, 1977.
4. Santoro J, Agarwal BN, Martinelli R, Wenger N, Levison ME: Pharmacology of cefaclor in normal volunteers and patients with renal failure. Antimicrob Agents Chemother **13:**951-954, 1978.

Effect of alprazolam on digoxin kinetics and creatinine clearance

Eight healthy men received a single, 1.25 mg dose of digoxin on two occasions, once in an otherwise drug-free control state and again while concurrently receiving alprazolam, 1.5 mg/day. There was no significant difference between control and alprazolam conditions in digoxin volume of distribution (11.0 vs. 11.2 L/kg), elimination $t_{1/2}$ (46 vs. 41 hours), or total clearance from serum (2.8 vs. 3.6 ml/min/kg). Alprazolam coadministration slightly reduced mean 96-hour urinary excretion of digoxin (37.6% vs. 30.9% of dose; $P < 0.01$), but there was no significant difference between treatment conditions in projected total cumulative excretion of digoxin (45.2% vs. 40.9% of dose) or in renal clearance of digoxin (1.23 vs. 1.44 ml/min/kg). Creatinine clearance also did not differ between the control and alprazolam conditions (164 vs. 142 ml/min). Thus therapeutic doses of alprazolam do not significantly alter digoxin clearance in healthy man. (Clin Pharmacol Ther 38:595-598, 1985.)

Hermann R. Ochs, M.D.,* David J. Greenblatt, M.D., and Birgitt Verburg-Ochs, M.D. *Bonn, Federal Republic of Germany, and Boston, Mass.*

This work is dedicated to Prof. Dr. med. F. Scheler on the occasion of his sixtieth birthday.

Alprazolam is a triazolobenzodiazepine derivative currently used as an anxiolytic drug.[5,6] Some evidence also suggests that alprazolam may have antidepressant and antipanic effects similar to those of tricyclic antidepressant derivatives.[5-7] Some antidepressants such as imipramine may have cardiac antiarrhythmic properties in common with traditional antiarrhythmics such as quinidine.[9,10] Quinidine and other antiarrhythmics are known to alter the pharmacokinetics of the cardiac glycoside digoxin, causing a reduction in the digoxin volume of distribution and total clearance.[8,14,16,19] This raises the possibility that alprazolam may have the potential to alter the pharmacokinetics of digoxin in man, as was suggested by a recent clinical report on alprazolam[23] as well as by some experimental data with other benzodiazepines.[1,2] Our present controlled study evaluated the influence of therapeutic doses of alprazolam on the pharmacokinetics of a single intravenous dose of digoxin and on creatinine clearance in healthy man.

From the Medizinische Universitätsklinik, University of Bonn, Bonn, and Tufts-New England Medical Center, Boston.

Supported in part by Grant No. OC 10/6-4 from Deutsche Forschungsgemeinschaft and by Grant No. MH-34223 from the United States Public Health Service.

Received for publication March 10, 1985; accepted Aug. 8, 1985.

Reprint requests to: Prof. Dr. med. H. R. Ochs, Marienkrankenhaus, Widumgasse 5, D-4770 Soest, Federal Republic of Germany.

*Present address: Marienkrankenhaus, Soest, Federal Republic of Germany.

METHODS

Eight healthy men 18 to 29 years old participated after giving informed consent. All were healthy, active, ambulatory adults without evidence of disease and receiving no other medications. Their mean (± SE) body weight was 69.6 ± 2.1 kg (range 56 to 78 kg).

Subjects participated in a single-dose, two-way crossover trial, with at least 4 weeks between doses. For each trial subjects received a single 1.25 mg iv dose of digoxin, and the sequence of the two trials was randomized. On one occasion, digoxin was given in the control state without drug coadministration. For the other trial, subjects took alprazolam, 0.5 mg po in the morning and 1.0 mg po at bedtime beginning 24 hours before digoxin dosing and continuing for the 4-day duration of the digoxin kinetic study. Because the mean alprazolam elimination $t_{1/2}$ in healthy young men is approximately 11 hours,[11,21] 24 hours of alprazolam dosing before digoxin dosing would be sufficient for the steady-state condition to be at least 75% achieved.[21]

For each digoxin trial, a 1.25 mg dose of injectable digoxin solution (Novodigal; Beiersdorf) was infused into an antecubital vein over 5 minutes. Venous blood samples were drawn into additive-free tubes before the dose and at the following times thereafter: 5, 15, 30, and 45 minutes and 1, 1.5, 2, 2.5, 3, 4, 6, 8, 12, 24, 48, 72, and 96 hours. Blood samples were allowed to clot and the serum was separated and frozen until as-

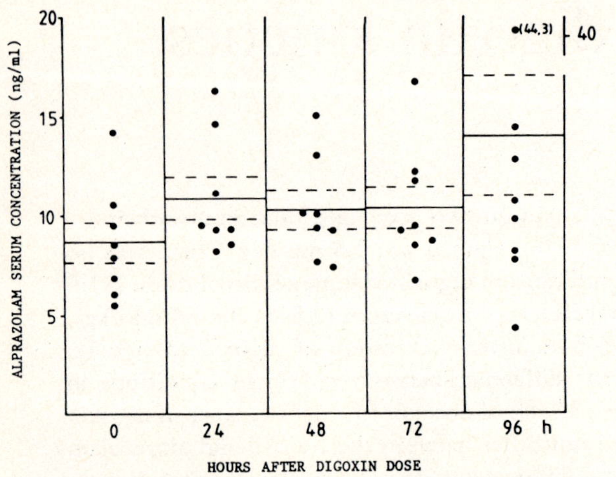

Fig. 1. Individual and mean (± SE) serum alprazolam concentrations during the digoxin-alprazolam coadministration trial.

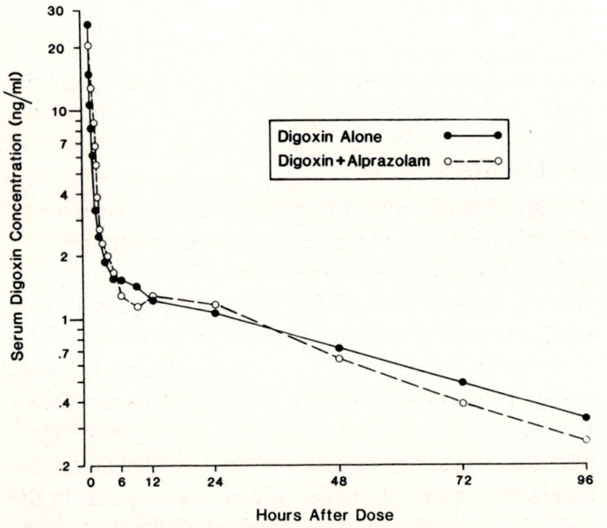

Fig. 2. Mean serum digoxin concentrations during the control trial and during coadministration of alprazolam.

sayed. A 96-hour urine collection, divided into four separate 24-hour intervals, began at the time of the infusion.

Digoxin concentrations in all serum and urine samples were determined by RIA.[13,22] The sensitivity limits are approximately 0.1 to 0.2 ng/ml serum, with a coefficient of variation for identical samples of 6.5% at 0.7 ng/ml (n = 20) and 5.4% at 2.0 ng/ml (n = 20). Compliance with the prescribed alprazolam regimen was verified by measurement of serum alprazolam concentrations[12] during the alprazolam-digoxin inter-

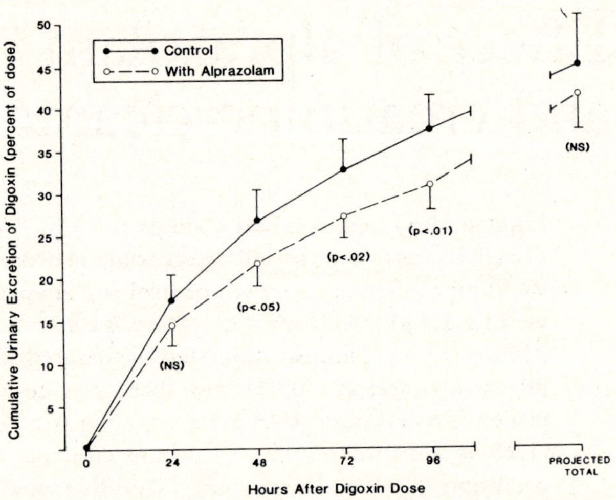

Fig. 3. Mean (± SE) cumulative urinary excretion of digoxin during the control trial and during alprazolam coadministration. Probabilities indicate level of significance of difference between the two conditions based on Student's paired t test.

action trial in samples drawn before the infusion and at 24, 48, 72, and 96 hours after the infusion.

Serum creatinine concentrations likewise were determined by an automatic analyzer in samples drawn before and 24, 48, and 72 hours after the infusion. Serum creatinine concentrations and urinary excretion of creatinine were used to determine creatinine clearance.

Digoxin serum concentrations after each trial were analyzed by iterative nonlinear least-squares regression techniques.[15,18] Concentrations were fit to a linear sum of two or three exponential terms. Exponents and infusion-corrected coefficients were used to calculate the following kinetic variables for digoxin: volume of the central compartment, total volume of distribution by the area method, elimination $t_{1/2}$, and total clearance.

The apparent excretion rate of immunoassayable digoxin was determined by linear regression analysis of a plot of the logarithm of the average interval excretion rate (ordinate) vs. collection interval midpoint (abscissa). The projected total cumulative excretion of immunoassayable digoxin from time zero to infinity was calculated as the sum of the actual 96-hour excretion plus the unexcreted quantity determined by extrapolation (the ratio of the projected instantaneous excretion rate at 96 hours divided by the excretion rate constant). Renal clearance of immunoassayable digoxin was calculated as the serum digoxin clearance multiplied by the projected cumulative total fraction of the dose recovered in the urine.

Differences between control and alprazolam coad-

Table I. Effect of alprazolam on digoxin kinetics and creatinine

	Control	*With alprazolam*	*Student's t*
Digoxin kinetics			
V_C (L/kg)	0.72 ± 0.12	0.71 ± 0.15	0.01
V_{area} (L/kg)	10.96 ± 1.32	11.23 ± 0.93	0.22
Elimination t½ (hr)	45.8 ± 4.9	41.3 ± 5.8	0.59
CL (ml/min/kg)	2.80 ± 0.22	3.56 ± 0.63	1.60
96-hr urinary excretion (% of dose)	37.6 ± 4.2	30.9 ± 3.0	3.66*
Projected total cumulative urinary excretion (% of dose)	45.2 ± 5.4	40.9 ± 4.1	1.13
CL_R (ml/min/kg)	1.23 ± 0.15	1.44 ± 0.27	0.80
Creatinine			
Serum creatinine (mg/dl)	0.76 ± 0.04	0.74 ± 0.05	2.12†
CL_{CR}			
ml/min	164 ± 16	142 ± 14	1.53
ml/min/kg	2.35 ± 0.19	2.04 ± 0.19	1.57

Data are $\overline{X}$ ± SE.
V_C = Volume of the central compartment; V_{area} = total volume of distribution; CL = total clearance; CL_R = renal clearance; CL_{CR} = creatinine clearance.
*$P < 0.01$; †$P < 0.1$.

ministration conditions were evaluated by Student's paired t test.

RESULTS

Serum alprazolam concentrations indicated good compliance with the prescribed alprazolam regimen (Fig. 1). Fig. 2 shows serum digoxin concentrations during the control period and during alprazolam dosing. There were no significant differences between the conditions in volume of the central compartment, total volume of distribution, elimination $t_{1/2}$, or total clearance. If anything, digoxin clearance was greater (although not significantly so) during alprazolam coadministration (Table I).

There was a small but significant reduction in the 96-hour urinary excretion of digoxin between control and alprazolam conditions (38% vs. 31% of dose; $P < 0.01$; Fig. 3). However, the projected total excretion of digoxin did not differ significantly between the two trials (45% vs. 41% of dose), nor was renal clearance of immunoassayable digoxin significantly different (1.23 vs. 1.44 ml/min/kg). Creatinine clearance was lower during alprazolam dosing, although differences between the conditions were not significant. Overall, renal clearance of creatinine and digoxin correlated positively ($r = 0.40$), but the correlation was not statistically significant.

DISCUSSION

Our present study in healthy men evaluated the influence of the coadministration of typical therapeutic doses of alprazolam on the kinetics of a single intravenous dose of digoxin and on creatinine clearance. Alprazolam doses were chosen to be within the range of those shown to be clinically effective for the treatment of anxiety.[3-6,20] Compliance with the alprazolam regimen was verified by daily measurement of serum alprazolam concentrations. Alprazolam coadministration had no significant influence on any of the kinetic variables for digoxin disappearance from serum. There was a tendency toward a reduction of creatinine clearance during alprazolam coadministration as compared with control, but the difference was not significant. Alprazolam did significantly reduce the 96-hour urinary excretion of digoxin, but there was no significant effect of alprazolam on the projected total excretion of digoxin or on digoxin renal clearance.

The pharmacokinetic profile of digoxin after single doses predicts the extent of drug accumulation and steady-state serum concentrations during multiple dosing.[17] Therefore, our results suggest that therapeutic doses of alprazolam should not influence steady-state digoxin concentrations during chronic therapy. Further studies are needed to evaluate the possibility of this interaction in more seriously ill patients and in those receiving higher doses of alprazolam.

We are grateful for the assistance of Elke Moritz, Monika Linden, and Jerold S. Harmatz.

References

1. Castillo-Ferrando JR, Carmona J: Étude pharmacocinetique de la digoxine en présence de diazepam et de clorazepam. J Pharmacol **12**:74-75, 1981.
2. Castillo-Ferrando JR, Prieto AC, de la Torre Brasas F: Effects of benzodiazepines on digoxin tissue concentra-

tions and plasma protein binding. J Pharm Pharmacol **35:**462-463, 1983.

3. Cohn JB: Multicenter double-blind efficacy and safety study comparing alprazolam, diazepam and placebo in clinically anxious patients. J Clin Psychiatry **42:**347-351, 1981.
4. Davison K, Farquharson RG, Khan MC, Majid A: A double blind comparison of alprazolam, diazepam and placebo in the treatment of anxious out-patients. Psychopharmacology **80:**308-310, 1983.
5. Dawson GW, Jue SG, Brogden RN: Alprazolam. A review of its pharmacodynamic properties and efficacy in the treatment of anxiety and depression. Drugs **27:**132-147, 1984.
6. Fawcett JA, Kravitz HM: Alprazolam: Pharmacokinetics, clinical efficacy, and mechanism of action. Pharmacotherapy **2:**243-254, 1982.
7. Feighner JP, Aden GC, Fabre LF, Rickels K, Smith WT: Comparison of alprazolam, imipramine, and placebo in the treatment of depression. JAMA **249:**3057-3064, 1983.
8. Fichtl B, Doering W: The quinidine-digoxin interaction in perspective. Clin Pharmacokinet **8:**137-154, 1983.
9. Glassman AH: Cardiovascular effects of tricyclic antidepressants. Ann Rev Med **35:**503-511, 1984.
10. Glassman AH, Bigger JT: Cardiovascular effects of therapeutic doses of tricyclic antidepressants. Arch Gen Psychiatry **38:**815-820, 1981.
11. Greenblatt DJ, Divoll M, Abernethy DR, Moschitto LJ, Smith RB, Shader RI: Alprazolam kinetics in the elderly: Relation to antipyrine disposition. Arch Gen Psychiatry **40:**287-290, 1983.
12. Greenblatt DJ, Divoll M, Shader RI: Automated gas chromatographic determination of plasma alprazolam concentrations. J Clin Psychopharmacol **3:**366-368, 1983.
13. Greenblatt DJ, Duhme DW, Koch-Weser J, Smith TW: Evaluation of digoxin bioavailability in single-dose studies. N Engl J Med **289:**651-654, 1973.
14. Nademanee K, Kannan R, Hendrickson J, Ookhtens M, Kay I, Singh BN: Amiodarone-digoxin interaction. J Am Coll Cardiol **4:**111-116, 1984.
15. Ochs HR, Bodem G, Bales G, Greenblatt DJ, Smith TW: Increased clearance of digoxin in rabbits during repeated administration. J Pharmacol Exp Ther **205:**516-524, 1978.
16. Ochs HR, Bodem G, Greenblatt DJ: Impairment of digoxin clearance by coadministration of quinidine. J Clin Pharmacol **21:**396-400, 1981.
17. Ochs HR, Greenblatt DJ, Bodem G: Single- and multiple-dose kinetics of intravenous digoxin. CLIN PHARMACOL THER **28:**340-345, 1980.
18. Ochs HR, Greenblatt DJ, Bodem G, Harmatz JS: Dose-independent pharmacokinetics of digoxin in humans. Am Heart J **97:**507-511, 1978.
19. Oyama Y, Fujii S, Kanda K, Akino E, Kawasaki H, Nagata M, Goto K: Digoxin-diltiazem interaction. Am J Cardiol **53:**1480-1481, 1984.
20. Rickels K, Csanalosi I, Greisman P, Cohen D, Werblowsky J, Ross HA, Harris H: A controlled clinical trial of alprazolam for the treatment of anxiety. Am J Psychiatry **140:**82-85, 1983.
21. Smith RB, Gwilt PR, Wright CE: Single- and multiple-dose pharmacokinetics of oral alprazolam in healthy smoking and nonsmoking men. Clin Pharm **2:**139-143, 1983.
22. Smith TW, Butler VP, Haber E: Determination of therapeutic and toxic serum digoxin concentrations by radoimmunoassay. N Engl J Med **281:**1212-1216, 1969.
23. Tollefson G, Lesar T, Grothe D, Garvey M: Alprazolam-related digoxin toxicity. Am J Psychiatry **141:**1612-1614, 1984.

Notes of the American Society for Clinical Pharmacology and Therapeutics

Status Report from the Council on Clinical Pharmacology, July 1985

Six years ago, duly appointed representatives of the American College of Clinical Pharmacology (ACCP), the American Society for Clinical Pharmacology and Therapeutics (ASCPT), and the American Society for Pharmacology and Experimental Therapeutics (ASPET) formed the Council on Clinical Pharmacology to explore mechanisms for certifying competence of physicians and nonphysicians in clinical pharmacology.[1,2]

After intensive discussions and careful consideration of all available options, the Council has developed a plan for a Certificate of Recognition in Clinical Pharmacology for nonphysicians and is developing a plan to form a Board of Clinical Pharmacology for certifying physicians.

The certification process for nonphysicians will probably be administered by the Council and will be based on satisfaction of various criteria relating to training in the discipline, publication of meritorious reports, involvement in training and regulatory affairs, and research in clinical pharmacology.

For physicians, the Council initially explored the establishment of a Certificate of Special Competency in Clinical Pharmacology for those clinical pharmacologists who hold Board Certification in Internal Medicine from the American Board of Internal Medicine (ABIM) within the American Board of Medical Specialties (ABMS). On May 13, 1983, the Council submitted a detailed application that the ABIM acknowledged as carefully prepared—one that followed a thoughtful, informed approach. However, after additional correspondence and careful consideration, our request (like others in recent years) was declined by the ABIM on October 2, 1984. It was suggested that we examine the model used by geneticists in establishing the American Board of Medical Genetics, Inc. in 1980. We understand that the American Board of Medical Genetics, Inc. has been well received and is a widely respected and efficient mechanism for certifying geneticists.

On December 8, 1984, the Council unanimously agreed to recommend to our three sponsoring societies (ACCP, ASCPT, and ASPET) that we develop a proposal for formation of an independent Board of Clinical Pharmacology to provide a certifying process for qualified physician clinical pharmacologists. Subsequently, the governing boards of the ACCP, ASCPT, and ASPET each agreed to support this recommendation fully and each society provided "seed" funds to initiate the process.

Several important working groups have been established for the purposes of developing this independent Board of Clinical Pharmacology. The working groups are as follows:

Financial Resources for Establishing the Board
Drs. Joseph R. Bianchine and Kazuo K. Kimura.

Establishment of a legal framework for the Board
Drs. Duncan E. Hutcheon, David T. Lowenthal, Joseph R. Bianchine, and Benjamin Calesnick

Credentialing of Candidates for the Board-Certifying Examination
Drs. Kazuo K. Kimura, Thomas P. Gibson, Joseph R. DiPalma, and Benjamin Calesnick

Development of a Board-Certifying Examination
Drs. Joseph R. DiPalma, W. Leigh Thompson, Harold F. Hailman, Donald S. Robinson, Darrell R. Abernethy, and Alexander Shephard

Accreditation of Training Programs
Drs. D. Craig Brater, Terrence F. Blaschke, David T. Lowenthal, and Carl C. Peck

If the Council's plan for an independent Board of Clinical Pharmacology is adopted by the constituent societies, it is anticipated that the first certifying examination administered by this Board will be offered in the spring of 1987.

Suggestions, comments, and offerings of assistance from interested individuals will be greatly appreciated, especially during the remainder of 1985, since it is anticipated that the actual formation of this Board and the implementation of the certifying process will be accomplished early in 1986.

Membership of the Council on Clinical Pharmacology
Joseph R. Bianchine, M.D., Ph.D., Chairman
Terrence F. Blaschke, M.D.
D. Craig Brater, M.D.
Benjamin Calesnick, M.D.
Joseph R. DiPalma, M.D.
William Forrest, M.D.
Thomas P. Gibson, M.D.
Harold F. Hailman, M.D., Ph.D.
Arthur H. Hayes, Jr., M.D.
Duncan E. Hutcheon, M.D.
Kazuo K. Kimura, M.D., Ph.D.
Louis Lemberger, M.D., Ph.D.
David T. Lowenthal, M.D.
Carl C. Peck, M.D.
W. Leigh Thompson, M.D., Ph.D.
Elliot S. Vesell, M.D.
Richard I. H. Wang, M.D., Ph.D.
Richard M. Weinshilboum, M.D.

References

1. Report of task force on clinical pharmacology certification. CLIN PHARM THER 1980;27:708-10.
2. Task force II report: Council on clinical pharmacology. CLIN PHARM THER 1980;27:827-8.

USAN Council

List No. 266

New Names

The following nonproprietary names for the compounds described have been adopted by the United States Adopted Names (USAN) Council, which is sponsored by the American Medical Association, the American Pharmaceutical Association, and the US Pharmacopeial Convention, Inc., in cooperation with the respective pharmaceutical manufacturers. The designation USAN (United States Adopted Name) distinguishes these formally adopted nonproprietary names from other names. The information given under the category Therapeutic Claim is based on the manufacturer's claims at the time of publication. Adoption of USAN does not imply endorsement of the claims or products by the AMA, the US Pharmacopeia, or the APhA.

In some instances, the drugs listed are available only from the manufacturer to properly qualified investigators for clinical study.

USAN — TUBULOZOLE HYDROCHLORIDE

Pronunciation — to͞o byo͞o′ lŏ zŏl′′

Therapeutic claim — antineoplastic (microtubule inhibitor)

Chemical names

(1) ethyl (±)-*cis*-[4-[[[2-(2,4-dichlorophenyl)-2-(1*H*-imidazol-1-ylmethyl)-1,3-dioxolan-4-yl]methyl]thio]phenyl]carbamate, monohydrochloride

(2) ethyl (±)-*cis*-*p*-[[[2-(2,4-dichlorophenyl)-2-(imidazol-1-ylmethyl)-1,3-dioxolan-4-yl]methyl]thio]carbanilate, monohydrochloride

Structural formula

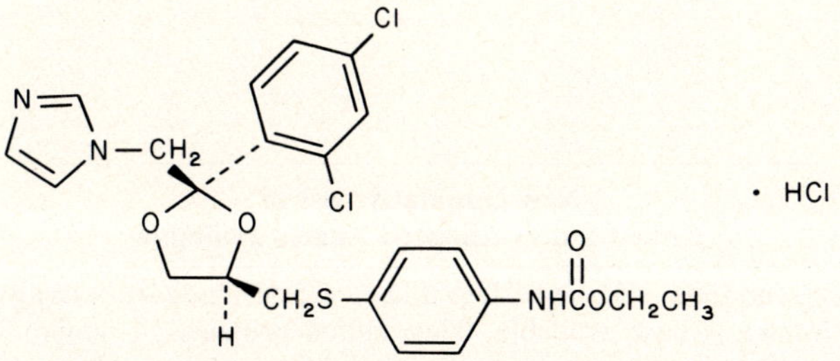

Molecular formula — $C_{23}H_{23}Cl_2N_3O_4S \cdot HCl$

Molecular weight — 544.88

Manufacturer — Janssen Pharmaceutica (Belgium)

Code designation — R 46,846

CAS registry No. — 83529-08-2

USAN — TEMOCILLIN

Pronunciation — tē′ mō sĭ′′ lĭn

Therapeutic claim — antibiotic

Chemical names

(1) [2*S*-(2α,5α,6α)]-6-[(carboxy-3-thienylacetyl)amino]-6-methoxy-3,3-dimethyl-7-oxo-4-thia-1-azabicyclo[3.2.0]heptane-2-carboxylic acid

(2) *N*-[(2*S*,5*R*,6*S*)-2-carboxy-6-methoxy-3,3-dimethyl-7-oxo-4-thia-1-azabicyclo[3.2.0]hept-6-yl]-3-thiophenemalonamic acid

Structural formula

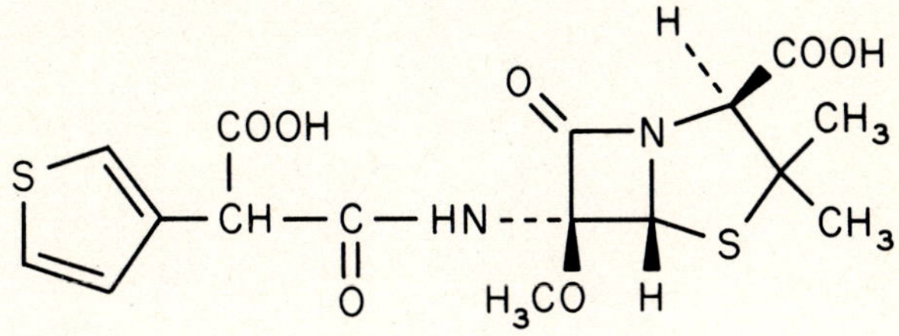

Molecular formula — $C_{16}H_{18}N_2O_7S_2$

Molecular weight — 414.45

Manufacturer — Beecham Pharmaceuticals (England)

CAS registry No. — 66148-78-5

NOTE: BRL 17421 is the code number for temocillin sodium.

USAN — NICOTINE POLACRILEX

Pronunciation — nĭk′′ ō tēn′ pŏl′′ ȧ krĭl′ ĕks

Therapeutic claim — an aid to help smokers give up smoking

Chemical names

(1) 2-methyl-2-propenoic aid polymer with diethenylbenzene, complex with *(S)*-3-(1-methyl-2-pyrrolidinyl)pyridine

(2) methacrylic acid polymer with divinylbenzene, complex with nicotine

Structural formula

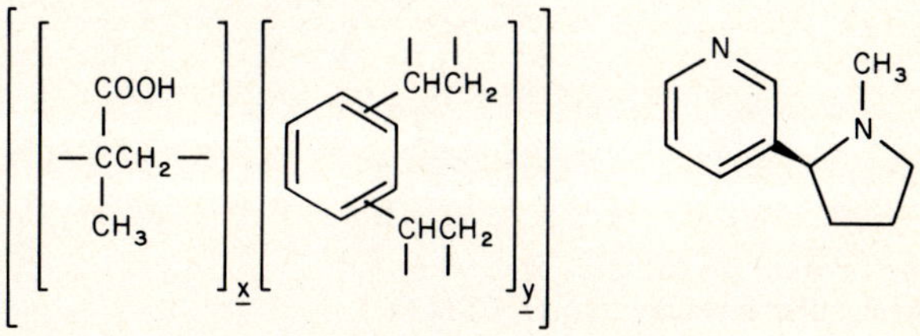

Molecular formula — $[(C_4H_6O_2)x(C_{10}H_{10})y]$ $(C_{10}H_{14}N_2)$

Trademark — Nicorette

Manufacturer — AB Leo

CAS registry No. — 96055-45-7

USAN	ACRIVASTINE
Pronunciation	ăk′ rĭ văs″ tēn
Therapeutic claim	antihistamine

Chemical names

(1) *(E,E)*-3-[6-[1-(4-methylphenyl)-3-(1-pyrrolidinyl)-1-propenyl]-2-pyridinyl]-2-propenoic acid

(2) *(E)*-6-[*(E)*-3-(1-pyrrolidinyl)-1-*p*-tolylpropenyl]-2-pyridineacrylic acid

Structural formula

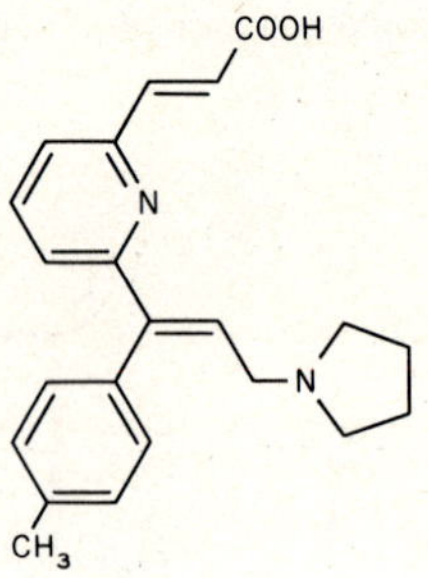

Molecular formula	$C_{22}H_{24}N_2O_2$
Molecular weight	348.44
Manufacturer	Burroughs Wellcome Co.
Code designation	BW 825C
CAS registry No.	87848-99-5

USAN	RECLAZEPAM
Pronunciation	rĕ klā′ zĕ păm
Therapeutic claim	sedative

Chemical names

(1) 2-[7-chloro-5-(2-chlorophenyl)-2,3-dihydro-1*H*-1,4-benzodiazepin-1-yl]-4(5*H*)-oxazolone

(2) 2-[7-chloro-5-(*o*-chlorophenyl)-2,3-dihydro-1*H*-1,4-benzodiazepin-1-yl]-2-oxazolin-4-one

Structural formula

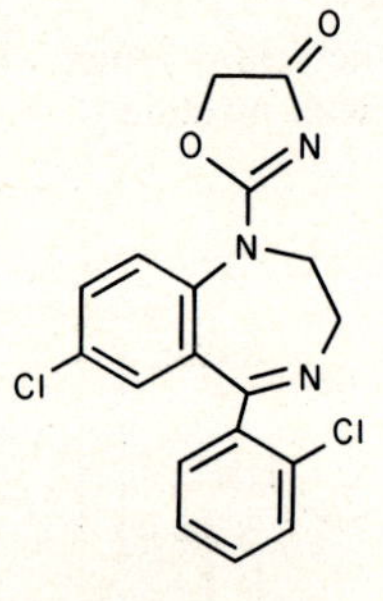

Molecular formula	$C_{18}H_{13}Cl_2N_3O_2$
Molecular weight	374.22
Manufacturer	G.D. Searle & Co.
Code designation	SC-33963
CAS registry No.	76053-16-2

USAN	NEFOCON A
Pronunciation	nē″ fō′ kŏn
Ingredient function	contact lens material (hydrophobic)

Chemical names

(1) methyl 2-methyl-2-propenoate polymer with 2-methyl-2-propenoic acid, 1,2-ethanediyl bis(2-methyl-2-propenoate), 3-[3,3,3-trimethyl-1,1-bis[(trimethylsilyl)oxy]disiloxanyl]propyl 2-methyl-2-propenoate and *N*-(1,1-dimethyl-3-oxobutyl)-2-propenamide

(2) methyl methacrylate polymer with methacrylic acid, ethylene dimethacrylate, 3-[3,3,3-trimethyl-1,1-bis(trimethylsiloxy)disiloxanyl]propyl methacrylate and *N*-(1,1-dimethyl-3-oxobutyl)acrylamide

Structural formula

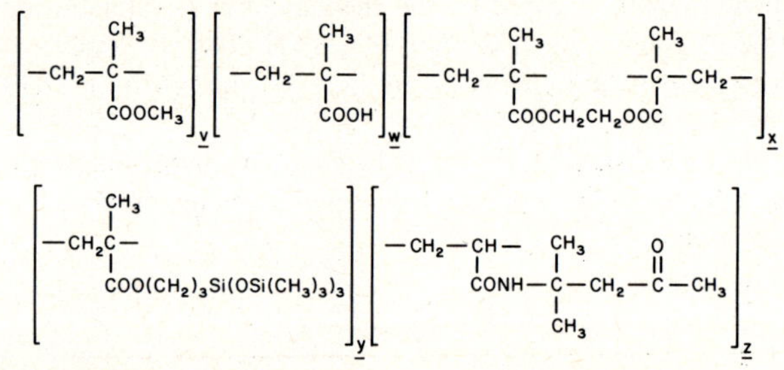

Molecular formula
$(C_5H_8O_2)v(C_4H_6O_2)w(C_{10}H_{14}O_4)x(C_{16}H_{38}O_5Si_4)y(C_9H_{15}NO_2)z$

Trademark	Ocusil
Manufacturer	Oculus Contact Lens Co.
CAS registry No.	91524-13-9

New cumulative list of United States Adopted Names available

The 1986 edition of *USAN and the USP Dictionary of Drug Names* is now available. This edition contains all nonproprietary names assigned by the United States Adopted Names Council since 1961, all international nonproprietary names, plus numerous code designations, synonyms, and trademarks. Each copy costs $54.95 and can be obtained from the USP Convention, Inc., Order Processing Department, 12601 Twinbrook Parkway, Rockville, MD 20852; telephone (301)881-0666.

CLINICAL PHARMACOLOGY & THERAPEUTICS
VOLUME 38 NUMBER 6 DECEMBER 1985

COMMENTARY

Clinical pharmacology: A personal perspective

Elliot S. Vesell, M.D. *Hershey, Pa.*

Harry Gold was the founding father of clinical pharmacology. He coined that term and performed the first placebo-controlled scientific studies of drug effects in man. A gifted investigator, Gold published pioneering studies on digitalis in 1929[1] long before modern drug assays became available and when many people considered experiments of drugs in man ethically and scientifically unjustifiable. To appreciate the legacy Gold left us, we should recall that his medical colleagues underestimated him and did not support his research or his vision of clinical pharmacology.[2]

Despite the fact that society and the medical profession now recognize the urgent need to investigate both new and old drugs in man, the path of academic clinical pharmacology is in some respects not much easier today than in the time of Harry Gold—only the nature of the problems has changed. In 1978 Franz Gross astutely characterized the pathway of contemporary academic clinical pharmacology as "thorny."[3] The formidable obstacles and difficulties that Gross identified remain and contribute to the recent exodus of many talented young investigators from the ranks of academic clinical pharmacology. (By academic I mean clinical pharmacology as practiced in medical schools. Although other institutions certainly qualify as academic, my comments are directed to the unique environments, responsibilities, and opportunities that prevail at medical schools with respect to patient care and clinical teaching.)

During this trying time for academic clinical pharmacology, it is encouraging to reflect on how much Gold achieved under adverse circumstances. Gold's influence lives on through his creativity and discoveries, his farsighted teachings on therapeutics, and his outstanding students, such as Walter Modell and Louis Lasagna. Gold inspired them and others to devote their lives to academic clinical pharmacology, to develop and expand the fundamental principles Gold propounded. All of us here today are indebted to Harry Gold.

From the Department of Pharmacology, The Pennsylvania State University College of Medicine.

1985 Harry Gold Award Address read before the American Society for Pharmacology and Experimental Therapeutics, Boston, Mass., Aug. 19, 1985.

Received for publication Aug. 19, 1985; accepted Aug. 26, 1985.

Reprint requests to: Dr. Elliot S. Vesell, M.D., Evan Pugh Professor and Chairman, Department of Pharmacology, The Pennsylvania State University College of Medicine, Hershey, PA 17033.

THE SIGNIFICANCE OF SCIENTIFIC TRADITION: TRANSMISSION OF SEMINAL CONCEPTS FROM ONE GENERATION TO ANOTHER

The recent establishment by the American Society for Pharmacology and Experimental Therapeutics of awards to honor pioneers in pharmacology such as Bernard Brodie, Louis Goodman, Alfred Gilman, Otto Krayer, and Gold is notable for several reasons. These awards help to remind present students not only of outstanding experiments of the past, but also of strong links between past and present in underlying concepts, principles, and achievements. Many students could profit from more knowledge about these discoveries. In some cases the actual discoveries, crucial as they may be, have less long-term impact than the personal influence and magnetism of a charismatic teacher who is responsible for the future development of a whole field through students and followers.

I have been asked to comment on my research pertaining to clinical pharmacology, but before relating the influence of Brodie and his laboratory on my work beginning in the mid-1960s, I must go back another decade to the period of the mid-1950s, when Detlev Bronk left Johns Hopkins University to transform Rockefeller Institute into Rockefeller University. The subsequent change in the orientation of Rockefeller University toward teaching made it possible for scientific novices such as me to work there. I was privileged to be assigned to Henry Kunkel's laboratory to perform studies in human biochemical genetics with Alexander Bearn. In the summer of 1956, at the impressionable age of 22, I found myself totally immersed in the rich scientific atmosphere that prevailed in the Kunkel laboratory.

Because a principal theme of this article is that the responses of human subjects to outside stimuli often depend on complex interactions among many host factors,[4] I should begin by explaining how this scientific environment at Rockefeller University influenced me. The environment in Kunkel's laboratory at that time was particularly stimulating. The focus of interest had turned from the study of enzymes in the diagnosis and management of liver disease to the role of immunologic mechanisms in causing collagen diseases. Autoimmunity as a pathogenetic mechanism was then an innovative concept because antibodies and γ-globulin were mysterious substances poorly understood and chemically uncharacterized. In addition to the farsighted and wise leadership of Kunkel, scientific discovery in that laboratory was facilitated by an unusually devoted group of gifted young investigators including, to name only a very few, Bearn, Edward Franklin, Gerry Edelman, Halsted Holman, Hans Muller Eberhard, and Ralph Williams. They befriended and helped me, a lowly first-year student from Harvard Medical School, to spend a summer in the laboratory. They encouraged me, showed me the ropes, and provided blood specimens from their patients. I was immensely impressed with the deep devotion and dedication of these young men. Experiments commonly continued until 2 or 3 o'clock in the morning, and the laboratory was busy on weekends. Seminars each Monday and daily ward rounds permitted frequent exchanges and heightened the opportunities to make rapid scientific advances. Fundamental discoveries emerged, including identification of the first autoantibodies in patients with disseminated lupus. Eventually a Nobel prize was awarded to a member of this laboratory for elucidation of the amino acid structure of the 7S γ-globulin molecule.

At Rockefeller University in the 1950s, all the staff members lunched together in a large room containing several dozen long, heavy, wooden tables. Each table comfortably accommodated eight people, a number appropriate for a vigorous discussion with general participation. To enhance opportunities for scientific exchange, we were requested to sit at a table with members of different laboratories. At first, acutely aware of my youth and inexperience, I tried to remain silent and unobserved, as my early luncheons seemed overwhelming and intimidating. But then one day a large man stood up on the opposite side of the table from me, leaned across the table, and offered me in a most friendly way his huge hand. "I'm Dick Shope," he said, "pleased to meet you. What's your name and where do you work?" That loosened things up considerably, and from then on I enjoyed the friendly spirit and free scientific interchange that prevailed at those lunches.

I had the opportunity over a period of three successive summers at Rockefeller University to become acquainted at such lunches with many scientists. I vividly recall Thomas Rivers, Frank Horsfall, Peyton Rous, William Stein, Stanford Moore, Eugene Opie, Herbert Gasser, Moses Kunitz, Lyman Craig, Maclyn McCarty, Vincent Dole, and Pete Ahrens. Talk was usually, but not always, scientific. If one wanted to change intellectual fare, lunch at Rene Dubos' table would be sure to turn up sharp insights into such topics as contemporary European economics or the seventeenth century French philosophes. Rene Dubos had a remarkable ability to draw original scientific generalizations from these seemingly unrelated topics. This stimulating environment fixed my determination to become an investigator; these men radiated a conviction that the scientific life was the one most worth pursuing. They were secure in what they did, and their productive lives inspired their students to follow in their footsteps.

Today some students seem aloof from that kind of charismatic persuasiveness, or at least appear not to be so influenced. Students should remain aware that seminal ideas and concepts transmitted from one generation to another are the basis for scientific continuity and progress. For example, all of us in Kunkel's laboratory used the technique of starch block electrophoresis to purify proteins. We knew that our chief had developed that convenient separation technique with Arne Tiselius while on a year sabbatical at Uppsala University in Sweden. In turn, Tiselius had discovered electrophoresis and produced the first electrophoresis apparatus. We were aware of long biochemical traditions in Sweden, Germany, and at Rockefeller University, where we knew who represented what school and viewpoint, as well as the precise line of descent for the concepts and research in a particular laboratory. As another example, Stein and Moore were trained at Rockefeller University by Max Bergmann, who in turn had worked with Emil Fischer in Berlin.

Medical and graduate students today need to realize the significance of such traditions. Knowledge of these intellectual pathways enriches our professional activities, deepens our commitment and dedication to the highest professional standards, and provides incentive for us to refine and transmit these standards to subsequent generations of students.

DISCOVERY OF MULTIPLE MOLECULAR FORMS OF LACTATE DEHYDROGENASE IN HUMAN SERUM AND TISSUES

To describe my contributions to clinical pharmacology, I need to tell how I came to work in pharmacogenetics. My experiments in the Kunkel laboratory gratified me primarily because they yielded reproducible results. This amazed me, because at medical school few of the experiments I performed in the laboratory of my biochemistry course worked. Yet at Rockefeller University I had a different experience. I attribute this to the extra time to plan, perform, and analyze each experiment and to the opportunity to repeat an experiment. By contrast, during a course students barely have time to complete one laboratory exercise before rushing on to another, often gaining an unsatisfactory impression and hence a false notion of research. The opportunity to design and execute an experiment under less constrained circumstances is an important aspect of research. In fact, the really appropriate design for a truly novel experiment, the one that provides the best insight or possibly a conceptual breakthrough, rarely occurs early in the study. It may come only after several months or years of work on a particular problem.

My mentor was Bearn, then a young human geneticist investigating Wilson's disease, a rare inborn error of metabolism characterized by abnormal copper disposition. The disease is crippling, chronic, and invariably fatal. Patients with Wilson's disease are deficient in ceruloplasmin, the serum protein that normally transports copper. As a result, copper accumulates in the liver, producing cirrhosis, and in the basal ganglia of the brain, causing spasticity, rigidity, dysarthria, and dysphagia. Bearn was interested in the identification of the nature of the abnormality in ceruloplasmin. Starch block electrophoresis revealed that ceruloplasmin was an α_2-globulin. Because ceruloplasmin binds copper, Bearn had given a tracer dose of ^{64}Cu to normal subjects and to patients with Wilson's disease to measure temporal changes in the distribution of ^{64}Cu. Soon after ^{64}Cu dosing the copper bound only to albumin. Later on, in normal subjects the albumin peak of ^{64}Cu diminished progressively as freshly synthesized ceruloplasmin bound the labeled copper. There were also corresponding elevations of the α_2-globulin peak in the normal subjects. In patients with Wilson's disease, however, no such redistribution was observed from albumin to α_2-globulin.

Because zinc is in the same group as copper in the periodic chart of the elements, I wondered whether zinc might also localize in the same serum fractions as copper. Bearn and I injected a tracer dose of ^{65}Zn into normal subjects (ourselves) and observed two peaks of radioactivity, one in the albumin and the other in the α_2-globulin, just as with ^{64}Cu. In my medical school biochemistry course I recalled that our professor, Bert Vallee, had told us that lactate dehydrogenase (LDH) was a zinc enzyme. Vallee was studying the function of zinc at the active site of several enzymes. Because total serum LDH activity was then of clinical interest as a test for myocardial infarction, the idea dawned on me to ask how a zinc enzyme such as LDH might localize in serum fractions. Would it appear in a single peak or in different peaks, perhaps in the same serum fractions as ^{65}Zn? This question was easily answered. We were surprised to observe three large peaks of LDH activity after electrophoretic separation of serum on starch blocks. In normal serum the distribution of total activity among the three main peaks was remarkably constant, but the distribution changed dramatically in serum from patients with myocardial infarction and leukemia. In patients with myocardial infarction, the α_1-

globulin peak of LDH activity increased as compared with the pattern in normal serum, whereas in patients with leukemia the α_2-globulin peak became differentially elevated.[5]

All the experienced enzymologists at Rockefeller University with whom I consulted, including Stein, Moore, Craig, and Kunitz, who with John Northrup had first crystallized an enzyme, were unanimous in declaring artifactual the heterogeneity of LDH activity that we observed in normal human serum. They believed that this heterogeneity arose from the relatively harsh conditions, i.e., 15 hours of electrophoresis at 400 V. The notion that the same enzyme could exist in multiple molecular forms in a cell or tissue to subserve different biochemical functions had not been considered in 1956 when these studies were performed. Although we were not able to disprove the argument that LDH heterogeneity was artifactual, being generated by conditions during electrophoresis, Bearn and I were convinced of its reality by the consistent changes in the LDH pattern in various disease states we had observed. Furthermore, we conceived of a rational biologic explanation for this changing pattern. Thus in 1957 we published our conviction that different tissues had distinctive patterns of LDH activity and that specific tissue patterns were reflected by the changing serum LDH distributions produced by diseases affecting these tissues.[5]

Two years later Markert[6] coined the term isozyme for multiple molecular forms of an enzyme that exist in a single cell or tissue. Today we accept the concept that many enzymes exist in such multiple molecular forms. Isozymes are recognized as a common mechanism used by nature to subserve a variety of metabolic functions. For example, isozymes of the hepatic mixed-function oxidases offer the organism the capacity to oxidize, and hence make highly diverse lipid-soluble xenobiotics more water soluble and therefore more easily excreted. This system, based on isozymes of cytochrome P-450, serves as a defense mechanism to enable removal of many different kinds of exogenous lipid-soluble chemicals. If vertebrates possessed only a single form of cytochrome P-450, we would all be incapable of mounting multiple metabolic attacks on such a diversity of exogenous chemicals, and hence we would be much more susceptible to toxicities.

Today, and for the past decade, the general biologic principle underlying isozymes is so well accepted that no one recalls the time when it was heretic. Perhaps the highest compliment that can be paid a scientist is to have his or her ideas pass from the stage at which no one accepts them to the stage at which they become so widely incorporated into scientific thought that they are taken as fundamental biologic truths. It may then be time to reexamine them to find, if not a fatal flaw, at least a significant deviation or exception.

TWIN STUDIES IN PHARMACOGENETICS

By the time I joined the Brodie laboratory at the National Institutes of Health in 1965, I had published approximately 70 papers on isozymes, focusing mainly on genetic, phylogenetic, and biochemical aspects. I had been trained as a human geneticist, having spent several years in the early 1960s as a staff member in Bearn's Laboratory of Heritable Diseases at Rockefeller University. Although I subsequently published several papers demonstrating the existence of isozymes of particular pharmacologic significance,[7-9] Brodie asked me to investigate not isozymes but the problem of why normal subjects have large interindividual variations in rates of drug elimination. Ironically, isozymes were again involved: The explanation eventually proved to be genetically controlled variations of different isozymes of cytochrome P-450. Brodie and his associates had developed reliable methods to separate drugs from their principal metabolites and used these methods to measure the concentrations of drugs and their principal metabolites in biologic fluids such as serum and urine. After the administration of single doses of many commonly used drugs, they quantitated rates of drug elimination and metabolite formation.

Brodie possessed an unusually brilliant, farsighted, and imaginative scientific mind. He was fascinated by the large pharmacokinetic variations that he had repeatedly observed for many different drugs in normal subjects. The extent of such variations among normal people was commonly ten- to twenty-fold, even for studies in only a dozen or so subjects. Brodie wanted to unravel the fundamental biologic explanation for these variations, and he expected me to apply formal genetic techniques to achieve this goal. Brodie had shown that for a particular drug, a given subject had a highly reproducible drug $t_{1/2}$. Why, then, were there such large differences in drug $t_{1/2}$ values between people? What mechanism maintained these extensive intersubject differences?

To explore this problem, I was fortunate in selecting a venerable technique in human genetics introduced in 1875 by Charles Darwin's cousin, Sir Francis Galton,[10] namely the twin method. Identical and fraternal twins constitute a unique resource because one can separate genetic from environmental contributions to large variations in quantitative, metric, and continuously distributed traits such as height, weight, blood pressure, and intelligence quotient. The twin method consists of comparison of the magnitude of variation for a trait within monozygotic (MZ) twins with that in dizygotic (DZ) twins. If genetic factors are mainly responsible for the large variations observed in that trait, then MZ twins will be much closer in their values than will DZ twins. However, if environmental factors predominate over genetic factors, then the correlation between MZ twins will be approximately the same as that between DZ twins.

A basic assumption of the method is that in critical respects the environments of MZ and DZ twins are similar. This assumption is necessary because in a valid experiment only one variable can be manipulated independently of all others. The variable that is changing in the twin paradigm is the genotype: MZ twins have identical genotypes, whereas the DZ twins share on average only half their genes, with the other half different. Therefore, if genetic constitution is to serve as the independent variable, the environment must be held constant. Under another experimental design, only MZ twins participate; thus genotype is held constant and differential environmental effects are investigated by comparison of pharmacokinetic values in MZ twins reared together with those reared apart. Because MZ twins reared apart are very rare, this attractive approach has not yet been used in pharmacogenetics. We tested our assumption that similar environments prevailed for our carefully selected MZ and DZ twins. Fortunately, our stringent selection criteria stood us in good stead, because according to several tests the environments of our MZ and DZ twins appeared to be very similar. Other critical aspects of these twin studies included selection of appropriate drugs, not only those whose elimination depended mainly on hepatic oxidative mechanisms, but those whose elimination rates after single oral doses would accurately reflect the activity of these hepatic enzymes.

The twin method had fallen into disrepute when we selected it. Standard texts in human genetics condemned twin studies because of numerous erroneous applications. Specifically, twins had been investigated to compare the incidence of all-or-none events, such as the presence or absence of disease. Such uses were occasionally invalid because they were too qualitative and statistically flawed and depended on a biased literature for twin ascertainment (i.e., the tendency is to report twins who are concordant, rather than discordant, for a disease).

Our experimental design and results demonstrated an unsuspected power and versatility of the twin method. Accurate and highly reproducible pharmacokinetic measurements in each twin indicated that the twin method could discriminate genetic from environmental causes of large interindividual pharmacokinetic variations. Now in pharmacogenetics, a twin study serves as the first part of a two-tier system.[11] If the twin study implicates genetic factors, a Mendelian mode of transmission can be identified by a second, more difficult step, a family study.[11] Should the twin study reveal that pharmacokinetic variation arises mainly from environmental factors, as in our twin investigation on conjugation of acetaminophen,[12] then family studies become unnecessary.

Results of our other twin studies of the sources of large pharmacokinetic variations in the oxidative metabolism of different drugs disclosed that genetic factors were primarily responsible. In MZ twins in whom there was no genetic variation, kinetic differences also vanished. However, in many, but not all, DZ twins large kinetic variations persisted. We observed this to be so for phenylbutazone,[13] antipyrine,[14] bishydroxycoumarin,[15] ethanol,[16] halothane,[17] and theophylline.[18] Others subsequently confirmed these conclusions in twin studies of nortriptyline,[19] phenytoin,[20] and amobarbital.[21]

The condition of the twins is critical in the interpretation of the results. All twins were normal and their hepatic drug metabolizing enzymes were neither markedly induced or inhibited; none took medications, smoked cigarettes, imbibed ethanol regularly, or took antifertility agents. Therefore, the results need to be qualified and limited to these particular conditions, specifically to normal unmedicated subjects under carefully controlled, uniform conditions. Under fluctuating, nonuniform conditions, the underlying genetic control of large pharmacokinetic variations could be masked by environmental factors that would be differentially operative. This would perturb the genetically set values of some, but not all, twins. Although twin studies cannot establish the Mendelian mode of transmission of a genetic factor, twin studies can implicate a genetic factor that requires family studies to elucidate. We have performed such family studies to explore a Mendelian hypothesis for both antipyrine[22] and theophylline.[18] Results suggest monogenic control of large pharmacokinetic variations for both drugs.

THE ANTIPYRINE TEST: EFFECTS OF HOST FACTORS ON HEPATIC DRUG METABOLISM

One of my main research efforts in clinical pharmacology has been to develop a safe, convenient, sensitive, and reproducible procedure to assess the impact of different environmental factors on the hepatic drug metabolizing capacity of normal subjects. The model drug approach, particularly with antipyrine, resulted from this effort.[23] Isozymes were again involved, because the antipyrine test reflects the activity of several hepatic cytochrome P-450 isozymes that metabolize antipyrine. The original antipyrine test consists of the measurement of plasma antipyrine concentrations after antipyrine dosing to subjects both before and after imposition of a single environmental change. The change in antipyrine clearance from the first to the second measurement is taken as an indication of the effect of the environmental factor on the hepatic drug metabolizing enzymes that biotransform antipyrine by three separate reactions. The test is both sensitive and safe. Use of each subject as control serves to reduce multiple host factors as contributions to kinetic change, such as all genetic factors and many environmental factors. Thus a single environmental factor, such as administration of a new drug, can be examined in virtual isolation from contributions made by all others. Dose-response curves can be generated for the factor, thereby permitting quantitative comparisons of the impact of different environmental factors on hepatic drug metabolism. Further refinement of the test involves measurement of the rates of formation or partial clearances of the three main antipyrine metabolites in each subject both before and after imposition of a single environmental change.[24,25] Each metabolite of antipyrine is produced by a genetically distinct cytochrome P-450. Because much more precise information is available from metabolite measurements, sharper insights into the nature of metabolic changes can be obtained than from the determination of antipyrine clearance alone.[26]

Approximately 200 reports of the antipyrine test have appeared in the literature to define effects of diverse environmental factors on hepatic drug metabolism in normal subjects. Many of these reports concern tests of the inducing or inhibiting potential of new and old drugs. In fact, the antipyrine test has become a standard industrial screen to determine whether a new drug affects a subject's capacity to eliminate other drugs. Other applications of the test have also been used to assess effects of the following factors on hepatic drug metabolism: drug interactions, dietary manipulations, diurnal variations, exercise, stress, fever, infection, and multiple disease states. Particularly appealing is the noninvasive character of one refinement in the test: Antipyrine concentrations can be measured in saliva, where they equal antipyrine concentrations in plasma.[27,28]

But any test has its limitations, and I have taken pains to point out numerous limitations of and unjustified expectations from the antipyrine test.[23] Nevertheless, several misconceptions about the test linger. No single drug substrate can serve adequately to predict the rate at which all others will be eliminated in a given subject. Therefore, drug substrates other than antipyrine need to be included if a more general picture is desired. However, very rigorous criteria must be fulfilled if changing peripheral concentrations of a model drug are to serve as a valid reflection of that drug's hepatic metabolism. Very few model chemicals besides antipyrine and aminopyrine satisfy the necessary requirements.[23] The main use of the antipyrine test is to assess for a given environmental factor, including a new drug, its capacity to enhance or diminish hepatic antipyrine metabolism.

For human subjects under both basal and disease conditions, the antipyrine test has provided an insight into the in vivo function of the hepatic antipyrine metabolizing enzymes. The generalizations that emerge from many studies with the antipyrine test are that these enzymes are exceedingly sensitive to perturbation by multiple environmental factors, but that under carefully controlled stable conditions their activity in a given subject is highly reproducible and genetically controlled. However, under changing environmental circumstances these activities fluctuate dramatically. Many host factors, including age, diet, disease, cigarette smoking, drug intake, ethanol consumption, and use of antifertility agents, can alter the activity of these enzymes. Fever, immunologic status, and the function of critical organs such as the heart, liver, and kidney can also affect these enzymes. Therefore, the capacity of many patients to eliminate drugs may be dynamically changing. A therapeutic dose of a drug at one stage of an illness may become a toxic or ineffective dose at another stage. These dynamic fluctuations in the hepatic drug metabolizing capacity constitute a formidable challenge to the physician, who must be prepared to detect such changes and adjust accordingly the dosage of drugs with low therapeutic indices. In making such decisions the physician can be helped by various tests, including measurements of drug concentrations in the patient's blood. At present there is no satisfactory substitute for close clinical observation of the patient, including careful scrutiny for signs of toxicity from each drug administered.

THE FUTURE OF CLINICAL PHARMACOLOGY

The mission of academic clinical pharmacology—improved pharmacotherapy through high standards of research, patient care, and teaching—is both laudable and necessary. These objectives, if fulfilled, should secure for our discipline a bright and successful future.

Yet, according to several criteria this success has eluded us. While I predict a bright future for academic clinical pharmacology in the United States, I am convinced that to attain success through realization of the potential and mission of academic clinical pharmacology, we need to take several difficult and challenging steps. We need to be more united on several fundamental issues. Strong, vigorous leadership is required, which means selfless leadership that will not accept the present unsatisfactory status quo. I agree with Gross[3] and others in attributing the present decline in academic clinical pharmacology in the United States primarily to our own policies and parochial attitudes. Also to blame are self-serving, shortsighted restrictions placed on the activities and resources of clinical pharmacology divisions by some turf-protecting medical school departments. I wish I could tell you that the many significant scientific advances in clinical pharmacology over the past decade would alone assure a bright future for our discipline. However, I would be less than candid if I left you with that impression.

Encouraging early signs of our mustering of unity and cooperation among clinical pharmacologists requisite for a bright future are the achievements of the Council on Clinical Pharmacology. This Council, composed of six delegates from each of the three principal societies that represent our discipline, has persevered admirably over the past 6 years to develop mechanisms for accreditation of expertise in clinical pharmacology. I urge you to support these efforts of the Council, all of whose principal recommendations were passed unanimously by its 18 members. One such recommendation has been to establish a Board Examination in Clinical Pharmacology for duly qualified physicians. Without such a board examination, I doubt that the mission of academic clinical pharmacology can be successful.

To illustrate how far we must go to attain the bright future our field merits and that I predict for it, I shall contrast the present unstable status of academic clinical pharmacology in our country to the relative stability and prosperity of the discipline in the United Kingdom. In the United Kingdom, therapeutics exists primarily as a patient care, service, and teaching specialty. In April of 1985 I visited 10 teaching hospitals in Great Britain under the auspices of the Frolich Visiting Professorship of the Royal Society of Medicine. I was amazed that in each of these teaching hospitals, therapeutics enjoyed the status of a separate, independent department. Most departments were small but were smoothly functioning autonomous units. Included in most of these departments were the following resources: three to five permanent professional staff, 1500 to 4000 square feet of space, and a medical service consisting of a number of patient beds, sometimes as many as 20 to 30. Every 4 to 6 days a therapeutics department "firm," a team composed of a consultant, registrars (residents), and medical students, admitted all medical patients requiring inpatient care who appeared during a 24-hour period at that particular teaching hospital. In addition, daily medical ward rounds were conducted by the staff of the department of therapeutics. Outpatient clinics were also scheduled twice each week, at which patients specifically referred for drug-related problems were examined and received therapy. Several medical students attended and learned from the professors of therapeutics, who devoted much time to individual student instruction generally conducted by the Socratic method. Under these conditions, therapeutics departments in the United Kingdom are designated very broad functions in patient care and clinical teaching.

As further reinforcement of the emphasis placed on clinical pharmacology as a distinct medical specialty in Britain, a large portion of the qualifying examination in medicine is devoted exclusively to clinical pharmacology. This impresses on all medical students the paramount importance of clinical pharmacology for the practice of medicine and hence the necessity that they learn thoroughly the material covered by this subject. In addition, a more advanced examination is available later in the course of a medical career to accommodate those qualified physicians who wish to be certified as specialists in therapeutics. These sequential examinations are cited as evidence of the existence in the United Kingdom of the requisite instruments to ensure adequate teaching and clinical practice of the discipline of clinical pharmacology.

By contrast to this well-organized system for the teaching and practice of clinical pharmacology in the United Kingdom, we in the United States have not structured academic clinical pharmacology in such a logical, sequential manner. Here it is conducted academically in a much less formal, more haphazard, and hence less stable way. For example, no consistent provisions are made in our medical schools for permanent, self-perpetuating divisions, much less departments, of clinical pharmacology. Several undesirable consequences of this loose-knit approach should be noted and the underlying causes corrected. One consequence is that when a clinical pharmacology division is dropped, usually because a key staff person departs (such as at Emory University, Massachusetts General Hospital, The University of Kansas, and The Pennsylvania State University), that division either becomes defunct or lies dormant for many years.

As a second consequence, many critical aspects of pharmacotherapeutics are not systematically or adequately taught in our medical schools. Either this information is learned individually and piecemeal by each physician during residency or thereafter, or it is never entirely acquired. This spotty method of teaching therapeutics has many undesirable consequences for patient care. At present, less than one fourth of our medical schools have active divisions of clinical pharmacology. Even fewer train clinical pharmacologists in such a regular manner that at least one emerges each year from the program. There are many examples of divisions of clinical pharmacology that were formed in our medical schools some years ago, thrived for a brief period, and then dissolved because of the departure of staff. As a result of such experiences, departments of medicine in our medical schools have become disillusioned with the discipline of clinical pharmacology. Chairpersons of departments of medicine have never fully appreciated the wide range of responsibilities that clinical pharmacologists are capable of assuming. Accordingly, the attitude of many such chairpersons toward clinical pharmacology has become negative or ambivalent.

As a third consequence, clinical pharmacology has thus far not been established as a legitimate medical subspecialty in the United States through development of a formal board examination like those offered in the United Kingdom and Sweden.

As a fourth consequence, it is not surprising that fewer bright young residents are attracted to academic clinical pharmacology than we would like or than the field needs for adequate growth and development. Nor is it surprising that clinical pharmacology has not benefitted from all the professional and financial incentives enjoyed by the other board-sanctioned medical subspecialties. In short, despite the great opportunities and the great need to improve pharmacotherapy, clinical pharmacology has not thrived in our academic institutions. Quite the reverse, to assure their professional and financial security our brightest graduates have usually elected to throw in their lot with more established specialties. The insecurity of those engaged in academic clinical pharmacology is further documented by a recent mass exodus of young, bright stars from our ranks. Most have left their posts as medical school clinical pharmacologists for industrial positions. Some remain in medical schools but in other capacities.

Diverse reasons have been offered for the failure of academic clinical pharmacology to thrive.[3] Some of these explanations are widely accepted, while others are controversial. Whatever the causes, it is clear that the present form and shape of academic clinical pharmacology in the United States reflect closely the concepts and viewpoints promulgated by many of us in the field. I refer to consistent rejection of the primary role of patient care and clinical teaching, both of which epitomize academic clinical pharmacology as practiced in the United Kingdom. By contrast, we in the United States feared that such time spent on clinical and teaching activities would detract from and even undermine our laboratory research. This strongly expressed attitude of most of our leading clinical pharmacologists prevented the institutionalization of academic clinical pharmacology as a patient care and clinical teaching subject in our medical schools. Instead, we have insisted that academic clinical pharmacology should exist primarily as a research activity within departments of medicine. So it does today; this decision and our present condition help to explain why in our clinical pharmacology training programs there is little time spent outside the laboratory and why these training programs are often vague and avoid the problems of a precise definition of what subject matter is required for a clinical pharmacologist.[29]

Even as a research speciality, academic clinical pharmacology has not thrived. Except for a very few academic programs, support from federal and industrial sources for research by academic clinical pharmacologists has not been sufficient for sustenance, much less growth. Scarcity of financial support for academic clinical pharmacologists has encouraged partisanship in the selection of young clinical pharmacologists for research career awards, membership in prestigous societies, and research grants.

This bias has not only prevented clinical pharmacology from attaining its potential in research, it has also limited opportunities for research in academic clinical pharmacology. To assure research survival, creativity, and vigor in the future, we need more funded training programs to enhance the attractiveness of clinical pharmacology so that more bright, young physicians will enter the field. To achieve these objectives, we require more centers of excellence for training in clinical pharmacology. I propose that over the next 5 years the pharmaceutic industry contribute a million dollars each to 20 outstanding medical schools to develop 20 new divisions of clinical pharmacology. These 20 leading schools should be selected from those now lacking such a division. Concurrently, National Institutes of Health support and matching funds from each medical school should be sought to help these new divisions perform their duties, including the development of new trainees and their own young faculty. Often overlooked is the urgent need for faculty development. The chairperson of the departments of pharmacology and medicine within each institution would take joint responsibility for implementation of the program with the assurance that a viable, new division of clinical pharmacology would be created. In the next decades a steady flow of creative clinical pharmacologists emanating from diverse academic programs is vital, not only to the pharmaceutic industry but also to the public health, in terms of the introduction of new drugs and the proper clinical use of existing drugs.

If we in the United States are to produce new academic clinical pharmacology divisions to provide for the future of our discipline after our recent heavy losses, fresh, progressive thinking and leadership are required. The success of the British model should show us how to plead more effectively the cause of academic clinical pharmacology in the United States. The example from Britain of a permanent, continuing department justified on the basis of the indispensible provision of patient care and clinical teaching should inspire us to incorporate these crucial features of academic clinical pharmacology into our system. I believe that with a few notable exceptions, these aspects have been either slighted or undervalued by most of our academic clinical pharmacology programs.

During the present period of major financial cutbacks, survival of most academic programs may depend on their provision of an urgently needed, indispensible service. While academic clinical pharmacology has such indispensible skills to offer (specifically, improved patient care through better pharmacotherapy), we as academic clinical pharmacologists have thus far selected another route: The pursuit of our own particular research interests. In my view, it is not yet too late to modify this course. Our problem is really an old one: The need to be needed. I believe we shall solve our problems, but much cooperation, effort, and leadership will be required.

References

1. Gold H, DeGraff AC. Studies on digitalis in ambulatory cardiac patients; elimination of digitalis in man. J Clin Invest 1929;6:613-26.
2. Modell W. Clinical pharmacology: reflections in my rearview mirror. CLIN PHARMACOL THER 1978;23:497-504.
3. Gross F. The thorny path of clinical pharmacology. CLIN PHARMACOL THER 1978;24:383-94.
4. Vesell ES. On the significance of host factors that affect drug disposition in man. CLIN PHARMACOL THER 1982; 31:1-7.
5. Vesell ES, Bearn AG. Localization of lactic acid dehydrogenase activity in serum fractions. Proc Soc Exp Biol Med 1957;94:96-9.
6. Markert CL, Moller F. Multiple forms of enzymes: tissues, ontogenetic, and species specific patterns. Proc Nat Acad Sci USA 1959;45:753-63.
7. Axelrod J, Vesell ES. Heterogeneity of N- and O-methyltransferases. Mol Pharmacol 1970;6:78-84.
8. Ross S, Weinshilboum RM, Molinnoff PB, Vesell ES, Axelrod J: Electrophoretic properties of dopamine β-hydroxylase in several tissues from three species. Mol Pharmacol 1972;8:50-8.
9. Cohn CK, Vesell ES, Axelrod J. Studies of a methionine activating enzyme. Biochem Pharmacol 1972;21:803-9.
10. Galton F. The history of twins as a criterion of the relative powers of nature and nurture. J Br Anthropol Inst 1875;5:391-406.
11. Vesell ES: Twin studies in pharmacogenetics. Human Genet 1978;1(suppl):19-30.
12. Nash RM, Stein L, Penno MB, Passananti GT, Vesell ES. Sources of interindividual variations in acetaminophen and antipyrine metabolism. CLIN PHARMACOL THER 1984;36:417-30.
13. Vesell ES, Page JG. Genetic control of drug levels in man: phenylbutazone. Science 1968;159:1479-80.
14. Vesell ES, Page JG. Genetic control of drug levels in man: antipyrine. Science 1968;161:72-3.
15. Vesell ES, Page JG. Genetic control of dicumarol levels in man. J Clin Invest 1968;47:2657-63.
16. Vesell ES, Page JG, Passananti GT. Genetic and environmental factors affecting ethanol metabolism in man. CLIN PHARMACOL THER 1971;12:192-201.
17. Cascorbi HF, Vesell ES, Blake DA, Hebrich M. Genetic and environmental influence on halothane metabolism in twins. CLIN PHARMACOL THER 1971;12:50-5.
18. Miller CA, Slusher LB, Vesell ES. Polymorphism of theophylline metabolism in man. J Clin Invest 1985;75: 1415-25.
19. Alexanderson B, Price Evans DA, Sjöqvist F: Steady state plasma levels of nortriptyline in twins: influence of genetic factors and drug therapy. Br Med J 1969;4: 764-8.
20. Andreasen PB, Froland A, Skovsted L, Andersen SA, Hauge M. Diphenylhydantoin half-life in man and its inhibition by phenylbutazone: the role of genetic factors. Acta Med Scand 1973;193:561-4.
21. Endreny L, Inaba T, Kalow W: Genetic study of amobarbital elimination based on its kinetics in twins. CLIN PHARMACOL THER 1977;20:701-14.
22. Penno MB, Vesell ES. Monogenic control of variations in antipyrine metabolite formation: new polymorphism of hepatic drug oxidation. J Clin Invest 1983;71:1698-1709.
23. Vesell ES. The antipyrine test in clinical pharmacology: conceptions and misconceptions. CLIN PHARMACOL THER 1979;26:275-86.

24. Danhof M, de Groot-van der Vis E, Breimer DD. Assay of antipyrine and its primary metabolites in plasma, saliva and urine by high performance liquid chromatography and some preliminary results in man. Pharmacology 1979;18:210-23.
25. Danhof M, Teunissen MWE, Breimer DD. 3-Hydroxymethyl antipyrine excretion in urine after an oral dose of antipyrine. Pharmacology 1982;24:181-4.
26. Slusher LB, Vesell ES. Cimetidine-induced reduction in gastrointestinal absorption of antipyrine and rate constants for formation of its metabolites. CLIN PHARMACOL THER 1984;35:568-75.
27. Welch RM, DeAngelis RL, Wingfield M, Farmer TW. Elimination of antipyrine from saliva as a measure of metabolism in man. CLIN PHARMACOL THER 1975;18:249-58.
28. Vesell ES, Passananti GT, Glenwright PA, Dvorchik BH. Studies on the disposition of antipyrine, aminopyrine, and phenacetin using plasma, saliva, and urine. CLIN PHARMACOL THER 1975;18:259-72.
29. Spector R, Vesell ES. Training programs in clinical pharmacology. J Clin Pharmacol 1980;20:309-15.

ORIGINAL ARTICLES

Inadequate aldosterone response to hyperkalemia during angiotensin converting enzyme inhibition in chronic renal failure

To assess the mechanism involved in hyperkalemia during angiotensin converting enzyme inhibition with captopril in chronic renal failure, captopril, 150 mg/day, was administered to 16 patients with hypertension with plasma creatinine levels between 1.6 and 12.4 mg/dl. After 4 weeks of therapy, plasma potassium levels increased from 3.9 ± 0.1 to 5.5 ± 0.2 mEq/L ($P < 0.001$) and the final plasma potassium levels correlated with plasma creatinine levels ($r = 0.67$; $P < 0.01$). In six patients with plasma creatinine levels ≥3 mg/dl, aldosterone excretion decreased after 4 weeks of captopril, from 7.5 ± 3.1 to 1.8 ± 0.5 μg/24 hr, whereas plasma renin activity increased from 0.6 ± 0.2 to 4.4 ± 1.1 ng/ml/hr ($P < 0.05$). This was associated with increases in plasma potassium levels from 3.9 ± 0.2 to 5.4 ± 0.4 mEq/L ($P < 0.005$) and a significant reduction in fractional excretion of potassium from an average of 34% to 25%. No significant changes in plasma creatinine levels were observed during therapy. There was a significant positive correlation between aldosterone excretion and the potassium excretion fraction ($r = 0.53$; $P < 0.01$). Increases in plasma potassium levels were not able to increase aldosterone excretion, although the greater the plasma potassium level attained, the smaller the reduction in aldosterone excretion ($r = 0.47$; $P < 0.05$). Our results indicate that adequate aldosterone production is essential to preserve potassium homeostasis in chronic renal failure. Moreover, angiotensin II appears necessary for an adequate aldosterone response to potassium stimulation. (Clin Pharmacol Ther 38:613-617, 1985.)

M. Teresa Zanella, M.D., Edilio Mattei, Jr., M.D., Sérgio A. Draibe, M.D., Claudio E. Kater, M.D., and Horácio Ajzen, M.D. *São Paulo, Brazil*

The orally active converting enzyme inhibitor captopril has been shown to be effective in the treatment of essential hypertension[2,4,5] and of the hypertension associated with chronic renal failure.[6] Potassium retention and increases in serum potassium levels have been reported during captopril therapy,[2] but overt hyperkalemia does not usually occur in patients with normal renal function.[2,14] However, we have observed that captopril may seriously compromise potassium homeostasis in patients with impaired renal function. Our observations are in agreement with reports that rapid rises in serum potassium levels and marked hyperkalemia may result from converting enzyme inhibition in chronic renal insufficiency.[7,14,16]

We evaluated the potassium-aldosterone relationship in patients with chronic renal failure during 4 weeks of captopril therapy to assess the role of aldosterone in the development of hyperkalemia in this condition.

From the Divisions of Nephrology and Endocrinology, Escola Paulista de Medicina.

Supported in part by Grant No. B/76/80/265/00/00 from FINEP, Brazil.

Received for publication March 23, 1985; accepted Aug. 8, 1985.

Reprint requests to: Maria Teresa Zanella, M.D., Escola Paulista de Medicina, Disciplina de Endocrinologia, Rua Botucatu no. 740, Caixa Posta 20.266, 04023, São Paulo SP, Brazil.

METHODS

Sixteen patients with hypertension and chronic renal failure were selected for captopril therapy. There were six women and 10 men, ranging in age from 12 to 63 years, with plasma creatinine levels varying between

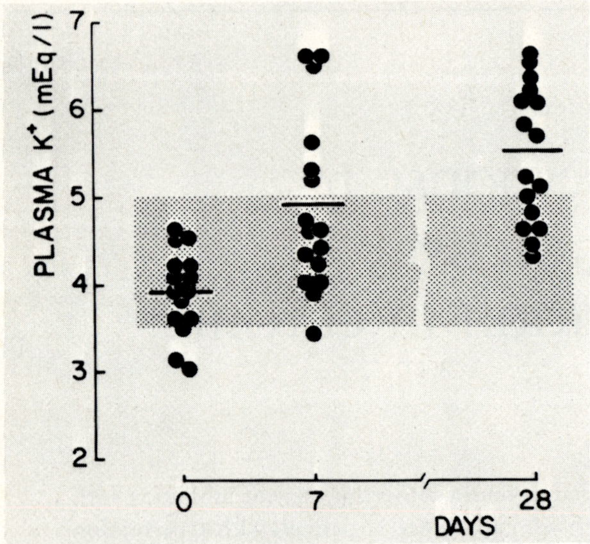

Fig. 1. Individual plasma potassium values in 16 patients with chronic renal failure before and 7 and 28 days after captopril therapy. *Shaded area* represents normal mean values ±2 SD.

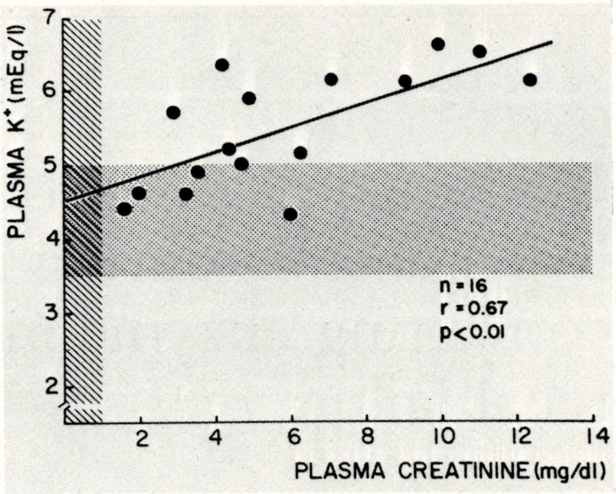

Fig. 2. Relationship between plasma creatinine and plasma potassium concentrations after 4 weeks of captopril therapy in 16 patients with chronic renal failure. *Shaded area* represents normal mean values ±2 SD.

1.6 and 12.4 mg/dl and plasma potassium levels <4.7 mEq/L. Fourteen had a diagnosis of chronic glomerulonephritis and two had renal interstitial disease. Patients with diabetes were not included in the study. All antihypertensive drugs were discontinued at least 1 week before the start of captopril dosing. Patients received captopril, 150 mg/day, for 4 weeks while maintaining their usual diet containing 100 to 200 mEq/day sodium and 30 to 50 mEq/day potassium. Blood pressure and plasma creatinine and potassium levels were determined before the start of therapy and 1 and 4 weeks thereafter. In six patients with plasma creatinine levels ≥3 mg/dl, plasma renin activity, levels of creatinine, sodium, and potassium, and urinary excretion of aldosterone, creatinine, and electrolytes were measured before and at weekly intervals during captopril dosing.

Plasma renin activity was estimated by RIA of generated angiotensin I.[15] Urinary aldosterone excretion was determined by measuring the 24-hour excretion of aldosterone-18-glucuronide by RIA[9] by use of a highly specific antiserum.* The urinary excretion of aldosterone-18-glucuronide has been shown to be a valid index of the aldosterone secretion rate in patients with chronic renal insufficiency.[12] Plasma and urine sodium, potassium, and creatinine levels were measured by routine methods.

All results are expressed as the $\overline{X}$ ± SE. Statistical significance was tested by ANOVA. Linear regression and correlation coefficients were determined by the method of least squares.

RESULTS

Captopril therapy resulted in a reduction of blood pressure in 10 of the 16 patients studied. For the group as a whole, mean arterial pressure decreased from a control value of 144 ± 6.3 to 123 ± 6.5 mm Hg ($P < 0.01$) after 7 days of captopril, and the reductions observed were sustained after 28 days of maintenance therapy. During captopril dosing there were no significant changes in plasma creatinine levels, and no patient had any acidemia.

Individual plasma potassium values during the study are shown in Fig. 1. All patients had basal plasma potassium levels <4.7 mEq/L. During therapy, plasma potassium levels rose consistently, exceeding 5.0 mEq/L in six of the 16 patients after 7 days of therapy. After 4 weeks every patient showed >0.5 mEq/L increments in plasma potassium levels, and hyperkalemia (plasma potassium level >5.0 mEq/L) was detected in 10 of the 16 patients. For the entire group, plasma potassium levels increased from 3.9 ± 0.1 to 5.5 ± 0.2 mEq/L ($P < 0.001$) after therapy. Fig. 2 shows the significant positive correlation between final plasma potassium and plasma creatinine levels during captopril dosing

*Provided by Dr. J. G. H. Vieira from the Hormone Laboratory at Escola Paulista de Medicina.

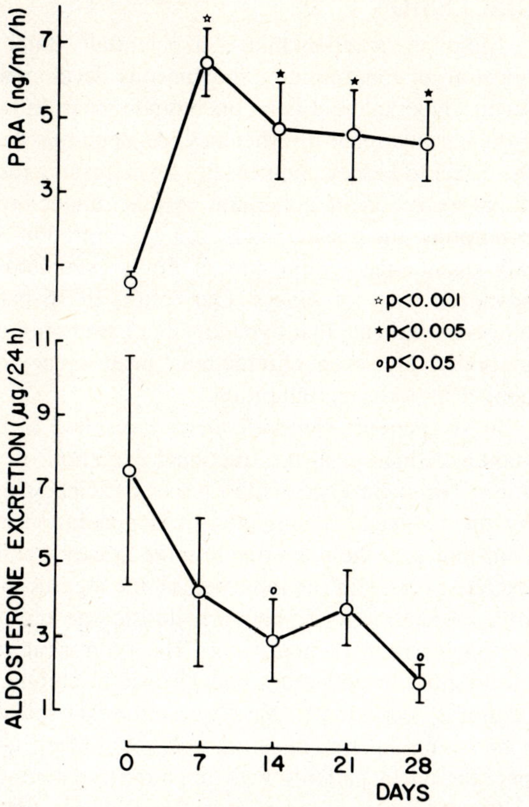

Fig. 3. Plasma renin activity *(PRA; top)* and aldosterone excretion *(bottom)* before and during 4 weeks of captopril therapy in six patients with chronic renal failure. Data are $\overline{X} \pm$ SE.

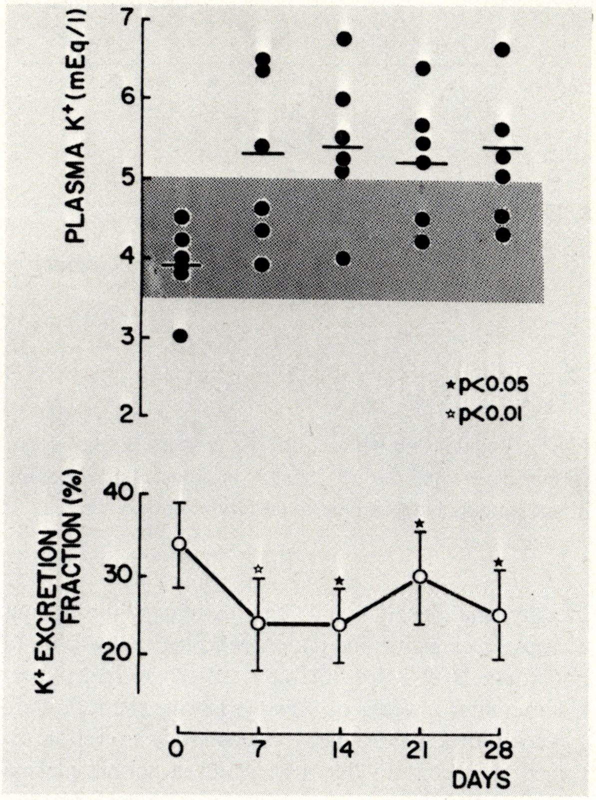

Fig. 4. Individual values of plasma potassium *(top)* and potassium excretion fraction *(bottom)* in six patients with chronic renal failure before and during 4 weeks of captopril therapy. *Shaded area* represents normal mean values ±2 SD.

(r = 0.67; P < 0.01). Although every patient demonstrated substantial increases in plasma potassium levels, values >6 mEq/L were found only among those with plasma creatinine levels >4 mg/dl.

Six patients had plasma potassium levels >6 mEq/L but no therapy for hyperkalemia was required. A plasma potassium level >6 mEq/L was detected after 7 days of captopril dosing in three patients who were monitored through frequent ECG recordings. After the first week of therapy, the plasma potassium level stabilized without any ECG sign of potassium toxicity. In the other three patients, plasma potassium levels just above 6 mEq/L were detected only after 3 weeks of therapy. Despite no evidence of potassium toxicity, captopril therapy was discontinued at the end of 4 weeks in all patients with plasma potassium levels >6 mEq/L. Other than hyperkalemia, no significant adverse effects were observed during the study.

Fig. 3 shows the effects of converting enzyme inhibition on plasma renin activity and aldosterone excretion in six patients who had creatinine clearances <40 ml/min. None had had high plasma renin activity before therapy. After 7 days of captopril dosing, plasma renin activity increased from 0.6 ± 0.2 to 6.5 ng/ml/hr (P < 0.001) and remained significantly higher than the basal values during therapy. After 7 to 14 days of captopril, aldosterone excretion decreased 30% to 80% in all patients. During the 2 subsequent weeks aldosterone excretion continued to fall in four patients, returning to basal values in the other two. For the entire group of patients, aldosterone excretion fell significantly from 7.5 ± 3.1 to 2.9 ± 1.1 μg/24 hr after 14 days of captopril dosing and remained low after 4 weeks of therapy.

In the above-mentioned series of six patients, captopril induced marked changes in plasma potassium levels (Fig. 4). The mean basal level of 3.9 ± 0.2 mEq/L increased to 5.3 ± 0.5 mEq/L after 7 days of

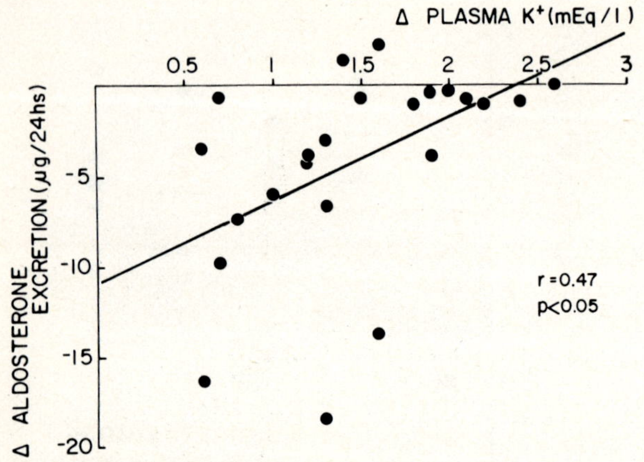

Fig. 5. Relationship between the net changes in plasma potassium levels and the net changes in aldosterone excretion in six patients with chronic renal failure during 4 weeks of captopril therapy.

therapy, and this high value was maintained throughout therapy. Except for one patient who had a low plasma potassium level before therapy, all others had hyperkalemia after 2 weeks of therapy. During the following 2 weeks, one patient whose aldosterone excretion returned to the basal value also achieved normal plasma potassium levels. The potassium level of the other patient whose aldosterone excretion also returned to the control value remained >6 mEq/L.

Urinary excretion of potassium decreased after 7 days of captopril therapy, but the changes were not statistically significant. However, the excretion fraction of potassium (the percentage of filtered potassium that is excreted) was significantly reduced by captopril. Before therapy, all six patients had elevated excretion fractions of potassium. As shown in Fig. 4, increases in plasma potassium levels were associated with pronounced decreases in the fractional excretion of potassium during captopril dosing.

Aldosterone excretion correlated positively with the excretion fraction of potassium ($r = 0.53$; $P < 0.01$) and negatively with plasma potassium level ($r = -0.37$; $P < 0.05$). Although every patient demonstrated marked rises in serum potassium levels, aldosterone excretion was always maintained near or below the basal values during therapy. However, the greater the rise in plasma potassium levels, the smaller the reduction in aldosterone excretion, as indicated by the positive correlation ($r = 0.47$; $P < 0.05$) shown in Fig. 5.

There were no significant changes in urinary volume, urinary sodium excretion, or in the excretion fraction of sodium during converting enzyme inhibition.

DISCUSSION

Although hyperkalemia is a potentially fatal complication of renal failure, spontaneous development of severe hyperkalemia is an uncommon event in nonoliguric chronic renal insufficiency. As nephrons are lost, the diseased kidney compensates by increasing the fractional excretion of potassium so that, under ordinary conditions, the plasma potassium concentration is usually maintained within normal limits even into a far advanced stage of illness. Our results in 16 patients, however, indicate that hyperkalemia commonly occurs in moderately severe chronic renal insufficiency during converting enzyme inhibition.

In six patients captopril therapy resulted in a substantial reduction in the fractional excretion of potassium. The occurrence of aldosterone deficiency induced by the blockade of angiotensin II generation clearly contributed to the impairment in the kidney's ability to excrete potassium, as indicated by the significant positive correlation found between aldosterone and the excretion fraction of potassium. The prominent role of aldosterone in potassium homeostasis in chronic renal failure is supported by the observation that spironolactone results in rises in serum potassium levels and hyperkalemia in patients with impaired renal function.[3] Although the presence of aldosterone seems important to sustain an enhanced potassium secretion by the residual nephrons in chronic renal failure, the magnitude of hyperkalemia induced by captopril seems to depend only slightly on the extent of aldosterone suppression. The low negative correlation between aldosterone excretion and plasma potassium levels indicates that other factors contribute to hyperkalemia in this condition. Because the final plasma potassium level correlated positively with the plasma creatinine level, it is plausible that factors related to the azotemic state itself contribute to the magnitude of hyperkalemia. The basal level of plasma potassium and the differences in sodium and potassium intake and in acid-base status among patients may also have influenced the final plasma potassium level. Although speculative, another contributory factor to hyperkalemia might be impairment in the extrarenal mechanism for potassium adaptation induced by chronic aldosterone deficiency.[1]

The influence of potassium on aldosterone production can be demonstrated by the positive correlation between the net changes in plasma potassium levels and the net changes in aldosterone excretion. This indicates that the stimulatory effect of potassium on aldosterone production may have masked the drops in aldosterone that would have resulted from the blockade of angiotensin II formation by captopril. However, despite marked degrees of hyperkalemia, aldosterone excretion remained below the basal values throughout captopril dosing. These observations suggest that, although hyperkalemia is to a certain extent a self-limited phenomenon, the plasma potassium level alone is not able to stimulate aldosterone fully for its own regulation during converting enzyme inhibition in chronic renal failure. The reasons for the inadequate aldosterone response to hyperkalemia in this condition are not clear. In normal subjects, hyperkalemia of the same magnitude as that observed in our patients is a powerful stimulus to aldosterone production.

Captopril dosing in chronic renal failure simulates the syndrome of hyporeninemic hypoaldosteronism, in which low levels of aldosterone are associated with hyperkalemia and impaired renal function.[8,12] Schambelan et al.[12,13] proposed that the inability to produce aldosterone in hyporeninemic hypoaldosteronism is a consequence of prolonged hyporeninemia. Similarly, captopril-induced angiotensin II deficiency might be implicated in the poor aldosterone response to hyperkalemia observed in our patients. This possibility is supported by the findings of Pratt et al,[11] who showed that captopril infusion in dogs blocks the stimulatory effect of potassium on aldosterone production. Furthermore, when angiotensin II and captopril were infused simultaneously, the adrenal responsiveness to potassium was restored. Also, in vitro the adrenal glomerulosa cells obtained from captopril-treated rats fail to produce aldosterone in response to potassium stimulation.[10]

Thus hyperkalemia develops frequently during converting enzyme inhibition in patients with moderate to severe chronic renal failure. Captopril-induced aldosterone deficiency and consequent reduction in the kidney's ability to excrete potassium are unequivocal contributory factors to the development of hyperkalemia in this condition. Furthermore, because aldosterone excretion remains suppressed during converting enzyme inhibition even in the presence of marked elevations in plasma potassium levels, angiotensin II may be necessary for effective potassium stimulation of aldosterone production.

References

1. Alexander EA, Levinsky NG: An extrarenal mechanism of potassium adaptation. J Clin Invest **47:**740-748, 1968.
2. Atlas SA, Case DB, Sealey J, Laragh J, McKinstry DN: Interruption of the renin-angiotensin system in hypertensive patients by captopril induces sustained reduction in aldosterone secretion, potassium retention, and natriuresis. Hypertension **1:**274-280, 1979.
3. Berl T, Katz FH, Henrich WL, Torrent A, Schrier RW: Role of aldosterone in the control of sodium excretion in patients with advanced chronic renal failure. Kidney Int **14:**228-235, 1978.
4. Bravo EL, Tarazi RC: Converting enzyme inhibition with an orally-active compound in hypertensive man. Hypertension **1:**39-46, 1979.
5. Brunner HR, Gavras H, Waeber B, Kershaw GR, Turini GA, Vukovich RA, McKinstry DN, Gavras I: Oral angiotensin converting enzyme inhibitor in long term treatment of hypertensive patients. Ann Intern Med **90:**19-23, 1979.
6. Brunner HR, Wauters JP, McKinstry D, Waeber B, Turini GA, Gavras H: Inappropriate renin secretion unmasked by captopril (SQ 14225) in hypertension of chronic renal failure. Lancet **2:**704-707, 1978.
7. Hamilton DV, Maidment G, Evans DB, Pryor JS: Captopril for refractory hypertension in patients with chronic renal failure and renal transplantation. J R Soc Med **74:**357-362, 1981.
8. Knochel JP: The syndrome of hyporeninemic hypoaldosteronism. Ann Rev Med **30:**145-153, 1979.
9. Langan J, Jackson R, Adlin EV, Channick BJ: A simple RIA for urinary aldosterone. J Clin Endocrinol Metab **38:**189-193, 1974.
10. Parkinson CA, Belton SJ, Pratt JH: The effect of captopril treatment on potassium-induced stimulation of aldosterone production in vitro. Endocrinology **114:**1567-1570, 1984.
11. Pratt JH: Role of angiotensin II in potassium-mediated stimulation of aldosterone secretion in the dog. J Clin Invest **70:**667-672, 1982.
12. Schambelan M, Sebastian A, Biglieri EG: Prevalence, pathogenesis and functional significance of aldosterone deficiency in hyperkalemic patients with chronic renal insufficiency. Kidney Int **17:**89-101, 1980.
13. Schambelan M, Stockigt JR, Biglieri EG: Isolated hypoaldosteronism in adults. A renin-deficiency syndrome. N Engl J Med **287:**573-578, 1972.
14. Textor SC, Bravo EL, Fouad FM, Tarazi RC: Hyperkalemia in azotemic patients during angiotensin-converting enzyme inhibition and aldosterone reduction with captopril. Am J Med **73:**719-725, 1982.
15. Vieira JGH, Noguti KD, Russo EMK, Maciel RMB: Radioimmunoassay for plasma renin activity: Methodologic aspects. Rev Bras Pat Clin (Por) **17:**195, 1981.
16. Warren SE, O'Connor DT: Hyperkalemia resulting from captopril administration. JAMA **244:**2551-2552, 1980.

Polymorphic dextromethorphan metabolism: Co-segregation of oxidative O-demethylation with debrisoquin hydroxylation

Dextromethorphan hydrobromide, 25 mg po, was given to 268 unrelated Swiss subjects to study urinary drug and metabolite profiles. Rates of *O*-demethylation yielding the main metabolite dextrorphan were expressed by the urinary dextromethorphan/dextrorphan metabolic ratio. We found a bimodal distribution of this parameter in our population study, which indicates that there are two phenotypes for dextromethorphan *O*-demethylation. The antimode at a metabolic ratio of 0.3 separated the poor metabolizer (PM; n = 23; prevalence of 9%) from extensive metabolizer (EM) phenotypes. Urinary output of dextrorphan was <6% of the dose in all PMs and was 50% in the 245 EMs. Pedigree analysis of 14 family studies revealed an autosomal-recessive transmission of deficient dextromethorphan *O*-demethylation. In these families, 37 heterozygous genotypes could be identified; however, through use of the urinary drug and metabolite analysis it was not possible to identify the heterozygous genotypes within the EM phenotype group. Co-segregation of dextromethorphan *O*-demethylation with debrisoquin 4-hydroxylation was also studied. Complete concordance of the two phenotypic assignments was obtained, with a Spearman rank correlation coefficient of $r_s = 0.78$ (n = 62; $P < 0.0001$) for dextromethorphan and debrisoquin metabolic ratios. Presumably the two drug oxidation polymorphisms are under the same genetic control. Thus the innocuousness and ubiquitous availability of dextromethorphan render it attractive for worldwide pharmacogenetic investigations in man. (CLIN PHARMACOL THER 38: 618-624, 1985.)

B. Schmid, Ph.D., J. Bircher, M.D., R. Preisig, M.D., and A. Küpfer, Ph.D.
Berne, Switzerland

Since the description of the genetic polymorphism of debrisoquin[19] and sparteine[8] metabolism, interest in the pharmacogenetics of oxidative drug metabolism has grown rapidly. In fact, hepatic handling of an increasing number of therapeutically important drugs was found to vary with this drug hydroxylation polymorphism.[7,14] Several clinically significant adverse drug reactions were found to be much more frequent in poor metabolizer (PM) than in extensive metabolizer (EM) phenotypes.[5,7,11] However, a major setback in the study of pharmacogenetics in man is that debrisoquin and sparteine are marketed only in a limited number of countries. Therefore, a test compound available worldwide would favor a more general application of pharmacogenetic investigations.

Recently, important interindividual differences in dextromethorphan *O*-demethylation were reported and a genetic basis was postulated.[21] With the phenotyped panel approach in 12 subjects of that study, a significant relationship between dextromethorphan *O*-demethylation and debrisoquin 4-hydroxylation could be established[17]; it was concluded that dextromethorphan *O*-demethylation to yield the main metabolite, dextrorphan, might provide a new procedure for the detection of EM and PM phenotypes of the debrisoquin type. We report herein the results of a European population study of 268 unrelated healthy subjects in which the 8-hour urinary dextromethorphan/dextrorphan metabolic ratio was studied. We also performed family

From the Department of Clinical Pharmacology, University of Berne.
Supported by the Swiss National Science Foundation.
Received for publication July 3, 1985; accepted July 23, 1985.
Reprint requests to: A. Küpfer, Ph.D., Department of Clinical Pharmacology, University of Berne, Murtenstrasse 35, CH-3010 Berne, Switzerland.

studies to assess the genetic basis of interindividual differences in the biotransformation of dextromethorphan.

METHODS

Dextromethorphan hydrobromide and dextrorphan were kindly supplied by G. Pfaff from H. Mack Pharmaceuticals. Hard gelatin capsules containing 25 mg dextromethorphan hydrobromide (corresponding to 19.3 mg or 71 μmol dextromethorphan base) were also manufactured by the same company. Dimetacrine hydrogentartrate (internal standard for GLC) was purchased from Siegfried Chemicals. Other chemicals were supplied by different commercial sources and were at least of American Chemical Society grade. For enzymatic hydrolysis, the β-glucuronidase/arylsulfatase of *Helix pomatia* was purchased from Boehringer Ingelheim.

For the population study, 268 normal healthy and drug-free subjects (138 men and 130 women, ranging in age from 20 to 74 years) gave informed consent. All subjects were unrelated residents of Switzerland. Women had to indicate their use of oral contraceptives, and all subjects were instructed to abstain from alcohol for 4 hours before and during the test. Subjects were requested to empty their bladder and to take a capsule of 25 mg dextromethorphan hydrobromide before bedtime. An 8-hour overnight urine collection was obtained. Samples were analyzed on arrival at the laboratory; dextromethorphan and dextrorphan were found to be stable at 4° C for at least 2 months.

We also carried out family studies to investigate the metabolism of dextromethorphan in first-degree relatives of dextromethorphan demethylation–deficient index cases (n = 6). Additional families (n = 13) previously analyzed by the Department of Pediatrics of the University of Zurich for various genetic markers were also investigated. Eight of these 13 families included members with deficient metabolism of dextromethorphan and were included in the pedigree analysis.

In the final part of the study, we investigated the cosegregation of dextromethorphan demethylation with debrisoquin hydroxylation in 50 subjects from either the population or family studies, as well as in 12 subjects previously phenotyped for debrisoquin hydroxylation.[17]

For analysis of drug and metabolite, 1 ml urine was diluted with 1 ml 0.1 mol/L acetate buffer at pH 5.0 and 50 μl of an aqueous solution containing 34 nmol dimetacrine (internal standard) were added in a screwtop test tube. Enzymatic hydrolysis of dextrorphan glucuronides was performed by the addition of 20 μl or 2000 Fishman units of β-glucuronidase/arylsulfatase. Microbial growth was prevented by 50 μl 0.6 mol/L aqueous sodium azide in the incubation mixture. Enzymatic hydrolysis was performed in a shaking bath at 37° C for 12 hours as previously established for complete cleavage of the conjugation products. Before extraction, 1 ml 1 mol/L glycine/sodium hydroxide buffer at pH 11.3 was added and dextromethorphan and dextrorphan were extracted into 5 ml ether by horizontal shaking for 15 minutes. The ether phase was evaporated to dryness under a gentle stream of nitrogen. The dry residue was dissolved in 20 μl of isoamyl alcohol and an aliquot of 3 to 4 μl was injected into a gas chromatograph with a nitrogen-sensitive thermionic detector.

Separation of all compounds was obtained on a 1.8 m glass column (2 mm id) packed with 3% XE-60 on Chromosorb WHP 80/100 mesh size (Supelco Inc.). Temperatures for the injection port, column oven, and detector were 250°, 200° (isothermal), and 250° C, respectively. The flow rates for nitrogen (carrier gas) and air and hydrogen (detector gases) were 36, 250, and 1.7 ml/min, respectively. These conditions resulted in retention times of 2.8, 5.8, and 9.0 minutes for dextromethorphan, dimetacrine, and dextrorphan, respectively. At 3.5 minutes a peak was noticed in 97% of all urine samples that could be identified as caffeine. Peak area integration was used in all analyses. The calibration curves were linear over the concentration ranges of 0.4 to 40 and 1.0 to 300 μmol/L for dextromethorphan and dextrorphan, respectively.

Intra-assay coefficients of variation were 1.4% (n = 6) for 13 μmol/L dextromethorphan and 2.5% (n = 6) for 230 μmol/L dextrorphan concentrations. Inter-assay coefficients of variation for 4 and 20 μmol/L dextromethorphan were 12% (n = 21) and 5% (n = 13), respectively. For 7 and 100 μmol/L dextrorphan concentrations, the respective values were 15% (n = 21) and 4% (n = 13). Recoveries of dextromethorphan and dextrorphan ranged from 90% to 100%. The signal-to-noise ratio allowed a minimum drug concentration analysis of 0.25 and 0.5 μmol/L for dextromethorphan and dextrorphan, respectively. These concentrations were therefore considered as limits of detection. Debrisoquin and 4-hydroxydebrisoquin in the 8-hour urine samples were analyzed by GLC after derivatization with acetylacetone.[18]

Analogous to the earlier proposed debrisoquin/4-hydroxydebrisoquin metabolic ratio, interindividual differences in rates of dextromethorphan metabolism were expressed by the metabolic ratio of urinary dextromethorphan/dextrorphan concentrations. In the semi-

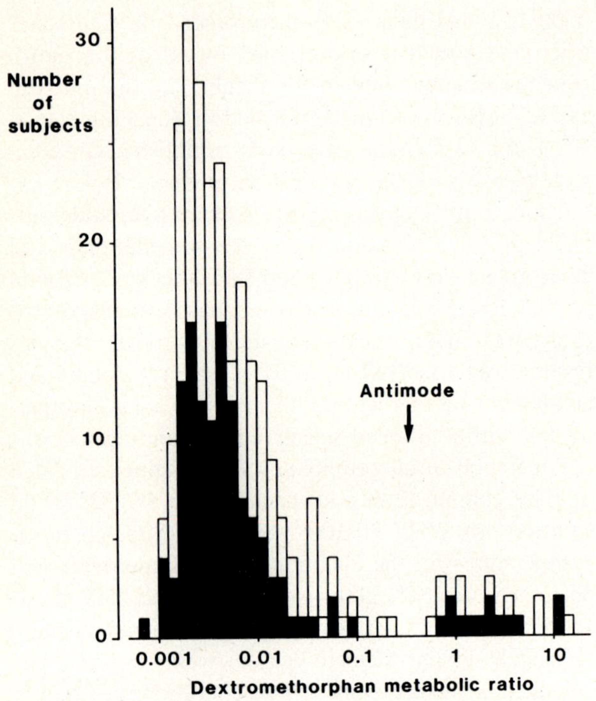

Fig. 1. Semilogarithmic frequency distribution histogram of the dextromethorphan/dextrorphan metabolic ratios in 8-hour urine samples of 130 female *(solid bars)* and 138 male *(open bars)* normal subjects after 71 μmol dextromethorphan by mouth. *Arrow* indicates the antimode at a metabolic ratio of 0.3.

logarithmic frequency distribution histogram, the mean values and the respective standard deviations were expressed by the medians and the differences between medians and the 84th (EMs) or the 16th (PMs) percentiles. The logarithms of these values were used to determine the antimode by density function analysis.[9,23] The intersection point of two density functions equals the antimode in a discontinuous frequency distribution histogram. Thus the mathematic description of the lower mode was set equal to the equation of the upper mode, and the logarithm of the metabolic ratio at the point of equal densities was calculated.

The two-tailed Student's t test was used for statistical analysis of group parameters. Conventional statistical procedures[13] were applied to calculate standard deviations and 95% confidence limits for the two allele frequencies and for the prevalencies of the two drug oxidation phenotypes.

RESULTS

Large interindividual differences were obvious in the urinary 8-hour excretion of dextrorphan, the major metabolite of dextromethorphan. In the most prominent cases, dextrorphan elimination was between 0.2% and 5.8% of the dose, whereas most subjects had 35% to 70% urinary recovery of this metabolite. An important difference in metabolic dextromethorphan disposition must be assumed, since the urinary outputs of unchanged dextromethorphan were approximately 10 times higher in urine samples from subjects with low dextrorphan output as compared with most of the urine samples from subjects with a large dextrorphan content.

Visual analysis of cumulative dextrorphan elimination in the form of a frequency distribution histogram revealed two distinct groups of subjects, those with urinary dextrorphan excretion >10% or <10% of the dose every 8 hours. The apparent bimodal distribution of dextrorphan elimination was further supported by the observation that none of the 268 subjects had dextrorphan excretion between 5.9% and 15.5% of the dose every 8 hours. Urinary dextrorphan concentrations also showed a bimodal distribution, and subjects with urinary dextromethorphan concentrations <14 μmol/L were identical to those excreting <5.9% of the dose in 8 hours, and vice versa. Therefore, a urinary concentration of 22 μmol/L was found tentatively to separate the two modes.

For more detailed analysis, the urinary dextromethorphan metabolic ratio was calculated to express interindividual differences in drug oxidation. Fig. 1 shows the semilogarithmic frequency distribution histogram of dextromethorphan metabolic ratios in all subjects. A bimodal distribution was found, with a gap between the metabolic ratios of 0.2 and 0.6. The antimode between EM and PM phenotypes was determined by density function analysis. In these calculations, only urine samples with measurable dextromethorphan concentrations were included and an antimode of 0.3 was calculated (Fig. 1). Subjects with metabolic ratios >0.3 were classified as PMs (n = 23 or 9% of the population; 95% confidence limits 6% to 12%), and the remaining subjects with metabolic ratios <0.3 were classified as EMs (n = 245 or 91% of the population; 95% confidence limits 88% to 106%). In 120 subjects with high urinary dextrorphan concentrations, the dextromethorphan concentrations were below the limit of detection in the currently used GLC system. In this situation, a concentration of 0.25 μmol/L was used to calculate the data for the frequency distribution histogram. By this method, metabolic ratios between 0.00078 and 0.0082 were obtained and their location in the histogram clearly shows that despite this simplification, no misclassification of drug oxidation phenotypes occurs.

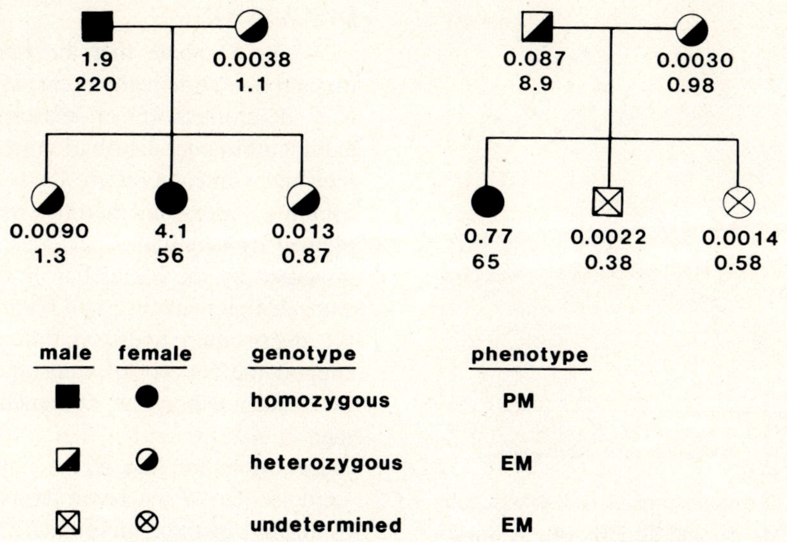

Fig. 2. Dextromethorphan *O*-demethylation pedigrees of EM and PM phenotypes. The *numbers* indicate dextromethorphan and debrisoquin metabolic ratios, respectively. The *left panel* shows the autosomal transmission of the defect and the *right panel* is compatible with the recessive trait of the allele coding for dextromethorphan *O*-demethylation deficiency.

Table I. Dextromethorphan and dextrorphan analysis in urine samples from 268 unrelated subjects after an oral dose of 71 μmol dextromethorphan

	PMs		*EMs*	
	Men	*Women*	*Men*	*Women*
No. of subjects	11	12	127	118
Age (yr)	33 ± 10	33 ± 12	35 ± 12	33 ± 12
Dextromethorphan output (μmol/8 hr)	2.3 ± 1.4*	2.5 ± 1.6*	0.34 ± 0.45†	0.20 ± 0.23
Dextrorphan output (μmol/8 hr)	1.3 ± 1.1*	1.2 ± 0.7*	37 ± 10	34 ± 8.4
Metabolic ratio	3.9 ± 4.1*	3.3 ± 3.7*	0.013 ± 0.028†	0.0069 ± 0.011

Data are $\overline{X}$ ± SD.
*Significantly different ($P < 0.0001$) from EMs irrespective of sex.
†Significantly different ($P < 0.05$) from female EMs.

Table I summarizes the results of dextromethorphan and dextrorphan analysis in urine of PM and EM phenotypes. Results have been calculated separately for male and female subjects. A 1.7-fold increase in dextromethorphan output and a correspondingly higher metabolic ratio was found in male EMs when compared with female EMs, but the cumulative urinary dextromethorphan excretions were the same in these subjects. By contrast, no sex differences were noted among the PMs.

The influence of age on dextromethorphan and dextrorphan could be ruled out by a comparison of the oldest (64 ± 4 years [$\overline{X}$ ± SD]; n = 8) and the youngest (22 ± 2 years; n = 8) sex-matched subjects. By the same approach, no significant influence of oral contraceptive use on dextromethorphan disposition was found in 24 women and no effect of smoking could be seen in matched subjects who did or did not smoke (n = 6).

For further investigation of the genetic basis of the observed bimodality of dextromethorphan *O*-demethylation, we phenotyped 24 first-degree relatives of six PM index cases in the population study. Eleven additional subjects could thus be classified as PMs. The 46% prevalence of subjects with deficient demethylation among first-degree relatives, compared with 9% in the unrelated population (χ^2 = 30; $P < 0.0001$), strongly supports the genetic basis of this deficiency in oxidative drug metabolism.

The mode of inheritance of dextromethorphan me-

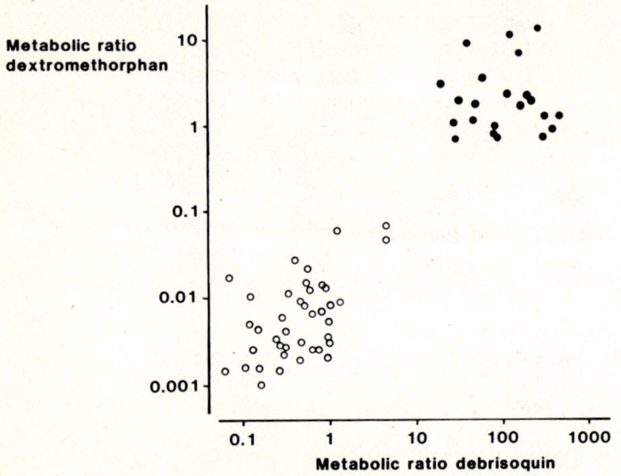

Fig. 3. Comparison of dextromethorphan and debrisoquin metabolic ratios in 40 EMs (○) and 22 PMs (●). A Spearman rank correlation coefficient of $r_s = 0.78$ ($n = 62$; $P < 0.0001$) was calculated and identical phenotypic assignments can be obtained irrespective of the test drug used.

tabolism was investigated in a total of 14 family pedigrees of deficient dextromethorphan demethylation phenotypes. All family studies are compatible with a Mendelian autosomal-recessive mode of transmission. Fig. 2 shows two representative drug oxidation pedigrees (additional information is available in the figure legend). In the same 14 families, 37 heterozygous genotypes could be identified by pedigree analysis. When these 37 cases were compared with the results of the population study (Table II), none of the parameters studied gave any indication by which the heterozygosity of these subjects could be established by the urinary drug and metabolite analysis.

The Mendelian model with one gene and two alleles can be applied to the population study, and the Hardy-Weinberg equilibrium allows calculation of the prevalences of homozygous and heterozygous EM phenotypes representing 50% and 41% of the population, respectively. The allele frequencies are 0.71 (95% confidence limits 0.66 to 0.75) and 0.29 (95% confidence limits 0.24 to 0.35) for the allele coding for extensive and defective dextromethorphan *O*-demethylation, respectively.

To establish the co-inheritance of defective debrisoquin hydroxylation with genetic dextromethorphan *O*-demethylation deficiency, we performed both tests in 62 subjects. As shown in Fig. 3, the genetic basis for both metabolic reactions seems to be identical, since 40 EMs and 22 PMs of either polymorphism exhibited identical phenotypes irrespective of the test compound used ($r_s = 0.78$; $n = 62$; $P < 0.0001$ for the metabolic ratios).

DISCUSSION

We have shown that the rates of hepatic dextromethorphan *O*-demethylation, as expressed by the urinary dextromethorphan/dextrorphan metabolic ratio, exhibit a bimodal distribution in a sample of 268 white men and women in Switzerland. The discontinuous distribution of dextromethorphan metabolism could be explained by hereditary mechanisms that are apparently governed by the Mendelian laws of genetic transmission. Pedigree analysis and complete concordance with the debrisoquin hydroxylation polymorphism further support the concept of autosomal-recessive control of the dextromethorphan *O*-demethylation deficiency in man.

Dextromethorphan is the nonopioid dextrorotatory stereoisomer of the levorotatory narcotic methorphan (*N*-methyl-methoxymorphinan) pharmacophore group. Because of its potent cough suppressant activity,[3,4] dextromethorphan was introduced in the early 1950s and was widely accepted thereafter. Because of its lack of addictive[12] and analgesic[3] properties, the drug became available without prescription as a safe antitussive over-the-counter drug even in pediatric practice.

An early account on dextromethorphan biotransformation was reported after the accidental oral intake of 180 mg dextromethorphan hydrobromide by a child and the discovery of the *O*-demethylated metabolite dextrorphan (approximately 45% of the dose) in a 24-hour urine sample.[25] Similar data were obtained by other investigators, and dextrorphan and additional *N*- or *N,O*-demethylated dextromethorphan metabolites have been described in human urine specimens.[26] The *O*-demethylated metabolite, dextrorphan, was found to be the major plasma constituent after oral dextromethorphan dosing.[22] In subsequent studies, pronounced hepatic first-pass metabolism of dextromethorphan[1,2,6] as well as unexplained interindividual differences of dextrorphan formation[10] were noted.

The potential importance of dextromethorphan metabolism in pharmacogenetic investigations became apparent when 12 subjects from a study of dextromethorphan pharmacokinetics[21] became available for debrisoquin phenotyping. In that study[17] we showed that the dispositions of dextromethorphan and debrisoquin are closely related and—by inference—hereditary factors are among the primary determinants of dextromethorphan metabolism. In six subjects of the same study, there was a highly significant correlation ($r_s = 0.94$; $P < 0.001$) between the urinary metabolic ratios of debrisoquin and the plasma $t_{1/2}$ values of dextromethorphan (ranging from 8 to 50 hours). This indicates that genetically controlled *O*-demethylation is also the main determinant of dextromethorphan pharmacoki-

Table II. Dextromethorphan and dextrorphan analysis in urine samples from PMs and EMs (population study) and from 37 known heterozygous genotypes of 14 family studies

	n	*Age (yr)*	*Dextromethorphan output (μmol/8 hr)*	*Dextrorphan output (μmol/8 hr)*	*Metabolic ratio*
PMs	23	33 ± 11	2.4 ± 1.5	1.2 ± 0.91	3.6 ± 3.8
EMs	245	34 ± 12	0.27 ± 0.36	35 ± 9.3	0.010 ± 0.022
Heterozygous genotypes	37	34 ± 20	0.39 ± 0.57*	32 ± 11*	0.014 ± 0.021*

Data are $\overline{X}$ ± SD.
*Significantly different (P < 0.0001) from PMs.

netics in man. Finally, the mephenytoin hydroxylation phenotypes were also determined and there was no indication for co-inheritance between mephenytoin and dextromethorphan metabolism in man.[16] From these data we concluded that dextromethorphan might be a new and specific drug candidate to assess genetic differences of the debrisoquin-type oxidative drug metabolism in man because it meets some essential prerequisites for a phenotype test drug, namely specificity, general availability, and innocuousness. Herein we tested the hypothesis that dextromethorphan might represent an alternative candidate for assigning the debrisoquin drug hydroxylation phenotype in normal subjects.

At the administered dextromethorphan dose of 20 mg po, this phenotype test drug was well tolerated in over 400 subjects. The validation of the experimental procedures was presented in a recent article[16] with respect to the dose dependency of dextromethorphan metabolism, duration of the urine collection period, and the pH dependency of dextromethorphan metabolic ratios. In our experimental protocol, a biologic repeatability of 94% could be reported for the dextromethorphan metabolic ratio.[16]

The bimodality of dextromethorphan metabolism could be established by use of the 8-hour urinary dextrorphan elimination as well as by the urinary dextromethorphan metabolic ratio (Fig. 1). In EMs, 50% of the administered dose can be recovered in urine after 8 hours in form of the *O*-demethylated metabolite dextrorphan, whereas in PMs only a total of 5% of the drug dose is eliminated. This 5% includes unchanged dextromethorphan, which accounts for more than two thirds of urinary drug elimination in PMs (Table I).

The consecutive administration of dextromethorphan and debrisoquin to a panel of EMs or PMs resulted in a clear bimodal distribution of the respective metabolic ratios in both studies (Fig. 3). When the antimodes of 0.3 for dextromethorphan and 12.6 for debrisoquin[15,24] are superposed on Fig. 3, the separation between the two drug hydroxylation phenotypes is clear. This approach was also used in family studies, in which the metabolic ratios of dextromethorphan and debrisoquin (Fig. 2) result in the same phenotypic and genotypic assignments for the various members of the family irrespective of the phenotype test drug used. The mutual genetic basis of dextromethorphan *O*-demethylation deficiency and debrisoquin 4-hydroxylation defect is further supported by the almost identical prevalence of the PM phenotypes in two separate studies, this one with dextromethorphan (8.6%; n = 268) and the other one with debrisoquin (9.9%; n = 221) as the test compound.[15]

In the family studies, special attention was given to the analysis of heterozygous phenotypes because a trimodality of dextromethorphan metabolism was suspected.[21] The hypothesis that heterozygous phenotypes might be identified without pedigree analysis was therefore pursued. However, as shown in Table II, the heterozygous EMs are not distinguishable from randomly selected EM phenotypes, at least by the currently used dextromethorphan test procedure. It must be noted, however, that the original hypothesis was based on dextromethorphan and dextrorphan concentrations in plasma. Under these conditions, a higher resolving power for interindividual differences might be anticipated, and the question of identifying heterozygous phenotypes with dextromethorphan as test compound awaits further clarification in a more elaborated experimental protocol.

In a separate investigation we used a syrup containing a comparable amount of dextromethorphan in combination with dexpanthenol and ammonium chloride, and found that this particular combination was also suitable for phenotyping. In addition, we tested four other commercial preparations containing dextromethorphan in combination with a nasal decongestant (pseudoephedrine), an antihistamine (mepyramine, chlorpheniramine), an expectorant (guaifenesin), an analgesic (acetaminophen), and ethanol in two EMs and two PMs to confirm the suitability of various drug combinations for the dextromethorphan phenotyping procedure. Thus for practical purposes, the dextromethorphan phenotyping protocol is the same for debrisoquin and dextromethorphan, except that the analysis of dextromethorphan and dextrorphan is faster and simpler than that for debrisoquin. A method for dextromethorphan and dextrorphan HPLC analysis has recently been published,[20] and the availability of several analytic methods in combination with the safety and general availability of dextromethorphan render this drug attractive for worldwide pharmacogenetic investigations.

We thank B. Flury, Ph.D., of the University of Berne for his expert advice with respect to population statistics and density function analysis.

References

1. Barnhart JW: The urinary excretion of dextromethorphan and three metabolites in dogs and humans. Toxicol Appl Pharmacol **55:**43-48, 1980.
2. Barnhart JW, Massad EN: Determination of dextromethorphan in serum by gas chromatography. J Chromatogr **163:**390-395, 1979.
3. Benson WM, Stefko PL, Randall LO: Comparative pharmacology of levorphan, racemorphan and dextrorphan and related methyl ethers. J Pharmacol Exp Ther **109:**189-200, 1953.
4. Cass LJ, Frederik WS: Evaluation of a new antitussive agent. N Engl J Med **249:**132-136, 1953.
5. Dayer P, Kubli A, Küpfer A, Courvoisier F, Balant L, Fabre J: Defective hydroxylation of bufuralol associated with side-effects of the drug in poor metabolisers. Br J Clin Pharmacol **13:**750-751, 1982.
6. Dixon R, Carbone JJ, Mohacsi E, Perry C: Dextromethorphan: Radioimmunoassay and pharmacokinetics in the dog. Res Commun Chem Pathol Pharmacol **22:**243-255, 1978.
7. Eichelbaum M: Defective oxidation of drugs: Pharmacokinetic and therapeutic implications. Clin Pharmacokinet **7:**1-22, 1982.
8. Eichelbaum M, Spannbrucker N, Steincke B, Dengler JH: Defective N-oxydation of sparteine in man: A new pharmacogenetic defect. Eur J Clin Pharmacol **16:**183-187, 1979.
9. Flury B, Riedwyl H: Angewandte multivariate Statistik. Stuttgart, 1983, G. Fischer Verlag.
10. Hinsvark ON, O'Brien J, Zazulak W, Amsel L, Giering JE: Drug analysis: Dextromethorphan, its disposition and determination. Pittsburg Conference on Analytical Chemistry and Applied Spectroscopy **9:**333, 1981.
11. Idle JR, Mahgoub A, Lancaster R, Smith RL: Hypotonic response to debrisoquine and hydroxylator phenotype. Life Sci **22:**979-984, 1978.
12. Isbell H, Fraser HF: Actions and addiction liabilities of dromoran derivatives in man. J Pharmacol Exp Ther **107:**524-530, 1953.
13. Islam SI, Idle JR, Smith RL: The polymorphic 4-hydroxylation of debrisoquine in a Saudi Arab population. Xenobiotica **10:**819-825, 1980.
14. Küpfer A, Preisig R: Inherited defects of hepatic drug metabolism. Semin Liv Dis **3:**341-354, 1983.
15. Küpfer A, Preisig R: Pharmacogenetics of mephenytoin: A new drug hydroxylation polymorphism in man. Eur J Clin Pharmacol **26:**753-759, 1984.
16. Küpfer A, Schmid B, Pfaff G: Pharmacogenetics of dextromethorphan O-demethylation in man. Xenobiotica. (In press.)
17. Küpfer A, Schmid B, Preisig R, Pfaff G: Dextromethorphan as a safe probe for debrisoquine hydroxylation polymorphism. Lancet **2:**517-518, 1984.
18. Lennard MS, Silas JH, Smith AJ, Tucker GT: Determination of debrisoquine and its 4-hydroxy metabolite in biological fluids by gas-chromatography with flame-ionization and nitrogen-selective detection. J Chromatogr **133:**161-166, 1977.
19. Mahgoub A, Idle JR, Dring LG, Lancaster R, Smith RL: Polymorphic hydroxylation of debrisoquine in man. Lancet **2:**584-586, 1977.
20. Park YH, Kullberg MP, Hinsvark ON: Quantitative determination of dextromethorphan and three metabolites in urine by reverse-phase high performance liquid chromatography. J Pharm Sci **73:**24-29, 1984.
21. Pfaff G, Briegel P, Lamprecht I: Inter-individual variation in the metabolism of dextromethorphan. Int J Pharm **14:**173-189, 1983.
22. Ramachander G, Williams FD, Emele JF: Determination of dextrorphan in plasma and evaluation of bioavailability of dextromethorphan hydrobromide in humans. J Pharm Sci **66:**1047-1048, 1977.
23. Riedwyl H: Angewandte mathematische Statistik. Bern, 1978, P. Haupt Verlag.
24. Price Evans DA, Mahgoub A, Sloan TP, Idle JR, Smith RL: A family and population study of the genetic polymorphism of debrisoquine oxidation in a white British population. J Med Genet **17:**102-105, 1980.
25. Versie R, Norfalaise A, Neven M, Malchair R: Toxicité et métabolisme du 3-méthoxy-N-methylmorphinane (Romilar) chez l'enfant. Ann Med Leg Criminol Police Sci **42:**561-565, 1962.
26. Willner K: Ausscheidung und Abbau von (+)-3-Methoxy-N-Methylmorphinan und seinen entmethylierten Derivaten beim Menschen. Drug Res **13:**26-29, 1963.

Effect of tolrestat on red blood cell sorbitol levels in patients with diabetes

The effect of the aldose reductase inhibitor, tolrestat, on red blood cell (RBC) sorbitol levels was studied in 23 patients with diabetes after oral dosing with tolrestat, 25 or 100 mg b.i.d. The mean (±SE) RBC sorbitol levels (measured 12 hours after the preceding dose) after 3, 7, and 13 days of dosing decreased after both dose levels. After 25 mg tolrestat the RBC sorbitol levels fell from 25.1 ± 4.0 to 20.0 ± 5.7 nmol/gm hemoglobin (21%) and after 100 mg tolrestat the level fell from 26.7 ± 3.7 to 11.4 ± 1.7 nmol/gm hemoglobin (57%; $P < 0.001$). This latter RBC sorbitol concentration is similar to levels in individuals without diabetes. At both dosage levels the maximum decrease in RBC sorbitol levels occurred after only 3 days of dosing. Tolrestat had no effect on plasma glucose or hemoglobin A_1 concentrations. The overall mean plasma unbound drug concentration measured 12 hours after 100 mg tolrestat (11.7 ± 3.0 ng/ml; 3.3×10^{-8} mol/L) was similar to the median inhibitory level (3×10^{-8} mol/L) of tolrestat for sorbitol accumulation in human RBCs incubated in a high-glucose medium. Our results demonstrate the systemic bioavailability of tolrestat and its aldose reductase inhibitory activity in erythrocytes of patients with diabetes. (Clin Pharmacol Ther 38:625-630, 1985.)

Philip Raskin, M.D., Julio Rosenstock, M.D., Patricia Challis, R.N., Steven Ryder, M.D., John F. Mullane, M.D., Ramona Gonzalez, Ph.D., David Hicks, Ph.D., Theodore Smith, Ph.D., and Dushan Dvornik, D.Sc.
Dallas, Tex., Princeton, N. J., and New York, N. Y.

The interest in drugs that inhibit aldose reductase (AR) was prompted when a role for AR was established in the pathogenesis of sugar cataracts.[21] Even more interest has been generated after the demonstration that the increased AR activity in hyperglycemia may also be involved in the development of other complications of long-term diabetes such as neuropathy.[7,24] This evidence is based on results, albeit variable, obtained in patients with diabetes who receive therapy with the AR inhibitors alrestatin,[5,10,11,13] sorbinil,[18,22,23,38] or ONO-2235.[16] Tolrestat (*N*-[[6-methoxy-5-(trifluoromethyl)-1-naphthalenyl]thioxomethyl]-*N*-methylglycine; AY-27,773) is a potent, structurally distinct AR inhibitor.[8,32] Pharmacokinetic studies in laboratory animals[2] and in man[15] have shown that tolrestat is well absorbed; has a serum $t_{1/2}$ ranging from 3 to 4 hours in mice, rats, and rabbits, 9 hours in monkeys, 11 hours in dogs, and 10 to 13 hours in patients with or without diabetes; and does not accumulate in the body.

In human red blood cells (RBCs), sorbitol is produced from glucose by the action of the enzyme AR.[3,27] The concentration of sorbitol in RBCs is related to the ambient plasma glucose concentration, which is always higher in patients with diabetes than in those without and thus cause elevated RBC sorbitol levels in patients with diabetes.[3,6,26,27,29,34] We describe the effectiveness of tolrestat in normalizing RBC sorbitol levels in patients with diabetes.

From the Department of Internal Medicine, The University of Texas Health Science Center at Dallas, Dallas, and Departments of Biochemistry and Clinical Research, Ayerst Laboratories, Princeton and New York.

Supported in part by National Institutes of Health Grant No. 5-MOI-RR00633 and by a grant from Ayerst Laboratories.

Presented in part at the United States–Japan Aldose Reductase Workshop, Honolulu, Hawaii, Nov. 28, 1984, and at the Forty-fifth Annual Meeting of The American Diabetes Association, Baltimore, Md., June 1985.

Received for publication May 8, 1985; accepted Aug. 6, 1985.

Reprint requests to: Philip Raskin, M.D., University of Texas Health Science Center at Dallas, 5323 Harry Hines Blvd., Dallas, TX 75235.

METHODS

Twenty-three patients (22 men and one woman) with stable insulin-dependent (n = 19) or noninsulin-dependent (n = 4) diabetes mellitus were studied. All had had diabetes for >4 months. Mean (±SD) age was 37.3 ± 12.4 years and mean weight was 72.7 ± 9.3 kg. All gave written informed consent before participation in the study. Except for required insulin or oral hypoglycemic drugs, patients did not receive any other medication, although occasional use of nonprescription

Table I. Plasma glucose and HbA_1 concentrations during tolrestat and placebo dosing

	Glucose (mg/dl)		*HbA_1 (%)*	
	Baseline	*Treatment*	*Baseline*	*Treatment*
Placebo (group I)	183 ± 20	213 ± 19	8.5 ± 0.5	8.6 ± 0.6
Tolrestat, 25 mg b.i.d. (group II)	192 ± 24	199 ± 36	8.5 ± 0.5	8.1 ± 0.6
Tolrestat, 100 mg b.i.d. (group III)	177 ± 25	177 ± 31	9.0 ± 0.7	8.4 ± 0.5

Data are $\overline{X}$ ± SE.

Table II. Plasma RBC sorbitol concentrations during tolrestat and placebo dosing

	RBC sorbitol (nmol/gm hemoglobin)		
		Tolrestat	
	Placebo (n = 8)	*25 mg b.i.d. (n = 8)*	*100 mg b.i.d. (n = 7)*
Baseline	23.1 ± 4.9	25.1 ± 4.0	26.7 ± 3.7
Treatment			
Day 3	23.2 ± 3.2	13.7 ± 4.3*	11.0 ± 1.8†
Day 7	24.5 ± 4.3	17.4 ± 4.2	10.3 ± 2.2
Day 13	28.9 ± 6.6	22.1 ± 8.2	12.2 ± 2.7*
Mean absolute 2-wk value	25.5 ± 4.0	20.0 ± 5.7	11.4 ± 1.7
Within-group comparison with baseline	P = 0.385	P = 0.091	P = 0.001
Change of baseline (%)‡	20.4 ± 13.8	−25.8 ± 11.3	−57.5 ± 3.2
Within-group comparison with baseline	P = 0.093	P = 0.042	P = 0.0015

Data are $\overline{X}$ ± SE.
*n = 5.
†n = 6.
‡Mean individual percentage change from baseline value.

drugs was permitted. All patients were studied in the General Clinical Research Unit of the University of Texas Health Science Center at Dallas. This was a single-center, double-masked, placebo-controlled, outpatient study with three parallel treatment groups. Before entry into the trial the patients were screened to identify those with elevated fasting RBC sorbitol concentrations. Blood samples for RBC sorbitol levels were drawn on 2 separate days and measurement of the fasting plasma glucose level and a glycosylated hemoglobin (HbA_1) measurement were also made. Patients were then randomly assigned to one of the three study groups for the duration of the 21-day study. During days 1 to 7, all patients received placebo; during days 8 to 21, patients in group I continued to receive placebo, while patients in groups II and III received tolrestat, 25 or 100 mg b.i.d., at 12-hour intervals, respectively. Each dosage form was taken by mouth 0.5 hours before breakfast and supper. All patients were examined on days 1, 8, 11, 15, and 21. Blood was drawn after an overnight fast but before the first daily drug dose (i.e., about 12 hours after the preceding dose) for the determination of glucose, HbA_1, RBC sorbitol, and tolrestat concentrations. For measurement of RBC sorbitol levels, the blood sample was drawn into a tube containing EDTA and was kept on ice. Two milliliters of blood was pipetted into a tube and centrifuged at 1500 rpm for 10 minutes at 4° C. The plasma was separated and the RBCs were frozen at −20° C until the samples were analyzed.

RBC sorbitol concentrations were determined by gas chromatography with flame ionization detection of the butylboronate derivative of sorbitol.[9,31] L-Iditol, used as internal standard, was prepared by borohydride reduction of L-sorbose[1] and was purified through its hexaacetyl derivative. After the addition of iditol (5 μg) the RBCs were thawed, and to eliminate glucose the samples were incubated with glucose oxidase solution (10 μg/ml; Sigma Type VII). The reaction was stopped with 0.5 ml trichloroacetic acid solution (50% w/v). Samples were centrifuged and the aqueous supernatant was washed twice with ether and then lyophilized. The residue was allowed to react for 20 minutes at room temperature with *n*-butyl boronic acid solution (0.2 ml; 50

mg/ml pyridine), dried, extracted with toluene, and washed with $CuSO_4$ solution and water. After evaporation, the residue was dissolved in 50 μl toluene and 5 μl was injected onto a 6 ft, 2 mm id coiled glass column packed with 3% OV-17 coated on a gas-chrom Q, 80-100 mesh (Applied Science Laboratories) in a Hewlett-Packard instrument (Series 5790) equipped with a Canlab recorder. Column, injector, and detector temperatures were 200°, 260°, and 350° C, respectively; the carrier gas was helium (22 ml/min); and the air and hydrogen flow rates to the detector were 220 and 40 ml/min, respectively. Linear calibration curves were obtained with the standards ($y = 0.227x - 0.011$; $r = 0.998$) and extracts of rat RBCs with added sorbitol ($y = 0.195x + 0.453$; $r = 0.996$). Because of incomplete relative recovery of sorbitol in RBC extracts as compared with pure standards, quantitation was done with extracts of normal rat RBCs with added sorbitol (5 μg) carried through the method with each set of samples (after correction for endogenous sorbitol). The mean (±SD) peak height ratio of sorbitol vs. iditol was 0.961 ± 0.019 (5 μg of each standard, on 11 different days, n = 3 for each day), and the coefficient of variation was 6.4%. RBCs were not washed because of the potential variation in sorbitol levels due to loss of cell lysis. The possibility of contamination of the RBCs with the sorbitol from the plasma is very small. Sorbitol levels in the plasma of normal subjects are about five times lower than those in RBCs[28] and they do not increase in with hyperglycemia.[17] Sorbitol concentrations in RBCs were expressed as nanomoles per gram of hemoglobin after correction in each patient for the mean hemoglobin concentration determined during the preselection and study periods. The assay has a limit of detection of 3 nmol/gm hemoglobin based on RBCs from 2 ml blood.

Tolrestat plasma concentrations were determined by HPLC[14] with a limit of detection of 0.1 μg/ml, based on 1 ml plasma.

HbA_1 was determined by ion exchange chromatography on thrice-washed RBCs after overnight incubation at 23° C to remove the labile fraction.

Results are expressed as the $\bar{X}$ ± SE. Between-group comparisons were made by a one-way ANOVA followed by the least significant difference method of multiple comparison. The comparison between the 25 and 100 mg tolrestat groups was two tailed, and their comparison with the placebo group was one tailed. Within-group comparison of absolute changes was by Student's t test for paired data. Within-group comparison of percentage changes in RBC sorbitol concentrations was based on a one sample Student's t test. All comparisons were made with $\alpha = 0.05$.[33]

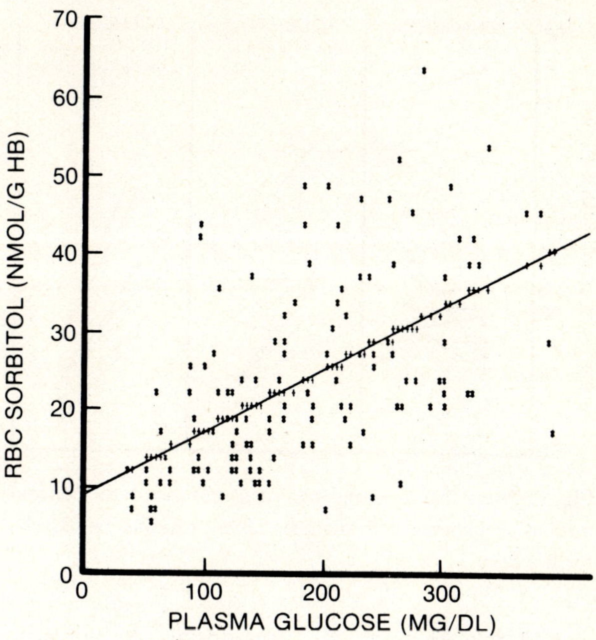

Fig. 1. Correlation of RBC sorbitol and plasma glucose concentrations in patients with diabetes during the preselection and placebo periods.

RESULTS

The study was completed with eight subjects each in groups I and II and with seven subjects in group III.

In none of the subjects was the mean plasma glucose concentration in the preselection and the placebo periods significantly different. Therefore, all plasma glucose concentrations determined before drug dosing were averaged to obtain the individual baseline values. As shown in Table I, the values for glucose and HbA_1 among the baseline and treatment periods for all groups were identical.

With respect to RBC sorbitol levels, because the mean concentrations in the placebo period were also not significantly different from those in the preselection period, all individual values obtained before tolrestat dosing (n = 5 to 8) were averaged to obtain the baseline value for each patient. The correlation between the plasma glucose concentration and baseline RBC sorbitol level is statistically significant ($r = 0.548$; $P < 0.0001$; $n = 159$; Fig. 1). A similar relationship has been reported in children[26] and adults[6,36] with diabetes.

The effect of tolrestat on RBC sorbitol levels was measured 12 hours after the preceding dose after 3, 7,

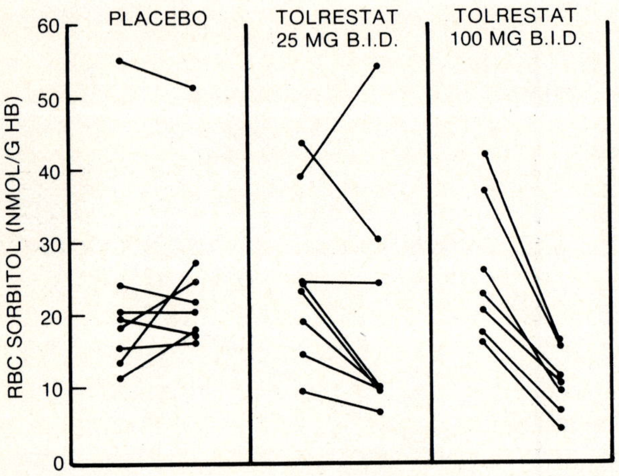

Fig. 2. Mean baseline and treatment RBC sorbitol concentrations in patients with diabetes taking tolrestat or placebo for 2 weeks.

and 13 days of twice-daily drug dosing. As shown in Table II, the maximal decrease in RBC sorbitol levels occurred at both dosages after 3 days of dosing. Values on those days were therefore averaged to obtain a mean value for the 2-week treatment period. Within-group comparison of the sorbitol concentrations indicates that the difference between baseline and the mean 2-week value is statistically significant for the 100 mg group ($P = 0.001$). The mean changes from baseline for the 25 and 100 mg groups ($P = 0.015$) and the 100 mg and placebo groups ($P = 0.0001$) also differed.

There was a relatively high variation in baseline RBC sorbitol levels in these patients, which resulted in varying absolute changes in RBC sorbitol levels. In view of these variations, we have also calculated the means of the individual percentage changes between the baseline and treatment RBC sorbitol concentrations. Within-group comparisons of mean individual percentage change from baseline were significant for both the 25 mg ($P = 0.042$) and 100 mg ($P = 0.0015$) groups. In addition, the differences between the mean individual percentage change from baseline are significant for the 25 mg ($P = 0.006$) and the 100 mg ($P < 0.0001$) group as compared with the placebo group, but not for the 25 mg vs. 100 mg group.

Tolrestat, 100 mg b.i.d., decreased the elevated RBC sorbitol level in all patients who received this dose, and at a dose of 25 mg the decrease occurred in six of eight subjects (Fig. 2). It is pertinent that one patient in the 25 mg tolrestat group with increased RBC sorbitol levesl (39%) had barely detectable tolrestat concentrations in the plasma at the time of RBC sobitol determination, suggesting that this patient failed to take the study drug.

Table III. Plasma tolrestat concentrations

	Tolrestat concentration (μg/ml)	
Day	*25 mg b.i.d.*	*100 mg b.i.d.*
0	ND	0.03 ± 0.02
3	0.48 ± 0.06	2.97 ± 1.00
7	0.44 ± 0.10	2.07 ± 0.15
13	0.40 ± 0.10	2.12 ± 0.34
Average	0.41 ± 0.07	2.43 ± 0.41

Data are $\bar{X}$ ± SE.
ND = Not detectable.

The mean plasma tolrestat concentrations measured 12 hours after the preceding dose after 3, 7, and 13 days of tolrestat dosing (Table III) indicate that steady state was attained by day 3. Theoretically,[12] based on a tolrestat $t_{1/2}$ of 10 to 13 hours;[15] and twice-daily dosing at 12-hour intervals, steady-state pharmacokinetics should have been attained after five to seven doses of tolrestat.

DISCUSSION

The mean fasting RBC sorbitol level of 24.9 ± 2.4 nmol/gm hemoglobin we found in these patients with diabetes is similar to reported values.[20,22,26,27] In accord with earlier reports,[6,26,36] the relationship between the fasting plasma glucose concentrations and the RBC sorbitol levels ($r = 0.548$) we measured during the preselection and placebo periods is statistically highly significant ($P < 0.0001$).

After 3 days of dosing, i.e., at a time when a pharmacokinetic steady state of tolrestat had been attained, tolrestat decreased the elevated RBC sorbitol level in each of the seven patients with diabetes who received tolrestat, 100 mg b.i.d. The amount of the decrease ranged from 43% to 72% (mean 59%), and the mean RBC sorbitol level decreased from 26.7 ± 3.7 to 11.0 ± 1.8 nmol/gm hemoglobin. It is important to note that, during the 2 weeks of dosing, tolrestat lowered the elevated RBC sorbitol levels to 11.0 ± 1.8 nmol/gm hemoglobin, a value comparable with that found in patients without diabetes (10 ± 1 nmol/gm hemoglobin).[25,26]

In those patients who took tolrestat, 25 mg b.i.d., the elevated RBC sorbitol levels were also decreased (16% to 58%) in four of five patients after 3 days of dosing, in seven of eight patients (20% to 66%) after 7 days of dosing, and in six of eight patients (25% to 59%) after 13 days of dosing. Because of the marked variation of baseline RBC sorbitol concentrations in three of these patients, the difference between the overall mean RBC level after 2 weeks of dosing and the predosing levels was not significant. The mean of the individual percentage changes from pretreatment (26%), however, does differ (P = 0.042).

The rapid response of RBC sorbitol to changes in plasma glucose concentration[17,34] and the relatively rapid fall of elevated RBC sorbitol levels induced by tolrestat indicate rapid uptake of glucose and tolrestat by the RBC.

The overall mean decrease in RBC sorbitol content of 58% found at steady state 12 hours after the preceding dose of 100 mg tolrestat was associated with an overall mean plasma tolrestat concentration of 2.43 ± 0.41 μg/ml. Based on a free fraction of 0.48%,[15] this corresponds to an unbound tolrestat concentration of 11.7 ± 3.0 ng/ml or 3.3×10^{-8} mol/L, a value similar to the median inhibitory level of 3×10^{-8} mol/L tolrestat for RBC sorbitol accumulation in human RBCs incubated in a glucose-rich medium.[8]

The fact that during the course of the study there were no changes observed in either fasting plasma glucose or HbA_1 levels suggests that the fall in RBC sorbitol content observed in the patients with diabetes who received tolrestat was due to inhibition of the conversion of glucose to sorbitol in the RBC. The evidence that accumulation of sorbitol in the RBC of patients with diabetes was controlled by three distinct AR inhibitors[16,20,22,27,37] supports the postulate that the sorbitol in human RBCs is formed by the action of AR.[27,35]

It is of interest that in the study of Malone et al.[27] in patients with diabetes, a significant reduction in RBC sorbitol levels was achieved with a 250 mg daily dose of sorbinil. In that study, the authors were able to show an 80% to 90% reduction in tissue sorbitol levels at a dose of 5 mg/kg in diabetic rats. In these diabetic animals RBC sorbitol levels correlated well with sorbitol level in lens and sciatic nerve. Others[30] have shown a significant decrease in RBC sorbitol levels in patients with diabetes after 200 mg[30] and even 100 mg[20] daily doses of sorbinil. Finally, Hotta et al.[16] reported a significant decrease in RBC sorbitol levels in patients with diabetes with clinical neuropathy after a 300 mg daily dose of ONO-2235. Certainly the most effective dose of tolrestat (200 mg/day) is in the same range as that of these other AR agents. In fact, because some effect on RBC sorbitol was seen at a dose of 50 mg/day, tolrestat may be slightly more potent.

Our results with tolrestat demonstrate the usefulness of monitoring RBC sorbitol levels in patients with diabetes who receive an AR inhibitor to establish systemic availability and AR inhibitory activity. Whether changes in the RBC sorbitol level reflect AR activity in other tissues that do not require insulin for glucose uptake is not clear. The pharmacodynamics of the response of the inhibitors of the AR enzyme in a given tissue depends on the intracellular interplay of several variables, such as rate of glucose uptake, rates of uptake and elimination of the AR inhibitor, and the rate of sorbitol elimination. Therefore, the pharmacodynamics of response to an AR inhibitor may not necessarily be the same in all tissue.[4,19]

The tolrestat and the placebo capsules were prepared by the Ayerst Clinical Supply Group, Rouses Point, N. Y. We thank Micheline Cartier, Nicole Marcouiller, Robert Piscina, Maria Foglio, and Diane Sawicki for their excellent technical assistance; Mrs. Bette Newton for secretarial assistance; and the staff and nurses of the General Clinical Research Unit.

References

1. Abel-Akher M, Hamilton JK, Smith F: The reduction of sugars with sodium borohydride. J Am Chem Soc **73:**4691, 1951.
2. Cayen MN, Hicks DR, Ferdinandi ES, Kraml M, Greselin E, Dvornik D: Metabolic disposition and pharmacokinetics of the aldose reductase inhibitor tolrestat in rats, dogs and monkeys. Drug Metab Dispos **13:**412-419, 1985.
3. Crabbe MJC, Basak Halder A: Affinity chromatography of bovine lens aldose reductase, and a comparison of some kinetic properties of the enzyme from lens and human erythrocyte. Biochem Soc Trans **8:**194-195, 1980.
4. Crabbe MJC, Bron AJ, Peckar CO, Petchey M, Ting H, Howard-Williams J: NADPH-oxidising activity in lens and erythrocytes in diabetic and nondiabetic patients with cataract. Br J Ophthalmol **67:**696-699, 1983.
5. Culebras A, Alio J, Herrera JL, Lopex-Fraile IP: Effect of an aldose reductase inhibitor on diabetic peripheral neuropathy. Arch Neurol **38:**133-134, 1981.
6. De Leeuw I, Vertommen J, De Winter P, Van Roelen W, Van Gaal L: Red blood sorbitol levels in normals and diabetics. Diabetologia **21:**263, 1981.
7. Dvornik D: Chronic complications of diabetes. *In* Hess HJ, editor: Annual reports in medicinal chemistry. New York, 1978, Academic Press, pp 159-166.
8. Dvornik D, Simard-Duquesne N, Greselin E, Dubuc J, Kraml M: AY-27,773: A novel orally active inhibitor of aldose reductase. Diabetes **32**(suppl 1):164A, 1983.
9. Eisenberg JRF: Cyclic butane boronic acid esters: Novel derivatives for the rapid separation of carbohydrates by gas. Carb Res **19:**135-139, 1971.
10. Fagius J, Jameson S: Effect of aldose reductase inhibitor treatment in diabetic polyneuropathy—A clinical neurophysiological study. J Neurosurg Psychiatry **44:**991-1001, 1981.
11. Gabbay KH, Spack N, Loo S, Hirsch H, Ackil AA: Aldose reductase inhibition: Studies in alrestatin. Metabolism **28**(suppl 1):471-476, 1979.

12. Gibaldi M, Perrier D: Pharmacokinetics, ed. 2. New York, 1982, Marcel Dekker Inc, p 124.
13. Handelsman DJ, Turtle JR: Clinical trial of an aldose reductase inhibitor in diabetic neuropathy. Diabetes **30:**459-464, 1981.
14. Hicks DR, Kraml M: Determination of tolrestat in serum and tissues. Ther Drug Monit **6:**328-333, 1984.
15. Hicks DR, Kraml M, Cayen MN, Dubuc J, Ryder S, Dvornik D: Tolrestat kinetics. CLIN PHARMACOL THER **36:**493-499, 1984.
16. Hotta N, Kakuta H, Kimura M, Fukasawa H, Koh N, Terashima H, Iida M, Sakamoto N: Experimental and clinical trial of aldose reductase inhibitor in diabetic neuropathy. Diabetes **32**(suppl 1):98A, 1983.
17. Hubinot C, Sener A, Malaisse WJ: Sorbitol content of plasma and erythrocytes during induced short-term hyperglycemia. Clin Biochem **14:**19-20, 1981.
18. Jaspan J, Maselli R, Herold K, Bartkus C: Treatment of severely painful diabetic neuropathy with an aldose reductase inhibitor: Relief of pain and improved somatic and autonomic nerve function. Lancet **2:**758-762, 1983.
19. Kikkawa R, Hatanaka I, Yasuda H, Kobayashi N, Shigeta Y, Terashima H, Morimura T, Tsuboshima M: Effect of a new aldose reductase inhibitor, *(E)*-3-carboxymethyl-5-[(2*E*)-methyl-3-phenylpropenylidene]rhodanine (ONO-2235) on peripheral nerve disorders in streptozotocin-diabetic rats. Diabetologia **24:**290-292, 1983.
20. Kilpelainen H, Puhakainen E, Saamanen AM, Lehtinen J, Riekkinen PJ: The effect of aldose reductase inhibitor (sorbinil®) on erythrocyte sorbitol concentration in diabetic neuropathy. J Neurochem **41:**S27, 1983.
21. Kinoshita JH: Mechanisms initiating cataract formation. Invest Ophthalmol **13:**713-724, 1974.
22. Lehtinen JM, Hyvonen SR, Uusitupa M, Puhakainen E: The effect of an aldose reductase inhibitor (sorbinil) on diabetic neuropathy. Diabetologia **27:**303A, 1984.
23. Lewin IG, O'Brien IAD, Morgan MH, Corrall RJM: Clinical and neurophysiological studies with the aldose reductase inhibitor, sorbinil, in symptomatic diabetic neuropathy. Diabetologia **26:**445-448, 1984.
24. Lipinski CA, Hutson NJ: Aldose reductase inhibitors as a new approach to the treatment of diabetic complications. *In* Baily DM, editor: Annual reports in medicinal chemistry. New York, 1984, Academic Press, pp 169-177.
25. Malone JI, Harvey RC, Putnam JC: Sorbitol, inositol and phosphatidylinositol (PI) elevated in diabetic red cells. The influence of sorbinil. Diabetes **32**(suppl 1):161A, 1983.
26. Malone JI, Knox G, Benford S, Tedesco TA: Red cell sorbitol: An indicator of diabetic control. Diabetes **29:**861-865, 1980.
27. Malone JI, Leavengood H, Peterson MJ, O'Brien MM, Page MG, Aldinger CE: Red blood cell sorbitol as an indicator of polyol pathway activity. Inhibition of sorbinil in insulin-dependent subjects. Diabetes **33:**45-49, 1984.
28. Morrison AD, Clements RS, Travis SB, Oski F, Winegrad AI: glucose utilization by the polyol pathway in human erythrocytes. Biochem Biophys Res Comm **40:**199-205, 1970.
29. Popp-Snijders C, Lomecky M, De Jong AP: Determination of sorbitol in erythrocytes of diabetic and healthy subjects by capillary gas chromatography. Clin Chim Acta **132:**83-89, 1983.
30. Popp-Snijders, Lomecky-Janousek MZ, Schouten JA, van der Veen EA: Myo-inositol and sorbitol in erythrocytes from diabetic patients before and after sorbinil treatment. Diabetologia **27:**514-516, 1984.
31. Rabinowitz MP, Reisberg P, Brodin J: GLC assay of sorbitol as cyclic n-butyl boronate. J Pharm Sci **63:**1601-1604, 1974.
32. Sestanj K, Bellini F, Fung S, Abraham M, Treasurywala A, Humber L, Simard-Duquesne N, Dvornik D: N-[[5-trifluoromethyl)-6-methoxy-1-naphthalenyl]thioxomethyl]N-methylglycine (Tolrestat) a potent orally active aldose reductase inhibitor. J Med Chem **27:**255-256, 1984.
33. Snedecor GW, Cochran WG: Statistical methods, ed 7. Ames, Iowa, 1980, Iowa State University Press, pp 83-102.
34. Somers G, Depoorter I, Sener A, Macaisse WJ: Sorbitol concentration in the plasma and erythrocytes of diabetic subjects. Diabetes Care **5:**319-321, 1982.
35. Travis SF, Morrison AD, Clements RS, Winegrad AI, Oski FA: Metabolic alterations in the human erythrocytes produced by increases in glucose concentration. J Clin Invest **50:**2104-2112, 1971.
36. Vertommen J, De Leeuw I, Rillaerts E, Gijsels M, Bekaert J: Discrepancy between insulin-dependent and non-insulin dependent diabetes in the interrelationship between red-blood-cell sorbitol and glycaemia. Diabetologia **27:**343A, 1984.
37. Wright J, Collier J, Stevenson P, English J, Passas R, Marks U: Sorbinil lowers erythrocyte sorbitol concentration in diabetes. Clin Sci **66:**44P, 1984.
38. Young RJ, Ewing DJ, Clark BF: A controlled trial of sorbinil, an aldose reductase inhibitor, in chronic painful diabetic neuropathy. Diabetes **32:**938-942, 1983.

Epidural and intrathecal opiates: Cerebrospinal fluid and plasma profiles in patients with chronic cancer pain

We studied the cerebrospinal fluid (CSF) and plasma concentration-time profiles of morphine, methadone, and β-endorphin after lumbar epidural or intrathecal injection in 17 patients with cancer. After epidural injection, all three drugs reached peak levels in lumbar CSF within 34 minutes that were 50 to 1300 times higher than free drug concentrations in plasma. The rate of decline of CSF levels correlated with drug lipid solubility (methadone [$t_{1/2}$ = 73 minutes] > morphine [126 minutes] > β-endorphin [317 minutes]). Plasma levels were comparable with those after intragluteal injection of the same dose. In four patients given intrathecal morphine or methadone, CSF at the C_{1-2} level contained high levels of morphine as early as 1 hour after injection, but levels of methadone were lower or undetectable. Three of 17 patients reported improved analgesia initially, but none were improved at 2 weeks after chronic therapy. We conclude that analgesia induced by intrathecal or epidural morphine injections is caused by drug acting at both spinal and supraspinal sites. The use of spinal opiates such as morphine is of limited value in patients whose pain is not adequately managed by high systemic doses of morphine-like drugs. (Clin Pharmacol Ther 38:631-641, 1985.)

Mitchell B. Max, M.D.,* Charles E. Inturrisi, Ph.D., Robert F. Kaiko, Ph.D., Patricia Y. Grabinski, Ph.D., Choh Hao Li, Ph.D., and Kathleen M. Foley, M.D.
New York, N. Y., and San Francisco, Calif.

Opiates applied to the spinal cord of animals inhibit the discharge of nociceptive neurons and produce analgesia by interacting with populations of spinal opiate receptors.[24,60,61] These findings have suggested a clinical application: Selective spinal opiate analgesia with few side effects is achievable assuming (1) that the degree of analgesia that can be produced by opiates affecting only spinal sites is clinically significant, and (2) that the drug remains relatively well localized at the spinal level after epidural or intrathecal injection, with minimal redistribution to the brain stem and cerebral opiate receptors that mediate nausea, dysphoria, sedation, and respiratory depression.

Although spinal administration of a number of opiates has been reported to give prolonged analgesia in postoperative patients[3,10,13,25,26,42,43] and in patients with chronic pain,[7,8,30,53,55] neither of the above assumptions has been adequately tested because little is known about the rate and degree of redistribution of various spinal opiates to the brain stem. The brisk absorption of epidural morphine[36,56] and meperidine[17] into systemic circulation, for example, may contribute to analgesia. Furthermore, there is evidence for significant ascent of drug injected in the lumbar region to the brain stem via spinal cerebrospinal fluid (CSF) pathways. The evidence includes the occurrence of nausea and vomiting in 15% to 35%[44,59] and of diffuse itching in 4%[44] of patients receiving postoperative epidural morphine, occasional respiratory depression 30 minutes after epidural meperidine[16] and 3 to 16 hours after epidural or

From the Department of Neurology and Analgesic Study Section, Memorial Sloan-Kettering Cancer Center and Departments of Neurology and Pharmacology, Cornell University Medical College, New York, and Hormone Research Laboratory, University of California Medical Center, San Francisco.

Supported in part by grants from the National Institute on Drug Abuse (Nos. DA 01707 and 01457), from the National Cancer Institute (No. CA32897), and by a Core Grant (No. CA-08748) and a National Research Service Award (No. 5F32 CA06997-02) from the National Cancer Institute.

Received for publication April 9, 1985; accepted Aug. 8, 1985.

Reprint requests to: Dr. Kathleen M. Foley, Department of Neurology, Memorial Sloan-Kettering Cancer Center, 1275 York Ave., New York, NY 10021.

*Postdoctoral fellow of the American Cancer Society. Present address: NIDR/NIH Pain Research Facility, National Institute of Dental Research, Building 10, Room 3C-403, Bethesda, MD 20892.

Table I. Clinical characteristics and analgesic responses of patients receiving epidural opiates

Patient No.	*Sex*	*Age (yr)*	*Weight (kg)*	*Site of pain/tumor type*	*Previous systemic analgesic*	*Epidural opiate*	*Pain relief*
1	M	60	50	Perirectal infiltration, colon carcinoma	Levorphanol, 12 mg po q3h	Methadone, 10 mg	Slight (1.5 hr)
						β-Endorphin, 5 mg	None
						Morphine, 30 mg	A lot (4.5 hr)
2	M	68	80	Lumbar plexus infiltration, bladder carcinoma	Hydromorphone, 32 mg po q2h	β-Endorphin, 5 mg	Moderate (2 hr)
						Morphine, 5 mg, and methadone, 5 mg	Moderate (1.5 hr)
						Morphine, 30 mg	None
3	M	59	70	Femur metastasis, colon carcinoma	Hydromorphone, 4 mg im q3h	β-Endorphin 5 mg, morphine, 7.5 mg, and methadone, 7.5 mg	Moderate (8 hr)
						Morphine, 15 mg	None
4	M	50	40	T_{12} epidural metastasis, maxillary cylindroma	Morphine, 220 mg po q3h	β-Endorphin, 5 mg	None
						Methadone, 10 mg	Moderate (2 hr)
5	M	35	80	Osteoid osteoma	Meperidine, 100 mg po q6h	β-Endorphin, 5 mg, morphine, 2.5 mg, and methadone, 2.5 mg	Slight (2 hr)
6	M	48	65	T_7 paravertebral metastasis, lung carcinoma	Methadone, 20 mg po q3h	β-Endorphin, 5 mg, and morphine, 5 mg	Slight (1 hr)
						Morphine, 15 mg	None
7	M	64	55	L_3 epidural metastasis, prostatic carcinoma	Morphine, 10 mg im q2h	Morphine, 5 mg	A lot (4 hr)
						Morphine, 7.5 mg	A lot (4 hr)
8	M	63	65	Chordoma L_5-S_5	Levorphanol, 28 mg po q3h	Morphine, 45 mg	Moderate (3 hr)
						Morphine, 90 mg	None
9	M	74	75	Lumbar plexus infiltration, colon carcinoma	Oxycodone, 5 mg po q3h	Morphine, 5 mg	Moderate (35 hr)
						Methadone, 5 mg	Moderate (4 hr)
10	F	58	53	Diffuse pelvic metastasis, colon carcinoma	Methadone, 30 mg iv q3h	Morphine, 50 mg	Moderate (2 hr)
						Morphine, 50 mg	Slight (2 hr)
11	F	62	60	Lumbar plexus infiltration, cervical carcinoma	Levorphanol, 8 mg po q3h	Morphine, 7.5 mg	A lot (8 hr)
						Morphine, 15 mg	A lot (9 hr)

M = Male; F = female.

intrathecal morphine,[6,11] and the spread of hypalgesia from lower to upper limbs by 3 hours and to the face by 6 to 9 hours after lumbar epidural morphine.[4]

The purpose of our study was to characterize the pharmacokinetics and rostral distribution of spinal opiate analgesics. Three opiates of differing lipid solubility—morphine, methadone, and β-endorphin—were injected into the lumbar epidural or intrathecal space in patients with localized chronic cancer pain. Distribution of drug into systemic circulation and into lumbar and high cervical (C_{1-2}) CSF was measured concurrent with changes in pain intensity.

METHODS

Patient selection. Seventeen patients with chronic pain in the low back, pelvis, and lower extremities followed by the Pain Service at Memorial Sloan-Kettering Cancer Center were selected for study because of pain that was poorly controlled or associated with significant side effects after varying doses of systemic opiate analgesics. All patients had normal hepatic and renal function, normal prothrombin and partial thromboplastin times, platelet counts >100,000/mm^3, and no evidence of sepsis. Sixteen of the 17 patients had well-defined cancer pain syndromes[14]; all had had extensive diagnostic evaluation, including myelography in all 17 and computed tomography scans in 16. Thirteen had tumor infiltration of the lumbar or sacral nerve roots or plexuses. Patients gave informed consent to spinal opiate dosing and to serial sampling of plasma or CSF. Eleven patients were given epidural opiates and seven received intrathecal opiates (patient 11 received both epidural and intrathecal opiates).

Lumbar epidural study

Catheter placement. Eleven patients had Teflon epidural catheters inserted via a 17-gauge Tuohy needle (Travenol Laboratories) at the L_{3-4} interspace (Table I). Catheter position was verified fluoroscopically by injecting 3 ml metrizamide, 500 mg/ml in saline solution. In 10 patients a thin stripe of contrast 3 to 4 vertebral segments long was seen in the epidural space. In one patient (no. 6) the opacified catheter was in the epidural

Table II. Clinical characteristics of patients receiving lumbar intrathecal opiates, levels of drug in CSF at $C_{1\text{-}2}$, and analgesic responses

Patient No.	Sex	Age (yr)	Weight (kg)	Tumor type	Previous systemic analgesic	Intrathecal opiate	$C_{1\text{-}2}$ CSF opiate: Concentration (ng/ml)	Time (min)	Analgesia
11	F	62	60	Lumbar plexus infiltration, cervical carcinoma	Levorphanol, 8 mg po q3h	Morphine, 7.5 mg	—	—	Moderate (6 hr)
12	F	59	50	Sacral plexus infiltration, colon carcinoma	Methadone, 5 mg po q4h	Morphine, 2 mg	4900	60	Moderate (2 hr)
13	M	33	45	L_3 paravertebral metastasis, lung carcinoma	Hydromorphine, 10 mg im q2h	Methadone, 5 mg	278	150	Slight (2 hr)
14	F	64	55	Sacral plexus infiltration, colon carcinoma	Codeine, 60 mg po q4h	Methadone, 2 mg	15	100	Moderate (3 hr)
15	M	31	80	Sacral plexus infiltration, colon carcinoma	Hydromorphone, 32 mg po q3h	Morphine, 2 mg, and	2035	315	Moderate (4 hr)
						methadone, 2 mg	Undetectable	315	
					Methadone, 20 mg po q4h	Morphine, 10 mg	—	—	Moderate (4 hr)
16	M	60	85	L_5 epidural metastasis, lung carcinoma	Methadone, 40 mg q4h	Morphine, 5 mg	—	—	Moderate (1 hr)
17	F	73	45	Lumbar plexus infiltration, colon carcinoma	Oxycodone, 10 mg q4h	Morphine, 1 mg	—	—	Slight (3 hr)

F = Female; M = male.

area near the intervertebral foramen; contrast streamed from the foramen to coat the psoas muscle but did not opacify the epidural space. The significance of this catheter position is discussed below.

Study protocol. In seven patients (nos. 1 through 6 and 9; Table I), the plasma and CSF pharmacokinetics of epidural morphine, methadone, and β-endorphin were studied. Each patient received two or three of these drugs through the epidural catheter, either sequentially or in combined injection, to facilitate pharmacokinetic comparison. Each drug was studied in six of the seven patients. Standard parenteral solutions of morphine and methadone were used, and human β-endorphin was synthesized.[27] Drugs were diluted to a volume of 5 ml in preservative-free sterile saline solution and were injected over 6 minutes; the midpoint of this period was considered the injection time for the drug kinetic study. The catheter was then flushed with 2 ml saline solution. Initial doses of morphine and methadone were generally chosen to approximate 25% to 50% of the patient's systemic drug dose based on previous clinical experience and on relative potency tables.[14,20] On the day of study, patients received their epidural study drug when they reported their pain as moderate or severe. Pain was measured by visual analog and categoric scales of pain intensity and pain relief.[54] Specially trained analgesic study nurses obtained these pain measurements serially; recorded blood pressure, pulse rate, respiratory rate, and side effects; and sampled blood through an intravenous catheter. In five patients, pupil size was recorded serially by a specially adapted Polaroid camera.[32] A 22-gauge spinal needle was inserted at the $L_{2\text{-}3}$ interspace, one vertebral level above the epidural catheter, just before epidural drug dosing. Samples of CSF (1 ml) were collected at 0, 7, 15, 30, 60, and 90 minutes; the needle was then removed and late samples were taken by repeated puncture at the same level. To compare the systemic absorption of epidural and intramuscular opiates, patients 1 and 5 were subsequently given intragluteal injections of the same dosage of opiate used in the epidural study; plasma was sampled serially after β-endorphin, 5 mg, in patient 1 and after morphine and methadone, 2.5 mg each, in patient 5.

Four other patients (7, 8, 10, and 11) who declined sampling of blood and CSF received epidural morphine alone in doses ranging as high as 90 mg. Pain intensity and pain relief were assessed hourly by visual analog and categoric scales.

Lumbar intrathecal study

Study protocol. Seven patients received lumbar intrathecal injections. Morphine alone was given to four patients, methadone alone was received by two, and both morphine and methadone were taken by one.

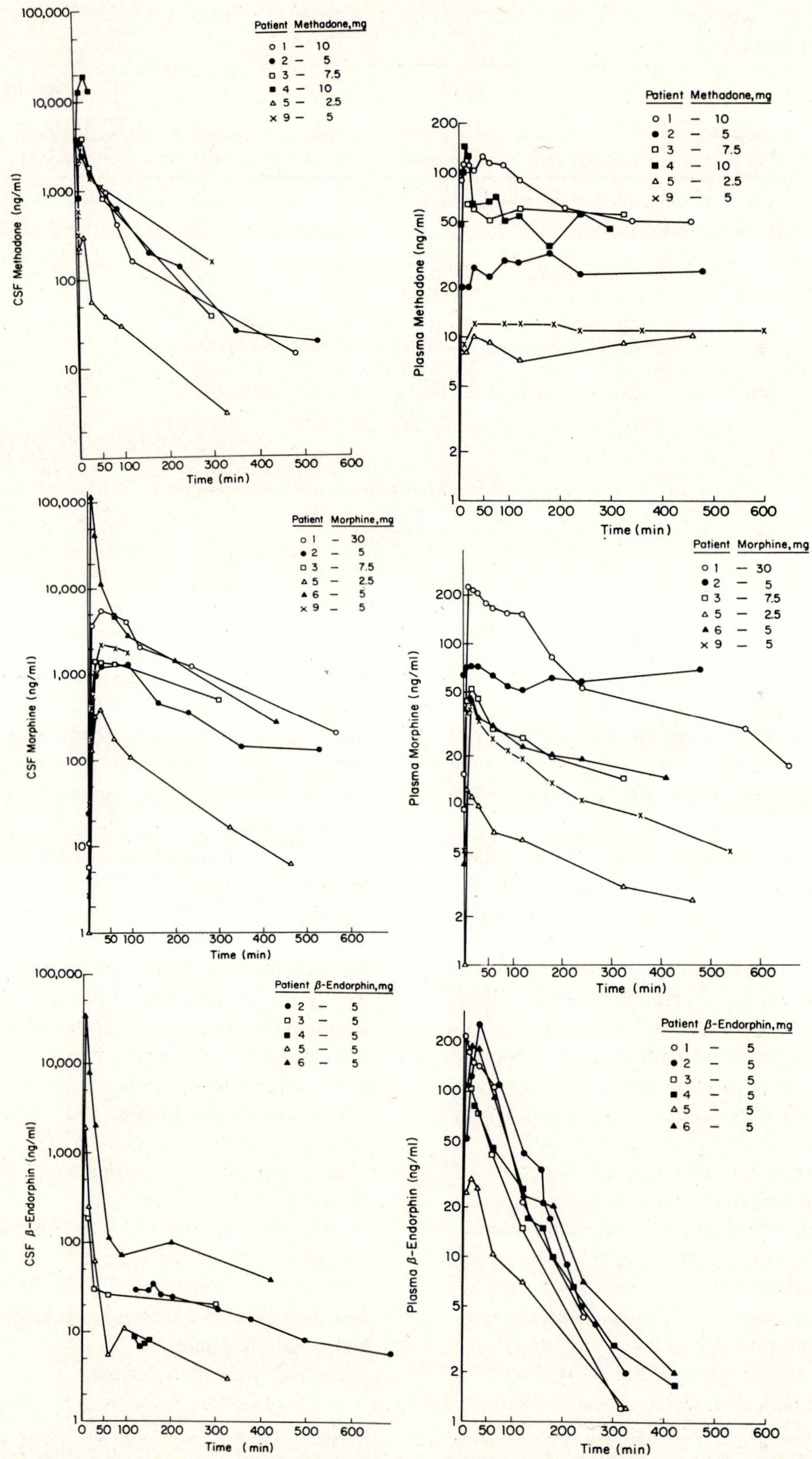

Fig. 1. Lumbar CSF *(left)* and plasma *(right)* opiate levels after lumbar epidural injection of methadone *(top)*, morphine *(middle)*, and β-endorphin *(bottom)*.

Table III. CSF and plasma pharmacokinetics of epidural opiates

	Time of peak concentration (min)				*Free drug concentration ratio**	*$t_{1/2}$ (min)*			
Drug	*CSF*		*Plasma*		*CSF/plasma*	*CSF*		*Plasma*	
Methadone	14.4	4.7	21	10	1301	73	24	ND	
Morphine	33.6	29.2	12	4	54	126	58	201	22
β-Endorphin	9.7	4.6	17	8	ND	317	305	51	11

Data are $\overline{X} \pm$ SD.
ND = Not determined.
*At CSF peak.

Drugs were administered through a 25-gauge spinal needle at L_{3-4} (Table II). Study drugs were injected in 2 ml saline solution followed by a 1 ml saline solution flush. Visual analog and categoric scales of pain intensity and pain relief were serially measured in all seven and plasma samples were collected in five for up to 8 hours. In each of four patients a single CSF sample was obtained by lateral cervical puncture at C_{1-2} under fluoroscopic guidance 1 to 5 hours after lumbar opiate injection to assess the spinal ascent of the drug from the lumbar injection site. The timing of high cervical sampling varied from patient to patient depending on availability of radiologic supervision and patient comfort.

Biofluid sampling and assays. Blood samples were centrifuged immediately after collection and both the plasma fraction and CSF samples were rapidly frozen and stored at −20° C. Plasma and CSF drug concentrations were determined by RIA. In a 0.05 ml sample volume, the lower limit of sensitivity is 3 ng/ml for the methadone RIA,[28] 0.3 ng/ml for the β-endorphin RIA,[21] and 1 ng/ml for the morphine RIA.[48] The methadone antiserum does not recognize the metabolites of methadone or any of the other systemic analgesics given to patients who received epidural methadone (see Table I). The morphine antiserum recognizes the major metabolite, morphine-3-glucuronide, with 6% cross-reactivity. β-Endorphin levels measured in biofluids after epidural injection were one to four orders of magnitude greater than the reported endogenous levels of β-endorphin.[21] By use of gel chromatography we established that the immunoreactive β-endorphin in plasma and CSF samples had the same chromatographic characteristics as the synthetic human β-endorphin administered to the patients. Plasma sampled from patients 60 minutes after drug dosing and pooled CSF samples from one patient taken at 30, 60, and 300 minutes after dosing were extracted and subjected to chromatography on a Bio-Gel P-60 column (Bio-Rad Laboratories) as described by Inturrisi et al.[21] Fifty-five percent of the plasma immunoreactivity and 90% of the CSF immunoreactivity eluted from the column as a single peak identical in elution position to that of authentic β-endorphin.

Determination of pharmacokinetic parameters. The elimination $t_{1/2}$ was estimated from a semilogarithmic plot of the terminal portion of the plasma or CSF drug concentration-time curve by the method of least squares. This phase of the curve has a slope equal to k/2.303, where k is the terminal elimination rate constant and $t_{1/2}$ = 0.693/k.

RESULTS

Lumbar epidural study

Pharmacokinetics. Fig. 1 shows the CSF and plasma profiles for methadone, morphine and β-endorphin after lumbar epidural administration. Note that peak levels in CSF are 50 to 500 times higher than simultaneous plasma levels. The rate of decline of CSF levels correlates with opiate lipid solubility (methadone > morphine > β-endorphin).

Six patients received epidural methadone in doses ranging from 2.5 to 10 mg. Methadone appeared in CSF and plasma in the first sample after dosing (2 to 7 minutes). The methadone concentration in both biofluids reached a peak at 15 to 20 minutes (Fig. 1; Table III), then CSF levels declined over the next 300 to 500 minutes while plasma methadone levels were sustained throughout the 600-minute sampling period.

Six patients received epidural morphine in doses ranging from 2.5 to 30 mg. The kinetics of morphine appearance in CSF and plasma (Fig. 1) were similar to those of methadone. In contrast to methadone, after reaching a peak, plasma morphine concentrations declined during the 600-minute sampling period. Patients 2, 3, and 9 took hydromorphone or oxycodone several hours before the study. These drugs cross-react with the morphine antibody. This did not significantly affect CSF values, as the predose levels were <2% of peak CSF morphine levels, but it did affect plasma morphine levels. Plasma data from patients 2 (who received hydromorphone, 32 mg po at 130 minutes; Fig. 1) and 3 are therefore excluded from calculations of plasma morphine kinetics.

The profiles of the six patients who received epidural β-endorphin at a dose of 5 mg (Fig. 1) are characterized by the rapid appearance of β-endorphin in CSF and plasma, followed by a rapid monoexponential decline in plasma levels and an apparent biexponential decline (rapid initial phase followed a slower secondary phase) in CSF levels.

Table III summarizes the pharmacokinetic data. Peak drug concentrations in CSF and plasma occurred at approximately the same time (10 to 30 minutes) after drug dosing. No significant difference could be demonstrated among the three drugs in their time to reach peak concentrations in either biofluid. In a previous study[23] we found the plasma methadone free fraction to average 0.12 in patients with cancer. Olsen et al.[38] reported the plasma morphine free fraction in normal subjects to be 0.65. Plasma protein binding and the free fraction for β-endorphin have not yet been determined. Assuming that the CSF drug concentration represents only free drug, it is possible from these data to calculate the CSF/plasma free drug concentration ratio for methadone and morphine at the time of peak CSF drug concentration. Table III indicates that the CSF/plasma free drug concentration ratio was nearly 25 times greater for methadone than for morphine.

Drug elimination from CSF, as expressed by the $t_{1/2}$, was most rapid for methadone and slowest for β-endorphin (Table III). Plasma elimination was most rapid for β-endorphin and slowest for methadone. Plasma methadone levels did not decline appreciably during the 600-minute sampling, so a reliable $t_{1/2}$ could not be calculated from these data (Fig. 1; Table III).

In patient 6, whose epidural catheter was seen in the epidural space with its tip near the neural foramen, CSF morphine and β-endorphin reached peak levels within 7 minutes that were six times higher than those of any other patient. This may have occurred because transdural passage of lipid-insoluble drugs is greatest across the nerve root sheath, which was directly apposed to the catheter tip,[2] or because the initial lumbar puncture may have caused a small rent in the dura around the needle through which the drug could rapidly reach the CSF.

In patient 5, plasma levels of methadone and morphine after epidural injection were similar to those after intramuscular injection (Fig. 2). In patient 1, levels of β-endorphin were higher during the first hour after epidural injection than after intramuscular injection.

Analgesia. The degree and duration of analgesia with epidural opiates were determined by a five-point categoric relief scale (none, slight, moderate, a lot, or complete relief; Table I). The 11 patients received 23 epidural opiate injections. Three patients got "a lot" of relief on one or more injections (median duration 4.5 hours), six patients had moderate relief (2 hours) as their best response, and two patients reported slight relief (1.5 hours). Although the epidural opiate dosage approached the previous systemic opiate dosage in most patients, only patients 9 and 11 reported that the epidural opiate provided better relief than their usual systemic analgesic. (These studies were designed primarily to assess drug distribution. Accordingly, several drugs were frequently injected in combination. We will make no attempt, therefore, to compare the specific analgesic effects of epidural or intrathecal morphine, methadone, and β-endorphin.)

Side effects. Six of the 11 patients had moderate discomfort at the injection site for 1 to 3 minutes after administration, and one other had lumbar itching for 1 hour. Four reported sleepiness at 30 minutes (three) or 2 hours (one) after injection, and one each reported transient light-headedness and dysphagia. Pupillary measurements were taken in patients 1, 2, 5, 6, and 9; significant miosis (≥0.5 mm) occurred only in patient 1, after 30 mg morphine. No patient developed respiratory depression or urinary retention.

Lumbar intrathecal study

Pharmacokinetics. CSF obtained at the C_{1-2} level contained high concentrations of morphine (4900 and 2035 ng/ml) at 60 and 315 minutes after lumbar intrathecal injection in two patients. C_{1-2} levels of methadone in three patients were 278 ng/ml, 12 ng/ml, and undetectable at 100, 150, and 315 minutes, respectively (Table II).

There was substantial uptake of intrathecal opiate into plasma. In patients 13 and 14, who received 10 mg morphine and 5 mg methadone, respectively, the peak level of morphine was 40 ng/ml at 15 minutes and that of methadone was 30 ng/ml at 30 minutes. These plasma levels and time courses are similar to those in Fig. 1 after epidural morphine or methadone. In three other patients given 1 to 2 mg doses, plasma levels were at or below the limits of detection.

Analgesia. Seven patients received either intrathecal morphine or methadone. Five patients reported moderate relief (median duration 3 hours), but three of these were still bedridden by pain. Two patients had slight relief for 2 and 3 hours, respectively. One patient (no. 16) reported the spinal drug to be more effective than the previous systemic therapy.

Side effects. Two of the seven patients noted sleepiness within 1 hour of drug injection. One patient had nausea and vomiting and two had sacral or total body itching. Neither respiratory depression nor urinary retention was observed.

DISCUSSION

The optimal design of spinal opiate therapy requires an understanding of how redistribution of spinally administered drugs to cerebral sites is affected by drug properties (lipid solubility, rate of metabolism, receptor affinity) and by the site and method of administration (epidural vs. intrathecal, bolus vs. constant infusion). While the pharmacokinetics of epidural opiates are complex[34] and our data are insufficient to develop a general pharmacokinetic model, these data provide an insight into the disposition of epidural opiates. After epidural injection, these three opiates readily crossed the dura to produce levels in lumbar CSF that were 30 to 2000 times the peak plasma levels. The times of peak concentrations in CSF for methadone and morphine (14 and 34 minutes) were similar to the times of maximal analgesia (17 and 37 minutes) observed by Bromage et al.[3] in postoperative patients. After reaching a peak, levels in CSF of the more polar drugs, β-endorphin and morphine, declined less rapidly than methadone levels; this is consistent with data in animals[52] and clinical impressions[59] that duration of analgesic action is longer for drugs with low lipid solubility, and with the study of Moore et al.[33] comparing the CSF kinetics of morphine and heroin.

Epidural drugs are rapidly taken up into systemic circulation by the rich plexus of epidural blood vessels. Like a number of local anesthetics,[29,46,51,57] the three opiates we studied reached peak levels in plasma within 10 to 20 minutes, and levels were comparable with those after intramuscular administration. Nordberg et al.[36,37] and Gustafsson et al.[19] reported similar results for the distribution of epidural morphine in CSF and plasma. This distribution of drug to brain stem and cerebral sites through systemic circulation may contribute to the analgesia and side effects of epidural opiates. This component is less significant with direct intrathecal injection, because vascular uptake of intrathecal drug is about half that of intramuscular or epidural drug[5] and because intrathecal injection permits the use of doses roughly one tenth the corresponding doses of epidural drug.

If we assume that the initial volume of distribution of a spinal opiate is approximately 15 ml,[33] the percentage of an epidural dose in CSF at the time of peak CSF opiate concentration can be estimated. This calculation reveals that at peak, the CSF of patients 2, 3, 5, and 9, who received equal doses of methadone and morphine, contained a mean (±SD) 0.75% ± 0.38% and 0.38% ± 0.17% of the respective epidural dose. Thus with epidural administration, less than 1% of the dose appears in the CSF, while a substantial fraction of the dose is absorbed into the systemic circulation.[17]

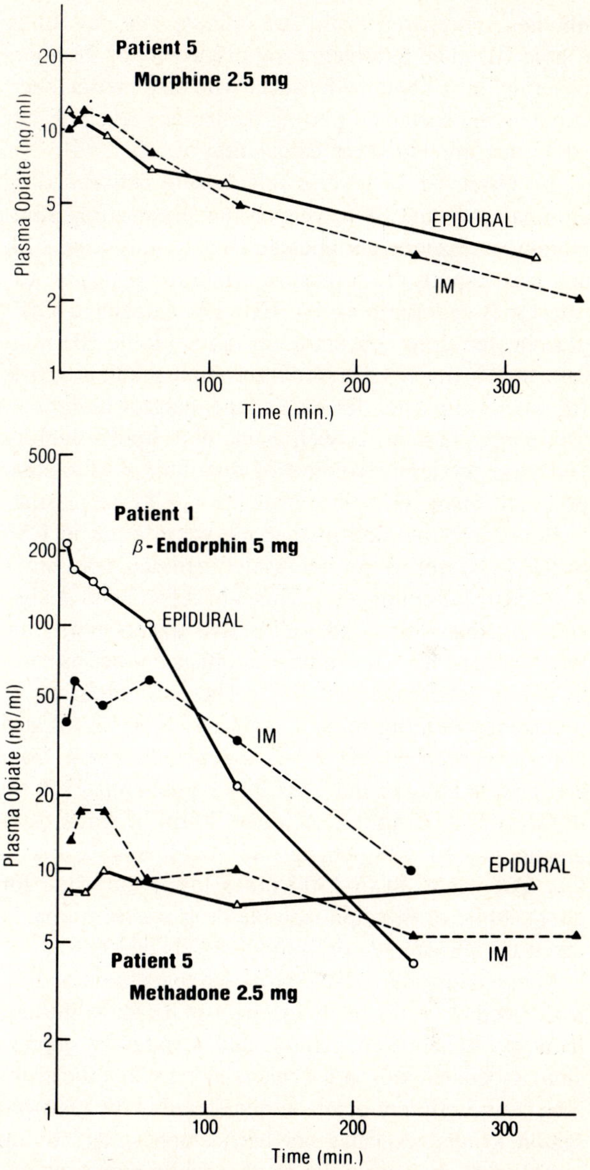

Fig. 2. Comparison of plasma opiate levels after epidural and intragluteal injections. Peak plasma levels after epidural injection may approach or exceed levels after an intramuscular (*IM*) dose.

The plasma elimination kinetics we observed are similar to those reported after intravenous administration of these opiates. Foley et al.[15] found the plasma $t_{1/2}$ for intravenous β-endorphin to be 37 minutes, compared with 51 minutes in our study. Stanski et al.[49] reported the plasma $t_{1/2}$ for intravenous morphine to average 177 minutes, compared with 201 minutes in our study (Table III). The relatively long plasma $t_{1/2}$ of 23 hours observed in patients with cancer who take methadone[23] explains the sustained plasma methadone levels in our study that precluded the calculation of a $t_{1/2}$.

We observed an inverse relationship between drug elimination from CSF and concurrent plasma drug elimination; methadone disappeared most rapidly from CSF and least rapidly from plasma, while the opposite was true for β-endorphin (Table III). The calculated CSF/plasma free drug concentration ratios (Table III) indicate that a much larger concentration gradient exists from CSF to plasma for methadone than for morphine. This large gradient, as well as the high lipid solubility and large systemic volume of distribution of methadone, all favor its rapid transfer from CSF to plasma.

Both morphine and methadone were found in CSF at the $C_{1\text{-}2}$ level, 3 cm below the medulla, between 1 and 5 hours after injection. This is in accord with studies showing that drugs and radioactive tracers reach the basal cisterna from the lumbar intrathecal space as early as 1 hour after injection.[12,45,47] The concentrations of morphine, 4900 ng/ml at 1 hour and 2030 ng/ml at 5 hours, approached the levels that would result from complete mixing of the 2 mg dose in the entire 140 ml of CSF (14,000 ng/ml) or in the 70 ml of spinal subarachnoid CSF (28,000 ng/ml). Methadone levels in $C_{1\text{-}2}$ CSF were 20 to 1000 times lower (adjusted for dose). Most of this lipid-soluble drug was presumably taken up into spinal cord blood vessels and tissue.

Many investigators have proposed that ascent of drug to the medulla is the likely mechanism for the vomiting, lethargy, generalized itching, and respiratory depression associated with spinal opiate therapy, but the probable contribution of opiate administered in the cisternal region to analgesia has not been emphasized. Yeung and Rudy[63] showed in the rat that while morphine applied only to the spinal cord or to periventricular sites caused some inhibition of responses to noxious stimuli, a far more potent inhibition followed injection of drug in both areas; this interaction was multiplicative rather than additive. If their model is valid for man, even the low cisternal concentrations of drug in the first hour after lumbar injection may significantly amplify effects at the local spinal site. Such potentiation will be greater for drugs of low lipid solubility, like morphine, that reach the high cervical area in significant amounts*; a larger proportion of lipid-soluble opiates, like methadone or heroin, will redistribute into tissue or systemic circulation during ascent in the spinal subarachnoid space.[33]

Because most studies of chronic spinal opiate dosing have used morphine, they give no information about the effectiveness of spinal opiate systems alone in controlling chronic pain in man. This could be better studied by a drug that is both lipid soluble (to minimize rostral redistribution via spinal CSF) and rapidly metabolized by the liver (to minimize systemic redistribution to the brain). Alternatively, a peptide that was degradable by neural tissue could be injected at the appropriate spinal segment.

The modest degree and short duration of analgesia described by our patients, despite high opiate levels in lumbar CSF, were disappointing and differ from reported experiences with spinal opiates in patients with chronic malignant pain.[7,8,30,31,40,41,55,64] Only three of 17 patients reported improved analgesia with spinal opiates, and no patients continued chronic spinal opiate therapy. Patient 9 reported 35 hours of relief after 5 mg epidural morphine. He had been taking only 5 mg oxycodone previously, however, and achieved good chronic analgesia with oral levorphanol. Patient 11 improved with epidural morphine, but when cauda equina compression developed 2 weeks later, even intrathecal morphine, 7.5 mg, did not permit leg movement; bilateral cordotomy was required to relieve her pain. After patient 14 responded well to intrathecal methadone, 2 mg, a lumbar subarachnoid catheter and subcutaneous Ommaya reservoir (Heyer-Schulte) were surgically implanted. For 4 days, 1 mg morphine every 24 hours provided good relief of perineal pain, but after 2 weeks even 4 mg morphine or 4 mg methadone became ineffective.

We suggest several reasons for this discrepancy between our results and those of other investigators. Our patients had received months of therapy with very high doses of systemic opiates before spinal injections (mean morphine dose 37 mg im every 4 hours); in other reports, previous narcotic exposure was lower or not specified. Spinal analgesic systems in animals[62] and man[18,53,58] develop marked tolerance after several days of exposure to high levels of intrathecal opiates. The use of agonists active at spinal δ-receptors, which remain sensitive in morphine-tolerant experimental animals, may be useful in this patient population.[9,35,39] Also, most of our patients had pain caused by extensive infiltration of nerve plexuses or spinal roots. Such "deafferentation pain" is not effectively relieved by opiates.[1] In most other reports of spinal opiate therapy in patients with cancer, the nature of the pain syndromes

*According to our preliminary studies, substantial cervical CSF levels of morphine also accompany chronic lumbar intrathecal infusions of morphine.

has not been defined. Furthermore, the placebo effect of a new and invasive therapy, as well as the effects of systemic uptake of epidural drug, may be mistaken for specific spinal opiate analgesia.

In summary, our studies demonstrate that epidural and intrathecal administration of opiates is associated with redistribution of drug to supraspinal sites through the CSF and the systemic circulation. Prior opiate exposure markedly reduces the efficacy of spinal opiate therapy in the patient with chronic cancer pain. Further pharmacokinetic and pharmacodynamic studies of a variety of opiates and peptides given by bolus or by continuous infusion are needed to approach the goal of selective spinal analgesia. While spinal morphine is now widely used in the treatment of chronic cancer pain, this lipid-insoluble drug has particularly brisk CSF redistribution to brain stem sites and the rationale for its advantages over systemic opiate therapy is not clear. We believe that physicians' lack of knowledge in the practical use of systemic opiates[22] and the unavailability of oral opiates for cancer pain in many countries[50] often lead to inappropriate use of spinal opiate therapies. These should be considered investigational techniques limited to patients with cancer who fail to achieve acceptable pain relief after trials with several systemic opiates.

References

1. Arnér S, Arnér B: Differential effects of epidural morphine in the treatment of cancer-related pain. Acta Anaesthesiol Scand **29**:32-36, 1985.
2. Bromage PR: Epidural analgesia. Philadelphia, 1978, WB Saunders Co, p 23.
3. Bromage PR, Camporesi E, Chestnut D: Epidural morphine for postoperative analgesia: A double-blind study. Anesth Analg (Cleve) **61**:236-240, 1982.
4. Bromage PR, Camporesi EM, Durant PAC, Nielsen CH: Rostral spread of epidural morphine. Anesthesiology **56**:931-936, 1982.
5. Chauvin M, Samii K, Schermann JM, Sandouk P, Bourdon R, Viars P: Plasma pharmacokinetics of morphine after i.m., extradural, and intrathecal administration. Br J Anesth **54**:843-848, 1982.
6. Christensen V: Respiratory depression after extradural morphine. Br J Anesth **52**:841, 1980.
7. Coombs DW, Saunders RL, Gaylor MS: Epidural narcotic infusion reservoir: Implantation technique and efficacy. Anesthesiology **56**:469-473, 1982.
8. Coombs DW, Saunders RL, Gaylor MS, Block AR: Relief of continuous chronic pain by intraspinal narcotic infusion via an implanted reservoir. JAMA **250**:2336-2339, 1983.
9. Coombs DW, Saunders RL, Lachance D, Savage S, Ragnarsson TS, Jensen LE: Intrathecal morphine tolerance: Use of intrathecal clonidine, DADLE, and intraventricular morphine. Anesthesiology **62**:358-363, 1985.
10. Cousins MJ, Mather LE: Intrathecal and epidural administration of opioids. Anesthesiology **61**:276-310, 1984.
11. Davies GK, Tolhurst-Cleaver CL, James TL: CNS depression from intrathecal morphine. Anesthesiology **52**:280, 1980.
12. DiChiro G: Movement of the cerebrospinal fluid in human beings. Nature **204**:290-291, 1964.
13. El-Baz NMI, Faber LP, Jensik RJ: Continuous epidural infusion of morphine for treatment of pain after thoracic surgery: A new technique. Anesth Analg (Cleve) **63**:757-764, 1984.
14. Foley KM: The management of pain of malignant origin. *In* Tyler HR, Dawson DM, editors: Current neurology, vol 2. Boston, 1981, Houghton Mifflin, pp 279-302.
15. Foley KM, Kourides IA, Inturrisi CE, et al: Beta-endorphin: Analgesic and hormonal effects in humans. Proc Natl Acad Sci USA **76**:5377-5381, 1979.
16. Glynn CJ, Mather LE, Cousins MJ, et al: Spinal narcotics and respiratory depression. Lancet **2**:356-357, 1981.
17. Glynn CJ, Mather LE, Cousins MJ, Graham JR, Wilson PR: Peridural meperidine in humans: Analgetic response, pharmacokinetics, and transmission into CSF. Anesthesiology **55**:520-526, 1981.
18. Greenberg HS, Taren J, Ensminger WD, Doan K: Benefit from and tolerance to continuous intrathecal infusion of morphine for intractable cancer pain. J Neurosurg **57**:360-364, 1982.
19. Gustafsson LL, Grell A-M, Garle M, Rane A, Schildt B: Kinetics of morphine in cerebrospinal fluid after epidural administration. Acta Anaesthesiol Scand **28**:535-539, 1984.
20. Inturrisi CE: Narcotic drugs. Med Clin N Am **66**:1061-1072, 1982.
21. Inturrisi CE, Alexopoulos G, Lipman R, Foley KM, Rossier J: Beta-endorphin: Immunoreactivity in the plasma of psychiatric patients receiving electroconvulsive treatment. Ann NY Acad Sci **398**:413-423, 1982.
22. Inturrisi CE, Foley KM: Narcotic analgesics in the management of pain. *In* Kuhar M, Pasternak G, editors: Analgesics. Neurochemical, behavioral and clinical perspectives. New York, 1984, Raven Press, pp 257-287.
23. Inturrisi CE, Foley KM, Kaiko RF, Houde RW: Disposition and effects of intravenous methadone in cancer patients. Pain **1**(suppl):99, 1981.
24. Kitahata LM, Collins JG: Spinal action of narcotic analgesics. Anesthesiology **54**:153-163, 1981.
25. Lanz E, Simko G, Theiss D, Glocke MH: Epidural buprenorphine—A double-blind study of postoperative analgesia and side effects. Anesth Analg (Cleve) **63**:593-598, 1984.
26. Lanz E, Theiss D, Riess W, Sommer U: Epidural morphine for postoperative analgesia: A double-blind study. Anesth Analg (Cleve) **61**:236-240, 1982.

27. Li CH, Yamashiro D, Tsen LF, Loh HH: Synthesis and analgesic activity of human beta-endorphin. J Med Chem **20:**325-328, 1977.
28. Ling GSF, Umans JG, Inturrisi CE: Methadone: Radioimmunoassay and pharmacokinetics in the rat. J Pharmacol Exp Ther **217:**147-151, 1981.
29. Lund PC, Covino BG: Distribution of local anesthetics in man following peridural anesthesia. J Clin Pharmacol **7:**324-329, 1967.
30. Magora F, Olshwang D, Eimerl D, et al: Observations on extradural morphine analgesia in various pain conditions. Br J Anaesth **52:**247-258, 1980.
31. Malone BT, Beye R, Walker J: Management of pain in the terminally ill by administration of epidural narcotics. Cancer **55:**438-440, 1985.
32. Marquardt WG, Martin WR, Jasinski DR: The use of the Polaroid camera in pupillography. Int J Addict **2:**301-304, 1973.
33. Moore A, Bullingham R, McQuay H, Allen M, Baldwin D, Cole A: Spinal fluid kinetics of morphine and heroin. Clin Pharmacol Ther **35:**40-45, 1984.
34. Moore RA, Bullingham RES, McQuay HJ, et al: Dural permeability to narcotics: In vitro determination and application to extradural administration. Br J Anesth **54:**1117-1128, 1982.
35. Moulin DE, Max MB, Kaiko RF, Inturrisi CE, Maggard J, Yaksh TL, Foley KM: The analgesic efficacy of D-ala^2-D-Leu^5-enkephalin in cancer patients with chronic pain. Pain. (In press.)
36. Nordberg G, Hedner T, Mellstrand T, Dahlstrom B: Pharmacokinetic aspects of epidural morphine analgesia. Anesthesiology **58:**545-551, 1983.
37. Nordberg G, Hedner T, Mellstrand T, Dahlstrom B: Pharmacokinetic aspects of intrathecal morphine analgesia. Anesthesiology **60:**448-454, 1984.
38. Olsen GD, Bennett WM, Porter GA: Morphine and phenytoin binding to plasma proteins in renal and hepatic failure. Clin Pharmacol Ther **17:**677-684, 1975.
39. Onofrio BM, Yaksh TL: Intrathecal delta-receptor ligand produces analgesia in man. Lancet **1:**1386-1387, 1983.
40. Onofrio BM, Yaksh TL, Arnold PG: Continuous low-dose intrathecal morphine administration in the treatment of chronic pain of malignant origin. Mayo Clin Proc **56:**516-520, 1981.
41. Poletti CE, Cohen AM, Todd DP, Ojemann RG, Sweet WH, Zervas NT: Cancer pain relieved by long-term epidural morphine with permanent indwelling systems for self-administration. J Neurosurg **55:**581-584, 1981.
42. Rawal N, Sjostrand U, Christoffersson E, Dahlstrom B, Arvill A, Rydman H: Comparison of intramuscular and epidural morphine for postoperative analgesia in the grossly obese: Influence on postoperative ambulation and pulmonary function. Anesth Analg (Cleve) **63:**583-592, 1984.
43. Rawal N, Sjostrand UH, Dahlstrom B, Nydahl P-A, Ostelius J: Epidural morphine for postoperative pain relief: A comparative study with intramuscular narcotic and intercostal nerve block. Anesth Analg (Cleve) **61:**93-98, 1982.
44. Reiz S, Westberg M: Side-effects of epidural morphine. Lancet **1:**203-204, 1980.
45. Rieselbach RE, DiChiro G, Freireich EG, Rall DP: Subarachnoid distribution of drugs after lumbar injection. N Engl J Med **267:**1273-1278, 1962.
46. Scott DB, Jebson PFR, Braid DP, Ortengren B, Frisch P: Factors affecting plasma levels of lignocaine and prilocaine. Br J Anaesth **44:**1040-1048, 1972.
47. Shapiro WR, Young DF, Mehta BM: Methotrexate: Distribution in cerebrospinal fluid after intravenous ventricular and lumbar injections. N Engl J Med **293:**161-166, 1975.
48. Spector S: Quantitative determination of morphine in serum by radioimmunoassay. J Pharmacol Exp Ther **178:**253-258, 1971.
49. Stanski DR, Greenblatt DJ, Lowenstein E: Kinetics of intravenous and intramuscular morphine. Clin Pharmacol Ther **24:**52-59, 1978.
50. Swerdlow M, Stjernswärd J: Cancer pain relief—An urgent problem. World Health Forum **3:**326-331, 1982.
51. Tucker GT, Moore DC, Bridenbaugh PO, Thompson GE: Systemic absorption of mepivicaine in commonly used regional block procedures. Anesthesiology **37:**277-287, 1972.
52. Tung AS, Yaksh TL: The antinociceptive effects of epidural opiates in the cat: Studies on their pharmacology and the effects of lipophilicity in spinal analgesia. Pain **12:**343-356, 1982.
53. Ventafridda V, Figliuzzi M, Tamburini M, et al: Clinical observation on analgesia elicited by intrathecal morphine in cancer patients. *In* Bonica JJ, editor: Advances in pain research and therapy. New York, 1979, Raven Press, pp 559-565.
54. Wallenstein SL, Heidrich G, Kaiko RF, Houde RW: Clinical evaluation of mild analgesics: The measurement of clinical pain. Br J Clin Pharmacol **10:**3195-3275, 1980.
55. Wang JK, Nauss LA, Thomas JE: Pain relief by intrathecally applied morphine in man. Anesthesiology **50:**149-151, 1979.
56. Weddel SJ, Ritter RR: Serum levels following epidural administration of morphine and correlation with relief of postsurgical pain. Anesthesiology **54:**210-214, 1981.
57. Wilkinson FG, Lund PC: Bupivicaine levels in plasma and cerebrospinal fluid following peridural administration. Anesthesiology **33:**482-486, 1971.
58. Woods WA, Cohen SE: High-dose epidural morphine in a terminally ill patient. Anesthesiology **56:**311-312, 1982.
59. Yaksh TL: Spinal opiate analgesia: Characteristics and principles of action. Pain **11:**293-346, 1981.
60. Yaksh TL: In vivo studies on spinal opiate receptor systems mediating antinociception. I. Mu and delta receptor profiles in the primate. J Pharmacol Exp Ther **226:**303-316, 1983.
61. Yaksh TL, Noueihed R: The physiology and pharma-

cology of spinal opiates. Ann Rev Pharmacol Toxicol **25:**433-462, 1985.
62. Yaksh TL, Reddy SVR: Studies in the primate on the analgetic effects associated with intrathecal actions of opiates, alpha-adrenergic agonists, and baclofen. Anesthesiology **54:**451-467, 1981.
63. Yeung JC, Rudy TA: Multiplicative interaction between narcotic agonisms expressed at spinal and supraspinal sites of antinociception action as revealed by concurrent intrathecal and intracerebroventricular injections of morphine. J Pharmacol Exp Ther **215:**633-642, 1980.
64. Zenz M, Scheale BS, Neuhaus R, Pipenbrock S, Hilfrich J: Long-term peridural morphine analgesia in cancer pain. Lancet **1:**91, 1981.

Food-induced changes in theophylline absorption from controlled-release formulations. Part II. Importance of meal composition and dosing time relative to meal intake in assessing changes in absorption

Theo-24 (G. D. Searle & Co.) is an ultra-slow-absorbing formulation of theophylline suitable for once-a-day dosing in slow and normal metabolizers of theophylline. Relative to fasting conditions, increased rate and extent of theophylline absorption occur when this product is administered immediately after a breakfast with a high fat content. Our study demonstrated that factors such as meal composition (fat content) or dosing time relative to meal intake can modify the high fat–induced changes in absorption. For consistent, slow absorption, patients taking high doses (≥900 mg) of Theo-24 once a day should take this product in the morning under fasting conditions or with a breakfast containing ≤10 gm fat. If a high-fat breakfast (>55 gm fat) is taken, then Theo-24 should be administered at least 1 hour before the meal. (Clin Pharmacol Ther 38:642-647, 1985.)

Aziz Karim, Ph.D., Thomas Burns, M.S., Denis Janky, M.S., and Aryeh Hurwitz, M.D. *Skokie, Ill., and Kansas City, Kan.*

A variety of formulation-dependent food-induced absorption changes[2] have been reported with controlled-release formulations of theophylline that have either pH-dependent[11] or pH-independent[4,5] in vitro dissolution characteristics. The absorption changes include a decrease in the rate,[6-8,10] decrease in the extent,[4,9] increase in the rate or extent,[3,5,11] and more erratic[6] absorption of theophylline. Recently, a marked increase in the rate and extent[3,11] of theophylline absorption from Theo-24 (G. D. Searle & Co.), an ultra-slow-absorbing formulation, was found when this product was taken immediately after a breakfast with a high fat content. The objective of our present investigation was to evaluate the importance of meal composition and dosing time relative to meal intake on the rate and extent of theophylline absorption from Theo-24.

From Searle Research & Development, Division of G. D. Searle & Co., Skokie, and Division of Clinical Pharmacology, University of Kansas Medical Center, Kansas City.

Preliminary results presented at the Third Annual Conference on Current Concepts in Biopharmaceutics and Clinical Trials, University of Maryland School of Pharmacy, Baltimore, Md., Oct. 2-4, 1984, and at the Searle Theophylline Symposium, Paradise Island, Bahamas, March 2-4, 1985.

Received for publication June 7, 1985; accepted July 25, 1985.

Reprint requests to: Aziz Karim, Ph.D., Searle Research & Development, Division of G. D. Searle & Co., 4901 Searle Pkwy., Skokie, IL 60077.

METHODS

Dosage form. Commercially available Theo-24 capsules (lot #1283-873) were used in both the meal composition and dosing time studies.

Subjects. Twelve healthy male nonsmokers with a mean (±SD) age of 24 ± 1 years, weight of 73.5 ± 6.2 kg and height of 176.8 ± 5.6 cm participated in the meal composition study, and 24 subjects with a mean (±SD) age of 26 ± 6 years, weight of 75.6 ± 7.4 kg and height of 177.5 ± 6.8 cm participated in the dosing time study. Subjects were judged healthy on the basis of history, physical examination, routine laboratory data, standard ECG, and blood pressure; all subjects weighed within ±10% of the ideal body weight for age and height. Study protocols were approved by Institutional Review Boards and each subject gave written informed consent.

Study designs. Alcohol- and xanthine-containing foods or beverages were prohibited for 48 hours before, during, and for 72 hours after each drug dosing. No medication other than theophylline was taken by the

Table I. Pharmacokinetic model-independent parameters of theophylline in 12 healthy male nonsmokers after single 900 mg doses of Theo-24 (three 300 mg capsules) taken while fasting and immediately after low-, medium-, and high-fat content breakfasts

Subject No.	C_{max} (μg/ml)				t_{max} (hr)				AUC(0-72) (μg · hr/ml)			
	F	L	M	H	F	L	M	H	F	L	M	H
1	7.1	4.4	6.1	15.4	14.0	16.0	12.0	8.0	231	186	186	283
2	7.9	9.6	7.3	12.2	12.0	10.0	14.0	16.0	233	193	155	272
3	5.6	7.5	5.3	7.5	10.0	8.0	8.0	16.0	137	164	146	149
4	8.3	8.1	9.4	13.5	10.0	28.0	10.0	28.0	275	248	285	332
5	8.5	12.0	14.9	16.7	28.0	12.0	16.0	24.0	284	320	342	407
6	8.2	6.2	5.9	9.5	10.0	12.0	10.0	28.0	238	214	201	227
7	6.6	9.1	5.8	14.0	16.0	10.0	16.0	8.0	157	189	158	190
8	12.4	5.8	7.6	10.1	10.0	16.0	14.0	12.0	256	156	189	245
9	6.7	6.4	7.6	17.1	8.0	16.0	10.0	10.0	308	168	231	329
10	7.5	7.4	8.2	13.4	16.0	10.0	14.0	10.0	254	254	297	358
11	9.1	11.3	6.5	16.4	10.0	10.0	10.0	14.0	243	255	168	294
12	8.8	8.9	7.6	9.9	12.0	10.0	14.0	14.0	182	216	227	183
$\overline{X}$	8.1*	8.1*	7.7*	13.0	13.0	13.2	12.3	15.7	233*	214*	216*	272
SD	1.7	2.3	2.6	3.2	5.4	5.4	2.7	7.2	51	48	63	77

F = Fasting; L = low-fat breakfast; M = medium-fat breakfast; H = high-fat breakfast.
*$P < 0.05$ compared with high-fat breakfast.

subjects from 1 week before each study until its completion.

The meal composition study was a four-way, randomized, balanced, crossover (7-day washout) study in which each of the 12 subjects received three 300 mg Theo-24 capsules under fasting and nonfasting conditions. In the latter case, Theo-24 was taken immediately after the standardized high-, medium-, and low-fat breakfasts described below:

The high fat breakfast included two slices of toasted white bread spread with butter, two eggs fried in butter, two slices of bacon, 2 oz hash-browned potatoes, and 8 oz whole milk (approximately 33 gm protein, 58 to 75 gm fat,* 58 gm carbohydrate; 870 to 1020 calories).

The medium-fat breakfast included one slice of toasted white bread spread with butter and jelly, 1 oz dry cereal (corn flakes), 8 oz skim milk, 6 oz orange juice, and one banana (approximately 17 gm protein, 8 gm fat, 103 gm carbohydrate; 583 calories).

The low-fat breakfast included one slice toasted white bread spread with jelly, 8 oz skim milk, and 6 oz orange juice (approximately 12 gm protein, 1 gm fat, 51 gm carbohydrate; 253 calories).

Under fasting conditions, subjects fasted overnight for at least 10 hours, fasted for an additional 4 hours after drug dosing, and then received the standardized high-fat breakfast.

*Because of different amounts of butter, the fat content in the dosing time and meal composition studies were 58 and 75 gm, respectively.

All doses were taken with 120 ml water. Dosing was done under observation at the clinical facility and standardized diet and activity were observed during the subjects' confinement.

Blood samples for determination of theophylline serum levels were drawn in Monovette tubes (Walter Sarstedt, Inc.) at 0 hours (immediately before dosing) and 1, 2, 3, 4, 6, 8, 10, 12, 14, 16, 24, 28, 32, 36, 40, 48, 52, 56, 60, and 72 hours after dosing.

The dosing time study was a four-way, randomized, balanced, crossover (7-day washout) study in which each of 24 subjects received three 300 mg Theo-24 capsules immediately after and at 0.5, 1.0, and 1.5 hours before the high-fat breakfast described previously.

Analytic techniques. Serum theophylline concentrations were determined by an enzyme immunoassay system (EMIT: Syva Co.). Between-day coefficients of variation ranged from 3% to 14% at serum concentrations of 0.6 to 20 μg/ml. Concentrations ≤0.6 μg/ml (detection limit) were considered as zero in all calculations.

Pharmacokinetic and statistical data analyses. Pharmacokinetic model-independent parameters including maximum serum concentration (C_{max}), time to maximum serum concentration (t_{max}), and the AUC (linear trapezoid method) were determined by a standard method.[1] Statistical comparisons of these parameters were made by univariate repeated-measures ANOVA. For the meal composition study the model included terms for individual subjects, meal composition, sequence of meal composition, and study period.

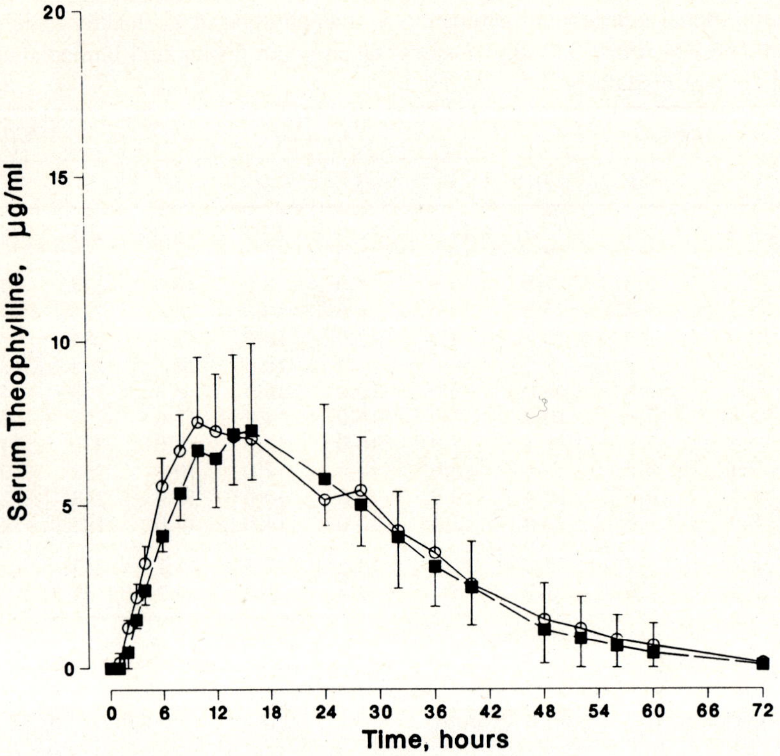

Fig. 1. Mean (± SD) serum theophylline concentration-time curves in 12 subjects after single 900 mg doses of Theo-24 (three 300 mg capsules) under fasting conditions (○) and immediately after a medium-fat breakfast (■).

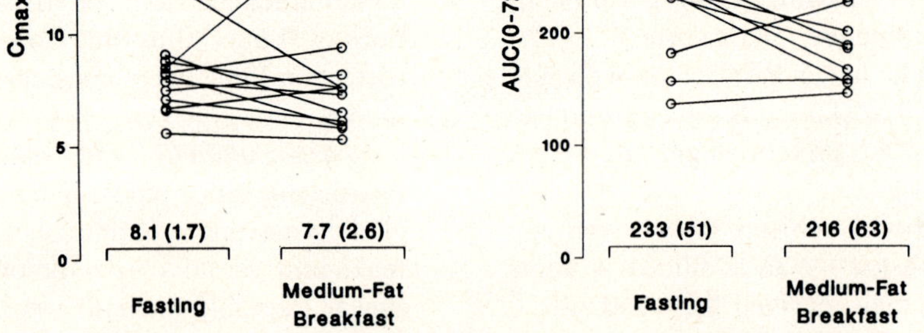

Fig. 2. Individual points and mean (SD) value of theophylline C_{max} and AUC(0-72) in 12 subjects after single 900 mg doses under fasting conditions and immediately after a medium-fat breakfast. *N.S.* = Not significant.

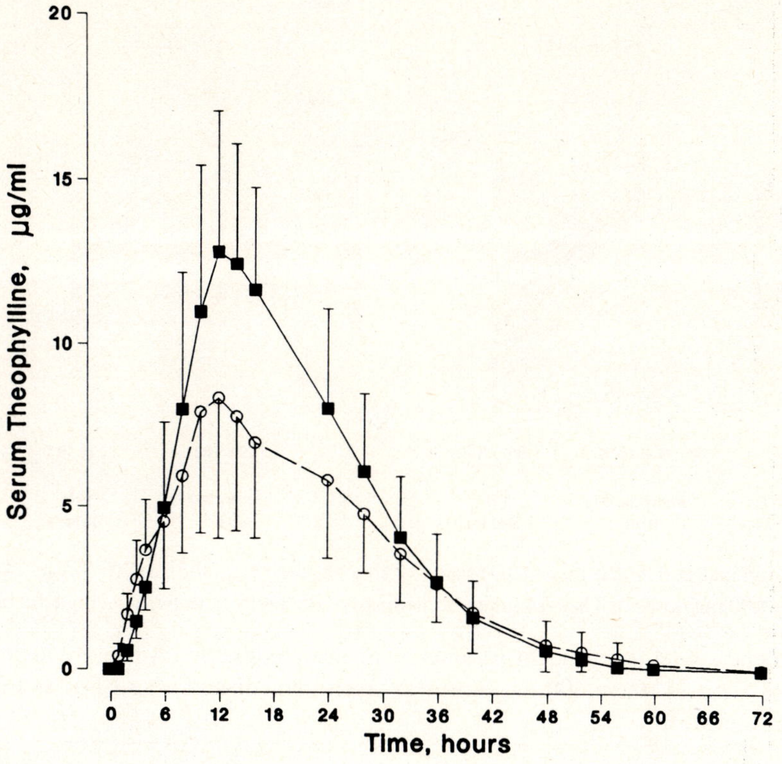

Fig. 3. Mean (± SD) serum theophylline concentration-time curves in 24 subjects after single 900 mg doses of Theo-24 (three 300 mg capsules) immediately after (■) and 1 hour before (○) a high-fat breakfast.

The model for the dosing time study included terms for individual subjects, dosing time, study period, and interaction of dosing time with study period. All statistical testing was performed at the 5% significance level. Data are reported as the $\overline{X} \pm SD$.

RESULTS

Meal composition study. Fig. 1 illustrates that the mean serum theophylline concentration-time curves were similar after a single 900 mg dose of Theo-24 taken under fasting conditions or immediately after a medium-fat breakfast. Differences in C_{max} were not significant when Theo-24 was given immediately after a low-fat breakfast (8.1 ± 2.3 μg/ml), a medium-fat breakfast (7.7 ± 2.6 μg/ml), and under fasting conditions (8.1 ± 1.7 μg/ml; Table I; Fig. 2). Each of these C_{max} values, however, was significantly different from that after the high-fat breakfast (13.0 ± 3.2 μg/ml). Relative to dosing immediately after a high-fat breakfast, C_{max} values were >30% lower in eight of 12 subjects taking Theo-24 immediately after the medium- or low-fat breakfasts. The t_{max} values did not differ significantly after any of the four treatments.

The AUC(0-72) values also did not differ significantly after dosing under fasting conditions (233 ± 51 μg · hr/ml) and immediately after low-fat (214 ± 48 μg · hr/ml) and medium-fat (216 ± 63 μg · hr/ml) breakfasts. Each one of these values, however, was significantly different from the AUC(0-72) after the high-fat breakfast (272 ± 77 μg · hr/ml). The power (1 − β) of the tests to detect a 20% difference relative to the fasting condition was 48% for C_{max}, 22% for t_{max}, and 98% for AUC(0-72) at $\alpha = 0.05$.

Dosing time study. Fig. 3 shows that the mean serum theophylline concentration-time curves were not similar when a single 900 mg dose of Theo-24 was given immediately after or 1 hour before a high-fat breakfast. A time-dependent decrease occurred in C_{max} values when Theo-24 was given immediately after (14.6 ± 3.1 μg/ml) or 0.5 (10.9 ± 3.4 μg/ml), 1.0 (9.4 ± 3.9 μg/ml; Fig. 4) and 1.5 (9.3 ± 3.4 μg/ml) hours before a high-fat breakfast (Table II). Relative to dosing immediately after a high-fat breakfast, C_{max} values decreased by >30% in 11, 14, and 16 of 24 subjects when Theo-24 was dosed 0.5, 1.0, and 1.5 hours, respectively, before this breakfast. The t_{max} values did not differ significantly after any of the four treatments.

The AUC(0-72) values differed significantly depend-

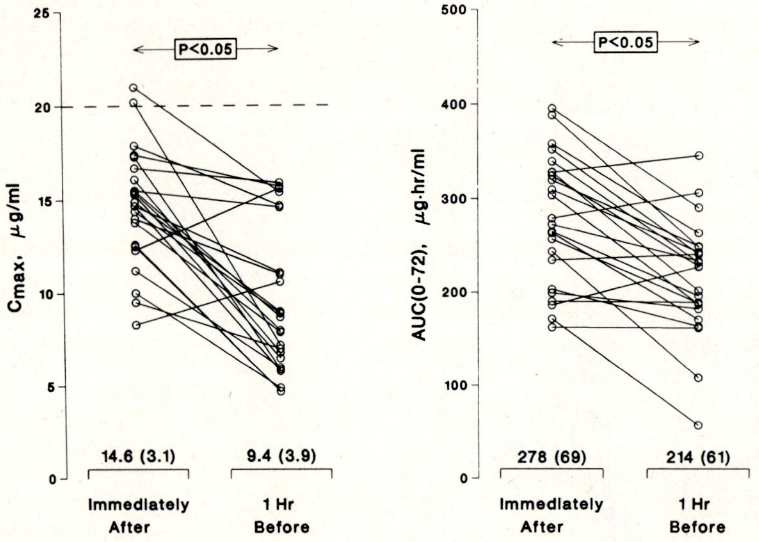

Fig. 4. Individual points and mean (SD) value of theophylline C_{max} and AUC(0-72) in 24 subjects after single 900 mg doses of Theo-24 given immediately after and 1 hour before a high-fat breakfast.

Table II. Pharmacokinetic model-independent parameters of theophylline in 24 healthy male nonsmokers after single 900 mg doses of Theo-24 (three 300 mg capsules) taken immediately after (0.0) and 0.5, 1.0, and 1.5 hours before a high-fat breakfast

Subject No.	C_{max} (µg/ml)				t_{max} (hr)				AUC(0-72) (µg · hr/ml)			
	0.0	0.5	1.0	1.5	0.0	0.5	1.0	1.5	0.0	0.5	1.0	1.5
13	10.0	10.6	4.9	9.2	8.0	6.0	4.0	8.0	171	161	57	147
14	17.9	12.4	14.7	8.9	14.0	14.0	12.0	24.0	279	278	306	232
15	12.6	5.1	4.7	6.2	10.0	10.0	10.0	10.0	190	190	189	185
16	12.5	6.4	4.7	6.4	12.0	14.0	12.0	14.0	203	177	163	190
17	9.5	7.9	7.0	6.7	12.0	12.0	8.0	12.0	162	160	161	125
18	17.3	7.0	5.9	17.3	14.0	16.0	28.0	12.0	352	259	240	329
19	14.7	14.8	5.8	7.4	16.0	14.0	24.0	16.0	324	343	227	232
20	16.1	10.3	6.8	9.8	12.0	12.0	8.0	12.0	328	271	201	290
21	20.2	11.0	7.2	6.8	12.0	10.0	12.0	8.0	265	183	196	198
22	16.7	16.1	15.9	9.4	16.0	10.0	12.0	14.0	395	325	290	242
23	14.7	10.8	11.1	12.3	10.0	12.0	10.0	10.0	309	310	242	266
24	17.4	16.8	15.7	11.3	10.0	12.0	10.0	8.0	328	326	345	277
25	11.2	5.6	6.0	4.6	8.0	14.0	10.0	6.0	243	175	108	104
26	21.0	13.1	15.4	9.1	12.0	10.0	12.0	16.0	358	265	263	271
27	15.5	8.8	8.7	10.1	10.0	28.0	14.0	12.0	388	301	248	317
28	14.9	13.9	9.0	6.7	10.0	12.0	10.0	14.0	199	241	182	120
29	14.4	11.4	8.9	17.2	10.0	14.0	10.0	12.0	304	212	187	271
30	13.8	14.2	7.9	8.3	24.0	24.0	24.0	24.0	320	327	249	245
31	8.3	9.5	10.6	6.3	24.0	16.0	24.0	8.0	186	228	227	158
32	14.0	10.1	11.0	9.6	24.0	14.0	24.0	24.0	272	289	233	260
33	12.3	12.9	15.6	6.9	14.0	16.0	12.0	12.0	234	285	240	214
34	15.4	9.8	8.0	11.0	10.0	10.0	14.0	24.0	339	275	232	422
35	15.5	7.9	14.6	15.1	10.0	12.0	10.0	10.0	257	232	188	230
36	15.3	16.1	6.5	7.4	12.0	10.0	16.0	12.0	263	221	170	187
$\overline{X}$	14.6	10.9*	9.4*	9.3*	13.1	13.4	13.8	13.4	278	251*	214*†	230*
SD	3.1	3.4	3.9	3.4	4.7	4.6	6.3	5.5	69	57	61	73

*$P < 0.05$ compared with 0-hour level.
†$P < 0.05$ compared with 0.5-hour level.

ing on whether Theo-24 was dosed immediately after (278 ± 69 μg · hr/ml) or 0.5 (251 ± 57 μg · hr/ml), 1.0 (214 ± 61 μg · hr/ml), and 1.5 (230 ± 73 μg · hr/ml) hours before the high-fat breakfast. The power of the tests to detect a 20% difference relative to dosing immediately after breakfast was >99% for AUC(0-72), 94% for C_{max}, and 65% for t_{max} at $\alpha = 0.05$.

DISCUSSION

Our study emphasizes the importance of standardizing experimental conditions when assessing food-induced absorption changes from controlled-release formulations of theophylline. Both the composition of the meal and dosing time relative to meal intake were found to be important factors affecting absorption. In the former case, the serum theophylline concentration-time curves were similar when Theo-24 was taken under fasting conditions or immediately after a low- to medium-fat breakfast. Enhancement in the rate and extent of theophylline absorption, however, occurred when Theo-24 was dosed immediately after a high-fat breakfast. In the subsequent study it was found that this enhancement of absorption was significantly lessened when Theo-24 was taken at least 1 hour before a high-fat breakfast.

Previous studies[3-5,11] have demonstrated that changes in absorption of controlled-release formulations induced by high-fat meals occur with products that differ in their mechanism of drug release, and with formulations that have pH-dependent or pH-independent in vitro dissolution characteristics. Ingestion of a high-fat meal is known to result in delayed gastric emptying and increased secretion of bile, pancreatic fluid, digestive enzymes, and gastric hormones. One or a combination of these factors is probably responsible for the absorption changes. From our findings it is apparent that the optimal condition to demonstrate food-induced absorption changes from a controlled-release formulation of theophylline, and possibly other drugs, is to administer the test preparation immediately after a high-fat (>55 gm fat) breakfast. In comparing food-induced absorption changes from different formulations of theophylline, it is therefore important to verify that the studies were done under similar experimental conditions.

The effect of meal composition and dosing time relative to meal intake on the absorption characteristics of theophylline should be assessed for all controlled-release formulations that are affected by food. In the case of Theo-24, our study demonstrates that to assure consistent, slow absorption, patients taking high doses (≥900 mg) once a day should take this product in the morning under fasting conditions or with a breakfast containing approximately ≤10 gm fat. If a high-fat breakfast (>55 gm fat) is taken, then the drug should be dosed at least 1 hour before the meal.

The clinical phase of the dosing time study was conducted at PharmaKinetics Laboratories (Baltimore, Md.) with Wallace A. Riley, M.D., as the principal investigator. Theophylline serum levels were determined in the Bioanalytical Department of G. D. Searle & Co. under the direction of Charles L. Jeuell, Ph.D.

References

1. Gibaldi M, Perrier D: Pharmacokinetics, ed 2. New York, 1982, Marcel Dekker, Inc.
2. Hendeles L, Iafrate RP, Weinberger M: A clinical and pharmacokinetic basis for the selection and use of slow release theophylline products. Clin Pharmacokinet **9:**95-135, 1984.
3. Karim A: Theophylline with food: Theo-24. Am Pharmacy **NS25:**4-5, 1985.
4. Karim A, Burns T, Wearley L, Streicher J, Palmer M: Food-induced changes in theophylline absorption from controlled-release formulations. Part I. Substantial increased and decreased absorption with Uniphyl tablets and Theo-Dur Sprinkle. CLIN PHARMACOL THER **38:**77-83, 1985.
5. Lagas M, Jonkman JHG: Greatly enhanced bioavailability of theophylline on postprandial administration of a sustained release tablet. Eur J Clin Pharmacol **24:**761-767, 1983.
6. Leeds NH, Gal P, Purohit AA, Walter JB: Effect of food on the bioavailability and pattern of release of a sustained-release theophylline tablet. J Clin Pharmacol **22:**196-200, 1982.
7. Osman MA, Patel RB, Irwin DS, Welling PG: Absorption of theophylline from enteric coated and sustained release formulations in fasted and non-fasted subjects. Biopharm Drug Dispos **4:**63-72, 1983.
8. Pedersen S: Delay in the absorption rate of theophylline from a sustained release theophylline preparation caused by food. Br J Clin Pharmacol **12:**904-905, 1981.
9. Pedersen S, Moller-Petersen J: Erratic absorption of a slow-release theophylline sprinkle product. Pediatrics **74:**534-538, 1984.
10. Thompson PJ, Kemp MW, McAllister WAC, Turner-Warwick M: Slow release theophylline in patients with airways obstruction with particular reference to the effects of food upon serum levels. Br J Dis Chest **77:**293-298, 1983.
11. Vaughan L, Milavetz G, Hill M, Weinberger M, Hendeles L: Food-induced dose-dumping of Theo-24, a "once-daily" slow-release theophylline product. Drug Intell Clin Pharm **18:**510, 1984.

Interaction of ibuprofen with the H-2 receptor antagonists ranitidine and cimetidine

The influences of cimetidine and ranitidine on single-dose ibuprofen kinetics were evaluated. Thirteen healthy subjects took a single, 600 mg oral dose of ibuprofen on three occasions: (1) in the control state without drug coadministration; (2) during concurrent dosing with cimetidine, 1.2 gm/day; and (3) during concurrent dosing with ranitidine, 150 mg twice daily. Compared with the control state, cimetidine increased the peak serum ibuprofen concentration (64 vs. 56 μg/ml), but the value during ranitidine dosing (57 μg/ml) was indistinguishable from the control value. There were no significant differences between control, cimetidine, and ranitidine conditions in ibuprofen elimination $t_{1/2}$ (2.1, 2.1, and 2.0 hours, respectively). Overall there was a significant difference among the control, cimetidine, and ranitidine conditions in ibuprofen oral clearance (52.8, 48.3, and 54.1 ml/min, respectively), but individual differences in cimetidine vs. control and between ranitidine vs. control were not statistically significant. The impairment of ibuprofen clearance by cimetidine is small, and ranitidine had no detectable effect on ibuprofen kinetics. These findings should be further validated during chronic dosing with ibuprofen. (Clin Pharmacol Ther 38:648-651, 1985.)

Hermann R. Ochs, M.D.,* David J. Greenblatt, M.D., Rita Matlis, B.S., and Jutta Weinbrenner, M.D. *Bonn, Federal Republic of Germany, and Boston, Mass.*

This work is dedicated to Prof. Dr. med. F. Scheler on the occasion of his sixtieth birthday.

Ibuprofen is a nonsteroidal anti-inflammatory drug extensively prescribed for the treatment of pain and inflammatory disorders.[10] Many individuals who require treatment with ibuprofen also receive H_2-receptor antagonists, because of either concurrent gastrointestinal disorders or the side effects associated with ibuprofen therapy. The H_2-antagonist cimetidine can cause a number of pharmacokinetic drug interactions, because it has the capacity to impair hepatic microsomal drug oxidizing capacity.[13,15,16] On the other hand, ranitidine has relatively little effect on drug oxidizing capacity,[2,9,12] and therefore produces few pharmacokinetic drug interactions. Our present study evaluated the influence of concurrent dosing with cimetidine and ranitidine on the pharmacokinetics of a single dose of ibuprofen in healthy subjects.

METHODS

Thirteen healthy subjects (10 men and three women) between 23 and 31 years old participated after giving written informed consent. All were healthy, active, ambulatory adults with no evidence of medical disease. Two of the women were taking oral contraceptive steroids, but otherwise subjects were taking no other medications.

Subjects participated in a single-dose, three-way crossover trial. On each occasion, a single 600 mg oral dose of ibuprofen (Dolorgiet GmbH) was taken in the fasting state. The three conditions of dosing were as follows: (1) Control, with no other drugs given; (2) concurrent dosing with cimetidine, 400 mg t.i.d., beginning 48 hours before ibuprofen dosing and continuing for the entire 15 hours of the ibuprofen kinetic study; and (3) concurrent dosing with ranitidine, 150 mg b.i.d., beginning 48 hours before ibuprofen dosing and continuing for the entire 15 hours of the ibuprofen kinetic study. At least 1 week elapsed between the three trials, the sequence of which was randomized.

From the Medizinische Universitätsklinik, University of Bonn, Bonn, and the Division of Clinical Pharmacology, Tufts-New England Medical Center, Boston.

Supported in part by Grant No. Oc 10/6-4 from Deutsche Forschungsgemeinschaft and Grant No. MH-34223 from the United States Public Health Service.

Received for publication May 10, 1985; accepted July 30, 1985.

Reprint requests to: Prof. Dr. med. H. R. Ochs, Marienkrankenhaus, Widumgasse 5, D-4770 Soest, Federal Republic of Germany.

*Present address: Marienkrankenhaus, Soest, Federal Republic of Germany.

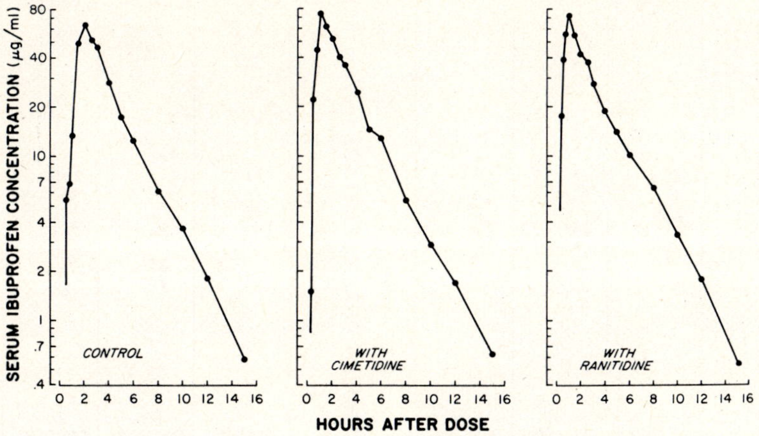

Fig. 1. Serum ibuprofen concentrations in a representative subject in the control state and during coadministration of cimetidine or ranitidine.

For each ibuprofen kinetic study, a single 600 mg oral dose of ibuprofen was taken after an overnight fast with 150 ml tap water. Subjects remained fasting until 3 hours after dosing. Venous blood samples were drawn into additive-free tubes before ibuprofen dosing and 0.25, 0.5, 0.75, 1, 1.5, 2, 2.5, 3, 4, 5, 6, 8, 10, 12, and 15 hours thereafter. Blood samples were allowed to clot and the serum was separated and frozen until analyzed.

Concentrations of ibuprofen in all serum samples were determined by HPLC.[7] All samples from a subject's set of three trials were extracted and analyzed together by use of the same calibration standards. Compliance with the prescribed cimetidine or ranitidine regimens was verified by HPLC[6] analysis of serum samples drawn before and 4, 8, and 12 hours after ibuprofen dosing to determine steady-state concentrations of cimetidine or ranitidine.

The slope (β) of the terminal log-linear phase of the serum ibuprofen concentration-time curve was determined by linear regression analysis. This was used to calculate the apparent elimination $t_{1/2}$ of ibuprofen. The AUC until the final detectable concentration was determined by the trapezoidal method and extrapolated to infinity by use of the ratio of the final concentration divided by β, to yield the total AUC. Apparent oral clearance (CL_o) of ibuprofen was determined as: CL_o = Dose/AUC, and apparent volume of distribution (V_{area}) was calculated as: $V_{area} = CL_o/\beta$. Because the absolute bioavailability of orally administered ibuprofen is not known, values of CL_o and V_{area} are termed "apparent" (calculations of true values would require knowledge of absolute systemic availability).

Overall differences in kinetic variables for ibuprofen across the three dosing conditions were evaluated by repeated-measures ANOVA. When significant differences were found, individual differences between control and cimetidine and between control and ranitidine conditions were evaluated by Dunnett's t test.

Table I. Steady-state serum concentrations of cimetidine and ranitidine

Time after ibuprofen dosing	*Cimetidine (μg/ml)*	*Ranitidine (ng/ml)*
Before	0.49 ± 0.19	109 ± 37
4 hr	1.12 ± 0.15	306 ± 44
8 hr	0.82 ± 0.12	189 ± 36
12 hr	0.92 ± 0.18	182 ± 25

Data are $\overline{X}$ ± SE.

RESULTS

Serum cimetidine and ranitidine concentrations indicated good compliance with the prescribed regimens (Table I). Concentrations at each sampling time were consistent with those encountered during usual clinical use of these doses.[14,16]

Fig. 1 shows serum ibuprofen concentrations in a representative subject in each of the three conditions. There were significant differences among conditions in the peak serum ibuprofen concentration (Table II). The peak serum levels in the control and ranitidine conditions were essentially identical (56 and 57 μg/ml), but the peak level during cimetidine coadministration (64 μg/ml) was significantly higher ($P < 0.05$) than that during the control condition. No significant differences were observed among the three conditions in the time of peak concentration (Table II).

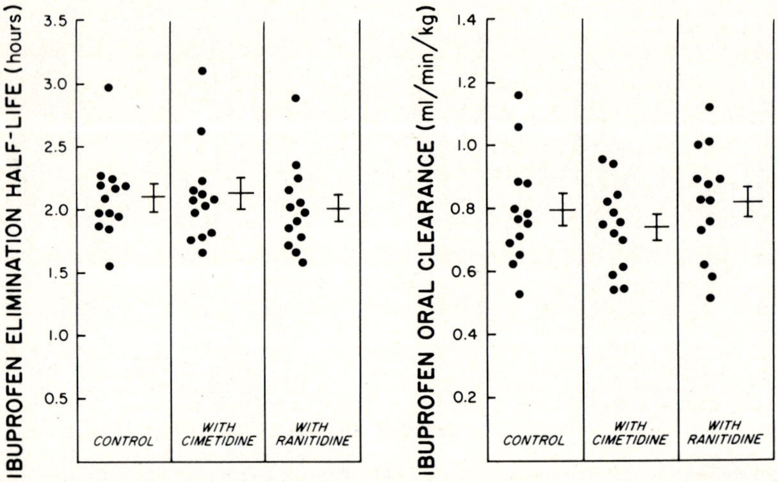

Fig. 2. Individual and mean (±SE) values of ibuprofen elimination $t_{1/2}$ *(left)* and CL_O *(right)* in the three dosing conditions (see Table II for statistical analysis).

Table II. Effect of cimetidine and ranitidine on ibuprofen kinetics

	Control	*Cimetidine*	*Ranitidine*	*F value**
Peak serum concentration (μg/ml)	56 ± 3	64 ± 3	57 ± 3	4.42†
Time of peak (hr after dose)	1.38 ± 0.15	1.33 ± 0.2	1.23 ± 0.2	0.25
Elimination $t_{1/2}$ (hr)	2.10 ± 0.09	2.11 ± 0.11	2.01 ± 0.10	1.39
Total AUC (μg/ml · hr)	203 ± 15	216 ± 13	196 ± 16	3.83‡
V_{area}				
L	9.4 ± 0.6	8.7 ± 0.5	9.2 ± 0.5	2.09
L/kg	0.14 ± 0.01	0.13 ± 0.01	0.14 ± 0.01	1.65
CL_O				
ml/min	52.8 ± 4.2	48.3 ± 2.8	54.1 ± 3.4	3.72‡
ml/min/kg	0.796 ± 0.048	0.736 ± 0.039	0.824 ± 0.049	3.87‡

Data are $\bar{X}$ ± SE.
*Degrees of freedom = 2,24 (ANOVA).
†P < 0.025.; ‡P < 0.05.

The three conditions did not differ significantly in ibuprofen elimination $t_{1/2}$ or V_{area} (Fig. 2; Table II). The conditions did differ ($P < 0.05$) in total AUC for ibuprofen and in ibuprofen CL_O, regardless of whether CL_O was corrected for body weight. Neither the cimetidine nor the ranitidine conditions individually differed from the control value based on Dunnett's t test. Inspection of the AUC and CL_O values indicates that control and ranitidine values were nearly identical. During cimetidine coadministration, the AUC increased and CL_O decreased relative to the control value, but the magnitude of the differences was small, with the mean CL_O during cimetidine dosing differing from the control value by <10%.

DISCUSSION

The potential pharmacokinetic interaction of nonsteroidal anti-inflammatory drugs with H_2-receptor antagonists is of considerable importance, since these two classes of drugs are among the most widely prescribed in the world and are very likely to be frequently coadministered. The capacity of cimetidine to impair hepatic drug oxidizing capacity is well established.[1,4-6,8,9,12,15,16] In some cases, the reduction in clearance of drugs influenced by this interaction can lead to considerable elevations in steady-state concentrations during multiple dosing, and sometimes these interactions have been of clinical importance.[15,16] In the case of ranitidine, a number of studies suggest that it does not impair drug oxidizing capacity to the same extent as does cimetidine,[2,9,12] and therefore is less likely to induce pharmacokinetic drug interactions.

The major metabolic pathway of ibuprofen in man involves a series of microsomal oxidative reactions.[11] One would predict that these metabolic reactions might be susceptible to impairment by cimetidine, but would be relatively spared during coadministration of ranitidine. We evaluated the effect of therapeutic doses, with verified therapeutic serum concentrations, of both cimetidine and ranitidine on the kinetics of a single dose of ibuprofen. Our findings indicated that ibuprofen kinetics were essentially identical between control and ranitidine dosing conditions, indicating a lack of a detectable pharmacokinetic interaction between these two drugs. The effects of cimetidine on ibuprofen kinetics also were minimal, consistent with an earlier report.[3] The peak serum ibuprofen concentration was increased during cimetidine dosing, but the small reduction in ibuprofen CL_0 during cimetidine dosing was not significant.

Our findings suggest that a pharmacokinetic interaction between single doses of ibuprofen and either cimetidine or ranitidine during usual clinical use is unlikely. Further studies are needed to evaluate this potential interaction during chronic dosing with ibuprofen.

We are grateful for the assistance of Monika Linden and Jerold S. Harmatz.

References

1. Abernethy DR, Greenblatt DJ, Divoll M, Ameer B, Shader RI: Differential effect of cimetidine on drug oxidation (antipyrine and diazepam) vs. conjugation (acetaminophen and lorazepam): Prevention of acetaminophen toxicity by cimetidine. J Pharmacol Exp Ther **224:**508-513, 1983.
2. Abernethy DR, Greenblatt DJ, Eshelman FN, Shader RI: Ranitidine does not impair oxidative or conjugative metabolism: Noninteraction with antipyrine, diazepam, and lorazepam. Clin Pharmacol Ther **35:**188-192, 1984.
3. Conrad KA, Mayersohn M, Bliss M: Cimetidine does not alter ibuprofen kinetics after a single dose. Br J Clin Pharmacol **18:**624-626, 1984.
4. Desmond PV, Patwardhan RV, Schenker S, Speeg KV: Cimetidine impairs elimination of chlordiazepoxide (Librium) in man. Ann Intern Med **93:**266-268, 1980.
5. Greenblatt DJ, Abernethy DR, Koepke HH, Shader RI: Interaction of cimetidine with oxazepam, lorazepam, and flurazepam. J Clin Pharmacol **24:**187-193, 1984.
6. Greenblatt DJ, Abernethy DR, Morse DS, Shader RI, Harmatz JS: Clinical importance of the interaction of diazepam and cimetidine. N Engl J Med **310:**1639-1643, 1984.
7. Greenblatt DJ, Arendt RM, Locniskar A: Ibuprofen pharmacokinetics: Use of liquid chromatography with radial compression separation. Arzneimittelforsch **33:**1671-1673, 1983.
8. Hardy BG, Zador IT, Golden L, Lalka D, Schentag JJ: Effect of cimetidine on the pharmacokinetics and pharmacodynamics of quinidine. Am J Cardiol **52:**172-175, 1983.
9. Henry DA, MacDonald IA, Kitchingman G, Bell GD, Langman MJS: Cimetidine and ranitidine: Comparison of effects on hepatic drug metabolism. Br Med J **281:**775-777, 1980.
10. Kantor TG: Ibuprofen. Ann Intern Med **91:**877-882, 1979.
11. Mills RFN, Adams SS, Cliffe EE, Dickenson W, Nicholson JS: The metabolism of ibuprofen. Xenobiotica **3:**589-598, 1973.
12. Powell JR, Rogers JF, Wargin WA, Cross RE, Eshelman FN: Inhibition of theophylline clearance by cimetidine but not ranitidine. Arch Intern Med **144:**484-486, 1984.
13. Puurunen J, Sotaniemi E, Pelkonen O: Effect of cimetidine on microsomal drug metabolism in man. Eur J Clin Pharmacol **18:**185-187, 1980.
14. Roberts CJC: Clinical pharmacokinetics of ranitidine. Clin Pharmacokinet **9:**211-221, 1984.
15. Sedman AJ: Cimetidine-drug interactions. Am J Med **76:**109-114, 1984.
16. Somogyi A, Gugler R: Clinical pharmacokinetics of cimetidine. Clin Pharmacokinet **8:**463-495, 1983.

Effect of single doses of cimetidine and ranitidine on the steady-state plasma levels of midazolam

H_2-Receptor antagonists may interfere with the pharmacokinetics of concomitantly administered drugs. Our study was designed to investigate whether cimetidine or ranitidine influence the disposition and sedative effect of midazolam. The effect of single oral doses of 800 mg cimetidine, 300 mg ranitidine, or placebo on the steady-state concentrations of midazolam was examined in a randomized crossover study in eight healthy subjects. A midazolam steady-state concentration was achieved by an intravenous bolus (0.05 mg/kg)-infusion (0.025 mg/kg/hr) technique. Plasma concentrations of midazolam, cimetidine, and ranitidine and the pharmacodynamic response to midazolam (choice reaction time, sedation index) were monitored throughout the 10-hour infusion. Cimetidine significantly increased the mean (± SD) steady-state plasma concentration of midazolam from 56.7 ± 7.8 to 71.3 ± 19.6 ng/ml ($P = 0.004$). In contrast, the steady-state midazolam concentration after ranitidine dosing (61.8 ± 6.8 ng/ml) did not differ significantly from that after placebo. No change in choice reaction time or sedation index was detected after cimetidine or ranitidine dosing. Nevertheless, in contrast to ranitidine, the recently advocated once-daily dosing of cimetidine has a potential for hepatic drug interaction that should be considered before its coadministration with drugs that have a narrow therapeutic index. (CLIN PHARMACOL THER 38:652-655, 1985.)

Ulrich Klotz, Ph.D., Pentti Arvela, Ph.D.,* and Bernd Rosenkranz, M.D.
Stuttgart, Federal Republic of Germany

The H_2-receptor antagonists cimetidine and ranitidine are among the most widely prescribed drugs. Both are now recommended for use in a single nocturnal dose for the treatment of peptic ulcer, because suppression of the nocturnal peaks in acid secretion seems to be the most important factor for therapeutic benefit.[6,9,13] Differences in the chemical structures of cimetidine and ranitidine are reflected in their different side effect profiles.[3,5] Especially important is the ability of cimetidine to bind to the cytochrome P-450 group of enzymes, thus impairing the hepatic metabolism of a great variety of drugs.[10,15] Surprisingly, one study reported that ranitidine significantly increased the oral bioavailability of midazolam,[4] a new rapidly eliminated benzodiazepine.[1,11] This alleged interaction might have resulted from an increase in the pH-dependent absorption of midazolam or to a decrease in the hepatic first-pass effect of this relatively high-clearance drug.

Our study was designed to assess whether cimetidine, 800 mg, and ranitidine, 300 mg, given as single doses have any significant effect on the hepatic metabolism of midazolam as assessed by their effect on the steady-state plasma concentration of intravenous midazolam and whether any such change is reflected as a parallel change in the pharmacodynamic effect of midazolam.

METHODS

Eight healthy men 24 to 46 years old weighing 62 to 85 kg who were taking no other drugs gave their written informed consent to participate. On three different occasions separated by at least 1 week, each subject received an intravenous bolus over 30 seconds of 0.05 mg/kg midazolam followed immediately by a constant infusion of 0.025 mg/kg/hr for 10 hours. A single oral dose of placebo, 800 mg cimetidine, and 300 mg ranitidine was given in random order 2 hours

From Dr. Margarete Fischer-Bosch-Institut für Klinische Pharmakologie.
Supported by the Robert Bosch Foundation, Stuttgart, West Germany.
Received for publication June 18, 1985; accepted Aug. 6, 1985.
Reprint requests to: U. Klotz, Ph.D., Dr. Margarete Fischer-Bosch-Institut für Klinische Pharmakologie, D-7000 Stuttgart 50, Auerbachstraße 112, Federal Republic of Germany.
*Fellow of the Alexander von Humbold Foundation, Bonn, West Germany. Present address: Department of Pharmacology, University of Oulu, Oulu, Finland.

after the start of the midazolam infusion. Blood samples (10 ml) were drawn before and 0.5, 1, 1.5, 2, 2.5, 3, 3.5, 4, 5, 6, 8, and 10 hours after the benzodiazepine injection. Plasma was separated and stored at −25° C until measurement of midazolam concentrations by a sensitive and specific gas chromatographic analysis[1,11] and of cimetidine and ranitidine concentrations by HPLC.[2] The peak of the only metabolite of midazolam detectable in plasma (α-hydroxymidazolam) in measurable concentrations (range 10 to 25 ng/ml during steady-state infusion) was well separated (retention time = 13.8 minutes) from that of unchanged midazolam (12 minutes).

At the time of blood sampling, the sedative effect of midazolam alone and in combination with each of the two H_2-receptor antagonists was assessed by a sedation index created from five visual analog scales and by measurement of choice reaction times (mean of 10 consecutive trials) by the Leeds psychomotor test (Zak). Before the study subjects underwent several training sessions with these tests to eliminate any learning effect during the study periods.

Pharmacodynamic test values and the steady-state plasma concentrations of midazolam 6, 8, and 10 hours after its intravenous administration by the bolus/infusion technique (4 to 8 hours after placebo, cimetidine, or ranitidine dosing) were compared statistically by the nonparametric Friedman test (overall effects) and subsequently by the Wilcoxon test (comparison of two groups). Individual values listed in the tables represent the mean value of the above three time points. The plasma AUC was calculated by the trapezoidal rule.

RESULTS

Steady-state plasma concentrations of midazolam were rapidly achieved by the bolus-infusion program used. After concomitant oral dosing with cimetidine, mean (±SD) plasma concentrations of midazolam increased by 26%, from 56.7 ± 7.8 to 71.3 ± 19.6 ng/ml (P = 0.004). In contrast, the steady-state plasma concentration of midazolam after ranitidine dosing did not differ significantly from placebo (Table I).

The rise in the plasma midazolam concentrations after cimetidine dosing was not associated with a measurable increase in its sedative effects (Table II). After the single oral doses of cimetidine and ranitidine, maximal plasma concentrations of both drugs were reached within 1.5 to 3 hours, and in some subjects a second peak was observed 3 to 6 hours after dosing. In general, plasma concentrations of cimetidine exceeded those of ranitidine by a factor of 4.5 to 5 (Table III).

Table I. Steady-state plasma levels of midazolam (ng/ml) during infusion

Subject	*Placebo*	*Cimetidine, 800 mg*	*Ranitidine, 300 mg*
U. K.	39.7	57.0	60.1
F. S.	62.8	104.4	59.8
B. R.	61.9	99.9	64.7
D. G.	58.9	65.0	76.8
T. F.	54.6	58.1	54.9
P. A.	59.8	68.5	63.7
U. W.	62.7	62.9	57.2
W. H.	53.2	54.7	57.0
$\bar{X}$ ± SD	56.7 ± 7.8	71.3 ± 19.6*	61.8 ± 6.9

χ^2(overall effect) = 7.75 (0.01 < P < 0.05).
*P = 0.004 (Wilcoxon test) compared with placebo.

DISCUSSION

Our pharmacodynamic and pharmacokinetic steady-state interaction study with midazolam as a probe drug with an intermediate high hepatic clearance (blood clearance in the range of 400 to 600 ml/min[1,11,12]) demonstrates that a single oral dose of 800 mg cimetidine impairs the hepatic elimination of the benzodiazepine. This can be concluded directly from the increase in the steady-state plasma midazolam concentrations, which are reciprocally related to its total body clearance. Apparently, there is no relationship between the plasma cimetidine concentration and the extent of inhibition of midazolam metabolism, because plasma concentrations of midazolam increased independent of the peak concentration and AUC of cimetidine (Tables I and III). The cimetidine-midazolam interaction (probably by competitive inhibition at the cytochrome P-450 binding sites) is rapid in onset; the increase in the steady-state plasma midazolam concentration was observed 4 to 8 hours after a single dose of the H_2-receptor antagonist. By the end of the 10-hour sampling period a new steady-state plateau of midazolam ($t_{1/2}$ about 2 hours[1,11]) had been approximately 90% achieved. The observed 26% increase in plasma midazolam concentrations might therefore represent an underestimation of the inhibitory potential of cimetidine, and slightly higher plasma midazolam concentrations would probably have been observed had sampling continued longer. In contrast, the single oral dose of 300 mg ranitidine had no significant effect on the steady-state plasma midazolam concentrations. This is in agreement with the large number of drug interaction studies in which no inhibition of drug metabolism by ranitidine could be demonstrated.[10,15]

Our investigation with intravenous midazolam might

Table II. Sedative effects of midazolam during its steady-state infusion and concomitant oral dosing with placebo, cimetidine, or ranitidine

	Reaction time 1 (msec)			*Reaction time 2 (msec)*			*Sedation index (cm)*		
Subject	*Placebo*	*Cimetidine*	*Ranitidine*	*Placebo*	*Cimetidine*	*Ranitidine*	*Placebo*	*Cimetidine*	*Ranitidine*
U. K.	386	431	402	549	611	587	24.4	35.8	27.1
F. S.	439	502	436	600	638	587	42.0	36.3	42.9
B. R.	348	332	344	448	435	438	38.8	34.7	28.7
D. G.	490	415	375	598	609	485	22.3	14.1	16.3
T. F.	563	535	534	736	705	680	17.1	13.4	14.2
P. A.	502	430	379	798	771	599	8.4	12.5	11.1
U. W.	378	490	358	608	749	506	26.0	31.0	29.4
W. H.	352	351	334	478	438	433	25.2	23.5	20.7
$\overline{X}$	432	448	395	602	620	539	25.5	25.2	23.8
SD	79	78	65	119	128	87	10.8	10.6	10.4

Table III. Maximal plasma concentrations and AUCs of both H_2-receptor antagonists after single oral doses

	Cimetidine, 800 mg		*Ranitidine, 300 mg*	
Subject	C_{max} *(μg/ml)*	*AUC(0-8) (μg/ml/hr)*	C_{max} *(μg/ml)*	*AUC(0-8) (μg/ml/hr)*
U. K.	3.03	14.4	0.62	2.9
F. S.	1.80	10.6	0.55	2.4
B. R.	2.33	8.0	0.53	2.0
D. G.	2.82	13.1	0.67	3.1
T. F.	2.23	9.8	0.80	3.8
P. A.	3.96	15.1	0.36	2.2
U. W.	2.43	13.2	0.39	1.9
W. H.	1.65	7.7	0.32	1.5
$\overline{X}$	2.53	11.5	0.53	2.5
SD	0.74	2.9	0.17	0.8

C_{max} = Maximum plasma concentration.

also clarify the mechanism of the reported ranitidine-induced increase in plasma midazolam concentrations after a single oral dose of 15 mg.[4] Midazolam has a water-soluble, open-ring structure that closes at pH levels >4.0, resulting in increased lipid solubility. Consequently, absorption from the stomach is probably facilitated and increased by any drug (e.g., H_2-receptor antagonists, antacids) that raises gastric pH. It is therefore possible that the previously reported ranitidine-midazolam interaction results from increased absorption of midazolam rather than from an effect on hepatic metabolism.

The pharmacodynamic response to infused midazolam showed considerable inter- and intraindividual variability during all three parts of the study (Table II). It is therefore not surprising that the increased plasma midazolam concentrations induced by cimetidine were not associated with measurable increases in sedative activity. In addition, within the measured concentration range the concentration-response curve might run very flat. Any sedation effect may also have been counterbalanced by the development of tolerance to the sedative effect of midazolam towards the end of the 10-hour infusion.

The lack of a pharmacodynamic interaction could be also due to central nervous system effects of the H_2-receptor antagonists, thus partly antagonizing the midazolam-induced sedation. However, two recent studies have clearly demonstrated that neither cimetidine nor ranitidine had any significant effects on performance, central nervous system function, or subjective assessment of mood.[14,16] Thus it is most unlikely that the effects of increased midazolam plasma levels were offset by stimulant effects of cimetidine or ranitidine.

Our study evaluated once-daily dosing with 800 mg cimetidine or 300 mg ranitidine and shows that these dosage regimens are similar to the multiple dosing scheme in terms of effects on the hepatic elimination of concomitantly administered drugs. This hepatic interaction with cimetidine should be kept in mind when drugs with a narrow therapeutic margin are given concurrently.

References

1. Allonen H, Ziegler G, Klotz U: Midazolam kinetics. CLIN PHARMACOL THER **30:**653-661, 1981.
2. Boutagy J, More DG, Munro IA, Shenfield GM: Simultaneous analysis of cimetidine and ranitidine in human plasma by HPLC. J Liquid Chromatogr **7:**1651-1664, 1984.
3. Editorial: Ranitidine or cimetidine. Ann Intern Med **99:**551-553, 1983.
4. Elwood RJ, Hildebrand PJ, Dundee JW, Collier PS: Ra-

nitidine influences the uptake of oral midazolam. Br J Clin Pharmacol **15:**743-745, 1983.

5. Feely J, Wormsley KG: H_2-receptor antagonists—cimetidine and ranitidine. Br Med J **286:**695-697, 1983.
6. Gledhill T, Howard OM, Buck M, Paul A, Hunt RH: Single nocturnal dose of an H_2-receptor antagonist for the treatment of duodenal ulcer. Gut **24:**903-908, 1983.
7. Henning N, Norpoth L: Die Magensekretion während des Schlafes. Dtsch Arch Klin Med **172:**558, 1932.
8. Howden CW, Jones DB, Hunt RH: Nocturnal doses of H_2 receptor antagonists for duodenal ulcer. Lancet **1:**647-648, 1985.
9. Ireland A, Gear P, Colin-Jones DG, Golding PL, Ramage JK, Williams PL, Leicester RJ, Smith CL, Ross G, Bamforth J, de Gara CJ, Gledhill T, Hunt RH: Ranitidine 150 mg twice daily vs 300 mg nightly in treatment of duodenal ulcers. Lancet **2:**274-276, 1984.
10. Klotz U, Reimann IW: Drug interactions through binding to cytochrome P-450: The experience with H_2-receptor blocking agents. Pharm Res **2:**59-62, 1984.
11. Klotz U, Ziegler G: Physiologic and temporal variation in hepatic elimination of midazolam. CLIN PHARMACOL THER **32:**107-112, 1982.
12. Klotz U, Reimann IW: Chronopharmacokinetic study with prolonged infusion of midazolam. Clin Pharmacokinet **9:**469-474, 1984.
13. Müller P, Simon B, Dammann H-G, Feurle G, Lichtwald K, Schmidt-Gayk H: Menschliche Säuresekretion unter täglich einmaliger Gabe von H_2-Blockern. Schweiz Med Wochenschr **114:**667-671, 1984.
14. Nicholson AN, Stone BM: The H_2-antagonists, cimetidine and ranitidine: Studies on performance. Eur J Clin Pharmacol **26:**579-582, 1984.
15. Powell JR, Donn KH: Histamine H_2-antagonist drug interactions in perspective: Mechanistic concepts and clinical implications. Am J Med **77**(suppl 5B):57-84, 1984.
16. Theofilopoulus N, Szabadi E, Bradshaw CM: Comparison of the effects of ranitidine, cimetidine and thioridazine on psychomotor function in healthy volunteers. Br J Clin Pharmacol **18:**135-144, 1984.

Computerized assessment of human neurotoxicity: Sensitivity to nitrous oxide exposure

We recently developed a flexible, portable, computer-based neurobehavioral evaluation system (NES) to standardize data collection in epidemiologic field studies of individuals at risk for neurobehavioral toxicity. The current study was performed to examine the system's sensitivity to subtle neurobehavioral impairment induced pharmacologically in normal subjects. Twelve men 18 to 36 years old were tested with the NES three times, in an initial training session followed by separate drug and control sessions in randomized order. During drug sessions subjects received a combination of 20% nitrous oxide and 80% oxygen through a nasal mask. In control sessions subjects received 100% oxygen. Nine NES tests evaluating psychomotor performance, visuospatial ability, memory, and mood were administered in approximately 40 minutes. Nitrous oxide exposure impaired performance on three tests: continuous performance, symbol-digit substitution, and finger tapping. Another test, pattern memory, showed a trend toward impairment, while the remainder were not affected by the drug. These data are consistent with previous reports that the threshold effect of nitrous oxide is a decrement in psychomotor speed. The findings indicate that our NES is sensitive to short-term impairment in central nervous system function of the type induced by a number of neuroactive agents. In view of its efficiency in data acquisition and analysis, computerized neurobehavioral testing appears to be a very promising method for evaluation of effects of a wide range of pharmacologic agents. (CLIN PHARMACOL THER 38:656-660, 1985.)

Benjamin D. Greenberg, Ph.D., Paul A. Moore, D.M.D., Ph.D., Richard Letz, Ph.D., and Edward L. Baker, M.D., M.P.H. *Boston, Mass.*

Neurobehavioral tests have long been recognized as powerful tools in the assessment of functional impairment in the central nervous system (CNS) produced by a variety of causes, including naturally occurring disease, head trauma, or exposure to neurotoxic agents.[9] One recent development that promises to enhance the utility and expand the uses of neurobehavioral testing (for example, in fields such as neurobehavioral toxicology) has been tests that can be administered by computer. As compared with traditional methods, a computer-based neurobehavioral evaluation system (NES) offers the advantages of standardization of testing conditions, ease of data acquisition, reduced need for extensive training of testing personnel, reduced potential for experimenter bias, extremely precise response measurement, and high subject or patient acceptance.[3,7] We recently developed one such system, described in detail elsewhere,[2] for use in epidemiologic studies of populations occupationally exposed to neurotoxic agents. This system is intended to be capable of detecting subclinical, subtle CNS functional impairment. It is not designed to provide information on localization of functional impairment or specific diagnoses.

Before testing systems such as our NES can win wide acceptance as research instruments, a number of questions about their utility must be satisfactorily answered. The most important of these are issues of the reliability and validity of an evaluation system.[1] Such systems should provide measures that are reliably obtained, stable over time, and correlate well with data obtained from standard nonautomated techniques. These issues are the subject of ongoing research.[3] Of course, a test system must also detect functional impairment with a reasonably high degree of sensitivity. The purpose of

From the Interdisciplinary Programs in Health and the Occupational Health Program, Harvard School of Public Health and Forsyth Dental Center.

Supported in part by National Institute of Dental Research Grant No. DE 07011 and by Environmental Protection Agency cooperative agreement No. CR 811896-01-0. B. D. G. was supported by Environmental Protection Agency Grant No. CR807809.

Received for publication June 16, 1985; accepted Aug. 8, 1985.

Reprint requests to: Dr. Richard Letz, Occupational Health Program, Harvard School of Public Health, 665 Huntington Ave., Boston, MA 02115.

our current study was to evaluate the sensitivity of the NES to a pharmacologic treatment producing subtle alteration in the functional status of the CNS. The treatment chosen was administration of a minimally suprathreshold dose of nitrous oxide, a safe, short-acting inhalation anesthetic with previously described CNS depressant properties.[6] Nitrous oxide is of particular interest as a test agent because of concern over possible occupational exposure to the drug among surgical and dental personnel,[10] and because its acute effects are analogous to those of CNS-depressant organic solvents used widely in industry.[11] Furthermore, demonstration of NES sensitivity to nitrous oxide would suggest potential utility of this system not only in epidemiologic field studies, but also in clinical research on neurobehavioral effects of a variety of drugs with varying modes of action.

METHODS

Subjects. Subjects were twelve men 18 to 36 years old ($\bar{X} \pm SD = 23 \pm 6.5$ years) who gave informed consent. The study was approved by the human subjects committee of the institution. Subjects were healthy and not taking any medication as determined by a medical history questionnaire. Subjects were undergraduate and graduate students and were paid for their participation.

Testing procedure. Each subject was tested on three separate occasions, beginning at the same time of day, over a 2-week period. Testing took place in an isolated room (82 ft^2) that was quiet and had moderately low fluorescent illumination. Before each session subjects were given a pretest questionnaire to identify conditions (e.g., acute illness) that might affect their performance. The first session was a training period during which subjects were given the tests while wearing a nasal mask through which gasses were administered as described below. In previous field studies we have observed that much of the improvement in performance on those tests suitable for repeated administration occurred between the first and second session. Therefore, a single training session was given before nitrous oxide administration and control sessions were given in counterbalanced order across subjects. Both the subject and the test administrator (B. D. G.) were unaware of treatment conditions.

Subjects were tested with the NES software developed by Baker et al.[2] and a portable microcomputer. The testing apparatus was brought to the laboratory on each test day; setup time was <5 minutes. The NES is a computer-based collection of neurobehavioral tests similar to nonautomated tests of human performance used widely in clinical neuropsychology and in epidemiologic investigations of possible neurobehavioral dysfunction produced by environmental exposure to neurotoxic agents.[7] The NES software is designed to run on IBM-compatible microcomputers. The system is flexible in that different subsets of the approximately 15 available tasks can be selected, and the difficulty of the tests can be adjusted depending on the purposes of a study.

Sessions began with a computer-presented orientation sequence during which subjects learned how to respond to the COMPAQ computer (COMPAQ Computer Corp.) using the numeric keys on the keyboard (the other keys were covered by an opaque acrylic template), two buttons, and a joystick (ORA Electronics). In addition, each separate task contained instructions and practice trials. The computer continually monitored the subjects' performance, interrupting with refresher instructions or a request to call the test administrator if a subject's error rate was high. Subjects rarely made sufficient errors for this to occur, and as a group had few questions about the testing procedure. The NES tests described below were presented for each session. Administration of the tests required approximately 40 minutes for each session. At the end of the second and third sessions, subjects were asked whether they thought they had received an active agent.

NES tests. Nine NES tests were selected for this study, listed below in order of administration and according to the aspect of CNS function they are primarily intended to evaluate. These tests and the rationale underlying their use are described in more detail elsewhere.[3]

Psychomotor performance. (1) Continuous performance test: In this test of sustained visual attention, subjects press a button in response to a large letter "S" appearing randomly as part of a 5-minute series of other letters that flash briefly on the display screen at the rate of one per second. Reaction times to the target stimuli and response errors are recorded. (2) Symbol-digit substitution test: In this task the subject is presented with nine pairs of symbols and digits at the top of the screen. The subject responds by matching digits to the nine symbols, which are reordered and appear at the bottom of the screen. The time taken to match digits to the appropriate symbols and the number of incorrect responses are recorded. After a practice trial, four sets of nine symbol-digit pairs are presented in succession. To avoid learning effects, the symbol-digit pairs are different between sets. (3) Finger tapping test: In this test of simple hand speed, subjects press a button with the index finger of the left hand as many times as possible in a 10-second interval, repeat this task with the

Table I. Effects of nitrous oxide on NES performance in normal subjects (n = 12)

	Training	*Control*	*Nitrous oxide*	*Paired t test*
Continuous performance test latency (msec)	445.8 ± 31.4	448.3 ± 31.5	464.8 ± 26.2	−2.97*
Symbol-digit (sec/symbol)	1.99 ± 0.32	1.87 ± 0.33	2.00 ± 0.32	−3.42†
Finger tapping (mean no.)	50.7 ± 11.6	54.9 ± 9.3	52.1 ± 7.3	3.18†
Pattern comparison latency (sec)	2.96 ± 0.57	2.41 ± 0.67	2.41 ± 0.66	0.00
Hand-eye coordination (root mean square error)	3.68 ± 1.09	3.30 ± 0.73	3.24 ± 0.29	0.56
Associate learning (no. correct)	5.27 ± 1.10	4.91 ± 1.97	4.82 ± 1.94	0.14
Associate recall (no. correct)	7.54 ± 1.37	5.72 ± 3.00	5.45 ± 2.58	0.30
Pattern memory (no. correct)	12.6 ± 1.6	12.9 ± 1.0	12.3 ± 2.2	1.12
Digit learning (no. correct)	2.25 ± 1.22	2.58 ± 2.58	2.25 ± 2.18	0.48

Data are $\overline{X} \pm SD$.
*$P < 0.01$, †$P < 0.005$ compared with control value.

right index finger, and then press two buttons (2 cm apart) alternately with the index finger of the preferred hand. This set of tapping trials is presented twice.

Visuospatial ability. (4) Pattern comparison test: The subject is presented with three patterns (each a 10 × 10 square array), two of which are identical, and asked to select the odd pattern. This task assesses visual organization ability, a cognitive function necessary in the perception of complex visual stimuli. For each trial response times and errors are recorded. (5) Hand-eye coordination test: Using a joystick modified to move in only one dimension, subjects trace a large sine-wave pattern on the display screen. The cursor is moved horizontally at a constant rate by the computer, while the subject controls only the cursor's vertical motion with the joystick. The average vertical deviation of the cursor from the pattern is recorded as the mean absolute error and root mean square error for each trial.

Memory. (6) Paired-associate learning test: This test is designed to evaluate short-term memory. Nine associations, in which a three-letter name is paired with a one-word occupation, are presented on the monitor for 2 seconds each with 1 second between pairs. The associations are presented three times in varying order. Subjects match jobs to the appropriate name from multiple choices after each presentation of the list. The number of correct responses is scored for each trial. To avoid learning effects across sessions, different associate pairs are presented in each test session. To evaluate memory encoding and intermediate recall, a multiple-choice matching trial with the same nine name-job associations is given near the end of the session. (In this study the retention interval was approximately 30 minutes.) The number of correct responses is scored for each of the immediate and delayed recall trials. (7) Pattern memory test: A test of short-term visual memory in which subjects are briefly presented a block-like pattern (like those used in the pattern comparison test) and then required to identify which of three subsequently presented patterns is identical to the original pattern. The similarity of the three test patterns to each other is increased over the fifteen trials, so that the choice between them becomes progressively more difficult. The number of correct responses and the response time are recorded for each trial. (8) Serial digit learning: This is a test of short-term memory and attention in which subjects are presented a series of 10 digits on the display screen at a rate of one per second. Upon completion they are asked to enter that series into the computer. The series is presented until two successive trials are performed perfectly, or at most 10 times. The number of correct digits entered on each trial is recorded. The series is changed for each test session to avoid learning effects.

Mood. (9) Mood scales: Subjects were asked to describe their mood during the 40-minute test session using a five-point scale to indicate the degree to which each of 25 adjectives presented described their emotional state. Responses to five items contributed equally to five mood scales: tension, depression, anger, fatigue, and confusion.

Drug administration. During drug sessions subjects received a combination of 20% nitrous oxide and 80% oxygen from a McKesson Analor 3C nitrous oxide inhalation sedation machine through a Brown Scavenging Mask (Narco Corporation). This dose is relatively low but above the threshold for neurobehavioral dysfunction.[10,12] The drug was administered and monitored by a licensed practitioner (P. A. M.). During the training and control sessions subjects received 100% oxygen. For all sessions the mask was given a peppermint scent to disguise possible odors of the administered gasses. In all cases, subjects began the first task after breathing through the mask for 10 minutes. As previously demonstrated, this is sufficient time for blood levels of nitrous oxide to stabilize under our experimental conditions.[10] After each session the mask was removed and subjects were monitored in air for at least 20 minutes until recovery was deemed complete.

Data analysis. All data were analyzed with SPSS personal computer software. Data for each behavioral measure were subjected to a t test for paired means. Because it was expected a priori that all effects of nitrous oxide would be in the direction of poorer performance, one-tailed probabilities were used. ANOVA and ANCOVA were performed to test for effects of order of drug administration and subjects' belief as to whether they received nitrous oxide.

RESULTS

Nitrous oxide significantly affected performance on three tests: the continuous performance task, symbol-digit substitution, and finger tapping (Table I). Summary measures for all three tasks showed slower performance during the nitrous oxide session than during the 100% oxygen session; that is, mean response time (of 60 trials) for the continuous performance task increased, the mean of the best two of four trials (expressed as seconds per correct symbol) for the symbol-digit substitution task increased, and the mean number of taps on the two trials when subjects alternated between buttons for the finger tapping test decreased. Performance of the other tasks (Table I) and measures of mood were not significantly affected by the dose of nitrous oxide used.

The pattern of scores across sessions was similar for most of the behavioral measures, with performance during the control (either the second or third) session better than during the training (first) session. This pattern was reversed for the associate learning and recall tests, in which poorer performance after the training session suggests a proactive interference effect (i.e., the learning of associate pairs on the first session may have interfered with subsequent acquisition of new associations). These trends illustrate the value of the training session in minimizing the potential increase in error variance resulting from a combination of the effects of repeated test presentation and drug administration.

Although our ability to assess the influence of other factors on subjects' performance was limited by the relatively small sample size, ANOVA of data for all three sessions indicated that order of treatment and subjects' belief as to whether they received an active agent had no significant influence on their performance. The subjective effects of nitrous oxide at the dose used were subtle; 25% of subjects receiving the drug believed they had received oxygen control. No subjects had excessive or idiosyncratic reactions to nitrous oxide.

DISCUSSION

Our current study was designed to assess the sensitivity of the NES in detecting neurobehavioral effects of exposure to a relatively low dose of nitrous oxide. Our observation that the continuous performance, symbol-digit substitution, and finger tapping tasks detected psychomotor impairment produced by 20% nitrous oxide are consistent with those of a number of previous studies[10,12] and indicate that the NES includes tests sensitive to the pharmacologic effects of this anesthetic. These findings may be particularly relevant to the intended use of the system in detecting neurobehavioral impairment in occupational settings. Disturbances in psychomotor functioning are frequently reported after exposure to a number of neurotoxins used in industry.[5] As discussed above, data on the effects of nitrous oxide may be especially helpful to research characterizing neurobehavioral effects of exposure to organic solvents that, like nitrous oxide, are CNS depressants and in some cases (e.g., 1,1,1-trichloroethane) were once used as inhalation anesthetics.[4]

While 20% nitrous oxide had significant effects on measures of psychomotor speed, the drug did not significantly affect performance on NES tasks designed to assess other neurobehavioral functions such as visuospatial ability (pattern recognition, hand-eye coordination), visual memory (pattern memory), verbal learning and memory (paired associates), and mood (mood scales). These findings are generally consistent with previous studies demonstrating that higher doses of nitrous oxide are required to affect such CNS functions as learning and memory consistently.[12] In addition, the sample size we used may have been too small to permit detection of subtle changes in cognitive performance suggested by the results, as there was a trend toward increased response latency in the pattern memory test. Further studies to assess the sensitivity of the various NES tests with higher nitrous oxide doses, other test agents, and larger subject groups would be useful.

Our findings are internally consistent, in that two tests sensitive to nitrous oxide exposure in this study correlated with each other when factor analysis was applied to data obtained in epidemiologic surveys of large populations. In those studies data from the continuous performance and symbol-digit tasks loaded heavily on a factor that appears related to psychomotor speed.* Although comparable field study data are not available for the finger tapping task, this test is also considered to measure psychomotor speed,[9] and a similar task has been demonstrated to be sensitive to nitrous

*Fidler AT: Unpublished observations, 1985.

oxide–induced impairment.[8] This internal consistency, together with the concordance noted above between our findings and previous work, mitigates a potential problem raised by the use of multiple comparisons in our statistical analysis (the possibility that some of the paired t tests reached statistical significance by chance). It therefore appears most likely that the effects we observed were not chance events but rather the result of the pharmacologic action of nitrous oxide.

These results provide evidence that a computer-based NES can reliably detect subtle psychomotor impairment induced by a CNS depressant (and presumably by other factors as well). The sensitivity of this system, coupled with the capability for rapid, efficient, and reliable data collection it provides, suggests that the NES holds promise for a variety of applications in epidemiologic, experimental, and clinical research. For example, as a monitor of CNS function, the NES may find application in assessing beneficial as well as toxic effects of drug therapy. While our experience with this system in the clinic does not suggest it should be used as a screening instrument, it does appear that the NES may be useful in monitoring the status of a variety of neurologic conditions (e.g., head trauma) in which severity would be expected to change over time. It is possible that the use of a common evaluation system in the laboratory, in clinical research, and in field studies could enhance progress in neurobehavioral toxicology by facilitating comparison of data obtained.

The NES software is currently available for scientific research purposes to members of the NES Users' Group at no charge. There are currently 23 users, and versions are available in English, French, Dutch, and Finnish. For information about joining the NES Users' Group, contact the last two authors.

References

1. American Psychological Association: Standards for Educational and Psychological Tests. Washington, DC, 1974, American Psychological Association.
2. Baker EL, Letz R, Fidler A: A computer-administered neurobehavioral evaluation system for occupational and environmental epidemiology: Rationale, methodology, and pilot study results. J Occupat Med **27:**206-212, 1985.
3. Baker EL, Letz RE, Fidler AT, Shalat S, Plantamura D, Lyndon M: A computer-based evaluation system for occupational and environmental epidemiology: Methodology and validation studies. Neurobehav Toxicol Teratol (In press.)
4. Dornette WHC, Jones JP: Clinical experiences with 1,1,1-trichloroethane. Anesth Analg (Cleve) **39:**249-254, 1960.
5. Feldman RG, Ricks NL, Baker EL: Neuropsychological effects of industrial toxins: A review. Am J Ind Med **1:**211-228, 1980.
6. Frankenhauser M, Berkman M: The susceptibility of intellectual functions to a depressant drug. Scand J Psychol **2:**93-99, 1961.
7. Hanninen H: Twenty-five years of behavioral toxicology within occupational medicine: A personal account. Am J Ind Med **7:**19-30, 1985.
8. Kortilla K, Gonheim MM, Jacobs L, Mewalt SP, Peterson RC: Time course of mental and psychomotor effects of 30 per cent nitrous oxide during inhalation and recovery. Anesthesiology **54:**220-226, 1981.
9. Lezak MD: Neuropsychological assessment. London, 1983, Oxford Press.
10. Moore PA: Psychomotor impairment due to nitrous oxide exposure. Anesth Prog **30:**72-75, 1983.
11. Norton S: Toxic responses of the central nervous system. *In* Doull J, Klaasen CD, Amdur MO, editors: Toxicology. New York, 1980, MacMillan.
12. Smith G, Shirley AW: A review of the effects of trace concentrations of anesthetics on performance. Br J Anaesth **50:**701-712, 1978.

The effect of renal function on enalapril kinetics

Enalapril maleate (MK-421), a nonmercapto-containing angiotensin converting enzyme (ACE) inhibitor, is converted in vivo to enalaprilat (MK-422), the active diacid. We evaluated serum profiles and urinary excretion of oral enalapril maleate in patients with renal disease (group I, creatinine clearance <3 ml/min, patients undergoing dialysis, n = 10; group II, creatinine clearance 10 to 79 ml/min, n = 9) compared with healthy subjects (group III, creatinine clearance >80 ml/min, n = 10). Group I received a 10 mg dose during a day while not receiving dialysis and a 10 mg dose 1 hour before dialysis 2 weeks later. Groups II and III received a single 10 mg dose. Blood samples and urine were collected for 48 hours. Impaired renal function resulted in elevated serum and plasma concentrations of enalapril maleate and decreased excretion rates and urinary recovery of enalapril maleate and enalaprilat. The data suggest an apparent increase in the extent of metabolism of enalapril maleate to enalaprilat or an increase in nonrenal elimination of unchanged enalapril maleate in renal disease compared with normal health. Enalaprilat was dialyzable. (Clin Pharmacol Ther 1985;38:661-6.)

D. T. Lowenthal, M.D., J. D. Irvin, M.D., Ph.D., D. Merrill, B.A., S. Saris, M.D., E. Ulm, Ph.D., S. Goldstein, M.D., M. Hichens, Ph.D., L. Klein, D.O., A. Till, Ph.D., and K. Harris, M.S. *Philadelphia and West Point, Pa.*

Enalapril maleate represents a new class of antihypertensive agents, the angiotensin converting enzyme inhibitors. The orally absorbed prodrug enalapril maleate is hydrolyzed in vivo to enalaprilat, an extremely potent inhibitor of converting enzyme.[1-4] Enalapril maleate is an effective antihypertensive[5-7] and can be useful in the treatment of congestive heart failure.[8-9]

Enalapril maleate is well absorbed and is rapidly and extensively hydrolyzed to enalaprilat.[10] After oral dosing of enalapril maleate to normal volunteers,[10,11] the mean urinary recovery of enalaprilat and total drug (enalaprilat plus enalapril) is approximately 40% and 60% of the administered enalaprilat equivalents, respectively. There is no detectable metabolism of enalapril beyond its hydrolysis to enalaprilat. Peak serum concentrations of enalapril occur approximately 1 hour after enalapril maleate dosing, with peak enalaprilat serum concentrations occurring 2 to 3 hours later. The average effective accumulation $t_{1/2}$ of enalaprilat in normal subjects is 11 hours.[12]

Our objective was to determine the influence of renal insufficiency on the serum profiles of enalaprilat and the urinary excretion of enalaprilat and total drug after a single oral dose of enalapril maleate. The effect of hemodialysis on serum enalaprilat concentrations was also determined in patients with severe renal insufficiency.

From Hahnemann University, Philadelphia, and Merck Sharp & Dohme Research Laboratories, West Point.

Received for publication April 8, 1985; accepted Aug. 20, 1985.

Reprint requests to: D. T. Lowenthal, M.D., 230 N. Broad St., Philadelphia, PA 19102.

METHODS

Subjects and dosage. There were three study groups. Group I consisted of 10 stable patients undergoing chronic hemodialysis with creatinine clearances of <3 ml/min. Group II consisted of nine patients with mild to moderate renal insufficiency, defined by creatinine clearances between 10 and 79 ml/min. Group III consisted of 10 normal, healthy subjects with creatinine clearances >80 ml/min. No participant had extrarenal disease and none were taking other medications except for dialysis-related medications such as vitamins, phosphate binders, and anticoagulants. One patient in group II was receiving immunosuppressive drugs after a successful renal transplantation (Table I).

Each participant took a single 10 mg tablet of enalapril maleate by mouth after an overnight fast.

Blood and urine sampling. Serial blood collections were drawn by venipuncture at 0.5, 1, 2, 3, 4, 6, 8, 12, 24, and 48 hours after dosing. Urine was collected in intervals of 0 to 4, 4 to 8, 8 to 12, 12 to 24, and 24 to 48 hours after drug dosing. Nine of the patients in group I were studied a second time and underwent he-

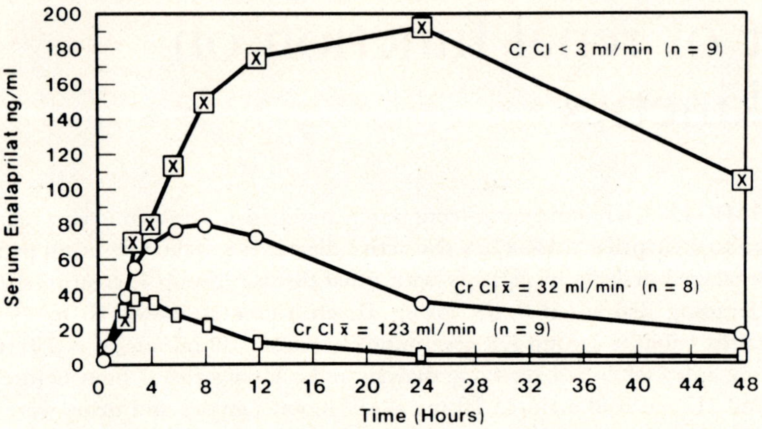

Fig. 1. Mean serum profiles of enalaprilat in patients with renal insufficiency (groups I and II) and in normal subjects (group III). *CrCl* = Creatinine clearance.

Table I. Demographic data

	No. of							Creatinine clearance
	Men	*Women*	*Whites*	*Blacks*	*Age (yr)*	*Height (in)*	*Weight (lb)*	*(ml/min)*
Group I (n = 10)	6	4	6	4	40.5 ± 20	67.9 ± 4.7	148.9 ± 25.8	<10
Group II (n = 9)	7	2	1	8	51.3 ± 22.3	67.9 ± 4.6	155.6 ± 44.0	32 ± 20
Group III (n = 10)	7	3	10	0	28.1 ± 4.9	69.3 ± 3.3	164.8 ± 24.8	123 ± 28

modialysis between the first and the fifth hour after taking enalapril maleate. During dialysis arterial and venous blood samples were collected each hour. At least 2 weeks elapsed between the first and second period of study. Samples were frozen at −20° C until analyzed.

Clinical observations. Subjects and patients were observed in the research unit for at least 12 hours after drug dosing and were monitored for blood pressure, heart rate, respiratory rate, and any adverse reactions. Most patients in group I received hemodialysis between 24 and 48 hours after drug dosing.

Physical examinations and laboratory studies were made on the morning of entry to the study period and were repeated before discharge from the unit and again 5 to 7 days after the treatment. In addition, a 12-lead ECG was obtained before entry and 5 to 7 days after the treatment.

Analytic procedure. Serum and urine samples from groups II and III were analyzed by RIA.[13] Because heparin, which is routinely given to patients undergoing dialysis, can interfere with the RIA, plasma samples from group I were analyzed by an enzymatic assay. The two methods have been shown to yield equivalent results.[10]

The RIA method[13] is specific for enalaprilat, but total drug (enalaprilat plus enalapril maleate) can be measured after hydrolysis of intact enalapril to enalaprilat with a rat liver homogenate preparation. Samples were assayed in triplicate with an interassay coefficient of variation of about 6% over most of the standard curve. The lower limit of measurement was 0.4 ng/ml for serum and 40 ng/ml for urine, with 15 μl serum and 15 μl of a 1:100 dilution of urine.

In the enzyme assay, enalaprilat was determined by the extent of inhibition observed in a standardized angiotensin converting enzyme assay.[14] Enalapril and enalaprilat were isolated from plasma by use of XAD-4 resin, with enalaprilat determined directly and total drug measured after hydrolysis of enalapril to enalaprilat in the isolate with 1N NaOH. The lower limit of measurement was 3 ng/ml as enalaprilat. Intra-assay variability estimated by Barrett's standard deviation of the difference between duplicates was 3.5% ± 0.44%. The interassay coefficient of variation was about 15%.

Statistical methods and participant exclusions. The difference between enalapril maleate therapy with and without dialysis in 0 to 6–hour AUC for the patients undergoing chronic hemodialysis (group I) was tested by the sign test. Differences between normal subjects and patients with stable renal insufficiency in AUC, urinary recovery, and urinary recovery rates were tested by a one-way ANOVA of the ranks. The analysis for the urinary recovery ratio was performed after a log transformation.

Table II. Enalaprilat plasma AUC for 0 to 6 hours after enalapril maleate dosing to patients in group I*

	AUC(0-6) (ng · hr/ml)	
Patient	*Without dialysis*	*With dialysis†*
IA	264	205
IB	321	245
IC	354	78
ID	493	149
IE	339	280
IF	517	327
IG	137	9
IH	194	121
II	466	—
IJ	226	90
Median‡	321	149

*Patients underwent dialysis for 4 hours beginning 1 hour after drug dosing.
†Significantly different ($P < 0.01$) from value without dialysis.
‡Excludes patient II.

Within-group changes in vital signs and laboratory parameters were tested by a paired t test. Results were corroborated by the Wilcoxon signed rank test for variables not meeting the normality assumption. Correlations of biopharmaceutic parameters with creatinine clearances were tested by the Spearman correlation coefficient. All tests were done at the $\alpha = 0.05$ level of significance.

One patient in group II was excluded from efficacy analyses because of ambiguous indicators of renal function (creatinine clearance was 86 ml/min but inulin clearance was 66 ml/min). Another was excluded from pharmacodynamic analyses because of a rebound increase in blood pressure at baseline resulting from discontinuation of other antihypertensive drugs. For purposes of analyses, patients in group II were subdivided into those with mild renal insufficiency (creatinine clearance of 62 and 63 ml/min [n = 2]) and those with moderate renal insufficiency (creatinine clearance between 9 and 31 ml/min [n = 6]). Analyses were performed on the total group and on the group with moderate renal insufficiency.

One normal subject in group III was excluded from efficacy analyses because of clinically and statistically abnormal urinary recovery and AUC values as compared with the other subjects.

RESULTS

Pharmacokinetic parameters. Fig. 1 shows the influence of renal function on enalaprilat serum (or plasma) profiles. From approximately 3 to 48 hours after oral enalapril maleate dosing, mean plasma concentrations of enalaprilat in patients with creatinine clearances <3 ml/min (group I) were markedly greater than serum concentrations in patients with creatinine clearances between 10 and 79 ml/min (group II) and subjects with creatinine clearances ≥80 ml/min (group III). Serum concentrations of enalaprilat were greater in group II than in group III throughout the 48-hour period of observation as well. In the normal subjects, the peak of the mean profile was attained at approximately 3 hours; in group II the peak was observed at approximately 8 hours, and in group I plasma concentrations continued to rise until 24 hours. Rates of absorption of enalapril, as evidenced by time to reach peak concentrations, were consistent among the three groups. Given the functionally anephric condition of patients in group I, the nearly 50% drop observed in the mean plasma profile for that group from 24 to 48 hours may be explained in part by the fact that patients received dialysis during that period.

In group I there were positive arteriovenous enalaprilat concentration differences during dialysis. The enalaprilat AUC from 0 to 6 hours was significantly lower for the dialysis treatment period than for the treat-

Table III. Enalaprilat serum AUC for 0 to 48 hours after enalapril maleate dosing in groups II and III

Patient or subject	*AUC(0-48) (ng · hr/ml)*
Group II	
IIA	417
IIB	1134
IIC	483
IID	1761
IIF	2435
IIG	2252
IIH	2546
III	4856
$\bar{X} \pm SD$	1986 ± 1430*
95% Confidence interval	790-3181
$\bar{X} \pm SD$†	2497 ± 1267*
95% Confidence interval†	1167-3828
Group III	
IIIA	444
IIIB	198
IIIC	412
IIID	444
IIIE	532
IIIF	366
IIIG	352
IIIH	299
IIII	278
IIIJ	258
$\bar{X} \pm SD$‡	409 ± 96
95% Confidence interval	335-483

*Significantly different ($P < 0.01$) from value in group III.
†Excluding patients IIA and IIC.
‡Excluding subject IIIB.

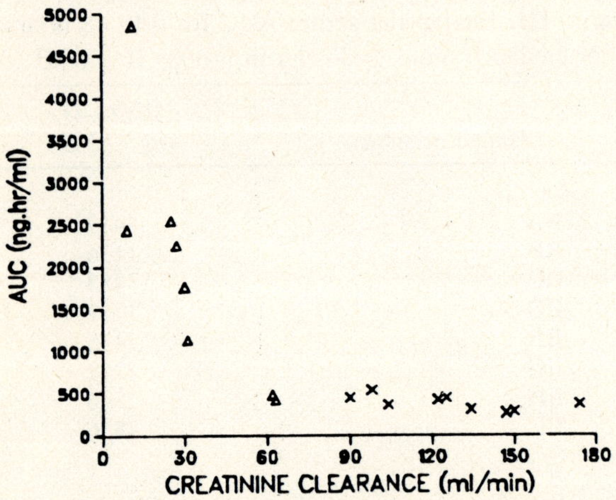

Fig. 2. Creatinine clearance vs. AUC(0-48) for enalaprilat. △ = Group II; X = group III.

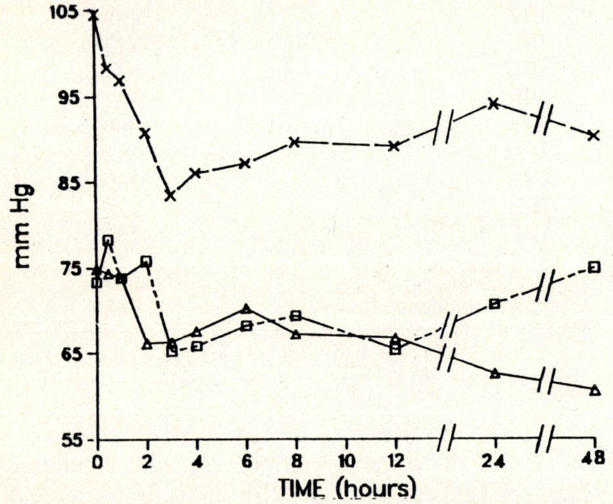

Fig. 3. Sitting diastolic blood pressure by time and group. △ = Group I (n = 9); X = group II (n = 7); □ = group III (n = 9).

ment period without dialysis for each patient in group I (Table II).

Enalaprilat AUCs from 0 to 48 hours for groups II and III are listed in Table III. Both the mean AUC for those patients in group II with moderate renal insufficiency (2497 ng · hr/ml) and the mean AUC for all of group II (1986 ng · hr/ml) were significantly greater than the mean AUC for group III (409 ng · hr/ml). There was a significant negative correlation between creatinine clearance and AUC for group II ($r = -0.93$; $P < 0.01$); no correlation was found between these parameters in group III (Fig. 2).

Mean 48-hour urinary recoveries of enalaprilat and total drug in groups II and III are listed in Table IV. The recovery of total drug was significantly less in group II (38%) than in group III (62%; $P < 0.01$). Recovery of enalaprilat was less in group II (30%) than in group III (40%), but not significantly so. The recovery ratio of enalaprilat/total drug, which serves as a rough approximation of the extent of hydrolysis of enalapril to enalaprilat, was significantly less ($P < 0.01$) in group III (0.64) than in group II (0.82).

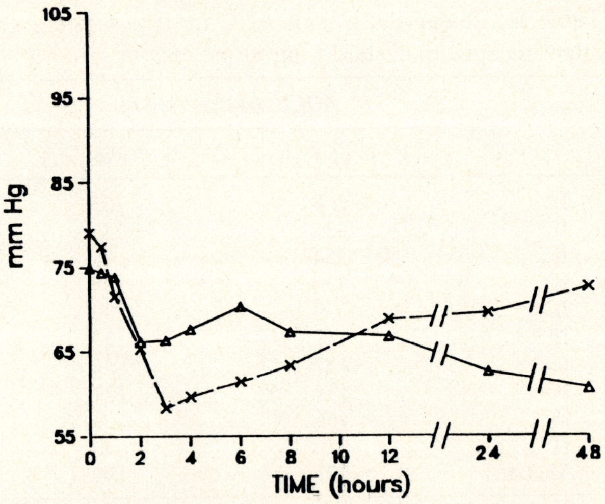

Fig. 4. Sitting diastolic blood pressure in group I with (△) and without (X) dialysis.

Table IV. 48-Hour urinary recovery (expressed as percent of administered enalaprilat)

	Enalaprilat	*Total drug*	*Enalaprilat/ total drug*
Group II			
Entire group	30 ± 13	38 ± 17*	0.82*
Subgroup†	30 ± 15	35 ± 19*	0.89*
Group III	40 ± 5	62 ± 8	0.64

*Significantly different ($P < 0.01$) from values in group III.
†Excluding patients IIA and IIC, who had creatinine clearances of 63 and 62 ml/min, respectively.

Table V lists the mean incremental urinary excretion rates for enalaprilat and total drug in groups II and III. The excretion rates of both were significantly greater in group III than in group II up to 8 hours after drug dosing; beyond 12 hours, excretion rates were significantly greater in group II.

Pharmacodynamic measurements. Consistent decreases were observed in blood pressure (Figs. 3 and 4) after 3 hours. Patients in group II had higher baseline values and therefore had the most significant changes. Mean pulse rates in group I increased consistently after

Table V. Urinary excretion rates (mg/hr) of enalaprilat and total drug

	Time period (hr)									
	0-4		*4-8*		*8-12*		*12-24*		*24-48*	
	ET	*TD*	*ET*	*TD*	*ET*	*TD*	*ET*	*TD*	*ET*	*TD*
Group II										
Entire group	55*	168*	112*	140*	80	87	63	63	17	17
Subgroup†	24*	77*	94*	124*	78	87	69‡	69‡	20‡	20‡
Group III	186	545	228	251	122	127	39	39	6.8	6.8

ET = Enalaprilat; TD = total drug.
*Significantly different ($P < 0.05$) from values in group III.
†Excluding patients IIA and IIC, who had creatinine clearances of 63 and 62 ml/min, respectively.
‡Significantly different ($P < 0.01$) from values in group III.

2 hours, but all changes were small and insignificant.

Adverse effects. Seven patients (six in group I and one in group II) and one subject reported clinical adverse experiences, with light-headedness (n = 3) and headache (n = 3) reported most frequently. One patient in group I developed moderate diarrhea during both testing periods and an episode of syncope after dialysis. In group I, one patient each reported headache, light-headedness, hypotension, and hot flashes during dialysis. The causes may be related both to increased plasma concentrations of drug (enalaprilat) and to the concomitant dialysis procedure. None of the adverse experiences were considered serious.

No adverse laboratory effects were reported. A decrease from baseline hemoglobin and hematocrit values was observed 5 to 7 days after treatment in group I (mean decrease from baseline of 1.98 gm/dl and 5.94 vol%, respectively after dialysis) and group III (mean decrease from baseline of 0.48 gm/dl and 0.73 vol%, respectively).

DISCUSSION

Our data support the safety of single doses of enalapril maleate in patients with varying degrees of renal insufficiency. Although six patients in group I reported adverse effects, none were severe or considered serious. Adverse experiences in five of the six patients occurred during or after the dialysis periods and are symptoms commonly associated with the dialysis procedure (syncope, headache, light-headedness, and hypotension), but they may also be drug related. The decrease in hemoglobin levels is not unexpected in patients undergoing chronic dialysis. The decrease in hemoglobin levels in the normal subjects (<1 gm/dl) was statistically but not clinically significant.

Serum and urinary recovery data for enalaprilat and total drug in group III were quite consistent with those previously reported for normal subjects after oral enalapril maleate.[11] The observed elevated serum concentrations of enalaprilat and the decreased urinary recovery of enalaprilat and total drug in patients with impaired renal function is not unexpected for a drug whose excretion is primarily renal.

Comparison of urinary recovery results in group II with those in group III suggests that renal impairment decreases the excretion rates of enalaprilat and enalapril, with a corresponding increase in the extent of hydrolysis of enalapril to enalaprilat or an increase in the elimination of enalapril by routes other than renal excretion or metabolism to enalaprilat (e.g., biliary excretion).

The significant correlation of AUC to creatinine clearance in group II and the lack of a correlation of these parameters in group III suggest that for creatinine clearances >60 ml/min there is little, if any, influence of kidney function on serum concentrations of enalaprilat. For creatinine clearances below approximately 60 ml/min, serum concentrations of enalaprilat are related to kidney function.

Evidence from studies in both animals and man point to the kidneys as the primary excretory route for enalaprilat.[4,10] For patients receiving dialysis, several lines of evidence argue that hemodialysis can serve this function. AUCs for the 6-hour period after enalapril maleate dosing were significantly higher in the period when dialysis was not being carried out (321 vs. 149 ng · hr/ml; $P < 0.01$). Concentrations of enalaprilat in plasma downstream from the dialyzer were lower than concentrations measured in samples drawn upstream. Patients who received dialysis between 24 and 48 hours after the enalapril maleate dose had significant drops in enalaprilat plasma concentrations compared with those patients in whom there was no dialysis.

In conclusion, enalapril maleate in a single, oral 10

mg dose appears safe and well tolerated in patients with mild to moderate and severe renal insufficiency. Impaired renal function, however, results in elevated serum or plasma concentrations of enalaprilat and reduced urinary excretion of enalaprilat and enalapril, with an apparent increase in the metabolism of enalapril to enalaprilat. Enalaprilat is dialyzable in patients with severe renal impairment.

The protracted blood pressure reduction in the patients with chronic renal failure (groups I and II) is possibly related to the elevated plasma enalaprilat concentrations. Plasma angiotensin converting enzyme concentrations are suppressed by enalapril.[15] Hypothetically, had enalaprilat levels been measured at 72 to 96 hours and found to be zero, the blood pressure reduction may have been related to angiotensin converting enzyme inhibition, tissue binding of drug to vascular smooth muscle, kinin-kininogen accumulation, or other factors. Therefore, for blood pressure control, lower doses or less frequent dosing of enalapril maleate may be indicated for patients with renal insufficiency than for those with normal renal function.

References

1. Biollaz J, Brunner HR, Gavras I, Waeber B, Gavras H. Antihypertensive therapy with MK-421: angiotensin II-renin relationships to evaluate efficacy of converting enzyme blockage. J Cardiovasc Pharmacol 1982;4:966-72.
2. Gross DM, Sweet CS, Ulm EH, et al. Antihypertensive activity of *N*-[*(S)-1*-(ethoxycarbonyl)-3-phenylpropyl-L-Ala-L-Pro] and its ethyl ester (MK-421) on angiotensin converting enzyme in vitro and angiotensin I pressor responses *in vivo*. J Pharmacol Exp Ther 1981;216:552-7.
3. Irvin JD, Till AE, Vlasses PH, et al. Bioavailability of enalapril maleate. Clin Pharmacol Ther 1984;35:248.
4. Patchett AA, Harris E, Tristam EW, et al. A new class of angiotensin converting enzyme inhibitors. Nature 1983;288:280-3.
5. Davies RO, Irvin JD, Kramsch DK, Walker JF, Moncloa F. Enalapril worldwide experience. Am J Med 1984;77:23-35.
6. Ferguson RK, Vlasses PH, Swanson BN, et al. Effects of enalapril, a new converting enzyme inhibitor, in hypertension. Clin Pharmacol Ther 1982;32:48-53.
7. Gavras H, Biollaz J, Waeber B, Brunner HR, Gavras I, Davies RO. Antihypertensive effect of the new oral angiotensin converting enzyme inhibitor "MK-421." Lancet 1981;2:543-7.
8. DiCarlo L Jr, Chatterjee K, Swedberg K, Atherton B, Curran D, Parmley W. MK-421: a new angiotensin converting enzyme inhibitor in chronic heart failure, acute and chronic hemodynamic response [Abstract 837]. Circulation 1982;66(suppl II):209.
9. Levine TB, Olivari MT, Cohn JH. Acute and long-term response to MK-421, a long acting oral converting enzyme inhibitor, in heart failure [Abstract 838]. Circulation 1982;66(suppl II):209.
10. Ulm EH. Enalapril maleate (MK-421), a potent, nonsulfhydryl angiotensin-converting enzyme inhibitor: absorption, disposition and metabolism in man. Drug Metab Rev 1983;14:99-110.
11. Ulm EH, Hichens M, Gomez HJ, et al. Enalapril maleate and a lysine analog (MK-521): disposition in man. Br J Clin Pharmacol 1982;14:357-62.
12. Till AE, Gomez HJ, Hichens M, et al. Pharmacokinetics of repeated single oral dose of enalapril maleate (MK-421) in normal volunteers. Biopharm Drug Dispos 1984;5:273-80.
13. Hichens M, Hand EL, Mulcahy WS. Radioimmunoassay for angiotensin converting enzyme inhibitors. Ligand 1981;4:43.
14. Tocco DJ, deLuna FA, Duncan AEW, Vassil TC, Ulm EH. The physiological disposition and metabolism of enalapril maleate in laboratory animals. Drug Metab Dispos 1982;10:15.
15. Lowenthal DT, Saris SD, Haratz A, Packer J, Porter RS, Conry K. The clinical pharmacology of antihypertensive drugs. J Hypertens 1984;2(suppl 2):13-24.

Effects of verapamil, diltiazem, and nifedipine on plasma levels and renal excretion of digitoxin

To determine whether verapamil, diltiazem, or nifedipine affect digitoxin kinetics, glycoside plasma concentrations and renal excretion were measured before and during steady-state dosing in 30 patients with cardiac insufficiency. The mean (±SD) digitoxin plasma concentration was 14.27 ± 3.66 ng/ml before and 18.15 ± 5.33 ng/ml during verapamil dosing in 10 patients over a period of 4 to 6 weeks. Renal digitoxin clearance was not influenced by verapamil, but total body clearance and extrarenal clearance of digitoxin were reduced by 27% and 29%, respectively. Diltiazem resulted in a 6% to 31% ($\bar{X}$ = 21%) increase in plasma digitoxin concentrations in five of 10 patients because of reduced extrarenal clearance of digitoxin. In contrast to verapamil, the concomitant dosing of nifedipine over 4 to 6 weeks did not alter digitoxin plasma levels or daily renal excretion. Based on these observations, the risk of digitalis intoxication after combined dosing with verapamil and digitoxin is much less pronounced than that after digoxin, and thus this glycoside is a valuable alternative. (CLIN PHARMACOL THER 38:667-673, 1985.)

J. Kuhlmann, M.D., Ph.D. *Würzburg, Federal Republic of Germany*

The simultaneous dosing of several drugs has become common in modern medicine. In addition to the desired effects, negative side effects must often be expected. These side effects cannot always be explained by the undesired effects of the individual substances. The correlation between undesirable drug actions and the number of drugs prescribed leads to the conclusion that undesirable interactions of several simultaneously prescribed drugs may be the underlying reason. Several investigations have demonstrated that concomitant dosing of the calcium antagonists verapamil or diltiazem may result in a clinically relevant rise in digoxin plasma levels, increasing the risk of digoxin overdosage.[2,8,10,18,19,23,26] A decrease in renal digoxin excretion because of additional drug intake is considered to be the main mechanism for this interaction. Because, contrary to that of digoxin, renal excretion of digitoxin is independent of renal function, this glycoside may possibly be an alternative if combined therapy with verapamil or diltiazem is necessary. The goal of this study was to examine the influence of therapeutic doses of the most frequently used calcium antagonists verapamil, diltiazem, and nifedipine on the pharmacokinetic behavior of digitoxin in a prospective clinical investigation.

From the Department of Internal Medicine, Medical Clinic of the University of Würzburg.

Presented in part at the Second World Conference on Clinical Pharmacology and Therapeutics, Washington, D.C., July 31-Aug. 5, 1983.

Received for publication May 8, 1985; accepted Aug. 20, 1985.

Reprint requests to: Prof. Dr. med. J. Kuhlmann, Institute of Clinical Pharmacology, Bayer AG, Aprather Weg, D-5600 Wuppertal 1, Federal Republic of Germany.

METHODS

Our subjects were 30 hospitalized patients with cardiac insufficiency (New York Heart Association stages II and III) with or without liver disease or renal insufficiency. Threshold values for our laboratory were 1.3 mg/dl for serum creatinine and 20 to 22 U/L for SGPT. Essential clinical data of the subjects are listed in Table I. All subjects had received stable oral digitoxin doses of 0.07 to 0.1 mg/day over several weeks before the study. Clinical indications for calcium antagonist therapy were coronary artery disease or hypertension inducing cardiac insufficiency requiring digitalis. All concomitant medication (nitrates or thiazide diuretics) was given in constant dosages throughout the studies. All subjects gave written informed consent to the protocol, which was approved by the ethical committee of the University of Würzburg.

To evaluate steady-state plasma glycoside concentrations, venous blood samples were drawn at least 5 days before and not less than every other day during simultaneous administration of 240 mg verapamil, 180 mg diltiazem, or 40 to 60 mg nifedipine daily for at least 4 to 6 weeks, always 24 hours after the daily digitoxin

Table I. Clinical data of the three groups during concurrent digitoxin dosing

Patient	*Age (yr)*	*Body weight (kg)*	*Sex*	*Serum creatinine (mg/dl)*	*CL_{CR} (ml/min/kg)*	*SGPT (U/L)*	*Albumin (gm/dl)*	*Diagnosis*
Verapamil								
B. P.	55	77	M	1.0	0.57	9	4.0	Card insuff, cor pulmon
S. C.	71	80	F	0.9	0.53	11	3.4	Card insuff, tachyarrhy
L. L.	72	65	F	0.8	1.11	10	4.8	Card insuff, tachyarrhy
B. I.	89	50	F	1.3	0.59	14	3.0	Card insuff
G. X.	75	51	F	1.1	0.88	17	4.3	Card insuff
Q. X.	77	92	M	1.1	1.29	11	4.2	Card insuff
P. E.	86	46	M	1.3	0.75	2	3.0	Card insuff, immunocytoma, chron bronchitis
B. T.	71	55	M	1.1	1.06	32	3.2	Card insuff, tachyarrhy, hepatocirrhosis
K. C.	75	74	M	3.5	0.37	13	4.1	Card insuff, plasmacytoma, DM with renal insuff
T. G.	69	68	F	0.8	1.09	21	4.2	Tachyarrhy
Diltiazem								
I. C.	77	57	F	0.8	0.97	16	3.9	Card insuff, malign lymph
N. T.	82	62	F	1.3	0.99	20	3.0	Card insuff, tachyarrhy
B. X.	67	102	M	1.2	0.65	26	4.1	Card insuff, artheroscl
B. L.	45	78	M	1.0	1.54	12	4.4	PT
F. T.	78	71	F	0.8	1.33	17	3.2	Card insuff, tachyarrhy, DM
N. N.	68	82	F	1.0	0.47	10	3.8	Card insuff, hyperlipoproteinemia
G. T.	71	84	M	1.0	1.84	9	3.5	Card insuff, artheroscl
B. N.	62	70	F	11.3	0.09	8	3.8	Card insuff, DM, glomerulosclerosis
S. I.	68	70	M	0.7	1.36	4	3.6	Card insuff, tachyarrhy
F. I.	62	77	M	1.5	0.64	20	3.3	Card insuff
Nifedipine								
G. I.	73	72	M	1.2	0.73	10	3.7	Card insuff, DM
I. C.	77	57	F	0.8	0.90	16	3.9	Card insuff, malign lymph
B. X.	67	102	M	1.2	0.75	26	4.1	Card insuff, artheroscl
F. X.	64	134	F	1.2	0.67	15	4.1	Card insuff, tachyarrhy
K. X.	57	84	F	1.1	0.81	9	4.4	Card insuff
S. I.	59	82	F	2.2	0.49	8	3.2	Card insuff, DM, chron pyelonephr
Q. B.	74	62	F	0.8	0.81	39	4.7	Card insuff, tachyarrhy, hepatocirrhosis
I. T.	68	88	F	6.3	0.12	20	2.9	Card insuff, DM, nephrosclerosis
B. C.	64	73	F	3.4	0.39	12	3.9	Card insuff, chron pyeloneph
F. L.	62	80	F	0.9	0.81	9	4.4	Card insuff, tachyarrhy

CL_{CR} = Creatinine clearance; M = male; Card insuff = cardiac insufficiency; cor pulmon = cor pulmonae; F = female; tachyarrhy = tachyarrhythmia; chron = chronic; DM = diabetes mellitus; insuff = insufficiency; malig lymph = malignant lymphoma; artheroscl = artherosclerosis; PT = paroxysmal tachycardia; pyelonephr = pyelonephritis.

dose and 8 to 12 hours after the last verapamil, diltiazem, or nifedipine dose at trough levels. Drug compliance was monitored daily. Twenty-four–hour urine specimens were collected daily in 18 subjects 5 days before and during dosing with verapamil (n = 7), diltiazem (n = 3), or nifedipine (n = 8) over 4 to 6 weeks.

Digitoxin concentrations in plasma and urine were determined by a ^{125}J-radioimmunoassay kit that gave only minimal cross-reaction between digitoxin and digoxin and the corresponding low carbohydrate metabolites.[14] Samples were stored at −20° C until analyzed. Urine samples were diluted with albumin buffer (bovine albumin, 1 gm/L, at pH 7.4) before measurement. All samples from a subject were measured on the same day in a calibrated plasma or urine series. The mean coefficient of variation, based on quadruplicate determinations with different assays ranging from 4.0 to 30.0 ng/ml, was 5%. In preliminary in vitro studies of plasma and urine from subjects taking verapamil, diltiazem, or nifedipine, there were no interactions between the glycoside and the calcium antagonists during the 24- or 48-hour incubation periods. The recovery of digitoxin was always >95% within the concentration range of 4.0 to 30.0 ng/ml.

Serum and urine creatinine concentrations were measured at least twice during each phase. Verapamil and diltiazem plasma concentrations were analyzed by gas chromatography, but there were no usual methods of

Table II. Plasma and renal excretion of digitoxin before and during verapamil dosing

Patient	*Digitoxin alone* Plasma (ng/ml)	*Digitoxin alone* Urine (μg/day)	*Digitoxin and verapamil, wk 1* Plasma (ng/ml)	*Digitoxin and verapamil, wk 1* Urine (μg/day)	*Digitoxin and verapamil, wk 2 to 6* Plasma (ng/ml)	*Digitoxin and verapamil, wk 2 to 6* Urine (μg/day)
B. P.	10.21 ± 0.41	17.70 ± 4.67	11.15 ± 0.45*	17.53 ± 4.05	12.13 ± 0.74*	22.05 ± 5.44
S. C.	17.33 ± 1.27	17.80 ± 7.48	19.70 ± 1.22*	18.13 ± 5.90	23.44 ± 1.05*	22.02 ± 4.28
L. L.	12.14 ± 2.50	22.25 ± 5.73	13.65 ± 1.30	15.52 ± 4.49	14.74 ± 1.38	20.47 ± 4.55
B. I.	19.08 ± 0.27	NM	20.58 ± 1.07	NM	22.10 ± 2.59	NM
G. X.	11.73 ± 0.97	19.84 ± 1.65	12.90 ± 2.20	21.95 ± 4.43	14.95 ± 0.79*	23.65 ± 1.82
Q. X.	15.17 ± 2.25	NM	18.79 ± 3.66	NM	22.87 ± 2.56*	NM
P. E.	12.75 ± 1.82	NM	15.07 ± 1.36	NM	14.51 ± 0.81	NM
B. T.	12.91 ± 0.91	13.67 ± 3.00	16.19 ± 2.98*	9.42 ± 0.99	25.38 ± 4.02*	9.09 ± 2.52
K. C.	10.52 ± 0.53	20.39 ± 1.08	10.24 ± 0.79	19.36 ± 3.35	10.50 ± 1.14	25.87 ± 1.92
T. G.	20.72 ± 1.09	18.34 ± 3.68	20.32 ± 0.36	11.86 ± 0.83	20.86 ± 2.63	14.01 ± 2.33
$\bar{X}$ ± SD	14.27 ± 3.66	18.57 ± 2.70	15.86 ± 3.85*	16.25 ± 4.35	18.15 ± 5.33*	19.59 ± 5.92

Data are $\bar{X}$ ± SD.
NM = Not measured.
*0.05 > P > 0.0001.

Table III. Plasma and renal excretion of digitoxin before and during diltiazem dosing

Patient	*Digitoxin alone* Plasma (ng/ml)	*Digitoxin alone* Urine (μg/day)	*Digitoxin and diltiazem, wk 1* Plasma (ng/ml)	*Digitoxin and diltiazem, wk 1* Urine (μg/day)	*Digitoxin and diltiazem, wk 2 to 6* Plasma (ng/ml)	*Digitoxin and diltiazem, wk 2 to 6* Urine (μg/day)
N. T.	14.65 ± 1.10	19.1 ± 3.8	16.13 ± 0.50	20.0 ± 1.6	18.34 ± 1.24*	18.0 ± 2.1
B. X.	13.62 ± 0.99	17.0 ± 3.0	20.79 ± 1.20	16.2 ± 2.1	17.78 ± 3.28*	17.2 ± 1.9
B. L.	12.90 ± 4.00	NM	13.90 ± 1.10	NM	15.05 ± 1.66	NM
G. T.	12.72 ± 1.77	NM	14.41 ± 0.92	NM	16.59 ± 0.63*	NM
F. I.	14.70 ± 0.70	NM	13.37 ± 1.22	NM	15.55 ± 2.39	NM
I. C.	13.72 ± 1.80	14.1 ± 1.8	13.13 ± 1.39	16.5 ± 3.5	14.01 ± 2.77	13.4 ± 2.1
N. N.	19.54 ± 0.79	NM	18.62 ± 0.82	NM	19.90 ± 1.15	NM
B. N.	23.12 ± 5.25	NM	23.00 ± 6.32	NM	22.53 ± 2.53	NM
S. I.	22.90 ± 2.21	NM	20.67 ± 1.68	NM	21.95 ± 1.09	NM
F. T.	20.34 ± 1.72	NM	24.77 ± 2.72	NM	18.38 ± 1.15	NM
$\bar{X}$ ± SD	16.82 ± 2.03	16.7 ± 2.9	17.88 ± 1.79	17.6 ± 2.4	18.01 ± 1.79	16.2 ± 2.0

Data are $\bar{X}$ ± SD.
NM = Not measured.
*0.05 > P > 0.01.

analysis available for determination of nifedipine plasma concentrations when the investigations were undertaken.

Arithmetic means, standard deviations, and coefficients of variation were calculated. Total digitoxin clearance (CL) was calculated as: $CL = (D \cdot F)/(C^{ss} \cdot \tau)$, where D is the dose required every dosage interval (τ) to maintain the steady-state digitoxin plasma concentration (C^{ss}) and F (0.95) is a correction factor for bioavailability of digitoxin. Renal digitoxin and creatinine clearances were calculated by dividing the amount of urinary digitoxin or creatinine excretion by the corresponding plasma concentrations. Extrarenal clearance of digitoxin was calculated as the difference between total body clearance and renal clearance. Differences between various kinetic parameters of digitoxin were evaluated by Student's paired t test.

RESULTS

Tables II to IV list plasma concentrations and daily urinary excretion of digitoxin in subjects receiving digitoxin alone and in combination with verapamil, diltiazem, or nifedipine.

In eight of 10 subjects the simultaneous dosing of

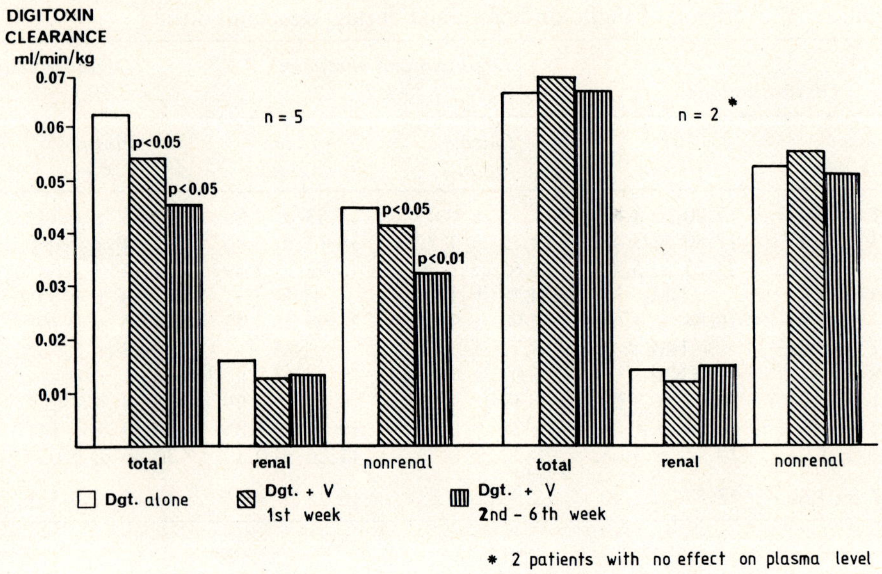

Fig. 1. Mean digitoxin clearance in seven subjects receiving maintenance digitoxin *(Dgt.)* doses before and during dosing with 240 mg verapamil *(V)*.

Table IV. Plasma and renal excretion of digitoxin before and during nifedepine dosing

	Digitoxin alone		*Digitoxin and nifedipine, wk 1*		*Digitoxin and nifedipine, wk 2 to 6*	
Patient	*Plasma (ng/ml)*	*Urine (μg/day)*	*Plasma (ng/ml)*	*Urine (μg/day)*	*Plasma (ng/ml)*	*Urine (μg/day)*
G. I.	20.28 ± 2.38	17.50 ± 4.05	13.28 ± 2.26	13.95 ± 5.22	18.27 ± 1.36	17.52 ± 2.92
I. C.	13.72 ± 1.80	14.10 ± 1.80	15.17 ± 2.26	20.95 ± 4.51	13.76 ± 0.68	18.11 ± 3.55
B. X.	13.62 ± 0.99	16.99 ± 2.95	14.97 ± 0.63	26.18 ± 1.25	17.03 ± 1.75	17.24 ± 6.15
F. X.	13.02 ± 1.62	24.20 ± 7.93	15.60 ± 1.72	29.93 ± 4.98	14.30 ± 1.02	28.33 ± 4.40
K. X.	12.03 ± 1.54	17.52 ± 0.56	13.47 ± 2.46	14.78 ± 5.32	13.90 ± 0.50	21.18 ± 2.00
S. I.	6.63 ± 0.71	25.95 ± 5.23	6.01 ± 0.45	26.84 ± 3.87	5.45 ± 0.29	26.77 ± 5.04
Q. B.	18.02 ± 1.17	18.90 ± 3.93	16.28 ± 0.77	16.98 ± 3.84	19.68 ± 2.09	21.85 ± 5.32
I. T.	11.18 ± 1.41	37.24 ± 6.36	8.03 ± 1.00	38.19 ± 5.30	9.05 ± 1.16	36.10 ± 10.78
B. C.	11.90 ± 2.88	NM	11.40 ± 1.20	NM	8.59 ± 1.78	NM
F. L.	18.60 ± 1.60	NM	18.52 ± 4.40	NM	21.53 ± 2.83	NM
$\overline{X}$ ± SD	13.90 ± 4.06	21.55 ± 7.45	13.27 ± 3.83	23.48 ± 8.38	14.16 ± 5.20	23.31 ± 6.62

Data are $\overline{X}$ ± SD.
NM = Not measured.

digitoxin and 240 mg verapamil daily led to a continuous rise in digitoxin plasma levels until a new steady state was reached after 2 to 3 weeks (Table II). In two subjects, however, there was no change in digitoxin plasma concentrations. Digitoxin plasma concentrations in the eight subjects were 35% (range 14% to 97%) higher than before verapamil dosing. The daily renal glycoside excretion was not significantly changed by verapamil coadministration. Whereas renal digitoxin clearance and endogenous creatinine clearance were not influenced by verapamil, total body clearance and extrarenal clearance of digitoxin were reduced 27% and 29% in subjects with plasma concentrations elevated by verapamil (Fig. 1; Table II).

Although there were considerable variations in verapamil plasma concentrations (range 50 to 450 ng/ml), there seems to be a direct correlation between the magnitude of the verapamil concentrations in plasma and the increase in digitoxin plasma levels. The two subjects without increased digitoxin concentrations after coadministration of verapamil also showed the lowest verapamil concentrations (50 to 100 ng/ml), while subject B. T., whose digitoxin levels doubled after verapamil dosing, also had the highest verapamil plasma concentrations of >400 ng/ml.

Concomitant diltiazem and digitoxin dosing increased steady-state digitoxin plasma levels in five of 10 subjects (mean 21%; range 6% to 31%). Renal excretion, which could be measured only in three subjects (I. C., N. T., B. X.), was not changed (Table III). Whereas renal digitoxin clearance and endogenous creatinine clearance were not influenced by diltiazem, total body clearance and extrarenal clearance of digitoxin were reduced in two of the five subjects in whom plasma concentrations were elevated by diltiazem and renal digitoxin excretion could be measured.

Individual diltiazem plasma concentrations varied greatly (range 23 to 168 ng/ml). There were no significant differences in subjects with or without diltiazem-induced changes in digitoxin plasma levels. The mean diltiazem plasma level in the five subjects with an elevated plasma digitoxin level was 45.8 ± 28 ng/ml, and it was 68.6 ± 57 ng/ml in the five subjects without a change in digitoxin plasma level.

In contrast to verapamil, the concomitant dosing of nifedipine did not alter steady-state plasma digitoxin levels or daily renal glycoside excretion (Table IV). Renal digitoxin clearance and endogenous creatinine clearance were not influenced by nifedipine, and total body clearance and extrarenal clearance of digitoxin were slightly but not significantly increased (Fig. 2; Table IV).

In all three groups there were no differences between subjects with and without impairment of kidney or liver function. There were no serious adverse reactions attributable to digitoxin, diltiazem, or nifedipine. One subject with doubled digitoxin levels after verapamil dosing showed a marked prolongation of the P-R interval, resulting in a primary or secondary atrioventricular block that disappeared after the digitoxin and verapamil doses were reduced.

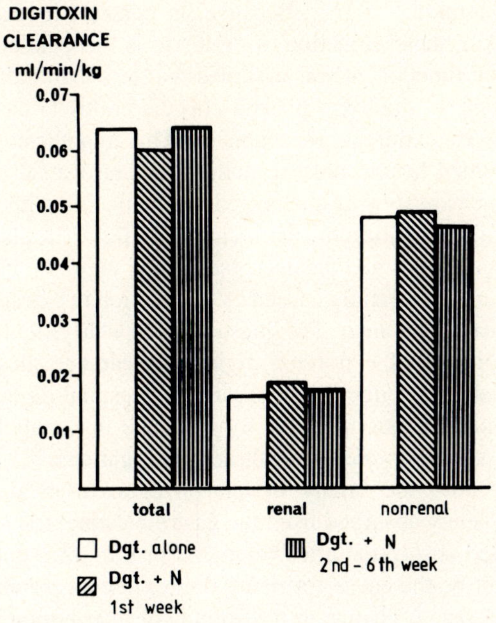

Fig. 2. Mean digitoxin clearance in subjects receiving maintenance digitoxin *(Dgt.)* doses before and during dosing with 40 to 60 mg nifedipine *(N)*.

DISCUSSION

Today, the combination of calcium antagonists and cardiac glycosides is widely used in the treatment of cardiac insufficiencies resulting from hypertension or coronary heart disease. During recent years many investigators have shown that concomitant dosing with verapamil and digoxin may result in a marked rise in digoxin plasma concentrations,[2,8,17,19,25] increasing the risk of digitalis intoxication.[27] According to Klein et al.,[8] 49 patients who received digoxin and verapamil for chronic atrial fibrillation showed a significant increase in digoxin plasma concentrations averaging 70%. Similar results were reported after combined therapy with digoxin and diltiazem.[18,22,25,26] Concomitant dosing with diltiazem and digoxin caused a significant increase in digoxin plasma levels of about 43% in eight of 12 subjects.[10] Contrary to this, digoxin plasma levels did not rise appreciably after the combined dosing of nifedipine and digoxin.[10,20,24] These reports show that the combination of verapamil and digitoxin may also result in a significant rise in digitoxin plasma levels under steady-state conditions. However, this increase, which amounts to a mean of 27%, is only half as high as that described for digoxin. Similar differences between digoxin and digitoxin were reported after studies of its interaction with quinidine.[1,4-7,11,21] In view of the great variability and the small number of subjects with a diltiazem-induced increase in digitoxin plasma level, it cannot be stated for certain that there is a clinically relevant pharmacokinetic interaction as is described for the combination with digoxin. In contrast, coadministration of nifedipine did not alter steady-state plasma digitoxin or digoxin levels or daily renal glycoside excretion.[13]

The reason for increasing digoxin plasma levels during concomitant dosing with quinidine or verapamil is mainly a decrease in renal excretion based on inhibition of active tubular secretion and possibly a rise in tubular reabsorption.[1,4,6,15,23,25] Because, in contrast to that of digoxin, the elimination of digitoxin is independent of kidney function, it was assumed that less than half the increase in digitoxin plasma concentrations is caused solely by extrarenal mechanisms. This hypothesis was confirmed by the present studies. Because renal digitoxin clearance was unchanged during dosing with verapamil and diltiazem, the increase in digitoxin plasma concentrations and the decrease in total digitoxin clearance must be mainly caused by a reduction in extrarenal digitoxin clearance. The question as to what extent this impairment of extrarenal digitoxin clearance may be caused by a reduction in biliary or intestinal digitoxin excretion or possibly also by a change in metabolism cannot be answered after these investigations.

Because the highly lipophilic digitoxin is almost completely absorbed from the gastrointestinal tract, increased absorption after verapamil or diltiazem dosing cannot be the cause for rising digitoxin concentrations in plasma. A change in the volume of distribution also seems unlikely, especially because alterations in bioavailability or volume of distribution of digitoxin were not observed during acute studies.[12]

Unlike verapamil, nifedipine does not influence the pharmacokinetics of digoxin and digitoxin. Therefore, different sites of pharmacokinetic interactions of these two calcium antagonists are assumed. Similar observations with regard to different sites of pharmacokinetic interactions were made with tiapamil and nicardipine, two new calcium antagonists of the verapamil or dihydropyridine type, respectively.[16] It is not known why only some and not all patients show an increase in plasma glycoside concentrations after diltiazem dosing.

In contrast to the case with digoxin, strict rules for a reduction in digitoxin dose during concomitant verapamil therapy cannot be set, because the elevation of digitoxin plasma levels is markedly less. Furthermore, the relatively slow rise in digitoxin plasma levels compared with those of digoxin may be advantageous, usually giving the physician enough time to adjust the digitoxin dose to suit clinical needs. The small increase in digitoxin plasma levels after diltiazem coadministration, however, is hardly of clinical significance. Because interactions resulting from impairment of renal excretion of digoxin appear to be much more frequent and are more dangerous than those after digitoxin dosing, digitoxin offers a valuable alternative.[3,9]

I thank Prof. Dr. E. Richter and Dr. G. Neurath for the verapamil and diltiazem determinations and Miss D. Schirmer for excellent technical assistance.

References

1. Belz GG, Aust PE, Doering W, Heinz M, Schneider B: Pharmacodynamics of a single dose of quinidine during chronic digoxin treatment. Eur J Clin Pharmacol **22:**111-117, 1982.
2. Belz GG, Doering W, Munkes R, Matthews J: Interaction between digoxin and calcium antagonists and antiarrhythmic drugs. CLIN PHARMACOL THER **33:**410-417, 1983.
3. Bussay H: The influence of quinidine and other agents on digitalis glycosides. Am Heart J **104:**289-302, 1982.
4. Doering W: Quinidine-digoxin interaction. Pharmacokinetics, underlying mechanism and clinical implications. N Engl J Med **301:**400-404, 1979.
5. Ejvinsson G: Effects of quinidine on plasma concentrations of digoxin. Br Med J **1:**279-280, 1978.
6. Hager WD, Fenster P, Mayersohn M, Perrier D, Graves P, Marcus FJ, Goldman S: Digoxin-quinidine interaction. Pharmacokinetic evaluation. N Engl J Med **300:**1238-1241, 1979.
7. Hooymans PM, Merkus FWHM: Effects of quinidine on plasma concentration of digoxin. Br Med J **2:**1022, 1978.
8. Klein HO, Lang R, Weiss E, DiSegni E, Libhaber C, Guerrero J, Kaplinsky E: The influence of verapamil on serum digoxin concentration. Circulation **65:**998-1003, 1982.
9. Kuhlmann J: Klinische Relevanz von Arzneimittelinteraktionen am Beispiel herzwirksamer Glykoside. Med Klin **79:**150-156, 1984.
10. Kuhlmann J: Effects of nifedipine and diltiazem on plasma levels and renal excretion of beta-acetyldigoxin. CLIN PHARMACOL THER **37:**150-156, 1985.
11. Kuhlmann J, Dohrmann M, Marcin S: Effects of quinidine on plasma level and renal excretion of digitoxin achieving steady state conditions. Naunyn Schmiedebergs Arch Pharmacol **325:**R85, 1984.
12. Kuhlmann J, Marcin S: Einfluβ von Verapamil auf Pharmakokinetik und Pharmakodynamik von Digitoxin beim Patienten. Verh Dtsch Ges Inn Med **90:**1395-1399, 1984.
13. Kuhlmann J, Marcin S, Frank KH: Pharmakokinetik und kardiale Wirksamkeit von β-Acetyldigoxin und Digitoxin unter einer Kombinationstherapie mit Nifedipin. Klin Wochenschr **62:**451-457, 1984.
14. Kuhlmann J, Pabst J: Eiweiβbindung und Hydroxylierungsrate von Digitoxin bei Niereninsuffizienz. Dtsch Med Wochenschr **107:**1551-1555, 1982.
15. Leahey EB Jr, Reiffel JA, Heissenbuttel KH, Drusin RE, Lovejoy W, Bigger JT Jr: Enhanced effect of digoxin during quinidine treatment. Arch Intern Med **139:**519-521, 1979.
16. Lessem J, Bellinetto A: Interaction between digoxin and the calcium antagonists nicardipine and tiapamil. Clin Ther 5:595-602, 1983.
17. Marcus FI, Fenster PE: Digoxin interactions with other cardiac drugs. J Cardiovasc Med **8:**25-29, 1983.

18. Oyama Y, Fujii S, Kanda K, Akino E, Kawasaki H, Nagata M, Goto K: Digoxin-diltiazem interaction. Am J Cardiol **53:**1480-1481, 1984.
19. Pedersen KE, Dorph-Pedersen A, Hvidt S, Klitgaard NA, Nielsen-Kudsk F: Digoxin-verapamil interaction. CLIN PHARMACOL THER **30:**311-316, 1981.
20. Pedersen KE, Dorph-Pedersen A, Hvidt S, Litgaard NA, Kjaer K, Nielsen-Kudsk F: Effect of nifedipine on digoxin kinetics in healthy subjects. CLIN PHARMACOL THER **32:**562-565, 1982.
21. Peters U, Risler T, Grabensee B, Falkenstein U, Kroukou Y: Interaktion von Chinidin und Digitoxin beim Menschen. Dtsch Med Wochenschr **105:**438-442, 1980.
22. Rameis H, Magometschnigg D, Ganzinger U: The diltiazem-digoxin interaction. CLIN PHARMACOL THER **36:** 183-189, 1984.
23. Schwartz JB, Keefe D, Kates RE, Harrison CD: Verapamil and digoxin: Another drug-drug interaction. Clin Res **29:**501A, 1981.
24. Schwartz JB, Rainzer A, Akers S: The effect of nifedipine on serum digoxin concentrations in patients. Am Heart J **107:**669-673, 1984.
25. Thiercelin JF, Hermann PH, Warrington S, Thénot JP, Morselli PL: Interaction study between digoxin and calcium antagonists: Verapamil and diltiazem. Presented at the Second World Conference on Clinical Pharmacology and Therapeutics, July 31-Aug. 5, 1983.
26. Yoshida A, Fujita M, Kurosawa N, Nioka M, Skichinohe T, Arakuwa M, Fakuda R, Owada E, Ito K: Effects of diltiazem on plasma level and urinary excretion of digoxin in healthy subjects. CLIN PHARMACOL THER **35:**681-685, 1984.
27. Zatuchni J: Verapamil-digoxin interaction. Am Heart J **108:**412-413, 1984.

Effect of etodolac in patients with moderate renal impairment compared with normal subjects

Twenty subjects (10 with normal renal function and 10 with moderate renal insufficiency) participated in an 8-day study to assess the effects of acute and chronic etodolac dosing on renal function. Subjects and patients were hospitalized and followed a controlled diet (150 mEq sodium, 60 to 80 mEq potassium) during the study. A 3-day drug-free period was followed by 4 days of etodolac, 200 mg b.i.d. Sodium balance and body weight remained unchanged in both groups. Modest reductions in renal function as measured by clearances of inulin and *p*-aminohippurate occurred acutely only in the patients with renal impairment. Chronic therapy resulted in no decrements in daily creatinine clearance. In an average effective anti-inflammatory dose, etodolac did not produce a sustained effect on renal function in either normal subjects or patients with moderate renal insufficiency. (CLIN PHARMACOL THER 1985;38:674-9.)

D. Craig Brater, M.D., Shirley A. Anderson, R.N., Debbie Brown-Cartwright, P.A., Robert D. Toto, M.D., Andrew Chen, M.S., and Ginette B. Jacob, M.D. *Dallas, Tex.*

Etodolac is a new nonsteroidal anti-inflammatory drug (NSAID) currently under clinical investigation. In laboratory animals it has substantial anti-inflammatory, analgesic, and antipyretic activity.[1] In man, etodolac in doses from 100 to 300 mg b.i.d. has been effective in the treatment of the symptoms of rheumatoid arthritis and osteoarthritis[2,3] and it is an effective analgesic for moderately severe postoperative and dental pain.[4-7] No unexpected patient complaints or laboratory abnormalities have been observed. The incidence of patient complaints related to the gastrointestinal system was similar to that in patients given placebo and was significantly lower than that in patients receiving aspirin.[8]

This class of drugs is known to have potential adverse renal effects.[9,10] Patients with decreased effective or actual circulating blood volume are at risk of acute renal ischemia when given NSAIDs.[11-28] In these clinical conditions, locally synthesized vasodilatory prostaglandins (PGs) counteract the vasoconstricting effects of angiotensin II and catecholamines and thereby maintain renal perfusion.[11-28] Inhibition of PG synthesis results in unopposed renal vasoconstriction and decrements in renal function.[11-28] Although the data are conflicting, it appears that either not all NSAIDs share this potential or that some have less propensity to inhibit renal PGs.[29] We therefore performed this study to assess the effects of etodolac on renal function in a susceptible patient group with doses sufficient to treat inflammatory conditions. Transient effects occurred in patients with chronic renal insufficiency but did not cause overall changes in renal homeostasis.

METHODS

Study design (Fig. 1). This was an open-label study in which participants were hospitalized in the General Clinical Research Center for 8 days. All potential participants had endogenous creatinine clearance measured within 2 weeks of the start of the study to document renal function. Participants were admitted to the Center 3 days before planned drug dosing to establish baseline values while following a controlled diet consisting of 150 mEq sodium and 60 to 80 mEq potassium per day. Fluids were allowed ad libitum, except for the controlled amounts on the days when clearances of inulin and *p*-aminohippurate (PAH) were determined.

Endogenous creatinine clearance and urinary electrolyte excretion were measured daily starting on the day of admission. On day 4, participants omitted breakfast and received a priming dose of inulin and PAH, followed by maintenance infusions to maintain steady-

From the Departments of Internal Medicine and Pharmacology, The University of Texas Health Science Center at Dallas, and Ayerst Laboratories.

Supported by Public Health Service Grants No. R01-AM27059, No. K04-AM00705, and No. M01-RR00633, and by a grant from Ayerst Laboratories.

Received for publication June 25, 1985; accepted Aug. 20, 1985.

Reprint requests to: D. C. Brater, M.D., Department of Pharmacology, The University of Texas Health Science Center at Dallas, 5323 Harry Hines Blvd., Dallas, TX 75235.

state serum concentrations of approximately 25 and 1.5 mg/dl, respectively. After a 45-minute equilibration period, three to four 20-minute baseline urine collections were obtained. Etodolac (200 mg) was taken by mouth and was followed by eight postdosing urine collections. Serum samples were drawn at the midpoint of each collection. Etodolac was then taken at 8 PM of day 4 and at 8 AM and 8 PM of days 5 to 7. On the morning of day 8, a repeat clearance study was performed as on day 4. At the start of the clearance study, participants drank a water load of 20 ml/kg. After each subsequent voiding, urinary losses were matched with oral water plus 1 ml/min for insensible losses.

Subjects. A total of 20 participants between the ages of 18 and 65 years who were within 20% of their ideal weight participated. Ten patients (seven men and three women) had moderately impaired renal function (endogenous creatinine clearance between 20 and 69 ml/min). These patients had no active multisystem disease or renal disease requiring acute treatment. Their demographic characteristics, diagnoses, level of renal function, and concomitant drugs are listed in Table I. They maintained their stable doses of all chronic medications. On days 4 and 8 diuretics were withheld until completion of the clearance studies. Renal function of the patients had been stable for at least 6 months, with no history of acute renal failure or intermittent dialysis within the past year. Ten normal men constituted the control group and were characterized as follows: Age = 27 ± 1 years ($\bar{X}$ ± SE); weight = 68 ± 3 kg; creatinine clearance = 134 ± 7 ml/min. They were receiving no medications, including nonprescription drugs.

Data analysis. During each clearance study, the effects of etodolac on clearances of inulin and PAH and on fractional excretions of electrolytes were assessed. Control values represent the mean of two to three stable collections during an established period of water diuresis as determined by values for urinary osmolality. Values for the effects of etodolac represent the mean of three collections: that representing peak effect as determined by the maximal decrease in sodium excretion and the collections immediately preceding and following this collection. Hence these three collections encompass the maximum effects of the drug, which occurred within 2.5 hours in all participants and in most at 90 minutes. On a daily basis, effects were assessed on 24-hour creatinine clearance and sodium and chloride excretion, on serum concentrations of creatinine and potassium, and on weight and blood pressure. Results of statistical analyses with paired Student's t tests were considered significant at a P level <0.05.

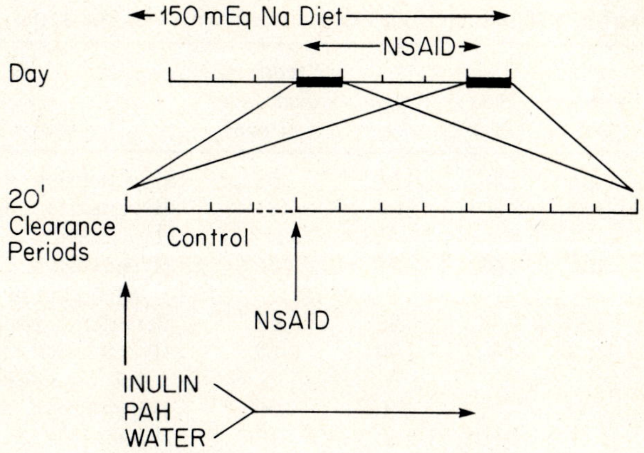

Fig. 1. Scheme of the study protocol.

RESULTS

The effects of etodolac on renal function were assessed in two ways: (1) The immediate effects of the NSAID were determined with the clearance studies performed with both initial exposure to the drug and on the fifth day of chronic dosing; and (2) daily serum and quantitative urine collections were obtained to assess effects of chronic dosing on overall renal homeostasis. In essence, then, we used both clearance and balance techniques to explore the effects of etodolac on renal function.

Clearance studies. Results of both the acute and chronic clearance studies are shown in Fig. 2. With the first dose of etodolac and with the morning dose on the fifth day of therapy, fractional excretions of all electrolytes and urinary volume decreased significantly in both the patients and the control subjects. The time at which the peak effect occurred in the patients was 90 ± 10 minutes in the acute study and 98 ± 11 minutes in the chronic study. This corresponds to the time of the peak serum concentration of etodolac.* Moreover, the relative decrements in electrolyte excretion were similar for patients and subjects. Importantly, it is also apparent from these data that the control values did not differ in the acute and chronic studies. Hence these data suggest that with each exposure to the drug there was a short-lived, reversible decrease in electrolyte and volume excretion. With a twice-daily dosing regimen, sufficient time elapsed for all parameters to return to baseline by the next dose.

While effects on urinary electrolyte and volume excretion were similar for patients and subjects, effects

*Brater DC, Anderson SA, Brown-Cartwright D, et al: Unpublished observations, 1985.

Table I. Characteristics of patients with chronic renal insufficiency

Patient No.	*Age (yr)*	*Weight (kg)*	*Creatinine clearance (ml/min)*	*Diagnoses*	*Concomitant drugs*
101	49	111	68	Hypertension, diabetes	Propranolol, hydralazine, furosemide, insulin
103	60	104	41	Hypertension, angina, gout	Diltiazem, allopurinol, nitroglycerin, isosorbide dinitrate, propranolol, furosemide
104	61	85	56	Hypertension, COPD, gout, osteoarthritis	Theophylline, amitriptyline, diphenhydramine, prazosin
106	58	56	63	Periarteritis nodosa, COPD	Hydrochlorothiazide
108	60	99	69	Hypertension, S/P CVA, S/P myocardial infarction	Allopurinol, minoxidil, propranolol, furosemide
109	72	110	39	Hypertension, diabetes, gout	Diphenhydramine, allopurinol, insulin, clonidine, hydralazine, furosemide
110	48	70	20	Hypertension	Ranitidine, nifedipine, furosemide
111	59	65	24	Hypertension, gout, COPD, osteoarthritis	Allopurinol, propranolol, clonidine, furosemide
113	54	91	52	Hypertension, S/P myocardial infarction, angina	Nifedipine, isosorbide dinitrate, dipyridamole, prazosin, atenolol, furosemide
114	68	65	36	Hypertension, gout, osteoarthritis	Allopurinol, hydralazine, nadolol, furosemide

COPD = Chronic obstructive pulmonary disease; S/P = status post; CVA = cerebrovascular accident.

on renal hemodynamics differed. Etodolac had no effect on the glomerular filtration rate or renal plasma flow in normal subjects but decreased both by approximately 30% with the first dose to the patients. With chronic dosing, etodolac again caused a decrease in renal hemodynamics in the patients, but the magnitude was less, approximately 20% and 15%, respectively, which was not statistically significant. Importantly, as occurred with electrolyte excretion, values for renal hemodynamics in the subjects were similar in both initial and chronic studies. This observation again implies that the decrements in renal hemodynamics observed in the patients with renal insufficiency are transient.

Balance studies. Fig. 3 shows daily values for participant weight, serum potassium and creatinine levels, urinary excretion of sodium and chloride, and creatinine clearance. Values during etodolac dosing did not differ from control values for any parameter. In addition, there were no effects on blood pressure during the study (data not shown). Hence, on a 24-hour basis, etodolac had no effect on renal function. This finding supports the implication from the clearance studies that effects of this NSAID on renal function are transient and that they dissipate quickly enough to cause no overall effects on renal hemodynamics or electrolyte homeostasis.

DISCUSSION

NSAIDs can affect the kidney in a number of ways, all of which presumably relate to inhibition of renal PG synthesis[9,10]: (1) Decreased sodium and water excretion over and above any effects on hemodynamics,[9,10] (2) decreased plasma renin activity with consequent hyporenin-hypoaldosteronism and increased serum potassium concentrations,[30,31] and (3) renal insufficiency most frequently of an ischemic nature.[11-28] The latter occurs in clinical settings associated with decreased actual or effective circulating blood volume, conditions in which homeostatic mechanisms result in increased concentrations of circulating vasoconstrictors including catecholamines, angiotensin II, and vasopressin.[11-28] To maintain renal perfusion in such settings, the kidney synthesizes vasodilating PGs, presumably PGI_2 and PGE_2. Their inhibition by NSAIDs can cause rapid deterioration of renal function.

Susceptible patient groups include those with cirrhosis,[11-16] congestive heart failure,[25] and renal insufficiency,[17-22,32] although it is possible that not all patients in this latter group may be at similar risk. For example, patients with lupus nephritis[19-22] or with nephrotic syndrome[17,18] appear to require increased renal PG synthesis to maintain renal hemodynamics. On the other hand, patients with renal insufficiency from hypertension, diabetes, or other causes probably do not have decreased actual or effective circulating volumes and may not require PGs to maintain renal perfusion. Hence we felt it important to explore whether etodolac adversely affects renal function in this patient population.

In addition, in studies of other NSAIDs in patients with renal insufficiency, the question has been raised that some NSAIDs such as sulindac may spare renal

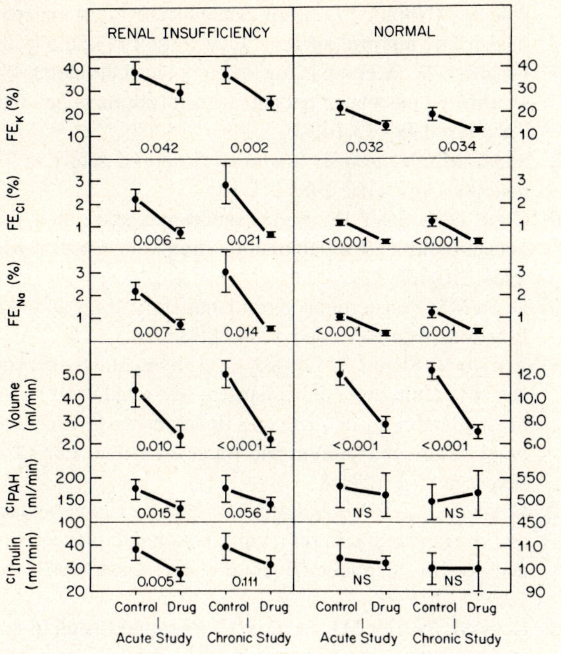

Fig. 2. Mean (±SE) effects of etodolac during both acute and chronic dosing evaluated by clearance techniques. P values are noted in the figure. *Cl* = Clearance; *FE* = fractional excretion; *NS* = not significant.

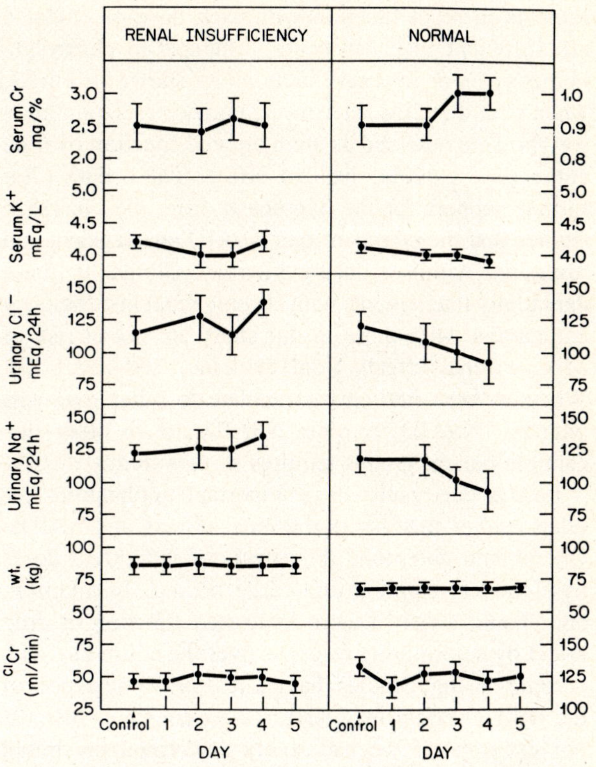

Fig. 3. Mean (±SE) effects of chronic etodolac dosing on daily participant creatinine clearances *(Cl_{Cr})*, weights *(wt)*, serum concentrations of potassium and creatinine *(Cr)*, and 24-hour urinary excretions of sodium and chloride.

PGs.[29] Consequently, it is important to explore this possibility with any new NSAID.

Lastly, no data address whether acute detrimental effects of any NSAID on renal function persist and extrapolate to chronic dosing. We felt it conceivable that compensatory mechanisms might be operative to normalize renal function after an initial insult. Our study, then, was designed to assess whether etodolac affected the kidney and if so, whether the effects persisted with chronic drug dosing.

In both the patients and the normal subjects of our study, etodolac had distinct effects on renal electrolyte and volume excretion. In the acute and the chronic clearance studies, etodolac decreased urinary volume and fractional excretion of all electrolytes within 2 hours, indicating an effect on tubular reabsorption of these electrolytes. This effect is similar to that previously reported with a number of different NSAIDs.[9,10] Of interest, however, is that the control values during the clearance study after chronic dosing are no different from those before exposure to etodolac. This finding indicates that complete recovery from these effects of etodolac occurs within a dosing interval.

Patients differed from the normal subjects in their renal hemodynamic response to etodolac. Subjects had no change in clearances of inulin or PAH with exposure to the NSAID. This observation is consistent with findings with other NSAIDs in normal subjects who are not sodium deprived.[26-28] In contrast, patients with renal insufficiency had decreases in the glomerular filtration rate and renal plasma flow of approximately 30% with the first exposure to etodolac. A similar phenomenon, although of lesser magnitude, occurred after chronic dosing. Similar to effects on solute handling, control values for renal hemodynamic parameters during the chronic clearance study did not differ from those before etodolac dosing. Hence full recovery of renal hemodynamics occurs within a dosing interval of etodolac.

In summary, the clearance studies clearly show effects of individual doses of etodolac, either acutely or chronically, on renal hemodynamics and on tubular reabsorption of solute. At the doses and dosing intervals we used, which are those projected for clinical use, recovery of function occurred. Whether higher doses or more frequent dosing would cause persistent effects is not known and is worthy of further study.

Of additional importance is whether the transient decrements in renal function with each dose of etodolac are sufficient to cause overall changes in electrolyte homeostasis or in renal function. As shown in Fig. 3, when renal function, electrolyte homeostasis, and body weight were assessed as an integrated function over an entire day, etodolac had no effect. These data offer further support for the hypothesis from the clearance studies that the effects of this NSAID are transient and reversible within a dosing interval. Clinically, these data imply that patients with chronic renal insufficiency comparable with those in our study are not at risk of adverse renal effects from etodolac, 200 mg b.i.d. Whether these findings extrapolate to other regimens with this NSAID, to other NSAIDs, or to other susceptible patient groups requires further study.

Lastly, our results have important implications for other studies that assess the renal effects of NSAIDs. One should determine the effects of individual doses by frequent sampling after drug dosing. In addition, one should assess a more integrated function of drug effect by determining response over the entire day with chronic dosing. Studies that address only one aspect of the NSAID effect may lead to erroneous conclusions. For example, if we had solely performed the initial clearance study, we would have concluded that etodolac had a substantial deleterious effect on renal function. In contrast, if we had only analyzed effects in terms of total daily urine collections, we might have concluded that etodolac had no effect on renal function. Clearly, neither conclusion in and of itself would have been correct. Future studies of this and other NSAIDs should assess both acute and chronic effects.

References

1. Martel RR, Klicius J. Anti-inflammatory and analgesic properties of etodolac in rats. Can J Physiol Pharmacol 1976;54:245-8.
2. Jacob GB, Hart KK, Mulane JF, Lutins S, Lee TY. Placebo-controlled study of etodolac and aspirin in the treatment of rheumatoid arthritis. Curr Ther Res 1983; 33:703-13.
3. Sanda M, Collins SH, Mahady J, Huth J, Krantz K. Three-month multicenter study of etodolac (Ultradol[R]) in patients with osteoarthritis of the hip. Curr Ther Res 1983;33:782-92.
4. Versichelen L, Bilsback P, Rolly G, Merlo M, Joubert L. Etodolac in post-surgical pain: a double-blind dose-ranging efficacy study with aspirin and placebo. Int J Clin Pharmacol Ther Toxicol 1982;20:236-9.
5. Gaston G, Mallow R, Frank J. The efficacy of etodolac for patients with pain following oral surgery. J Oral Maxill Surg 1984;42:362-6.
6. Hutton CE. The effectiveness of 100 and 200 mg of etodolac (Ultradol[R]), aspirin, and placebo in patients with pain following oral surgery. Oral Surg 1983;56:575-80.
7. Friedrich E. A comparison of etodolac (Ultradol[R]) with aspirin and placebo in patients with episiotomy pain. Curr Ther Res 1983;33:100-7.
8. Sanda M, Zuchero D, Shand D. Etodolac: safety in 992 patients. Adv Ther 1985;2:1-10.
9. Clive DM, Stoff JS. Renal syndromes associated with nonsteroidal anti-inflammatory drugs. N Engl J Med 1984;310:563-72.
10. Dunn MJ. Nonsteroidal antiinflammatory drugs and renal function. Ann Rev Med 1984;35:411-28.
11. Arroyo V, Planas R, Gaya J, et al. Sympathetic nervous activity, renin-angiotensin system and renal excretion of prostaglandin E_2 in cirrhosis. Relationship to functional renal failure and sodium and water excretion. Eur J Clin Invest 1983;13:271-8.
12. Boyer TD, Zia P, Reynolds TB. Effect of indomethacin and prostaglandin A_1 on renal function and plasma renin activity in alcoholic liver disease. Gastroenterology 1979;77:215-22.
13. Levy M, Wexler MJ, Fechner C. Renal perfusion in dogs with experimental hepatic cirrhosis: role of prostaglandins. Am J Physiol 1983;245:F521-9.
14. Zambraski EJ, Dunn MJ. Importance of renal prostaglandins in control of renal function after chronic ligation of the common bile duct in dogs. J Lab Clin Med 1984;103:549-59.
15. Zipser RD, Hoefs JC, Speckart PF, Zia PK, Horton R. Prostaglandins: modulators of renal function and pressor resistance in chronic liver disease. J Clin Endocrinol Metab 1979;48:895-900.
16. Zipser RD, Little T, Ziperovich H, Duke R. The role of arachidonic acid metabolites in the functional renal impairment associated with liver disease. In: Dunn MJ, Patrono C, Cinotti GA, eds. Prostaglandins and the kidney. Biochemistry, physiology, pharmacology and clinical applications. New York: Plenum Publishing Corp, 1983:263-74.
17. Kleinknecht C, Broyer M, Gubler M-C, Palcoux J-B. Irreversible renal failure after indomethacin in steroid-resistant nephrosis. N Engl J Med 1981;302:691.
18. Tiggeler RGWL, Hulme B, Wijdeveld PGAB. Effect of indomethacin on glomerular permeability in the nephrotic syndrome. Kidney Int 1979;16:312-21.
19. Kimberly RP, Gill JR Jr, Bowden RE, Keiser HR, Plotz PH: Elevated urinary prostaglandins and the effects of aspirin on renal function in lupus erythematosus. Ann Intern Med 1978;89:336-41.
20. Kimberly RP, Plotz PH. Aspirin-induced depression of renal function. N Engl J Med 1977;296:418-24.
21. Kimberly RP. Renal prostaglandins in systemic lupus erythematosus. Lancet 1978;2:553-5.
22. Rasmussen S, Petersen J, Nielsen IL, Christensen P, Hilden T. Effect of acetylsalicylic acid on renal function in systemic lupus erythematosus. Eur J Clin Pharmacol 1982;23:505-8.

23. Fink MP, MacVittie TJ, Casey LC. Effects of nonsteroidal anti-inflammatory drugs on renal function in septic dogs. J Surg Res 1984;36:516-25.
24. Henrich WL, Anderson RJ, Berns AS, McDonald KM, Paulsen PJ, Berl T, Schrier RW. The role of renal nerves and prostaglandins in control of renal hemodynamics and plasma renin activity during hypotensive hemorrhage in the dog. J Clin Invest 1978;61:744-50.
25. Oliver JA, Sciacca RR, Pinto J, Cannon PJ. Participation of the prostaglandins in the control of renal blood flow during acute reduction of cardiac output in the dog. J Clin Invest 1981;67:229-37.
26. Muther RS, Bennett WM. Effects of aspirin on glomerular filtration rate in normal humans. Ann Intern Med 1980;92:386-7.
27. Muther RS, Potter DM, Bennett WM. Aspirin-induced depression of glomerular filtration rate in normal humans: role of sodium balance. Ann Intern Med 1981;94:317-21.
28. Oliver JA, Pinto J, Sciacca RR, Cannon PJ. Increased renal secretion of norepinephrine and prostaglandin E_2 during sodium depletion in the dog. J Clin Invest 1980;66:748-56.
29. Ciabattoni G, Cinotti GA, Pierucci A, et al. Effects of sulindac and ibuprofen in patients with chronic glomerular disease. Evidence for the dependence of renal function on prostacyclin. N Engl J Med 1984;310:279-83.
30. Tan SY, Shapiro R, Franco R, Stockard H, Mulrow PJ. Indomethacin-induced prostaglandin inhibition with hyperkalemia. Ann Intern Med 1979;90:783-5.
31. Tan SY, Shapiro R, Franco R, Stockard H, Mulrow PJ. Indomethacin-induced prostaglandin inhibition with hyperkalemia. A reversible cause of hyporeninemic hypoaldosteronism. Ann Intern Med 1979;90:783-5.
32. Kirschenbaum MA, Serros ER. Effect of prostaglandin inhibition on glomerular filtration rate in normal and uremic rabbits. Prostaglandins 1981;22:245-54.

A simple method for the estimation of glomerular filtration rate by gentamicin pharmacokinetics during routine drug monitoring in the newborn

Assessment of the glomerular filtration rate (GFR) in the newborn is often imprecise because of difficulties in urine collection and because the plasma creatinine level, the traditional marker of renal function, is influenced by many factors in this age group. Gentamicin is given to most preterm infants for suspected or proved sepsis. This drug is eliminated almost entirely by the kidney and its rate of elimination parallels the GFR. We calculated gentamicin pharmacokinetic parameters ($t_{1/2}$, volume of distribution, and clearance) from three consecutive concentration-time points (trough, peak, and next trough levels) in 38 newborn infants. Creatinine clearance was measured by the conventional method. Both $t_{1/2}$ ($r = 0.74$; $P < 0.001$) and gentamicin clearance ($r = 0.77$; $P < 0.001$) correlated well with measured creatinine clearance. There was no correlation between these variables and urine output. Gentamicin elimination $t_{1/2}$ and clearance are useful indices of GFR in the newborn infant and can be easily calculated during routine therapeutic drug monitoring. (CLIN PHARMACOL THER 38:680-685, 1985.)

Gideon Koren, M.D.,* Andrew James, M.D., and Max Perlman, M.D.
Toronto, Ontario, Canada

Various methods have been described for the estimation of the glomerular filtration rate (GFR) in newborn infants.[2] These have been based on either endogenous physiologic markers such as plasma creatinine (C_{CR}) levels,[16] or exogenous substances that are eliminated entirely by glomerular filtration,[7] such as inulin. There are various methodologic problems with measurements of GFR based on C_{CR} in the newborn infant.[2] Similarly, several methods based on inulin have been shown to be inaccurate in this age group.[7]

The aminoglycoside gentamicin is given to many neonates for suspected or proved Gram negative bacterial infections. In our neonatal intensive care unit, 80% of the preterm infants receive therapy with gentamicin or other aminoglycosides, and this figure is comparable with data from other units.[1] As gentamicin is eliminated almost entirely by the kidney, both its clearance and elimination rates depend on the GFR in neonates, children, and adults.[6,11,18] Thus gentamicin may be an ideal exogenous marker for estimation of the GFR in the newborn. Moreover, unlike inulin, gentamicin is repeatedly administered to the neonate, and because of its potential toxicity its serum concentrations are routinely monitored. Therefore, serial estimations of the GFR in the neonate may be easily obtained by a method based on gentamicin as an exogenous marker of glomerular function.

In the present study we used a simple pharmacokinetic model for the calculation of gentamicin clearance (CL) and elimination $t_{1/2}$ based on serum concentrations of gentamicin measured as part of our routine therapeutic drug monitoring. We compared CL and $t_{1/2}$ with creatinine clearance (CL_{CR}) in the same patients and suggest a simple method for the clinical application of this technique.

From the Divisions of Clinical Pharmacology and Neonatal Intensive Care Unit, The Research Institute, The Hospital for Sick Children and Departments of Pediatrics and Pharmacology, University of Toronto.

Received for publication May 1, 1985; accepted Aug. 26, 1985.

Reprint requests to: Dr. G. Koren, M.D., Division of Clinical Pharmacology, The Hospital for Sick Children, 555 University Ave., Toronto, Ontario M5G 1X8, Canada.

*Fellow of the Medical Research Council of Canada.

METHODS

Thirty-eight neonates in the neonatal intensive care unit at The Hospital for Sick Children in Toronto participated in the study, which was approved by the hospital's Committee for Human Experimentations. There were 15 full-term ($\overline{X} \pm SE = 40 \pm 1$ weeks gestational age; body weight 2.98 ± 0.125 kg) and 23 pre-

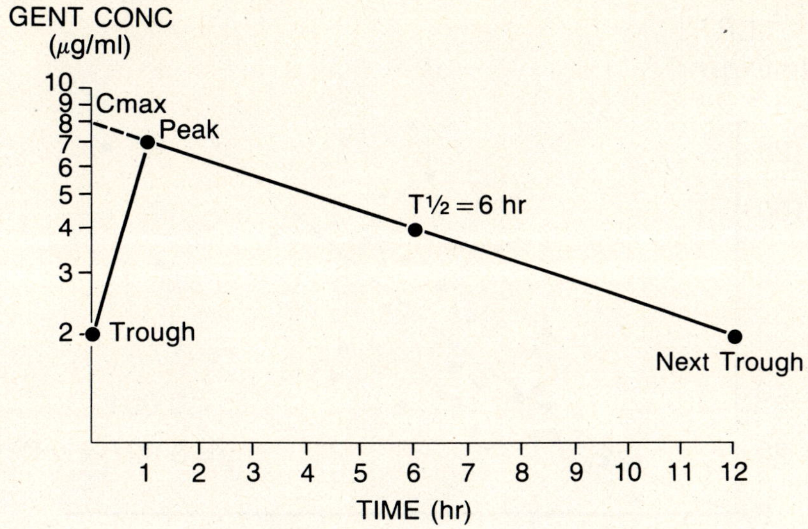

Fig. 1. Graphic estimation of gentamicin *(GENT)* $t_{1/2}$, V_{area}, and CL from trough, peak, and next trough serum concentrations (see Appendix for formulas).

term infants (29.8 ± 1 weeks gestational age; body weight 1.4 ± 0.1 kg). As part of their management, gentamicin was administered intravenously in a dose range of 1.25 to 3.2 mg/kg twice daily (in most instances) or once daily (in some infants of very low birth weight) at a rate of 5 to 16 ml/hr. The full delivery of the gentamicin dose was controlled by an infusion pump.

Three determinations of gentamicin serum concentration were performed: (a) before a dose (trough); (b) within 0.5 hour after the end of the dose (peak); and (c) before the next dose (next trough). Serum concentrations of gentamicin were analyzed by the EMIT method (Syva Diagnostics). The coefficient of variation of this test in our laboratory is <5%.

The three concentration-time points were drawn on semilogarithmic paper (Fig. 1; Appendix). In a one-compartment open model of gentamicin pharmacokinetics,[8,15] the elimination $t_{1/2}$ was calculated from the peak and next trough points. Back extrapolation of the line connecting peak and the next trough yields the maximal theoretic concentration at time zero (C_{max}).

The distribution volume of gentamicin (V_{area}) was calculated by two different methods. According to one formula (method A)[15]:

$$V_{area} = \frac{k_o(1 - e^{-k_e \cdot t'})}{k_e(C_{max} - C_0 \cdot e^{-k_e \cdot t'})}$$

where k_o is the infusion rate of the dose, t' is the infusion period (duration of constant-rate delivery of the dose), k_e is the elimination rate constant, and C_0 is the trough level. This formula corrects for the amount of drug eliminated during the infusion. Gentamicin pharmacokinetics calculated by this method[12] are essentially similar to values calculated by more concentration-time points fit into a two-compartment open model.[13]

Additionally, a simplified formula (method B) was tested that may be used by the clinician who has no access to the above program. If one assumes that the drug is delivered within 3 to 30 minutes, then only a negligible portion of the dose could be eliminated during the infusion time. The gentamicin V_{area} can then be calculated as: V_{area} = Dose (mg)/(C_{max} − trough).

The gentamicin CL was calculated as: CL = (V_{area} 0.69)/$t_{1/2}$.

To determine CL_{CR}, urine was collected for 24 hours at the day of the gentamicin determinations and assessed for creatinine concentration by the Kodak Ektachem analyzer (Eastman Kodak Inc.). At the middle of the study day, blood was drawn for the determination of C_{CR} (Creatinine Analyzer 2; Beckman Instruments, Inc.), thus correcting for a potential physiologic decrease in C_{CR} within the study day.[16]

The correlations among gentamicin CL, $t_{1/2}$, daily urine output, C_{CR}, and CL_{CR} were studied by least-squares regression analysis. Both linear and nonlinear equations were tested. Results are expressed as the $\overline{X}$ ± SE.

RESULTS

There was good correlation between gentamicin CL and CL_{CR}. Method A, which corrects for the infusion

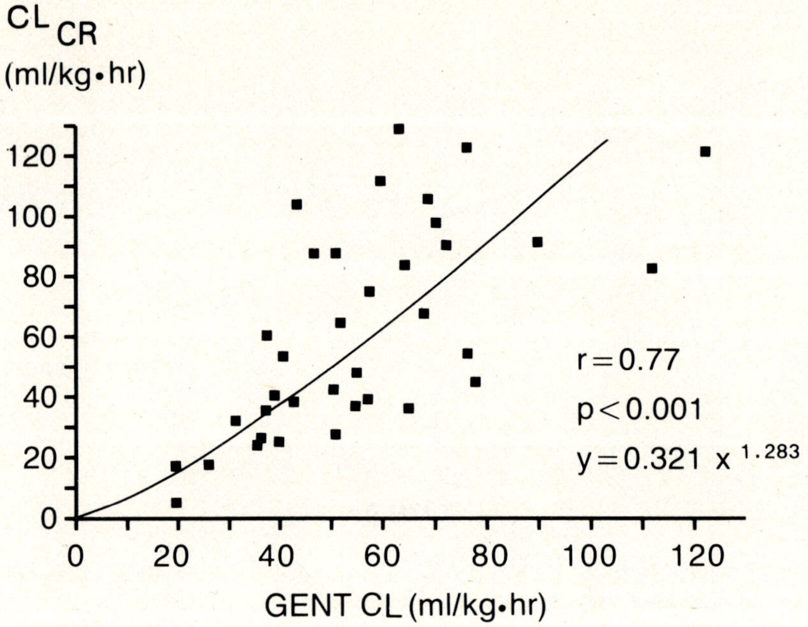

Fig. 2. Correlation between gentamicin *(GENT)* CL and CL_{CR} in newborns.

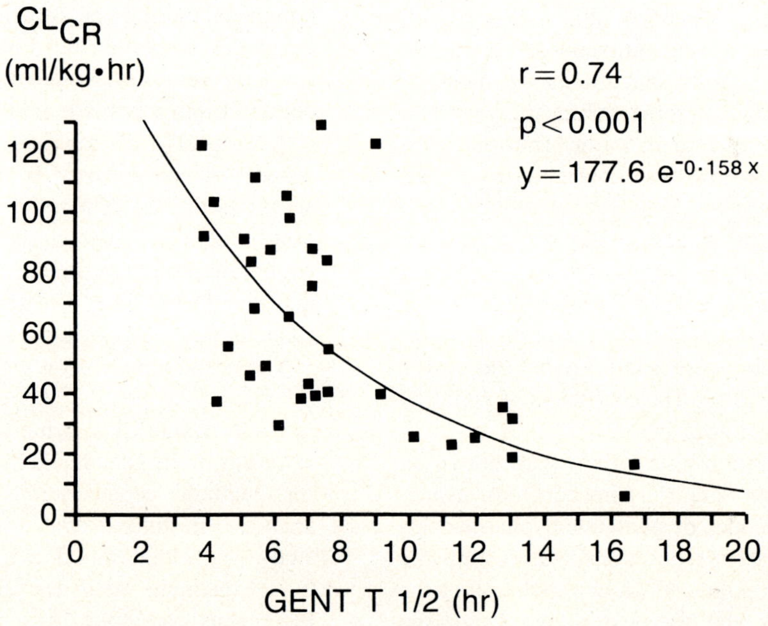

Fig. 3. Correlation between gentamicin *(GENT)* $t_{1/2}$ and CL_{CR} in newborns.

time, has the regression line: $CL_{CR} = 0.332 \cdot CL^{1.283}$ ($r = 0.77$; $P < 0.001$; Fig. 2). Method B for the calculation of V_{area}, which assumes negligible elimination of gentamicin during the infusion period, yielded similar values of V_{area} ($r = 0.98$; $P < 0.001$) because of the rapid delivery of the drug (3 to 8 minutes).

There was good correlation between CL_{CR} and the gentamicin $t_{1/2}$ (Fig. 3) according to the formula: $CL_{CR} = 177.6 \cdot e^{-0.158\ t_{1/2}}$ ($r = 0.74$; $P < 0.001$). The correlation between C_{CR} and CL_{CR} could be best described by the equation: $CL_{CR} = 3210 \cdot C_{CR}^{-1.039}$ $r = 0.77$; $P < 0.001$; Fig. 4).

The gentamicin V_{area} was similar in preterm and full-term infants (514 ± 44 and 508 ± 50 ml/kg, respec-

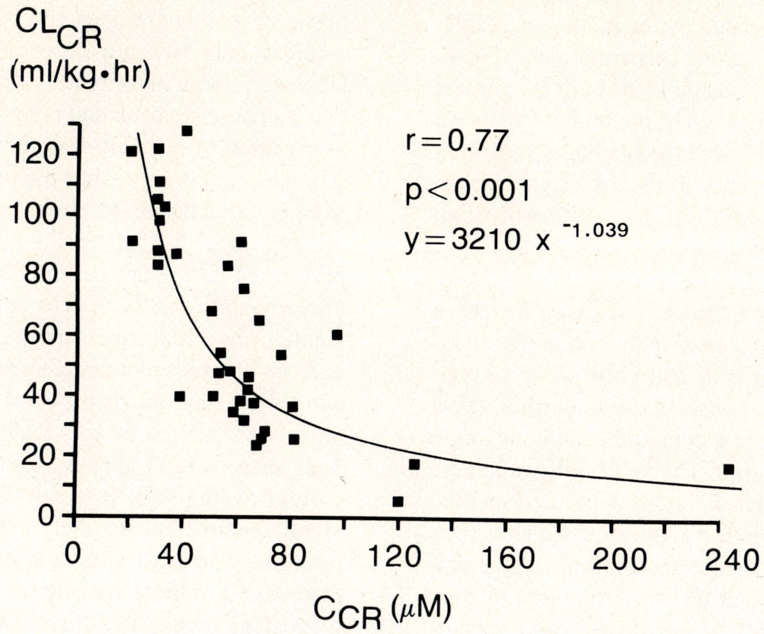

Fig. 4. Correlation between C_{CR} and CL_{CR} in newborns.

Table I. Translation of calculated gentamicin CL or $t_{1/2}$ into CR_{CL} in newborns

Calculated gentamicin CL range (ml/kg · hr)	0-25	26-40	41-60	>60
Predicted CL_{CR} (ml/kg · hr)	16 ± 10	35.7 ± 14	58.4 ± 26	88.5 ± 30
Calculated gentamicin $t_{1/2}$ range (hr)	>10	6-10	4-6	<4
Predicted CL_{CR} (ml/kg · hr)	22.8 ± 10	69 ± 33	78.9 ± 29	106.3 ± 15

Data are $\overline{X}$ ± SD.

tively). There was a significant correlation between the gentamicin CL and $t_{1/2}$ ($r = 0.77$; $P < 0.001$) but no correlation between V_{area} and $t_{1/2}$.

An estimation of GFR based on our data from either CL or $t_{1/2}$ is presented in Table I.

DISCUSSION

The currently available methods for the estimation of GFR that obviate urine collection in the newborn are often imprecise.[2] Completely voided and accurately timed urine collections for calculation of inulin clearance or CL_{CR} are difficult and often impossible. Physiologic markers that are used in older children and adults are not applicable in the newborn. At birth the neonatal C_{CR} is equivalent to the maternal C_{CR}.[3,17] The subsequent reduction in C_{CR} depends on the load of maternal creatinine, the neonatal creatinine production, and the rate of creatinine excretion.[2] Thus C_{CR} does not present a steady-state value during the first weeks of life and may not accurately reflect GFR. BUN levels are influenced by GFR, tubular reabsorption, hydration, and nutritional status and do not correlate well with GFR in the newborn.[5] Coulthard[7] examined the accuracy of methods based on inulin as an exogenous marker of GFR in the newborn, and has demonstrated that a constant infusion of inulin over a period of at least 24 hours is necessary to obtain a reliable estimate of GFR.

The association between gentamicin and renal function is important, because the drug is eliminated almost entirely by the kidney and one of its major side effects is impairment of renal function.[14] Consequently, renal function has to be assessed carefully during prolonged gentamicin therapy, with appropriate adjustment of the dose or the dose interval.[14] The potential of gentamicin to serve as an exogenous marker for GFR has not been assessed previously. Theoretically, this aminoglycoside has the ideal qualities for the purpose: (1) It is in current clinical use and is administered to many newborns; (2)

it is almost entirely eliminated by the kidney in a GFR-dependent fashion[6]; (3) serum concentrations of gentamicin are routinely measured in current clinical practice[14]; (4) with current assay methods there is no known cross-reactivity between gentamicin and other compounds in the blood; and (5) the use of gentamicin as an exogenous marker of GFR does not involve additional intervention or expense.

In our present study a good correlation was demonstrated between gentamicin CL and CL_{CR}. We chose to compare CL with CL_{CR} rather than with inulin clearance, because the former is the currently accepted clinical tool and because we considered it both impractical and unethical to undertake a continuous 24-hour inulin infusion in these newborns.[7] The values of gentamicin CL, V_{area}, and $t_{1/2}$ calculated by this simplified method are similar to pharmacokinetic values calculated by a two-compartment open model and multiple concentration-time points.[13] The fact that the simplified method for the calculation of V_{area} (method B) yields results very similar to the more sophisticated calculation (method A) indicates that calculation of V_{area} can be readily done by the physician on semilogarithmic paper without losing much sensitivity (Fig. 1). However, the simplified method demands a rapid infusion (3 to 15 minutes) of gentamicin, as the model assumes that the elimination of the dose during the infusion time is negligible. This is feasible even in the infant with an extremely low birth weight. If a dose of 2 mg gentamicin from a stock solution of 10 mg/ml is to be given to an infant weighing 800 gm who is receiving parenteral fluid at a rate of 3 ml/hr, then this dose is delivered within 4 minutes.

The correlation between the gentamicin $t_{1/2}$ and CL_{CR} is of special interest, because it suggests that the $t_{1/2}$ may yield a sufficiently accurate estimation of GFR for the clinician. The elimination $t_{1/2}$ is influenced by both clearance and V_{area} according to the formula: $t_{1/2} = (V_{area} \cdot 0.69)/CL$.[8] Because V_{area} is independent of GFR and there is no correlation between the gentamicin V_{area} and $t_{1/2}$, the elimination $t_{1/2}$ may be used to predict GFR. Our results demonstrate the known hyperbolic relationship between C_{CR} and CL_{CR}. This means that the reciprocal of plasma creatinine levels (and not C_{CR} itself) has a linear relationship with CL_{CR}. Clinicians often base their estimation of GFR in newborns on the urine output. Our results suggest that such an attempt may be futile.

The described calculations of both gentamicin CL and $t_{1/2}$ are simple, can be performed by the physician within a few minutes, and can be repeated several times during the patient's hospitalization. Three concentration-time points are needed for the calculation of CL, whereas only two are necessary to generate the $t_{1/2}$. However, some investigators have calculated CL from two points only (peak and next trough levels) under the assumption of a steady-state level after at least 3 days of unchanged dosage; thus the predose level is assumed to be equal to the next trough level.[10] When three points are available, the calculations described above can be performed during any given dose without necessitating a steady-state condition. The application of the method we describe is not necessarily confined to the newborn, and can be used in other age groups, both pediatric and adult. However, the distribution and elimination of gentamicin are altered by age, fever, burns, cystic fibrosis, liver disease with ascites, anemia, obesity, and concurrent dosing with β-lactam antibiotics.[14] Therefore, kinetic parameters are likely to be altered by these confounding variables and cannot be easily extrapolated from one group of patients to another. Other aminoglycosides such as tobramycin and amikacin could also be used to estimate GFR with the same technique after the relationship between their CL, $t_{1/2}$, and GFR is characterized.

APPENDIX

As shown in Fig. 1, the $t_{1/2}$ (the time taken for the concentration to decrease by one half) is derived from the line connecting the measured peak and the next trough concentrations. In the example in the figure, the $t_{1/2}$ is 6 hours. When this line is back extrapolated to time zero, the y-intercept yields the C_{max}. V_{area} can then be calculated as: V_{area} = Intravenous dose/(C_{max} − trough). For example, if the dose is 2 mg/kg, then

$$V_{area} = \frac{2 \text{ mg/kg}}{(8 \text{ mg/L} - 2 \text{ mg/L})} = 0.33 \text{ L/kg}.$$

CL is calculated as: $CL = (0.69 \cdot V_{area})/t_{1/2}$. In this example,

$$CL = \frac{0.69 \cdot 0.33 \text{ L/kg}}{6 \text{ hours}} = 38 \text{ mg/kg/hr}.$$

References

1. Aranda JV, Cohen S, Neims AH: Drug utilization in a newborn intensive care unit. J Pediatr **89**:315-317, 1976.
2. Arant BS Jr: Estimating glomerular filtration rate in infants. J Pediatr **104**:890-892, 1984.
3. Arant BS Jr: The newborn kidney. *In* Rudolph AJ, editor: Pediatrics, ed 17. New York, 1982, Appleton-Century-Crofts, p 1154.
4. Arant BS Jr, Edelmann CM Jr, Spitzer A: The congruence of creatinine and inulin clearances in children: Use of the Technicon AutoAnalyzer. J Pediatr **81**:559-561, 1972.
5. Avery GB: Neonatology. Philadelphia, 1975, JB Lippincott, p 493.

6. Balant L, Fabre J: Renal failure, drug pharmacokinetics and drug action. *In:* Gibaldi M, Prescott L, editors: Handbook of clinical pharmacokinetics. New York, 1983, ADIS Health Science Press, pp 213-234.
7. Coulthard CG: Comparison of methods of measuring renal function in preterm babies using inulin. J Pediatr **102:**923-930, 1983.
8. Gibaldi M, Perrier D: Pharmacokinetics, ed 2. New York, 1982, Marcel Dekker, Inc, pp 1-27, 331.
9. Goldsmith DI: Clinical and laboratory evaluation of renal function. *In:* Edelman CM Jr, editor: Pediatric kidney disease. Boston, 1978, Little, Brown, pp 213-224.
10. Kelman AW, Thomson AH, Whiting B, Bryson SM, Steedman AD, Mawer GE, Samba-Donga LA: Estimation of gentamicin clearance and volumes of distribution in neonates and young children. Br J Clin Pharmacol **18:**685-692, 1984.
11. Kildoo C, Modanlou HD, Kamat SU, Harralson A, Hodding J: Developmental patterns of gentamicin kinetics in very low birth weight sick children. Dev Pharmacol Ther **7:**345-356, 1984.
12. Koren G, Leeder S, Harding L, MacLeod SM: Optimization of gentamicin therapy in very low birth weight infants. Pediatr Pharmacol **5:**79-88, 1985.
13. Landers S, Berry PL, Kearns GL, Kaplan SL, Rudolph AJ: Gentamicin disposition and effect on development of renal function in the very low birth weight infant. Dev Pharmacol Ther **7:**285-302, 1984.
14. Lauermann M, Barza M: Why monitor serum levels of gentamicin. *In:* Gibaldi M, Prescott L, editors: Handbook of clinical pharmacokinetics. New York, 1983, ADIS Health Science Press, pp 164-179.
15. Sawchuk RJ, Zaske DE, Cipolle RJ, Wargin WA, Strate RG: Kinetic model for gentamicin dosing with the use of individual patient parameters. CLIN PHARMACOL THER **21:**362-369, 1977.
16. Schwartz GJ, Feld LG, Langford DJ: A simple estimate of glomerular filtration rate in full term infants during the first year of life. J Pediatr **104:**849-856, 1984.
17. Sertel H, Scopes I: Rates of creatinine clearance in babies less than 1 week of age. Arch Dis Child **48:**717-720, 1973.
18. Sininavin S, McCracken GH, Nelson JD: Determining gentamicin dosage in infants and children with renal failure. J Pediatr **96:**331-334, 1980.

Effect of aminoglycosides on the disposition of thyroid hormones and thyroglobulin

Our study was designed to confirm the potential effects of three aminoglycosides on the disposition of thyroid hormones. Twenty-seven patients diagnosed with either cellulitis (n = 19), chronic osteitis (n = 4), or an abscess (n = 4) were selected. Thirteen patients received tobramycin, 60 to 100 mg iv q. 8 h., plus cloxacillin, 1 gm iv q. 4 h.; seven patients received netilmicin, 40 to 120 mg iv q. 8 h., plus cloxacillin, 1 gm iv q. 4 h.; and seven patients received either cloxacillin, 1.5 gm iv q. 4 h., or cefoperazone, 2 to 4 gm iv q. 12 h. for at least 7 days. Another group of six normal subjects received neomycin, 0.5 gm po q. 6 h. for 7 days. All these subjects had normal thyroid function before antibiotic dosing and none had thyroid function abnormalities. Tobramycin and cloxacillin/cefoperazone did not influence thyroid function. Netilmicin decreased the total serum concentrations of triiodothyronine (T_3) from 114 ± 9 to 75 ± 7 ng/dl ($P < 0.01$), probably because of increased clearance, as the T_3 free fraction increased from 0.43% ± 0.02% to 0.49% ± 0.02% ($P < 0.05$). Thyroxine (T_4) and reverse T_3 (rT_3) levels were not affected. Neomycin decreased T_3 levels from 104 ± 8 to 92 ± 7 ng/dl ($P < 0.05$) and the serum concentrations of thyroglobulin from 17.3 ± 2.0 to 11.7 ± 2.0 ng/ml ($P < 0.001$). Because T_4 and rT_3 levels did not change, our results suggest that neomycin may have directly affected the gland. We conclude that some aminoglycosides can alter the disposition of thyroid hormones. (CLIN PHARMACOL THER 38:686-691, 1985.)

Patrick du Souich, M.D., Ph.D.,* Cesar Pison, M.D., Louise Pedneault, M.D., Pierre Larochelle, M.D., Ph.D., Richard Morisset, M.D., Carlos Vega, M.D., Denis Phaneuf, M.D., and Michel Poisson, M.D. *Montreal, Quebec, Canada*

These results constitute an effort to document a phenomenon repeatedly observed in the Infectious Diseases Service of the Hôpital Hôtel-Dieu de Montréal. The medical staff of this service has observed that certain patients during their hospitalization show pronounced decreases in the plasma levels of T_3. In these patients, the usual causes known to affect thyroid function were absent, and interestingly most of them were receiving aminoglycosides.

Normal thyroid hormonogenesis and hormone release include complex steps modulated by multiple regulatory mechanisms. Furthermore, the disposition of the released hormones (T_4, T_3, and rT_3) is also controlled by numerous factors.[31] The diversity of intermediate steps from thyroid stimulation to hormone effect suggests that there are many possible ways to deregulate thyroid function. Indeed, a great number of xenobiotics do affect thyroid function through very different mechanisms.[22] Therefore, there was a definite possibility that aminoglycosides could also influence thyroid function. We prospectively studied the influence of three amino-

Abbreviations

k_e	Elimination rate constant
PTU	Propylthyouracil
rT_3	Reverse triiodothyronine
Tg	Thyroglobulin
TSH	Thyrotropin
TRH	Thyrotropin-releasing hormone
T_4	Thyroxine
T_4f	Free thyroxine concentration
T_3	Triiodothyronine
T_3f	Free triiodothyronine concentration

From the Division of Clinical Pharmacology, Service of Nuclear Medicine and Service of Infectious Diseases, Departments of Medicine, Radiology, and Pharmacology, Hôpital Hôtel-Dieu de Montréal and University of Montreal.

Received for publication June 6, 1985; accepted Aug. 26, 1985.

Reprint requests to: Dr. Patrick du Souich, Département de pharmacologie, Faculté de médecine, Université de Montréal C.P. 6128, Succursale "A", Montréal, Québec H3C 3J7, Canada.

*Research Scholar of the Fonds de la Recherche en Santé du Québec.

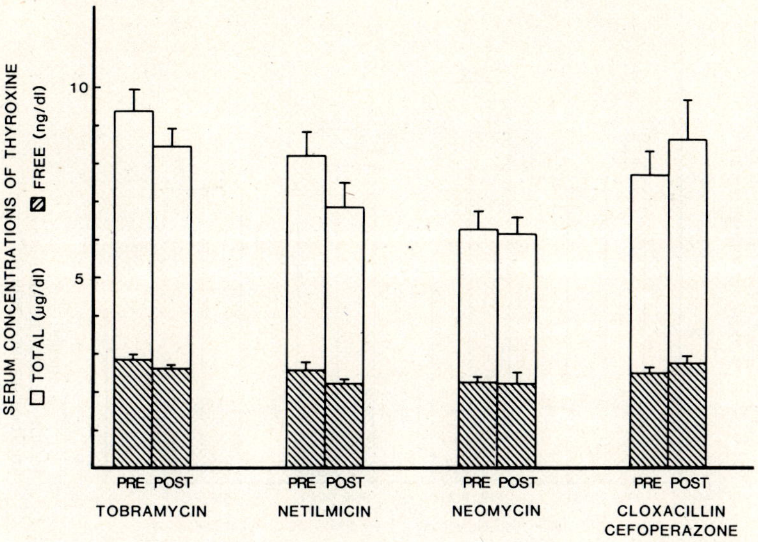

Fig. 1. Average (± SE) serum concentrations of total T_4 and T_4f before and after antibiotic dosing for 1 week.

glycosides on thyroid function in normal subjects and in hospitalized patients.

METHODS

Subjects. Patients were selected from among those hospitalized in the infectious Diseases Service of the Hôpital Hôtel-Dieu de Montréal. Inclusion criteria were normal thyroid function, age <70 years, a normal record of nutrition and weight, and the presence of an infectious disease requiring antibiotic therapy for at least 7 days. Patients with fever or chronic diseases such as depression or liver or renal failure or those taking drugs known to alter thyroid function (i.e., propranolol, dexamethasone, amiodarone, PTU, and radiocontrast agents) were excluded from study.

Twenty-seven patients (16 men and 11 women) between 21 and 68 years old ($\overline{X}$ = 42.5 years) were randomly selected. Thirteen of these patients had cellulitis alone, six had cellulitis complicated by tubular lymphangitis, four had chronic osteitis, and four had an infected cyst or an abscess. Of these subjects, 13 received tobramycin, 60 to 100 mg iv q. 8 h., plus cloxacillin, 1 gm iv q. 4 h.; seven patients received netilmicin, 40 to 120 mg iv q. 8 h., plus cloxacillin, 1 gm iv q. 4 h.; and of the other seven patients, three received cloxacillin, 1.5 gm iv q. 4 h., and four received cefoperazone, 2 to 4 gm iv q. 12 h. The doses of the antibiotics were selected by the attending physician according to individual needs.

Before the start of antibiotic therapy, renal and liver function were assessed by SMAC-20 testing in all patients. Thyroid function was estimated from serum concentrations of T_4, T_4f, T_3, T_3f, rT_3, Tg, and TSH before and after 7 days of antibiotic therapy.

Another group of six healthy nonsmoking men 19 to 38 years old ($\overline{X}$ = 24 years) received neomycin, 0.5 gm po q. 6 h., for 7 days. All subjects appeared normal based on clinical examination and routine diagnostic test results. Before and after the antibiotic, the TRH stimulation test was performed. For this purpose, after two control blood samples were drawn at −15 and 0 minutes, subjects received TRH, 400 ng iv, in 60 seconds. Blood samples were then drawn 8, 12, 15, 20, 30, 60, 90, 120, and 180 minutes after the injection. In all these blood samples, including the two control samples (−15 and 0), the same parameters as listed above were estimated to assess thyroid function.

Assay procedures. Serum total T_4 and T_3 were measured by RIA as described elsewhere.[5] Levels of T_4f and T_3f were determined by equilibrium dialysis according to the method of Ekins and Ellis.[13] Levels of rT_3 in serum were measured by RIA.[20] Serum TSH levels were measured by RIA as described by Pekary et al.[25] Finally, Tg was determined in unextracted sera by double-antibody RIA as described by Van Herle et al.[18]

Calculations. The TSH k_e after the TRH stimulation test before and after neomycin dosing was determined by regression analyses of the terminal phase of the plasma decay data (i.e., by multiplying the slope by 2.303). The rate of TSH secretion was estimated by linear regression analysis of the logarithm of the resid-

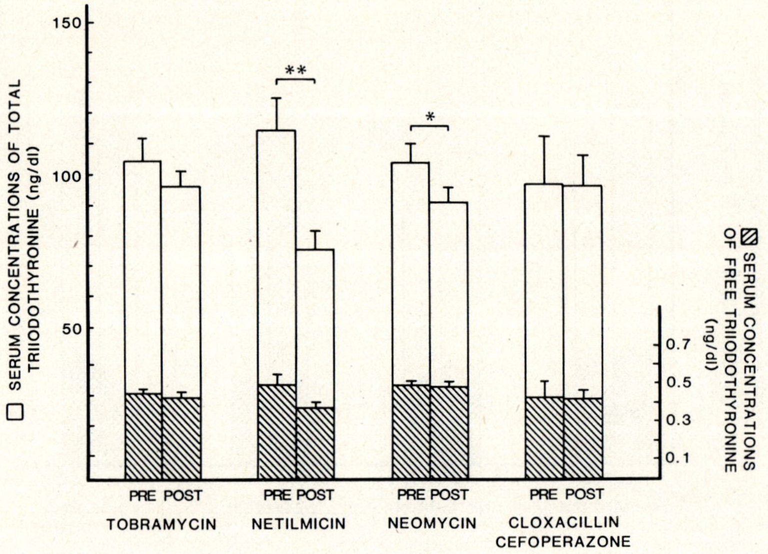

Fig. 2. Average (±SE) serum concentrations of total T_3 and T_3f before and after antibiotic dosing for 1 week. *P < 0.05; **P < 0.01.

Table I. Influence of aminoglycosides and cloxacillin/cefoperazone on the serum concentrations of rT_3, Tg, and TSH before and after dosing

	rT_3 (pg/ml)	Tg (ng/ml)	TSH (μU/ml)
Tobramycin (n = 13)			
Before	184 ± 25	15.4 ± 2.1	3.25 ± 0.80
After	150 ± 14	14.1 ± 1.4	4.79 ± 1.47
Netilmicin (n = 7)			
Before	260 ± 58	22.1 ± 5.9	5.4 ± 3.2
After	257 ± 91	19.7 ± 4.5	6.9 ± 3.9
Neomycin (n = 6)			
Before	173 ± 15	17.3 ± 2.0	1.13 ± 0.15
After	167 ± 12	11.7 ± 2.0*	1.25 ± 0.17
Cloxacillin/cefoperazone (n = 7)			
Before	†	14.8 ± 3.6	2.05 ± 0.42
After	†	14.4 ± 2.5	2.90 ± 0.38

Data are $\overline{X}$ ± SE.
*P < 0.001.
†Not measured.

ual concentration values of the secretion phase. In both instances it was assumed that secretion of TSH by the hypophysis is of very short duration, and is in fact instantaneous. If TSH secretion is not instantaneous, the k_e values we present would be underestimated. The plasma hormone AUC was calculated by the trapezoidal rule.

The results before the start of antibiotic dosing were compared with those after antibiotic therapy by a paired t test. The critical limit of significance was P = 0.05.

In vitro studies. To test the possibility that neomycin affects the conversion of T_4 to T_3 in peripheral tissues, in vitro studies were performed. Homogenates of rat liver were used to incubate T_4 alone (2.5 μmol/L) or in combination with PTU (1 mmol/L) or neomycin (0.005 mmol/L). These operations were done according to the technique described by Chopra et al.[8] The concentration of neomycin was selected with the knowledge that there is no accumulation of this class of antibiotics in the liver.[14,24] We assumed that the maximum tissue concentrations would be equal to plasma peak concentrations (5 μg/ml). The selected concentrations of T_4 and PTU were those used by Chopra et al.[8]

RESULTS

As shown in Fig. 1, aminoglycoside dosing for 7 days did not significantly affect the serum concentrations of T_4 or T_4f. As a result, the free fraction of T_4 remained constant. By contrast, these antibiotics did appear to influence T_3 serum concentrations (Fig. 2). Tobramycin showed only a tendency to decrease T_3 serum concentrations, but the effects of netilmicin (P < 0.01) and neomycin (P < 0.05) were much more pronounced. On the other hand, cloxacillin and cefoperazone had no effect on T_3 serum concentrations. As shown in the same figure, T_3f serum concentrations remained fairly constant or decreased proportionally less than total T_3 serum concentrations. As a result, the T_3 free fraction increased significantly after netilmicin dosing (0.43% ± 0.02% to 0.49% ± 0.02%; P < 0.05), but showed only a slight increase after neomycin dosing (0.47% ± 0.01% to 0.50% ± 0.02%).

Neither the rT_3 serum concentrations nor the levels of TSH were influenced by antibiotic dosing. Interest-

Table II. Effect of neomycin, 2 gm/day for 7 days, on TRH stimulation test in six normal subjects

	Before neomycin	*After neomycin*
T_4 AUC (μg · min/dl)	1,131 ± 66	1,159 ± 86
ΔT_4 peak concentrations (%)	12 ± 4	19 ± 2*
T_3 AUC (ng · min/dl)	20,698 ± 1,688	19,610 ± 1,857
ΔT_3 peak concentrations (%)	40 ± 4	47 ± 5*
rT_3 AUC (ng · min/ml)	33,152 ± 5,338	32,539 ± 2,940
ΔrT_3 peak concentrations (%)	2 ± 1	7 ± 4
Tg AUC (ng · min/ml)	3,084 ± 474	2,201 ± 574*
ΔTg peak concentrations (%)	10 ± 7	14 ± 8

Data are $\bar{X}$ ± SE.
*$P < 0.05$.

ingly, the levels of Tg decreased significantly in the subjects who received neomycin (Table I).

In response to TRH, the rate of secretion of TSH was not significantly influenced by neomycin (0.0798 ± 0.0058 vs. 0.0883 ± 0.070 minutes^{-1}), nor were TSH peak serum concentrations (9.7 ± 1.6 vs. 8.8 ± 1.8 μU/ml). On the other hand, the estimated apparent rate of TSH elimination decreased from 0.0109 ± 0.0008 to 0.0094 ± 0.0008 minutes^{-1} ($P < 0.05$). The values of TSH AUC were not affected by neomycin. Although neomycin did not influence the T_4 AUC, the increment in T_4 peak concentrations was significantly higher (Table II). Furthermore, despite the fact that T_3 levels before the TRH test were significantly lowered by neomycin, T_3 AUC values in response to TRH (Fig. 2) were almost identical, indicating that the response of the thyroid apparently increased after neomycin dosing. After TRH testing, peak T_3 values increased by 40% ± 4% before neomycin and by 47% ± 5% after neomycin ($P < 0.05$). Interestingly, the stimulation of Tg secretion by TRH via TSH did not mask the decrease in Tg induced by neomycin. After stimulation with TRH, the rT_3 response was not influenced by neomycin (Table II).

The in vitro studies showed that PTU decreased the formation of T_3 and rT_3 from T_4. Neomycin did not appear to affect the in vitro conversion of T_4 (Table III).

Table III. Effect of neomycin on the conversion of T_4 into T_3 and rT_3 in rat liver homogenate compared with PTU

	T_3 (ng/ml)	*rT_3 (ng/dl)*
Thyroxine (2.5 μmol/L)	5.16 ± 0.39	9.51 ± 0.63
Thyroxine and PTU	2.19 ± 0.27	0.97 ± 0.09
Thyroxine and neomycin	5.71 ± 0.78	12.76 ± 1.07

Data are $\bar{X}$ ± SE of the results from triplicate determinations in individual liver homogenates of five rats.

DISCUSSION

Our data demonstrate that some aminoglycosides do affect thyroid function. The fact that patients in the same environment with similar diseases who receive cloxacillin or cefoperazone did not show any change in thyroid function reinforces our findings. It is also obvious that the effects of aminoglycosides differ from drug to drug. At the doses used, netilmicin and neomycin (but not tobramycin) modified the disposition of thyroid hormones. Even the effects of the two former antibiotics differed from one another, in that neomycin depressed serum concentrations of both T_3 and Tg.

Netilmicin decreased the serum T_3 concentrations without affecting T_4 or rT_3 concentrations. Because T_4 and T_4f levels remained constant, TSH levels did not increase. Interestingly, netilmicin did not affect T_3f, so the T_3 free fraction increased significantly. Thus we may speculate that netilmicin affects thyroid function by interfering with T_3 protein binding and increasing the T_3 free fraction and T_3 clearance. This mechanism may explain why T_4 and rT_3 were not modified. The competition of drugs with thyroid hormones for the same binding sites has been described for other compounds (for more details see Robbins et al.[27]). In general, most drugs compete with T_4 for binding sites; however, that does not exclude the possibility that aminoglycosides decrease T_3 binding alone. In fact, it is logical that T_3 binding would be more influenced than would T_4 binding, because the affinity constants of thyroid binding globulin, prealbumin, and albumin for T_3 are much lower than those for T_4.[17]

The explanation of how neomycin decreases T_3 and Tg levels is more complex and probably includes several mechanisms of action. As a first possibility, neomycin was given orally and in healthy subjects the amount absorbed does not exceed 6% of the dose.[3,21] Because a large amount of neomycin is eliminated in the stool, it is highly likely that the colonic bacterial flora may be affected, which in turn would limit T_3 deconjugation and interfere with its reabsorption. Consequently, T_3 clearance could increase.[15,16,28] Although we cannot confirm this hypothesis, we do not believe it is the only possible mechanism explaining the decrease in T_3 levels. Because T_3 concentrations are theoretically at steady state, a decrease of 12% indicates a proportional increase in clearance; however, the relative importance of conjugated T_3 in the enterohepatic circulation cannot justify such an increase in clearance. On the other hand, if neomycin was to modify significantly the enterohepatic cycle of T_3, we should expect that T_4 serum concentrations would also be affected, because the T_4 conjugation and enterohepatic cycle are quantitatively more important than the T_3 conjugation and enterohepatic cycle.[28] Because T_4 serum concentrations remained stable (Fig. 1), we must conclude that any effect of neomycin on the enterohepatic cycle of T_3 must be of minor importance.

As a second possibility, neomycin may have a direct effect on the thyroid gland. After neomycin dosing for 7 days, Tg levels fell by 32% (Table I). Very little is known about the role and disposition of Tg, but it is possible that this decrease is a result of decreased thyroid secretion or of increased catabolism. Although we have no clear explanation for such changes, we speculate that because neomycin has an inhibitory effect on protein synthesis at the initiation step in the ribosomes,[2] it may also inhibit the synthesis of Tg. There is no actual information to support an increased catabolism of Tg by neomycin.

Another possible mechanism explaining the decrease in both T_3 and Tg levels is based on the fact that thyroid iodide transport appears to depend on the Na^+-K^+ adenosine triphosphatase system,[32,33] which has been recently demonstrated to be inhibited by neomycin.[23] If such a mechanism is operating, we may wonder why T_4 serum levels were not affected. It is possible that serum T_4 changes may have been partially masked because of its long $t_{1/2}$ (9 days).

The TRH stimulation test performed after 7 days of neomycin dosing showed minor changes in TSH kinetics. However, after this test, the increase in T_4 and T_3 peak serum concentrations was significantly greater after than before neomycin, suggesting that neomycin affected thyroid function. However, this modification does not give us any information on the mechanisms of action explaining these changes. Finally, the in vitro studies showed that neomycin had no effect on the hepatic conversion of T_4 to T_3 and rT_3, which supports the hypothesis that in vivo this drug affects thyroid function essentially through a direct effect on the gland (although we cannot completely discard an effect on the T_3 enterohepatic cycle). Further studies are necessary to confirm such a hypothesis and to explain the selective effect of neomycin on T_3.

The effect of netilmicin and neomycin on thyroid function differs significantly from that of other drugs. PTU,[29] propranolol,[6] trimethoprim,[12] dexamethasone,[11] and amiodarone[4] all appear to block the conversion of T_4 to T_3 by inhibiting 5′-monodeiodination. As a consequence, T_3 levels decrease rapidly. The blockade of 5′-monodeiodination also results in a decrease in rT_3 clearance and, therefore, in an increase in serum levels of this hormone. In our studies, rT_3 levels always remained unchanged, indicating that the mechanism of action of aminoglycosides differs from that described for these drugs.

Finally, it is important to mention that aminoglycosides do not appear to interfere with the RIAs we used to measure the thyroidal hormones.[1]

The antithyroid activity of aminoglycosides may not be clinically relevant in patients with an intact hypothalamus or hypophysis thyroid gland axis. In such patients this interaction would not entail any serious clinical consequences. However, in situations in which the serum concentrations of T_3 tend to be low, such as in older patients,[19] patients with diabetes,[26] fasting patients,[30] those in febrile states,[9] those with hepatic cirrhosis[10] or renal failure,[7] and those taking exogenous T_4, the effect of aminoglycosides could be of clinical importance, particularly when dosed for long periods. Clinicians should be aware of the potential effects of these drugs on thyroid function.

References

1. Berger SA, Sowinski S: Lack of influence of some antibiotics on various thyroid hormone assays. Clin Chem **28:**1240-1241, 1982.
2. Betina V: The chemistry and biology of antibiotics. Nauta WT, Rekker RF, editors: New York, 1983; Elsevier Scientific Publishing Company, vol 5, pp 421-429.
3. Breen KJ, Bryant RE, Levinson JD, Schenker S: Neomycin absorption in man. Ann Intern Med **76:**211-218, 1972.
4. Burger A, Dinichert D, Nicod P, Jenny M, Lemarchand-Beraud T, Valloton MB: Effect of amiodarone on serum T_3, rT_3, T_4 and thyrotropin. A drug influencing peripheral metabolism of thyroid hormones. J Clin Invest **58:**255-259, 1976.
5. Challand GS, Ratcliffe WA, Ratcliffe JG: Semiautomated radioimmunoassay for total serum thyroxine and triiodothyronine. Clin Chem Acta **60:**25-29, 1975.
6. Chambers JB, Pittman CS, Suda AK: The effects of propranolol on thyroxine metabolism and triiodothyro-

nine production in man. J Clin Pharmacol **22:**110-116, 1982.

7. Chopra IJ, Chopra U, Smith SR, Reza M, Solomon DH: Reciprocal changes in serum concentrations of 3,3′,5′-triiodothyronine (reverse T_3) and 3,3′,5-triiodothyronine (T_3) in systemic illness. J Clin Endocrinol Metab **41:**1043-1049, 1975.
8. Chopra IJ, Chua-Teco GN, Eisenberg JB, Wiersinga WM, Solomon DH: Structure-activity relationships of inhibition of hepatic monodeiodination of thyroxine to 3,5,3′-triiodothyronine by thiouracil and related compounds. Endocrinology **110:**163-168, 1982.
9. Chopra IJ, Solomon DH, Chopra U, Wu SY, Fisher DA, Nakamura Y: Pathways of metabolism of thyroid hormones. Recent Prog Horm Res **34:**521-567, 1978.
10. Chopra IJ, Solomon DH, Chopra U, Young RT, Chua-Teco GN: Alterations in circulating thyroid hormones and thyrotropin in hepatic cirrhosis: Evidence for euthyroidism despite subnormal serum triiodothyronine. J Clin Endocrinol Metab **39:**501-511, 1974.
11. Chopra IJ, Williams DE, Orgiazzi J, Solomon DH: Opposite effects of dexamethasone on serum concentrations of rT_3 and T_3. J Clin Endocrinol Metab **41:**911-920, 1975.
12. Cohen HN, Pearson DWM, Thomson JA, Ratcliffe WA, Beastall GH: Trimetroprim and thyroid function. Lancet **1:**676-677, 1981.
13. Ekins RP, Ellis SM: The radioimmunoassay of free thyroid hormones in serum. *In* Robbins T, Bravermann LE, editors: Thyroid research. Amsterdam, 1976, Excerpta Medica, pp 597-600.
14. Fabre J, Rudhardt M, Blanchard P, Regamey C: Persistence of isomicin and gentamicin in renal cortex and medulla compared with other organs and serum of rats. Kidney Int **10:**444-449, 1976.
15. Flock EV, Bollman JL, Grindlay JH: Conjugates of triiodothyronine and its metabolites. Endocrinology **67:**419-429, 1960.
16. Flock EV, Bollman JL, Grindlay JH, McKenzie BF: Metabolites of radioactive L-thyroxine and L-triiodothyronine. Endocrinology **61:**461-473, 1957.
17. Gershangorn MC, Glinoer D, Robbins J: Transport and metabolism of thyroid hormones. *In* de Visscher M, editor: The thyroid gland. New York, 1980, Raven Press, pp 81-121.
18. Van Herle AJ, Uller RP, Matthews NL, Brown J: Radioimmunoassay for measurement of thyroglobulin in human serum. J Clin Invest **52:**1320-1327, 1973.
19. Herrmann J, Heinen E, Kroll HJ, Rudorff KH, Kruskemper HL: Thyroid function and thyroid hormone metabolism in elderly people. Low T_3-syndrome in old age? Klin Wochenschr **59:**315-323, 1981.
20. Hufner M, Grussendorf M: Radioimmunoassay for 3,3′,5′-triiodothyronine. Clin Chim Acta **69:**497-504, 1976.
21. Kunin CM, Chalmers TC, Leevy CM, Sebastyen SC, Lieber CS, Finland M: Absorption of orally administered neomycin and kanamycin. N Engl J Med **262:**380-385, 1960.
22. Langer P, Greer MA: Antithyroid substances and naturally occurring goitrogens. Basel, 1977, S Karger AG.
23. Lipsky JJ, Lietman PS: Neomycin inhibition of adenosine triphosphatase: Evidence for a neomycin-phospholipid interaction. Antimicrob Agents Chemother **18:**532-535, 1980.
24. Luft FC, Kleit SA: Renal parenchimal accumulation of aminoglycoside antibiotics in rats. J Infect Dis **130:**656-659, 1974.
25. Pekary AE, Hershman JM, Parlow AF: A sensitive and precise radioimmunoassay for human thyroid-stimulating hormone. J Clin Endocrinol Metab **41:**676-684, 1977.
26. Pittman CS, Suda AK, Chambers JB, McDaniel HG, Ray GY, Preston BK: Abnormalities of thyroid hormone turnover in patients with diabetes mellitus before and after insulin therapy. J Clin Endocrinol Metab **48:**854-860, 1979.
27. Robbins J, Rall JE, Gorden P: The thyroid and iodine metabolism. *In* Boundy PK, Rosenberg JE, editors: Metabolic control and disease. Philadelphia, 1980, WB Saunders Co, pp 1325-1343.
28. Taurog A: Conjugation and excretion of thyroid hormone. Brookhaven Symp Biol **7:**111-136, 1954.
29. Taurog A: The mechanism of action of the thioureylene antithyroid drugs. Endocrinology **98:**1031-1046, 1976.
30. Vagenakis AG, Portnay GI, O'Brian JT, Rudolph M, Arky RA, Ingbar SH, Braverman LE: Effect of starvation on the production and metabolism of thyroxine and triiodothyronine in euthyroid obese patients. J Clin Endocrinol Metab **45:**1305-1309, 1977.
31. de Visser M: The thyroid gland. New York, 1980, Raven Press.
32. Wolff J, Halmi NS: Thyroidal iodide transport. V. The role of Na^+-K^+–activated, ouabain-sensitive adenosintriphosphatase activity. J Biol Chem **238:**847-851, 1963.
33. Wolf J, Maurey JR: Cardiac glycosides and thyroidal iodide transport. Nature **182:**957, 1958.

Sulbactam kinetics and excretion into breast milk in postpartum women

We gave intravenous infusions of sulbactam, a β-lactamase inhibitor, in combination with ampicillin or cephalothin to women 2 days after cesarean section delivery. The elimination $t_{1/2}$ was 1.0 hours, the volume of distribution at steady state was 268 ml/kg, and renal clearance was 295 ml/min. These values are similar to those in normal young men and in surgical patients and suggest that dose regimens of sulbactam will not need adjustment in the postpartum period. Sulbactam concentrations in breast milk averaged 0.5 μg/ml, a value similar to that of several β-lactam antibiotics. (Clin Pharmacol Ther 1985;38:692-6.)

George Foulds, Ph.D., R. David Miller, M.D., Anthony K. Knirsch, M.D., and Lauri D. Thrupp, M.D. *Groton, Conn., and Orange, Calif.*

The kinetics of many drugs are altered in pregnancy and in labor.[1,2] The changes in drug kinetics in pregnant women are related to major increases in both plasma volume and the glomerular filtration rate at term. Decreases in both the elimination $t_{1/2}$ and peak serum concentrations (C_{max}) are frequently noted in women who are pregnant as compared with those in women who are not pregnant. For ampicillin, such changes have been attributed to an increase in the apparent volume of distribution (V_{area}) and renal clearance (CL_R) of drug in pregnant women as compared with values in the same women after their return to a nonpregnant state (cessation of lactation and restoration of the normal menstrual cycle).[3,4] Similarly, the $t_{1/2}$ of ampicillin was decreased late in pregnancy,[5] and ampicillin kinetics may also be altered during labor.[6-8]

Sulbactam is a β-lactam with very little intrinsic antimicrobial activity. When combined with ampicillin or other β-lactam antibiotics, however, sulbactam extends their spectrum of activity through the irreversible inhibition of enzymes that would otherwise hydrolyze the antibiotic.[9-12] Because sulbactam kinetics in normal subjects are very similar to those of ampicillin,[13-15] with which it is combined for the treatment of infections, and because ampicillin kinetics are altered in pregnancy and in the puerperium, we compared the kinetics of sulbactam in postpartum women with those in normal subjects to determine if there is a need for dose adjustment in the early postpartum period.

From the Central Research Division, Pfizer, Inc., Groton, and University of California Irvine Medical Center, Orange.

Received for publication Feb. 17, 1985; accepted Aug. 28, 1985.

Reprint requests to: George Foulds, Ph.D., Central Research Division, Pfizer, Inc., Groton, CT 06340.

METHODS

Patients. Patients who failed to respond to doses of 2 gm cephalothin every 4 hours or 2 gm ampicillin every 6 hours administered to prevent postpartum sepsis were selected for participation. These patients, most of whom had undergone a cesarean section delivery, continued their cephalothin or ampicillin dosing regimens and also received 500 mg or 1 gm sulbactam, infused intravenously over 20-minute intervals every 6 hours, starting an average (±SD) of 2.1 ± 0.93 days (range 0.99 to 4.33 days) after delivery. After one of the sulbactam doses (the first dose in nine patients, the second dose in one patient, and the third dose in two patients), sequential serum samples were drawn (from six patients after 1 gm doses and from six patients after 0.5 gm doses). Samples were analyzed for sulbactam and were subjected to kinetic analysis. A few serum samples were drawn from the other patients. Additionally, urine samples were collected from 10 patients and milk was collected with a breast pump at random times between the first and thirteenth doses from 11 patients (68 samples) and were assayed for sulbactam. The efficacy of sulbactam in combination with ampicillin or cephalothin in the study from which these patients were chosen has been reported.[16]

Assays. Sulbactam assays were by gas chromatography of the methyl ester with detection by mass spectrometry.[15] The method is highly specific, free from interference by ampicillin or cephalothin, and rapid. Assays were compared with standard curves of sulbactam in control media (human serum, urine, or milk).

Kinetics. Kinetics were examined by standard methods.[17,18] The apparent steady-state volume of distribution (V_{ss}) was calculated with the use of a noncompartmental method[19,20]: $V_{ss} = \text{Dose} \times \text{AUMC}/\text{AUC}^2$,

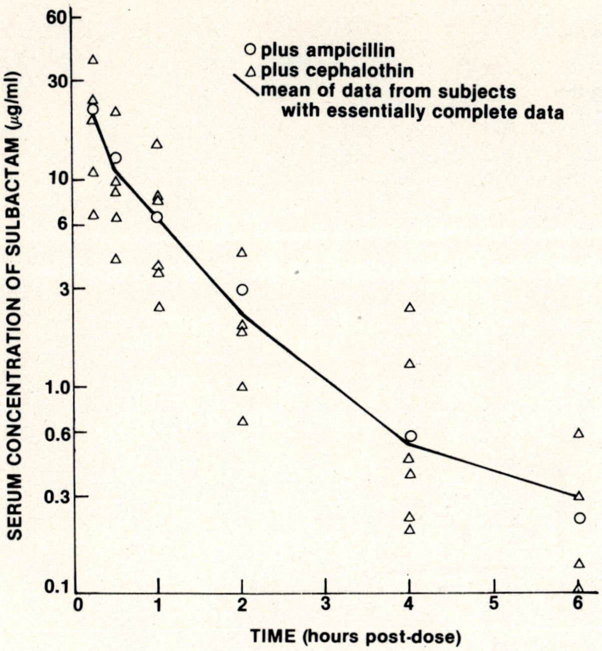

Fig. 1. Serum concentrations of sulbactam after 20-minute infusions of 0.5 gm to postpartum women.

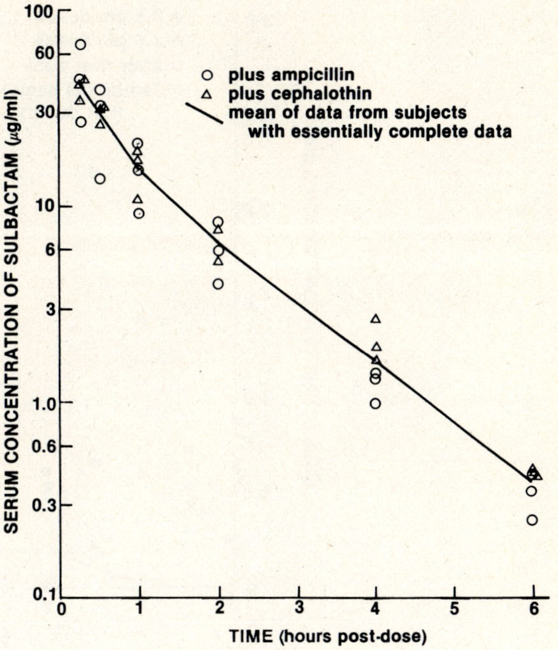

Fig. 2. Serum concentrations of sulbactam after 20-minute infusions of 1 gm to postpartum women.

Table I. Sulbactam AUC, C_{max}, and $t_{1/2}$ after 20-minute infusions to postpartum women

Combination therapy	*Co-drug dose (gm)*	*Patient No.*	*AUC* (μg · hr/ml)*	*C_{max}† (μg/ml)*	*$t_{1/2}$‡ (hr)*
0.5 gm sulbactam with					
Ceph	2	1	9.9	9.0	1.00
Ceph	2	3	52.9	44.6	1.47
Ceph	2	4	16.9	17.9	0.73
Ceph	2	5	25.4	22.4	1.04
Ceph	2	6	20.9	27.7	1.75
Ceph	1	12	28.7	26.7	1.03
$\overline{X}$			25.8	24.7	0.95§
1.0 gm sulbactam with					
Ceph	2	7	70.4	56.7	1.08
Ceph	2	9	61.6	68.3	1.12
Ceph	2	10	63.7	48.6	0.97
Ceph	2	17	45.5	58.0	0.97
Amp	1	18	88.7	106.7	0.89
Amp	2	19	66.4	55.6	0.85
$\overline{X}$			66.0	65.6	0.98

Ceph = Cephalothin; Amp = ampicillin.
*AUC(0-∞), including projected C_{max}.
†Projected from concentrations observed 0.25 and 1.0 hours after dosing.
‡Between 1 and 6 hours after the infusion.
§Excluding patients 3 and 6.

where AUMC is the area under the first-moment curve (concentration × time vs. time).

Unless otherwise indicated, data are reported as the $\overline{X}$ ± SD.

RESULTS

Serum concentrations of sulbactam after 500 mg infusions are shown in Fig. 1. Although individual values for all patients are shown, mean values were calculated

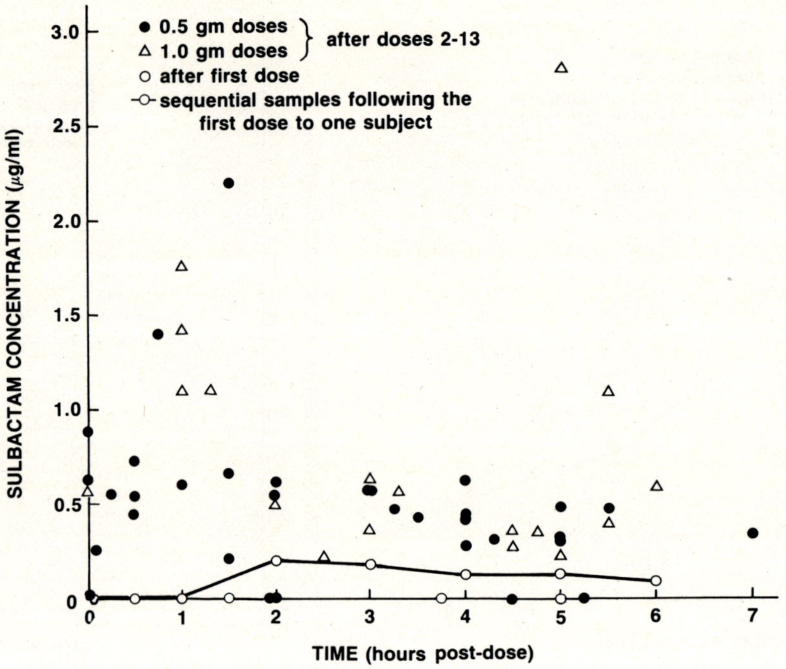

Fig. 3. Sulbactam concentrations in human milk after combination therapy with sulbactam and either cephalothin or ampicillin in postpartum women.

Table II. Concentrations of sulbactam in breast milk after infusions of sulbactam with cephalothin to postpartum women: Samples obtained >8 hours after last dose

Patient No.	*Time after dosing (hr)*	*Sulbactam concentration (µg/ml)*
1	10.5	0.38
	19.2	0.13
	49.0	ND
2	12.0	1.2
4	12.0	0.67
	20.0	0.47
	20.5	0.31

ND = None detected (<0.1 µg/ml).

only from data in patients with essentially complete data (n = 6). The mean of the highest observed concentrations after an 0.5 gm dose (15 minutes after infusion) was 19 µg/ml, and that observed after 1 gm doses to six patients was 44 µg/ml (Fig. 2). The projected C_{max}, $t_{1/2}$, and AUC values for sulbactam in these women are summarized in Table I. The sulbactam $t_{1/2}$ was approximately 1 hour. High concentrations of sulbactam were found in the urine (mean = 481 ± 272 µg/ml; range 181 to 955 µg/ml). Recovery (from 0 to 6 hours) from 10 patients averaged 54% ± 15.9% (range 36% to 83%) of a single dose. The mean concentration in milk samples taken between 0 and 8 hours after dosing was 0.52 µg/ml, with the greatest single observed concentration of 2.8 µg/ml (Fig. 3). There was little apparent difference in sulbactam concentrations in milk after the 0.5 or 1.0 gm doses, except perhaps within the first 2 hours after dosing. Peak concentration appears to occur within 2 hours. In one patient from whom sequential samples were drawn each hour after the first dose of 1 gm sulbactam, the peak concentration occurred 2 hours after dosing and concentrations declined with a $t_{1/2}$ of 2.4 hours. After 8 hours, concentrations remained low and appeared to decline (Table II).

The serum concentration-time data fit well to the two-compartment open model, with an $r^2 \geq 0.992$ for 11 of the patients. Data for one patient were fit equally well by a one-compartment model. The mean apparent volume of distribution of the central compartment (V_c; serum and rapidly equilibrating tissues) was approximately 180 ml/kg, and the apparent whole body volume of distribution was approximately 450 ml/kg (Table III). Approximately 40% of the drug was in the central compartment in the postdistributive phase. Mean CL_R was 222 ± 173 ml/min (n = 8). Total clearance of the drug (CL) as calculated by two methods (CL = Dose/AUC and CL = $k_{10} \times V_c$, with excellent agreement between the methods) was 295 mg/min. The V_{ss}, calculated including the projected C_{max} at

Table III. Apparent volumes of distribution, fraction of drug in central compartment, distribution rates, and intrinsic elimination rates after intravenous doses of sulbactam to postpartum women (two-compartment open model)

Patient No.	V_C *(ml/kg)*	*Total volume (ml/kg)*	f_C	k_{12} *(hr⁻¹)*	k_{21} *(hr⁻¹)*	k_{10} *(hr⁻¹)*
0.5 gm sulbactam						
1	281	694	0.40	1.18	1.53	1.82
3	132	307	0.43	0.62	1.11	1.46
4	415	649	0.64	0.27	1.32	1.31
6	99	694	0.14	0.52	0.51	2.99
12	216	464	0.46	0.68	1.27	1.47
$\bar{X}$ (n = 5)	229	562	0.41	0.65	1.15	1.81
1.0 gm sulbactam						
7	150	313	0.48	0.36	0.84	1.05
9	114	396	0.29	0.83	0.89	1.93
10	229	316	0.73	0.15	1.09	0.94
17	77	471	0.16	2.53	1.13	3.89
18	63	209	0.30	1.11	1.23	2.54
19*	—	269	—	—	—	—
$\bar{X}$ (n = 5)	127	341	0.39	1.00	1.04	2.07
Overall $\bar{X}$ (n = 10)	178	451	0.40	0.83	1.09	1.94

*One-compartment model.

the end of the infusion (Table I), was approximately 18.1 L (268 mg/kg). This value was in reasonable agreement with the value calculated from the two-compartment model in 10 patients (309 ml/kg).

DISCUSSION

After 20-minute infusions of sulbactam, the projected C_{max} values (25 μg/ml after a 500 mg dose and 66 μg/ml after a 1 gm dose) were similar to those in healthy young men.[14] Also, the sulbactam $t_{1/2}$ values in the postpartum women were similar to those in healthy young men. Excretion in urine was the major route of sulbactam elimination, with CL_R of 220 ml/min. CL was 290 ml/min, a value similar to that of normal young men and surgical patients (Table IV). The sulbactam V_{ss} (268 ml/kg) was similar to that in normal men (246 ml/kg; Table IV), suggesting that equal dose regimens will produce serum concentrations in postpartum women similar to or only slightly less than those in normal men. Additionally, V_{ss} in the postpartum women was similar to that in surgical patients (283 ml/kg). The differences in V_{ss} and in CL_R between postpartum women and healthy young men were not significant (Welch's test[22]).

It is well known that most drugs pass into breast milk to a measurable extent. The excretion of sulbactam into human milk was low, with a mean concentration of only 0.52 μg/ml. The concentrations of sulbactam in milk were similar to those of other β-lactams such as ampicillin (0.07 μg/ml after 500 mg po doses[23]), amoxicillin (0.8 μg/ml after 1 gm po doses[24]), cephalothin (0.5 μg/ml after 1 gm iv doses[24]), and cefoperazone (0.3 μg/ml after 1 gm im doses[25]). Sulbactam did not persist in milk, as little sulbactam was found in samples of milk obtained more than 8 hours after the last dose. The maximum probable exposure of a nursing infant to sulbactam in mother's milk was estimated by assuming an intake of approximately 4 oz (30 ml) milk per feeding for six feedings per day and by multiplying this value by the maximum observed sulbactam concentration of 2.8 μg/ml. For a 3 kg infant, the estimated maximum exposure of 2 mg/day or 0.7 mg/kg/day amounts to <1% of the typical adult exposure of 80 mg/kg/day. Thus it may be safe for an infant to continue to nurse while the mother is receiving sulbactam.

The high serum and urine concentrations of sulbactam and its rapid distribution and effective penetration

Table IV. Comparison of total body clearance and V_{ss} of sulbactam in postpartum women with values in healthy young men[14] and surgical patients[21]

	Healthy men	*Postpartum women*	*Surgical patients*
V_{ss} (ml/kg)			
$\bar{X}$	246	268	283
SD	40	108	79
n	40	12	11
Total clearance (ml/min)			
$\bar{X}$	262	295	311
SD	59	96	72
n	40	11	11

into extravascular fluid in animals[26] and into blister fluid and peritoneal fluid in man[13,27] suggest that sulbactam in combination with ampicillin or other β-lactam antibiotics may be useful in the prevention and treatment of infections during the postpartum period.

We thank Mr. R. H. Allen, Ms. D. R. Brennan, and Mr. S. C. McNeill for their analytic assistance.

References

1. Nation RL. Drug pharmacokinetics in childbirth. In: Gibaldi M, Prescott L, eds. Handbook of clinical pharmacokinetics. New York: ADIS Health Science Press, 1983:18-43 (section II).
2. Philipson A. Pharmacokinetics of antibiotics in pregnancy and labour. In: Gibaldi M, Prescott L, eds. Handbook of clinical pharmacokinetics. New York: ADIS Health Science Press, 1983:44-57 (section II).
3. Assael BM, Como ML, Miraglia M, Pardi G, Sereni F. Ampicillin kinetics in pregnancy. Br J Clin Pharmacol 1979;8:286-8.
4. Philipson A. Pharmacokinetics of ampicillin during pregnancy. J Infect Dis 1977;136:370-6.
5. Bastert G, Wallhauser KH, Wernicke K, Muller WG. Pharmakokinetische Untersuchungen zum Ubertritt von Antibiotika in das Fruchtwasser am Ende der Schwangerkeit. 1. Teil: Ampicillin. Z Geburtshife Perinatol 1973;177:330-9.
6. Bray RE, Boe RW, Johnson WL. Transfer of ampicillin into fetus and amniotic fluid from maternal plasma in late pregnancy. Am J Obstet Gynecol 1966;96:938-42.
7. Hirsh HA, Dreher E, Perrochet A, Schmid E. Transfer of ampicillin to the fetus and amniotic fluid during continuous infusion (steady state) and by repeated single intravenous injections to the mother. Infection 1974;2:207-12.
8. von Voigt R, Schroder S, Meinhold P, Zenner I, Noschel H. Klinische Untersuchungen zum Einfluss von Schwangerschaft und Geburt auf die Pharmakokinetik von ampizillin. Zentralbl Gynakol 1978;100:701-5.
9. English AR, Retsema JA, Girard AE, Lynch JE, Barth WE. CP-45,899, a beta-lactamase inhibitor that extends the antibacterial spectrum of beta-lactams: initial bacteriological characterization. Antimicrob Agents Chemother 1978;14:414-9.
10. Retsema JA, English AR, Girard AE. CP-45,899 in combination with penicillin or ampicillin against penicillin-resistant *Staphylococcus, Haemophilus influenzae* and *Bacteroides*. Antimicrob Agents Chemother 1980;17: 615-22.
11. Retsema JA, Schelkly WV, Girard AE, English AR. Beta-lactamase inhibitor CP-45,899 (sulbactam) mode of action against a type III beta-lactamase and synergy effects with cephalosporins. Drugs Exp Clin Res 1981; 7:255-61.
12. Wise R, Andrews JM, Bedford KA. Clavulanic acid and CP-45,899: a comparison of their *in vitro* activity in combination with penicillins. J Antimicrob Chemother 1980;6:197-206.
13. Brown RN, Wise R, Andrews JM, Hancox J. Comparative pharmacokinetics and tissue penetration of sulbactam and ampicillin after concurrent intravenous administration. Antimicrob Agents Chemother 1982;21:565-7.
14. Foulds G, Knirsch AK, Stankewich JP, Weidler DR. The parenteral kinetics of ampicillin/sulbactam in man. Int J Clin Pharmacol Res 1985;5:79-86.
15. Foulds G, Stankewich JP, Marshall DC, et al. Pharmacokinetics of sulbactam in humans. Antimicrob Agents Chemother 1983;23:692-9.
16. Miller RD, Thrupp LD, Meskin DJ, et al. Evaluation of sulbactam in patients with postpartum infections [Abstract no WO 59/11]. Vienna, Austria: Thirteenth International Congress of Chemotherapy, Aug. 28-Sept. 2, 1983.
17. Gibaldi M, Perrier D. Pharmacokinetics. 2nd ed. New York: Marcel Dekker, Inc., 1983.
18. Wagner JR. Fundamentals of clinical pharmacokinetics. Hamilton, Ill.: Drug Intelligence Publications, 1975.
19. Benet LZ, Galeazzi RL. Noncompartmental determination of the steady-state volume of distribution. J Pharm Sci 1979;68:1071-4.
20. Perrier D, Mayersohn M. Noncompartmental determination of the steady-state volume of distribution for any mode of administration. J Pharm Sci 1982;71:372-3.
21. Gill MA, Kern JW, Chenella FC, et al. Pharmacokinetics of parenteral sulbactam in patients with appendicitis. Ther Drug Monitor 1984;6:428-31.
22. Gans DJ. Use of a preliminary test in comparing two sample means. Commun Statist Simula Computa 1981;B10:163-74.
23. Lohmeyer H, Halfpap E. Pharmakokinetische Untersuchungen und Klinsche Erfahrungen mit Ampicillin bei der Behandlung von Infectionen des Urogenitaltrakts der Frau. Z Geburtschilfe Gynaekol 1965;164:184-202.
24. Kafetyis DA, Siafas CA, Georgakopoulos PA, Papadatos CJ. Passage of cephalosporins and amoxicillin into the breast milk. Acta Paediatr Scand 1981;70:285-8.
25. Ueda Y, ed. New drug symposium I, T-1551 (cefoperazone). Fukuoka City, Japan: The Twenty-seventh General Congress of Japan Society of Chemotherapy, June 7, 1979:74-82.
26. English AR, Girard D. Distribution of a combination of the β-lactamase inhibitor CP-45,899 and ampicillin into serum and extravascular fluid in mice and rats [Abstract no A37]. Dallas, Tex: Twenty-first Annual Meeting of the American Society for Microbiology, March 1-6, 1981.
27. Wise R, Donovan IA, Andrews JM, Drumn J, Bennet S. Penetration of sulbactam and ampicillin into peritoneal fluid. Antimicrob Agents Chemother 1983;24:290-2.

Age, sex, and nitrazepam kinetics: Relation to antipyrine disposition

Forty healthy men and women 19 to 80 years old received a single 10 mg oral dose of the 7-nitro benzodiazepine nitrazepam. Nitrazepam plasma concentrations were measured during the next 72 hours. Among men, the elderly had a larger volume of distribution (V_{area}) than did younger subjects (1.96 vs. 1.63 L/kg; $P < 0.05$); because clearance did not change with age (0.84 vs. 0.95 ml/min/kg), the prolonged $t_{1/2}$ in elderly men (28 vs. 20 hours; $P < 0.01$) was a result of the larger V_{area}. Elderly and young women did not differ in nitrazepam V_{area} (2.58 vs. 2.55 L/kg), $t_{1/2}$ (26 vs. 27 hours), or total clearance (1.19 vs. 1.09 ml/min/kg). The nitrazepam free fraction in plasma (18% to 19% unbound) was not related to age or sex. Among 18 subjects who also received antipyrine, the clearance of nitrazepam and antipyrine were not correlated ($r = 0.23$). Thus age minimally influences nitrazepam clearance (accomplished mainly by nitroreduction), which in turn is not significantly related to antipyrine oxidizing capacity. (CLIN PHARMACOL THER 1985;38:697-703.)

David J. Greenblatt, M.D., Darrell R. Abernethy, M.D., Ph.D., Ann Locniskar, B.S., Hermann R. Ochs, M.D.,* Jerold S. Harmatz, B.A., and Richard I. Shader, M.D. *Boston, Mass., Houston, Tex., and Bonn, Federal Republic of Germany*

Nitrazepam (see structure) is a 7-nitrobenzodiazepine derivative extensively used as a hypnotic agent. Its principal metabolic pathway in man involves initial nitroreduction at the 7 position, yielding 7-aminonitrazepam, followed by acetylation to yield 7-acetamidonitrazepam (see structure).[1-4] Both of these metabolites have minimal pharmacologic activity.[5] The two metabolic products appear in urine in free and conjugated forms, and on the average account for >50% of an oral dose.[1,4] Thus nitroreduction accounts for the most important fraction of nitrazepam clearance.

Previous studies have demonstrated impaired clearance and a prolonged elimination $t_{1/2}$ associated with the aging process for a number of benzodiazepines biotransformed by hepatic microsomal oxidation, including diazepam,[6-11] chlordiazepoxide,[12,13] desmethyldiazepam,[14-16] desalkylflurazepam[17] (formed from its precursor flurazepam), clobazam,[18,19] alprazolam,[20] triazolam,[21] midazolam,[22] and brotizolam.[23] In some studies the impairment of benzodiazepine oxidation with aging has been relatively sex specific, being more evident in men than in women.[14,16-20,22] However, impaired benzodiazepine oxidation in the elderly has not been found in every study,[24-26] with results apparently dependent on the study design, number of participants, and characteristics of the particular study population including sex composition, presence of concurrent illness, and other concurrent drugs. In contrast to the influence of age on benzodiazepine oxidation, the aging process appears to have little if any effect on the clearance of benzodiazepines biotransformed principally by conjugation, including oxazepam,[27-29] lorazepam,[30,31] temazepam,[26,32] and lormetazepam.[33]

The influence of age on the pharmacokinetics of drugs biotransformed by nitroreduction is not completely established, in part because relatively few drugs biotransformed by this pathway can be safely studied in man. Nitrazepam and clonazepam are two such drugs that can be given to man. Previous studies of nitrazepam kinetics in the elderly[34-36] suggest that the volume of distribution of nitrazepam relative to total weight might increase with increasing age, thereby leading to a prolonged $t_{1/2}$. However, nitrazepam clearance appears not to be related to age. These studies are not necessarily definitive, because sex as well as age may importantly influence the capacity for drug metabolism. Our present

From the Division of Clinical Pharmacology, Tufts-New England Medical Center, Boston; the Section on Hypertension/Clinical Pharmacology, Baylor College of Medicine, Houston; and the Medizinische Universitätsklinik, University of Bonn, Bonn.

Supported in part by Grants No. MH-34223 and No. AM-MH-32050 from the United States Public Health Service and by Grant No. Oc 10/6-4 from Deutsche Forschungsgemeinschaft, Federal Republic of Germany.

Received for publication July 12, 1985; accepted Sept. 12, 1985.

Reprint requests to: David J. Greenblatt, M.D., Division of Clinical Pharmacology, Box 1007, Tufts-New England Medical Center, 171 Harrison Ave., Boston, MA 02111.

*Present address: Marienkrankenhaus, Soest, Federal Republic of Germany.

NITRAZEPAM 7-AMINO NITRAZEPAM 7-ACETAMIDO NITRAZEPAM

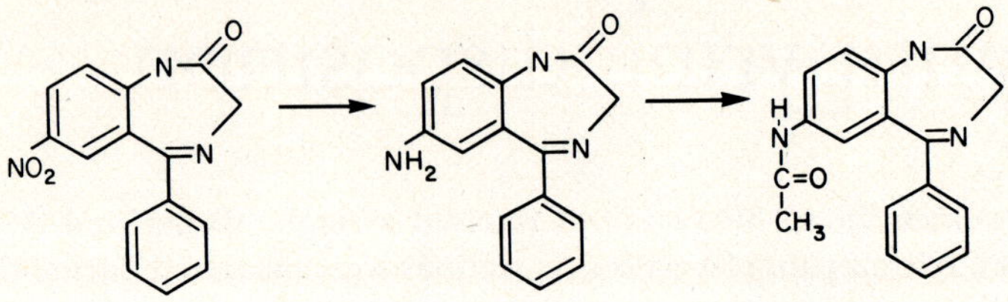

Nitrazepam and its principal metabolites

Table I. Effect of age and sex on nitrazepam kinetics

	Young men	*Young women*	*Elderly men*	*Elderly women*
Subject characteristics				
n	8	12	11	9
Age (yr)	35 ± 1.6	27 ± 1.9	67 ± 1.9*	69 ± 5.8*
Weight (kg)	69 ± 1.4	56 ± 2.0	79 ± 2.2*	58 ± 1.6
Plasma albumin (gm/dl)	4.4 ± 0.07	4.3 ± 0.05	4.2 ± 0.06	4.3 ± 0.09
Total (free plus bound) nitrazepam				
Peak plasma concentration (ng/ml)	161 ± 27	101 ± 12	164 ± 24	138 ± 12
Time of peak (hr after dose)	0.84 ± 0.16	2.4 ± 0.5	0.81 ± 0.11	0.9 ± 0.3†
Elimination $t_{1/2}$ (hr)	20 ± 1.3	27 ± 1.4	28 ± 1.5*	26 ± 1.9
Volume of distribution				
L	112 ± 8	143 ± 12	156 ± 9*	149 ± 10
L/kg	1.63 ± 0.13	2.55 ± 0.16	1.96 ± 0.09†	2.58 ± 0.15
Total clearance				
ml/min	66 ± 2.6	61 ± 4.9	67 ± 6.5	68 ± 6.2
ml/min/kg	0.95 ± 0.04	1.09 ± 0.06	0.84 ± 0.07	1.19 ± 0.11
Unbound nitrazepam				
Free fraction (% unbound)	17.8 ± 0.4	17.9 ± 0.5	18.9 ± 0.4	19.0 ± 0.3
Volume of distribution				
L	634 ± 49	801 ± 66	822 ± 44†	783 ± 52
L/kg	9.2 ± 0.8	14.4 ± 1.0	10.4 ± 0.4	13.6 ± 0.8
Free clearance				
ml/min	368 ± 14	344 ± 30	352 ± 32	360 ± 31
ml/min/kg	5.3 ± 0.2	6.2 ± 0.4	4.4 ± 0.3	6.3 ± 0.6

Data are $\bar{X}$ ± SE.
*$P < 0.01$, †$P < 0.05$, ‡$P < 0.025$ (Student's t test) compared with values in young subjects of same sex.

study was therefore undertaken to evaluate the effect of age and sex on the pharmacokinetics of a single oral dose of nitrazepam in healthy subjects.

METHODS

Subjects and procedure. Forty healthy men and women participated after giving written informed consent. They were divided into four similarly sized groups of young men, young women, elderly men, and elderly women (Table I). All young subjects (aged 19 to 44 years) were healthy, active, ambulatory adults with no history of medical disease and receiving no other drugs. The young women were not receiving oral contraceptives. Elderly subjects (aged 60 to 80 years) were likewise healthy, ambulatory adults without active medical disease. One elderly man had mild essential hypertension controlled with a diuretic, and an elderly woman was receiving digoxin and a diuretic because of ischemic heart disease. For both subjects the conditions were fully compensated and stable.

Subjects fasted overnight before and for 3 hours after nitrazepam dosing, after which they resumed their normal diet. A single 10 mg oral dose of nitrazepam (two 5 mg tablets) was taken with 100 to 200 ml tap water. Venous blood samples were drawn from an indwelling butterfly cannula kept open by a slow infusion of phys-

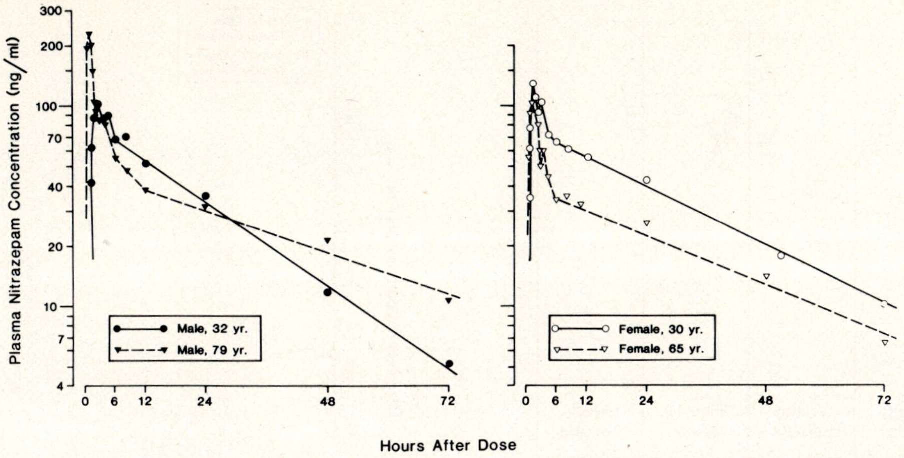

Fig. 1. Plasma concentration-time curves for nitrazepam in a representative young man, young woman, elderly man, and elderly woman.

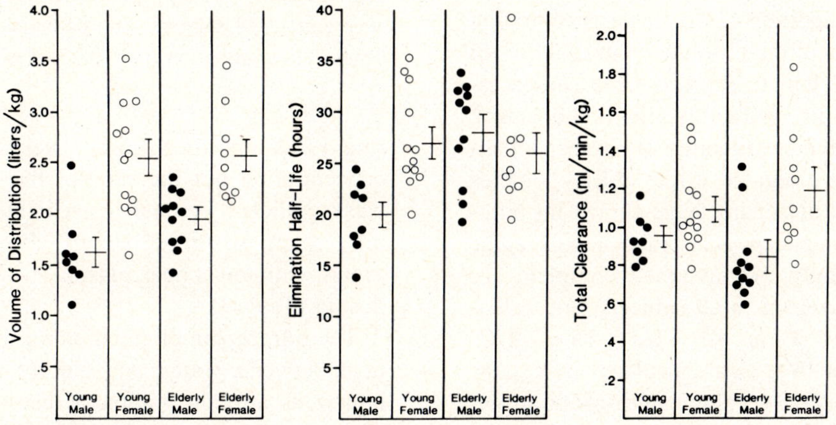

Fig. 2. Individual and mean (±SE) nitrazepam volume of distribution, elimination $t_{1/2}$, and total clearance in relation to age and sex.

iologic saline solution or from a separate venipuncture into heparinized tubes before dosing and at the following times thereafter: 5, 10, 15, 30, and 45 minutes and 1, 1.5, 2, 2.5, 3, 4, 6, 8, 12, 24, 48, and 72 hours. Blood samples were centrifuged and the plasma was separated and frozen until assayed.

Chemical analysis. Concentrations of nitrazepam in all samples were determined without derivitization by GC with electron-capture detection.[37] The sensitivity limit is approximately 3 to 5 ng/ml sample.

For each subject, the extent of nitrazepam binding to plasma protein was determined in a single sample drawn in the nonfasting state. To duplicate 1 ml aliquots of plasma were added 4.3 nCi/ml ^{14}C-nitrazepam (52 μCi/mg). The extent of binding was determined by equilibrium dialysis for 18 hours at 37° C.[38] Although not specifically evaluated for nitrazepam, the plasma binding of 10 other benzodiazepines, including the closely related derivative flunitrazepam, is concentration independent up to total plasma concentrations of 10,000 ng/ml.[38] Accordingly, concentration-independence was assumed for nitrazepam binding and only one sample was dialyzed per subject.

Kinetic and statistical analysis. For each subject the terminal log-linear phase of the plasma nitrazepam concentration-time curve was identified visually, and the slope (β) was determined by regression analysis. This was used to calculate the elimination $t_{1/2}$. The AUC until the final detectable plasma nitrazepam concentration was determined by the trapezoidal method and extrap-

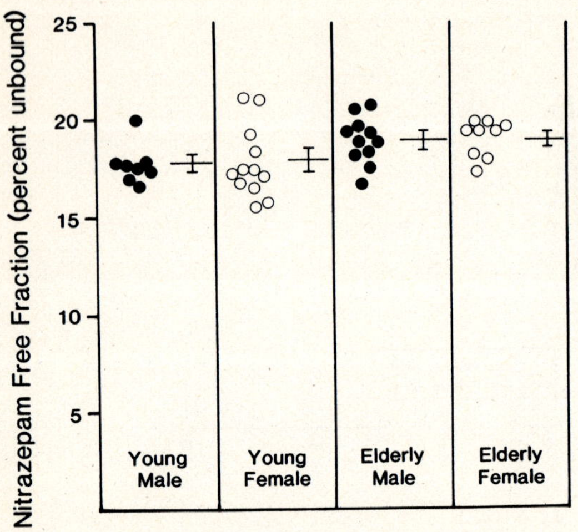

Fig. 3. Individual and mean (±SE) nitrazepam free fraction in relation to age and sex.

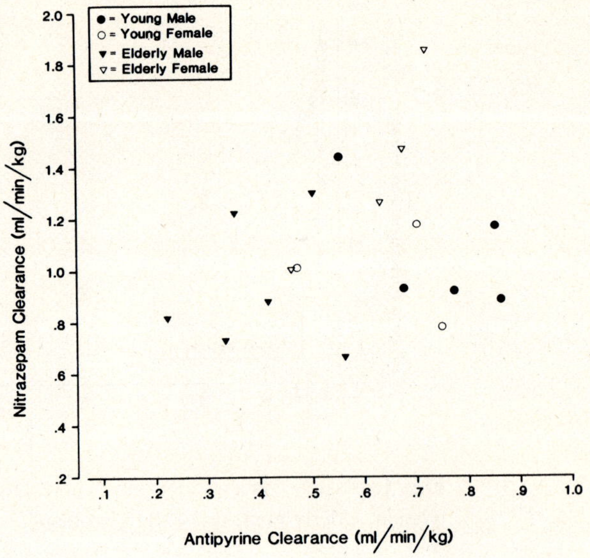

Fig. 4. Relation of antipyrine clearance and nitrazepam clearance among 18 subjects who participated in studies of both drugs. The correlation (r = 0.23) was not significant.

olated to infinity by addition of the final concentration divided by β. Studies of the absolute bioavailability of nitrazepam in young human subjects have shown essentially 100% systemic availability after oral dosing.[39] Although the absolute bioavailability of nitrazepam has not been specifically evaluated in the elderly, studies of lorazepam[30,40] and diazepam[6] have shown no influence of age on the completeness of oral benzodiazepine absorption. Accordingly, we assumed complete absorption of oral nitrazepam in all subjects, and calculated oral clearance (CL_o) as: CL_o = Dose/AUC. Volume of distribution (V_{area}) was calculated as: $V_{area} = CL_o/\beta$. For each subject, the volume of distribution and the clearance of total (free plus bound) nitrazepam was divided by that subject's free fraction to yield corresponding values of unbound volume of distribution and unbound (free) clearance. Differences in nitrazepam pharmacokinetic parameters between young and elderly subjects of the same sex were evaluated by Student's independent t test.

RESULTS

Young and elderly women were comparable with respect to body weight and plasma albumin concentration (Table I). Among men, the young and elderly were comparable with respect to plasma albumin levels, but elderly men were significantly heavier than the young men.

Fig. 1 shows representative plasma concentration-time curves for nitrazepam in young and elderly subjects of both sexes. Nitrazepam was rapidly absorbed from the gastrointestinal tract. The overall peak plasma nitrazepam concentration averaged 141 ng/ml, occurring 1.2 hours after dosing. Neither the peak plasma concentration nor the time of the peak concentration was significantly related to age in men. Among women, nitrazepam was more slowly absorbed in the young group, with lower peak plasma levels reached later after dosing (Table I).

The nitrazepam elimination $t_{1/2}$ was essentially identical between young and elderly women (27 vs. 26 hours), as were the volume of distribution and total oral clearance regardless of whether these variables were corrected for total body weight (Fig. 2). Because plasma protein binding of nitrazepam was similar between young and elderly women (Fig. 3), conclusions were the same if unbound volume of distribution and free clearance were used to compare the groups.

Among men, the nitrazepam elimination $t_{1/2}$ was significantly longer in the elderly subjects (28 vs. 20 hours; $P < 0.01$). However, this was apparently attributable to an increase in the volume of distribution rather than to a reduction in total metabolic clearance. Nitrazepam volume of distribution in general was smaller in men than in women regardless of age, but increased significantly with age in men (Fig. 2). This difference was partly attributable to the higher body weights in elderly men; after correction for total weight, the magnitude of the age-related difference in the volume of distribution was smaller (Table I). Oral clearance of nitrazepam was not significantly different between young and elderly men, regardless of whether clearance was cor-

Table II. Correlation coefficients* of antipyrine clearance and nitrazepam clearance among 18 subjects who participated in studies of both drugs

	Nitrazepam clearance			
	Total (free plus bound)		*Unbound (free)*	
	ml/min	*ml/min/kg*	*ml/min*	*ml/min/kg*
Antipyrine clearance				
ml/min	0.01		0.15	
ml/min/kg		0.23		0.34

*For n = 18, d.f. = 16; $P < 0.05$ when $r > 0.468$.

rected for body weight. The nitrazepam free fraction in plasma was slightly, but not significantly, higher in elderly than in young men (Fig. 3). After individual differences in binding were taken into account, conclusions about the relation of age to volume of distribution and clearance of unbound nitrazepam were similar to those based on the volume of distribution and clearance of total nitrazepam.

Eighteen subjects had previously participated in pharmacokinetic studies of antipyrine.[20,21,41] There was no significant relationship between total clearance of antipyrine and that of nitrazepam (Fig. 4; Table II).

DISCUSSION

Considerable data exist on the influence of age on the pharmacokinetics of benzodiazepines biotransformed by hepatic microsomal oxidation or by glucuronide conjugation. However, much less is known about the pharmacokinetics of nitroreduced benzodiazepines such as nitrazepam and clonazepam. Some studies have suggested alterations in distribution without a significant change in clearance of the nitroreduced benzodiazepine nitrazepam in association with the aging process,[35,36] but the potential confounding effects of sex, disease processes, or use of other drugs have not been completely excluded. We assessed the kinetics of a single oral dose of nitrazepam in healthy young and elderly subjects of both sexes. Because a parenteral preparation of nitrazepam is not available, we evaluated the kinetics of oral nitrazepam. Age-related alterations in absolute bioavailability of oral nitrazepam could possibly have influenced comparisons between age groups in kinetic variables such as volume of distribution and clearance. However, this seems unlikely because the absolute bioavailability of oral nitrazepam in young subjects is essentially complete,[39] and because the completeness of absorption of other benzodiazepines studied to date[6,30,40] is independent of age.

As in the case of benzodiazepines transformed principally by oxidation, there was no effect of age on the kinetic properties of nitrazepam among women. Among men, the nitrazepam volume of distribution was consistently smaller than in women regardless of age. This probably reflects the differing body habitus between men and women, with increased distribution of nitrazepam relative to total body weight in the female population because of the greater fraction of total weight accounted for by adipose tissue. Nonetheless, in the men there was an increased nitrazepam volume of distribution with age, which may also reflect a relative increase in adipose tissue, consistent with a higher body weight in the elderly than in the young men. The prolonged elimination $t_{1/2}$ associated with age in men resulted mainly from increased distribution, because changes in nitrazepam clearance with age in men were small. None of our findings were significantly influenced by plasma protein binding, inasmuch as neither age nor sex influenced nitrazepam binding. Consistent with previous reports,[2] nitrazepam is a rapidly absorbed benzodiazepine, reaching peak plasma concentrations within 90 minutes of oral dosing.

The marker compound antipyrine has been widely used as an index of drug oxidizing capacity.[42-44] A series of studies[20,41] of a design similar to the present one has suggested that the capacity of a given person to biotransform antipyrine is reasonably consistent with the same individual's capacity to clear or eliminate benzodiazepine derivatives similarly biotransformed by microsomal oxidation, including diazepam, desmethyldiazepam, desalkylflurazepam, and alprazolam. However, our study demonstrated little relationship between the clearances of antipyrine and of nitrazepam among 18 subjects who participated in studies of both drugs. This suggests that different mechanisms underlie individual variations in nitrazepam clearance, biotransformed principally by nitroreduction, as opposed to the control of benzodiazepine oxidizing capacity. This is consistent with reports that the oxidative inhibitor cimetidine, known to produce large impairment in the clearance of oxidized benzodiazepines,[45-50] had only a small influence on the clearance of nitrazepam in man.[51]

References

1. Kangas L. Urinary elimination of nitrazepam and its main metabolites. Acta Pharmacol Toxicol 1979;45:16-19.
2. Kangas L, Breimer DD. Clinical pharmacokinetics of nitrazepam. Clin Pharmacokinet 1981;6:346-66.
3. Rieder J, Wendt G. Pharmacokinetics and metabolism of the hypnotic nitrazepam. In: Garattini S, Mussini E, Randall LO, eds. The benzodiazepines. New York: Raven Press, 1973:99-127.
4. Sawada H, Shinohara K. On the urinary excretion of nitrazepam and its metabolites. Arch Toxicol 1971; 28:214-21.
5. Randall LO, Kappell B. Pharmacological activity of some benzodiazepines and their metabolites. In: Garattini S, Mussini E, Randall LO, eds. The benzodiazepines. New York: Raven Press, 1973:27-51.
6. Divoll M, Greenblatt DJ, Ochs HR, Shader RI. Absolute bioavailability of oral intramuscular diazepam: effect of age and sex. Anesth Analg (Cleve) 1983;62:1-8.
7. Greenblatt DJ, Allen MD, Harmatz JS, Shader RI. Diazepam disposition determinants. CLIN PHARMACOL THER 1980;27:301-12.
8. Kanto J, Maenpaa M, Mantyla R, Sellman R, Valovirta E. Effect of age on the pharmacokinetics of diazepam given in conjunction with spinal anesthesia. Anesthesiology 1979;51:154-9.
9. Klotz U, Avant GR, Hoyumpa A, Schenker S, Wilkinson GR. The effects of age and liver disease on the disposition and elimination of diazepam in adult man. J Clin Invest 1975;55:347-59.
10. Macklon AF, Barton M, James O, Rawlins MD. The effect of age on the pharmacokinetics of diazepam. Clin Sci 1980;59:479-83.
11. Ochs HR, Greenblatt DJ, Divoll M, Abernethy DR, Feyerabend H, Dengler HJ. Diazepam kinetics in relation to age and sex. Pharmacology 1981;23:24-30.
12. Roberts RK, Wilkinson GR, Branch RA, Schenker S. Effect of age and parenchymal liver disease on the disposition and elimination of chlordiazepoxide (Librium). Gastroenterology 1978;75:479-85.
13. Shader RI, Greenblatt DJ, Harmatz JS, Franke K, Koch-Weser J. Absorption and disposition of chlordiazepoxide in young and elderly male volunteers. J Clin Pharmacol 1977;17:709-18.
14. Allen MD, Greenblatt DJ, Harmatz JS, Shader RI. Desmethyldiazepam kinetics in the elderly after oral prazepam. CLIN PHARMACOL THER 1980;28:196-202.
15. Klotz U, Müller-Seydlitz P. Altered elimination of desmethyldiazepam in the elderly. Br J Clin Pharmacol 1979;7:119-20.
16. Shader RI, Greenblatt DJ, Ciraulo DA, Divoll M, Harmatz JS, Georgotas A. Effect of age and sex on disposition of desmethyldiazepam formed from its precursor clorazepate. Psychopharmacology 1981;75:193-7.
17. Greenblatt DJ, Divoll M, Harmatz JS, MacLaughlin DS, Shader RI. Kinetics and clinical effects of flurazepam in young and elderly noninsomniacs. CLIN PHARMACOL THER 1981;30:475-86.
18. Greenblatt DJ, Divoll M, Puri SK, Ho I, Zinny MA, Shader RI. Clobazam kinetics in the elderly. Br J Clin Pharmacol 1981;12:631-6.
19. Greenblatt DJ, Divoll M, Puri SK, Ho I, Zinny MA, Shader RI. Reduced single-dose clearance of clobazam in elderly men predicts increased multiple-dose accumulation. Clin Pharmacokinet 1983;8:83-94.
20. Greenblatt DJ, Divoll M, Abernethy DR, Moschitto LJ, Smith RB, Shader RI. Alprazolam kinetics in the elderly: relation to antipyrine disposition. Arch Gen Psychiatr 1983;40:287-90.
21. Greenblatt DJ, Divoll M, Abernethy DR, Moschitto LJ, Smith RB, Shader RI. Reduced clearance of triazolam in old age: relation to antipyrine oxidizing capacity. Br J Clin Pharmacol 1983;15:303-9.
22. Greenblatt DJ, Abernethy DR, Locniskar A, Harmatz JS, Limjuco RA, Shader RI. Effect of age, gender, and obesity on midazolam kinetics. Anesthesiology 1984; 61:27-35.
23. Jochemsen R, Nandi KL, Corless D, Wesselman JGJ, Breimer DD. Pharmacokinetics of brotizolam in the elderly. Br J Clin Pharmacol 1983;16:299s-307s.
24. Avram MJ, Fragen RJ, Caldwell NJ. Midazolam kinetics in women of two age groups. CLIN PHARMACOL THER 1983;34:505-8.
25. MacLeod SM, Giles HG, Bengert B, Liu FF, Sellers EM. Age- and gender-related differences in diazepam pharmacokinetics. J Clin Pharmacol 1979;19:15-9.
26. Smith RB, Divoll M, Gillespie WR, Greenblatt DJ. Effect of subject age and gender on the pharmacokinetics of oral triazolam and temazepam. J Clin Pharmacol 1983;3:172-6.
27. Greenblatt DJ, Divoll M, Harmatz JS, Shader RI. Oxazepam kinetics: effects of age and sex. J Pharmacol Exp Ther 1980;215:86-91.
28. Ochs HR, Greenblatt DJ, Otten H. Disposition of oxazepam in relation to age, sex, and cigarette smoking. Klin Wochenschr 1981;59:899-903.
29. Shull HJ, Wilkinson GR, Johnson R, Schenker S. Normal disposition of oxazepam in acute viral hepatitis and cirrhosis. Ann Intern Med 1976;84:420-5.
30. Greenblatt DJ, Allen MD, Locniskar A, Harmatz JS, Shader RI. Lorazepam kinetics in the elderly. CLIN PHARMACOL THER 1979;26:103-13.
31. Kraus JW, Desmond PV, Marshall JP, Johnson RF, Schenker S, Wilkinson GR. Effects of aging and liver disease on disposition of lorazepam. CLIN PHARMACOL THER 1978;24:411-9.
32. Divoll M, Greenblatt DJ, Harmatz JS, Shader RI. Effect of age and gender on disposition of temazepam. J Pharm Sci 1981;70:1104-7.

33. Hümpel M, Nieuweboer B, Milius W, Hanke H, Wendt H. Kinetics and biotransformation of lormetazepam. II. Radioimmunologic determinations in plasma and urine of young and elderly subjects: first-pass effect. Clin Pharmacol Ther 1980;28:673-9.
34. Holm V, Melander A, Wahlin-Boll E. Influence of food and of age on nitrazepam kinetics. Drug Nutr Interact 1982;1:307-11.
35. Jochemsen R, Van Beusekom BR, Spoelstra P, Janssens AR, Breimer DD. Effect of age and liver cirrhosis on the pharmacokinetics of nitrazepam. Br J Clin Pharmacol 1983;15:295-302.
36. Kangas L, Iisalo E, Kanto J, et al. Human pharmacokinetics of nitrazepam: effect of age and diseases. Eur J Clin Pharmacol 1979;15:163-70.
37. Locniskar A, Greenblatt DJ, Ochs HR. Simplified GC assay of underivatized nitrazepam in plasma. J Chromatogr 1985;337:131-5.
38. Moschitto LJ, Greenblatt DJ. Concentration-independent plasma protein binding of benzodiazepines. J Pharm Pharmacol 1983;35:179-80.
39. Jochemsen R, Hogendoorn JJH, Dingemanse J, Hermans J, Boeijinga JK, Breimer DD. Pharmacokinetics and bioavailability of intravenous, oral, and rectal nitrazepam in humans. J Pharmacokinet Biopharm 1982;10:231-45.
40. Greenblatt DJ, Shader RI, Franke K, et al. Pharmacokinetics and bioavailability of intravenous, intramuscular and oral lorazepam in humans. J Pharm Sci 1979;68:57-63.
41. Greenblatt DJ, Divoll M, Abernethy DR, Harmatz JS, Shader RI. Antipyrine kinetics in the elderly: prediction of age-related changes in benzodiazepine oxidizing capacity. J Pharmacol Exp Ther 1982;220:120-6.
42. Breimer DD. Interindividual variations in drug disposition—clinical implications and methods of investigation. Clin Pharmacokinet 1983;8:371-7.
43. Stevenson IH. Factors influencing antipyrine elimination. Br J Clin Pharmacol 1977;4:261-5.
44. Vesell ES. The antipyrine test in clinical pharmacology: conceptions and misconceptions. Clin Pharmacol Ther 1979;26:275-86.
45. Abernethy DR, Greenblatt DJ, Divoll M, Ameer B, Shader RI. Differential effect of cimetidine on drug oxidation (antipyrine and diazepam) versus conjugation (acetaminophen and lorazepam): prevention of acetaminophen toxicity by cimetidine. J Pharmacol Exp Ther 1983;224:508-13.
46. Abernethy DR, Greenblatt DJ, Divoll M, Moschitto LJ, Harmatz JS, Shader RI. Interaction of cimetidine with the triazolobenzodiazepines alprazolam and triazolam. Psychopharmacology 1983;80:275-8.
47. Desmond PV, Patwardhan RV, Schenker S, Speeg KV. Cimetidine impairs elimination of chlordiazepoxide (Librium) in man. Ann Intern Med 1980;93:266-8.
48. Divoll M, Greenblatt DJ, Abernathy DR, Shader RI. Cimetidine impairs clearance of antipyrine and desmethyldiazepam in the elderly. J Am Geriatr Soc 1982;30:684-9.
49. Greenblatt DJ, Abernethy DR, Morse DS, Shader RI, Harmatz JS. Clinical importance of the interaction of diazepam and cimetidine. N Engl J Med 1984;310:1639-43.
50. Klotz U, Reimann I. Influence of cimetidine on the pharmacokinetics of desmethyldiazepam and oxazepam. Eur J Clin Pharmacol 1980;18:517-20.
51. Ochs HR, Greenblatt DJ, Gugler R, Müntefering G, Locniskar A, Abernethy DR. Cimetidine impairs nitrazepam clearance. Clin Pharmacol Ther 1983;34:227-30.

Notes of the American Society for Clinical Pharmacology and Therapeutics

A Letter to the Members

This note contains updates on some of the developing issues.

First, the survey with regards to Board Certification has been completed as of Aug. 31, 1985. Twenty-five percent of the membership of the American Society for Clinical Pharmacology and Therapeutics (ASCPT) responded. This equates to 455 responses, with 68% in favor of a required certification examination for physicians and 60% in favor of some kind of certification process for nonphysicians also. At the first and second Task Force meetings of the Council on Clinical Pharmacology, it was considered that nonphysicians should receive a certificate of recognition indicating their ongoing activity and performance in clinical pharmacology. The actual completion of a written examination for nonphysicians would, therefore, be unnecessary. However, written certification for physicians would be administered by a separate board in clinical pharmacology. Hopefully, the first of these examinations would be given sometime in 1987. Because the American Board of Internal Medicine has looked upon applications for new subspecialty examinations with disfavor, the Council has elected to have an independent board in clinical pharmacology. It is apparent that there is a mandate from the ASCPT to proceed along these lines. Once the actual processes for physicians and nonphysicians have been delineated, membership of the ASCPT will be appraised for comments and voting.

Second, at the end of January 1986, David Nierenberg, M.D., Director of Clinical Pharmacology at Dartmouth Medical College in Hanover, N. H., will be hosting a small plenary workshop on teaching techniques in clinical pharmacology. This initial gathering will be a means of setting guidelines for teaching medical students, house staff, and graduate physicians. It will also serve as a springboard for the symposium to be held at the annual meeting of the ASCPT in Washington, D.C., in March 1986.

Third, Dr. Ed Sellers, Chairman of the Ad Hoc Committee on Alcohol and Drug Dependence and Past President of ASCPT, will be meeting with his committee in February. They will hopefully prepare a position paper on this issue to submit to the Board at the annual meeting.

Fourth, Marcus Reidenberg, M.D., Immediate Past President of the ASCPT, has been working on a program whereby ASCPT will be sponsoring the submission of our JOURNAL to underprivileged countries. This will expose those professionals to international contributions in clinical pharmacology. There will be more about this in future issues.

Fifth, please remember the 3rd World Conference on Clinical Pharmacology in Stockholm, Sweden, July 27-Aug. 1, 1986. The call for abstracts is due by Feb. 15, 1986.

Finally, make your reservations now for the ASCPT's eighty-seventh annual meeting on March 20-22, 1986, at the Sheraton Washington Hotel in Washington, D.C. A hotel reservation form and preregistration card are found on pages 723 and 724 of this issue.

Best wishes, and I hope to see you all in Washington in March.

David T. Lowenthal, M.D.
President, ASCPT

USAN Council

List No. 267

New Names

The following nonproprietary names for the compounds described have been adopted by the United States Adopted Names (USAN) Council, which is sponsored by the American Medical Association, the American Pharmaceutical Association, and the US Pharmacopeial Convention, Inc., in cooperation with the respective pharmaceutical manufacturers. The designation USAN (United States Adopted Name) distinguishes these formally adopted nonproprietary names from other names. The information given under the category Therapeutic Claim is based on the manufacturer's claims at the time of publication. Adoption of USAN does not imply endorsement of the claims or products by the AMA, the US Pharmacopeia, or the APhA.

In some instances, the drugs listed are available only from the manufacturer to properly qualified investigators for clinical study.

USAN SALMETEROL

Pronunciation săl mĕ′ tĕ rōl

Therapeutic claim bronchodilator

Chemical names

(1) (±)-4-hydroxy-α^1-[[[6-(4-phenylbutoxy)hexyl]amino]methyl]-1,3-benzenedimethanol

(2) (±)-4-hydroxy-α^1-[[[6-(4-phenylbutoxy)hexyl]amino]methyl]-*m*-xylene-α,α′-diol

Structural formula

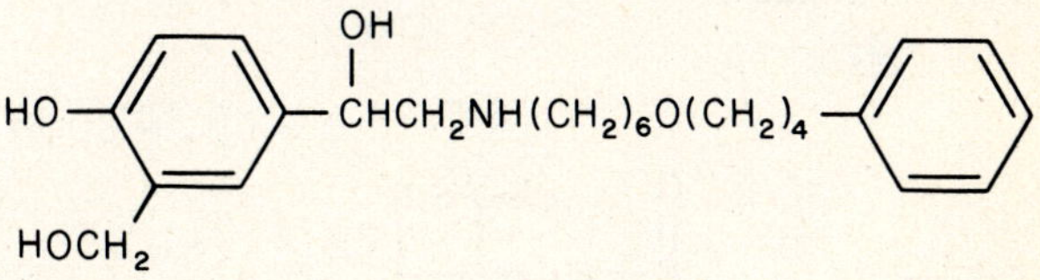

Molecular formula $C_{25}H_{37}NO_4$

Molecular weight 415.59

Manufacturer Glaxo (England)

Code designation GR 33343 X

CAS registry No. 89365-50-4

USAN FELODIPINE

Pronunciation fĕ lō′ dĭ pēn

Therapeutic claim vasodilator

Chemical name

ethyl methyl 4-(2,3-dichlorophenyl)-1,4-dihydro-2,6-dimethyl-3,5-pyridinedicarboxylate

Structural formula

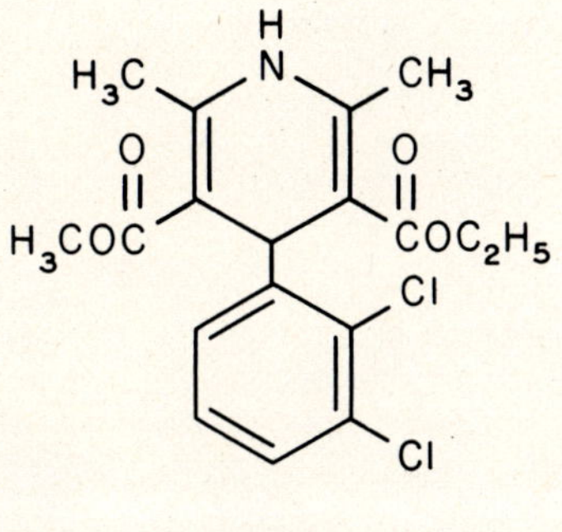

Molecular formula $C_{18}H_{19}Cl_2NO_4$

Molecular weight 384.26

Manufacturer Astra Pharmaceutical Production AB (Sweden)

Code designation H 154/82

CAS registry No. 72509-76-3

USAN ENPROFYLLINE

Pronunciation ĕn prō′ fĭ lĭn

Therapeutic claim bronchodilator

Chemical names

(1) 3,7-dihydro-3-propyl-1*H*-purine-2,6-dione

(2) 3-propylxanthine

Structural formula

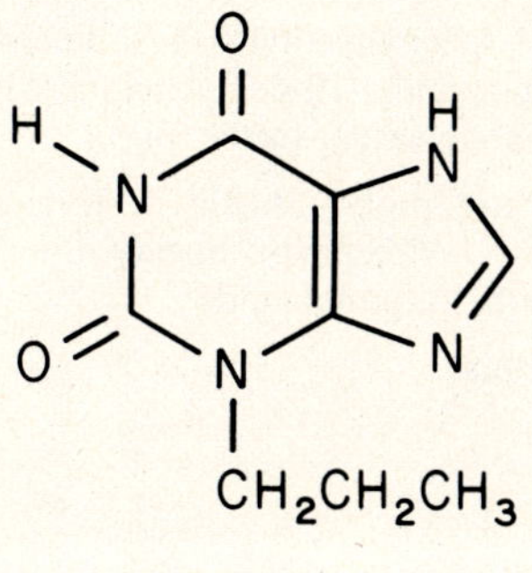

Molecular formula $C_8H_{10}N_4O_2$

Molecular weight 194.2

Manufacturer Astra Pharmaceutical Production AB (Sweden)

Code designation D 4028

CAS registry No. 41078-02-8

USAN	OXIMONAM
Pronunciation	ŏks′ ĭ mō″ năm
Therapeutic claim	antibiotic

Chemical names

(1) [2*S*-[2α,3β(*Z*)]]-[[3-[[(2-amino-4-thiazolyl)(methoxyimino)acetyl]amino]-2-methyl-4-oxo-1-azetidinyl]oxy]acetic acid

(2) [[(2*S*,3*S*)-3-[(2-amino-4-thiazolyl)glyoxylamido]-2-methyl-4-oxo-1-azetidinyl]oxy]acetic acid, 3[2]-(*Z*)-(*O*-methyloxime)

Structural formula

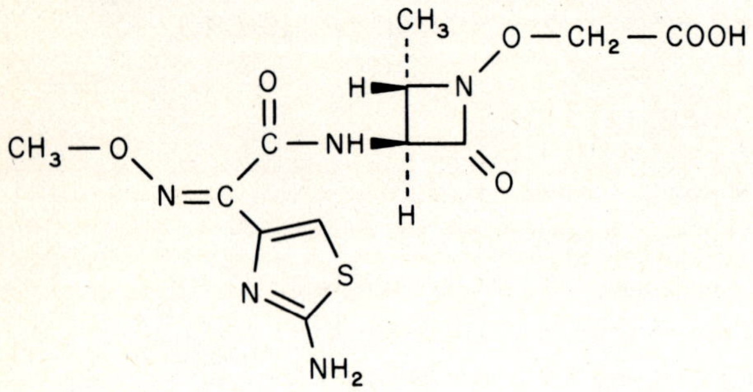

Molecular formula	$C_{12}H_{13}N_5O_6S$
Molecular weight	357.34
Manufacturer	E. R. Squibb & Sons, Inc.
Code designation	SQ 82629
CAS registry No.	90898-90-1

USAN	OXIMONAM SODIUM
Pronunciation	ŏks′ ĭ mō″ năm
Therapeutic claim	antibiotic

Chemical names

(1) sodium [2*S*-[2α,3β(*Z*)]]-[[3-[[(2-amino-4-thiazolyl)(methoxyimino)acetyl]amino]-2-methyl-4-oxo-1-azetidinyl]oxy]acetate

(2) sodium [[(2*S*,3*S*)-3-[(2-amino-4-thiazolyl)glyoxylamido]-2-methyl-4-oxo-1-azetidinyl]oxy]acetate, 3[2]-(*Z*)-(*O*-methyloxime)

Structural formula

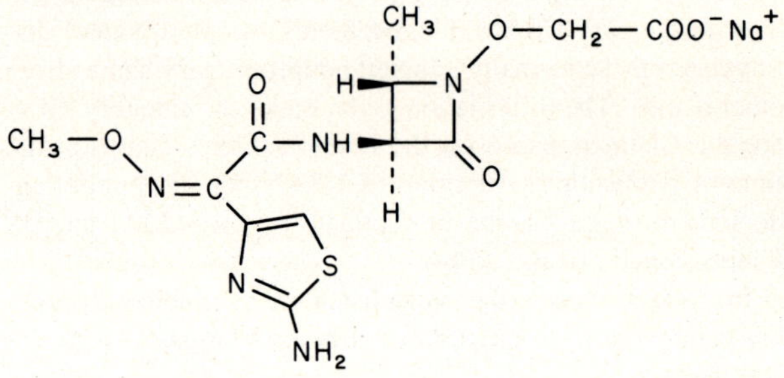

Molecular formula	$C_{12}H_{14}N_5NaO_6S$
Molecular weight	379.33
Manufacturer	E. R. Squibb & Sons, Inc.
Code designation	SQ 82629
CAS registry No.	90849-08-4

USAN	HISTRELIN
Pronunciation	hĭs trĕl′ ĭn
Therapeutic claim	LHRH agonist

Chemical names

(1) 6-[1-(phenylmethyl)-D-histidine]-9-(*N*-ethyl-L-prolinamide)-10-deglycinamideluteinizing hormone-releasing factor (pig)

(2) 5-oxo-L-prolyl-L-histidyl-L-tryptophyl-L-seryl-L-tyrosyl-*N*$^{\tau}$-benzyl-D-histidyl-L-leucyl-L-arginyl-*N*-ethyl-L-prolinamide

Structural formula

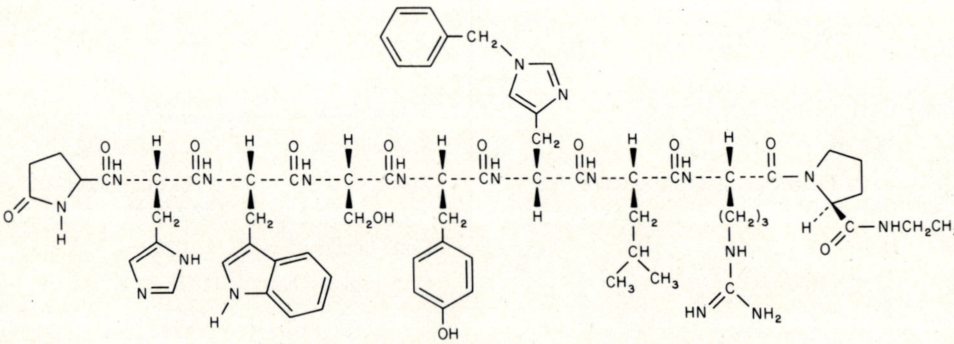

Molecular formula	$C_{66}H_{86}N_{18}O_{12}$
Molecular weight	1323.53
Manufacturer	Ortho Pharmaceutical Corporation
Code designation	ORF 17070
CAS registry No.	76712-82-8

Index to volume 38

Author index

A

Abernethy DR, 342, 697
Abraham PA, 31
Ajayi AA, 560
Ajzen H, 613
Akagi K, 290
Albin HC, 285
Alradi AO, 495
Alván G, 241, 394
Ambre JJ, 318
Anderson SA, 674
Anslow JA, 533
Anton RF, 52
Apicella M, 150
Araujo P, 533
Aronoff GR, 212
Arvela P, 652
Atkinson AJ Jr, 318
Atkinson RL, 419

B

Bachofen H, 96
Baker EL, 656
Baliga G, 266
Barnes JS, 258
Bayliff CD, 457
Beguin J, 549
Benet LZ, 121, 481
Berger A, 28
Berglund G, 188
Berke LK, 419
Berthelin C, 549
Besnard M, 549
Bibbs ML, 419
Bigelow GE, 219
Bigot M-C, 549
Bircher J, 618
Bodey GP, 134
Bongaerts MCM, 301
Bosso JA, 121
Bouchet JL, 285
Boutagy J, 371
Bowsher DJ, 318
Branch RA, 402, 414
Brater DC, 674
Brittain DC, 590
Brown-Cartwright D, 674
Bugiardini R, 101
Burckart GJ, 296
Burns T, 77, 642
Byington RP, 509

C

Cafarell R, 150
Calimlim JF, 177
Calissendorff B, 37
Camí J, 336
Campbell BC, 560
Carruthers SG, 495
Carson JL, 359
Challis P, 625
Chen A, 674
Chiang W-T, 37
Chow MJ, 318
Christiaanse JC, 301
Clarke J, 266
Cohen AF, 381
Collins JM, 45
Conrad KA, 331
Crawford MH, 538
Crivelli AM, 96
Cunci R, 439

D

Dahlqvist R, 37
Danan G, 439
Darke A, 533
Davies RO, 65
Davis R, 12
Dayer P, 488
Debruyne D, 549
Demotes-Mainard FM, 285
de Prost D, 171
de Simone G, 434
de Torres S, 336
DeVane CL, 586
DiPette DJ, 199
Dommisse CS, 586
Draibe SA, 613
Drake CR, 419
du Souich P, 686
Dvornik D, 625

E

Echizen H, 71
Eckfeldt JH, 157
Edgar B, 205
Edwards KDG, 313
Egan B, 519
Eichelbaum M, 71
Ellis GM Jr, 572
Emilsson H, 37
Erill S, 365
Erlinger S, 439
Eshelman FN, 157
Evans RR, 199

F

Fasano ML, 434
Faure G, 6
Feldman RD, 350
Ferrara LA, 434
Ferraro JC, 199
Ferrini D, 101
Fine RL, 45
Finley DK, 157
Fischer LJ, 350
Fischman MW, 318
Fleming JJ, 409
Flowers OV, 273
Foley KM, 631
Folgering HTM, 428
Fortner G, 273
Foulds G, 692
Freeman DJ, 56
Fujishima M, 462
Furberg CD, 509

G

Gagliardi R, 434
Galeazzi RL, 96, 140
Galvani M, 101
Gebhard RL, 157
George CF, 387
Gerber JG, 258
Goldberg MJ, 350
Goldstein S, 661
Gonzalez R, 625
Gore R, 195
Goto F, 402
Grabinski PY, 631
Graham DY, 65
Greenberg BD, 656
Greenblatt DJ, 595, 648, 697
Gridelli C, 101
Guerot C, 171
Guerra D, 336
Gugger M, 96

H

Hakala TR, 296
Haley NJ, 164
Halstenson CE, 31
Hamilton M, 381
Hardy BG, 457
Harmatz JS, 697
Harris K, 661
Hasegawa J, 306
Hawes EM, 128
Hayashi K, 462
Hedner T, 188
Hermens WAJJ, 469
Herskovic JE, 450
Hichens M, 661
Hicks D, 625
Hirakata H, 462

July, pp 1-120; August, pp 121-240; September, 241-358; October, 359-480; November, 481-602; December, 603-724.

Hirose T, 590
Ho DH, 134
Hobbes J, 371
Hoffman D, 164
Hofkamp HG, 301
Holmes GI, 65
Holtzman JL, 157
Honc F, 251
Hooper JW, 533
Hori R, 290
Hunninghake DB, 313
Hunter T, 228
Hurwitz A, 642

I

Inturrisi CE, 631
Irvin JD, 661
Iselius L, 394
Isles AF, 89

J

Jacob GB, 674
Jacqz E, 402
Jamali F, 325
James A, 680
Janicke D, 150
Janky D, 642
Jarvik ME, 450
Jasinski DR, 544
Jenkins JF, 45
Johansson L, 205
Johnson SL, 331
Johnsson G, 205
Judson BA, 572
Juhl RP, 525
Julius S, 519
Jusko WJ, 150

K

Kaiko RF, 631
Kaiser DL, 419
Kamiya A, 290
Karim A, 77, 642
Karsenty F, 171
Kassem N, 503
Kater CE, 613
Kauffman R, 183
Keane WF, 31
Keirns JJ, 278
Kendall C, 28
Kennedy GT, 538
Kershaw RA, 251
Kilpatrick SJ, 273
Kinsella TJ, 45
Klecker RW, 45
Klein L, 661
Klotz U, 652
Knirsch AK, 692
Kochak GM, 251
Korchinski ED, 128
Koren G, 680
Koshakji RP, 579
Kradjan WA, 12
Krantz KD, 28
Kroboth PD, 525
Kronbach T, 488
Kuhlmann J, 667
Küpfer A, 414, 618

L

Labetalol/Hydrochlorothiazide Multicenter Study Group, 24
Lacouture PG, 183
Lai AA, 586
Laizure SC, 586
Lammers J-WJ, 428
Langendijk PNJ, 121
Larochelle P, 686
Lasagna L, 177
Lauterburg BH, 566
LeBlanc B, 134
Lenzi S, 101
LeRoy AA, 359
Letz R, 656
Levy G, 6
Li CH, 631
Liebson IA, 219
Liedholm H, 475 (letter)
Lin ET, 306
Lindsten J, 394
Littman GS, 16
Locker B, 549
Locniskar A, 697
Löfberg I, 205
Louik C, 183
Lovejoy FH Jr, 183
Lowenthal DT, 661
Ludden TM, 475 (letter), 538
Lundborg P, 205

M

MacDougall B, 228
MacGregor TR, 278
MacLeod SM, 89
Magnusson A, 37
Mahachai V, 325
Malè P-J, 488
Maloy JW, 503
Mann MA, 572
Mari L, 101
Maronde RF, 503
Martin M, 199
Martin WS, 533
Martin-Dupont C, 285
Matlis R, 648
Mattei E Jr, 613
Matzek KM, 278
Matzke GR, 31
Max MB, 631
Mayersohn M, 331
McAllister CB, 402
McBurney A, 409
McCabe EJ, 60
McGourty JC, 409
McKay G, 128
McIntyre KM, 509
McLean A, 475 (letter)
Medakovic M, 503
Meeran MK, 60
Meier UT, 488
Melander A, 475 (letter)
Merkus FWHM, 469
Merrill D, 661
Meyer UA, 488
Micalizzi E, 195
Midha KK, 128
Miller RD, 692
Mitchell AA, 183
Mitchell JR, 566
Mitenko PA, 228
Montay G, 439
Moore PA, 656
Morisset R, 686
Morse G, 150
Morse ML, 359
Morton A, 52
Motomura K, 462
Mottonen LR, 157
Moulin M, 549
Mullane JF, 625
Musselman D, 195

N

Nakamura K, 402
Nakano H, 290
Nelson G, 266
Netter P, 6
Neu HC, 590
Neubig R, 519
Nies AS, 258
Nihira H, 290
Nurmi A-K, 443

O

Ochs HR, 595, 648, 697
Ohchi N, 462
Okumura K, 290
Omae T, 462
Onoyama K, 462
Overdiek HWPM, 469
Owen JA, 228

P

Paladine JA, 52
Palmer M, 77
Park GD, 350
Patterson SE, 423
Peck AW, 381
Pedneault L, 686
Perlman M, 680
Persson B, 188
Pettersson A, 188
Phaneuf D, 686
Philipson R, 381
Piontek K, 150
Pison C, 686
Pitkäjärvi T, 443
Poisson M, 686
Presig R, 618
Preston KL, 219, 544
Procknal JA, 6
Ptachcinski RJ, 296
Puddu P, 101
Pyykönen M-L, 443

R

Rakhit A, 251
Raskin P, 625
Ray WA, 402
Regårdh CG, 205
Regent MC, 6
Reid JL, 560
Reidenberg MM, 2
Reilly CS, 579
Reilly PA, 325
Reinhardt LA, 273
Renwick AG, 387
Riddell JG, 554
Roberts DG, 258
Rolston K, 134
Rönn O, 205
Rose JE, 450
Rosenkranz B, 652
Rosenstock J, 625

Rosenthal JT, 296
Rothbard RL, 84
Roy SD, 128
Rubin PC, 560
Ruo TI, 318
Ryder S, 625

S

San L, 336
Saris S, 661
Saucedo R, 365
Schenck-Gustafsson K, 37
Schmid B, 618
Schneider BE, 16
Schramm NT, 572
Schreiner BF, 84
Schwartz JB, 342
Schwartz ML, 457
Scully BE, 590
Sepkovic DW, 164
Seppälä E, 443
Shader RI, 697
Shanks RG, 554
Shapiro S, 183
Sharp T, 28
Sheiner LB, 481
Shenfield GM, 371
Shepherd AMM, 475 (letter)
Silas JH, 409
Silke B, 266
Sitar DS, 228
Sjöqvist F, 394
Sjöval J, 241
Sloan RS, 212
Slomka M, 195
Smallridge RC, 12
Smith CV, 566
Smith JL, 65
Smith PC, 121
Smith RB, 525
Smith T, 625
Smith V-E, 60
Solé A, 336
Sopko GS, 313
Sörgel F, 306
Soro S, 434
Spector R, 350
Spino M, 89
Spruance SL, 56
Steiner E, 394
Stewart JT, 586
Stitzer ML, 109
Stoehr GP, 525
St-Pierre MV, 89
Straehl P, 140
Streeter WC, 273
Streicher J, 77
Strom BL, 359
Strong HA, 387
Strong JM, 45

T

Tartiere J, 549
Tashchian A, 572
Taylor RJ, 296
Taylor SH, 266
Tesoro A, 89
Thomas RW, 52
Thomassin C, 549
Thomson ABR, 325
Thrupp LD, 692
Till A, 661
Todd EL, 342, 566
Tollemeto D, 101
Tomooka S, 462
Tosiello RL, 313
Toto RD, 674
Trilling Y, 450
Tsuruda H, 462

U

Ugena B, 336
Ulm E, 661

V

van den Ende A, 278
van Herwaarden CLA, 428
van Marion WF, 301
van Ouwerkerk W, 301
van Tol RGL, 278
van Wayjen RGA, 278
Vapaatalo H, 443
Vega C, 686
Venkataramanan R, 296
Verburg-Ochs B, 595
Verma P, 12
Verma SP, 266
Vesell ES, 603
Vincon GA, 285
Vlachakis ND, 503
Vogelgesang B, 71
Vokonas PS, 509
von Bahr C, 37

W

Wagner WE, 251
Waldes L, 251
Walker BR, 16
Walle T, 509
Walshe J, 150
Ward JW, 409
Warner NJ, 387
Wearley L, 77
Weinbrenner J, 648
Wenerstron G, 56
Westerlund D, 241
White WB, 60
Wilkin JK, 273
Wilkinson GR, 402
Williams FL, 419
Williams RL, 306
Wood AJJ, 579
Wood M, 579
Wynder EL, 164

Y

Yaffe SJ, 183
Yeo E, 134
Ylitalo P, 443
Yu PN, 84

Z

Zacny JP, 109
Zanella MT, 613
Zerbe GO, 258

Subject index

A

Acebutolol
Circulatory effects of intravenous and oral acebutolol in acute myocardial infarction (Silke et al), 266

Acifran
Controlled trial of acifran in type II hyperlipoproteinemia (Hunninghake et al), 313

Acyl glucuronides
Effect of probenecid on the formation and elimination of acyl glucuronides: Studies with zomepirac (Smith et al), 121

Acrivastine
Acrivastine (USAN List No. 266), 602
The acute effects of acrivastine (BW825C), a new antihistamine, compared with triprolidine on measures of central nervous system performance and subjective effects (Cohen et al), 381

Adverse reaction(s)
A study of adverse reaction algorithms in a drug surveillance program (Louik et al), 183

Age
Age, sex, and nitrazepam kinetics: Relation to antipyrine disposition (Greenblatt et al), 697
Effects of age and disease on the pharmacokinetics and pharmacodynamics of sulindac (Sitar et al), 228
Gastrointestinal absorption as a function of age: Xylose absorption in healthy adults (Johnson et al), 331
Salicylate kinetics in old age (Netter et al), 6

Alacepril
Pharmacokinetics of a new angiotensin I converting enzyme inhibitor (alacepril) after oral dosing in fasting or fed states (Onoyama et al), 462

Alcohol
Effect of acute alcohol consumption on lithium kinetics (Anton et al), 52

Aldosterone
Inadequate aldosterone response to hyperkalemia during angiotensin converting enzyme inhibition in chronic renal failure (Zanella et al), 613

Algorithm(s)
A new dosing regimen in renal insufficiency: Application to cephalexin (Hori et al), 290
A study of adverse reaction algorithms in a drug surveillance program (Louik et al), 183

Alpha-receptor(s)
Evaluation and application of the linear variable differential transformer technique for the assessment of human dorsal hand vein alpha-receptor activity (Alradi and Carruthers), 495
Pharmacologic reduction of sympathetic drive increases platelet alpha-2–receptor number (Egan et al), 519

Alprazolam
Effect of alprazolam on digoxin kinetics and creatinine clearance (Ochs et al), 595

American Society for Clinical Pharmacology and Therapeutics
A letter to the Members, 704
A message from the President, 235
Donors, 478
Status report from the Council on Clinical Pharmacology, July 1985, 599

Amfilcon A
Amfilcon A (USAN List No. 262), 117

Aminoglycosides
Effect of aminoglycosides on the disposition of thyroid hormones and thyroglobulin (du Souich et al), 686

Amoxycillin
Dose-dependent absorption of amoxycillin and bacampicillin (Sjövall et al), 241

Analgesia
Reassessment of verbal and visual analog ratings in analgesic studies (Littman et al), 16

Analog scales
Reassessment of verbal and visual analog ratings in analgesic studies (Littman et al), 16

Angiotensin
Enalaprilat, an intravenous angiotensin-converting enzyme inhibitor, in hypertensive crises (DiPette et al), 199
Inadequate aldosterone response to hyperkalemia during angiotensin converting enzyme inhibition in chronic renal failure (Zanella et al), 613
Pharmacokinetics of a new angiotensin I converting enzyme inhibitor (alacepril) after oral dosing in fasting or fed states (Onoyama et al), 462

July, pp 1-120; August, pp 121-240; September, 241-358; October, pp 359-480; November, pp 481-602; December, pp 603-724.

Antagonist(s)
Effects of the calcium antagonist tiapamil on pulmonary gas exchange in patients with chronic obstructive pulmonary disease who receive salbutamol (Gugger et al), 96
Interaction of ibuprofen with the H-2 receptor antagonists ranitidine and cimetidine (Ochs et al), 648
Antihistamine
The acute effects of acrivastine (BW825C), a new antihistamine, compared with triprolidine on measures of central nervous system performance and subjective effects (Cohen et al), 381
Antihypertensive effect
Inhibition of prostaglandin synthesis by indomethacin interacts with the antihypertensive effect of atenolol (Ylitalo et al), 443
Antipyrine
Age, sex, and nitrazepam kinetics: Relation to antipyrine disposition (Greenblatt et al), 697
Arthroscopy
Prilocaine in arthroscopy: Clinical pharmacokinetics and rational use (Debruyne et al), 549
Asthma
Ventilatory effects of atenolol and bevantolol in asthma (Lammers et al), 428
Astifilcon A
Astifilcon A (USAN List No. 265), 480
Atenolol
Effects of betaxolol, propranolol, and atenolol on isoproterenol-induced beta-adrenoceptor responses (Riddell and Shanks), 554
Inhibition of prostaglandin synthesis by indomethacin interacts with the antihypertensive effect of atenolol (Ylitalo et al), 443
Ventilatory effects of atenolol and bevantolol in asthma (Lammers et al), 428
Atropine
Atropine serum concentrations after multiple inhaled doses of atropine sulfate (Kradjan et al), 12

B

Bacampicillin
Dose-dependent absorption of amoxycillin and bacampicillin (Sjövall et al), 241
Baclofen
The pharmacokinetics of baclofen derived from intestinal infusion (Kochak et al), 251
Bactericide
The pharmacokinetics and bactericidal characteristics of oral cefixime (Brittain et al), 590
Beta-adrenoceptor(s)
Effects of betaxolol, propranolol, and atenolol on isoproterenol-induced beta-adrenoceptor responses (Riddell and Shanks), 554
Beta-blocker(s)
Biologic determinants of propranolol disposition: Results from 1308 patients in the Beta-blocker Heart Attack Trial (Walle et al), 509
Pharmacokinetics and beta-blocking effects of timolol in poor and extensive metabolizers of debrisoquin (McGourty et al), 409
Ultra-short-acting beta-blockade: A comparison with conventional beta-blockade (Reilly et al), 579
Betaxolol
Effects of betaxolol, propranolol, and atenolol on isoproterenol-induced beta-adrenoceptor responses (Riddell and Shanks), 554
Benzodiazepine
Pharmacodynamic evaluation of the benzodiazepine-oral contraceptive interaction (Kroboth et al), 525
Bevantolol
Ventilatory effects of atenolol and bevantolol in asthma (Lammers et al), 428
Blood flow
Prostaglandins and nicotinate-provoked increase in cutaneous blood flow (Wilkin et al), 273
Blood loss
Fecal blood loss during isoxicam and piroxicam administration for 28 days (Hooper et al), 533
Blood pressure
Effects of chronic nitrendipine on casual (office) and 24-hour ambulatory blood pressure (White et al), 60
Books received
Book received, 358
Breast milk
Sulbactam kinetics and excretion into breast milk in postpartum women (Foulds et al), 692
Bupropion
Pharmacokinetics of bupropion and its major basic metabolites in normal subjects after a single dose (Laizure et al), 586
Butylated hydroxytoluene
Treatment of recurrent herpes simplex labialis with topical butylated hydroxytoluene (Freeman et al), 56

C

Cancer
Epidural and intrathecal opiates: Cerebrospinal fluid and plasma profiles in patients with chronic cancer pain (Max et al), 631
Cannabinoid
Excretion patterns of cannabinoid metabolites after last use in a group of chronic users (Ellis et al), 572
Captopril
Effect of naloxone on the actions of captopril (Ajayi et al), 560

Caucasian
Interethnic differences in genetic polymorphism of debrisoquin and mephenytoin hydroxylation between Japanese and Caucasian populations (Nakamura et al), 402
Cefixime
The pharmacokinetics and bactericidal characteristics of oral cefixime (Brittain et al), 590
Cefotaxime
Cefotaxime and desacetyl cefotaxime kinetics in renal impairment (Matzke et al), 31
Pharmacokinetics of intravenous and intraperitoneal cefotaxime in chronic ambulatory peritoneal dialysis (Albin et al), 285
Central nervous system
The acute effects of acrivastine (BW825C), a new antihistamine, compared with triprolidine on measures of central nervous system performance and subjective effects (Cohen et al), 381
Cephalexin
A new dosing regimen in renal insufficiency: Application to cephalexin (Hori et al), 209
Cerebrospinal fluid
Epidural and intrathecal opiates: Cerebrospinal fluid and plasma profiles in patients with chronic cancer pain (Max et al), 631
Cetirizine hydrochloride
Cetirizine hydrochloride (USAN List No. 262), 117
Charcoal
Lack of effect of oral activated charcoal on imipramine clearance (Goldberg et al), 350
Chronic obstructive pulmonary disease
Effects of the calcium antagonist tiapamil on pulmonary gas exchange in patients with chronic obstructive pulmonary disease who receive salbutamol (Gugger et al), 96
Cigarette(s)
Cigarette smoking as a risk for cardiovascular disease. Part VI. Compensation with nicotine availability as a single variable (Haley et al), 164
Transdermal nicotine reduces cigarette craving and nicotine preference (Rose et al), 450
Cimetidine
Effect of single doses of cimetidine and ranitidine on the steady-state plasma levels of midazolam (Klotz et al), 652
Interaction of ibuprofen with the H-2 receptor antagonists ranitidine and cimetidine (Ochs et al), 648
Lack of interaction between verapamil and cimetidine (Abernethy et al), 342
Lack of pharmacokinetic interaction between cimetidine and pirenzepine (Jamali et al), 325
Ciramadol
Hemodynamic and respiratory effects of dezocine, ciramadol, and morphine (Rothbard et al), 84
Oral ciramadol in the treatment of postoperative pain (Lasagna and Calimlim), 177
Cirrhosis
Pefloxacin kinetics in cirrhosis (Danan et al), 439
Clavulanic acid
Clinical pharmacology of timentin (ticarcillin and clavulanic acid) (Bodey et al), 134
Clinical pharmacology
Clinical pharmacology: A personal perspective (Vesell), 603
Clinical pharmacology of 5-iodo-2′-deoxyuridine and 5-iodouracil and endogenous pyrimidine modulation (Klecker et al), 45
Clinical pharmacology of timentin (ticarcillin and clavulanic acid) (Bodey et al), 134
The discipline of clinical pharmacology (Reidenberg), 2
Clonidine
Efficacy of clonidine and of methadone in the rapid detoxification of patients dependent on heroin (Camí et al), 336
Pharmacokinetics of transdermally delivered clonidine (MacGregor et al), 278
Self-administration of clonidine, oxazepam, and hydromorphone by patients undergoing methadone detoxification (Preston et al), 219
Cocaine
Kinetics of cocaine distribution, elimination, and chronotropic effects (Chow et al), 318
Colon
Sulindac metabolism: The importance of an intact colon (Strong et al), 387
Computer(s)
Computerized assessment of human neurotoxicity: Sensitivity to nitrous oxide exposure (Greenberg et al), 656
The computerized on-line Medicaid pharmaceutical analysis and surveillance system: A new resource for postmarketing drug surveillance (Strom et al), 359
Continuous ambulatory peritoneal dialysis
Moxalactam epimer disposition in patients undergoing continuous ambulatory peritoneal dialysis (Morse et al), 150
Pharmacokinetics of intravenous and intraperitoneal cefotaxime in chronic ambulatory peritoneal dialysis (Albin et al), 285
Contraceptive(s)
Interactions between ethanol and oral contraceptive steroids (Hobbes et al), 371
Creatinine
Effect of alprazolam on digoxin kinetics and creatinine clearance (Ochs et al), 595
Cyclosporine
Cyclosporine kinetics in renal transplantation (Ptachcinski et al), 296

D

Debrisoquin
A family study of genetic and environmental factors determining polymorphic hydroxylation of debrisoquin (Steiner et al), 394
Interethnic differences in genetic polymorphism of debrisoquin and mephenytoin hydroxylation between Japanese and Caucasian populations (Nakamura et al), 402
Metabolism of methoxyphenamine in extensive and poor metabolizers of debrisoquin (Roy et al), 128
Pharmacokinetics and beta-blocking effects of timolol in poor and extensive metabolizers of debrisoquin McGourty et al), 409
Polymorphic dextromethorphan metabolism: Co-segregation of oxidative O-demethylation with debrisoquin hydroxylation (Schmid et al), 618

Demethylation
Polymorphic dextromethorphan metabolism: Co-segregation of oxidative O-demethylation with debrisoquin hydroxylation (Schmid et al), 618

Desacetyl cefotaxime
Cefotaxime and desacetyl cefotaxime kinetics in renal impairment (Matzke et al), 31

Detoxification
Efficacy of clonidine and of methadone in the rapid detoxification of patients dependent on heroin (Camí et al), 336
Self-administration of clonidine, oxazepam, and hydromorphone by patients undergoing methadone detoxification (Preston et al), 219

Dextromethorphan
Polymorphic dextromethorphan metabolism: Co-segregation of oxidative O-demethylation with debrisoquin hydroxylation (Schmid et al), 618

Dezocine
Assessment of dezocine for morphine-like subjective effects and miosis (Jasinski and Preston), 544
Hemodynamic and respiratory effects of dezocine, ciramadol, and morphine (Rothbard et al), 84

Diabetes
Effect of tolrestat on red blood cell sorbitol levels in patients with diabetes (Raskin et al), 625

Digitoxin
Effects of verapamil, diltiazem, and nifedipine on plasma levels and renal excretion of digitoxin (Kuhlmann), 667

Digoxin
Effect of alprazolam on digoxin kinetics and creatinine clearance (Ochs et al), 595

Diltiazem
Effects of verapamil, diltiazem, and nifedipine on plasma levels and renal excretion of digitoxin (Kuhlmann), 667

Disease
Cigarette smoking as a risk for cardiovascular disease. Part VI. Compensation with nicotine availability as a single variable (Haley et al), 164
Effects of age and disease on the pharmacokinetics and pharmacodynamics of sulindac (Sitar et al), 228
Effects of the calcium antagonist tiapamil on pulmonary gas exchange in patients with chronic obstructive pulmonary disease who receive salbutamol (Gugger et al), 96

Disopyramide
Kinetics and dynamics of disopyramide and its dealkylated metabolite in healthy subjects (Chiang et al), 37

Dosing regimen (see algorithm)

Drug marketing
Premarketing observational studies of population pharmacokinetics of new drugs (Sheiner and Benet), 481
The computerized on-line Medicaid pharmaceutical analysis and surveillance system: A new resource for postmarketing drug surveillance (Strom et al), 359

E

Enalapril
The effect of renal function on enalapril kinetics (Lowenthal et al), 661

Enalaprilat
Enalaprilat, an intravenous angiotensin-converting enzyme inhibitor, in hypertensive crises (DiPette et al), 199

Enprofylline
Enprofylline (USAN List No. 267), 705

Environment
A family study of genetic and environmental factors determining polymorphic hydroxylation of debrisoquin (Steiner et al), 394

Enzyme
Enalaprilat, an intravenous angiotensin converting enzyme inhibitor, in hypertensive crises (DiPette et al), 199
Inadequate aldosterone response to hyperkalemia during angiotensin converting enzyme inhibition in chronic renal failure (Zanella et al), 613
Pharmacokinetics of a new angiotensin I converting enzyme inhibitor (alacepril) after oral dosing in fasting or fed states (Onoyama et al), 462

Epimer
Moxalactam epimer disposition in patients undergoing continuous ambulatory peritoneal dialysis (Morse et al), 150

Ethanol
The effects of several weeks of ethanol consumption on ethanol kinetics in normal men and women (Holtzman et al), 157
Interactions between ethanol and oral contraceptive steroids (Hobbes et al), 371

Ethnic differences
Interethnic differences in genetic polymorphism of debrisoquin and mephenytoin hydroxylation between Japanese and Caucasian populations (Nakamura et al), 402

Etodolac
Effect of etodolac in patients with moderate renal impairment compared with normal subjects (Brater et al), 674

Errata
Alpha-methyldopa disposition in mothers with hypertension and in their breast-fed infants (White et al), 317
Tolrestat kinetics (Hicks et al), 317

F

Feces
Fecal blood loss during isoxicam and piroxicam administration for 28 days (Hooper et al), 533

Felodipine
Felodipine (USAN List No. 267), 705
Felodipine kinetics in healthy men (Edgar et al), 205

Flestolol sulfate
Flestolol sulfate (USAN List No. 262), 118

Food
Concomitant food intake does enhance the bioavailability and effect of hydralazine (Melander et al), 475 (letter)
Food induced changes in theophylline absorption from controlled-release formulations (Karim et al)
I. Substantial increased and decreased absorption with Uniphyl tablets and Theo-Dur Sprinkle, 77
II. Importance of meal composition and dosing time relative to meal intake in assessing changes in absorption, 642

Fosarilate
Fosarilate (USAN List No. 264), 357

Furegrelate sodium
Furegrelate sodium (USAN List No. 264), 356

G

Gastric (see stomach)
Gastrointestinal (see stomach, intestine)

Genetics
A family study of genetic and environmental factors determining polymorphic hydroxylation of debrisoquin (Steiner et al), 394
Interethnic differences in genetic polymorphism of debrisoquin and mephenytoin hydroxylation between Japanese and Caucasian populations (Nakamura et al), 402

Gentamicin
A simple method for the estimation of glomerular filtration rate by gentamicin pharmacokinetics during routine drug monitoring in the newborn (Koren et al), 680

Glomerular filtration rate
A simple method for the estimation of glomerular filtration rate by gentamicin pharmacokinetics during routine drug monitoring in the newborn (Koren et al), 680

H

Hand vein
Evaluation and application of the linear variable differential transformer technique for the assessment of human dorsal hand vein alpha-receptor activity (Alradi and Carruthers), 495

Heart
Biologic determinants of propranolol disposition: Results from 1308 patients in the Beta-blocker Heart Attack Trial (Walle et al), 509
Cigarette smoking as a risk for cardiovascular disease. Part VI. Compensation with nicotine availability as a single variable (Haley et al), 164
Determinants of systemic availability of oral hydralazine in heart failure (Crawford et al), 538
Effects of d,l-verapamil on atrioventricular conduction in relation to its stereoselective first-pass metabolism (Echizen et al), 71

Hemostasis
Pentosane polysulfate: The effect on hemostasis of a continuous 3-day infusion (de Prost et al), 171

Heroin
Efficacy of clonidine and of methadone in the rapid detoxification of patients dependent on heroin (Camí et al), 336

Herpes simplex labialis
Treatment of recurrent herpes simplex labialis with topical butylated hydroxytoluene (Freeman et al), 56

Histamine
Interaction of ibuprofen with the H-2 receptor antagonists ranitidine and cimetidine (Ochs et al), 648
Morphine-induced skin wheals: A possible model for the study of histamine release (Saucedo and Erill), 365

Histrelin
Histrelin (USAN List No. 267), 706

Hormones
Effect of aminoglycosides on the disposition of thyroid hormones and thyroglobulin (du Souich et al), 686

Hydralazine
Concomitant food intake does enhance the bioavailability and effect of hydralazine (Melander et al), 475 (letter)
Determinants of systemic availability of oral hydralazine in heart failure (Crawford et al), 538

Hydrazine
Oxidation of hydrazine metabolites formed from isoniazid (Lauterburg et al), 566

Hydrochlorothiazide
Labetalol and hydrochlorothiazide in hypertension (Labetalol/Hydrochlorothiazide Multicenter Study Group), 24

Hydromorphone
Self-administration of clonidine, oxazepam, and hydromorphone by patients undergoing methadone detoxification (Preston et al), 219

Hydroxylation
A family study of genetic and environmental factors determining polymorphic hydroxylation of debrisoquin (Steiner et al), 394
Interethnic differences in genetic polymorphism of debrisoquin and mephenytoin hydroxylation between Japanese and Caucasian populations (Nakamura et al), 402
Mephenytoin hydroxylation polymorphism: Characterization of the enzymatic deficiency in liver microsomes of poor metabolizers phenotyped in vivo (Meier et al), 488
Polymorphic dextromethorphan metabolism: Co-segregation of oxidative O-demethylation with debrisoquin hydroxylation (Schmid et al), 618
Stereoselective mephobarbital hydroxylation cosegregates with mephenytoin hydroxylation (Küpfer and Branch), 414

Hyperkalemia
Inadequate aldosterone response to hyperkalemia during angiotensin converting enzyme inhibition in chronic renal failure (Zanella et al), 613

Hyperlipoproteinemia
Controlled trial of acifran in type II hyperlipoproteinemia (Hunninghake et al), 313

Hypertension
Antihypertensive and cardiovascular effects of nitrendipine: A controlled study vs. placebo (Ferrara et al), 434
Enalaprilate, an intravenous angiotensin-converting enzyme inhibitor, in hypertensive crises (DiPette et al), 199
Labetalol and hydrochlorothiazide in hypertension (Labetalol/Hydrochlorothiazide Multicenter Study Group), 24
Losulazine, a new antihypertensive (Gore et al), 195
Treatment of arterial hypertension with ketanserin in mono- and combination therapy (Pettersson et al), 188

I

Ibuprofen
Interaction of ibuprofen with the H-2 receptor antagonists ranitidine and cimetidine (Ochs et al), 648

Icotidine
Icotidine (USAN List No. 265), 480

Iloprost
Myocardial ischemia induced by prostacyclin and iloprost (Bugiardini et al), 101

Imipramine
Lack of effect of oral activated charcoal on imipramine clearance (Goldberg et al), 350

Indolapril hydrochloride
Indolapril hydrochloride (USAN List No. 265), 480

Indomethacin
Inhibition of prostaglandin synthesis by indomethacin interacts with the antihypertensive effect of atenolol (Ylitalo et al), 443

Infarction
Circulatory effects of intravenous and oral acebutolol in acute myocardial infarction (Silke et al), 266

Inhalation (see specific drug)

Inhibition
Enalaprilat, an intravenous angiotensin converting enzyme inhibitor, in hypertensive crises (DiPette et al), 199
Inadequate aldosterone response to hyperkalemia during angiotensin converting enzyme inhibition in chronic renal failure (Zanella et al), 613
Pharmacokinetics of a new angiotensin I converting enzyme inhibitor (alacepril) after oral dosing in fasting or fed states (Onoyama et al), 462

Interaction(s)
Inhibition of prostaglandin synthesis by indomethacin interacts with the antihypertensive effect of atenolol (Ylitalo et al), 443
Interaction of ibuprofen with the H-2 receptor antagonists ranitidine and cimetidine (Ochs et al), 648
Interactions between ethanol and oral contraceptive steroids (Hobbes et al), 371
Lack of interaction between verapamil and cimetidine (Abernethy et al), 342
Lack of pharmacokinetic interaction between cimetidine and pirenzepine (Jamali et al), 325

Intestine
Gastrointestinal absorption as a function of age: Xylose absorption in healthy adults (Johnson et al), 331
The pharmacokinetics of baclofen derived from intestinal infusion (Kochak et al), 251

5-Iodo-2′-deoxyuridine
Clinical pharmacology of 5-iodo-2′-deoxyuridine and 5-iodouracil and endogenous pyrimidine modulation (Klecker et al), 45

5-Iodouracil
Clinical pharmacology of 5-iodo-2′-deoxyuridine and 5-iodouracil and endogenous pyrimidine modulation (Klecker et al), 45

Ischemia
Myocardial ischemia induced by prostacyclin and iloprost (Bugiardini et al), 101

Isoniazid
Oxidation of hydrazine metabolites formed from isoniazid (Lauterburg et al), 566

Isoproterenol
Effects of betaxolol, propranolol, and atenolol on isoproterenol-induced beta-adrenoceptor responses (Riddell and Shanks), 554

Isosorbide dinitrate
Isosorbide dinitrate bioavailability, kinetics, and metabolism (Straehl and Galeazzi), 140

Isoxicam
Fecal blood loss during isoxicam and piroxicam administration for 28 days (Hooper et al), 533

J

Japanese
Interethnic differences in genetic polymorphism of debrisoquin and mephenytoin hydroxylation between Japanese and Caucasian populations (Nakamura et al), 402

K

Ketanserin
Treatment of arterial hypertension with ketanserin in mono- and combination therapy (Pettersson et al), 188

Kidney
A new dosing regimen in renal insufficiency: Application to cephalexin (Hori et al), 209
A simple method for the estimation of glomerular filtration rate by gentamicin pharmacokinetics during routine drug monitoring in the newborn (Koren et al), 680
Cefotaxime and desacetyl cefotaxime kinetics in renal impairment (Matzke et al), 31
Cyclosporine kinetics in renal transplantation (Ptachcinski et al), 296
Effect of etodolac in patients with moderate renal impairment compared with normal subjects (Brater et al), 674
Effects of verapamil, diltiazem, and nifedipine on plasma levels and renal excretion of digitoxin (Kuhlmann), 667
Inadequate aldosterone response to hyperkalemia during angiotensin converting enzyme inhibition in chronic renal failure (Zanella et al), 613
Nitrendipine kinetics in normal and impaired renal function (Aronoff and Sloan), 212
Sulindac is not renal sparing in man (Roberts et al), 258
The effect of renal function on enalapril kinetics (Lowenthal et al), 661

L

Labetalol
Labetalol and hydrochlorothiazide in hypertension (Labetalol/Hydrochlorothiazide Multicenter Study Group), 24
Pharmacodynamics of intravenous labetalol and follow-up therapy with oral labetalol (Vlachakis et al), 503

Lamotrigine
Lamotrigine (USAN List No. 264), 356

Linear variable differential transformer
Evaluation and application of the linear variable differential transformer technique for the assessment of human dorsal hand vein alpha-receptor activity (Alradi and Carruthers), 495

Lithium
Effect of acute alcohol consumption on lithium kinetics (Anton et al), 52

Liver
Mephenytoin hydroxylation polymorphism: Characterization of the enzymatic deficiency in liver microsomes of poor metabolizers phenotyped in vivo (Meier et al), 488

Losulazine
Losulazine, a new antihypertensive (Gore et al), 195

Lung
Effects of the calcium antagonist tiapamil on pulmonary gas exchange in patients with chronic obstructive pulmonary disease who receive salbutamol (Gugger et al), 96

Lupitidine hydrochloride
Lupitidine hydrochloride (USAN List No. 263), 237

M

Maduramicin
Maduramicin (USAN List No. 263), 238

Medicaid
The computerized on-line Medicaid pharmaceutical analysis and surveillance system: A new resource for postmarketing drug surveillance (Strom et al), 359

Mephenytoin
Interethnic differences in genetic polymorphism of debrisoquin and mephenytoin hydroxylation between Japanese and Caucasian populations (Nakamura et al), 402
Mephenytoin hydroxylation polymorphism: Characterization of the enzymatic deficiency in liver microsomes of poor metabolizers phenotyped in vivo (Meier et al), 488
Stereoselective mephobarbital hydroxylation cosegregates with mephenytoin hydroxylation (Küpfer and Branch), 414

Mephobarbital
Stereoselective mephobarbital hydroxylation cosegregates with mephenytoin hydroxylation (Küpfer and Branch), 414

Metabolism
Effects of d,l-verapamil on atrioventricular conduction in relation to its stereoselective first-pass metabolism (Echizen et al), 71
Excretion patterns of cannabinoid metabolites after last use in a group of chronic users (Ellis et al), 572
Isosorbide dinitrate bioavailability, kinetics, and metabolism (Straehl and Galeazzi), 140
Kinetics and dynamics of disopyramide and its dealkylated metabolite in healthy subjects (Chiang et al), 37
Metabolism of methoxyphenamine in extensive and poor metabolizers of debrisoquin (Roy et al), 128
Oxidation of hydrazine metabolites formed from isoniazid (Lauterburg et al), 566
Pharmacokinetics of bupropion and its major basic metabolites in normal subjects after a single dose (Laizure et al), 586
Polymorphic dextromethorphan metabolism: Co-segregation of oxidative O-demethylation with debrisoquin hydroxylation (Schmid et al), 618
Sulindac metabolism: The importance of an intact colon (Strong et al), 387

Temporal variation in the disposition of theophylline and its metabolites (St-Pierre et al), 89
Metabolite(s) (see metabolism, specific drug)
Methadone
Efficacy of clonidine and of methadone in the rapid detoxification of patients dependent on heroin (Camí et al), 336
Self-administration of clonidine, oxazepam, and hydromorphone by patients undergoing methadone detoxification (Preston et al), 219
Methoxyphenamine
Metabolism of methoxyphenamine in extensive and poor metabolizers of debrisoquin (Roy et al), 128
Midazolam
Effect of single doses of cimetidine and ranitidine on the steady-state plasma levels of midazolam (Klotz et al), 652
Miosis
Assessment of dezocine for morphine-like subjective effects and miosis (Jasinski and Preston), 544
Morphine
Assessment of dezocine for morphine-like subjective effects and miosis (Jasinski and Preston), 544
Hemodynamic and respiratory effects of dezocine, ciramadol, and morphine (Rothbard et al), 84
Morphine-induced skin wheals: A possible model for the study of histamine release (Saucedo and Erill), 365
Motion sickness
Influence of transdermal scopolamine on motion sickness during 7 days' exposure to heavy seas (van Marion et al), 301
Moxalactam
Moxalactam epimer disposition in patients undergoing continuous ambulatory peritoneal dialysis (Morse et al), 150
Mucosa
Nonsteroidal anti-inflammatory effect of sulindac sulfoxide and sulfide on gastric mucosa (Graham et al), 65

N

Naloxone
Effect of naloxone on the actions of captopril (Ajayi et al), 560
Naltrexone
Effects of long-term therapy with naltrexone on body weight in obesity (Atkinson et al), 419
Napamezole hydrochloride
Nepamezole hydrochloride (USAN List No. 264), 357
Nefocon A
Nefocon A (USAN List No. 266), 602
Neurotoxicity
Computerized assessment of human neurotoxicity: Sensitivity to nitrous oxide exposure (Greenberg et al), 656
Newborn
A simple method for the estimation of glomerular filtration rate by gentamicin pharmacokinetics during routine drug monitoring in the newborn (Koren et al), 680
Nicotinate
Prostaglandins and nicotinate-provoked increase in cutaneous blood flow (Wilkin et al), 273
Nicotine
Cigarette smoking as a risk for cardiovascular disease. Part VI. Compensation with nicotine availability as a single variable (Haley et al), 164
Transdermal nicotine reduces cigarette craving and nicotine preference (Rose et al), 450
Nicotine polacrilex
Nicotine polacrilex (USAN List No. 266), 601
Nifedipine
Effects of verapamil, diltiazem, and nifedipine on plasma levels and renal excretion of digitoxin (Kuhlmann), 667
Nitrazepam
Age, sex, and nitrazepam kinetics: Relation to antipyrine disposition (Greenblatt et al), 697
Nitrendipine
Antihypertensive and cardiovascular effects of nitrendipine: A controlled study vs. placebo (Ferrara et al), 434
Effects of chronic nitrendipine on casual (office) and 24-hour ambulatory blood pressure (White et al), 60
Nitrendipine kinetics in normal and impaired renal function (Aronoff and Sloan), 212
Nitrous oxide
Computerized assessment of human neurotoxicity: Sensitivity to nitrous oxide exposure (Greenberg et al), 656
Nonsteroidal anti-inflammatory drugs
Nonsteroidal anti-inflammatory effect of sulindac sulfoxide and sulfide on gastric mucosa (Graham et al), 65
Notes
A note from the Co-Editor, 1
Notes of the ASCPT (see American Society for Clinical Pharmacology)

O

Obesity
Effects of long-term therapy with naltrexone on body weight in obesity (Atkinson et al), 419
Opiate(s)
Epidural and intrathecal opiates: Cerebrospinal fluid and plasma profiles in patients with chronic cancer pain (Max et al), 631
Oral contraceptive(s)
Pharmacodynamic evaluation of the benzodiazepine–oral contraceptive interaction (Kroboth et al), 525
Oxazepam
Self-administration of clonidine, oxazepam, and hydromorphone by patients undergoing methadone detoxification (Preston et al), 219

Oxidation
Oxidation of hydrazine metabolites formed from isoniazid (Lauterburg et al), 566
Oximonam
Oximonam (USAN List No. 267), 706
Oximonam sodium (USAN List No. 267), 706

P

Pain
Epidural and intrathecal opiates: Cerebrospinal fluid and plasma profiles in patients with chronic cancer pain (Max et al), 631
Oral ciramadol in the treatment of postoperative pain (Lasagna and Calimlim), 177
Pefloxacin
Pefloxacin kinetics in cirrhosis (Danan et al), 439
Pelrinone hydrochloride
Pelrinone hydrochloride (USAN List No. 262), 118
Pentobarbital
Pharmacokinetics of high-dose pentobarbital in severe head trauma (Bayliff et al), 457
Pentopril
Pentopril (USAN List No. 262), 118
Pentosane polysulfate
Pentosane polysulfate: The effect on hemostasis of a continuous 3-day infusion (de Prost et al), 171
Pirenzepine
Lack of pharmacokinetic interaction between cimetidine and pirenzepine (Jamali et al), 325
Piroxicam
Fecal blood loss during isoxicam and piroxicam administration for 28 days (Hooper et al), 533
Platelet(s)
Pharmacologic reduction of sympathetic drive increases platelet alpha-2–receptor number (Egan et al), 519
Polybutester
Polybutester (USAN List No. 263), 238
Postpartum women
Sulbactam kinetics and excretion into breast milk in postpartum women (Foulds et al), 692
Potassium chloride
Endoscopic evaluation of slow-release potassium chloride preparations (Kendall et al), 28
Prilocaine
Prilocaine in arthroscopy: Clinical pharmacokinetics and rational use (Debruyne et al), 549
Probenecid
Effect of probenecid on the formation and elimination of acyl glucuronides: Studies with zomepirac (Smith et al), 121
Propranolol
Biologic determinants of propranolol disposition: Results from 1308 patients in the Beta-blocker Heart Attack Trial (Walle et al), 509
Effects of betaxolol, propranolol, and atenolol on isoproterenol-induced beta-adrenoceptor responses (Riddell and Shanks), 554
Prostacyclin
Myocardial ischemia induced by prostacyclin and iloprost (Bugiardini et al), 101
Prostaglandin(s)
Inhibition of prostaglandin synthesis by indomethacin interacts with the antihypertensive effect of atenolol (Ylitalo et al), 443
Prostaglandins and nicotinate-provoked increase in cutaneous blood flow (Wilkin et al), 273
Pulmonary (see lung)

Q

Quadazocine mesylate
Quadazocine mesylate (USAN List No. 264), 356
Quinapril hydrochloride
Quinapril hydrochloride (USAN List No. 263), 237

R

Ranitidine
Effect of single doses of cimetidine and ranitidine on the steady-state plasma levels of midazolam (Klotz et al), 652
Interaction of ibuprofen with the H-2 receptor antagonists ranitidine and cimetidine (Ochs et al), 648
Recainam
Recainam hydrochloride (USAN List No. 264), 357
Recainam tosylate (USAN List No. 265), 479
Reclazepam
Reclazepam (USAN List No. 266), 602
Red blood cells
Effect of tolrestat on red blood cell sorbitol levels in patients with diabetes (Raskin et al), 625
Remoxipride
Remoxipride (USAN List No. 262), 117
Renal (see kidney)
Reviewers
List of reviewers to volume 37, 477
Rifapentine
Rifapentine (USAN List No. 263), 237

S

Salbutamol
Effects of the calcium antagonist tiapamil on pulmonary gas exchange in patients with chronic obstructive pulmonary disease who receive salbutamol (Gugger et al), 96
Salicylate
Salicylate kinetics in old age (Netter et al), 6
Salmeterol
Salmeterol (USAN List No. 267), 705

Scopolamine
Influence of transdermal scopolamine on motion sickness during 7 days' exposure to heavy seas (van Marion et al), 301
Sex
Age, sex, and nitrazepam kinetics: Relation to antipyrine disposition (Greenblatt et al), 697
Smoking
Cigarette smoking as a risk for cardiovascular disease. Part VI. Compensation with nicotine availability as a single variable (Haley et al), 164
Effects of smoke deprivation interval on puff topography (Zacny and Stitzer), 109
Spironolactone
New insights into the pharmacokinetics of spironolactone (Overdiek et al), 469
Steroids
Interactions between ethanol and oral contraceptive steroids (Hobbes et al), 371
Stomach
Gastrointestinal absorption as a function of age: Xylose absorption in healthy adults (Johnson et al), 331
Nonsteroidal anti-inflammatory effect of sulindac sulfoxide and sulfide on gastric mucosa (Graham et al), 65
Sulbactam
Sulbactam kinetics and excretion into breast milk in post-partum women (Foulds et al), 692
Sulindac
Effects of age and disease on the pharmacokinetics and pharmacodynamics of sulindac (Sitar et al), 228
Nonsteroidal anti-inflammatory effect of sulindac sulfoxide and sulfide on gastric mucosa (Graham et al), 65
Sulindac is not renal sparing in man (Roberts et al), 258
Sulindac metabolism: The importance of an intact colon (Strong et al), 387
Surfilcon A
Surfilcon A (USAN List No. 265), 479
Sympathetic system
Pharmacologic reduction of sympathetic drive increases platelet alpha-2–receptor number (Egan et al), 519

T

Temocillin
Temocillin (USAN List No. 266), 601
Temporal variation
Temporal variation in the disposition of theophylline and its metabolites (St-Pierre et al), 89
Terazosin
Terazosin kinetics after oral and intravenous doses (Patterson), 423
Theophylline
Food-induced changes in theophylline absorption from controlled-release formulations (Karim et al)
I. Substantial increased and decreased absorption with Uniphyl tablets and Theo-Dur Sprinkle, 77
II. Importance of meal composition and dosing time relative to meal intake in assessing changes in absorption, 642
Temporal variation in the disposition of theophylline and its metabolites (St-Pierre et al), 89
Thyroid
Effect of aminoglycosides on the disposition of thyroid hormones and thyroglobulin (du Souich et al), 686
Thyroglobulin
Effect of aminoglycosides on the disposition of thyroid hormones and thyroglobulin (du Souich et al), 686
Tiapamil
Effects of the calcium antagonist tiapamil on pulmonary gas exchange in patients with chronic obstructive pulmonary disease who receive salbutamol (Gugger et al), 96
Ticarcillin
Clinical pharmacology of timentin (ticarcillin and clavulanic acid) (Bodey et al), 134
Timentin
Clinical pharmacology of timentin (ticarcillin and clavulanic acid) (Bodey et al), 134
Timolol
Pharmacokinetics and beta-blocking effects of timolol in poor and extensive metabolizers of debrisoquin (McGourty et al), 409
Tolrestat
Effect of tolrestat on red blood cell sorbitol levels in patients with diabetes (Raskin et al), 625
Transplantation
Cyclosporine kinetics in renal transplantation (Ptachcinski et al), 296
Transdermal (see specific drug)
Trauma
Pharmacokinetics of high-dose pentobarbital in severe head trauma (Bayliff et al), 457
Triamterene
Oral triamterene disposition (Sörgel et al), 306
Triprolidine
The acute effects of acrivastine (BW825C), a new antihistamine, compared with triprolidine on measures of central nervous system performance and subjective effects (Cohen et al), 381
Trospectomycin sulfate
Trospectomycin sulfate (USAN List No. 262), 118
Tubulozole hydrochloride
Tubulozole hydrochloride (USAN List No. 266), 601

V

Verapamil
Effects of d,1-verapamil on atrioventricular conduction in relation to its stereoselective first-pass metabolism (Echizen et al), 71

Effects of verapamil, diltiazem, and nifedipine on plasma levels and renal excretion of digitoxin (Kuhlmann), 667
Lack of interaction between verapamil and cimetidine (Abernethy et al), 342
Viprostol
Viprostol (USAN List No. 264), 357

W

Wheals
Morphine-induced skin wheals: A possible model for the study of histamine release (Saucedo and Erill), 365

X

Xylose
Gastrointestinal absorption as a function of age: Xylose absorption in healthy adults (Johnson et al), 331

Z

Zomepirac
Effect of probenecid on the formation and elimination of acyl glucuronides: Studies with zomepirac (Smith et al), 121